NURSING CARE PLANS

Guidelines for Planning and Documenting Patient Care
Edition 3

Marilynn E. Doenges, RN, BSN, MA, CS
Clinical Specialist
Adult Psychiatric/Mental Health Nursing
Private Practice
Instructor
Beth-El College of Nursing
Colorado Springs, Colorado

Mary Frances Moorehouse, RN, CCP, CCRN, CRRN
Nurse Consultant
TNT-RN Enterprises
Colorado Springs, Colorado

Alice C. Geissler, RN, BSN, CCRN, CRRN
Director of Nurses
National Medical Care-Home Care Division
Colorado Springs, Colorado

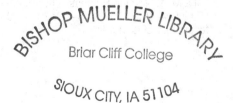
F. A. DAVIS COMPANY • PHILADELPHIA

F.A. Davis Company
1915 Arch Street
Philadelphia, PA 19103

Printed in the United States of America

Last digit indicates print number: 10 9 8 7 6 5 4 3 2 1

Publisher, Nursing: Robert G. Martone
Production Editor: Crystal S. McNichol
Cover Design by: Steven R. Morrone

As new scientific information becomes available through basic and clinical research, recommended treatments and drug therapies undergo changes. The author(s) and publisher have done everything possible to make this book accurate, up to date, and in accord with accepted standards at the time of publication. The authors, editors, and publisher are not responsible for errors or omissions or for consequences from application of the book, and make no warranty, expressed or implied, in regard to the contents of the book. Any practice described in this book should be applied by the reader in accordance with professional standards of care used in regard to the unique circumstances that may apply in each situation. The reader is advised always to check product information (package inserts) for changes and new information regarding dose and contraindications before administering any drug. Caution is especially urged when using new or infrequently ordered drugs.

Library of Congress Cataloging-in-Publication Data

Doenges, Marilynn E., 1922–
Nursing care plans: guidelines for planning and documenting patient care/Marilynn E. Doenges, Mary Frances Moorhouse, Alice C. Geissler.—3rd ed.
    p. cm.

    Rev. ed. of: Nursing care plans/Marilynn E. Doenges . . . [et al.]. 2nd ed. c1989.
    Includes bibliographical references and index.
    ISBN 0-8036-2662-2 (softbound: alk. paper)
1. Nursing care plans. I. Moorhouse, Mary Frances, 1947– . II. Geissler, Alice C., 1946– . III. Title.
[DNLM: 1. Nursing Process—handbooks. 2. Patient Care Planning—handbooks. WY 39 D651nc]
RT49.D64 1993   610.73—dc20   DNLM/DLC
for Library of Congress

92-48304
CIP

KEY TO ESSENTIAL TERMINOLOGY

PATIENT ASSESSMENT DATA BASE

Provides an overview of the more commonly occurring etiology and coexisting factors associated with a specific medical/surgical diagnosis as well as the signs/symptoms and corresponding diagnostic findings.

NURSING PRIORITIES

Establishes a general ranking of needs/concerns on which the Nursing Diagnoses are ordered in constructing the plan of care. This ranking would be altered according to the individual patient situation.

DISCHARGE GOALS

Identifies generalized statements that could be developed into short-term and intermediate goals to be achieved by the patient before being "discharged" from nursing care. They may also provide guidance for creating long-term goals for the patient to work on after discharge.

NURSING DIAGNOSES

The general problem/concern (Diagnosis) is stated without the distinct cause and signs/symptoms, which would be added to create a patient diagnostic statement when specific patient information is available. For example, when a patient displays increased tension, apprehension, quivering voice, and focus on self, the nursing diagnosis of Anxiety could be stated: Anxiety, severe, related to unconscious conflict, threat to self-concept as evidenced by statements of increased tension, apprehension; observations of quivering voice, focus on self.

In addition, diagnoses identified within these guides for planning care as actual or high risk can be changed or deleted and new diagnoses added, depending entirely on the specific patient information.

MAY BE RELATED TO/POSSIBLY EVIDENCED BY

These lists provide the usual/common reasons (etiology) why a particular problem may occur with probable signs/symptoms, which would be used to create the "related to" and "evidenced by" portions of the *patient diagnostic statement* when the specific patient situation is known.

When a high-risk (formerly "potential") diagnosis has been identified, signs/symptoms have not yet developed and therefore are not included in the nursing diagnosis statement. However, interventions are provided to prevent progression to an *actual* problem. The exception to this occurs in the nursing diagnosis *Violence, high risk for,* which has possible indicators that suggest the patient may be at risk.

DESIRED OUTCOMES/EVALUATION CRITERIA—PATIENT WILL

These give direction to patient care as they identify what the patient or nurse hopes to achieve. They are stated in general terms to permit the practitioner to modify/individualize them by adding time lines and individual patient criteria so they become "measurable." For example, "Patient will appear relaxed and report anxiety is reduced to a manageable level within 24 hours."

ACTIONS/INTERVENTIONS

Activities are divided into independent and collaborative and are ranked in this book from most to least common. When creating the individual plan of care, interventions would normally be ranked to reflect the patient's specific needs/situation. In addition, the division of independent/collaborative is arbitrary and is actually dependent of the individual nurse's capabilities and hospital/community standards.

RATIONALE

Although not commonly appearing in patient plans of care, rationale has been included here to provide a pathophysiologic basis to assist the nurse in deciding about the relevance of a specific intervention for an individual patient situation.

NURSING DIAGNOSES (THROUGH 10TH NANDA CONFERENCE) 1992

Activity Intolerance
Activity Intolerance, high risk for
Adjustment impaired
Airway Clearance, ineffective
Anxiety [specify level]*
Aspiration, high risk for
Body Image disturbance
Body Temperature, altered, high risk for
Bowel Incontinence
Breastfeeding, effective
Breastfeeding, ineffective
Breastfeeding, interrupted
Breathing Pattern, ineffective
Cardiac Output, decreased
Caregiver Role Strain
Caregiver Role Strain, high risk for
Communication, impaired verbal
Constipation
Constipation, colonic
Constipation, perceived
Coping, defensive
Coping, Individual, ineffective
Decisional Conflict (specify)
Denial, ineffective
Diarrhea
Disuse Syndrome, high risk for
Diversional Activity deficit
Dysreflexia
Family Coping, ineffective, compromised
Family Coping, ineffective, disabling
Family Coping, potential for growth
Family Processes, altered
Fatigue
Fear
Fluid Volume deficit [active loss]*
Fluid Volume deficit [regulatory failure]*
Fluid Volume deficit, high risk for
Fluid Volume excess
Gas Exchange, impaired
Grieving, anticipatory
Grieving, dysfunctional
Growth and Development, altered
Health Maintenance, altered
Health-Seeking Behaviors (specify)
Home Maintenance Management, impaired
Hopelessness
Hyperthermia
Hypothermia
Incontinence, functional
Incontinence, reflex
Incontinence, stress
Incontinence, total
Incontinence, urge
Infant Feeding Pattern, ineffective
Infection, high risk for
Injury, high risk for
Knowledge Deficit [Learning need]* (specify)

Noncompliance [Compliance, altered]* (specify)
Nutrition, altered, less than body requirements
Nutrition, altered, more than body requirements
Nutrition, altered, high risk for more than body requirements
Oral Mucous Membrane, altered
Pain [acute]
Pain, chronic
Parental Role Conflict
Parenting, altered
Parenting, altered, high risk for
Peripheral Neurovascular dysfunction, high risk for
Personal Identity disturbance
Physical Mobility, impaired
Poisoning, high risk for
Post-trauma Response
Powerlessness
Protection, altered
Rape trauma Syndrome
Rape trauma Syndrome: compound reaction
Rape trauma Syndrome: silent reaction
Relocation Stress Syndrome
Role Performance, altered
Self-care Deficit, feeding, bathing/hygiene, dressing/grooming, toileting
Self-esteem, chronic low
Self-esteem disturbance
Self-esteem, situational low
Self-mutilation, high risk for
Sensory-perceptual alterations (specify): visual, auditory, kinesthetic, gustatory, tactile, olfactory
Sexual dysfunction
Sexuality Patterns, altered
Skin Integrity, impaired
Skin Integrity, impaired: high risk for
Sleep Pattern disturbance
Social Interaction, impaired
Social Isolation
Spiritual Distress (distress of the human spirit)
Spontaneous Ventilation, inability to sustain
Suffocation, high risk for
Swallowing impaired
Therapeutic Regimen (Individuals), ineffective management of
Thermoregulation, ineffective
Thought Processes, altered
Tissue Integrity, impaired
Tissue Perfusion, altered (specify): cerebral, cardiopulmonary, renal, gastrointestinal, peripheral
Trauma, high risk for
Unilateral Neglect
Urinary Elimination, altered
Urinary Retention [acute/chronic]*
Ventilatory Weaning Response, dysfunctional (DVWR)
Violence, high risk for, directed at self/others

---

* [Author recommendations]

To our spouses, children, parents, and friends, who much of the time have had to manage without us while we work as well as cope with our struggles and frustrations.

The Doenges families: Dean, Jim, Barbara, and Bob Lanza; David, Monita, Matthew, and Tyler; John, Holly Sponaugle, Nicole, and Kelsey; and the Daigle family, Nancy, Jim, Jennifer, and Jonathan.

The Moorhouse family: Jan, Paul, Jason, Alexa, and Ellaina Ward.

The Geissler family: especially Bill, who patiently waits; and in loving memory of my mother, Norma Loughmiller, who was my biggest promoter in my early days of writing.

To our FAD family, especially Bob Martone, Ruth De George, Herb Powell, and Crystal McNichol, whose support is so vital to the completion of a project of this magnitude.

To the nurses we are writing for, who daily face the challenge of caring for the acutely ill patient and are looking for a practical way to organize and document this care. We believe that nursing diagnosis and these guides will help.

Finally, to the late Mary Lisk Jeffries, who initiated the original project. The memory of our early friendship and struggles remains with us. We miss her and wish she were here to see the growth of the profession and how nursing diagnosis has contributed to the process.

PREFACE

One of the most significant achievements in the health care field during the past 20 years has been the emergence of the nurse as an active coordinator and initiator of patient care. While the transition from help-mate to health care professional has been painfully slow and is not yet complete, the importance of the nurse within the system can no longer be denied or ignored. Today's nurse designs nursing care interventions that will move the total patient toward the goal of improved health.

The current state of the theory of Nursing Process, Diagnosis, and Intervention has been brought to the clinical setting to be implemented by the nurse. This book gives definition and direction to the development and use of individualized nursing care. The book is not an end in itself therefore, but it is a beginning for the future growth and development of the profession.

Professional care standards, physicians, and patients will continue to increase expectations for nurses' performance as each day brings advances in the struggle to understand the mysteries of normal body function and human response to actual and potential health problems. With this increased knowledge comes greater responsibility for the nurse. To meet these challenges competently, the nurse must have up-to-date physical assessment skills and a working knowledge of pathophysiologic concepts concerning the more common diseases/conditions presented on a general medical/surgical unit. This book is a tool, a means of attaining that competency.

In the past, plans of care were viewed principally as learning tools for students and seemed to have little relevance after graduation. However, the need for a written format to communicate and document individualized patient care has been recognized in all care settings. In addition, governmental regulations and third-party payor requirements have created the need to validate the appropriateness of the care provided, as well as the need to justify patient care charges and staffing patterns. Thus, although the student's "case studies" were too cumbersome to be practical in the clinical setting, the patient plan of care meets the aforementioned identified needs. The practicing nurse, as well as the nursing student, will welcome this text as a ready reference in clinical practice. The book is designed for use in the acute medical/surgical setting and is organized by systems for easy reference. Rationales (which state not only why an intervention is important but also provide a brief related pathophysiology, when applicable) enhance the reader's understanding of the intervention. This information also serves as a catalyst for thought in planning and evaluating the care being rendered.

Chapter 1 discusses some current issues and trends affecting the nursing profession. An overview of cultural, community, sociologic, and ethical concepts impacting on the nurse is included. The important concept of cooperation and coordination with other health care professionals is integrated throughout the plans of care.

Chapter 2 reviews the historic use of the nursing process in formulating plans of care and the nurse's role in the delivery of that care. Nursing diagnosis is discussed to assist the nurse in understanding its role in the nursing process.

Chapter 3 discusses construction of the plan of care and the use and adaptation of the guides for planning care presented in this book. A nursing-based assessment tool is presented to aide the nurse to make the transition from theory to practice. Finally, a sample patient situation with data base and corresponding plan of care are included.

Chapters 4 through 17 present guides for planning care that include information from multiple disciplines to assist the nurse to provide holistic care. Each plan of care is developed by identifying nursing diagnoses with "related to" and "evidenced by" factors that provide an explanation of patient problems/needs. Each plan includes a patient assessment data base (presented in a nursing format) and associated diagnostic studies. After the data base is collected, nursing priorities are sifted from the information to help focus and structure the patient care provided. Discharge goals are also listed to identify which general goals should be accomplished by the time of discharge from acute care. In addition, mean length of stay has been identified to provide a general idea of time constraints for achieving discharge goals. Desired patient outcomes are stated in behavioral terms that can be measured to evaluate the patient's progress and the effectiveness of care provided. The interventions are designed to assist with problem resolution. Rationales for these actions are provided to enable the nurse to decide whether the intervention applies to a particular patient situation. Additional information is provided to assist the nurse in identifying and planning for rehabilitation as the patient progresses toward discharge.

As a final note, this book is not intended to be a procedure manual, and efforts have been made to avoid detailed descriptions of techniques/protocols that might be viewed as individual/regional in nature. Instead, the reader is referred to a procedure manual/standards of care book for in-depth direction for these concerns.

CONTRIBUTORS

Joseph T. Burley, RN, MNEd
Instructor
College of Nursing
University of Florida
Gainesville, Florida

Nancy Lea Carter, RN, BSN, MA
Clinical Nurse, Orthopedics
Presbyterian Medical Center
Albuquerque, New Mexico

Elizabeth Hagge, RN, BS
Clinical Supervisor, Retired
Penrose/St. Francis Healthcare System
Colorado Springs, Colorado

Judith Halley, RNC, BSN
Clinical Nurse
Burn Center
Penrose/St. Francis Healthcare System
Colorado Springs, Colorado

Christie A. Hinds, RN, NP
Director
HIV Patient Care
FHL Health Care, Inc.
Colorado Springs, Colorado

Laura Teigen Johnson, BSN, CNOR
Clinical Educator
Surgery
Penrose Community Hospital
Colorado Springs, Colorado

Von Matheny, RN
Acute/Long-Term Care
Fort Morgan, Colorado

Rebecca F. Murray, RN, MOT
Home Health Care Nurse
Colorado Springs, Colorado

Leslie Stimpson-Smith, RN, BSN
Utilization Review
Penrose/St. Francis Healthcare System
Colorado Springs, Colorado

Barbara Thomas, RN, BSN, C
Director of Partial Hospitalization and Residential
    Treatment Program
Cedar Springs Psychiatric Hospital
Colorado Springs, Colorado

Linda Wienerman
West Linn, Oregon

Anne Zobec, RN, MS, CS, OCN
Clinical Nurse Specialist
Medical/Surgical/Oncology
Penrose/St. Francis Healthcare System
Colorado Springs, Colorado

SPECIAL RECOGNITION

R. Matthew Reveille, MD
Assistant Professor of Medicine
Division of Gastroenterology
University of Colorado Health Sciences Center
Denver, Colorado

CONTENTS IN BRIEF

INDEX OF NURSING DIAGNOSES
appears on pages 1103–1108

INDEX OF NURSING DIAGNOSES appears on pages 1103–1108

A table of contents including Nursing Diagnoses follows.

INDEX OF NURSING DIAGNOSES appears on pages 1103–1108

DETAILED CONTENTS

INDEX OF NURSING DIAGNOSES
appears on pages 1103–1108

INDEX OF NURSING DIAGNOSES appears on pages 1103–1108

INDEX OF NURSING DIAGNOSES appears on pages 1103–1108

INDEX OF NURSING DIAGNOSES appears on pages 1103–1108

INDEX OF NURSING DIAGNOSES appears on pages 1103–1108

INDEX OF NURSING DIAGNOSES appears on pages 1103–1108

INDEX OF NURSING DIAGNOSES appears on pages 1103–1108

INDEX OF NURSING DIAGNOSES appears on pages 1103–1108

INDEX OF NURSING DIAGNOSES appears on pages 1103–1108

ISSUES AND TRENDS IN MEDICAL/SURGICAL NURSING

The entire field of health care is changing, and nowhere are these changes occurring at a more rapid rate than in the acute care arena. Here, nurses offer direct assistance to both patients and families who are dealing with illness or injury. This provides a tremendously exacting and exciting challenge for the nurse. The responsibility for coordinating this care requires planning and documentation that clearly identifies problems and interventions, as well as short- and long-range health care planning for individuals and families.

In this changing arena, what lies ahead? In 1989, we noted seven major trends that we believed would have a lasting impact on nursing and patient care. These were:

1. Decreasing health care dollars
2. Quantification of nursing care costs
3. Reduced length of stay
4. Increasing reliance on high technology
5. Requirement for advanced nursing knowledge
6. Need for collaboration and communication
7. Innovations in care planning through computerization

Those monitoring these trends (as well as the staff nurse providing direct care) can testify that these trends have indeed had, and continue to have, a profound effect on the profession and the practice of nursing.

Decreasing Health Care Dollars

Implementation of prospective reimbursement beginning with Medicare patients shifted the focus of health care to cost containment. Hospitals have responded to decreased dollars by reducing the number of beds and staff. In addition, although patients' hospitalizations are shorter, patients are sicker, resulting in escalated nursing care needs and workloads. This has required that nursing redefine minimum standards of care while still maintaining and providing effective nursing care. As a result of these changes, the nurse must function more efficiently. As never before, the patient plan of care must reflect preparation for meeting patient needs and standards of care within the restrictions of time limitations and fewer resources.

In 1989, we asked: "How shall allocation of a fixed number of resources to many possible users be determined? Beyond that, who will decide who receives the benefits purchased with these scarce dollars?" In partial answer to that question, the American Nurses Association (ANA), in conjunction with more than 60 other nursing organizations, released *Nursing's Agenda for Health Care Reform,* (1991). This document identifies a basic core of essential health care services which nursing believes should be available to all individuals, and presents a framework to meet present and future health care needs. The reader is urged to contact the ANA at 1-800-637-0323 to acquire a copy of the *Agenda* and other ANA publications of interest.

Quantification of Nursing Care Costs

The profession's attention is thus focused on the cost of providing nursing care to patients within the setting of prospective reimbursement, fewer dollars, limited time, and reduced beds and staff. Quantification of nursing's contribution to patient care can be used to determine the cost of providing care to specific patients. Quantifying nursing time requires the identification of the level of nursing care necessary for each patient, which can be used for direct "billing" of services rendered. In those hospitals already billing for nursing services, the patient plan of care is an integral part of the justification of nursing care costs.

Describing the work of nursing has been an ongoing challenge since the beginning of our profession. The *what* and *how* of the work of nursing has been explained in part in a number of existing publications which help to operationalize the work of nursing. The 1980 ANA's *Nursing: A Social Policy Statement* described nursing as the diagnosis and treatment of human responses to actual or potential health problems. The North American Nursing Diagnosis Association's (NANDA) development of a taxonomy (1989) provided a beginning classification schema to categorize and classify nursing diagnostic labels. NANDA's definition of nursing diagnosis (1990) further clarified the second step of the nursing process (i.e., problem identification/diagnosis). The ANA *Standards of Clinical Nursing Practice,* (1991) describes the patient care process and identifies standards for professional performance (Table 1-1).

The advancement of knowledge continues with the US Department of Health and Human Services' Agency for Health Care Policy and Research (AHCPR) whose purpose is to enhance the quality, appropriateness, and effectiveness of health care services and access to these services. To this end, multidisciplinary panels of clinicians (including nurses) have begun the arduous process of creating clinical practice guidelines addressing specific patient care situations. These guidelines are intended to assist health care providers in the prevention, diagnosis, treatment, and management of clinical conditions. They provide a resource by which patient care can be evaluated, the provider held accountable, and reimbursement justified. At this printing, four clinical practice guidelines are published and available free of charge. These are

- *Acute Pain Management: Operative or Medical Procedures and Trauma*
- *Urinary Incontinence in Adults*
- *Pressure Ulcers*
- *Sickle Cell Anemia*

Also, in 1992, the *Iowa Intervention Project: Nursing Interventions Classification* (NIC) moved our focus to the content and process of nursing care by identifying and standardizing some of the direct care activities nurses perform.

Reduced Length of Stay

The provision of personalized care must be planned and provided with continuity as the quantity of care time decreases. Many patients who leave the hospital earlier are still in need of health care. Hospitals are responding to this need by creating transitional care floors/beds, creating their own health care agencies, or hiring hospital-based coordinators to work with private home health care agencies. Nurses are assuming a larger portion of responsibility for ensuring that patients are discharged on time according to their diagnosis related group (DRG) classification. Aggressive discharge planning must begin on admission to the medical/surgical unit and incorporate knowledge of hospital and community resources available for the patient.

To facilitate early but safe discharge and to ensure continuity of care, many traditional unit boundaries are loosening. Nursing-case managers follow patients from admission to the general care units through discharge into the community in an effort to achieve optimal outcomes. An effectively coordinated plan of care can help ensure continuity of care between the health care system and the home or agency accepting transfer.

TABLE 1–1. Standards of Clinical Nursing Practice*

Standards of Care

1. Assessment: The nurse collects client health data.
2. Diagnosis: The nurse analyzes the assessment data in determining diagnoses.
3. Outcome identification: The nurse identifies expected outcomes individualized to the client.
4. Planning: The nurse develops a plan of care that prescribes interventions to attain expected outcomes.
5. Implementation: The nurse implements the interventions identified in the plan of care.
6. Evaluation: The nurse evaluates the client's progress toward attainment of outcomes.

Standards of Professional Performance

1. Quality of Care: The nurse systematically evaluates the quality and effectiveness of nursing practice.
2. Performance Appraisal: The nurse evaluates his or her own nursing practice in relation to professional practice standards and relevant statutes and regulations.
3. Education: The nurse acquires and maintains current knowledge in nursing practice.
4. Collegiality: The nurse contributes to the professional development of peers, colleagues, and others.
5. Ethics: The nurse's decisions and actions on behalf of clients are determined in an ethical manner.
6. Collaboration: The nurse collaborates with the client, significant others, and health care providers in providing client care.
7. Research: The nurse uses research findings in practice.
8. Resource utilization: The nurse considers factors related to safety, effectiveness, and cost in planning and delivering client care.

*Measurement criteria have also been developed for each standard and are included in the document *Standards of Clinical Nursing Practice,* 1991, available form the American Nurses Association.

Increasing Reliance on High Technology

In the "hostile" environment of a litigious society, the practice of *defensive* medicine has resulted in increased dependency on sophisticated diagnostic technology and treatment interventions. Several years ago before "high tech/high touch" became a trendy phrase, nurses expressed concern that the patient was in danger of being lost among the tubes, monitors, and machines as complex technology became an increasingly larger part of health care. This led nurses to advocate for patient individuality, the holistic concept of "mind-soul-body" interaction, and heightened awareness of ethical issues such as the quality of life/right to die dilemma. Inclusion of these concepts and consideration of the individual's cultural/socioeconomic background can facilitate achieving balance between technologic advances and human needs.

Requirement for Advanced Nursing Knowledge

Intensive nursing interventions are required to deal with increased patient acuity in the face of shorter lengths of stay within the medical/surgical environment. The nurse needs greater clinical expertise, maturity, critical thinking ability, assertiveness, and patient management skills to handle these increased responsibilities.

Nursing specialty certification programs share common goals: to provide consumer protection, to enhance nursing knowledge and competency, to increase nursing autonomy, and to strengthen collaboration. Certification acknowledges the nurse's attainment of predetermined standards established by the certifying group, and thus takes on importance in this cost-conscious era as managers seek to hire competent professionals. In addition, this type of credentialing can provide a framework for reimbursement by third-party payors.

Need for Collaboration and Communication

As health care delivery becomes more complex and more economically centered, the need for communication and collaboration among health care professionals is intensified. Only through collaboration between departments, services, and facilities can medical professionals deliver the most efficient and comprehensive care. The nurse, as the primary coordinator of overall patient care, strives to ensure that this takes place.

Interdepartmental communication and collaboration may take the form of a patient care conference. Information obtained from these conferences is incorporated into the overall plan of care by the nurse, who works as a liaison between health care providers. Thus, the plan of care serves as the vehicle for and documentation of ongoing communication between nurses and other disciplines.

Patients and families, assuming responsibility for themselves (internal locus-of-control), are also participating in more decisions concerning the level and amount of health care they desire. Their moral and ethical concerns, such as no code/living will decisions, with date, time, and names of those participating should be included in the plan of care. This provides legal and ethical documentation of the decision making/communication process.

Innovations in Planning Care Through Computerization

Many nurses believe that their limited time can be better spent at the bedside giving patient care rather than filling out paperwork. The use of written plans of care reflecting only functional divisions of tasks and duties perpetuates the notion that plans of care are "busy work," unrelated to caregiving. Restructuring plans of care to use nursing models increases usage and provides succinct documentation, demonstrating the relationship between planning and documentation. Institutions using computers report increased numbers of plans of care being generated and maintained than occurred previous to computerization. In fact, computerized systems have had a favorable impact on the process, as nurses may quickly enter, display, update, evaluate, and print a plan of care, thus improving the quality of record keeping.

Most computerized systems use standardized patient plans of care, which reflect accepted standards of care for particular medical/nursing problems. Many use the nursing diagnoses accepted for testing by NANDA. Because computerized plans reflect a wealth of varied nursing knowledge and experience, they allow even novice practitioners to formulate effective care strategies. Standardized care plans also serve as "memory joggers" to nurses caring for patients not usually seen in their area of clinical practice, thus providing information to promote effective practice. In addition, they provide all nurses with an efficient means of developing comprehensive, continuously updated, individualized, and legible plans of care for each patient.

Conclusion

Rapid changes in the health care environment, with continuous technologic advances, increasing severity of illness, budget constraints, and expanding nursing knowledge, have greatly increased the responsibilities facing today's nurse. To fulfill these responsibilities, planning and documentation of care are essential to satisfy patient needs and meet legal obligations. Documentation of the impact of nursing on patient care also provides information for continuing care needs, legal concerns, and payment.

What lies ahead for nursing and care planning? Definitely, a tremendously exciting and exacting challenge!

Bibliography

Books

Bulechek, FM and McCloskey, JC: Nursing Interventions: Essential Nursing Treatments, ed 2. Mosby Year Book, St Louis, 1992.
McCloskey, JC and Bulechek, GM: Iowa Intervention Project: Nursing Interventions Classification (NIC). Mosby Year Book, St Louis, 1992.
Taxonomy I—with Official Nursing Diagnoses. North American Nursing Diagnosis Association, St. Louis, 1990.

Articles

Fagin, CM: Nursing's value proves itself. AJN 20(10):17, 1990.
Jacox, AK, Pillar, B, and Redman, BK: A classification of nursing technology. Nursing Outlook 38:81, 1990.
Kerr, M, et al: Development of definitions for Taxonomy II. Nursing Diagnosis 3(2):65, 1992.
Kerr, M, et al: From Taxonomy I to Taxonomy II. Nursing Diagnosis 2(4):313, 1991.
Loomis, ME and Conco, D: Patient's perceptions of health, chronic illness, and nursing diagnoses. Nursing Diagnosis 2(3):162, 1991.
Mallison, MB: Ninety years through nursing's lens. AJN 20(19):44, 1992.
Meyer, C: Bedside computer charting: Inching toward tomorrow. AJN 22(4):38, 1992.
Mitchell, GJ: Nursing diagnosis: An ethical analysis. Image: Journal of Nursing Scholarship 23(2):99, 1991.
Moriarty, M: Ten years later. RN August 1992, p 44.
Nornhold, P, Bailey, M, and Barrick, B, et al: 90 predictions for the 90's. Nursing 90 20(1):35, 1990.
Pillar, B, Jacox, AK, and Redman, BK: Technology: Its assessment and nursing. Nursing Outlook 38:16, 1990.

CHAPTER 2

THE NURSING PROCESS

Nursing care is a key factor in patient survival and in the maintenance, rehabilitative, and preventive aspects of health care. To this end, the nursing profession has identified a problem-solving process that "combines the most desirable elements of the art of nursing with the most relevant elements of systems theory, using the scientific method" (Shore, 1988).

This nursing process was introduced in the 1950s as a three-step process of *assessment, planning,* and *evaluation* based on the scientific method of observing, measuring, gathering data, and analyzing the findings. Years of study, use, and refinement have led nurses to the expansion of the nursing process to five concrete steps (assessment, problem identification, planning, implementation, and evaluation) which provide an efficient method of organizing thought processes for clinical decision making. These five steps are central to nursing actions and the delivery of higher quality, individualized patient care in any setting. The nursing process is included in the conceptual framework of all nursing curricula and is accepted as part of the legal definition of nursing in the Nurse Practice Acts of most states.

When a patient enters the health care system, the nurse, using the steps of the nursing process, collects data, identifies problems/needs (nursing diagnoses), establishes goals, identifies outcomes, and chooses nursing interventions to achieve these outcomes and goals. After interventions have been carried out, the nurse evaluates the effectiveness of the plan of care in reaching the desired outcomes and goals by determining whether or not the problems have been resolved. If some of the identified problems remain unresolved at the time of discharge, plans must be made for further assessment, additional problem identification, alteration of outcomes and goals, and/or changes of interventions in the home care setting.

Although we use the terms assessment, problem identification, planning, implementation, and evaluation as separate, progressive steps, they are, in reality, interrelated elements. Together, they form a continuous circle of thought and action throughout the patient's contact with the health care system. Figure 2–1 gives some idea of how this cycling process works. The nursing process, combining all of the skills of critical thinking, creates a method of active problem-solving that is both dynamic and cyclic.

The critical element for providing effective planned nursing care is its relevance as identified in patient assessments. According to the American Nurses Association *Standards of Clinical Nursing Practice* (ANA, 1991), patient assessment is required in the following areas: physical, psychologic, sociocultural, spiritual, cognitive, functional abilities, development, economic, and lifestyle. These assessments, combined with the results of medical findings and diagnostic studies, are documented in the patient data base and form a strong basis for developing the patient's plan of care.

Patient Data Base

Assessment includes data collected through the history-taking interview, physical assessment, laboratory and diagnostic studies, and review of prior records.

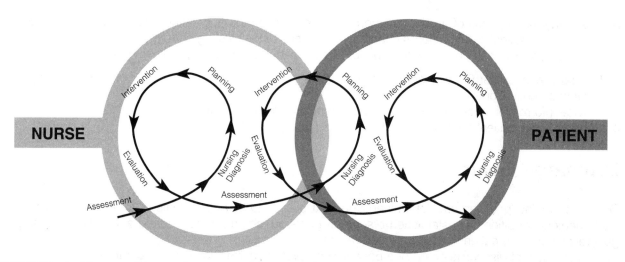

FIGURE 2–1. Diagram of the nursing process. The steps of the nursing process are interrelated, forming a continuous circle of thought and action that is both dynamic and cyclic.

In this book each selected medical condition has an accompanying patient data base which includes subjective ("may report") and objective ("may exhibit") data. The patient data base is organized within the 13 categories of the Diagnostic Divisions. A sample medical/surgical assessment tool, definitions of the divisions, and a patient situation are included in Chapter 3.

INTERVIEWING

Interviewing provides data the nurse obtains from the patient and significant others through conversation and observation. The data may be collected during one or more contact periods and should include all relevant data. Organizing and updating this data assists in the ongoing identification of patient care needs and nursing diagnoses. All participants in the interview process need to know that collected data is used in planning the patient's care.

PHYSICAL ASSESSMENT

During this aspect of information gathering, the nurse exercises perceptual and observational skills, using the senses of sight, hearing, touch, and smell. The duration and depth of any physical assessment depends on the current condition of the patient and the urgency of the situation but usually includes *inspection, palpation, percussion,* and *auscultation.* In this book the physical assessment data are presented within the patient data base as *objective* data.

LABORATORY AND DIAGNOSTIC STUDIES

Laboratory and diagnostic studies are included as part of the data-gathering process. The nurse needs to be aware of significant test results that require reporting to the physician and/or initiation of specific nursing interventions. Some tests are used to diagnose disease, whereas others are useful in following the course of a disease or in adjusting therapies. In many cases, the relationship of the test to the pathologic physiology is clear, but in other cases it is not. This is the result of the interrelationship between various organs and body systems. Interpretation of diagnostic test results should be integrated with the history and physical findings.

Nursing Priorities

In this book, nursing priorities are listed in a certain order to facilitate the ranking of selected associated nursing diagnoses that appear in the care-plan guides. In any given patient situation, nursing priorities differ on the basis of specific patient need and can vary from minute to minute. A nursing diagnosis that is a priority today may be less of a priority tomorrow depending on the fluctuating physical and psychosocial condition of the patient or the patient's changing responses to the existing condition.

An example of nursing priorities for a patient diagnosed with severe hypertension would include:

1. Maintain/enhance cardiovascular functioning.
2. Prevent complications.
3. Provide information about disease process, prognosis, and treatment regimen.
4. Support active patient control of condition.

Discharge Goals

Once the nursing priorities are determined, the next step is to establish goals of treatment. In this book each medical condition has established *discharge goals,* which are broadly stated and reflect the desired general status of the patient on discharge or transfer.

An example of discharge goals for a patient with severe hypertension would include:

1. Blood pressure within acceptable limits for individual.
2. Cardiovascular and systemic complications prevented/minimized.
3. Disease process/prognosis and therapeutic regimen understood.
4. Necessary lifestyle/behavioral changes initiated.

Nursing Diagnosis (Problem Identification)

Nursing diagnoses are a uniform way of identifying, focusing on, and dealing with specific patient needs and responses to actual and high risk problems. Nursing diagnosis labels provide a format for expressing the problem identification portion of the nursing process. The current working definition of nursing diagnosis developed by the North American Nursing Diagnosis Association (NANDA) is presented in Box 2–1.

Box 2–1. NANDA Working Definition of Nursing Diagnosis

Nursing diagnosis is a clinical judgment about individual, family, or community responses to actual and potential health problems/life processes. Nursing diagnoses provide the basis for selection of nursing interventions to achieve outcomes for which the nurse is accountable.

There are several steps involved in the process of problem identification. Integrating these steps provides a systematic approach to accurately identifying nursing diagnoses.

1. Collecting a patient data base (nursing interview, physical assessment, and laboratory and diagnostic studies) combined with information collected by other health care providers.
2. Reviewing and analyzing the patient data.
3. Synthesizing the gathered patient data as a whole and then labeling your clinical judgment about the patient's response to these actual or high risk problems.
4. Comparing and contrasting the relationships among your clinical judgments against NANDA documented related factors and defining characteristics for the selected nursing diagnosis. This step is crucial to choosing the appropriate nursing diagnosis label to be used in creating a specific patient diagnostic statement.
5. Combining the nursing diagnosis with the related factors and defining characteristics to create the patient diagnostic statement. For example, the diagnostic statement for a paraplegic patient with a decubitus ulcer could read: Skin Integrity, impaired, related to pressure, circulatory impairment, and decreased sensation evidenced by draining wound, sacral area.

The nursing diagnosis is as correct as the present data will allow because it is supported by the immediate data collected. It documents what the patient's situation is at the present time and should reflect changes as they occur in the patient's condition. Accurate problem identification and diagnostic labeling provide the basis for selecting nursing interventions.

The nursing diagnosis may be a physical or a psychosocial response. Physical nursing diagnoses can include those that pertain to physical processes, such as circulation (Altered Tissue Perfusion); ventilation (Impaired Gas Exchange); and elimination (Constipation). Psychosocial nursing diagnoses can include those that pertain to the mind (Altered Thought Processes); emotion (Fear); or lifestyle/relationship (Altered Role Performance). Unlike medical diagnoses, nursing diagnoses change as the patient progresses through various stages of illness/maladaptation to resolution of the problem or to the conclusion of the condition. Each decision the nurse makes is time-dependent and, with additional information gathered at a later point in time, decisions may change. For example, the initial problems/needs for a patient undergoing cardiac surgery may be Pain, Cardiac Output, Airway Clearance, and High Risk for Infection. As the patient progresses, problems/needs will likely shift to Activity Intolerance, Knowledge Deficit, and Role Performance.

Desired Patient Outcomes

A desired patient outcome is defined as the result of nursing interventions and patient responses that are achievable, desired by the patient and/or caregiver, and attainable within a defined time period, given the present situation and resources. These desired outcomes are the measurable steps toward achieving the previously established discharge goals. Useful desired patient outcomes must:

1. Be specific.
2. Be realistic.
3. Be measurable.
4. Indicate a definite time frame for achievement.
5. Consider patient's desires and resources.

Desired patient outcomes are written by listing items and/or behaviors which can be observed and monitored to determine whether or not an acceptable outcome has been achieved within a specified time frame. Action verbs and time frames are used, e.g., "patient will ambulate, using cane, within 48 hours of surgery." These time frames are dependent on the patient's projected or anticipated length of stay, often determined by diagnosis related group (DRG) classification and considering the presence of complications or extenuating circumstances (e.g., age).

When outcomes are properly written, they provide direction for planning and validating the selected nursing interventions. Consider the two following patient outcomes: "Identifies individual nutritional needs within 36 hours" and "Formulates a dietary plan based on identified nutritional needs within 72 hours."

Based on the clarity of these outcomes, the nurse can select nursing interventions to ensure that the patient's dietary knowledge is assessed, individual needs identified, and nutritional education presented.

Nursing Actions/Interventions

Nursing interventions are prescriptions for specific behaviors expected from the patient and/or actions to be carried out by nurses. Nursing actions/interventions are selected to assist the patient in achieving the stated desired patient outcomes and discharge goals. The expectation is that the prescribed behavior will benefit the patient and family in a predictable way, related to the identified problem and chosen outcomes. These interventions have the intent of individualizing care by meeting a specific patient need and should incorporate identified patient strengths when possible.

Nursing interventions should be specific and clearly stated, beginning with an action verb. Qualifiers of *how, when, where, time/frequency,* and *amount* provide the content of the planned activity. For example, "Assist as needed with self-care activities each morning." "Record respiratory and pulse rates before, during, and after activity." "Measure intake/output hourly." "Active-listen patient's concerns regarding diagnosis."

This book divides the nursing interventions/actions into *independent* (nurse-initiated) and *collaborative* (initiated by other care providers). Examples of these two different professionally initiated actions are:

Independent: Provide calm, restful surroundings, minimize environmental activity/noise, and limit numbers of visitors and length of stay.

Collaborative: Administer antianxiety medication as indicated.

Rationale

Although rationales do not appear on agency plans of care, they are included to assist the student and practicing nurse in associating the pathophysiologic and/or psychologic principles with the selected nursing intervention.

DOCUMENTING THE NURSING PROCESS

In general, the goals of the documentation system are to:

- Facilitate the quality of patient care.
- Ensure documentation of progress with regard to patient-focused outcomes.
- Facilitate interdisciplinary consistency and the communication of treatment goals and progress.

Two recent publications provide the nurse with guidelines for documenting the nursing process and support the need for a written (or computer-generated) plan of care. As previously noted, the Standards of Care (*Standards of Clinical Nursing Practice,* ANA 1991) ". . . delineate care that is provided to all clients of nursing services," and each standard includes a measurement criteria addressing documentation. In addition, the Nursing Care Standards (Joint Commission on Accreditation of Health Care Organizations [JCAHO], 1992) also focus our attention on documentation as presented in Table 2–1. These revised standards delineate the professional responsibilities of all registered nurses and provide criteria to assist in measuring achievement of identified standards.

From a nursing focus, documentation provides a record of the use of the nursing process for the delivery of individualized patient care. The initial *assessment* is recorded in the patient history or database. The *diagnosis* of patient problems/needs, and the *planning* of patient care are recorded in the plan of care. The *implementation* of the plan is recorded in progress notes and/or flow sheets. The evaluation of care is documented in the progress notes and/or plan of care.

The maintenance of a medical record is one of the most essential requirements for accreditation of health care facilities by JCAHO and/or other credentialing and licensing agencies. JCAHO standards state that the medical record be documented accurately and in a timely manner. Therefore, the importance of completing notes on schedule and in a manner which facilitates retrieval of data should be emphasized.

Documentation is not only a requirement for accreditation but is a permanent record of what happens with each patient. It is a legal requirement in any health care setting. In our society, with its many lawsuits and aggressive malpractice emphasis, all aspects of the medical record may be important for legal documentation. The plan of care that has been developed for a particular patient serves as a framework or outline for the charting of administered care. Progress notes and flow sheets therefore reflect implementation of the treatment plan by documenting that appropriate actions have been carried out, precautions taken, and so on. Both the implementation of interventions and progress toward the measurable outcomes need to be documented in the progress notes. They should be written in a clear and objective fashion and in a manner which reflects progress toward desired measurable outcomes with the use of planned staff interventions. These notations also need to be date and time specific and be signed by the person making the entry. Any errors in the document must be crossed out with one line so that it is still legible, identified by the author as "error," and then initialed. White-outs or cross-outs that make the information unreadable are not acceptable, as they could be construed to mean that the individual or facility is trying to alter facts.

The medical record is also the primary source of providing proof of services, which is a necessary piece of maintaining revenues. Third-party payors are insistent that the *why, when, where, how, what,* and *who* of services be clearly documented. Absence of such documentation may result in termination of funding for individual patients and therefore termination of treatment. Therefore, progress notes must document what is happening to the patient during all phases of illness, treatment, and recovery. It is important to record information and observations, which will assist both the oncoming nurse and other patient care providers in maintaining the continuity of planned care. Table 2–2 provides examples of information to be documented in the patient's record.

There are several charting formats that are currently used for documentation (e.g., problem-oriented medical record [POMR]; FOCUS® Charting). Regardless of the form you use, entries should be concise and consistent in style and format to avoid confusion and to comply with existing agency policies and procedures. Examples of documentation formats are included in Chapter 3.

TABLE 2–1. A Sample Portion of One Nursing Care Standard from JCAHO

NC.1. Patients receive nursing care based on a documented assessment of their needs.
    NC.1.3.4. The patient's medical record includes documentation of:
        NC.1.3.4.1 The initial assessments and reassessments
        NC.1.3.4.2 The nursing diagnosis and/or patient care needs
        NC.1.3.4.3 The interventions identified to meet the patient's nursing care needs
        NC.1.3.4.4 The nursing care provided
        NC.1.3.4.5 The patient's response to, and the outcomes of, the care provided
        NC.1.3.4.6 The abilities of the patient and/or, as appropriate, his or her significant other to manage continuing care needs after discharge

TABLE 2–2. Contents of a Progress Note

- Unsettled or unclear problems or issues which need to be dealt with, including attempts to contact other patient care providers
- Noteworthy incidents or interviews involving the patient that would benefit from a more detailed recording
- Other pertinent data such as notes on phone calls, home visits, and family interactions
- Additional critical incident data such as seemingly significant or revealing statements made by the patient; an insight you have into a patient's patterns of behavior; patient injuries; the use of any special treatment procedure; or other major events such as episodes of pain, respiratory distress, panic attacks, medication reactions, or suicidal comments
- Administered care, activities, or observations if not recorded elsewhere on flow sheets (physician visits, completion of ordered tests, prn medications, and so on)

Summary

This book is intended to facilitate the application of the nursing process and the use of nursing diagnosis in medical/surgical patients. Each care plan guide was designed to provide generalized information on the associated medical condition. The guides can be modified by either using portions of the information provided or adding additional patient care information to the existing guides. The care plan guidelines were developed using the NANDA recommendations except in a few examples where the authors believed more clarification and enhancement were required. The ongoing controversy on the validity of the NANDA approved nursing diagnosis, Knowledge Deficit, is one example where further clarification was added. The term "Learning Need" has been added to the nursing diagnoses Knowledge Deficit. For example, for the patient with severe hypertension, a nursing diagnosis was developed with the following label: Knowledge Deficit [Learning Need] regarding condition, prognosis, and treatment plan.

We recognize that not all of the NANDA approved nursing diagnoses have been used in these care plan guides but we hope that these guides will assist you in determining your patient's needs, outcomes, and nursing interventions.

Chapter 3 will assist you in applying and adapting theory to practice.

Bibliography

American Nurses Association: Nursing: A social policy statement. Pub code NP-63 3SM, 12/80, Kansas City, 1980.
American Nurses Association: Standards of nursing practice. Pub code NO-41 10M 1:77, Kansas City, 1973.

Books

Alfaro, RA: Application of Nursing Process: A Step-by-Step Guide to Care Planning, ed 2. JB Lippincott, Philadelphia, 1990.
Cox, HC, et al: Clinical Applications of Nursing Diagnosis. Williams & Wilkins, Baltimore, 1989.
Doenges, ME and Moorhouse, MF: Application of Nursing Process and Nursing Diagnosis: An Interactive Text. FA Davis, Philadelphia, 1992.
Lampe, SS: Focus® Charting: Creative Nursing Management, ed 4. Minneapolis, MN, 1986.

Articles

Dolan, M: Why nurses and doctors should be partners in diagnosis. Nursing90 20(11):41, 1990.
Mosher, C, Cronk, P, and Kidd, A, et al: Upgrading practice with critical pathways. AJN 22(1):41, 1992.
Radwin, LE: Research on diagnostic reasoning in nursing. Nursing Diagnosis 1(2):70–77, 1990.

CHAPTER 3
APPLYING THEORY TO PRACTICE

In the previous chapter, we discussed the theory of nursing process, incorporating nursing diagnosis. In this chapter, given the formative stage of nursing diagnosis, the nurse is encouraged to investigate and learn, in order to tailor the plan of care to the individual patient. The plans of care presented here are guides for the nurse in the use of this process. They are designed to give the nurse a sampling of information about general patient situations and to identify many factors that may or may not need to be given consideration in caring for any particular patient.

Patient assessment is the foundation on which identification of individual needs, responses, and problems is based. To facilitate this step of the nursing process, we have constructed an assessment tool using a nursing focus instead of the more familiar medical approach ("review of systems"). To achieve this nursing focus, we used the North American Nursing Diagnosis Association (NANDA) nursing diagnoses (Table 3–1) grouped in related categories entitled "Diagnostic Divisions" (Table 3–2), which reflect a blending of theories, primarily Maslow's Hierarchy of Needs and a self-care philosophy. As data are collected, the divisions serve to direct the nurse to the appropriate corresponding nursing diagnosis labels. Because these divisions are based on human responses/needs and are not specific "systems," information may be recorded in more than one area. For this reason, the nurse is encouraged to collect as much data as possible before choosing the nursing diagnosis that best reflects the patient's situation. The results (synthesis) of the collected data are written concisely (patient diagnostic statements).

Nursing priorities and diagnoses are arranged in a general order that can be altered to fit the individual patient. Each nursing diagnosis has been provided with a list of etiologic/risk factors ("may be related to" or "risk factors may include") and defining characteristics or signs/symptoms ("possibly evidenced by") which the nurse may select from or add to, to accurately represent the patient's situation.

Desired patient outcomes are then identified to facilitate choosing appropriate interventions and to serve as evaluators of both nursing care and patient response. These outcomes also form the framework for documentation.

Interventions are designed to specify the action of the nurse, the patient, and/or significant other(s). They are not all inclusive, because such basic nursing actions as "bathe the patient" or "notify the physician of changes" have been left out. It is expected that these are included in routine patient care. Sometimes controversial issues or treatments are presented for the sake of information and/or because alternate therapies may be used in different care settings or geographic locations.

In addition to achieving physiologic stability, interventions need to promote movement toward independence. An important aspect of the self-care philosophy is the involvement of patients in their own care. Information is given at the level of the individual's understanding and ability so as to encourage participation in decisions about care and outcomes whenever possible. This promotes patient responsibility, negating the idea that health care providers control patient lives.

To assist you in visualizing the tailoring of a care plan guide, a specific Patient Situation (p 23) is provided as an example of data collection and care plan construction. As you review the patient assessment data base, you can see the etiologic/risk factors and defining characteristics that were used to formulate the patient diagnostic statements. Time lines were added to specific patient outcomes to reflect anticipated length of stay and individual patient/nurse expectations. Interventions are based on the concerns and needs identified by the patient and nurse during data collection, as well as physician orders. Although not normally included in a plan of care, rationales are included in this sample for the purpose of explaining or clarifying the choice of interventions and enhancing the nurse's learning. Finally, to complete the learning experience, samples of documentation based on the patient situation are presented.

TABLE 3-1. Nursing Diagnoses (Through 10th NANDA Conference) 1992

Activity Intolerance
Activity Intolerance, high risk for
Adjustment impaired
Airway Clearance, ineffective
Anxiety [specify level]*
Aspiration, high risk for
Body Image disturbance
Body Temperature, altered, high risk for
Bowel Incontinence
Breastfeeding, effective
Breastfeeding, ineffective
Breastfeeding, interrupted
Breathing Pattern, ineffective
Cardiac Output, decreased
Caregiver Role Strain
Caregiver Role Strain, high risk for
Communication, impaired verbal
Constipation
Constipation, colonic
Constipation, perceived
Coping, defensive
Coping, ineffective, individual
Decisional Conflict (specify)
Denial, ineffective
Diarrhea
Disuse Syndrome, high risk for
Diversional Activity deficit
Dysreflexia
Family Coping, compromised
Family Coping, disabling
Family Coping, potential for growth
Family Processes, altered
Fatigue
Fear
Fluid Volume deficit [active loss]*
Fluid Volume deficit [regulatory failure]*
Fluid Volume deficit, high risk for
Fluid Volume excess
Gas Exchange, impaired
Grieving, anticipatory
Grieving, dysfunctional
Growth and Development, altered
Health Maintenance, altered
Health-Seeking Behaviors (specify)
Home Maintenance Management, impaired
Hopelessness
Hyperthermia
Hypothermia
Incontinence, functional
Incontinence, reflex
Incontinence, stress
Incontinence, total
Incontinence, urge
Infant Feeding Pattern, ineffective
Infection, high risk for
Injury, high risk for
Knowledge Deficit [Learning need]* (specify)
Noncompliance [Compliance, altered]* (specify)

Nutrition, altered, less than body requirements
Nutrition, altered, more than body requirements
Nutrition, altered, high risk for more than body requirements
Oral Mucous Membrane, altered
Pain
Pain, chronic
Parental Role Conflict
Parenting, altered
Parenting, altered, high risk for
Peripheral Neurovascular dysfunction, high risk for
Personal Identity disturbance
Physical Mobility, impaired
Poisoning, high risk for
Posttrauma Response
Powerlessness
Protection, altered
Rape-trauma Syndrome
Rape-trauma Syndrome: compound reaction
Rape-trauma Syndrome: silent reaction
Relocation Stress Syndrome
Role Performance, altered
Self-care Deficit, feeding, bathing/hygiene, dressing/grooming, toileting
Self-esteem, chronic low
Self-esteem disturbance
Self-esteem, situational low
Self-mutilation, high risk for
Sensory-perceptual alterations (specify): visual, auditory, kinesthetic, gustatory, tactile, olfactory
Sexual dysfunction
Sexuality Patterns, altered
Skin Integrity, impaired
Skin Integrity, impaired: high risk for
Sleep Pattern disturbance
Social Interaction, impaired
Social Isolation
Spiritual Distress (distress of the human spirit)
Spontaneous Ventilation, inability to sustain
Suffocation, high risk for
Swallowing impaired
Therapeutic Regimen (Individuals), ineffective management of
Thermoregulation, ineffective
Thought Processes, altered
Tissue Integrity, impaired
Tissue Perfusion, altered (specify): (cerebral, cardiopulmonary, renal, gastrointestinal, peripheral)
Trauma, high risk for
Unilateral Neglect
Urinary Elimination, altered patterns
Urinary Retention [acute/chronic]*
Ventilatory Weaning Response, dysfunctional (DVWR)
Violence, high risk for, directed at self/others

*[Author recommendations].

TABLE 3–2. Nursing Diagnoses Organized According to Diagnostic Divisions

After data are collected and areas of concern/need identified, the nurse is directed to the Diagnostic Divisions to review the list of nursing diagnoses that fall within the individual categories. This will assist the nurse in choosing the specific diagnostic label to describe the data accurately. Then, with the addition of etiology (when known) and signs and symptoms, the patient diagnostic statement emerges.

Activity/rest—Ability to engage in necessary/desired activities of life (work and leisure) and to obtain sleep/rest.

    Activity Intolerance
    Activity Intolerance, high risk
    Disuse Syndrome, high risk for
    Diversional Activity deficit
    Fatigue
    Sleep Pattern disturbance

Circulation—Ability to transport oxygen and nutrients necessary to meet cellular needs.

    Cardiac Output, decreased
    Dysreflexia
    Tissue Perfusion, altered, (specify): renal, cerebral, cardiopulmonary, gastrointestinal, peripheral

Ego Integrity—Ability to develop and use skills and behaviors to integrate and manage life experiences.

    Adjustment, impaired
    Anxiety (specify level)
    Body Image disturbance
    Coping, defensive
    Coping ineffective, Individual
    Decisional Conflict (specify)
    Denial, ineffective
    Fear
    Grieving, anticipatory
    Grieving, dysfunctional
    Hopelessness
    Personal Identity Disturbance
    Posttrauma Response
    Powerlessness
    Rape-trauma Syndrome
    Rape-trauma Syndrome: compound reaction
    Rape-trauma Syndrome: silent reaction
    Relocation Stress Syndrome
    Self-esteem, chronic low
    Self-esteem disturbance
    Self-esteem, situational low
    Spiritual Distress (distress of the human spirit)

Elimination—Ability to excrete waste products.

    Bowel Incontinence
    Constipation
    Constipation, colonic
    Constipation, perceived
    Diarrhea
    Incontinence, functional
    Incontinence, reflex
    Incontinence, stress
    Incontinence, total
    Incontinence, urge
    Urinary Elimination, altered patterns
    Urinary Retention [acute/chronic]

Food/Fluid—Ability to maintain intake of and use nutrients and liquids to meet physiologic needs.

    Breastfeeding, effective
    Breastfeeding, ineffective
    Breastfeeding, interrupted
    Fluid Volume deficit [active loss]
    Fluid Volume deficit [regulatory failure]

Fluid Volume deficit, high risk for
Fluid Volume excess
Infant Feeding Pattern, ineffective
Nutrition, altered, less than body requirements
Nutrition, altered, more than body requirements
Nutrition, altered, high risk for more than body requirements
Oral Mucous Membranes, altered
Swallowing, impaired
Hygiene—Ability to perform activities of daily living.
   Self-care deficit: feeding, bathing/hygiene, dressing/grooming,
     toileting.
Neurosensory—Ability to perceive, integrate, and respond to internal and external cues.
   Peripheral Neurovascular dysfunction, high risk for
   Sensory-perceptual alterations (specify): visual, auditory, kinesthetic, gustatory, tactile, olfactory
   Thought Processes, altered
   Unilateral Neglect
Pain/Comfort—Ability to control internal/external environment to maintain comfort.
   Pain [acute]
   Pain, chronic
Respiration—Ability to provide and use oxygen to meet physiologic needs.
   Airway Clearance, ineffective
   Aspiration, high risk for
   Breathing Pattern, ineffective
   Gas Exchange, impaired
   Spontaneous Ventilation, inability to sustain
   Ventilatory Weaning Response, dysfunctional (DVWR)
Safety—Ability to provide safe, growth promoting environment.
   Body Temperature, altered, potential
   Health Maintenance, altered
   Home Maintenance Management, impaired
   Hyperthermia
   Hypothermia
   Infection, high risk for
   Injury, high risk for
   Physical Mobility, impaired
   Poisoning, high risk for
   Protection, altered
   Self-mutilation, high risk for
   Skin Integrity, impaired
   Skin Integrity, impaired, potential
   Suffocation, high risk for
   Thermoregulation, ineffective
   Tissue Integrity, impaired
   Trauma, high risk for
   Violence, high risk for, directed at self/others
Sexuality [Component of Ego Integrity and Social Interaction]—Ability to meet requirements/characteristics
of male/female role.
   Sexual dysfunction
   Sexuality Patterns, altered
Social Interaction—Ability to establish and maintain relationships.
   Caregiver Role Strain
   Caregiver Role Strain, high risk for
   Communication, impaired verbal
   Family Coping, compromised
   Family Coping, disabling
   Family Coping, potential for growth
   Family Processes, altered
   Parental Role conflict
   Parenting, altered
   Parenting, altered, high risk for
   Role Performance, altered

Social Interaction, impaired
Social Isolation
Teaching/Learning—Ability to incorporate and use information to achieve healthy lifestyle/optimal wellness
Growth and Development, altered
Health Seeking Behaviors (specify)
Knowledge deficit [learning need] (specify)
Noncompliance [Compliance, altered] (specify)
Therapeutic Regimen (Individuals), ineffective management

ADULT MEDICAL/SURGICAL ASSESSMENT TOOL _____

This is a suggested tool for development by an individual or institution to create a data base reflecting Diagnostic Divisions of Nursing Diagnoses. Although the divisions are alphabetized for ease of presentation, they can be prioritized or rearranged to meet individual needs.

GENERAL INFORMATION

Name: _____

Age: _____ DOB: _____ Sex: _____ Race: _____

Admission date: _____ Time: _____ From: _____

Source of information: _____ Reliability (1–4 with 4 = very reliable): _____

ACTIVITY/REST

Reports (Subjective)

Occupation: _____ Usual activities/hobbies: _____

Leisure time activities: _____

Feelings of boredom/dissatisfaction: _____

Limitations imposed by condition: _____

Sleep: Hours: _____ Naps: _____ Aids: _____

    Insomnia: _____ Related to: _____

    Rested upon awakening: _____

    Other: _____

Exhibits (Objective)

Observed response to activity: Cardiovascular: _____

                        Respiratory: _____

Mental status (i.e., withdrawn/lethargic): _____

Neuromuscular assessment: _____

    Muscle mass/tone: _____

    Posture: _____ Tremors: _____

    ROM: _____ Strength: _____

    Deformity: _____

CIRCULATION

Reports (Subjective)

History of: Hypertension: _____ Heart trouble: _____

         Rheumatic fever: _____ Ankle/leg edema: _____

         Phlebitis: _____ Slow healing: _____

         Claudication: _____

Extremities: Numbness: _____ Tingling: _____

Cough/hemoptysis: _____

Change in frequency/amount of urine: _____

Exhibits (Objective)

BP: R and L: Lying/sitting/standing: _____

    Pulse pressure: _____ Auscultatory gap: _____

Pulse (palpation): Carotid: _____ Temporal: _____

                Jugular: _____ Radial: _____

                Femoral: _____ Popliteal: _____

                Posttibial: _____ Dorsalis pedis: _____

Cardiac (palpation):

    Thrill: _____ Heaves: _____

Heart sounds: Rate: _____ Rhythm: _____ Quality: _____

    Friction rub: _____ Murmur: _____

Breath sounds: Vascular bruit: _____ Jugular vein distention: _____

Extremities: Temperature: _____ Color: _____

    Capillary refill: _____

    Homan's sign: _____ Varicosities: _____

    Nail abnormalities: _____

    Distribution/quality of hair: _____

Color: _____ Mucous membranes: _____ Lips: _____

    Nail beds: _____ Conjunctiva: _____ Sclera: _____

    Diaphoresis: _____

EGO INTEGRITY

Reports (Subjective)

Stress factors: _____

Ways of handling stress: _____

Financial concerns: _____

Relationship status: _____

Cultural factors: _____

Religion: _____ Practicing: _____

Lifestyle: _____ Recent changes: _____

Feelings: Helplessness: _____ Hopelessness: _____

    Powerlessness: _____

Exhibits (Objective)

Emotional status (check those that apply):

    Calm: _____ Anxious: _____ Angry: _____

    Withdrawn: _____ Fearful: _____ Irritable: _____

    Restive: _____ Euphoric: _____

Observed physiologic response(s): _____

ELIMINATION

Reports (Subjective)

Usual bowel pattern: _____ Laxative use: _____

Character of stool: _____ Last bowel movement: _____

History of bleeding: _____   Hemorrhoids: _____

Constipation: _____   Diarrhea: _____

Usual voiding pattern: _____   Incontinence/when: _____

    Urgency: _____   Frequency: _____   Retention: _____

Character of urine: _____

Pain/burning/difficulty voiding: _____

History of kidney/bladder disease: _____

Diuretic use: _____

Exhibits (Objective)

Abdomen: Tender: _____   Soft/firm: _____

    Palpable mass: _____   Size/girth: _____

    Bowel sounds: _____

Hemorrhoids: _____

Bladder palpable: _____   Overflow voiding: _____

FOOD/FLUID

Reports (Subjective)

Usual diet (type): _____   Number of meals daily: _____

Last meal/intake: _____   Dietary pattern: _____

Loss of appetite: _____   Nausea/vomiting: _____

Heartburn/indigestion: _____   Related to: _____   Relieved by: _____

Allergy/Food intolerance: _____

Mastication/swallowing problems: _____

    Dentures: _____

Usual weight: _____   Changes in weight: _____

Diuretic use: _____

Exhibits (Objective)

Current weight: _____   Height: _____   Body build: _____

Skin turgor: _____   Mucous membranes moist/dry: _____

Edema: General: _____   Dependent: _____

    Periorbital: _____   Ascites: _____

Jugular vein distention: _____

Thyroid enlarged: _____   Hernia/masses: _____   Halitosis: _____

Condition of teeth/gums: _____

Appearance of tongue: _____

    Mucous membranes: _____

Bowel sounds: _____

Breath sounds: _____

Urine S/A or Chemstix: _____

HYGIENE

Reports (Subjective)

Activities of daily living: Independent/dependent: _____

    Mobility: _____   Feeding: _____

Hygiene: _____ Dressing: _____

Toileting: _____

Preferred time of bath: _____

Equipment/prosthetic devices required: _____

Assistance provided by: _____

Exhibits (Objective)

General appearance: _____

Manner of dress: _____ Personal habits: _____

Body odor: _____ Condition of scalp: _____

Presence of vermin: _____

NEUROSENSORY

Reports (Subjective)

Fainting spells/dizziness: _____

Headaches: Pain location: _____ Frequency: _____

Tingling/numbness/weakness (location): _____

Stroke (residual effects): _____

Seizures: _____ Type: _____ Aura: _____ Frequency: _____

    Postical state: _____ How controlled: _____

Eyes: Vision loss: _____ Last examination: _____

    Glaucoma: _____ Cataract: _____

Ears: Hearing loss: _____ Last examination: _____

Epistaxis: _____ Sense of smell: _____

Exhibits (Objective)

Mental status: _____

    Oriented/disoriented: Time: _____

                      Place: _____

                       Person: _____

    Alert: _____ Drowsy: _____ Lethargic: _____

    Stuporous: _____ Comatose: _____

    Cooperative: _____ Combative: _____ Delusions: _____

    Hallucinations: _____ Affect (describe): _____

Memory: Recent: _____ Remote: _____

Glasses: _____ Contacts: _____ Hearing aids: _____

Pupil size/reaction: R/L: _____

Facial droop: _____ Swallowing: _____

Handgrasp/release: R/L: _____ Posturing: _____

Deep tendon reflexes: _____ Paralysis: _____

PAIN/DISCOMFORT

Reports (Subjective)

Location: _____ Intensity (1–10 with 10 most severe): _____ Frequency: _____

Quality: _____ Duration: _____ Radiation: _____

Precipitating factors: _____

How relieved, associated factors: _____

Exhibits (Objective)

Facial grimacing: _____ Guarding affected area: _____

Emotional response: _____ Narrowed focus: _____

RESPIRATION

Reports (Subjective)

Dyspnea, related to cough/sputum: _____

History of bronchitis: _____ Asthma: _____

    Tuberculosis: _____ Emphysema: _____

    Recurrent pneumonia: _____

    Exposure to noxious fumes: _____

Smoker: _____ Pack/d: _____ Number of years: _____

Use of respiratory aids: _____ Oxygen: _____

Exhibits (Objective)

Respiratory: Rate: _____ Depth: _____ Symmetry: _____

Use of accessory muscles: _____ Nasal flaring: _____

Fremitis: _____

Breath sounds: _____

Egophony: _____

Cyanosis: _____ Clubbing of fingers: _____

Sputum characteristics: _____

Mentation/restlessness: _____

SAFETY

Reports (Subjective)

Allergies/sensitivity: _____ Reaction: _____

Previous alteration of immune system: _____ Cause: _____

History of sexually transmitted disease (date/type): _____

High-risk behaviors: _____ Testing: _____

Blood transfusion/number: _____ When: _____

    Reaction described: _____

History of accidental injuries: _____

Fractures/dislocations: _____

Arthritis/unstable joints: _____

Back problems: _____

Changes in moles: _____ Enlarged nodes: _____

Impaired vision, hearing: _____

Prosthesis: _____ Ambulatory devices: _____

Exhibits (Objective)

Temperature: _____ Diaphoresis: _____

Skin integrity: _____

    Scars: _____ Rashes: _____

    Lacerations: _____ Ulcerations: _____

    Ecchymosis: _____ Blisters: _____

    Burns: (degree/percent): _____ Drainage: _____

Mark location of above on diagram:

General strength: _____ Muscle tone: _____

    Gait: _____ Range of motion: _____

    Paresthesia/paralysis: _____

    Results of cultures, immune system testing: _____

SEXUALITY: (Component of Social Interaction)ï

Sexually active: _____ Use of condoms: _____ Sexual concerns/

difficulties: _____ Recent change in frequency/interest: _____

Female

Reports (Subjective)

Age at menarche: _____ Length of cycle: _____ Duration: _____

Last menstrual period: _____ Menopause: _____

Vaginal discharge: _____ Bleeding between periods: _____

Practices breast self-examination/mammogram: _____ Last PAP smear: _____

Exhibits (Objective)

Breast examination: _____

Genital warts/lesions: _____

Male

Reports (Subjective)

Penile discharge: _____ Prostate disorder: _____

Circumcised: _____ Vasectomy: _____

Practices self-examination: _____ Breast/testicles: _____

Last proctoscopic/prostate examination: _____

Exhibits (Objective)

Examination: _____ Breast/penis/testicles: _____

Genital warts/lesions: _____

SOCIAL INTERACTIONS

Reports (Subjective)

Marital status: _____ Years in relationship: _____

    Living with: _____

    Concerns/stresses: _____

Extended family: _____

Other support person(s): _____

Role within family structure: _____

Problems related to illness/condition: _____

Change in speech: Use of communication aids: _____

    Laryngectomy present: _____

Exhibits (Objective)

Speech: Clear: _____ Slurred: _____

    Unintelligible: _____ Aphasic: _____

    Unusual speech pattern/impairment: _____

    Use of speech aids: _____

Verbal/nonverbal communication with family/SO(s): _____

_____

Family interaction (behavioral) pattern: _____

TEACHING/LEARNING

Reports (Subjective)

Dominant language (specify): _____ Literate: _____

Education level: _____

Learning disabilities (specify): _____

Cognitive limitations: _____

Health beliefs/practices: _____

Special health care concerns (e.g., impact of religious/cultural practices): _____

Familial risk factors (indicate relationship): _____

    Diabetes: _____ Tuberculosis: _____

    Heart disease: _____ Strokes: _____

    High BP: _____ Epilepsy: _____

    Kidney disease: _____ Cancer: _____

    Mental illness: _____ Other: _____

Prescribed medications (circle last dose):

Drug	Dose	Times	Take regularly	Purpose
_____	_____	_____	_____	_____
_____	_____	_____	_____	_____
_____	_____	_____	_____	_____

Nonprescription drugs: OTC drugs: _____

    Street drugs: _____ Tobacco: _____ Smokeless tobacco: _____

Use of alcohol (amount/frequency): _____

Admitting diagnosis per physician: _____

Reason for hospitalization per patient: _____

History of current complaint: _____

Patient expectations of this hospitalization: _____

Previous illnesses and/or hospitalizations/surgeries: _____

_____

Evidence of failure to improve: _____

Last complete physical examination: _____

Discharge Plan Considerations

DRG projected mean length of stay: _____

Date information obtained: _____

1. Anticipated date of discharge: _____

2. Resources available: Persons: _____

    Financial: _____

3. Anticipated changes in living situation after discharge: _____

4. Areas that may require alteration/assistance: _____

Food preparation: _____ Shopping: _____

Transportation: _____ Ambulation: _____

Medication/IV therapy: _____ Treatments: _____

Wound care: _____ Supplies: _____

Self-care assistance (specify): _____

Physical layout of home (specify): _____

Homemaker/maintenance assistance (specify): _____

Living facility other than home (specify): _____

PATIENT SITUATION: Diabetes Mellitus _____

Mr. R.S., a noninsulin dependent diabetic (NIDDM, Type II) for 5 years, presented to his physician's office with a nonhealing ulcer of 3 weeks' duration on his left foot. Laboratory studies at the doctor's office revealed blood sugar of 256/fingerstick and urine clinitest of 1% small.

ADMITTING PHYSICIAN'S ORDERS

Culture/sensitivity and Gram stain of foot ulcer.
Random blood sugar on admission and fingerstick BG.
Blood sugar q6h × 24 hours, then daily.
CBC, electrolytes, glycosylated Hb in AM.
Chest x-ray and ECG in AM.
Humulin N insulin 15 U q AM, sc. Begin insulin instruction for self-care.
Dicloxacillin 500 mg po, q6h, start after culture obtained.
Darvon 65 mg q4h prn, pain.
Diet—2400 calories ADA/3 meals with 2 snacks.
Up in chair ad lib with feet elevated.
Foot cradle for bed.
Betadine soak L foot tid x 15 minutes, then cover with dry sterile dressing.
Vital signs qid.

PATIENT ASSESSMENT DATA BASE

Name: R. S. Informant: Patient. Reliability (Scale 1–4): 3.
Age: 64. DOB: 5/3/27. Race: Caucasian. Sex: M.
Admission date: 6/28/91 Time: 7 PM From: Home.

ACTIVITY/REST

Reports (Subjective):	Occupation: Farmer.
	Usual activities/hobbies: Reading, playing cards. "Don't have time to do much. Anyway I'm too tired most of the time to do anything after the chores."
	Limitations imposed by illness: "Have to watch what I order if I eat out."
	Sleep: Hours: 6–8 h/night. Naps: No. Aids: No.
	Insomnia: "Not unless I drink coffee after supper."
	Usually feels rested when awakens at 4:30 AM.
Exhibits (Objective):	Observed response to activity: Favors L foot when walking.
	Mental status: Alert/active.
	Neuromuscular assessment: Muscle mass/tone: bilaterally equal/firm.
	Posture: Erect. ROM: Full.
	Strength: Equal 3 extremities/favors L leg currently.

CIRCULATION

Reports (Subjective):	Slow healing: lesion L foot, 3 weeks.
	Extremities: Numbness/tingling: "My feet feel cold and tingly when I walk a lot."
	Cough/character of sputum: Occasional/white.
	Change in frequency/amount of urine: Yes, voiding more lately.

Exhibits (Objective):	Peripheral pulses: Radials 3+, popliteal, dorsalis, posttibial, pedal, all 1+.

Exhibits (Objective):

Peripheral pulses: Radials 3+, popliteal, dorsalis, posttibial, pedal, all 1+.

BP: R: Sit: 140/86. Lying: 146/90. Stand: 138/90.
  L: Sit: 138/88. Lying: 142/88. Stand: 138/84.

Pulse: Apical: 86. Radial: 86. Quality: Strong. Rhythm: Regular.

Chest auscultation: Few rhonchi clear with cough, no murmurs/rubs.

JVD: -0-.

Extremities: Temperature: Feet cool bilat/remainder warm.
  Color—skin: Legs pale. Capillary refill: Slow both feet.
  Homan's sign: -0-. Varicosities: Few enlarged superficial veins (both calves).
    Nails: Toenails thickened, yellow, brittle. Distribution and quality of hair: Coarse hair to ankles, none on toes.
  Color—general: Ruddy face/arms. Mucous membranes/lips: Pink.
  Nail beds: Blanch well. Conjunctiva and sclera: White.

EGO INTEGRITY

Reports (Subjective):

Report of stress factors: "Normal farmer's problems: weather, pests, bankers, and so on."

Ways of handling stress: "I get busy with the chores and talk things over with my livestock; they listen real good."

Financial concerns: No insurance and needs to hire someone while in hospital.

Relationship status: Married.

Cultural factors: Rural/agrarian.

Religion: Protestant/practicing.

Lifestyle: Middle class/self-sufficient farmer.

Recent changes: -0-.

Feelings: "I'm in control of most things, except the weather and this diabetes."

Exhibits (Objective):

Emotional status: Calm.

Other: Concerned regarding possible therapy change "from pills to shots."

Observed physiologic response(s): Occasionally sighs deeply/frowns, shrugs shoulders.

ELIMINATION

Reports (Subjective):

Usual bowel pattern: Most every PM.

Last bowel movement: Last night. Character of stool: Firm/brown.

Bleeding: -O-. Hemorrhoids: -0-. Constipation: Occasional.

Laxative used: Hot prune juice.

Urinary: No problems. Character of urine: Pale yellow.

Exhibits (Objective):

Abdomen tender: No. Soft/Firm: Soft. Palpable mass: None.

Bowel sounds: Active all 4 quads.

FOOD/FLUID

Reports (Subjective):

Usual diet (type): 2400 ADA (occasionally "cheats with dessert, but my wife watches it pretty closely"). Number of meals daily: 3.

Dietary Pattern: Breakfast: Fruit juice, toast, ham, coffee. Lunch: Meat, potatoes, vegetables, fruit, milk. Dinner: Meat sandwich, soup, fruit, coffee. Snack: milk/crackers at HS. Usual beverage: Skim milk, 2–3 cups decaf coffee. Drinks a *lot* of water.

	Last meal/intake: Dinner: roast beef sandwich, vegetable soup, pear with cheese, decaf coffee.
	Loss of appetite: "Never, but lately I don't feel as hungry as usual."
	Nausea/Vomiting: -O-. Food Allergies: None.
	Heartburn/food intolerance: Cabbage causes gas.
	Mastication/swallowing problems: No. Dentures: Upper; partial.
	Usual weight: 175 lb.
	Recent changes: Has lost about 3 lb this month.
	Diuretic therapy: No.
Exhibits (Objective):	Wt: 171 lb. Ht: 5'10". Build: Stocky. Skin turgor: Good/leathery.
	Appearance of tongue: Midline, pink. Mucous membranes: Pink, intact.
	Condition of teeth/gums: Good; (no problem with bleeding).
	Breath sounds: Few rhonchi cleared with cough.
	Bowel sounds: Active all 4 quads.
	Urine Chemstix: 1%/small. Fingerstick: 256.

HYGIENE

Reports (Subjective):	Activities of daily living: Independent in all areas.
	Preferred time of bath: PM.
Exhibits (Objective):	General appearance: Clean, shaven, short hair.
	Hands: Rough and dry. Scalp and eyebrows: Scaly white patches.

NEUROSENSORY

Reports (Subjective):	Headache: "Occasionally behind my eyes when I worry too much."
	Tingling/Numbness: Feet, occasionally.
	Eyes: Vision loss, far-sighted. Examination: 2 years ago.
	Ears—Hearing loss: R: "Some" L: No (Has not been tested).
	Nose: Epistaxis: -O-. Sense of smell: No problems.
Exhibits (Objective):	Mental status: Alert, oriented to time, place, person. Affect: Concerned. Memory: Remote and recent; clear and intact.
	Speech: Clear/coherent.
	Pupil reaction: PERLA. Glasses: Reading. Hearing Aid: No.
	Handgrip/release: Strong/equal.

PAIN/DISCOMFORT

Reports (Subjective):	Location: lateral aspect, heel of L foot.
	Intensity (0–10): 2–3. Quality: Dull ache.
	Frequency/Duration: "Seems like all the time." Radiation: No.
	Precipitating factors: Shoes, walking. How relieved: ASA, not helping.
	Other complaints: Sometimes has back pain following chores/heavy lifting relieved by ASA/linament.
Exhibits (Objective):	Facial grimacing: When lesion border palpated.
	Guarding affected area: Pulls foot away. Narrowed focus: No.
	Emotional response: Tense, irritated.

RESPIRATORY

**Reports
(Subjective):**

Dyspnea: -O-. Cough: Occasional morning cough, white sputum.

Emphysema: -O-. Bronchitis: -O-. Asthma: -O-. Tuberculosis: -0-.

Smoker: Filters. Packs/day: 1/2. Number of years: 40+.

Use of respiratory aids: -O-.

**Exhibits
(Objective):**

Respiratory rate: 22. Depth: Good. Symmetry: Equal, bilateral.

Auscultation: Few rhonchi, clear with cough.

Cyanosis: -O-. Clubbing of fingers: -O-.

Sputum characteristics: None at present.

Mentation/restlessness: Alert/oriented/relaxed.

SAFETY

**Reports
(Subjective):**

Allergies: -0-. Blood transfusions: -0-.

Sexually transmitted disease: None.

Fractures/dislocations: L clavicle, 1962, fell getting off tractor.

Arthritis/unstable joints: "Think I've got some in my knees."

Back problems: Occasional lower back pain.

Vision impaired: Requires glasses for reading (far-sighted).

Hearing impaired: Slightly, compensates by turning "good ear" toward speaker.

**Reports
(Objective):**

Temperature: 99.4, oral.

Skin integrity: Impaired L foot. Scars: R Ing, surgical.

Rashes: -O-. Bruises: -O-. Lacerations: -0-. Blisters: -0-.

Ulcerations: Medial aspect L foot, 2.5 cm diameter, approximately 3 mm deep, draining small amount cream color/pink tinged matter, no odor noted.

Strength (general): Equal all extremities. Muscle tone: Firm.

ROM: Good. Gait: Favors L foot. Paresthesia/Paralysis: -O-.

SEXUALITY

**Reports
(Subjective):**

Penile discharge: -O-. Prostate disorder: -O-. Vasectomy: -O-.

Last proctoscopic examination: 2 years ago. Prostate examination: 1 year ago.

Practice self-examination: Breast/testicles: No.

Problems/complaints: "I don't have any problems, but you'd have to ask my wife if there are any complaints."

**Exhibits
(Objective):**

Examination—Breast: No masses. Testicles: Deferred. Prostate: Deferred.

SOCIAL INTERACTIONS

**Reports
(Subjective):**

Marital status: Married, 40 years. Living with: Wife.

Report of problems: None.

Extended family: 1 daughter lives in town (30 miles away); 1 daughter married/grandson, living out of state.

Other: Several couples; he and wife play cards/socialize 2 or 3 times a month.

Role: Works farm alone; husband/father/grandfather.

Report of problems related to illness/condition: None until now.

Coping behaviors: "My wife and I have always talked things out. You know the 11th commandment is Thou shalt not go to bed angry."

Exhibits (Objective):	Speech: Clear, intelligible.
	Verbal/Nonverbal communication with family/SO(s): Speaks quietly with wife, looking her in the eye; relaxed posture.
	Family interaction patterns: Wife sitting at bedside, relaxed, both reading paper, making occasional comments to each other.

TEACHING/LEARNING

Reports (Subjective):

Dominant language: English. Literate: Yes.

Education level: 2 years of college.

Health beliefs/practices: "I take care of the minor problems and only see the doctor when something's broken."

Familial risk factors/relationship:
Diabetes: Maternal uncle. Tuberculosis: Brother died age 27.
Heart Disease: Father died age 78, heart attack.
Strokes: Mother died age 81. High BP: Mother.

Prescribed medications:

Drug	Dose	Schedule	Time/last dose	Purpose
Orinase	250 mg	8 AM/6 PM	Last dose 6 PM today	Diabetes

Home urine glucose monitoring: "Stopped several months ago when I ran out of TesTape. It was always negative anyway."

Takes medications regularly: Yes.

Nonprescription (OTC) drugs: Occasionally ASA.

Use of alcohol (amount/frequency): Socially, occasionally beer.

Admitting Diagnosis (physician): Hyperglycemia and ulcer L foot.

Reason for hospitalization (patient): Sore on foot and "My sugar is up."

History of current complaint: "Three weeks ago, I got a blister on my foot from breaking in my new boots. It got sore so I lanced it, but it isn't getting any better."

Patient's expectations of this hospitalization: "Clear up this infection and control my diabetes."

Other relevant illness and/or previous hospitalizations/surgeries: 1965 R Ing. hernia repair.

Evidence of failure to improve: Lesion L foot, 3 weeks.

Last physical examination: Complete 1 year ago, office follow up 3 months ago.

Discharge Considerations (as of 6/28):

Anticipated discharge: 7/1/91 (3 days).

Resources: Person: Wife. Financial: "If this doesn't take too long to heal, we got some savings to cover things."

Anticipated lifestyle changes: None.

Assistance needed: May require farm help for several days. Learn new medication regimen and wound care.

SAMPLE PLAN OF CARE: Diabetes Mellitus

PATIENT DIAGNOSTIC STATEMENT:	SKIN INTEGRITY, IMPAIRED, related to pressure, altered metabolic state, circulatory impairment, and decreased sensation evidenced by draining wound L foot.
DESIRED OUTCOMES— PATIENT WILL:	Demonstrate correction of metabolic state as evidenced by blood sugar within normal limits within 36 hours.
	Be free of purulent drainage within 48 hours.
	Display signs of healing with wound edges clean/pink within 60 hours.

ACTIONS/INTERVENTIONS	RATIONALE
Obtain culture of wound drainage on admission.	Identifies pathogens and therapy of choice.
Administer dicloxacillin 500 mg po q6h, starting 10 PM. Observe for signs of hypersensitivity, i.e., pruritus, urticaria, rash.	Treatment of infection/prevention of complications. Food interferes with drug absorption requiring scheduling around meals. Although no prior history of penicillin reaction, it may occur at any time.
Soak foot in room temperature sterile water with betadine solution tid × 15 minutes.	Local germicidal effective for surface wounds.
Assess wound with each dressing change.	Provides information about effectiveness of therapy and identifies additional needs.
Massage area around wound site.	Stimulates circulation and delivery of white blood cells, fibroblasts, and nutrients required for healing and removal of phagocytized debris.
Dress wound with dry sterile dressing. Use paper tape.	Keeps wound clean/minimizes cross-contamination. Adhesive tape may be abrasive to fragile tissues.
Administer 15 U Humulin N insulin sc q AM after daily laboratory sample drawn.	Treats underlying metabolic dysfunction, reducing hyperglycemia and promoting healing.

PATIENT DIAGNOSTIC STATEMENT:	Acute pain related to physical agent (wound L foot) evidenced by verbal report of discomfort and guarding behavior.
DESIRED OUTCOMES— PATIENT WILL:	Report pain is minimized/relieved within 48 hours.
	Ambulate normally, full weight bearing by discharge.

ACTIONS/INTERVENTIONS	RATIONALE
Determine pain characteristics through patient's description.	Establishes baseline for assessing improvement/ changes.

ACTIONS/INTERVENTIONS

Place foot cradle on bed/encourage use of loose fitting slipper, when up.

Administer Darvon 65 mg po q4h as needed. Document effectiveness.

RATIONALE

Avoids direct pressure to area of injury, which could result in vasoconstriction/increased pain.

Provides relief of discomfort when unrelieved by other measures.

PATIENT DIAGNOSTIC STATEMENT:	TISSUE PERFUSION, ALTERED, peripheral related to decreased arterial flow evidenced by decreased pulses, pale/cool feet, thick brittle nails, numbness/tingling of feet "when walks a lot."
DESIRED OUTCOMES— PATIENT WILL:	Verbalize understanding of relationship between chronic disease (diabetes mellitus) and circulatory changes. Demonstrate awareness of safety factors/proper foot care within 72 hours.

ACTIONS/INTERVENTIONS

Elevate feet when up in chair. Avoid long periods with feet dependent.

Assess for signs of dehydration. Monitor intake/output. Encourage oral fluids.

Instruct patient to avoid constricting clothing/socks and ill-fitting shoes.

Reinforce safety precautions regarding use of heating pads, hot water bottles/soaks.

Discuss complications of disease that result in vascular changes, i.e.; ulceration, gangrene, muscle or bony structure changes.

Review proper foot care as outlined in teaching plan.

RATIONALE

Minimizes interruption of blood flow, reduces venous pooling.

Glycosuria may result in dehydration reducing circulating volume and further alteration of peripheral perfusion.

Compromised circulation and decreased pain sensation may precipitate or aggravate tissue breakdown.

Heat increases metabolic demands on compromised tissues. Vascular insufficiency alters pain sensation increasing risk of injury.

Proper control of diabetes mellitus may not prevent complications but may minimize severity of effect.

Altered perfusion of lower extremities may lead to serious/persistent complications at the cellular level.

PATIENT DIAGNOSTIC STATEMENT:	LEARNING NEED REGARDING DIABETIC CONDITION, related to misinterpretation of information and/or lack of recall evidenced by inaccurate follow-through of instructions regarding home glucose monitoring and foot care and failure to recognize signs/symptoms of hyperglycemia.
DESIRED OUTCOMES— PATIENT WILL:	Verbalize basic understanding of disease process and treatment within 48 hours. Perform procedure of home glucose monitoring and insulin administration correctly within 72 hours. Explain reasons for actions within 72 hours.

ACTIONS/INTERVENTIONS	RATIONALE
Determine patient's level of knowledge, priorities of learning needs, desire/need for including wife in instruction.	Establishes baseline and direction for teaching/planning. Involvement of wife, if desired, will provide additional resource for recall/understanding and may enhance patient's follow through.
Provide teaching guide, "Understanding your Diabetes" 6/29 AM. Show film "Diabetes and You" 6/29 4 PM when wife is visiting. Include in group teaching session 6/30 AM. Review information and obtain feedback from patient and wife.	Provides different methods for accessing/reinforcing information and enhances opportunity for learning/understanding.
Discuss factors related to/altering diabetes control, e.g., stress, illness, exercise.	Drug therapy/diet may need to be alterated in response to both short- and long-term stressors.
Review signs/symptoms of hyperglycemia, (e.g., fatigue, nausea/vomiting, polyuria/dypsia). Discuss how to prevent and evaluate this situation, and when to seek medical care. Have patient identify appropriate interventions.	Recognition/understanding of these signs/symptoms and timely intervention will aid patient in avoiding recurrences and preventing complications.
Review and provide information about necessity for routine examination of feet, and proper foot care, e.g., daily inspection for injuries, pressure areas, corns, calluses; proper nail cutting; daily washing. Tell patient to avoid going barefoot and to wear loose fitting socks and properly fitting shoes (break new shoes in gradually); if foot injury/skin break occurs, wash with soap and water, cover with sterile dressing. Inspect wound and change dressing daily. Report redness, swelling, or presence of drainage.	Reduces risk of tissue injury, promotes understanding and prevention of stasis ulcer formation and wound healing difficulties.
Instruct regarding prescribed insulin therapy:	May be a temporary treatment of hyperglycemia with infection, or may be permanent replacement of oral hypoglycemic.
Humulin N Insulin, sc;	Intermediate-acting insulin generally lasts 18–28 hours, with peak effect 6–12 hours.
Keep vial in current use at room temperature, store extra vials in refrigerator;	Refrigeration prevents wide fluctuations in temperature prolonging the drug shelf-life; can impede absorption.
Roll bottle and invert to mix. Do not shake vigorously;	Vigorous shaking may create foam which can interfere with accurate dose withdrawal and may damage the insulin molecule.
Rotate injection sites/provide diagram.	Minimizes tissue damage and improves absorption of medication.
Demonstrate, then observe patient in drawing insulin into syringe, reading syringe markings, and administering dose. Assess for accuracy.	May require several instruction sessions and practice before patient and wife feel comfortable drawing up and injecting medication.
Instruct in signs/symptoms of insulin reaction/hypoglycemia, i.e., fatigue, nausea, headache, hunger, sweating, irritability, shakiness, anxiety, difficulty concentrating.	Knowing what to watch for and appropriate treatment, such as grape juice for immediate response/cheese for sustained effect, may prevent/minimize complications.

ACTIONS/INTERVENTIONS	RATIONALE
Review "Sick Day Rules," For example, call the doctor if too sick to eat normally/stay active; take insulin as ordered; keep record as noted on Sick Day Guide.	Understanding of necessary actions in the event of mild/severe illness promotes competent self-care and reduces risk of hyper/hypoglycemia.
Instruct patient/SO in fingerstick glucose monitoring and observe their demonstrations of the procedure.	Patient was using urine sugar monitoring, which is now replaced by more accurate blood glucose monitoring.
Recommend patient maintain record of fingerstick testing, insulin dosage/site, unusual physiologic response, dietary intake.	Provides accurate record for review by caregivers for assessment of therapy effectiveness.
Refer to dietician for consultation regarding diet.	Calories are unchanged on new orders but have been redistributed to 3 meals and 2 snacks. Dietary choices (e.g., increased vitamin C) may enhance healing.
Discuss other health care issues, e.g., smoking habits, self-monitoring for cancer (breasts/testicles), and reporting changes in general well-being.	Encourages patient involvement, awareness, and responsibility for own health; promotes wellness.

EVALUATION

As nursing care is provided, ongoing assessments determine the patient's response to therapy and progress toward accomplishing the desired outcomes. This activity serves as the feedback and control part of the nursing process, through which the status of the individual patient diagnostic statement is judged to be resolved, continuing, or requires revision.

This process is visualized in Figure 3–1. Observation of Mr. R.S's wound reveals that edges are clean and pink and drainage is scant. Therefore, he is progressing *toward* achieving wound healing, and this problem will continue to be addressed although no revision in the treatment plan is required at this time.

DOCUMENTATION

There are several charting formats that have been used for documentation. These include block notes, with a single entry covering an entire shift (e.g., 7–3 PM); narrative timed notes (e.g., 8:30 AM, ate all of breakfast); and the problem-oriented medical record system (POMR or PORS) using the SOAP/SOAPIER approach, to name a few. The latter can provide thorough documentation, but it was designed by physicians for episodic care and requires that the entries be tied to a patient problem identified from a problem list.

A new system format created by nurses for documentation of frequent/repetitive care is FOCUS® Charting. It was designed to encourage looking at the patient from a positive rather than a negative (or problem-oriented) perspective by using precise documentation to record the nursing process. Recording of assessment, interventions, and evaluation information in a Data, Action, and Response (DAR) format facilitates tracking and following what is happening to the patient at any given moment. Charting focuses on patient and nursing concerns. The focal point is patient status and the associated nursing care. The Focus is always stated in a way that reflects the *patient's* concern/need rather than reflecting a nursing task or medical diagnosis. Thus, the focus can be a patient problem/concern or nursing diagnosis; signs/symptoms of potential importance (e.g., fever, dysrhythmia, edema); a significant event or change in status; or specific standards of care/hospital policy. Based on the patient situation of Mr. R.S., the following examples of documentation are provided:

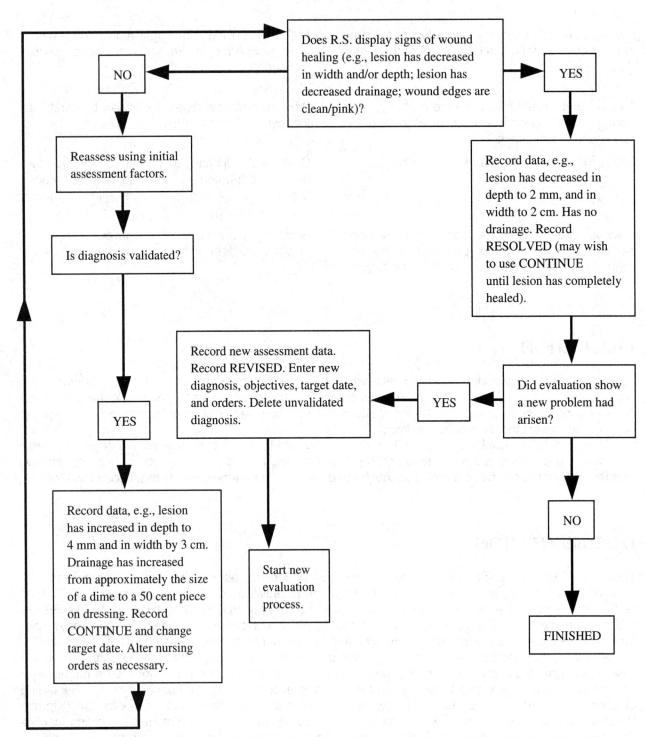

Figure 3–1. Outcome-based evaluation of the patient's response to therapy. (Adapted from Cox, HC, et al: Clinical Applications of Nursing Diagnosis. Williams & Wilkins, Baltimore, 1989.)

Date	Time	Number/Problem	Soap Format
6/30/91	1400	#1 (Skin Integrity)	S: "That hurts" (when tissue surrounding wound is palpated). O: Scant amount serous drainage on dressing. Wound borders pink. No odor present. A: Wound shows early, signs of healing, free of infection. P: To continue skin care per care plan.
6/28/91	2100	#2 (Pain)	S: "Dull, throbbing pain in left foot." States there is no radiation to other areas. O: Muscles tense. A: Persistent pain. P: Foot cradle placed on bed. Darvon 65 mg given po. Signed: M Sickus, RN

Other examples of documentation:

Date	Time	Focus®	Focus: DAR Format
6/30/91	1400	Skin Integrity, L foot	D: Scant amount serous drainage on dressing, wound borders pink, no odor present, denies discomfort except with direct palpation of surrounding tissue. A: Betadine soak as ordered. Lateral aspect of L foot massaged gently. Sterile dressing applied with paper tape. R: Wound clean, no drainage present. Signed: E. Moore, RN

The following is an example of documentation of a patient need/concern that currently does not require identification as a patient problem (nursing diagnosis) or inclusion in the plan of care and therefore not easily documented in the SOAP format:

Date	Time	Focus®	Focus: DAR Format
6/29/91	2020	Gastric distress	D: Awakened, reports "indigestion/burning sensation" with hand over epigastric area. Skin warm/dry, color pink, vital signs unchanged. A: Given Mylanta 30 ml po. Head of bed elevated approximately 15 degrees. R: Reports pain relieved. Appears relaxed, resting quietly. Signed: E. Moore, RN

CHAPTER 4

CARDIOVASCULAR

Hypertension: Severe

Hypertension is defined by the Joint National Committee on Detection, Evaluation and Treatment of High Blood Pressure (JNC) as pressure greater than 140/90 mm Hg and is classified according to the degree of severity, ranging from high normal BP to malignant hypertension. It is categorized as primary/essential (constituting approximately 90% of all cases) or secondary, occurring as a result of an identifiable, often correctable pathologic condition.

RELATED CONCERNS:

Cerebrovascular Accident, p 290
Myocardial Infarction, p 80
Psychosocial Aspects of Acute Care, p 899
Renal Failure, p 618
Valvular Heart Disease, p 102

PATIENT ASSESSMENT DATA BASE

ACTIVITY/REST

May report:	Weakness, fatigue, shortness of breath, sedentary lifestyle.
May exhibit:	Elevated heart rate.
	Change in heart rhythm.
	Tachypnea.

CIRCULATION

May report:	History of hypertension, atherosclerosis, valvular/coronary artery heart disease and cerebrovascular disease.
	Episodes of palpitations, perspiration.
May exhibit:	Elevated BP (serial elevated measurements are necessary to confirm diagnosis).
	Postural hypotension (may be related to drug regimen).
	Pulse: Bounding carotid, jugular, radial pulsations; pulse disparities, e.g., femoral delay as compared with radial or brachial pulsation; absence of/diminished popliteal, posterior tibial, pedal pulses.

Apical pulse: PMI possibly displaced and/or forceful.

Rate/rhythm: Tachycardia, various dysrhythmias.

Heart sounds: Accentuated S_2 at base; S_3 (early CHF); S_4 (rigid left ventricle/left ventricular hypertrophy).

Murmurs of valvular stenosis.

Vascular bruits audible over carotid, femoral, or epigastrium (artery stenosis).

JVD (venous congestion).

Extremities: Discoloration of skin, cool temperature (peripheral vasoconstriction); capillary refill possibly slow/delayed (vasoconstriction).

Skin—Pallor, cyanosis, and diaphoresis (congestion, hypoxemia); flushing (pheochromocytoma).

EGO INTEGRITY

May report:
History of personality changes, anxiety, depression, euphoria, or chronic anger (may indicate cerebral impairment).

Multiple stress factors (relationship, financial, job-related).

May exhibit:
Mood swings, restlessness, narrowed attention span, outbursts of crying.

Emphatic hand gestures, tense facial muscles (particularly around the eyes), quick physical movement, expiratory sighs, accelerated speech pattern.

ELIMINATION

May report:
Past or present renal insult (e.g., infection/obstruction or past history of kidney disease).

FOOD/FLUID

May report:
Food preferences, which may include high-salt, high-fat, high-cholesterol foods (e.g., fried foods, cheese, eggs); licorice; high caloric content.

Nausea, vomiting.

Recent weight changes (gain/loss).

History of diuretic use.

May exhibit:
Normal weight or obesity.

Presence of edema (may be generalized or dependent); venous congestion, JVD; glycosuria (almost 10% of hypertensive patients are diabetic).

NEUROSENSORY

May report:
Fainting spells/dizziness.

Throbbing, suboccipital headaches (present on awakening and disappearing spontaneously after several hours).

Episodes of numbness and/or weakness on one side of the body.

Visual disturbances (diplopia, blurred vision).

Episodes of epistaxis.

May exhibit:
Mental status: Changes in alertness, orientation, speech pattern/ content, affect, thought process, or memory.

Motor responses: Decreased strength hand grip and/or deep tendon reflexes.

Optic retinal changes: From mild sclerosis/arterial narrowing to marked retinal and sclerotic changes with edema or papilledema, exudates, and hemorrhages dependent on severity/duration of hypertension.

PAIN/DISCOMFORT

May report:
Angina (coronary artery disease/cardiac involvement).

Intermittent pain in legs/claudication (indicative of arteriosclerosis of lower extremity arteries).

Severe occipital headaches as previously noted.

Abdominal pain/masses (pheochromocytoma).

RESPIRATION
(Generally associated with advanced cardiopulmonary effects of sustained/severe hypertension.)

May report:
Dyspnea associated with activity/exertion.

Tachypnea, orthopnea, paroxysmal nocturnal dyspnea.

Cough with/without sputum production.

Smoking history.

May exhibit:
Respiratory distress/use of accessory muscles.

Adventitious breath sounds (crackles/wheezes).

Cyanosis.

SAFETY

May report/ exhibit:
Impaired coordination/gait.

Transient episodes of unilateral paresthesia.

Postural hypotension.

TEACHING/LEARNING

May report:
Familial risk factors: Hypertension, atherosclerosis, heart disease, diabetes mellitus, cerebrovascular/kidney disease.

Ethnic/racial risk factors, e.g., African-American, Southeast Asian.

Use of birth control pills or other hormones; drug/alcohol use.

Discharge Plan Considerations:
DRG projected mean length of stay: 4.2 days.

Assistance with self-monitoring of BP.

Alterations in medication therapy.

DIAGNOSTIC STUDIES

Hemoglobin/hematocrit: Not diagnostic but assesses relationship of cells to fluid volume (viscosity) and may indicate risk factors such as hypercoagulability, anemia.

BUN/creatinine: Provides information about renal perfusion/function.

Glucose: Hyperglycemia (diabetes mellitus is a precipitator of hypertension) may result from elevated catecholamine levels (increases hypertension).

Serum potassium: Hypokalemia may indicate the presence of primary aldosteronism (cause) or be a side effect of diuretic therapy.

Serum calcium: Elevation may contribute to hypertension.

Serum cholesterol and triglycerides: Elevated level may indicate predisposition for/presence of atheromatous plaquing (cardiovascular effect).

Thyroid studies: Hyperthyroidism may lead/contribute to vasoconstriction and hypertension.

Serum/urine aldosterone level: To assess for primary aldosteronism (cause).

Urinalysis: Blood, protein, glucose suggest renal dysfunction and/or presence of diabetes.

Urine VMA (catecholamine metabolite): Elevation may indicate presence of pheochromocytoma (cause); 24-hour urine VMA may be done for assessment of pheochromocytoma if hypertension is intermittent.

Uric acid: Hyperuricemia has been implicated as a risk factor for the development of hypertension.

Urine steroids: Elevation may indicate hyperadrenalism, pheochromocytoma or pituitary dysfunction, Cushing's syndrome; renin levels may also be elevated.

IVP: May identify cause of hypertension, e.g., renal parenchymal disease, renal/ureteral calculi.

Chest x-ray: May demonstrate obstructing calcification in valve areas; deposits in and/or notching of aorta; cardiac enlargement.

CT scan: Assesses for cerebral tumor, CVA, encephalopathy, or to rule out pheochromocytoma.

ECG: May demonstrate enlarged heart, strain patterns, conduction disturbances. *Note:* Broad, notched P wave is one of the earliest signs of hypertensive heart disease.

NURSING PRIORITIES

1. Maintain/enhance cardiovascular functioning.
2. Prevent complications.
3. Provide information about disease process/prognosis and treatment regimen.
4. Support active patient control of condition.

DISCHARGE GOALS

1. BP within acceptable limits for individual.
2. Cardiovascular and systemic complications prevented/minimized.
3. Disease process/prognosis and therapeutic regimen understood.
4. Necessary lifestyle/behavioral changes initiated.

NURSING DIAGNOSIS:	CARDIAC OUTPUT, DECREASED, HIGH RISK FOR
Risk factors may include:	Increased afterload, vasoconstriction.
	Myocardial ischemia.
	Ventricular hypertrophy/rigidity.
Possibly evidenced by:	[Not applicable; presence of signs and symptoms establishes an actual diagnosis.]
DESIRED OUTCOMES/ EVALUATION CRITERIA— PATIENT WILL:	Participate in activities that reduce BP/cardiac workload.
	Maintain BP within individually acceptable range.
	Demonstrate stable cardiac rhythm and rate within patient's normal range.

ACTIONS/INTERVENTIONS	RATIONALE
Independent	
Monitor BP. Measure in both arms/thighs for initial evaluation. Use correct cuff size and accurate technique.	Comparison of pressures provides a more complete picture of vascular involvement/scope of problem. Severe hypertension is classified in the adult as a diastolic pressure elevation to 130; progressive diastolic readings above 130 are considered first accelerated, then malignant. Systolic hypertension also is an established risk factor for cerebrovascular disease and ischemic heart disease when diastolic pressure is 90–115.

ACTIONS/INTERVENTIONS	RATIONALE

Independent

Note presence, quality of central and peripheral pulses.

Bounding carotid, jugular, radial and femoral pulses may be observed/palpated. Pulses in the legs may be diminished, reflecting effects of vasoconstriction (increased SVR) and venous congestion.

Auscultate heart tones and breath sounds.

S_4 is common in severely hypertensive patients due to the presence of atrial hypertrophy (increased atrial volume/pressure). Development of S_3 indicates ventricular hypertrophy and impaired functioning. Presence of crackles, wheezes may indicate pulmonary congestion secondary to developing or chronic heart failure.

Observe skin color, moisture, temperature, and capillary refill time.

Presence of pallor, cool, moist skin and delayed capillary refill time may be due to peripheral vasoconstriction or reflect cardiac decompensation/decreased output.

Note dependent/general edema.

May indicate heart failure, renal or vascular impairment.

Provide calm, restful surroundings, minimize environmental activity/noise. Limit the number of visitors and length of stay.

Helps to reduce sympathetic stimulation; promotes relaxation.

Maintain activity restrictions, e.g., bed/chair rest; schedule periods of uninterrupted rest; assist patient with self-care activities as needed.

Reduces stress and tension that affect blood pressure and the course of hypertension.

Provide comfort measures, e.g., back and neck massage, elevation of head.

Decreases discomfort and may reduce sympathetic stimulation.

Instruct in relaxation techniques, guided imagery, distractions.

Can reduce stressful stimuli, produce calming effect, thereby reducing BP.

Monitor response to medications to control blood pressure.

Response to "stepped" drug therapy (consisting of diuretics, sympathetic inhibitors and vasodilators) is dependent on both the individual and synergistic effects of the drugs. Because of side effects, it is important to use the fewest number and lowest dosage of medications.

Collaborative

Administer medications as indicated, e.g.:
Thiazide diuretics, e.g., chlorothiazide (Diuril); hydrochlorothiazide (Esidrix/HydroDIURIL); bendroflumethiazide (Naturetin);

Thiazides may be used alone or in association with other drugs to reduce BP in patients with relatively normal renal function. These diuretics potentiate other antihypertensive agents by limiting fluid retention.

Loop diuretics, e.g., furosemide (Lasix); ethacrynic acid (Edecrin); bumetanide (Burmex);

These drugs produce marked diuresis by inhibiting resorption ot sodium and chloride and are effective antihypertensives, especially in patients who are resistant to thiazides or have renal impairment.

Potassium-sparing diuretics, e.g., spironolactone (Aldactone); triamterene (Dyrenium); amilioride (Midamor);

May be given in combination with a thiazide diuretic to minimize potassium loss.

ACTIONS/INTERVENTIONS	RATIONALE
Collaborative	
Sympathetic inhibitors, e.g., propranolol (Inderal); metoprolol (Lopressor); atenolol (Tenormin); nadolol (Corgard); methyldopa (Aldomet); reserpine (Serpasil); clonidine (Catapres);	Specific actions of these drugs vary, but they generally reduce BP through the combined effect of decreased total peripheral resistance, reduced cardiac output, inhibited sympathetic activity, and suppression of renin release.
Vasodilators, e.g., minoxidil (Loniten); hydralazine (Apresoline); calcium channel blockers, e.g., nifedipine (Procardia); verapamil (Calan);	May be necessary to treat severe hypertension when a combination of a diuretic and a sympathetic inhibitor has not sufficiently controlled BP. Vasodilation of healthy cardiac vasculature and increased coronary blood flow are secondary benefits of vasodilator therapy.
Antiadrenergic agents: α-1 blockers prazosin (Minipress); tetazosin (Hytrin);	Act on blood vessels to keep them from constricting.
Adrenergic neuron blockers: guanadrel (Hyloree); quanethidine Ismelin); reserpine (Serpasil);	Reduces arterial and venous constriction activity at the sympathetic nerve endings.
Centrally acting adrenergic inhibitors: clonidine; (Catapress); guanabenz (Wytension); methyldopa (Aldomet);	These drugs increase sympathetic stimulation of vasomotor center to reduce peripheral arterolar resistance.
Direct-acting oral vasodilators: hydralazine (Apresoline); minoxidil; (Loniten);	Relax vascular smooth muscle.
Direct-acting parenteral vasodilators: diazoxide (Hyperstat); nitroprusside; (Nipride, Nitropess).	These are given intravenously for management of hypertensive emergencies.
Ganglion blockers, e.g., guanethidine (Ismelin); trimethaphan (Arfonad). ACE inhibitor, e.g., captopril (Capoten).	The use of an additional sympathetic inhibitor may be required (for its cumulative effect) when other measures have failed to control BP and patient cooperation with the therapeutic regimen has been verified.
Implement fluid and dietary sodium restrictions as indicated.	These restrictions can manage fluid retention with associated hypertensive response, thereby decreasing myocardial workload.
Prepare for surgery, when indicated.	When hypertension is due to the presence of pheochromocytoma, removal of the tumor will correct condition.

NURSING DIAGNOSIS: **ACTIVITY INTOLERANCE**

May be related to:	Generalized weakness.
	Imbalance between oxygen supply and demand.
Possibly evidenced by:	Verbal report of fatigue or weakness.
	Abnormal heart rate or BP response to activity.
	Exertional discomfort or dyspnea.
	ECG changes reflecting ischemia; dysrhythmias.

DESIRED OUTCOMES/ EVALUATION CRITERIA— PATIENT WILL:	Participate in necessary/desired activities.
	Report a measurable increase in activity tolerance.
	Demonstrate a decrease in physiologic signs of intolerance.

ACTIONS/INTERVENTIONS

Independent

Assess the patient's response to activity, noting pulse rate over 20 bpm above resting rate; marked increase in BP during/after activity (systolic pressure increase of 40 mm Hg or diastolic pressure increase of 20 mm Hg); dyspnea or chest pain; excessive fatigue and weakness; diaphoresis; dizziness or syncope.

Instruct patient in energy-saving techniques, e.g., using chair when showering, sitting to brush teeth or comb hair, carrying out activities at a slower pace.

Encourage progressive activity/self-care when tolerated. Provide assistance as needed.

RATIONALE

The stated parameters are helpful in assessing physiologic responses to the stress of activity and, if present, are indicators of overexertion associated with the activity level.

Energy-saving techniques reduce the energy expenditure, thereby assisting in equalization of oxygen supply and demand.

Gradual activity progression prevents a sudden increase in cardiac workload. Providing assistance only as needed encourages independence in performing activities.

NURSING DIAGNOSIS:	PAIN, [ACUTE], HEADACHE
May be related to:	Increased cerebral vascular pressure.
Possibly evidenced by:	Reports of throbbing pain located in suboccipital region, present on awakening, and disappearing spontaneously after being up and about.
	Reluctance to move head, rubbing head, avoidance of bright lights and noise, wrinkled brow, clenched fists.
	Reports of stiffness of neck, dizziness, blurred vision, nausea, and vomiting.
DESIRED OUTCOMES/ EVALUATION CRITERIA— PATIENT WILL:	Report pain/discomfort is relieved/controlled.
	Verbalize methods that provide relief.
	Follow prescribed pharmacologic regimen.

ACTIONS/INTERVENTIONS

Independent

Maintain bed rest during acute phase.

RATIONALE

Minimizes stimulation/promotes relaxation.

ACTIONS/INTERVENTIONS	RATIONALE

Independent

Provide nonpharmacologic measures for relief of headache, e.g., cool cloth to forehead; back and neck rubs; quiet, dimly lit room; relaxation techniques (guided imagery, distraction); and diversional activities.

Measures that reduce cerebral vascular pressure and which slow/block sympathetic response are effective in relieving headache and associated complications.

Eliminate/minimize vasoconstricting activities that may aggravate headache, e.g., straining at stool, prolonged coughing, bending over.

Activities that increase vasoconstriction accentuate the headache in the presence of increased cerebral vascular pressure.

Assist patient with ambulation as needed.

Dizziness and blurred vision frequently are associated with headache. The patient may also experience episodes of postural hypotension.

Provide liquids, soft foods, frequent mouth care if nosebleeds occur or nasal packing has been done to stop bleeding.

Promotes general comfort. Nasal packing may interfere with swallowing or require mouth breathing, leading to stagnation of oral secretions and drying mucous membranes.

Collaborative

Administer medications as indicated:
  Analgesics;

Reduces/controls pain and decreases stimulation of the sympathetic nervous system.

  Antianxiety e.g., lorazepam (Ativan), diazepam (Valium).

May aid in the reduction of tension and discomfort that is intensified by stress.

NURSING DIAGNOSIS:	NUTRITION, ALTERED, MORE THAN BODY REQUIREMENTS
May be related to:	Excessive intake in relation to metabolic need.
	Sedentary lifestyle.
	Cultural preferences.
Possibly evidenced by:	Weight 10%–20% over ideal for height and frame.
	Triceps skin fold greater than 15 mm in men and 25 mm in women (maximum for age and sex).
	Reported or observed dysfunctional eating patterns.
DESIRED OUTCOMES/ EVALUATION CRITERIA— PATIENT WILL:	Identify correlation between hypertension and obesity.
	Demonstrate change in eating patterns (e.g., food choices, quantity, and so on), to attain desirable body weight with optimal maintenance of health.
	Initiate/maintain individually appropriate exercise program.

ACTIONS/INTERVENTIONS	RATIONALE
Independent	
Assess patient understanding of direct relationship between hypertension and obesity.	Obesity is an added risk with high blood pressure because of the disproportion between fixed aortic capacity and increased cardiac output associated with increased body mass.
Discuss necessity for decreased caloric intake and limiting intake of fats, salt, and sugar as indicated.	Faulty eating habits contribute to atherosclerosis and obesity, which predispose to hypertension and subsequent complications, e.g., stroke, kidney disease, heart failure. Excessive salt intake expands the intravascular fluid volume and may damage kidneys, which can further aggravate hypertension.
Determine patient's desire to lose weight.	Motivation for weight reduction is internal. The individual must want to lose weight, or program most likely will not succeed.
Review usual daily caloric intake and dietary choices.	Identifies current strengths/weaknesses in dietary program. Aids in determining individual need for adjustment/teaching.
Establish a realistic weight reduction plan with the patient, e.g., 1 lb weight loss/wk.	Reducing one's caloric intake by 500 calories daily theoretically yields a weight loss of 1 lb/wk. Slow reduction in weight is therefore indicative of fat loss with muscle sparing and generally means a change in eating habits.
Encourage patient to maintain a diary of food intake including when and where eating takes place and the circumstances and feelings around which the food was eaten.	Provides a data base for both the adequacy of nutrients eaten, as well as the emotional conditions of eating. Helps to focus attention on factors which patient has control over/can change.
Instruct and assist in appropriate food selection, avoiding foods high in saturated fat (butter, cheese, eggs, ice cream, meat), and cholesterol (fatty meats, egg yolks, whole dairy products, shrimp, organ meats).	Avoiding foods high in saturated fat and cholesterol is important in preventing progressing atherogenesis.
Collaborative	
Refer to dietitian as indicated.	Provides counseling and assistance with meeting individual dietary needs.

NURSING DIAGNOSIS:	COPING, INDIVIDUAL, INEFFECTIVE
May be related to:	Situational/maturational crisis.
	Multiple life changes.
	Inadequate relaxation.
	Inadequate support systems.
	Little or no exercise.
	Poor nutrition.

Unmet expectations.

Work overload.

Unrealistic perceptions.

Inadequate coping methods.

Possibly evidenced by: Verbalization of inability to cope or ask for help.

Inability to meet role expectations/basic needs or problem-solve.

Destructive behavior toward self; overeating, lack of appetite; excessive smoking/drinking, proneness to alcohol abuse.

Chronic fatigue/insomnia; muscular tension; frequent head/neck aches; chronic worry/irritability/anxiety/emotional tension, depression.

DESIRED OUTCOMES/ EVALUATION CRITERIA— PATIENT WILL: Identify ineffective coping behaviors and consequences.

Verbalize awareness of own coping abilities/strengths.

Identify potential stressful situations and take steps to avoid/modify them.

Demonstrate the use of effective coping skills/methods.

ACTIONS/INTERVENTIONS	RATIONALE
Independent	
Assess effectiveness of coping strategies by observing behaviors, e.g., ability to verbalize feelings and concerns, willingness to participate in the treatment plan.	Adaptive mechanisms are necessary to appropriately alter one's lifestyle, deal with the chronicity of hypertension, and integrate prescribed therapies into daily living.
Note reports of sleep disturbances, increasing fatigue, impaired concentration, irritability, decreased tolerance of headache, inability to cope/problem-solve.	Manifestations of maladaptive coping mechanisms may be indicators of repressed anger and have been found to be major determinants of diastolic BP.
Assist patient to identify specific stressors and possible strategies for coping with them.	Recognition of stressors is the first step in altering one's response to the stressor.
Include patient in planning of care and encourage maximum participation in treatment plan.	Involvement provides the patient with an ongoing sense of control, improves coping skills, and can enhance cooperation with therapeutic regimen.
Encourage patient to evaluate life priorities/goals. Ask questions such as, "Is what you are doing getting you what you want?"	Focuses patient's attention on reality of present situation relative to patient's view of what is wanted. Strong work ethic, need for "control," and outward focus may have led to lack of attention to personal needs.
Assist patient to identify and begin planning for necessary lifestyle changes. Assist to adjust, rather than abandon personal/family goals.	Necessary changes should be realistically prioritized to avoid being overwhelmed and feeling powerless.

NURSING DIAGNOSIS:	KNOWLEDGE DEFICIT [LEARNING NEED], REGARDING CONDITION, TREATMENT PLAN
May be related to:	Lack of knowledge/recall.
	Information misinterpretation.
	Cognitive limitation.
	Denial of diagnosis.
Possibly evidenced by:	Verbalization of the problem.
	Request for information.
	Statement of misconception.
	Inaccurate follow-through of instructions; inadequate performance of procedures.
	Inappropriate or exaggerated behaviors, e.g., hostile, agitated, apathetic.
DESIRED OUTCOMES/ EVALUATION CRITERIA— PATIENT WILL:	Verbalize understanding of disease process and treatment regimen.
	Identify drug side effects and possible complications that necessitate attention.
	Maintain BP within normal parameters.

ACTIONS/INTERVENTIONS	RATIONALE
Independent	
Assess readiness and blocks to learning. Include SO.	Misconceptions and denial of the diagnosis because of longstanding feelings of well-being may interfere with patient/SO willingness to learn about disease, progression, and prognosis. If the patient does not accept the reality of a life condition requiring continuing treatment, lifestyle/behavioral changes will not be initiated/sustained.
Define and state the limits of normal BP. Explain hypertension and its effects on the heart, blood vessels, kidneys, and brain.	Provides basis for understanding elevations of BP and clarifies frequently used medical terminology. Understanding that high BP can exist without symptoms is central to enabling patient to continue treatment even when feeling well.
Avoid saying "normal" BP, and use the term "well-controlled" when describing patient's BP within desired limits.	Because treatment for hypertension is life-long, conveying the idea of "control" helps the patient to understand the need for continued treatment/medication.
Assist the patient in identifying modifiable cardiovascular risk factors, e.g., obesity, diet high in saturated fats and cholesterol, sedentary lifestyle, smoking, alcohol intake (more than 2 oz/d on a regular basis), stressful lifestyle.	These risk factors have been shown to contribute to hypertension and cardiovascular and renal disease.

44

ACTIONS/INTERVENTIONS	RATIONALE

Independent

Problem-solve with patient to identify ways in which appropriate lifestyle changes can be made to reduce the above factors.

Risk factors may accelerate the disease process or exacerbate symptoms. Changing "comfortable/ usual" behavior patterns can be very stressful. Support, guidance, and empathy can enhance the patient's success in accomplishing these tasks.

Discuss importance of eliminating smoking and assist patient in formulating a plan to quit smoking.

Nicotine increases catecholamine discharge, resulting in increased heart rate, BP, and vasoconstriction; reducing tissue oxygenation; and increasing the myocardial workload.

Reinforce the importance of cooperation with treatment regimen and keeping follow-up appointments.

Lack of cooperation is a common reason for failure of antihypertensive therapy. Therefore, ongoing evaluation for patient compliance is critical to successful treatment. Effective therapy reduces the incidence of stroke, heart failure, renal impairment, and possibly MI.

Instruct and demonstrate technique of BP self-monitoring. Evaluate patient's hearing, visual acuity, manual dexterity, and coordination.

Teaching the patient or SO to monitor the BP is reassuring to the patient, as it provides visual/positive reinforcement for patient efforts.

Help patient to develop a simple, convenient schedule for taking medications.

Individualizing medication schedule to fit the patient's personal habits/needs may facilitate cooperation with long-term regimen.

Explain prescribed medications along with their rationale, dosage, expected and adverse side effects, and idiosyncrasies, e.g.;

Adequate information and understanding that side effects (e.g., mood changes, initial weight gain, dry mouth) are common and often subside with time enhances cooperation with treatment plan.

Diuretics: Take daily dose (or larger dose) in the early morning;

Scheduling minimizes nighttime urination.

Weigh self on a regular schedule and record;

Primary indicator of effectiveness of diuretic therapy.

Avoid/limit alcohol intake;

The combined vasodilating effect of alcohol and the volume-depleting effect of a diuretic greatly increases the risk of orthostatic hypotension.

Notify physician if unable to tolerate food or fluid;

Dehydration can develop rapidly if intake is poor and patient continues to take a diuretic.

Antihypertensives: Take prescribed dose on a regular schedule, avoid skipping, altering, or making up doses, and do not discontinue without notifying the health care provider; rise slowly from a lying to standing position, sitting for a few minutes before standing. Sleep with the head slightly elevated.

Abruptly discontinuing drug causes rebound hypertension that may lead to severe complications.

Measures reduce severity of orthostatic hypotension associated with the use of vasodilators and diuretics.

Suggest frequent position changes, leg exercises when lying down.

Decreases peripheral venous pooling that may be potentiated by vasodilators and prolonged sitting/ standing.

Recommend avoiding hot baths, steam rooms, and saunas and concomitant use of alcoholic beverages.

Prevents unnecessary vasodilation with dangerous side effect of syncope and hypotension.

ACTIONS/INTERVENTIONS	RATIONALE

Independent

Instruct the patient to consult health care provider before taking other prescription or nonprescription medication.

Precaution is important in preventing potentially dangerous drug interactions. Any drug that contains a sympathetic nervous stimulant may increase BP or may counteract antihypertensive effects.

Instruct patient about increasing intake of foods/fluids high in potassium, e.g., oranges, bananas, figs, dates, tomatoes, potatoes, raisins, apricots, Gatorade, fruit juices; and those high in calcium, e.g., low fat milk, yogurt or calcium supplements, as indicated.

Diuretics can deplete potassium levels. Dietary replacement is more palatable than drug supplements and may be all that is needed to correct deficit. Some studies show that 400–2000 mg of calcium/d can lower systolic and diastolic BP. Correcting mineral deficiencies can also affect BP.

Review signs/symptoms requiring notification of health care provider, e.g., headache present on awakening; sudden and continued increase of BP; chest pain/shortness of breath; irregular/increased pulse rate; significant weight gain (2 lb/d or 5 lb/wk) or peripheral/abdominal swelling; visual disturbances; frequent, uncontrollable nose bleeds; depression/ emotional lability; severe dizziness or episodes of fainting, muscle weakness/cramping, nausea/vomiting; excessive thirst, decreased libido/ impotence.

Early detection of developing complications of, decreased effectiveness of, or adverse reactions to drug regimen allows for timely intervention.

Explain rationale for prescribed dietary regimen (usually a diet low in sodium, saturated fat, and cholesterol).

Excess saturated fats, cholesterol, sodium, alcohol, and calories have been defined as nutritional risks in hypertension. A low-fat and high polyunsaturated-fat diet reduces BP, possibly through prostaglandin balance, in both normotensive and hypertensive people.

Help patient to identify sources of sodium intake, (e.g., table salt, salty snacks, processed meats and cheeses, sauerkraut, sauces, canned soups and vegetables, baking soda, baking powder, monosodium glutamate). Stress importance of reading ingredient labels of foods and OTC drugs.

Two years on a moderately low salt diet may be sufficient to control mild hypertension or reduce the amount of medication required.

Encourage patient to decrease or eliminate caffeine, e.g., coffee, tea, cola, chocolate.

Caffeine is a cardiac stimulant and may adversely affect cardiac function/reserves.

Stress importance of planning/accomplishing daily rest periods.

Alternating rest and activity increases tolerance to activity progression.

Recommend that patient monitor own physiologic response to activity (e.g., pulse rate, shortness of breath); report a decreased tolerance to activity; and stop activity that causes chest pain, shortness of breath, dizziness, extreme fatigue, or weakness.

The patient's involvement in monitoring his or her own activity tolerance is vital to safely resuming and/or modifying activities of daily living.

Encourage patient to establish an individual exercise program incorporating aerobic exercise (walking, swimming) within the patient's capabilities. Stress the importance of avoiding isometric activity.

Besides helping to lower BP, aerobic activity aids in toning the cardiovascular system. Isometric exercise can increase serum catecholamine levels, further elevating BP.

ACTIONS/INTERVENTIONS	RATIONALE

Independent

Demonstrate application of ice pack to the back of the neck and pressure over the distal third of nose, and recommend that patient lean the head forward, if nose bleed occurs.

Nasal capillaries may rupture as a result of excessive vascular pressure. Cold and pressure constrict capillaries, which slows or halts bleeding. Leaning forward reduces the amount of blood that is swallowed.

Provide information regarding community resources and support the patient in making lifestyle changes. Initiate a referral if indicated.

Community resources such as the American Heart Association, "coronary clubs," stop smoking clinics, alcohol rehabilitation, weight loss programs, stress management classes, and counseling services may be helpful to the patient's efforts to initiate and maintain lifestyle changes.

Congestive Heart Failure: Chronic _____

Failure of the left and/or right chambers of the heart results in inability to provide sufficient output to meet tissue needs and causes the development of pulmonary and systemic congestion. Despite diagnostic and therapeutic advances, CHF continues to be associated with high morbidity and mortality.

RELATED CONCERNS:

Cardiac Surgery, p 113
Digitalis Toxicity, p 62
Dysrhythmias, p 94
Psychosocial Aspects of Acute Care, p 899

PATIENT ASSESSMENT DATA BASE

ACTIVITY/REST

May report: Fatigue/exhaustion progressing throughout the day.

Insomnia.

Chest pain with activity.

Dyspnea at rest or with exertion.

May exhibit: Restlessness, mental status changes, e.g., lethargy.
Vital sign changes with activity.

CIRCULATION

May report: History of hypertension, recent/acute multiple MIs, previous episodes of CHF, valvular heart disease, cardiac surgery, endocarditis, SLE, anemia, septic shock.

Swelling of feet, legs, abdomen, "belt too tight" (right-sided failure).

May exhibit: BP: May be low (pump failure); normal (mild or chronic CHF); or high (fluid overload/increased SVR).

Pulse pressure: May be narrow, reflecting reduced stroke volume.

Heart rate: Tachycardia (left-sided failure).

Heart rhythm: Dysrhythmias, e.g., atrial fibrillation, premature ventricular contractions/tachycardia, heart blocks.

Apical pulse: PMI may be diffuse and displaced inferiorly to the left.

Heart sounds: S_3 (gallop) is diagnostic; S_4 may occur; S_1 and S_2 may be softened.

Systolic and diastolic murmurs may indicate the presence of valvular stenosis or insufficiency.

Pulses: Peripheral pulses diminished; alteration in strength of beat may be noted; central pulses may be bounding, e.g., visible jugular, carotid, abdominal pulsations.

Color: Ashen, pale, dusky, cyanotic.

Nailbeds: Pale or cyanotic with slow capillary refill.

Liver: Enlarged/palpable, positive hepatojugular reflex.

Breath sounds: Crackles, rhonchi.

Edema: May be dependent, generalized, or pitting, especially in extremities; JVD.

EGO INTEGRITY

May report: Anxiety, apprehension, fear.

Stress related to illness/financial concerns (job/cost of medical care).

May exhibit: Various behavioral manifestations, e.g., anxiety, anger, fearful, irritable.

ELIMINATION

May report: Decreased voiding, dark urine.

Night voiding (nocturia).

Diarrhea/constipation.

FOOD/FLUID

May report: Loss of appetite.

Nausea/vomiting.

Significant weight gain.

Lower extremity swelling.

Tight clothing/shoes.

Diet high in salt/processed foods, fat, sugar, and caffeine.

Use of diuretics.

May exhibit: Rapid weight gain.

Abdominal distention (ascites); edema (general, dependent, brawn, pitting).

HYGIENE

May report: Fatigue/weakness, exhaustion during self-care activities.

May exhibit: Appearance indicative of neglect of personal care.

NEUROSENSORY

May report: Weakness, dizziness, fainting episodes.

May exhibit: Lethargy, confusion, disorientation.

Behavior changes, irritability.

PAIN/DISCOMFORT

May report: Chest pain, chronic or acute angina.

Right upper abdominal pain (RVF).

Muscle aches.

May exhibit: Nervousness, restlessness.

Narrowed focus (withdrawal).

Guarding behavior.

RESPIRATION

May report: Dyspnea on exertion, sleeping sitting up, or with several pillows.

Cough with/without sputum production.

History of chronic lung disease.

Use of respiratory aids, e.g., oxygen or medications.

May exhibit: Respirations: Tachypnea; shallow, labored breathing; use of accessory muscles, nasal flaring.

Cough: Dry/hacking/nonproductive or may be gurgling with/without sputum production.

Sputum: May be blood-tinged, pink/frothy (pulmonary edema).

Breath sounds: May be diminished, with bibasilar crackles and wheezes.

Mentation: May be diminished; lethargy; restlessness.

Color: Pallor or cyanosis.

SAFETY

May exhibit: Changes in mentation.

Loss of strength/muscle tone.

Skin excoriations.

SOCIAL INTERACTION

May report: Decreased participation in usual social activities.

TEACHING/LEARNING

May report: Use/misuse of cardiac medications, e.g.; β-blockers, calcium channel blockers.

Recent/recurrent hospitalizations.

May exhibit: Evidence of failure to improve.

Discharge Plan Considerations: **DRG projected mean length of stay: 8.2 days.**

Assistance with shopping, transportation, self-care needs, homemaker/maintenance tasks.

Alteration in medication use/therapy.

Changes in physical layout of home.

DIAGNOSTIC STUDIES

ECG: Ventricular or atrial hypertrophy, axis deviation, ischemia, and damage patterns may be present. Dysrhythmias, e.g., tachycardia, atrial fibrillation, frequent PVCs may be present. Persistent ST/T segment elevation 6 weeks or more after myocardial infarction suggests presence of ventricular aneurysm (may cause cardiac dysfunction/failure).

Sonograms (echocardiogram, doppler echocardiogram): May reveal enlarged chamber dimensions, alterations in valvular function/structure, or areas of decreased ventricular contractility.

Heart Scan: (Multigated acquisition [MUGA]): Measures ejection fraction and estimates wall motion.

Cardiac catheterization: Abnormal pressures are indicative and help differentiate right versus left-sided heart failure, and valve stenosis or insufficiency. Also assess patency of coronary arteries. Contrast injected into the ventricles reveals abnormal size and ejection fraction/altered contractility.

Chest x-ray: May show enlarged cardiac shadow reflecting chamber dilatation/hypertrophy, or changes in blood vessels reflecting increased pulmonary pressure. Abnormal contour, e.g., bulging of left cardiac border, may suggest ventricular aneurysm.

Liver enzymes: Elevated in liver congestion/failure.

Electrolytes: May be altered due to fluid shifts/decreased renal function, diuretic therapy.

Pulse oximetry: Oxygen saturation may be low, especially when acute CHF is imposed on COPD or chronic CHF.

ABGs: Left ventricular failure is characterized by mild respiratory alkalosis (early) or hypoxemia with an increased PCO_2 (late).

BUN, creatinine: Elevated BUN suggests decreased renal perfusion. Elevation of both BUN and creatinine is indicative of renal failure.

Serum albumin/transferrin: May be decreased as a result of reduced protein intake or reduced protein synthesis in congested liver.

CBC: May reveal anemia, polycythemia, or dilutional changes indicating water retention. WBCs may be elevated, reflecting recent/acute MI, pericarditis, or other inflammatory or infectious states.

Sedimentation rate (ESR): May be elevated, indicating acute inflammatory reaction.

Thyroid studies: Increased thyroid activity suggests thyroid hyperactivity as precipitator of CHF.

NURSING PRIORITIES

1. Improve myocardial contractility/systemic perfusion.
2. Reduce fluid volume overload.
3. Prevent complications.
4. Provide information about disease/prognosis, therapy needs and prevention of recurrences.

DISCHARGE GOALS

1. Cardiac output adequate for individual needs.
2. Complications prevented/resolved.
3. Optimum level of activity/functioning attained.
4. Disease process/prognosis and therapeutic regimen understood.

NURSING DIAGNOSIS:	CARDIAC OUTPUT, DECREASED
May be related to:	Altered myocardial contractility/inotropic changes.
	Alterations in rate, rhythm, electrical conduction.
	Structural changes (e.g., valvular defects, ventricular aneurysm).
Possibly evidenced by:	Increased heart rate (tachycardia); dysrhythmias; ECG changes.
	Changes in BP (hypotension/hypertension).
	Extra heart sounds (S_3, S_4).
	Decreased urine output.
	Diminished peripheral pulses.
	Cool, ashen skin; diaphoresis.
	Orthopnea, crackles, JVD, liver engorgement, edema.
	Chest pain.
DESIRED OUTCOMES/ EVALUATION CRITERIA— PATIENT WILL:	Display vital signs within acceptable limits (dysrhythmias absent/controlled) and free of symptoms of failure (e.g., hemodynamic parameters within normal limits, urinary output adequate).
	Report decreased episodes of dyspnea, angina.
	Participate in activities that reduce cardiac workload.

ACTIONS/INTERVENTIONS	RATIONALE
Independent	
Auscultate apical pulse; assess heart rate, rhythm; (Document dysrhythmia if telemetry available).	Tachycardia is usually present (even at rest) to compensate for decreased ventricular contractility. PACs, PAT, MAT, PVCs, and AF are common dysrhythmias associated with CHF although others may also occur. *Note:* Intractable ventricular dysrhythmias unresponsive to medication suggest ventricular aneurysm.
Note heart sounds.	S_1 and S_2 may be weak because of diminished pumping action. Gallop rhythms are common (S_3 and S_4), produced as blood flows into noncompliant/distended chambers. Murmurs may reflect valvular incompetence/stenosis.
Palpate peripheral pulses.	Decreased cardiac output may be reflected in diminished radial, popliteal, dorsalis pedis, and posttibial pulses. Pulses may be fleeting or irregular to palpation, and pulsus alternans (strong beat alternating with weak beat) may be present.
Monitor BP.	In early, moderate, or chronic CHF, BP may be elevated due to increased SVR. In advanced CHF, the body may no longer be able to compensate, and profound/irreversible hypotension may occur.
Inspect skin for pallor, cyanosis.	Pallor is indicative of diminished peripheral perfusion secondary to inadequate cardiac output, vasoconstriction, and anemia. Cyanosis may develop in refractory CHF. Dependent areas are often blue or mottled as venous congestion increases.
Monitor urine output, noting decreasing output and dark/concentrated urine.	Kidneys respond to reduced cardiac output by retaining water and sodium. Urine output is usually decreased during the day because of fluid shifts into tissues but may be increased at night as fluid returns to circulation when patient is recumbent.
Assess changes in sensorium, e.g., lethargy, confusion, disorientation, anxiety, and depression.	May indicate inadequate cerebral perfusion secondary to decreased cardiac output.
Provide rest semirecumbent in bed or chair. Assist with physical care as indicated.	Physical rest should be maintained during acute or refractory CHF to improve efficiency of cardiac contraction and to decrease myocardial oxygen demand/consumption and workload.
Provide for psychologic rest by quiet environment; explaining medical/nursing management; helping patient avoid stressful situations, listening/responding to expressions of feelings/fears.	Emotional stress produces vasoconstriction, which elevates BP and increases heart rate/work.
Provide bedside commode. Have patient avoid activities eliciting a Valsalva response, e.g., straining during defecation, holding breath during position changes.	Commode use decreases work of getting to bathroom or struggling to use bedpan. Valsalva maneuver causes vagal stimulation followed by rebound tachycardia, which further compromises cardiac function/output.
Elevate legs, avoiding pressure under knee. Encourage active/passive exercises. Increase ambulation/activity as tolerated.	Decreases venous stasis and may reduce incidence of thrombus/embolus formation.

ACTIONS/INTERVENTIONS	RATIONALE

Independent

Check for calf tenderness, diminished pedal pulse, swelling, local redness, or pallor of extremity.

Reduced cardiac output, venous pooling/stasis, and enforced bedrest increases risk of thrombophlebitis.

Withhold digitalis preparation and notify physician if marked changes occur in cardiac rate or rhythm or signs of digitalis toxicity occur.

Incidence of toxicity is high (20%) because of narrow margin between therapeutic and toxic ranges. Digoxin may have to be discontinued in the presence of toxic drug levels, a slow heart rate, or low potassium level.

Collaborative

Administer supplemental oxygen by nasal cannula/mask as indicated.

Increases available oxygen for myocardial uptake to combat effects of hypoxia/ischemia.

Administer medications as indicated:

A variety of medications may be used to increase stroke volume, improve contractility, and reduce congestion.

Diuretics, e.g., furosemide (Lasix); ethacrynic acid (Edecrin); bumetanide (Bumex); spironolactone (Aldactone);

Type and dosage of diuretic depends on degree of heart failure and state of renal funtion. Preload reduction is most useful in treating patients with a relatively normal cardiac output accompanied by congestive symptoms. Loop diuretics block chloride reabsorption, thus interfering with the reabsorption of sodium and water.

Vasodilators, e.g., nitrates (Nitro-Dur, Isordil); arteriodilators, e.g., hydralazine (Apresoline); combination drugs, e.g., prazosin (Minipress);

Vasodilators are used to increase cardiac output, reducing circulating volume (venodilators) and decreasing systemic vascular resistance (arteriodilators), thereby reducing ventricular workload.

Digoxin (Lanoxin);

Increases force of myocardial contraction and slows heart rate by decreasing conduction velocity and prolonging refractory period of the AV junction to increase cardiac efficiency/output.

Captopril (Capoten); lisinopril (Prinivil); enalapril (Vasotec);

ACE inhibitors may be used to control heart failure by inhibiting angiotensin conversion in the lungs and reduce vasoconstriction, SVR, and BP.

Morphine sulfate;

Decreases vascular resistance and venous return reducing myocardial workload. Allays anxiety and breaks the feedback cycle of anxiety/catecholamine release/anxiety.

Tranquilizers/sedatives;

Promotes rest/relaxation reducing oxygen demand and myocardial workload. *Note:* There is an "on-trial" oral analogue of amrinone (Inocor) a positive inotropic agent, called milrinone, which may be suitable for long-term use.

Anticoagulants, e.g., low-dose heparin; warfarin (Coumadin).

May be used prophylactically to prevent thrombus/emboli formation in presence of risk factors such as venous stasis, enforced bed rest, cardiac dysrhythmias, and history of previous thrombolic episodes.

Administer IV solutions, restricting total amount as indicated. Avoid saline solutions.

Because of existing elevated left ventricular pressure, patient may not tolerate increased fluid vol-

ACTIONS/INTERVENTIONS	RATIONALE
Collaborative	
	ume (preload). CHF patients also excrete less sodium, which causes fluid retention and increases myocardial workload.
Monitor/replace electrolytes.	Fluid shifts and use of diuretics can alter electrolytes (especially potassium and chloride), which affect cardiac rhythm and contractility.
Monitor serial ECG and chest x-ray changes.	ST segment depression and T wave flattening can develop because of increased myocardial oxygen demand, even if no coronary artery disease is present. Chest x-ray may show enlarged heart and changes of pulmonary congestion.
Monitor laboratory studies, e.g., BUN, creatinine;	Elevation of BUN/creatinine reflects kidney hypoperfusion/failure.
Liver function studies (AST, LDH);	AST/LDH may be elevated due to liver congestion and indicate need for smaller dosages of medications that are detoxified by the liver.
PT/APTT/coagulation studies.	Measures changes in coagulation processes or effectiveness of anticoagulant therapy.
Prepare for insertion/maintain pacemaker, if indicated.	May be necessary to correct bradydysrhythmias unresponsive to drug intervention, which can aggravate congestive failure/produce pulmonary edema.
Prepare for surgery as indicated.	Congestive failure due to ventricular aneurysm or valvular dysfunction may require aneurysectomy or valve replacement to improve myocardial contractility/function.

NURSING DIAGNOSIS:	**ACTIVITY INTOLERANCE**
May be related to:	Imbalance between oxygen supply/demand.
	Generalized weakness.
	Prolonged bed rest/immobility.
Possibly evidenced by:	Weakness, fatigue.
	Changes in vital signs, presence of dysrhythmias.
	Dyspnea.
	Pallor.
	Diaphoresis.
DESIRED OUTCOMES/ EVALUATION CRITERIA— PATIENT WILL:	Participate in desired activities; meet own self-care needs.
	Achieve measurable increase in activity tolerance, evidenced by reduced fatigue and weakness and vital signs within acceptable limits during activity.

ACTIONS/INTERVENTIONS	RATIONALE

Independent

Check vital signs before and immediately after activity, especially if patient is on vasodilators, diuretics, or β-blockers.

Orthostatic hypotension can occur with activity because of medication effect (vasodilation); fluid shifts (diuresis); or compromised cardiac function.

Document cardiopulmonary response to activity. Note tachycardia, dysrhythmias, dyspnea, diaphoresis, pallor.

Compromised myocardium/inability to increase stroke volume during activity may cause an immediate increase in heart rate and oxygen demands, thereby aggravating weakness and fatigue.

Assess for other precipitators/causes of fatigue, e.g., treatments, pain, medications.

Fatigue is a side effect of some medications (β-blockers, tranquilizers, and sedatives). Pain and stressful regimens also extract energy and produce fatigue.

Evaluate accelerating activity intolerance.

May denote increasing cardiac decompensation rather than overactivity.

Provide assistance with self-care activities as indicated. Intersperse activity periods with rest periods.

Meets patient's personal care needs without undue myocardial stress/excessive oxygen demand.

Collaborative

Implement graded cardiac rehabilitation/activity program.

Gradual increase in activity avoids excessive myocardial workload/oxygen consumption. Strengthens and improves cardiac function under stress, if cardiac dysfunction is not irreversible.

NURSING DIAGNOSIS:	**FLUID VOLUME, EXCESS**
May be related to:	Reduced glomerular filtration rate (decreased cardiac output)/increased ADH production, and sodium/water retention.
Possibly evidenced by:	Orthopnea, S_3 heart sound.
	Oliguria, edema, JVD, positive hepatojugular reflex.
	Weight gain.
	Hypertension.
	Respiratory distress, abnormal breath sounds.
DESIRED OUTCOMES/ EVALUATION CRITERIA— PATIENT WILL:	Demonstrate stabilized fluid volume with balanced intake and output, breath sounds clear/clearing, vital signs within acceptable range, stable weight, and absence of edema.
	Verbalize understanding of individual dietary/fluid restrictions.

ACTIONS/INTERVENTIONS	RATIONALE
Independent	
Monitor urine output, noting amount and color, as well as time of day when diuresis occurs.	Urine output may be scanty and concentrated (especially during the day) because of reduced renal perfusion. Recumbency favors diuresis; therefore urine output may be increased at night/during bed rest.
Monitor/calculate 24-hour intake and output balance.	Diuretic therapy may result in sudden/excessive fluid loss (hypovolemia) even though edema/ascites remains.
Maintain chair or bedrest in semi-Fowler's position during acute phase.	Recumbency increases glomerular filtration and decreases production of ADH, thereby enhancing diuresis.
Establish fluid intake schedule, incorporating beverage preferences when possible. Give frequent mouth care/ice chips as part of fluid allotment.	Involving patient in therapy regimen may enhance sense of control and cooperation with restrictions.
Weigh daily.	Documents changes in/resolution of edema in response to therapy. A gain of 5 lb represents approximately 2 L of fluid. Conversely, diuretics can result in rapid/excessive fluid shifts and weight loss.
Assess for distended neck and peripheral vessels. Inspect dependent body areas for edema with/without pitting; note presence of generalized body edema (anasarca).	Excessive fluid retention may be manifested by venous engorgement and edema formation. Peripheral edema begins in feet/ankles (or dependent areas) and ascends as failure worsens. Pitting edema is generally obvious only after retention of at least 10 lb of fluid. Increased vascular congestion (associated with right-sided heart failure) eventually results in systemic tissue edema.
Change position frequently. Elevate feet when sitting. Inspect skin surface, keep dry and provide padding as indicated. (Refer to ND: Skin Integrity, impaired, high risk for, p. 58.)	Edema formation, slowed circulation, altered nutritional intake and prolonged immobility/bed rest are cumulative stressors which affect skin integrity and require close supervision/preventive interventions.
Auscultate breath sounds, noting decreased and/or adventitious sounds, e.g., crackles, wheezes. Note presence of increased dyspnea, tachypnea, orthopnea, paroxysmal nocturnal dyspnea, persistent cough.	Excess fluid volume often leads to pulmonary congestion. Symptoms of pulmonary edema may reflect acute left-sided heart failure. Right-sided heart failure's respiratory symptoms (dyspnea, cough, orthopnea) may have slower onset but are more difficult to reverse.
Investigate complaints of sudden extreme dyspnea/air hunger, need to sit straight up, sensation of suffocation, feelings of panic or impending doom.	May indicate development of complications (pulmonary edema/embolus) and differs from orthopnea and paroxysmal nocturnal dyspnea in that it develops much more rapidly and requires immediate intervention.
Monitor BP and CVP (if available).	Hypertension and elevated CVP suggests fluid volume excess and may reflect developing/increasing pulmonary congestion, heart failure.
Assess bowel sounds. Note complaints of anorexia, nausea, abdominal distention, constipation.	Visceral congestion (occurring in progressive CHF), can alter gastric/intestinal function.

ACTIONS/INTERVENTIONS	RATIONALE
Independent	
Provide small, frequent easily digestible meals.	Reduced gastric motility can adversely affect digestion and absorption. Small, frequent meals may enhance digestion/prevent abdominal discomfort.
Measure abdominal girth, as indicated.	In progressive right-sided heart failure, fluid may shift into the peritoneal space, causing increasing abdominal girth (ascites).
Encourage verbalization of feelings regarding limitations.	Expression of feelings/concerns may decrease stress/anxiety, which is an energy drain and can contribute to feelings of fatigue.
Palpate for hepatomegaly. Note complaints of right upper quadrant pain/tenderness.	Advancing heart failure leads to venous congestion, resulting in abdominal distention, liver engorgement, and pain. This can alter liver function and impair/prolong drug metabolism.
Note increased lethargy, hypotension, muscle cramping.	Signs of potassium and sodium deficits that may occur due to fluid shifts and diuretic therapy.
Collaborative	
Administer medications as indicated:	
Diuretics, e.g., furosemide (Lasix); bumetanide (Bumex);	Increases rate of urine flow and may inhibit reabsorption of sodium/chloride in the renal tubules.
Thiazides with potassium-sparing agents, e.g., spironolactone (Aldactone);	Promotes diuresis without excessive potassium losses.
Potassium supplements, e.g., K Dur.	Replaces potassium that is lost as a common side effect of diuretic therapy, which can adversely affect cardiac function.
Maintain fluid/sodium restrictions as indicated.	Reduces total body water/prevents fluid reaccumulation.
Consult with dietitian.	May be necessary to provide diet acceptable to patient that meets caloric needs within sodium restriction.
Monitor chest x-ray.	Reveals changes indicative of increase/resolution of pulmonary congestion.
Assist with rotating tourniquets/phlebotomy, dialysis, or ultrafiltration as indicated.	Although not frequently used, mechanical fluid removal may be carried out to rapidly reduce circulating volume, especially in pulmonary edema refractory to other therapies.

NURSING DIAGNOSIS:	GAS EXCHANGE, IMPAIRED, HIGH RISK FOR
Risk factors may include:	Alveolar-capillary membrane changes, e.g., fluid collection/shifts into interstitial space/alveoli.
Possibly evidenced by:	[Not applicable; presence of signs and symptoms establishes an actual diagnosis.]

ACTIONS/INTERVENTIONS	RATIONALE

Independent

Auscultate breath sounds noting crackles, wheezes.	Reveals presence of pulmonary congestion/collection of secretions indicating need for further intervention.
Instruct patient in effective coughing, deep breathing.	Clears airways and facilitates oxygen delivery.
Encourage frequent position changes.	Helps prevent atelectasis and pneumonia.
Maintain chair/bedrest with head-of-bed elevated 20 to 30 degrees, semi-Fowler's position. Support arms with pillows.	Reduces oxygen consumption/demands and promotes maximal lung inflation.

Collaborative

Monitor/graph serial ABGs, pulse oximetry.	Hypoxemia can be severe during pulmonary edema. Compensatory changes are usually present in chronic CHF.
Administer supplemental oxygen as indicated.	Increases alveolar oxygen concentration, which may correct/reduce tissue hypoxemia.
Administer medications as indicated:	
Diuretics, e.g., furosemide (Lasix);	Reduces alveolar congestion, enhancing gas exchange.
Bronchodilators, e.g., aminophylline.	Increases oxygen delivery by dilating small airways and exerts mild diuretic effect to aid in reducing pulmonary congestion.

NURSING DIAGNOSIS:	SKIN INTEGRITY, IMPAIRED, HIGH RISK FOR
Risk factors may include:	Prolonged bed rest.
	Edema, decreased tissue perfusion.
Possibly evidenced by:	[Not applicable; presence of signs and symptoms establishes an actual diagnosis.]
DESIRED OUTCOMES/ EVALUATION CRITERIA— PATIENT WILL:	Maintain skin integrity.
	Demonstrate behaviors/techniques to prevent skin breakdown.

ACTIONS/INTERVENTIONS	RATIONALE
Independent	
Inspect skin, noting skeletal prominences, presence of edema, areas of altered circulation/pigmentation, or obesity/emaciation.	Skin is at risk because of impaired peripheral circulation, physical immobility, and alterations in nutritional status.
Massage reddened or blanched areas.	Improves blood flow, minimizing tissue hypoxia.
Reposition frequently in bed/chair, assist with active/passive range of motion exercises.	Improves circulation/reduces time any one area is deprived of blood flow.
Provide frequent skin care, minimize contact with moisture/excretions.	Excessive dryness or moisture damages skin and hastens breakdown.
Check fit of shoes/slippers and change as needed.	Dependent edema may cause shoes to fit poorly, increasing risk of pressure and skin breakdown on feet.
Avoid intramuscular medication.	Interstitial edema and impaired circulation impede drug absorption and predispose to tissue breakdown/development of infection.
Collaborative	
Provide alternating pressure/eggcrate mattress, sheep skin, elbow/heel protectors.	Reduces pressure to skin, may improve circulation.

NURSING DIAGNOSIS:	**KNOWLEDGE DEFICIT [LEARNING NEED], REGARDING CONDITION, TREATMENT REGIMEN**
May be related to:	Lack of understanding/misconceptions about interrelatedness of cardiac function/disease/failure.
Possibly evidenced by:	Questions.
	Statements of concern/misconceptions.
	Recurrent, preventable episodes of CHF.
DESIRED OUTCOMES/ EVALUATION CRITERIA— PATIENT WILL:	Identify relationship of ongoing therapies (treatment program) to reduction of recurrent episodes and prevention of complications.
	List signs/symptoms that require immediate intervention.
	Identify own stress/risk factors and some techniques for handling.
	Initiate necessary lifestyle/behavioral changes.

ACTIONS/INTERVENTIONS	RATIONALE
Independent	
Discuss normal heart function. Include information regarding patient's variance from normal function. Explain difference between heart attack and CHF.	Knowledge of disease process and expectations can facilitate adherence to prescribed treatment regimen.

ACTIONS/INTERVENTIONS	RATIONALE
Independent	
Reinforce treatment rationale.	Patient may believe it is acceptable to alter post-discharge regimen when feeling well and symptom-free or when feeling below par, which can increase the risk of exacerbation of symptoms. Understanding of regimen, medications, and restrictions may augment cooperation with control of symptoms.
Discuss importance of being as active as possible without becoming exhausted and to rest between activities.	Excessive physical activity can further weaken the heart, exacerbating failure.
Discuss importance of sodium limitation. Provide list of sodium content of common foods that are to be avoided/limited. Encourage reading of labels on food and drug packages.	Dietary intake of sodium above 3 g/d will offset diuretic effect. Most common source of sodium is table salt and obviously salty foods, although canned soups/vegetables, luncheon meats, and dairy products also may contain high levels of sodium.
Discuss medications, purpose and side effects. Provide both oral and written instructions.	Understanding therapeutic needs and importance of prompt reporting of side effects can prevent occurrence of drug-related complications. Anxiety may block comprehension of input or details and patient/SO may refer to written material at later date to refresh memory.
Recommend taking diuretic early in morning.	Provides adequate time for drug effect before bedtime to prevent/limit interruption of sleep.
Instruct and receive return demonstration of ability to take and record daily pulse and when to notify health care provider, e.g., pulse above/below preset rate, changes in rhythm/regularity.	Promotes self-monitoring of condition/drug effect. Early detection of changes allows for timely intervention and may prevent complications, such as digitalis toxicity.
Explain and discuss patient's role in control of risk factors (e.g., smoking) and precipitating or aggravating factors, (e.g., high salt diet, inactivity/overexertion, exposure to extremes in temperature).	Adds to body of knowledge and permits patient to make informed decisions regarding control of condition and prevention of recurrence/complications. Smoking potentiates vasoconstriction; sodium intake promotes water retention/edema formation; improper balance between activity/rest and exposure to extremes in temperature may result in exhaustion/increased myocardial workload and increased risk of respiratory infections.
Review signs/symptoms that require immediate medical attention, e.g., rapid weight gain, edema, shortness of breath, increased fatigue, cough, hemoptysis, fever.	Self-monitoring increases patient responsibility in health maintenance and aids in prevention of complications, e.g., pulmonary edema, pneumonia.
Provide opportunities for patient/SO to ask questions, discuss concerns and to make necessary lifestyle changes.	Chronicity and recurrent/debilitating nature of CHF often exhausts coping abilities and supportive capacity of both patient and SO, leading to depression.

ACTIONS/INTERVENTIONS	RATIONALE

Independent

Stress importance of reporting signs/symptoms of digitalis toxicity, e.g., development of GI and visual disturbances, changes in pulse rate/rhythm, worsening of congestive failure.

Early recognition of developing complications and involvement of health care provider may prevent toxicity/hospitalization.

Collaborative

Refer to community resources/support groups and Visiting Nurse Association as indicated.

May need additional assistance with self-monitoring/home management.

Digitalis Toxicity

Upwards of 15% of all patients receiving digitalis preparations will develop toxicity sometime during their course of therapy.

RELATED CONCERNS:

Congestive Heart Failure, p 48
Dysrhythmias, p 94
Psychosocial Aspects of Acute Care, p 899

PATIENT ASSESSMENT DATA BASE

ACTIVITY/REST

May report:	Insomnia, fatigue.
May exhibit:	Exertional dyspnea, fatigue, weakness.
	Abnormal pulse/blood pressure response to activity.

CIRCULATION

May report:	History of recent/acute myocardial infarction, congestive heart failure.
	Changes in usual heart rate/rhythm.
May exhibit:	Excessive slowing of pulse (increasing degrees of AV block).
	Characteristic ECG changes (see diagnostic studies).
	Dysrhythmias: Frequent premature beats, ventricular bigeminy, PAT.

EGO INTEGRITY

May report:	Feelings of helplessness/hopelessness, or powerlessness.
May exhibit:	Irritability, restlessness, agitation.
	Confusion, depression, delirium, psychosis (with high serum levels).

ELIMINATION

May report:	Use of diuretics.
	Diarrhea.
May exhibit:	Decreased urine output.
	Dependent edema.

FOOD/FLUID

May report:	Loss of appetite.
	Nausea, vomiting.
	Dietary restrictions affecting electrolyte balance.
	Changes in weight.
	Use of diuretics.
May exhibit:	Changes in weight/decrease in muscle mass, subcutaneous fat.
	Signs of altered fluid balance (excess or deficit).

NEUROSENSORY

May report: Visual disturbances, e.g., double vision, blurry vision, flickering lights, yellow/green tint to vision, colored dots.

Vertigo, faintness.

Seizure activity.

Headache.

May exhibit: Disorientation.

Restlessness.

Irritability, confusion, agitation/combative behavior.

Slurred speech.

Hallucinations, psychoses.

Seizures.

PAIN/DISCOMFORT

May report: Chest/abdominal pain.

May exhibit: Guarding/distraction behaviors.

Self-focusing.

Autonomic responses (changes in vital signs).

SAFETY

May exhibit: Muscle weakness.

Vision impairment.

TEACHING/LEARNING

May report: Improper use of digitalis; concurrent use of drugs/substances that may lead to increased digitalis effect/toxicity; interactions, e.g., thiazide or loop diuretics, steroids, Quinidine, nifedipine, verapamil, β-blockers, thyroid hormones, caffeine.

Evidence of failure to improve.

Discharge Plan Considerations: **DRG projected mean length of stay: 2.6 days.**

Alteration in medication use/therapy.

DIAGNOSTIC STUDIES

Serum digoxin/digitoxin level: Usually elevated above therapeutic range of particular preparation.

ECG: Prolonged P-R interval, dysrhythmias, and heart blocks are associated with digitalis toxicity. Other changes (T wave and ST segment depression) characteristically produced by the therapeutic digitalis effect on the heart can mimic ischemic changes.

Electrolytes: Imbalance in potassium, magnesium, and calcium are known to aggravate digitalis toxicity.

NURSING PRIORITIES

1. Document current digitalis therapy and usage.
2. Prevent/control dysrhythmias.
3. Correct/maintain fluid balance.
4. Educate patient/SO regarding proper drug usage, signs/symptoms of developing toxicity.

DISCHARGE GOALS

1. Cardiac rate/rhythm within patient's expected range.
2. Free of signs and symptoms of digitalis toxicity.
3. Adequate fluid balance maintained.
4. Cognitive/perceptual abilities improved.
5. Digitalis regimen, and what/when to report to health care provider understood.

NURSING DIAGNOSIS:	CARDIAC OUTPUT, DECREASED
May be related to:	Altered myocardial contractility.
	Alterations in rate, rhythm, electrical conduction.
	Long half-life and narrow therapeutic range of digitalis preparation used.
	Patient's age, organ function, amount of muscle mass, nutritional status, electrolyte/acid-base balance.
	Concurrent use of other medications.
Possibly evidenced by:	Dysrhythmias.
	Changes in mentation.
	Worsening of congestive heart failure.
	Elevated serum digitalis levels.
DESIRED OUTCOMES/ EVALUATION CRITERIA— PATIENT WILL:	Demonstrate heart rate and rhythm within patient's expected range with absence/control of dysrhythmias.
	Maintain usual mentation.

ACTIONS/INTERVENTIONS	RATIONALE
Independent	
Assess/monitor blood pressure.	Dysrhythmias can reduce blood pressure and promote tissue hypoxia, which can worsen digitalis toxicity.
Palpate radial pulse, noting rate and regularity. Auscultate apical pulse, noting rate/rhythm and presence of extra heart sounds.	Rapid irregular pulse/heart rate or excessively slow pulse/heart rate may indicate digitalis toxicity. Extra heart sounds (i.e., S_3) are common in the presence of congestive heart failure.
Monitor/document cardiac rhythm.	Numerous dysrhythmias can occur, including several which are life-threatening. PVCs are common, with possible bigeminal and trigeminal rhythms. Digitalis-induced tachydysrhythmias can lead to potentially lethal ventricular dysrhythmias.
Evaluate for presence of dependent/generalized edema, increased jugular venous distention/hepatojugular reflux. Auscultate breath sounds noting development of crackles.	Digitalis toxicity has been found to be responsible for deterioration of preexisting CHF and/or development of heart failure during digitalization. In severe/refractory CHF, altered cardiac binding of dig-

ACTIONS/INTERVENTIONS

Independent

Investigate changes in sensorium and behavior, e.g., confusion, restlessness, agitation, delirium.

Note presence of gastrointestinal symptoms, e.g., vomiting, diarrhea, abdominal discomfort.

Identify factors that may alter drug absorption/excretion (e.g., small bowel disease, cirrhosis, hyperthyroidism; use of certain drugs, e.g., barbiturates, Dilantin).

Note concomitant use of drugs which increase potential for digitalis toxicity or dysrhythmias.

Collaborative

Monitor serum digoxin (Lanoxin) or digitoxin (Crystodigin) level.

Monitor laboratory studies that may be impacted by digitalis preparations, e.g., electrolytes, BUN, creatinine, liver function studies.

Administer potassium, calcium, and magnesium as indicated.

Administer other appropriate antidysrhythmia medications, e.g., Lidocaine, propanalol, and procanamide.

Prepare patient for transfer to critical care unit, as indicated.

RATIONALE

italis may result in toxicity even with previously appropriate drug doses.

Although psychic disturbances may be the result of decreased cardiac output, drug effect, or electrolyte imbalance, they could indicate developing pathology unrelated to drug toxicity/electrolyte imbalance.

May be direct effect of drug toxicity or reflect altered electrolytes or cardiac output/organ perfusion.

Digitalis absorption, half-life, and effectiveness may be reduced by these factors thereby necessitating higher dosage of digitalis to achieve desired effect. When any of these factors change without alteration in digitalis dosage, toxicity can occur. Diminished renal/liver function and loss of body fat/muscle mass may slow drug metabolism, necessitating reduction in drug dosage.

Quinidine can double serum digitalis level and Verapamil can increase digitalis level by 60%; some antibiotics can increase digitalis level by 10%–40%. Thiazide and loop diuretics, steroids and laxatives, (which potentiate potassium, calcium, and magnesium loss) increase potential for digitalis toxicity. Propanolol (Inderal), other β-blockers, and thyroid preparations also fall in this category.

Digoxin has a narrow therapeutic serum range, with toxicity occurring at levels greater than 2.4 ng/ml. Laboratory levels are evaluated in conjunction with clinical manifestations and ECG to determine individual therapeutic levels/resolution of toxicity.

Abnormal levels of potassium, calcium, or magnesium increase heart's sensitivity to digitalis. Impaired kidney function can cause Lanoxin (mainly excreted by the kidney) to accumulate to toxic levels. Crystodigin levels (mainly excreted by the bowel) are affected by impaired liver function.

Returning these electrolytes to normal may correct many dysrhythmias.

May be necessary to maintain/improve cardiac output.

Patients with digitalis toxicity frequently require intensive monitoring until therapeutic levels have been restored. Because all digitalis preparations

ACTIONS/INTERVENTIONS

Collaborative

Prepare patient for insertion of temporary pacemaker if indicated.

RATIONALE

have long serum half-lives, stabilization can take several days.

May be required on rare occasions to maintain adequate heart rate until digitalis levels are within therapeutic range.

NURSING DIAGNOSIS:	FLUID VOLUME DEFICIT/EXCESS, HIGH RISK FOR
Risk factors may include:	Gastrointestinal side effects of digitalis toxicity, e.g., nausea/vomiting, diarrhea.
	Continued use of diuretics in face of reduced intake.
	Excess sodium/fluid retention.
	Decreased plasma proteins/malnutrition.
Possibly evidenced by:	[Not applicable; presence of signs and symptoms establishes an actual diagnosis.]
DESIRED OUTCOMES/ EVALUATION CRITERIA— PATIENT WILL:	Demonstrate stabilized fluid volume with balanced intake/output, stable weight, vital signs within patient's norms, and absence of edema.
	Verbalize relief from nausea and absence of vomiting/diarrhea.

ACTIONS/INTERVENTIONS

Independent

Monitor intake/output. Calculate fluid balance, noting insensible losses. Weigh as indicated.

Evaluate skin turgor, mucous membrane moisture, presence of dependent/generalized edema.

Monitor vital signs (blood pressure, pulse and respiratory rate). Auscultate breath sounds, noting presence of crackles.

Review fluid requirements. Establish 24-hour schedule and routes to be used. Ascertain patient beverage/food preferences.

Eliminate noxious sights and smells from the environment. Provide frequent oral hygiene.

Instruct patient to take fluids and food slowly as indicated.

RATIONALE

Direct evaluators of fluid status. Sudden changes in weight suggest fluid loss/retention.

Indirect indicators of fluid status/resolution of imbalance.

Fluid deficits may be manifested by hypotension and tachycardia, as heart tries to maintain cardiac output. Fluid excess/developing failure may be manifested by hypertension, tachycardia, tachypnea, crackles, respiratory distress.

Dependent on situation, fluids may be restricted or forced. Providing information involves patient in formulating schedule with individual preferences and enhances a sense of control and cooperation with regimen.

May reduce stimulation of the vomiting center.

May reduce occurrence of vomiting when nauseated.

ACTIONS/INTERVENTIONS

Collaborative

Provide IV fluids via control device.

Administer antiemetics, e.g., prochlorperazine maleate (Compazine), trimethobenzamide (Tigan), as indicated.

Monitor laboratory studies as indicated, e.g., Hb/Hct, BUN/Cr, plasma proteins, electrolytes.

RATIONALE

Fluids may be needed to prevent dehydration, although fluid restrictions may be required if the patient is in CHF.

May be helpful in reducing nausea/vomiting (considered to be central, rather than gastric in origin) enhancing fluid/food intake.

Evaluates hydration status, renal function and causes/effects of imbalance.

NURSING DIAGNOSIS:	THOUGHT PROCESSES, ALTERED, HIGH RISK FOR
Risk factors may include:	Physiologic effects of toxicity/reduced cerebral perfusion.
Possibly evidenced by:	[Not applicable; presence of signs and symptoms establishes an actual diagnosis.]
DESIRED OUTCOMES/ EVALUATION CRITERIA— PATIENT WILL:	Regain/maintain usual mentation.

ACTIONS/INTERVENTIONS

Independent

Assess/investigate changes in mentation/sensorium. Talk to family members about patient's usual mentation.

Stay with/arrange for companion when patient is severely agitated.

Explain procedures, repeatedly if indicated. Reorient to surroundings as needed.

Provide emotional support to the patient/SO. Discuss temporary nature of recent changes in mentation.

Collaborative

Administer supplemental oxygen if indicated.

RATIONALE

The elderly patient may already have problems in mentation associated with age, cerebral vascular impairment, and/or multiple system failure in addition to digitalis toxicity. Information from the family concerning usual mentation is helpful in understanding the patient's progress in resolution of the toxic state. Exaggerated symptoms usually resolve as digitalis level returns to therapeutic range.

Protects patient from bodily harm until more normal functioning is regained.

May reduce agitation/anxiety, promoting sense of security as toxicity clears.

Provides reassurance and reduces level of fear in stressful situation.

May be helpful in improving level of mentation/ thought processes, especially in the presence of severe heart disease, CHF, or acid-base imbalance.

NURSING DIAGNOSIS:	KNOWLEDGE DEFICIT [LEARNING NEED], REGARDING CONDITION, TREATMENT NEEDS
May be related to:	Lack of information/misconceptions concerning specific digitalis therapy or ways to monitor safety/effectiveness of therapy.
Possibly evidenced by:	Failure to follow prescribed regimen.
	Failure to recognize toxic side effects.
DESIRED OUTCOMES/ EVALUATION CRITERIA— PATIENT WILL:	Verbalize understanding of why drug is needed, how it interacts with other drugs, and importance of maintaining prescribed regimen.
	Demonstrate how to count pulse rate.
	Recognize signs of digitalis overdose and developing CHF and what to report to physician.
	Relate individual drug prescription to be followed after discharge.

ACTIONS/INTERVENTIONS	RATIONALE

Independent

Explain why digitalis preparation is needed, e.g., to strengthen heart muscle contraction and to correct irregular heartbeat.	Understanding need for using potentially dangerous drug may enhance compliance with therapeutic regimen.
Explain patient's specific type of digitalis.	Reduces confusion due to digitalis preparations varying in name (although they may be similar), dosage strength, and onset and duration of action.
Instruct patient not to change dose for any reason, not to omit dose, not to increase dose or take extra doses, and to contact doctor if more than one dose is omitted.	Alterations in drug regimen can reduce therapeutic effects/result in toxicity and cause complications.
Show patient how to count pulse for 1 full minute. Have patient demonstrate. Instruct patient to contact doctor before taking dose if pulse is below or above predetermined levels or is more irregular/regular as appropriate.	Digitalis may potentiate/cause dangerous dysrhythmias, impairing cardiac output/patient safety. Note: Patients with atrial dysrhythmias (e.g., AF) may display a more regular pulse as digitalis toxicity develops and AV block increases.
Advise patient that digitalis may react with any other drug(s) (e.g., barbiturates, neomycin, quinidine) presently taken and to provide physician with information that digitalis is taken whenever new medications are prescribed. Advise patient not to take OTC drugs (e.g., laxatives, antidiarrheals, antacids, cold remedies, diuretics) without first checking with the pharmacist or physician.	Knowledge may help prevent dangerous drug interactions.
Provide information and have the patient/SO verbalize understanding of toxic signs/symptoms to report to the physician.	Nausea, vomiting, diarrhea, unusual drowsiness, confusion, very slow or very fast irregular pulse, thumping in chest, double/blurred vision, yellow/

ACTIONS/INTERVENTIONS	RATIONALE

Independent

green tint or halos around objects, flickering color forms or dots, and altered color perception are warning signs that patient should be aware of and report to physician immediately.

Provide written instructions to take home. Involve SO in education.

Patient teaching card listing important facts in large, readable print and simple terms can minimize misinterpretation and may enhance cooperation with treatment regimen.

Collaborative

Arrange for visiting nurse/ home assistance if responsible SO is not readily available.

If elderly patient lives alone and/or is visually or cognitively impaired, home follow-up is essential to reduce risk of overdose.

Angina Pectoris

The classic symptom of coronary artery disease is angina—pain caused by inadequate flow of oxygen to the myocardium. Angina has three major forms, (1) stable (caused by effort of short duration and relieved easily); (2) unstable (longer lasting, more severe, may not be relieved by rest or nitroglycerin); and (3) variant (chest pain at rest with ECG changes).

RELATED CONCERNS:

Cardiac Surgery, p 113
Congestive Heart Failure, p 48
Dysrhythmias, p 94
Myocardial Infarction, p 80
Psychosocial Aspects of Acute Care, p 899
Valvular Heart Disease, p 102

PATIENT ASSESSMENT DATA BASE

ACTIVITY/REST

May report:
Sedentary lifestyle, weakness.

Fatigue, feeling incapacitated after exercise.

Chest pain with exertion.

Being awakened with chest pain.

May exhibit:
Exertional dyspnea.

CIRCULATION

May report:
History of heart disease, hypertension, obesity.

May exhibit:
Tachycardia, dysrhythmias.

Blood pressure normal, elevated, or decreased.

Heart sounds: May be normal; late S_4 or transient late systolic murmur (papillary muscle dysfunction) may be evident during pain.

Moist, cool, pale skin/mucous membranes in presence of vasoconstriction.

FOOD/FLUID

May report:
Nausea, "heartburn"/epigastric distress with eating.

Diet high in cholesterol/fats, salt, caffeine, liquor.

May exhibit:
Belching, gastric distention.

EGO INTEGRITY

May report:
Stressors of work, family, others.

May exhibit:
Apprehension, uneasiness.

PAIN/DISCOMFORT

May report:
Substernal, anterior chest pain that may radiate to jaw, neck, shoulders, and upper extremities (to left side more than right).

Quality: Varies; mild to moderate, heavy pressure, tightness, squeezing, burning.

Duration: Usually less than 15 minutes, rarely more than 30 minutes (average 3 minutes).

Precipitating factors: Pain may be related to physical exertion or great emotion, such as anger or sexual arousal; exercise in weather extremes; or may be unpredictable and/or occur during rest.

Relieving factors: Pain may be responsive to particular relief mechanisms (e.g., rest, antianginal medications).

New or ongoing chest pain which has changed in frequency, duration, character or predictability (i.e., unstable, variant, Prinzmetal's).

May exhibit: Facial grimacing, placing fist over midsternum, rubbing left arm, muscle tension, restlessness.

Autonomic responses, e.g., tachycardia, blood pressure changes.

RESPIRATION

May report: Dyspnea with exertion.

History of smoking.

May exhibit: Respirations: Increased rate/rhythm and alteration in depth.

TEACHING/LEARNING

May report: Family history of heart disease, hypertension, stroke, diabetes.

Use/misuse of cardiac, hypertensive, or OTC drugs.

Regular alcohol use, illicit drug use, e.g., cocaine, amphetamines.

Discharge Plan Considerations: **DRG projected mean length of stay: 3.8 days.**

Alteration in medication use/therapy.

Assistance with homemaker/maintenance tasks.

Changes in physical layout of home.

DIAGNOSTIC STUDIES

Cardiac enzymes/isoenzymes, usually WNL: Elevation indicates myocardial damage.

ECG: Usually normal when patient at rest but flattening or depression of the ST segment of T wave signifies ischemia. Transient ST elevation or decrease greater than 1 mm during pain with no abnormalities when pain-free demonstrates transient myocardial ischemia. Dysrhythmias and heart block may also be present.

24-hour ECG monitoring (Holter): Done to see whether pain episodes correlate with ST segment changes. ST depression without pain is highly indicative of ischemia.

Chest x-ray: Usually normal; however, infiltrates may be present reflecting cardiac decompensation or pulmonary complications.

Pco_2, potassium and myocardial lactate: May be elevated during anginal attack (all play a role in myocardial ischemia and may perpetuate it).

Serum cholesterol/triglycerides: May be elevated (CAD risk factor).

Echocardiogram: May reveal abnormal valvular action as cause of chest pain.

Paced stress-atrial tachycardia: May show ST segment change. LVEDP may rise or remain static with ischemia. Rise with chest pain or ST change is diagnostic of ischemia.

Nuclear imaging studies: Thallium 201: Ischemic regions appear as areas of decreased thallium uptake.

Multigated imaging (MUGA): Evaluates specific and general ventricle performance, regional wall motion, and ejection fraction.

Cardiac catheterization with angiography: Indicated in patients with known ischemic disease with angina, or incapacitating chest pain, in patients with cholesteremia and familial heart disease who are experiencing chest pain, and in patients with abnormal resting ECGs. Abnormal results are present in valvular disease, altered contractility, ventricular failure, and circulatory abnormalities. Note: 10% of patients with unstable angina have normal-appearing coronary arteries.

Ergonovine (Ergotrate) injection: Patients who have angina at rest may demonstrate hyperspastic coronary vessels. (Patients with resting angina usually experience chest pain, ST elevation, or depression and/or pronounced rise in LVEDP, fall in systemic systolic pressure, and/or high-grade coronary artery narrowing. Some patients may also have severe ventricular dysrhythmias.)

NURSING PRIORITIES

1. Relieve/control pain.
2. Prevent/minimize development of myocardial complications.
3. Provide information about disease process/prognosis and treatment.
4. Support patient/SO in initiating necessary lifestyle/behavioral changes.

DISCHARGE GOALS

1. Achieves desired activity level; meets self-care needs with minimal or no pain.
2. Free of complications.
3. Disease process/prognosis and therapeutic regimen understood.
4. Participating in treatment program, behavioral changes.

NURSING DIAGNOSIS:	PAIN [ACUTE]
May be related to:	Decreased myocardial blood flow.
	Increased cardiac workload/oxygen consumption.
Possibly evidenced by:	Reports of pain varying in frequency, duration, and intensity (especially as condition worsens).
	Narrowed focus.
	Distraction behaviors (moaning, crying, pacing, restlessness).
	Autonomic responses, e.g., diaphoresis, blood pressure and pulse rate changes, pupillary dilation, increased/decreased respiratory rate.
DESIRED OUTCOMES/ EVALUATION CRITERIA— PATIENT WILL:	Verbalize/demonstrate relief of pain.
	Report anginal episodes decreased in frequency, duration, and severity.

ACTIONS/INTERVENTIONS	RATIONALE

Independent

Instruct patient to notify nurse immediately when chest pain occurs.

Pain and decreased cardiac output may stimulate the sympathetic nervous system to release excessive amounts of norepinephrine, which increases platelet aggregation and release of thromboxane A_2. This potent vasoconstrictor causes coronary artery spasm which can precipitate, complicate, and/or prolong an anginal attack. Unbearable pain may cause vasovagal response, decreasing BP and heart rate.

ACTIONS/INTERVENTIONS	RATIONALE
Independent	
Assess and document patient response/effects of medication.	Provides information about disease progression. Aids in evaluating effectiveness of interventions and may indicate need for change in therapeutic regimen.
Identify precipitating event, if any; frequency, duration, intensity, and location of pain.	Helps differentiate this chest pain and aids in evaluating possible progression to unstable angina. (Stable angina usually lasts 3–5 minutes while unstable angina is more intense and may last up to 45 minutes.)
Observe for associated symptoms, e.g., dyspnea, nausea/vomiting, dizziness, palpitations, desire to micturate.	Decreased cardiac output (which may occur during ischemic myocardial episode) stimulates sympathetic/parasympathetic nervous system, causing a variety of vague aches/sensations that patient may not identify as related to anginal episode.
Evaluate reports of pain in jaw, neck, shoulder, arm, or hand (typically on left side).	Cardiac pain may radiate, e.g., pain is often referred to more superficial sites served by the same spinal cord nerve level.
Place patient at complete rest during anginal episodes.	Reduces myocardial oxygen demand to minimize risk of tissue injury/necrosis.
Elevate head of bed if patient is short of breath.	Facilitates gas exchange to decrease hypoxia and resultant shortness of breath.
Monitor heart rate/rhythm.	Unstable angina patients have an increased risk of acute life-threatening dysrhythmias, which occur in response to ischemic changes and/or stress.
Monitor vital signs every 5 minutes during anginal attack.	Blood pressure may rise initially due to sympathetic stimulation, then fall if cardiac output is compromised. Tachycardia also develops in response to sympathetic stimulation and may be sustained as a compensatory response if cardiac output falls.
Stay with patient who is experiencing pain or appears anxious.	Anxiety releases catecholamines which increase myocardial workload and can escalate/prolong ischemic pain. Presence of nurse can reduce feelings of fear and helplessness.
Maintain quiet, comfortable environment; restrict visitors as necessary.	Mental/emotional stress increases myocardial workload.
Provide light meals. Have patient rest for 1 hour after meals.	Decreases myocardial workload associated with work of digestion, reducing risk of anginal attack.
Collaborative	
Provide supplemental oxygen as indicated.	Increases oxygen available for myocardial uptake/reversal of ischemia.
Administer antianginal medication(s) promptly as indicated:	
Nitroglycerine: Sublingual (Nitrostat), buccal or oral tablets, sublingual spray;	Nitroglycerin has set the standard for treating and preventing anginal pain for more than 100 years. Today it is still the cornerstone of antianginal therapy. Rapid vasodilator effect lasts 10–30 minutes and can be used prophylactically to prevent, as

73

ACTIONS/INTERVENTIONS	RATIONALE
Collaborative	
	well as abort, anginal attacks. *Note:* May enhance vasospastic angina.
Sustained release tablets, caplets, patches, transmucosal ointment, chewable tablets (long-acting), e.g., Nitro-Dur, Transderm-Nitro, isosorbide (Isordil, Sorbitrate);	Reduces frequency and severity of attack by producing prolonged/continuous vasodilation. May cause headache, dizziness, lightheadedness, symptoms which usually pass quickly. If headache is intolerable, alteration of dose or discontinuation of drug may be necessary.
β-blockers, e.g., atenolol (Tenormin); nadolol (Corgard); metroprolol (Lopressor), propranolol (Inderal);	Reduces angina by reducing the heart's workload. (Refer to ND: Cardiac Output, decreased, below.)
Analgesics, i.e., acetaminophen (Tylenol);	Usually sufficient analgesia for relief of headache caused by dilatation of cerebral vessels in response to nitrates.
Morphine sulphate.	Potent narcotic analgesic that has several beneficial effects, e.g., causes peripheral vasodilation and reduces myocardial workload; has a sedative effect to produce relaxation; interrupts the flow of vasoconstricting catecholamines and thereby effectively relieves severe chest pain. MS is given IV for rapid action and because decreased cardiac output compromises peripheral tissue absorption.
Monitor serial ECG changes.	Ischemia during anginal attack may cause transient ST segment depression or elevation and T wave inversion. Serial tracings verify ischemic changes which may disappear when patient is painfree and are also baseline with which to compare later pattern changes.

NURSING DIAGNOSIS:	CARDIAC OUTPUT, DECREASED
May be related to:	Inotropic changes (transient/prolonged myocardial ischemia, effects of medications).
	Alterations in rate/rhythm and electrical conduction.
Possibly evidenced by:	Changes in hemodynamic readings.
	Dyspnea.
	Restlessness.
	Decreased tolerance for activity; fatigue.
	Diminished peripheral pulses.
	Cool/pale skin.
	Change in mental status.
	Continued chest pain.

DESIRED OUTCOMES/ EVALUATION CRITERIA— PATIENT WILL:	Report/display decreased episodes of dyspnea, angina, and dysrhythmias. Demonstrate increased activity tolerance. Participate in behaviors/activities that reduce the workload of the heart.

ACTIONS/INTERVENTIONS	RATIONALE
Independent	
Monitor vital signs, e.g., heart rate, BP.	Tachycardia may be present because of pain, anxiety, hypoxemia, and reduced cardiac output. Changes may also occur in BP (hypertension or hypotension) because of cardiac response.
Evaluate mental status, noting development of confusion, disorientation.	Reduced perfusion of the brain can produce observable changes in sensorium.
Note skin color and presence/quality of pulses.	Peripheral circulation is reduced when cardiac output falls, giving the skin a pale or gray color (depending on level of hypoxia) and diminishing the strength of peripheral pulses.
Auscultate breath sounds and heart sounds. Listen for murmurs.	S_3, S_4, or crackles can occur with cardiac decompensation or some medications (especially β-blockers). Development of murmurs may reveal a valvular cause for chest pain, e.g., aortic stenosis, mitral stenosis, or papillary muscle rupture.
Maintain bedrest in position of comfort during acute episodes.	Decreases oxygen consumption/demand reducing myocardial workload and risk of decompensation.
Provide for adequate rest periods. Assist with/perform self-care activities, as indicated.	Conserves energy, reduces cardiac workload.
Stress importance of avoiding straining/bearing down, especially during defecation.	Valsalva maneuver causes vagal stimulation, reducing heart rate (bradycardia), which may be followed by rebound tachycardia, both of which may impair cardiac output.
Encourage immediate reporting of pain for prompt administration of medications as indicated.	Timely interventions can reduce oxygen consumption and myocardial workload and may prevent/minimize cardiac complications.
Monitor for and document effects of/adverse response to medications, noting BP, heart rate and rhythm, (especially when giving combination of calcium antagonists, β-blockers, and nitrates).	Desired effect is to decrease myocardial oxygen demand by decreasing ventricular stress. Drugs with negative inotropic properties can decrease perfusion to an already ischemic myocardium. Combination of nitrates and β-blockers may have cumulative effect on cardiac output.
Assess for signs and symptoms of CHF.	Angina is only a symptom of underlying pathology causing myocardial ischemia. Disease may compromise cardiac function to point of decompensation.
Collaborative	
Administer supplemental oxygen as needed.	Increases oxygen available for myocardial uptake

ACTIONS/INTERVENTIONS	RATIONALE
Collaborative	to improve contractility, reduce ischemia, and lactic acid levels.
Administer medications, as indicated:	
Calcium channel blockers, e.g.: diltiazem (Cardizem); nifedipine (Procardia); verapamil (Calan);	Although differing in mode of action, calcium channel blockers play a major role in preventing and terminating ischemia induced by coronary artery spasm and in reducing vascular resistance, thereby decreasing BP and cardiac workload.
β-blockers, e.g., atenolol (Tenormin); nadolol (Corgard); propranolol (Inderal); esmolol (Brebivbloc).	These medications decrease cardiac workload by reducing heart rate and systolic BP. *Note:* Overdosage produces cardiac decompensation.
Discuss purpose and prepare for stress testing and cardiac catheterization, when indicated.	Stress testing provides information about the health/strength of the ventricles, which is useful in determining appropriate levels of activity. Angiography may be indicated to identify areas of coronary artery obstruction/damage that may require surgical intervention.
Prepare for surgical intervention (PTCA, valve replacement, CABG), if indicated.	PTCA has become a fairly common procedure in the last 15 years. PTCA increases coronary blood flow by compression of atheromatous lesions and dilatation of the vessel lumen in an occluded coronary artery. This procedure may be preferred over the more invasive cardiac surgery (CABG). CABG is recommended when testing confirms myocardial ischemia as a result of left main coronary artery disease or symptomatic three-vessel disease.
Prepare for transfer to critical care unit if condition warrants.	Profound/prolonged chest pain with decreased cardiac output reflects development of complications requiring more intense/emergency interventions.

NURSING DIAGNOSIS:	**ANXIETY (SPECIFY LEVEL)**
May be related to:	Situational crises.
	Threat to *self-concept* (altered image/abilities).
	Underlying pathophysiologic response.
	Threat to or change in health status (disease course which can lead to further compromise, debility, even death).
	Negative self-talk.
Possibly evidenced by:	Expressed concern regarding changes in life events.
	Increased tension/helplessness.

Apprehension, uncertainty, restlessness.

Association of diagnosis with loss of healthy body image, loss of place/influence.

View of self as noncontributing member of family/society.

Fear of death as an imminent reality.

DESIRED OUTCOMES/ EVALUATION CRITERIA— PATIENT WILL:

Verbalize awareness of feelings of anxiety and healthy ways to deal with them.

Report anxiety is reduced to a manageable level.

Express concerns about effect of disease on lifestyle, position within family and society.

Demonstrate effective coping strategies/problem-solving skills.

ACTIONS/INTERVENTIONS	RATIONALE

Independent

Explain purpose of tests and procedures, e.g., stress testing.

Reduces anxiety attributable to fear of diagnosis and prognosis.

Promote expression of feelings and fears, e.g., denial, depression, and anger. Let patient/SO know these are normal reactions. Note statements of concern, e.g., "Heart attack is inevitable."

Unexpressed feelings may create internal turmoil and affect self-image. Verbalization of concerns reduces tension, verifies level of coping, and facilitates dealing with feelings. Presence of negative self-talk can increase level of anxiety and may contribute to exacerbation of angina attacks.

Encourage family and friends to treat patient as before.

Reassures patient that role in the family and business has not been altered.

Tell patient the medical regimen has been designed to reduce/limit future attacks and increase cardiac stability.

Encourages patient to test symptom control (e.g., no angina with certain levels of activity), to increase confidence in medical program, and integrate abilities into perceptions of self.

(Refer to CP: "Psychosocial Aspects of Acute Care" for additional considerations, p 899).

Collaborative

Administer sedatives, tranquilizers, as indicated.

May be desired to help patient to relax until physically able to reestablish adequate coping strategies.

NURSING DIAGNOSIS:	**KNOWLEDGE DEFICIT [LEARNING NEED], REGARDING CONDITION, TREATMENT NEEDS**
May be related to:	Lack of exposure.
	Inaccurate/misinterpretation of information.
	Unfamiliarity with information resources.
Possibly evidenced by:	Questions.

DESIRED OUTCOMES/ EVALUATION CRITERIA— PATIENT WILL:	Request for information. Statement of concerns. Inaccurate follow-through of instructions. Participate in learning process. Assume responsibility for own learning, looking for information and asking questions. Verbalize understanding of condition/disease process and treatment. Participate in treatment regimen. Initiate necessary lifestyle changes.

ACTIONS/INTERVENTIONS	RATIONALE

Independent

Review pathophysiology of condition. Stress need for preventing anginal attacks.	Patients with angina need to learn why it occurs and what they can do to control it. This is the focus of therapeutic management in order to reduce likelihood of myocardial infarction.
Encourage avoidance of factors/situations that may precipitate anginal episode, e.g., emotional stress, physical exertion, ingestion of large/heavy meal, exposure to extremes in environmental temperature.	May reduce incidence/severity of ischemic episodes.
Assist patient/SO to identify sources of physical and emotional stress and discuss ways that they can be avoided.	This is a crucial step in limiting/preventing anginal attacks.
Review importance of weight control, cessation of smoking, dietary changes, and exercise.	Knowledge of the significance of risk factors provides patient with opportunity to make needed changes.
Encourage patient to follow prescribed reconditioning program; caution to avoid exhaustion.	Fear of triggering attacks may cause patient to avoid participation in activity that has been prescribed to enhance recovery (increase myocardial strength and form collateral circulation).
Discuss impact of illness on desired lifestyle and activities, including work, driving, sexual activity, and hobbies. Provide information, privacy, or consultation, as indicated.	Patient may be reluctant to resume/continue usual activities because of fear of anginal attack/death. Patient should take nitroglycerine prophylactically before any activity that is known to precipitate angina.
Demonstrate/encourage patient to monitor own pulse during activities, schedule/simplify activities, avoid strain.	Allows patient to identify those activities that can be modified to avoid cardiac stress and stay below the anginal threshold.
Discuss steps to take when anginal attacks occur, e.g., cessation of activity, administration of prn medication, use of relaxation techniques.	Being prepared for an event takes away the fear that patient will not know what to do if attack occurs.

ACTIONS/INTERVENTIONS	RATIONALE
Independent	
Review prescribed medications for control/prevention of anginal attacks.	Angina is a complicated condition which often requires the use of many drugs given to decrease myocardial workload, improve coronary circulation, and control the occurrence of attacks.
Stress importance of checking with physician prior to taking OTC drugs.	OTC drugs may potentiate or negate prescribed medications.
Discuss ASA as indicated.	May be given prophylactically on a daily basis to decrease platelet aggregation and improve coronary circulation.
Review symptoms to be reported to physician, e.g., increase in frequency/duration of attacks, changes in response to medications.	Knowledge of expectations can avoid undue concern for insignificant reasons or delay in treatment of important symptoms.
Discuss importance of follow-up appointments.	Angina is a symptom of progressive coronary artery disease which should be monitored and may require occasional adjustment of treatment regimen.

Myocardial Infarction _____

Myocardial infarction (MI) is caused by reduced blood flow through one or more of the coronary arteries, resulting in myocardial ischemia and necrosis.

RELATED CONCERNS:

Angina Pectoris, p 70
Congestive Heart Failure, p 48
Dysrhythmias, p 94
Inflammatory Cardiac Conditions, p 126
Psychosocial Aspects of Acute Care, p 899
Thrombophlebitis, p 135

PATIENT ASSESSMENT DATA BASE

ACTIVITY/REST

May report:	Weakness, fatigue, loss of sleep.
	Sedentary lifestyle, sporadic exercise schedule.
May exhibit:	Tachycardia, dyspnea with rest/activity.

CIRCULATION

May report:	History of previous MI, coronary artery disease, CHF, BP problems, diabetes mellitus.
May exhibit:	BP: May be normal or increased/decreased; postural changes may be noted from lying to sitting/standing.
	Pulse: May be normal; full/bounding, or weak/thready quality with delayed capillary refill; irregularities (dysrhythmias) may be present.
	Heart sounds: Extra heart sounds: S_3/S_4 may reflect cardiac failure/decreased ventricular contractility, or compliance.
	Murmurs: If present, may reflect valvular insufficiency or papillary muscle dysfunction.
	Friction rub: Suggests pericarditis.
	Heart rate: May be abnormal (tachycardia, bradycardia).
	Heart rhythm: Can be regular or irregular.
	Edema: Jugular vein distention, peripheral/dependent edema, generalized edema, crackles may be present with cardiac/ventricular failure.
	Color: Pallor or cyanosis/mottling of skin, nailbeds, mucous membranes, and lips may be noted.

EGO INTEGRITY

May report:	Denial of significance of symptoms/presence of condition.
	Fear of dying, feelings of impending doom.
	Anger at inconvenience of illness/"unnecessary" hospitalization.
	Worry about family, job, finances.
May exhibit:	Denial, withdrawal, anxiety, lack of eye contact.
	Irritability, anger, combative behavior.
	Focus on self/pain.

ELIMINATION

May exhibit: Normal or decreased bowel sounds.

FOOD/FLUID

May report: Nausea, loss of appetite, belching, indigestion/heartburn.

May exhibit: Decreased skin turgor; dry/diaphoretic skin.
Vomiting.
Weight change.

HYGIENE

**May report/
exhibit:**   Difficulty performing care tasks.

NEUROSENSORY

May report: Dizziness, fainting spells in or out of bed (upright or at rest).

May exhibit: Changes in mentation.
Weakness.

PAIN/DISCOMFORT

May report: Sudden onset chest pain (may/may not be associated with activity), unrelieved by rest or nitroglycerin. (Athough most pain is deep and visceral, 20% of the MIs are painless).

Location: Typically anterior chest, substernal, precordium; may radiate to arms, jaws, face. May have atypical location such as epigastrium, elbow, jaw, abdomen, back, neck.

Quality: Crushing, constricting, viselike, squeezing, heavy, steady.

Intensity: Usually 10 on a scale of 1–10; may be "worst pain ever experienced."

Note: Pain may be absent in postoperative patients, those with diabetes mellitus, or hypertension, or the elderly.

May exhibit: Facial grimacing, changes in body posture.
Crying, groaning, squirming, stretching.
Withdrawal, loss of eye contact.
Autonomic responses: Changes in heart rate/rhythm, BP, respirations, skin color/moisture, level of consciousness.

RESPIRATION

May report: Dyspnea with/without exertion, nocturnal dyspnea.
Cough with/without sputum production.
History of smoking, chronic respiratory disease.

May exhibit: Increased respiratory rate, shallow/labored breathing.
Pallor or cyanosis.
Breath sounds: Clear or crackles/wheezes.
Sputum: Clear, pink-tinged.

SOCIAL INTERACTION

May report: Recent stress, e.g., work, family.

Difficulty coping with current stressors, e.g., illness, hospitalization.

May exhibit: Difficulty resting quietly, overemotional responses (intense anger, fear).

Withdrawal from family.

TEACHING/LEARNING

May report: Family history of heart disease/MI, diabetes, stroke, hypertension, peripheral vascular disease.

Use of tobacco.

Discharge Plan Considerations: **DRG projected length of stay: 7.3 days; (2–4 days/CCU).**

Assistance with food preparation, shopping, transportation, homemaking/maintenance tasks; physical layout of home.

DIAGNOSTIC STUDIES

ECG: Shows S-T wave elevation, signifying ischemia; depressed or inverted T wave, indicating injury; and presence of Q waves, signifying necrosis.

Cardiac enzymes and isoenzymes: CPK-MB (isoenzyme found in heart muscle) elevates within 4–6 hours, peaks in 12–20 hours, returns to normal in 36–48 hours. *LDH* elevates within 12–24 hours, peaks within 24–48 hours, and may take as long as 10–14 days to return to normal. *AST* (aspartate aminotransferase) elevations (less reliable/specific) occur in 6–12 hours, peak in 24 hours, return to normal in 3–4 days.

Electrolytes: Imbalances can alter conduction and can compromise contractility, e.g., hypokalemia/hyperkalemia.

WBC: Leukocytosis (10,000–20,000) usually appears on the second day after MI due to inflammatory process.

Sedimentation rate: Rises on second to third day after MI, indicating inflammation.

Chemistry profiles: May be abnormal depending on acute/chronic abnormal organ function/perfusion.

ABGs/pulse oximetry: May indicate hypoxia or acute/chronic lung disease processes.

Serum cholesterol/triglycerides: Elevation may reflect arteriosclerosis as a cause for MI.

Chest x-ray: May be normal or show an enlarged cardiac shadow suggestive of CHF or ventricular aneurysm.

Echocardiogram: May be done to determine dimensions of chambers, septal/ventricular wall motion, and valve configuration/function.

Nuclear imaging studies:

Thallium: Evaluates myocardial blood flow and status of myocardial cells, e.g., location/extent of acute/previous MI.
Technetium: Accumulates in ischemic cells outlining necrotic area(s).

Cardiac blood imaging/MUGA: Evaluates specific and general ventricular performance, regional wall motion, and ejection fraction (blood flow).

Coronary angiography: Visualizes narrowing/occlusion of coronary arteries and is usually done in conjunction with measurements of chamber pressures and assessment of left ventricular function (ejection fraction). Procedure is not usually done in acute phase of MI unless angioplasty/emergency heart surgery is imminent.

Digital subtraction angiography (DSA): Technique used to visualize status of arterial bypass grafts and to detect peripheral artery disease.

Nuclear magnetic resonance (NMR): Allows visualization of blood flow, cardiac chambers/intraventricular septum, valves, vascular lesions, plaque formations, areas of necrosis/infarction, and blood clots.

Exercise stress test: Determines cardiovascular response to activity (often done in conjunction with thallium imaging in the recovery phase).

NURSING PRIORITIES

1. Relieve pain, anxiety.
2. Reduce myocardial workload.
3. Prevent/detect and assist in treatment of life-threatening dysrhythmias or complications.
4. Promote cardiac health, self-care.

DISCHARGE GOALS

1. Chest pain absent/controlled.
2. Heart rate/rhythm sufficient to sustain adequate cardiac output/tissue perfusion.
3. Achievement of activity level sufficient for basic self-care.
4. Anxiety reduced/managed.
5. Disease process, treatment plan, and prognosis understood.

NURSING DIAGNOSIS:	PAIN, [ACUTE]
May be related to:	Tissue ischemia secondary to coronary artery occlusion.
Possibly evidenced by:	Complaints of chest pain with/without radiation.
	Facial grimacing.
	Restlessness, changes in level of consciousness.
	Changes in pulse, BP.
DESIRED OUTCOMES/ EVALUATION CRITERIA— PATIENT WILL:	Verbalize relief/control of chest pain.
	Demonstrate use of relaxation techniques.
	Display reduced tension, relaxed manner, ease of movement.

ACTIONS/INTERVENTIONS	RATIONALE
Independent	
Monitor/document characteristics of pain, noting verbal reports, nonverbal cues, and hemodynamic response (e.g., moaning, crying, restlessness, diaphoresis, clutching chest, rapid breathing, BP/ heart rate changes).	Variation of appearance and behavior of patients in pain may present a challenge in assessment. Most patients with an acute MI appear ill, distracted, and focused on pain. Verbal history and deeper investigation of precipitating factors should be postponed until pain is relieved. Respirations may be increased as a result of pain and associated anxiety, while release of stress induced catecholamines will increase heart rate and BP.
Obtain full description of pain from patient including location; intensity (0–10); duration; quality (dull/crushing); and radiation.	Pain is a subjective experience and must be described by the patient. Assist patient to quantify pain by comparing it to other experiences.
Review history of previous angina, anginal equivalent, or MI pain. Discuss family history if pertinent.	May differentiate current pain from preexisting patterns, as well as identify complications such as extension of infarction, pulmonary embolus, or pericarditis.

ACTIONS/INTERVENTIONS	RATIONALE
Independent	
Instruct patient to report pain immediately.	Delay in reporting pain hinders pain relief/may require increased dosage of medication to achieve relief. In addition, severe pain may induce shock by stimulating the sympathetic nervous system, thereby creating further damage and interfering with diagnostics and relief of pain.
Provide quiet environment, calm activities, and comfort measures (e.g., dry/wrinkle-free linens, backrub). Approach the patient calmly and with confidence.	Decreases external stimuli, which may aggravate anxiety and cardiac strain and limit coping abilities and adjustment to current situation.
Assist/instruct in relaxation techniques, e.g., deep/slow breathing, distraction behaviors, visualization, guided imagery.	Helpful in decreasing perception of/response to pain. Provides a sense of having some control over the situation, increase in positive attitude.
Check vital signs before and after narcotic medication.	Hypotension/respiratory depression can occur as a result of narcotic administration. These problems may increase myocardial damage in presence of ventricular insufficiency.
Collaborative	
Administer supplemental oxygen by means of nasal cannula or face mask, as indicated.	Increases amount of oxygen available for myocardial uptake and thereby may relieve discomfort associated with tissue ischemia.
Administer medications as indicated, e.g.:	
Antianginals, e.g., nitroglycerin (Nitro-Bid, Nitrostat, Nitro-Dur);	Nitrates are useful for pain control by coronary vasodilating effects, which increase coronary blood flow and myocardial perfusion. Peripheral vasodilation effects reduce the volume of blood returning to the heart (preload), thereby decreasing myocardial work and oxygen demand.
β-blockers, e.g., atenolol (Tenormin); pindolol (Visken); propranolol (Inderal);	Important second-line agents for pain control through effect of blocking sympathetic stimulation, thereby reducing heart rate, systolic BP, and myocardial oxygen demand. May be given alone or with nitrates. *Note:* β-blockers may be contraindicated if myocardial contractility is severely impaired, because negative inotropic properties can further reduce contractility.
Analgesics, e.g., morphine, meperidine (Demerol);	Although IV morphine is the usual drug of choice, other injectable narcotics may be used in acute phase/recurrent chest pain unrelieved by nitroglycerin to reduce severe pain, provide sedation, and decrease myocardial workload. IM injections should be avoided, if possible, because they can alter the CPK diagnostic indicator and are not well absorbed in underperfused tissue.
Calcium channel blockers, e.g., verapamil (Calan); diltiazem (Cardizem); nifedipine (Procardia);	Vasodilation effects can increase coronary blood flow, encourage collateral circulation, and reduce preload and myocardial oxygen demands. Some of these agents also have antidysrhythmic properties.

ACTIONS/INTERVENTIONS	RATIONALE
Collaborative	
PTCA angioplasty, also called balloon angioplasty.	This procedure is employed to open partially blocked coronary arteries before they become totally blocked. The mechanism seems to include a combination of vessel stretching and plaque compression.

NURSING DIAGNOSIS:	ACTIVITY INTOLERANCE
May be related to:	Imbalance between myocardial oxygen supply and demand.
	Presence of ischemia/necrotic myocardial tissues.
	Cardiac depressant effects of certain drugs (β-blockers, antidysrhythmics).
Possibly evidenced by:	Alterations in heart rate and BP with activity.
	Development of dysrhythmias.
	Changes in skin color/moisture.
	Exertional angina.
	Generalized weakness.
DESIRED OUTCOMES/ EVALUATION CRITERIA— PATIENT WILL:	Demonstrate measurable/progressive increase in tolerance for activity with heart rate/rhythm and BP within patient's normal limits and skin warm, pink, dry.
	Report angina absent/controlled within time-frame for administered medications.

ACTIONS/INTERVENTIONS	RATIONALE
Independent	
Record/document heart rate, rhythm, and BP changes before, during, after activity, as indicated. Correlate with reports of chest pain/shortness of breath. (Refer to ND: Cardiac Output, decreased high risk for, p. 88.)	Trends determine patient's response to activity and may indicate myocardial oxygen deprivation that may require decrease in activity level/return to bedrest, changes in medication regimen, use of supplemental oxygen.
Promote rest (bed/chair) initially. Limit activity on basis of pain/hemodynamic response. Provide nonstress diversional activities.	Reduces myocardial workload/oxygen consumption, reducing risk of complications (e.g., extension of MI).
Limit visitors and/or visiting by patient, initially.	Lengthy/involved conversations can be very taxing for the patient; however, periods of quiet visitation can be therapeutic.
Instruct patient to avoid increasing abdominal pressure, e.g., straining during defecation.	Activities that require holding the breath and bearing down (Valsalva maneuver) can result in bradycardia, temporarily reduced cardiac output, and rebound tachycardia with elevated BP.

ACTIONS/INTERVENTIONS

Independent

Explain pattern of graded increase of activity level, e.g., getting up in chair when there is no pain, progressive ambulation, and resting for 1 hour after meals.

Review signs/symptoms reflecting intolerance of present activity level or requiring notification of nurse/physician.

Collaborative

Refer to cardiac rehabilitation program.

RATIONALE

Progressive activity provides a controlled demand on the heart, increasing strength and preventing overexertion.

Palpitations, pulse irregularities, development of chest pain, or dyspnea may indicate need for changes in exercise regimen or medication.

Provides continued support/additional supervision and participation in recovery and wellness process.

NURSING DIAGNOSIS:	ANXIETY/FEAR, SPECIFY LEVEL
May be related to:	Threat to or change in health and socioeconomic status.
	Threat of loss/death.
	Unconscious conflict about essential values, beliefs, and goals of life.
	Interpersonal transmission/contagion.
Possibly evidenced by:	Fearful attitude.
	Apprehension, increased tension, restlessness, facial tension.
	Uncertainty.
	Feelings of inadequacy.
	Somatic complaints/sympathetic stimulation.
	Focus on self, expressions of concern about current events.
	Fight (e.g., belligerent attitude) or flight behavior.
DESIRED OUTCOMES/ EVALUATION CRITERIA— PATIENT WILL:	Recognize feelings.
	Identify causes, contributing factors.
	Verbalize reduction of anxiety/fear.
	Demonstrate positive problem-solving skills.
	Identify/use resources appropriately.

ACTIONS/INTERVENTIONS

Independent

Identify and acknowledge patient's perception of threat/situation. Encourage expressions of and

RATIONALE

Coping with pain and emotional trauma of an MI is difficult. Patient may fear death and/or be anxious

ACTIONS/INTERVENTIONS	RATIONALE
Independent	
do not deny feelings of anger, grief, sadness, fear, etc.	about immediate environment. Ongoing anxiety (related to concerns about impact of heart attack on future lifestyle, matters left unattended/unresolved, and effects of illness on family) may be present in varying degrees for some time and may be manifested by symptoms of depression.
Note presence of hostility, withdrawal, and/or denial (inappropriate affect or refusal to comply with medical regimen).	Research into survival rates between type A/type B individuals and the impact of denial has been ambiguous. However, studies show some correlation between degree/expression of anger or hostility and an increased risk for MI.
Maintain confident manner (without false reassurance).	Patient and SO can be affected by the anxiety/uneasiness displayed by health team members. Honest explanations can alleviate anxiety.
Observe for verbal/nonverbal signs of anxiety and stay with patient. Intervene if patient displays destructive behavior.	Patient may not express concern directly, but words/actions may convey sense of agitation, aggression, and hostility. Intervention can help patient to regain control of own behavior.
Accept but do not reinforce use of denial. Avoid confrontations.	Denial can be beneficial in decreasing anxiety but can postpone dealing with the reality of the current situation. Confrontation can promote anger and increase use of denial, reducing cooperation and possibly impeding recovery.
Orient patient/SO to routine procedures and expected activities. Promote participation when possible.	Predictability and information can decrease anxiety for patient.
Answer all questions factually. Provide consistent information; repeat as indicated.	Accurate information about the situation reduces fear, strengthens patient-nurse relationship, and assists patient/SO to deal realistically with situation. Attention span may be short, and repetition of information helps with retention.
Encourage patient/SO to communicate with one another, sharing questions and concerns.	Sharing information elicits support/comfort and can relieve tension of unexpressed worries.
Provide rest periods/uninterrupted sleep time, quiet surroundings, with patient controlling type, amount of external stimuli.	Conserves energy and enhances coping abilities.
Support normality of grieving process, including time necessary for resolution.	Can provide reassurance that feelings are normal response to situation/perceived changes.
Provide privacy for patient and SO.	Allows needed time for expression of feelings, relief of anxiety, and the establishing of more adaptive behaviors.
Encourage independence, self-care, and decision making within accepted treatment plan.	Increased independence from staff promotes self-confidence and reduces feelings of abandonment that can accompany transfer from coronary unit/discharge from hospital.
Encourage discussion about postdischarge expectations.	Helps patient/SO identify realistic goals, thereby reducing risk of discouragement in face of the reality of limitations of condition/pace of recuperation.

87

ACTIONS/INTERVENTIONS	RATIONALE
Collaborative	
Administer antianxiety/hypnotics as indicated, e.g., diazepam (Valium); flurazepam (Dalmane); lorazepam (Ativan).	Promotes relaxation/rest and reduces feelings of anxiety.

NURSING DIAGNOSIS:	CARDIAC OUTPUT, DECREASED, HIGH RISK FOR
Risk factors may include:	Changes in rate, rhythm, electrical conduction.
	Reduced preload/increased SVR.
	Infarcted/dyskinetic muscle, structural defects, e.g., ventricular aneurysm, septal defects.
Possibly evidenced by:	[Not applicable; presence of signs and symptoms establishes actual diagnosis.]
DESIRED OUTCOMES/ EVALUATION CRITERIA— PATIENT WILL:	Maintain hemodynamic stability, e.g., BP, cardiac output within normal range, adequate urinary output, decreased/absent dysrhythmias.
	Report decreased episodes of dyspnea, angina.
	Demonstrate an increase in activity tolerance.

ACTIONS/INTERVENTIONS	RATIONALE
Independent	
Auscultate BP. Compare both arms and obtain lying, sitting, and standing pressures when able.	Hypotension may occur related to ventricular dysfunction, hypoperfusion of the myocardium, and vagal stimulation. However, hypertension is also a common phenomenon, possibly related to pain, anxiety, catecholamine release, and/or preexisting vascular problems. Orthostatic (postural) hypotension may be associated with complications of infarct, e.g., CHF.
Evaluate quality and equality of pulses, as indicated.	Decreased cardiac output results in diminished weak/thready pulses. Irregularities suggest dysrhythmias, which may require further evaluation/monitoring.
Note development of S_3, S_4;	S_3 is usually associated with CHF, but it may also be noted with mitral insufficiency (regurgitation) and left ventricular overload that can accompany severe infarction. S_4 may be associated with myocardial ischemia, ventricular stiffening, and pulmonary or systemic hypertension.
Presence of murmurs/rubs.	Indicates disturbances of normal blood flow within the heart, e.g., incompetent valve, septal defect, or vibration of papillary muscle/chordae tendonae (complication of MI). Presence of rub with an infarction is also associated with inflammation, e.g., pericardial effusion and pericarditis.

ACTIONS/INTERVENTIONS	RATIONALE
Independent	
Auscultate breath sounds.	Crackles reflecting pulmonary congestion may develop because of depressed myocardial function.
Monitor heart rate and rhythm. Document dysrhythmias via telemetry.	Heart rate and rhythm respond to medication and activity, as well as developing complications/dysrhythmias (especially premature ventricular contractions or progressive heart blocks), which could compromise cardiac function or increase ischemic damage. Acute or chronic atrial flutter/fibrillation may be seen with coronary artery or valvular involvement and may or may not be pathologic.
Note response to activity and promote rest appropriately. (Refer to ND: Activity Intolerance, p. 85.)	Overexertion increases oxygen consumption/demand and can compromise myocardial function.
Provide bedside commode if unable to use bathroom facilities.	Attempts at using bedpan can be exhausting and psychologically stressful, thereby increasing oxygen demand and cardiac workload.
Provide small/easily digested meals. Restrict caffeine intake, e.g., coffee, chocolate, cola.	Large meals may increase myocardial workload and cause vagal stimulation resulting in bradycardia/ectopic beats. Caffeine is a direct cardiac stimulant that can increase heart rate.
Have emergency equipment/medications available.	Sudden coronary occlusion, lethal dysrhythmias, extension of infarct, or unrelenting pain are situations that may precipitate cardiac arrest, requiring immediate life-saving therapies/transfer to critical care unit.
Collaborative	
Administer supplemental oxygen, as indicated.	Increases amount of oxygen available for myocardial uptake, reducing ischemia and resultant dysrhythmias.
Maintain IV/hep-lock access as indicated.	Patent line is important for administration of emergency drugs in presence of persistent dysrhythmias or chest pain.
Review serial ECGs.	Provides information regarding progression/resolution of infarction, status of ventricular function, electrolyte balance, and effects of drug therapies.
Review chest x-ray.	May reflect pulmonary edema related to ventricular dysfunction.
Monitor laboratory data: e.g., cardiac enzymes, ABGs, electrolytes.	Enzymes monitor resolution/extension of infarction. Presence of hypoxia indicates need for supplemental oxygen. Electrolyte imbalance, e.g., hypokalemia/hyperkalemia adversely affects cardiac rhythm/contractility.
Administer antidysrhythmic drugs as indicated.	Dysrhythmias are usually treated symptomatically, except for PVCs, which are often treated prophylactically.
Assist with insertion/maintain pacemaker, when used.	Pacing may be a temporary support measure during acute/healing phase or may be needed permanently if infarction severely damages conduction system.

NURSING DIAGNOSIS:	TISSUE PERFUSION, ALTERED, HIGH RISK FOR
Risk factors may include:	Reduction/interruption of blood flow, e.g., vasoconstriction, hypovolemia/shunting, and thromboembolic formation.
Possibly evidenced by:	[Not applicable; presence of signs and symptoms establishes an actual diagnosis.]
DESIRED OUTCOMES/ EVALUATION CRITERIA— PATIENT WILL:	Demonstrate adequate perfusion as individually appropriate, e.g., skin warm and dry, peripheral pulses present/ strong, vital signs within patient's normal range, patient alert/oriented, balanced intake/output, absence of edema, free of pain/discomfort.

ACTIONS/INTERVENTIONS	RATIONALE
Independent	
Investigate sudden changes or continued alterations in mentation, e.g., anxiety, confusion, lethargy, stupor.	Cerebral perfusion is directly related to cardiac output and is also influenced by electrolyte/acid-base variations, hypoxia, or systemic emboli.
Inspect for pallor, cyanosis, mottling, cool/clammy skin. Note strength of peripheral pulse.	Systemic vasoconstriction resulting from diminished cardiac output may be evidenced by decreased skin perfusion and diminished pulses. (Refer to ND: Cardiac Output, decreased, high risk for, p. 88.)
Assess for Homans' sign (pain in calf on dorsiflexion), erythema, edema.	Indicators of deep vein thrombosis.
Encourage active/passive leg exercises, avoidance of isometric exercises.	Reduces venous stasis, enhancing venous return and decreasing risk of thrombophlebitis. However, isometric exercises can adversely affect cardiac output by increasing myocardial work and oxygen consumption.
Instruct patient in application/periodic removal of antiembolic hose, when used.	Limits venous stasis, improves venous return and reduces risk of thrombophlebitis in patient who is limited in activity.
Monitor respirations, note work of breathing.	Cardiac pump failure may precipitate respiratory distress. However, sudden/continued dyspnea may indicate thromboembolic pulmonary complications.
Assess gastrointestinal function, noting anorexia, decreased/absent bowel sounds, nausea/vomiting, abdominal distention, constipation.	Reduced blood flow to mesentery can produce gastrointestinal dysfunction, e.g., loss of peristalsis. Problems may be potentiated/aggravated by use of analgesics, decreased activity, and dietary changes.
Monitor intake, note changes in urine output. Record specific gravity as indicated.	Decreased intake/persistent nausea may result in reduced circulating volume, which negatively impacts perfusion and organ function. Specific gravity measurements reflect hydration status and renal function.

ACTIONS/INTERVENTIONS

Collaborative

Monitor laboratory data, e.g., ABGs, BUN, creatinine, electrolytes.

Administer medications as indicated, e.g.:

Heparin/warfarin sodium (Coumadin);

Cimetidine (Tagamet); ranitidine (Zantac); antacids.

Prepare for/assist with administration of thrombolytic agents, t-PA, streptokinase; transfer to critical care, and other measures as indicated.

RATIONALE

Indicators of organ perfusion/function.

Low-dose heparin may be given prophylactically in high-risk patients (e.g., atrial fibrillation, obesity, ventricular aneurysm, or history of thrombophlebitis) to reduce risk of thrombophlebitis or mural thrombus formation. Coumadin is the drug of choice for long-term/postdischarge anticoagulant therapy.

Reduces or neutralizes gastric acid, preventing discomfort and gastric irritation, especially in presence of reduced mucosal circulation.

In the event of infarct extension, or new MI, thrombolytic therapy is the treatment of choice (when initiated within 6 hours) to dissolve the clot (if that is the cause of the MI) and restore perfusion of the myocardium.

NURSING DIAGNOSIS:	FLUID VOLUME, EXCESS, HIGH RISK FOR
Risk factors may include:	Decreased organ perfusion (renal). Increased sodium/water retention. Increased hydrostatic pressure or decreased plasma proteins (sequestering of fluid in interstitial space/tissues).
Possibly evidenced by:	[Not applicable; presence of signs and symptoms establishes an actual diagnosis.]
DESIRED OUTCOMES/ EVALUATION CRITERIA— PATIENT WILL:	Maintain fluid balance as evidenced by BP within patient's normal limits. Absence of peripheral/venous distention and dependent edema. Lungs clear and weight stable.

ACTIONS/INTERVENTIONS

Independent

Auscultate breath sounds for presence of crackles.

Note JVD, development of dependent edema.

Measure intake/output, noting decrease in output, concentrated appearance. Calculate fluid balance.

RATIONALE

May indicate pulmonary edema secondary to cardiac decompensation.

Suggests developing congestive failure/fluid volume excess.

Decreased cardiac output results in impaired kidney perfusion, sodium/water retention, and re-

91

ACTIONS/INTERVENTIONS	RATIONALE
Independent	
	duced urine output. Recurrent positive fluid balance in presence of other symptoms suggests volume excess/cardiac failure.
Weigh daily.	Sudden changes in weight reflect alterations in fluid balance.
Maintain total fluid intake at 2000 ml/24 h within cardiovascular tolerance.	Meets normal adult body fluid requirements but may require alteration/restriction in presence of cardiac decompensation.
Collaborative	
Provide low sodium diet/beverages.	Sodium enhances fluid retention and should therefore be restricted.
Administer diuretics, e.g., furosemide (Lasix); hydralazine (Apresoline); spirolactone with hydrochlorothiazide (Aldactazide).	May be necessary to correct fluid overload. Drug choice is usually dependent on acute/chronic nature of symptoms.
Monitor potassium as indicated.	Hypokalemia can limit effectiveness of therapy and can occur with use of potassium-depleting diuretics.

NURSING DIAGNOSIS:	**KNOWLEDGE DEFICIT [LEARNING NEED], REGARDING CONDITION, TREATMENT NEEDS**
May be related to:	Lack of factual information regarding cardiac functioning/implications of heart disease and future health status.
	Need for lifestyle changes.
	Unfamiliarity with postdischarge therapy/self-care needs.
Possibly evidenced by:	Statements of concern/misconceptions, questions.
	Development of preventable complications.
DESIRED OUTCOMES/ EVALUATION CRITERIA— PATIENT WILL:	Verbalize understanding of own heart disease, treatment plan, purpose of medications, and side effects/adverse reactions.
	Relate symptoms that require immediate attention.
	Identify/plan for necessary lifestyle changes.

ACTIONS/INTERVENTIONS	RATIONALE
Independent	
Assess patient/SO level of knowledge and ability/desire to learn.	Necessary for creation of individual instruction plan. Reinforces expectation that this will be a "learning experience." Verbalization identifies misunderstandings and allows for clarification.

ACTIONS/INTERVENTIONS	RATIONALE
Independent	
Be alert to signs of avoidance, e.g., changing subject away from information being presented or extremes of behavior (withdrawal/euphoria).	Natural defense mechanisms such as anger, denial of significance of situation can block learning, affecting patient's response and ability to assimilate information. Changing to a less formal/structured style may be more effective until patient/SO is ready to accept/deal with current situation.
Present information in varied learning formats, e.g., programmed books, audio/visual tapes, question/answer sessions, group activities.	Using multiple learning methods enhances retention of material.
Reinforce explanations of risk factors, dietary/activity restrictions, medications, and symptoms requiring immediate medical attention.	Provides opportunity for patient to retain information and to assume control/participate in rehabilitation program.
Encourage identification/reduction of individual risk factors, e.g., smoking/alcohol consumption, obesity.	These behaviors/chemicals have direct adverse effect on cardiovascular function and may impede recovery, increase risk for complications.
Warn against isometric activity, Valsalva maneuver, and activities requiring arms positioned above head.	These activities greatly increase cardiac work/myocardial oxygen consumption and may adversely affect myocardial contractility/output.
Review programmed increases in levels of activity. Educate patient regarding gradual resumption of activities, e.g., walking, work, recreational and sexual activity. Provide guidelines for gradually increasing activity and instruction regarding target heart rate and pulse taking, as appropriate.	Gradual increase in activity increases strength and prevents overexertion, may enhance collateral circulation, and allows return to normal lifestyle.
Identify alternate activities for "bad weather" days, such as measured walking in house or shopping mall.	Provides for continuing daily activity program.
Review signs/symptoms requiring reduction in activity and notification of health care provider.	Pulse elevations beyond established limits, development of chest pain, or dyspnea may require changes in exercise and medication regimen.
Stress importance of follow-up care and identify community resources/support groups, e.g., cardiac rehabilitation programs, "Coronary Clubs," smoking cessation clinics.	Emphasizes that this is an ongoing/continuing health problem for which support/assistance is available postdischarge.
Emphasize importance of contacting physician if chest pain, change in anginal pattern, or other symptoms recur.	Timely evaluation/intervention may prevent complications.
Stress importance of reporting development of fever in association with diffuse/atypical chest pain (pleural, pericardial) and joint pain.	Post-MI complication of pericardial inflammation (Dressler's syndrome) requires further medical evaluation/intervention.

Dysrhythmias _____

Cardiac dysrhythmias are changes in heart rate and rhythm caused by abnormal electrical conduction or automaticity. Dysrhythmias vary in severity and in their effects on cardiac function, which is partially influenced by the site of origin (ventricular or supraventricular).

RELATED CONCERNS:

Congestive Heart Failure, p 48
Digitalis Toxicity, p 62
Inflammatory Cardiac Conditions, p 126
Myocardial Infarction, p 80
Psychosocial Aspects of Acute Care, p 899

PATIENT ASSESSMENT DATA BASE

ACTIVITY/REST

May report: Weakness, generalized and exertional fatigue.

May exhibit: Changes in heart rate/BP with activity/exercise.

CIRCULATION

May report: History of previous/acute MI (90%–95% experience dysrhythmias), cardiomyopathy, CHF, valvular heart disease, hypertension.

History of pacemaker insertion.

Pulse: Fast, slow, or irregular; palpitations, skipped beats.

May exhibit: BP changes, e.g., hypertension or hypotension during episodes of dysrhythmia.

Pulses: May be irregular, e.g., skipped beats; pulsus alternans (regular strong beat/weak beat); bigeminal pulse (irregular strong beat/weak beat).

Pulse deficit (difference between apical pulse and radial pulse).

Heart sounds: Irregular rhythm, extra sounds, dropped beats.

Skin: Color and moisture changes, e.g., pallor, cyanosis, diaphoresis (heart failure, shock).

Edema: Dependent, generalized, JVD (in presence of heart failure).

Urine output: Decreased if cardiac output is severely diminished.

EGO INTEGRITY

May report: Feeling nervous (certain tachydysrhythmias), sense of impending doom.

Stressors related to current medical problems.

May exhibit: Anxiety, fear, withdrawal, anger, irritability, crying.

FOOD/FLUID

May report: Loss of appetite, anorexia.

Food intolerance (with certain medications).

Nausea/vomiting.

Changes in weight.

May exhibit: Changes in weight.
Edema.

94

Changes in skin moisture/turgor.
Respiratory crackles.

NEUROSENSORY

May report: Dizzy spells, fainting, headaches.

May exhibit: Mental status/sensorium changes, e.g., disorientation, confusion, loss of memory; changes in usual speech pattern/consciousness, stupor, coma.

Behavioral changes, e.g., combativeness, lethargy, hallucinations.

Pupil changes (equality and reaction to light).

Loss of deep tendon reflexes with life-threatening dysrhythmias (ventricular tachycardia, severe bradycardia).

PAIN/DISCOMFORT

May report: Chest pain, mild to severe, which may or may not be relieved by antianginal medication.

May exhibit: Distraction behaviors, e.g., restlessness.

RESPIRATION

May report: Chronic lung disease.

History of or current tobacco use.

Shortness of breath.
Coughing (with/without sputum production).

May exhibit: Changes in respiratory rate/depth during dysrhythmia episode.

Breath sounds: Adventitious sounds (crackles, rhonchi, wheezing) may be present indicating respiratory complications, such as left heart failure (pulmonary edema) or pulmonary thromboembolic phenomena.

Hemoptysis.

SAFETY

May exhibit: Fever.

Skin rashes (medication reaction).

Inflammation, erythema, edema (superficial thrombosis).

Loss of muscle tone/strength.

TEACHING/LEARNING

May report: Familial risk factors, e.g., heart disease, stroke.

Use/misuse of prescribed medications, e.g., heart medications (digitalis); anticoagulants (Coumadin); or OTC medications, e.g., cough syrup and analgesics containing ASA.

Lack of understanding about disease process/therapeutic regimen.

Evidence of failure to improve, e.g., recurrent/intractable dysrhythmias that are life-threatening.

Discharge Plan Considerations: **DRG projected mean length of stay: 3.2 days.**
Alteration of medication use/therapy.

95

DIAGNOSTIC STUDIES:

ECG: Demonstrates patterns of ischemic injury and conduction aberrance. Reveals type/source of dysrhythmia and effects of electrolyte imbalances and cardiac medications.

Holter monitor: Extended ECG tracing (24 hours) may be desired to determine which dysrhythmias may be causing specific symptoms when patient is active (home/work). May also be used to evaluate pacemaker function/antidysrhythmia drug effect.

Chest x-ray: May show enlarged cardiac shadow due to ventricular or valve dysfunction.

Myocardial imaging scans: May demonstrate ischemic/damaged myocardial areas that could impede normal conduction or impair wall motion and pumping capabilities.

Exercise stress test: May be done to demonstrate exercise-induced dysrhythmias.

Electrolytes: Elevated or decreased levels of potassium, calcium, and magnesium can cause dysrhythmias.

Drug screen: May reveal toxicity of cardiac drugs, presence of street drugs, or suggest interaction of drugs, e.g., digitalis, quinidine, and so on.

Thyroid studies: Elevated or depressed serum thyroid levels can cause/aggravate dysrhythmias.

Sedimentation rate: Elevation may indicate acute/active inflammatory process, e.g., endocarditis, as a precipitating factor for dysrhythmias.

ABGs/pulse oximetry: Hypoxemia can cause/exacerbate dysrhythmias.

NURSING PRIORITIES

1. Prevent/treat life-threatening dysrhythmias.
2. Support patient/SO in dealing with anxiety/fear of potentially life-threatening situation.
3. Assist in identification of cause/precipitating factors.
4. Review information regarding condition/prognosis/treatment regimen.

DISCHARGE GOALS

1. Free of life-threatening dysrhythmias and complications of impaired cardiac output/tissue perfusion.
2. Anxiety reduced/managed.
3. Disease process, therapy needs, and prevention of complications understood.

NURSING DIAGNOSIS:	CARDIAC OUTPUT, DECREASED, HIGH RISK FOR
Risk factors may include:	Altered electrical conduction. Reduced myocardial contractility.
Possibly evidenced by:	[Not applicable; presence of signs and symptoms establishes an actual diagnosis.]
DESIRED OUTCOMES/ EVALUATION CRITERIA— PATIENT WILL:	Maintain/achieve adequate cardiac output as evidenced by BP/pulse within normal range, adequate urinary output, palpable pulses of equal quality, usual level of mentation. Display reduced frequency/absence of dysrhythmia(s). Participates in activities that reduce myocardial workload.

ACTIONS/INTERVENTIONS	RATIONALE
Independent	
Palpate pulses (radial, carotid, femoral, dorsalis	Differences in equality, rate, and regularity of

ACTIONS/INTERVENTIONS	RATIONALE

Independent

pedis) noting rate, regularity, amplitude (full/ thready), and symmetry. Document presence of pulsus alternans, bigeminal pulse, or pulse deficit.

pulses are indicative of the effect of altered cardiac output on systemic/peripheral circulation.

Auscultate heart sounds noting rate, rhythm. Note presence of extra heart beats, dropped beats.

Specific dysrhythmias are more clearly detected audibly than by palpation. Hearing extra heart beats or dropped beats helps identify dysrhythmias in the unmonitored patient.

Monitor vital signs and assess adequacy of cardiac output/tissue perfusion. Report significant variations in BP/pulse rate equality, respirations, changes in skin color/temperature, level of consciousness/sensorium, and urine output during episodes of dysrhythmias.

Although not all dysrhythmias are considered life-threatening, immediate treatment to terminate dysrhythmia may be required in the presence of alterations in cardiac output and tissue perfusion.

Determine type of dysrhythmia and document with rhythm strip (if cardiac/telemetry monitoring is available):

Useful in determining need for/type of intervention required.

Tachycardia;

Tachycardia can occur in response to stress, pain, fever, infection, coronary artery blockage, valvular dysfunction, hypovolemia, hypoxia, or as a result of decreased vagal tone or increased sympathetic nervous system activity with the release of catecholamines. Persistent tachycardia may worsen underlying pathology in patients with ischemic heart disease because of shortened diastolic filling time and increased oxygen demands.

Bradycardia;

Bradycardia is common in patients with acute MI (especially inferior) and is the result of excessive parasympathetic activity, blocks in conduction to the SA or AV nodes, or loss of automaticity of the heart muscle. Patients with severe heart disease may not be able to compensate for a slow rate by increasing stroke volume. Therefore, decreased cardiac output, CHF, and potentially lethal ventricular dysrhythmias may occur.

Atrial dysrhythmias;

PACs can occur as a response to ischemia and are normally harmless but can precede or precipitate AF. Acute and chronic atrial flutter and/or fibrillation can occur with coronary artery or valvular disease and may or may not be pathologic. Rapid atrial flutter/fibrillation reduces cardiac output as a result of incomplete ventricular filling (shortened cardiac cycle) and increased oxygen demand.

Ventricular dysrhythmias;

PVCs or VPBs reflect cardiac irritability and are commonly associated with MI, digitalis toxicity, coronary vasospasm, and misplaced temporary pacemaker leads. Frequent, multiple, or multifocal PVCs result in diminished cardiac output and may lead to potentially lethal dysrhythmias, e.g., VT or sudden death/cardiac arrest from ventricular flutter/fibrillation. Note: Intractable ventricular dys-

97

ACTIONS/INTERVENTIONS	RATIONALE
Independent	rhythmias unresponsive to medication may reflect ventricular aneurysm.
Heart blocks.	Reflect altered transmission of impulses through normal conduction channels (slowed, altered) which may be the result of MI, coronary artery disease with reduced blood supply to SA or AV nodes, drug toxicity, and sometimes cardiac surgery. Progressing heart block is associated with slowed ventricular rates, decreased cardiac output, and potentially lethal ventricular dysrhythmias or cardiac standstill.
Provide calm/quiet environment. Review reasons for limitation of activities during acute phase.	Reduces stimulation and release of stress-related catecholamines, which cause/aggravate dysrhythmias and vasoconstriction and increase myocardial workload.
Demonstrate/encourage use of stress management behaviors, e.g., relaxation techniques, guided imagery, slow/deep breathing.	Promotes patient participation in exerting some sense of control in a stressful situation.
Investigate reports of chest pain, documenting location, duration, intensity, and relieving/aggravating factors. Note nonverbal pain cues, e.g., facial grimacing, crying, changes in BP/heart rate.	Reasons for chest pain are variable and depend on underlying cause of dysrhythmias. However, chest pain may indicate ischemia due to decreased myocardial perfusion or increased oxygen need (impending/evolving MI).
Be prepared for/initiate CPR as indicated.	Development of life-threatening dysrythmias requires prompt intervention to prevent ischemic damage/death.
Collaborative	
Monitor laboratory studies, e.g.: Electrolytes;	Imbalance of electrolytes such as potassium, magnesium, and calcium, adversely affects cardiac rhythm and contractility.
Drug levels.	Reveals therapeutic/toxic level of prescription medications or street drugs which may affect/contribute to presence of dysrhythmias.
Administer supplemental oxygen as indicated.	Increases amount of oxygen available for myocardial uptake, which decreases irritability caused by hypoxia.
Administer medications as indicated:	Dysrhythmias are generally treated symptomatically, except for ventricular prematures, which may be treated prophylactically in acute MI.
Potassium;	Correction of hypokalemia may be sufficient to terminate some ventricular dysrhythmias.
Antidysrhythmics:	
Group Ia, e.g.: disopyramide (Norpace); procainamide (Pronestyl); quinidine (Ouinaglute);	These drugs increase action potential, duration, and effective refractory period, and decrease membrane responsiveness. Useful for treatment of atrial and ventricular premature beats, repetitive dysrhythmias (e.g., atrial tachycardias and atrial

ACTIONS/INTERVENTIONS

Collaborative

RATIONALE

flutter/fibrillation). *Note:* Myocardial depressant effects may be potentiated when used in conjunction with any drugs possessing similar properties.

Group Ib, e.g.: lidocaine (Xylocaine); phenytoin (Dilantin); tocainide (Tonocard); mexiletine (Mexitil);

These drugs shorten duration of refractory period, and their action depends on the tissue affected and the level of extracellular potassium. Drugs of choice for ventricular dysrhythmias, they are also effective for automatic and reentrant dysrhythmias and digitalis-induced dysrhythmias. *Note:* These drugs may aggravate myocardial depression.

Group Ic, e.g., encainide (Enkaid); flecainide (Tambocor); propafenone (Rythnol);

These drugs slow conduction by depressing SA node automaticity and decreasing conduction velocity through the atria, ventricles, and Purkinje fibers. They suppress and prevent all types of ventricular dysrhythmias. *Note:* Propafenone can worsen or cause new dysrhythmias, a tendency called the "proarrhythmic effect."

Group II, e.g.: propranolol (Inderal); nadolol (Corgard); acebutolol (Monitan); esmolol (Brevibloc);

β-adrenergic blockers have antiadrenergic properties and decrease automaticity. Therefore, they are useful in the treatment of dysrhythmias occurring because of SA and AV node dysfunction (e.g., supraventricular tachycardias, atrial flutter or fibrillation). *Note:* These drugs may exacerbate bradycardia and cause myocardial depression, especially when combined with drugs with similar properties.

Group III e.g.: bretylium tosylate (Bretylol); amiodarone;

These drugs prolong refractory period and action potential duration. They are used to terminate ventricular fibrillation, especially when lidocaine/pronestyl is not effective.

Group IV e.g.: verapamil (Calan); nifedipine (Procardia); diltiazem (Cardizem);

Calcium antagonists slow conduction time through the AV node to decrease ventricular response in supraventricular tachycardias, atrial flutter/fibrillation.

Others, e.g.: atropine sulfate, isoproterenol (Isuprel); cardiac glycosides: digitalis (Lanoxin).

Useful in treating bradycardia by increasing SA and AV conduction and enhancing automaticity. Cardiac glycosides may be used alone or in combination with other antidysrhythmic drugs to reduce ventricular rate in presence of uncontrolled/poorly tolerated atrial tachycardias or flutter/fibrillation.

Prepare for/assist with elective cardioversion.

May be used in atrial fibrillation or certain unstable dysrhythmias to restore normal heart rate/relieve symptoms of heart failure.

Assist with insertion/maintain pacemaker function.

Temporary pacing may be necessary to accelerate impulse formation or override tachydysrhythmias and ectopic activity in order to maintain cardiovascular function until spontaneous pacing is restored or permanent pacing is initiated.

ACTIONS/INTERVENTIONS	RATIONALE
Collaborative	
Insert/maintain IV access.	Patent access line may be required for administration of emergency drugs.
Prepare for invasive diagnostic procedures/surgery as indicated.	Differential diagnosis of underlying cause may be required to formulate appropriate treatment plan. Resection of ventricular aneurysm may be required to correct intractable ventricular dysrhythmias unresponsive to medical therapy. CABG may be indicated to enhance circulation to myocardium and conduction system.
Prepare for/assist with automatic implantable cardioverter or defibrillator (AICD) when indicated.	This device may be surgically implanted in those patients with recurrent, life-threatening ventricular dysrhythmias despite carefully tailored drug therapy.

NURSING DIAGNOSIS:	KNOWLEDGE DEFICIT [LEARNING NEED], REGARDING CAUSE/TREATMENT OF CONDITION
May be related to:	Lack of information/misunderstanding of medical condition/therapy needs.
	Unfamiliarity with information resources.
	Lack of recall.
Possibly evidenced by:	Questions.
	Statement of misconception.
	Failure to improve on previous regimen.
	Development of preventable complications.
DESIRED OUTCOMES/ EVALUATION CRITERIA— PATIENT WILL:	Verbalize understanding of condition, treatment regimen, and function of pacemaker (if used).
	List desired action and possible adverse side effects of medications.
	Correctly perform necessary procedures and explain reasons for actions.
	Relate signs of pacemaker failure.

ACTIONS/INTERVENTIONS	RATIONALE
Independent	
Review normal cardiac function/electrical conduction.	Provides a knowledge base to understand individual variations and to understand reasons for therapeutic interventions.
Explain/reinforce specific dysrhythmia problem and therapeutic measures to patient/SO.	Ongoing/updated information (e.g., whether or not the problem is resolving or may require long-term

ACTIONS/INTERVENTIONS

Independent

Identify adverse effects/complications of specific dysrhythmias, e.g., fatigue, dependent edema, progressing changes in mentation, vertigo.

Instruct/document teaching regarding medications. Include why the drug is needed (desired action); how and when to take the drug; what to do if a dose is forgotten (dosage and usage information); expected side effects or possible adverse reactions/interactions with other prescribed/OTC drugs or substances (alcohol, tobacco); as well as what and when to report to the physician.

Encourage development of regular exercise routine, avoiding overexertion. Identify signs/symptoms requiring immediate cessation of activities, e.g., dizziness, lightheadedness, dyspnea, chest pain.

Review individual dietary needs/restrictions, e.g., potassium, caffeine.

Provide information in written form for patient/SO to take home.

Instruct patient in proper pulse-taking technique. Encourage daily recording of pulse before medication/during exercise. Identify situations requiring immediate medical intervention.

Review safety precautions, techniques to evaluate/maintain pacemaker or AICD function, and symptoms requiring medical interventions.

Review procedures to terminate PAT e.g., carotid/sinus massage, Valsalva maneuver, if appropriate.

RATIONALE

control measures) can decrease anxiety associated with the unknown and prepare patient/SO to make necessary lifestyle adaptations. Educating the SO may be especially important if the patient is elderly, visually or hearing impaired, or unable or even unwilling to learn/follow instructions. Repeated explanations may be needed, because anxiety and/or bulk of new information can block/limit learning.

Dysrhythmias may decrease cardiac output manifested by symptoms of developing cardiac failure/altered cerebral perfusion. Tachydysrhythmias may also be accompanied by debilitating anxiety/feelings of impending doom.

Information necessary for patient to make informed choices and to manage medication regimen.

When dysrhythmias are properly managed, normal activity should not be affected. Exercise program is useful in improving overall cardiovascular well-being.

Depending on specific problem, patient may need to increase dietary potassium, such as when potassium depleting diuretics are used. Caffeine may be limited to prevent cardiac excitation.

Follow-up reminders may enhance patient's understanding and cooperation with the desired regimen. Written instructions are a helpful resource when patient is not in direct contact with health care team.

Continued self-observation/monitoring provides for timely intervention to avoid complications. Medication regimen may be altered or further evaluation may be required when heart rate varies from desired rate or pacemaker's preset rate.

Promotes self-care, provides for timely interventions to prevent serious complications. Instructions/concerns will be dependent on function and type of device, as well as the patient's condition and presence/absence of family or caregivers.

On occasion, these procedures may be deemed necessary in some patients to restore regular rhythm/cardiac output in emergency situations.

Valvular Heart Disease

Valvular heart disease results from mechanical defects of the heart valves, and whether congenital or acquired, can result in narrowing of the valve opening (stenosis) or incomplete closure of the valve. Either type will impair cardiac output. The main types are aortic stenosis (AS), insufficiency (AI), mitral stenosis (MS), insufficiency (MI); prolapse (MVP); tricuspid stenosis (TS), insufficiency (TI); pulmonic stenosis (PS), insufficiency (PI).

RELATED CONCERNS:

Angina Pectoris, p 70
Cardiac Surgery, p 113
Congestive Heart Failure, p 48
Dysrhythmias, p 94
Inflammatory Cardiac Conditions, p 126
Psychosocial Aspects of Acute Care, p 899

PATIENT ASSESSMENT DATA BASE

ACTIVITY/REST

May report:
Weakness, fatigue.

Dizziness, fainting spells.

Dyspnea on exertion, palpitations.

Sleep disturbance (orthopnea, paroxysmal nocturnal dyspnea, nocturia, night sweats).

May exhibit:
Tachycardia, alterations in BP.

Effort syncope.

Tachypnea, dyspnea.

CIRCULATION

May report:
History of predisposing conditions, e.g., rheumatic fever, subacute bacterial endocarditis, streptococcal infection; hypertension, congenital conditions (e.g., atrial-septal defect, Marfan's syndrome), chest trauma, pulmonary hypertension.

History of heart murmur, palpitations.

Hoarseness, hemoptysis.

Cough, with/without sputum production.

May exhibit:
Systolic BP decreased (late AS).

Pulse pressure: Narrowed (AS); widened (AI).

Carotid pulse: Slow with small pulse volume (AS); bounding, with visible arterial pulsations (AI).

Apical pulse: PMI forceful and displaced downward and to the left (MI); forceful and displaced laterally (AI).

Thrills: Diastolic thrill at apex (MS). Systolic thrill at base (AS). Diastolic thrill along left sternal border; systolic thrill in jugular notch and along carotid arteries (AI).

Heaves: Apical heave during systole (AS).

Heart sounds: Loud S_1, opening snap (MS). Diminished or absent S_1, wide splitting of S_2, development of S_3, S_4 (severe MI). Systolic ejection click (AS). Systolic click, accentuated by standing/squatting (MVP).

Rate: Tachycardia (MVP); resting tachycardia (MS).

Rhythm: Irregular, atrial fibrillation (MS and MI). Dysrhythmias and first degree AV block (AS).

Murmurs: Diastolic murmur in pulmonic area (PI). Low-pitched, rumbling diastolic murmur (MS). Systolic murmur heard best at apex (MR). Systolic murmur heard best at base with radiation to neck (AS). Systolic murmur at lower left sternal border (PS) increasing during inspiration (TI). Diastolic murmurs (blowing), high-pitched and heard best at base (AI). Diastolic murmur at lower left sternal border increasing with inspiration (TS).

JVD: May be present in the presence of right ventricular failure (AI, AS, MI, TI, MS).

Color/cyanosis: Skin warm, damp, and flushed (AI). Capillary beds flush and pale with each pulse (AI).

EGO INTEGRITY

May exhibit: Signs of anxiety, e.g., restlessness, pallor, diaphoresis, trembling, narrowed focus.

FOOD/FLUID

May report: Dysphagia (chronic MI).

Changes in weight.

Use of diuretics.

May exhibit: Generalized or dependent edema.

Hepatomegaly and ascites (MS, MI, TI).

Warm, flushed and damp skin (AI).

Labored, wet, and noisy respirations with audible crackles and wheezes.

NEUROSENSORY

May report: Episodes of dizziness/fainting related to exertion.

PAIN/DISCOMFORT

May report: Chest pain, angina (AS, AI).

Nonanginal/atypical chest pain (MVP).

RESPIRATION

May report: Dyspnea (exertional, orthopnea, paroxysmal, nocturnal). Persistent or nocturnal cough (may/may not be productive of sputum).

May exhibit: Tachypnea.

Adventitious breath sounds (crackles and wheezes).

Frothy, blood-tinged sputum (pulmonary edema).

Restlessness/apprehension (in the presence of pulmonary edema).

SAFETY

May report: Recent infectious process/sepsis, radiation chemotherapy.

Recent dental care (cleaning, fillings, and so on.)

May exhibit: Need for oral/dental care.

TEACHING/LEARNING

May report: Recent/chronic use of IV drugs (illicit).

Discharge Plan Considerations: **DRG projected mean length of stay: 4.9 days.**
Assistance with self-care needs, homemaker/maintenance tasks.
Alteration in medication therapy.
Physical layout of home.

DIAGNOSTIC STUDIES

Radionuclide studies (MUGA): Determines resting and exercise ventricular ejection fractions.

Cardiac catheterization: Provides the following diagnostic information:

MS: Pressure gradient (in diastole) between the left atrium and left ventricle across the mitral valve, decreased valve orifice (1.5 cm), elevated left atrial, pulmonary artery, and right ventricular pressures; low cardiac output.
MI: Back flow of contrast media through the mitral valve during systole, elevated left atrial and pulmonary artery pressures.
AS: Increased pressure gradient in systole across the aortic valve, increased LVEDP.
AI: Back flow of contrast media through the aortic valve during diastole, increased LVEDP.
TS: Increased pressure gradient across valve, increased right atrial pressure, low cardiac output.
TI: Back flow of contrast media through tricuspid valve, elevated right atrial pressure, normal or decreased cardiac output.
PS: Decreased valve orifice, increased right ventricular pressure, decreasd pulmonary artery pressure.
PI: Increased right ventricular pressure, back flow of contrast media through valve.

Left ventriculography: Used to demonstrate mitral cusp prolapse (MVP).

ECG:

MI: Left atrial and ventricular hypertrophy; sinus tachycardia, premature atrial contractions, atrial-fibrillation.
MVP: T-wave abnormalities.
MS: Left atrial enlargement, right ventricular hypertrophy, chronic atrial fibrillation.
AS: Atrial and ventricular arrhythmias; left atrial hypertrophy, right ventricular hypertrophy, right axis deviation; ST/T wave changes, conduction defects (first degree AV block, left bundle branch block).
AI: Left ventricular hypertrophy; atrial fibrillation present if congestive failure is severe.
TS: Right atrial hypertrophy, right or left ventricular hypertrophy; atrial fibrillation.
TI: Right atrial or ventricular hypertrophy, atrial fibrillation.
PS: Right atrial and ventricular hypertrophy, right axis deviation, atrial fibrillation.
PI: Right ventricular and possibly atrial dilation.

Chest x-ray:

MS: Enlarged right ventricle and left atrium, increased vasculature, signs of pulmonary congestion/edema.
MI: Calcification of the mitral annulus, dilation of cardiac chambers; increased vascularity in the upper lung lobe, signs of pulmonary edema.
AS: Aortic and left ventricular dilation/hypertrophy; aortic valve calcification.
AI: Left ventricular enlargement; dilated ascending aorta.
TS: Right atrial enlargement.
TI: Right atrial and ventricular enlargement.
PI: Right ventricular enlargement; dilation of pulmonary artery.

Echocardiograms: Two dimensional and Doppler echocardiography can confirm valvular problems, i.e.:

MS: Left atrial enlargement, altered movement of valve leaflets.
MI: Left atrial enlargement, hyperdynamic left ventricle, prolapse of mitral valve leaflet.
AS: Restricted movement of aortic valve.
AI: Left ventricular dilation, calcification or vegetation on the aortic valve, enlargement of the aortic root of ascending aorta.

MVP: Leaflets bulge posteriorly into left atrium during ventricular systole.
TS: Right atrial dilation, altered movement of tricuspid valve leaflets.
TI: Right atrial dilation, prolapse of tricuspid valve leaflet.

NURSING PRIORITIES

1. Maintain adequate cardiac output.
2. Maintain and/or increase activity tolerance.
3. Relieve/control pain.
4. Provide information about disease process, management, and prevention of complications.

DISCHARGE GOALS

1. Free of signs/symptoms of cardiac decompensation.
2. Meeting self-care needs with improved activity tolerance.
3. Pain/discomfort minimized/controlled.
4. Disease process, management, and prevention of complications understood.

NURSING DIAGNOSIS:	**CARDIAC OUTPUT, DECREASED**
May be related to:	Alteration in preload/increased atrial pressure and venous congestion.
	Alteration in afterload/increased LVEDP and SVR.
	Alteration in electrical conduction, rate/rhythm.
	Left ventricular outflow obstruction.
Possibly evidenced by:	Variations in hemodynamic parameters.
	Dysrhythmias/ECG changes.
	Dyspnea, crackles.
	JVD.
	Cold, clammy skin.
	Cyanosis/pallor of skin and mucous membranes.
	Oliguria/anuria.
	Weak peripheral pulses.
	Fatigue, exhaustion.
DESIRED OUTCOMES/ EVALUATION CRITERIA— PATIENT WILL:	Report/display decreased episodes of dyspnea, chest pain, and dysrhythmias.
	Participate in activities that reduce cardiac workload.
	Demonstrate increased activity tolerance.
	Identify early signs of cardiac decompensation, ways to alter activities and when to seek help.

ACTIONS/INTERVENTIONS	RATIONALE
Independent	
Monitor BP, apical pulse, peripheral pulses.	Clinical indicators of the adequacy of cardiac output. Monitoring enables early detection/treatment of decompensation.
Monitor cardiac rhythm as indicated.	Dysrhythmias are common in patients with valve disease. Atrial dysrhythmias are most common, due to increased atrial pressures and volumes. Conduction abnormalities can also occur, e.g., with aortic valve disease, because of reduced coronary artery perfusion.
Promote/encourage bedrest with head of bed elevated to 45 degrees.	Reduces blood volume returning to the heart (preload), which improves oxygenation, reducing dyspnea and cardiac strain.
Assist with activities as indicated (e.g., walking) when patient is able to be out of bed.	Gradual resumption of activities prevents overtaxing of cardiac reserves.
Discuss/demonstrate techniques of stress management. (Refer to ND: Anxiety, p. 109.)	Reduction of anxiety can reduce sympathetic cardiac stimulation and workload.
Collaborative	
Administer supplemental oxygen as indicated. Monitor ABGs/pulse oximetry.	Provides optimal oxygen for myocardial uptake in an attempt to compensate for increasing oxygen demand.
Administer medications as indicated, e.g., antidysrhythmics; inotropic drugs; vasodilators; diuretics.	Treatment of atrial and ventricular dysrhythmias is specific to underlying condition and symptomatology but is aimed at sustaining/enhancing cardiac efficiency/output. Vasodilators are used to decrease hypertension by reducing systemic vascular resistance (afterload). This reduces regurgitation and outflow resistance. Diuretics decrease circulating volume (preload), which reduces BP across dysfunctional valve, thereby improving cardiac function and reducing venous congestion.
Prepare for surgical intervention as indicated.	Replacement of diseased/compromised valve(s) may be necessary to enhance cardiac output or control/reverse cardiac decompensation.

NURSING DIAGNOSIS:	FLUID VOLUME, EXCESS, HIGH RISK FOR
Risk factors may include:	Altered glomerular filtration.
	Increased fluid and sodium retention.
Possibly evidenced by:	[Not applicable; presence of signs and symptoms establishes an actual diagnosis.]
DESIRED OUTCOMES/ EVALUATION CRITERIA— PATIENT WILL:	Demonstrate balanced intake and output, stable weight, vital signs within normal range, and absence of edema.
	Verbalize understanding of individual dietary/fluid restrictions.

ACTIONS/INTERVENTIONS	RATIONALE

Independent

Monitor intake and output, note fluid balance (positive or negative). Weigh daily.

Important in ongoing assessment of cardiac and kidney function and effectiveness of diuretic therapy. Continued positive fluid balance (intake greater than output) and weight gain reflect worsening cardiac failure.

Auscultate breath and heart sounds.

Adventitious breath sounds (crackles) may indicate the onset of acute pulmonary edema or reflect chronic CHF. An audible S_3 is one of the first clinical findings associated with cardiac decompensation. It may be transient (acute pulmonary congestive failure) or permanent (chronic or advancing heart and organ failure associated with severe valvular disease).

Assess for jugular venous distension/elevation of CVP.

Clinical indicator of right-sided heart failure and systemic congestion present in advanced valvular (2 or 3 valve) disease.

Monitor BP.

Hypertension is a common result of certain valvular disorders, e.g., aortic stenosis. However, increases in BP above patient's usual range may indicate fluid volume excess, especially if it occurs suddenly, along with signs of pulmonary congestion.

Note reports of dyspnea, orthopnea. Evaluate presence/degree of edema (dependent/generalized).

Development/resolution of symptoms reflects status of fluid balance and effectiveness of therapy.

Explain purpose of fluid/sodium restriction to patient/SO. Involve in planning fluid intake schedule/choosing appropriate diet.

May enhance patient cooperation. Provides some sense of control in face of enforced limitations.

Collaborative

Administer diuretics, e.g., furosemide (Lasix), ethacrynic acid (Edecrin) as indicated.

Inhibits reabsorption of sodium/chloride, which enhances fluid excretion, and reduces total body water excess and pulmonary edema.

Monitor serum electrolytes, particularly potassium. Provide potassium-rich diet and potassium supplement, if indicated.

Electrolyte values change in response to diuresis and alterations in oxygenation and metabolism. Hypokalemia predisposes the patient to further cardiac rhythm disturbance.

Administer IV fluids via control device.

Intravenous pump prevents inadvertent excess administration of fluid.

Restrict fluids as indicated (both oral and intravenous).

May be necessary to decrease extracellular fluid volume/edema.

Provide sodium restricted diet as indicated.

Decreases fluid retention.

NURSING DIAGNOSIS:	TISSUE PERFUSION, ALTERED, REGARDING CONDITION, TREATMENT NEEDS
May be related to:	Interruption of arterial-venous flow, e.g., systemic emboli (mitral valve involvement) or venous thrombosis (venous stasis, decreased activity).

107

Possibly evidenced by:	[Not applicable; presence of signs and symptoms establishes an actual diagnosis.]
DESIRED OUTCOMES/ EVALUATION CRITERIA— PATIENT WILL:	Maintain/demonstrate improved tissue perfusion as individually appropriate.

Refer to CP: Inflammatory Cardiac Conditions, ND: Tissue Perfusion, altered, high risk for, p 131.

NURSING DIAGNOSIS:	**PAIN, [ACUTE], HIGH RISK FOR**
Risk factors may include:	Ischemia of myocardial tissues. Stretching of left atrium.
Possibly evidenced by:	[Not applicable; presence of signs and symptoms establishes an actual diagnosis.]
DESIRED OUTCOMES/ EVALUATION CRITERIA— PATIENT WILL:	Report pain is relieved/controlled. Verbalize methods that provide relief.

ACTIONS/INTERVENTIONS	RATIONALE
Independent	
Investigate reports of chest pain and compare with previous episodes. Use pain scale (0–10) for rating intensity. Note verbal/nonverbal expressions of pain, autonomic response to pain (diaphoresis, BP and pulse changes, increased or decreased respiratory rate).	Differentiation of symptoms is necessary to identify causes of pain. Behaviors and changes in vital signs help determine the degree/presence of discomfort the patient is experiencing, especially when patient denies presence of pain.
Evaluate response to medication.	Useful in establishing drug therapy and dosage. *Note:* Pain that is unrelieved or increased with nitrates may indicate MVP, which is associated with atypical/ nonanginal chest pain.
Provide restful environment and limit activity as needed.	Activities which increase myocardial oxygen demands (e.g., sudden exertion, stress, heavy meals, cold exposure) may precipitate chest pain.
Instruct patient in appropriate response to angina (e.g., stopping angina-producing activity, resting, and taking appropriate antianginal medication).	Ceasing activity reduces oxygen demands and cardiac workload and often stops angina.
Collaborative	
Administer vasodilators, e.g., nitroglycerin, nifedipine, (Procardia), as indicated.	Medications given to enhance myocardial circulation (vasodilation) reduce angina associated with ischemic myocardium.

108

NURSING DIAGNOSIS:	ACTIVITY INTOLERANCE
May be related to:	Imbalance between oxygen supply and demand (decreased/fixed cardiac output).
Possibly evidenced by:	Verbal report of fatigue or weakness.
	Abnormal heart rate or BP in response to activity.
	Exertional discomfort or dyspnea.
DESIRED OUTCOMES/ EVALUATION CRITERIA— PATIENT WILL:	Demonstrate a measurable increase in activity tolerance.
	Identify factors that influence activity tolerance and reduce those with a negative effect.

ACTIONS/INTERVENTIONS	RATIONALE
Independent	
Assess patient's tolerance to activity using the following parameters: pulse rate >20 bpm above resting rate; marked increase in BP, dyspnea, or chest pain; excessive fatigue and weakness; diaphoresis; dizziness; or syncope.	The stated parameters reflect the patient's physiologic response to the stress of activity and are indicators of the degree of overexertion/cardiac compromise.
Assess readiness for increased activity, e.g., reduction in fatigue/weakness, stable BP/pulse rate, increased interest in activities and self-care.	Physiologic stability at rest is essential prior to progressing the individual's activity level.
Encourage progression in activity/self-care as tolerated.	Myocardial oxygen consumption during various activities may exceed the amount of oxygen available. Gradual activity progression prevents a sudden increase in cardiac workload.
Provide assistance as needed and suggest use of shower chair, sitting to brush teeth/hair, and so on.	Energy-saving techniques reduce the energy expenditure and thereby assist in equalizing oxygen supply and demand.
Encourage patient to participate in alternating rest periods with activity.	Such scheduling increases tolerance to activity progression and prevents fatigue.

NURSING DIAGNOSIS:	ANXIETY [SPECIFY LEVEL]
May be related to:	Threat to/change in health status (chronicity of disease).
	Physiologic effects.
	Situational crisis (hospitalization/absence from family).
Possibly evidenced by:	Sympathetic stimulation, cardiovascular excitation, restlessness, insomnia.
	Increased tension, apprehension.
	Increased helplessness.

DESIRED OUTCOMES/ EVALUATION CRITERIA— PATIENT WILL:	Uncertainty. Fear of unspecified consequences. Focus on self. Expressed concerns regarding changes in life events. Verbalize awareness of feelings of anxiety. Report anxiety reduced/controlled. Appear relaxed. Demonstrate behaviors to manage stress.

ACTIONS/INTERVENTIONS	RATIONALE
Independent	
Identify/evaluate patient's perception of the threat represented by the situation.	Aids in defining the scope of the problem and choice of interventions.
Monitor physical responses, e.g., palpitations, tachycardia, repetitive movements, restlessness.	Helpful in determining degree of anxiety as well as cardiac status. Useful in evaluating congruency of verbal and nonverbal responses.
Provide comfort measures (e.g., shower/ bath, back rub, position change).	Helps to redirect attention and promotes relaxation, enhancing coping abilities.
Coordinate time for rest and diversional activities appropriate for condition.	Provides a sense of control for patient to manage some aspects of treatment (e.g., care activities, private time). Reduces fatigue, enhances energy level.
Encourage ventilation of feelings about disease— its effect on lifestyle and future health status. Assess the effectiveness of coping with stressors.	Adaptive mechanisms are necessary to cope with the chronicity of valvular heart disease and to appropriately alter one's lifestyle, integrating prescribed therapies into daily living.
Include patient/SO in planning care and encourage maximum participation in treatment plan.	Involvement will help focus patient's attention in a positive manner and provide a sense of control.
Instruct patient in relaxation techniques, e.g., deep breathing, guided imagery, progressive relaxation.	Provides a means of altering response to anxiety, refocuses attention, promotes relaxation enhancing coping abilities.

NURSING DIAGNOSIS:	KNOWLEDGE DEFICIT [LEARNING NEED], REGARDING CONDITION, TREATMENT NEEDS
May be related to:	Lack of exposure to information about valvular heart disease. Misconceptions/misinterpretation of information.
Possibly evidenced by:	Request for information. Statement of concerns.

DESIRED OUTCOMES/ EVALUATION CRITERIA— PATIENT WILL:	Inappropriate or exaggerated behaviors, e.g., excessive anxiety, agitation (particularly in MVP). Inaccurate follow-through of instruction. Verbalize understanding of disease process, treatment regimen, and potential complications. Identify behaviors/lifestyle changes to prevent complications. Recognize need for cooperation and follow-up care.

ACTIONS/INTERVENTIONS	RATIONALE
Independent	
Explain basic pathophysiology of valve abnormality.	The patient should have a basic understanding of own valve abnormality and the hemodynamic consequences of the defect as a basis for explaining rationale for various aspects of treatment.
Explain medication rationale, dosage, side effects, and importance of taking as prescribed, e.g., diuretics, antidysrhythmics, inotropic agents, vasodilators.	May enhance cooperation with drug therapy and prevent unauthorized discontinuation of medication and/or adverse drug interactions.
Instruct the patient taking a diuretic to take daily dose (or larger dose) in the morning.	Scheduling minimizes nighttime urination/interruption of sleep.
Recommend monitoring own weight and maintaining a record. Encourage reporting weight gain of 2 lb in 1 day or 5 lb in 1 week; swelling of ankles, feet, or abdomen; weight loss of > 5 lb in 1 week.	Weight is a primary indicator of the effectiveness of diuretic therapy and should be measured on a regular basis for monitoring trends.
Stress importance of reporting excessive thirst, severe dizziness, or episodes of fainting.	May indicate a need to evaluate electrolyte status (specifically potassium) and/or alter medication regimen.
Instruct and have patient demonstrate skill in self-monitoring of pulse if the patient is discharged on digitalis.	Any change in pulse rate (typically below 60 bpm in adults) and rhythm (onset of irregularity) may be an indication of digitalis toxicity and should be reported to the physician for evaluation.
Discuss safety precautions which will minimize orthostatic hypotension if the patient is discharged on vasodilators, e.g., rise slowly from a lying to standing position and sit for a few minutes before standing; avoid prolonged standing; wear support stockings when up and around; avoid hot baths, steam rooms, and saunas.	Measures help to minimize untoward side effects of vasodilation and enhance postural adjustments in BP (may prevent syncope/falls).
Explain rationale for the prescribed dietary regimen (usually a diet low in sodium).	Increased sodium results in water retention and increased cardiac workload.
Discuss with patient need to balance activity and rest. Explain importance of consistency in activity/exercise.	A consistent, appropriately paced activity program is best to minimize deconditioning and fatigue while preventing overexertion, which can increase cardiac workload/decompensation.

ACTIONS/INTERVENTIONS	RATIONALE

Independent

Provide instructions on appropriate activity regimen: regular low intensity exercise, e.g., walking program (stable/asymptomatic patients); self-care activities, active or assisted range-of-motion, and energy saving techniques (symptomatic patients).	Activity regimen needs to be individualized, as some patients tolerate only range-of-motion exercises while others participate in more active programs.
Instruct patient to (1) monitor own physiologic response to activity, e.g., pulse rate, shortness of breath; (2) stop activity that causes chest pain, shortness of breath, dizziness, or extreme fatigue or weakness; (3) report decreased tolerance to activity.	The patient's involvement in monitoring own activity tolerance is vital to safely resuming and/or modifying activities of daily living.
Stress importance of informing health care provider of effort syncope or chest pain.	These are indicative of intolerance to activity, which is related to inadequate cardiac output/worsening valve dysfunction.
Provide information concerning significance of endocarditis.	Patients with valvular heart disease are at risk for endocarditis (due to the adherence of infected vegetations on cardiac structures), which can lead to further valvular scarring, retraction of leaflets, and loss of function requiring surgical intervention.
Instruct the patient requiring antithrombotic therapy in the purpose, dosage, and side effects of the medication prescribed, e.g., warfarin (Coumadin); dipyridamole (Persantine); and ASA.	The patient with an enlarged left atrium, chronic atrial fibrillation, and certain prosthetic valves is at increased risk for embolization, and therefore may be discharged on anticoagulant medications.
Reinforce the importance of taking the anticoagulant according to physician instructions and routinely reporting to laboratory for prothrombin times.	Drugs need to be taken at the same time every day to maintain therapeutic level. The therapeutic range for Coumadin is based on patient prothrombin time.
Identify the most common signs of early bleeding, e.g., develops bruises without trauma. Stress importance of reporting bleeding to health care provider.	Prompt evaluation and intervention may prevent more serious complications.
Instruct patient to avoid OTC medications, use electric shaver rather than blade razors, floss and brush teeth gently, cut nails carefully, and avoid straining at stool.	Anticoagulant action is affected by many OTC products. Attention to safety measures will help minimize the risk of traumatic bleeding.
Stress importance of maintaining a minimum fluid intake of 2500 ml/d (unless contraindicated).	This will help to prevent increased blood viscosity, which leads to hypercoagulability and potentiates thrombus formation.
Review necessary dietary modification.	Alcohol and foods high in vitamin K alter the prothrombin time and should be avoided.
Encourage patient to wear an identification bracelet/tag.	Alerts emergency personnel that patient is taking anticoagulants.
Identify/refer to community resources and support group.	Chronic nature of condition may affect ability to meet self-care needs/home maintenance management, increasing risk of social isolation/depression.

Cardiac Surgery: Coronary Artery Bypass Graft; Valve Replacement [Postoperative Care]

The goal of treatment for heart disease is to maximize cardic output. Surgically, this may be done by improving myocardial muscle function and blood flow through coronary artery bypass grafting and/or replacement of defective valves.

RELATED CONCERNS:

Angina Pectoris, p 70
Congestive Heart Failure, p 48
Dysrhythmias, p 94
Hemothorax/Pneumothorax, p 195
Myocardial Infarction, p 80
Psychosocial Aspects of Acute Care, p 899
Pulmonary Embolism, p 174
Surgical Intervention, p 918
Valvular Heart Disease, p 102

PATIENT ASSESSMENT DATA BASE

The preoperative data presented here are dependent on the specific disease process and underlying cardiac condition/reserve.

ACTIVITY/REST

May report:
History of exercise intolerance.

Generalized weakness, fatigue.

Inability to perform expected/usual life activities.

May exhibit:
Abnormal heart rate, BP changes with activity.

Exertional discomfort or dyspnea.

ECG changes/dysrhythmias.

CIRCULATION

May report:
History of recent/acute MI, three (or more) vessel coronary artery disease, valvular heart disease, hypertension.

May exhibit:
Variations in BP, heart rate/rhythm.

Dysrhythmias/ECG changes.

Abnormal heart sounds: S_3/S_4 murmurs.

Pallor/cyanosis of skin or mucous membranes.

Cool/cold, clammy skin.

Edema, JVD.

Diminished peripheral pulses.

Crackles.

Restlessness/other changes in mentation or sensorium (severe cardiac decompensation).

EGO INTEGRITY

May report:
Feeling scared/apprehensive, helpless.

Distress over current events (anger/fear).
Fear of death/eventual outcome of surgery, possible complications.
Fear about changes in lifestyle/role functioning.

May exhibit: Apprehension.
Restlessness.
Insomnia/sleep disturbance.
Facial/general tension.
Withdrawal/lack of eye contact.
Crying.
Focus on self, hostility, anger.
Changes in heart rate, BP, breathing patterns.

FOOD/FLUID

May report: Change in weight.
Loss of appetite.
Abdominal pain, nausea/vomiting.
Change in urine frequency/amount.

May exhibit: Weight gain/loss.
Dry skin, poor skin turgor.
Postural hypotension.
Diminished/absent bowel sounds.
Edema (generalized, dependent, pitting).

NEUROSENSORY

May report: Fainting spells, vertigo.

May exhibit: Changes in orientation or usual response to stimuli.
Restlessness.
Irritability.
Apathy.
Exaggerated emotional responses.

PAIN/COMFORT

May report: Chest pain, angina.
Postoperative:
Incisional discomfort.
Pain/paresthesia of shoulders, arms, hands, legs.

May exhibit: *Postoperative:*
Guarding.
Facial mask of pain.
Grimacing.
Distraction behaviors.
Moaning.
Restlessness.
Changes in BP/pulse/respiratory rate.

RESPIRATION

May report: Shortness of breath.

Postoperative:

Inability to cough or take a deep breath.

May exhibit: *Postoperative:*

Decreased chest expansion.

Splinting/muscle guarding.

Dyspnea (normal response to thoracotomy).

Areas of diminished or absent breath sounds (atelectasis).

Anxiety.

Changes in ABGs/pulse oximetry.

SAFETY

May report: Infectious episode with valvular involvement.

May exhibit: *Postoperative:* Oozing/bleeding from chest or donor site incisions.

TEACHING/LEARNING

May report: Familial risk factors of diabetes, heart disease, hypertension, strokes.

Use of various cardiovascular drugs.

Failure to improve.

Discharge Plan Considerations: **DRG projected mean length of stay: 11.2 days.**

Assistance with food preparation, shopping, transportation, self-care needs and homemaker/home maintenance tasks.

DIAGNOSTIC STUDIES (POSTOPERATIVE)

Hemoglobin/hematocrit: Decreased Hb reduces oxygen-carrying capacity and indicates need for red blood cell replacement. Elevation of Hct suggests dehydration/need for fluid replacement.

Coagulation studies: Various studies may be done (e.g., platelet count, bleeding and clotting time) to determine possible problems before surgery.

Electrolytes: Imbalances (hyperkalemia/hypokalemia, hypernatremia/hyponatremia, and hypocalcemia) can affect cardiac function and fluid balance.

ABGs: Identifies oxygenation status/effectiveness of respiratory function and acid/base balance.

Pulse oximetry: Noninvasive measure of oxygenation at tissue level.

BUN/creatinine: Reflects adequacy of renal and liver perfusion/function.

Amylase: Elevation is occasionally seen in high-risk patients, e.g., those with heart failure undergoing valve replacement.

Glucose: Fluctuations may occur due to preoperative nutritional status, presence of diabetes/organ dysfunction rate of dextrose infusions.

Cardiac enzymes/isoenzymes: Elevated in the presence of acute, recent, or perioperative MI.

Chest x-ray: Reveals heart size and position, pulmonary vasculature, and changes indicative of pulmonary complications (e.g., atelectasis). Verifies condition of valve prosthesis and sternal wires, position of pacing leads, intravascular/cardiac lines.

ECG: Identifies changes in electrical/mechanical function such as might occur in immediate postoperative phase, acute/perioperative MI, valve dysfunction, and/or pericarditis.

Cardiac angiography: Abnormal chamber pressures and pressure gradients across valves are present with

115

valve disease. Findings in coronary artery disease include occlusions of arteries, impaired coronary perfusion, and possible wall-motion abnormalities.

Nuclear studies: (e.g., thallium 201, DPY-thallium/Persantine).Heart scans demonstrate coronary artery disease, heart chamber dimensions, and presurgical/postsurgical functional capabilities.

NURSING PRIORITIES

1. Support hemodynamic stability/ventilatory function.
2. Promote relief of pain/discomfort.
3. Promote healing.
4. Provide information about postoperative expectations and treatment regimen.

DISCHARGE GOALS

1. Activity tolerance adequate to meet self-care needs.
2. Pain alleviated/managed.
3. Complications prevented/minimized.
4. Incisions healing.
5. Postdischarge medications, exercise, diet, therapy understood.

NURSING DIAGNOSIS:	CARDIAC OUTPUT, DECREASED, HIGH RISK FOR
Risk factors may include:	Decreased myocardial contractility secondary to temporary factors (e.g., ventricular wall surgery, recent MI, response to certain medications/drug interactions).
	Decreased preload (hypovolemia).
	Alterations in electrical conduction (dysrhythmias).
Possibly evidenced by:	[Not applicable; presence of signs and symptoms establishes an actual diagnosis.]
DESIRED OUTCOMES/ EVALUATION CRITERIA— PATIENT WILL:	Report/display decreased episodes of angina and dysrhythmias.
	Demonstrate an increase in activity tolerance.
	Participate in activities that maximize/enhance cardiac function.

ACTIONS/INTERVENTIONS	RATIONALE
Independent	
Monitor/document trends in heart rate and BP, especially noting hypertension. Be aware of specific systolic/diastolic limits defined for patient.	Tachycardia is a common response to discomfort and anxiety, inadequate blood/fluid replacement, and the stress of surgery. However, sustained tachycardia increases cardiac workload and can decrease effective cardiac output. Hypertension can occur (fluid excess or preexisting condition) placing stress on suture lines of new grafts and

ACTIONS/INTERVENTIONS	RATIONALE
Independent	
	changing blood flow/pressure within heart chambers and across valves, with increased risk for various complications. Hypotension may result from fluid deficit, dysrhythmias, heart failure/shock.
Monitor/document cardiac dysrhythmias. Observe patient response to dysrhythmias, e.g., drop in BP.	Life-threatening dysrhythmias can occur due to electrolyte imbalance, myocardial ischemia, or alterations in the heart's electrical conduction. Decreased cardiac output and hemodynamic compromise occurring with dysrhythmias require prompt intervention.
Observe for changes in usual mental status/orientation/body movement or reflexes, e.g., onset of confusion, disorientation, restlessness, reduced response to stimuli, stupor.	May indicate decreased cerebral blood flow or oxygenation as a result of diminished cardiac output (sustained or severe dysrhythmias, low BP, heart failure, or thromboembolic phenomena).
Record skin temperature/color, and quality/equality of peripheral pulses.	Warm, pink skin and strong, equal pulses are general indicators of adequate cardiac output.
Measure/document intake, output, and fluid balance.	Useful in determining fluid needs or identifying fluid excesses which can compromise cardiac output/oxygen consumption.
Schedule uninterrupted rest/sleep periods. Assist with self-care activities.	Prevents fatigue/overexhaustion and excessive cardiovascular stress.
Monitor graded activity program. Note patient response, vital signs before/during/after activity, development of dysrhythmias.	Regular exercise stimulates circulation/cardiovascular tone and promotes feeling of well-being. Progression of activity is dependent on cardiac tolerance.
Evaluate presence/degree of anxiety/emotional duress. Encourage the use of relaxation techniques, e.g., deep breathing, diversional activities.	Excessive/escalating emotional reactions can affect vital signs and systemic vascular resistance, eventually affecting cardiac function.
Inspect for JVD, peripheral or dependent edema, congestion in lungs, shortness of breath, change in mental status.	May be indicative of heart failure (acute or chronic).
Investigate complaints of angina/severe chest pain, accompanied by restlessness, diaphoresis, ECG changes.	Although not a common complication of CABG, perioperative or postoperative MI can occur.
Investigate/report profound hypotension (unresponsive to fluid challenge), tachycardia, distant heart sounds, stupor/coma.	Development of cardiac tamponade can rapidly progress to cardiac arrest due to inability of the heart to fill adequately for effective cardiac output. Note: This is a relatively rare life-threatening complication that usually occurs in the immediate postoperative period but can occur later in the recovery phase.
Review serial ECGs.	Most frequently done to follow the progress in normalization of electrical conduction patterns/ventricular function after surgery or to identify complications, e.g., perioperative MI.

117

ACTIONS/INTERVENTIONS	RATIONALE
Independent	
Administer IV fluids/blood transfusions as indicated.	IV fluids may be discontinued prior to discharge from the intensive care unit, or one line (central/peripheral) may remain in place for fluid replacement and/or emergency cardiac medications. Red blood cell replacement may be indicated on occasion to restore/maintain adequate circulating volume and enhance oxygen-carrying capacity.
Administer supplemental oxygen as indicated.	Promotes maximal oxygenation, which can reduce cardiac workload, aid in resolving myocardial ischemia and dysrhythmias.
Administer electrolytes and medications as indicated, e.g., electrolyte solutions/potassium, antidysrhythmics, β-blockers, digitalis, diuretics, anticoagulants.	Patient needs are variable, depending on type of surgery (CABG or valve replacement), response to surgical intervention, and preexisting conditions (e.g., general health, age, type of heart disease). Electrolytes, antidysrhythmics, and other heart medications may be required on a short-term or long-term basis to maximize cardiac contractility/output.
Maintain surgically placed pacing wires (atrial/ventricular), and initiate pacing if indicated.	May be required to support cardiac output in presence of conduction disturbances (severe dysrhythmias) which compromise cardiac function.

NURSING DIAGNOSIS:	PAIN [ACUTE], [DISCOMFORT]
May be related to:	Sternotomy (mediastinal incision) and/or donor site (leg/arm incision).
	Myocardial ischemia (acute MI, angina).
	Tissue inflammation/edema formation.
	Intraoperative nerve trauma.
Possibly evidenced by:	Reports of incisional discomfort/pain, paresthesia, pain in hand, arm, shoulder.
	Anxiety, restlessness, irritability.
	Distraction behaviors.
	Increased heart rate.
DESIRED OUTCOMES/ EVALUATION CRITERIA— PATIENT WILL:	Verbalize relief/absence of pain.
	Demonstrate relaxed body posture, ability to rest/sleep appropriately.
	Differentiate surgical discomfort from angina/preoperative heart pain.

ACTIONS/INTERVENTIONS	RATIONALE
Independent	
Encourage patient to report type, location, and intensity of pain, rating on a scale of 0–10. Ask the patient how this compares with preoperative chest pain.	Pain is perceived, manifested, and tolerated individually. It is important for the patient to differentiate incisional pain from other types of chest pain, e.g., angina. Many CABG patients do not experience severe discomfort in chest incision and may complain more often of donor site incision discomfort. Severe pain in either area should be investigated further for possible complications.
Observe for anxiety, irritability, crying, restlessness, sleep disturbances.	These nonverbal cues may indicate the presence/degree of pain being experienced.
Monitor vital signs.	Heart rate usually increases with pain, although a bradycardiac response can occur in a severely diseased heart. BP may be elevated slightly with incisional discomfort but may be decreased or unstable if chest pain is severe and/or myocardial damage is occurring.
Identify/promote position of comfort using adjuncts as necessary.	Pillows/blanket rolls are useful in supporting extremities, maintaining body alignment, and splinting incisions to reduce muscle tension/promote comfort.
Provide comfort measures (e.g., back rubs, position changes), assist with self-care activities and encourage diversional activities as indicated.	May promote relaxation/redirect attention and reduce analgesic dosage needs/frequency.
Schedule care activities to balance with adequate periods of sleep/rest.	Rest and sleep are vital for cardiac healing (balance between oxygen demand and consumption), and can enhance coping with stress and discomfort.
Identify/encourage use of behaviors such as guided imagery, distractions, visualizations, deep breathing.	Relaxation techniques aid in management of stress, promote sense of well-being, may reduce analgesic needs, and promote healing.
Tell patient that it is acceptable, even preferable, to request analgesics as soon as discomfort becomes noticeable.	Presence of pain causes muscle tension, which can impair circulation, slow healing process, and intensify pain.
Medicate prior to procedures/activities as indicated.	Patient comfort and cooperation in respiratory treatments, ambulation, and procedures (e.g., removal of chest tubes, pacemaker wires and suture removal) are facilitated by prior analgesic administration.
Investigate reports of pain in unusual areas (e.g., calves of legs, abdomen) or vague complaints of discomfort, especially when accompanied by changes in mentation, vital signs, respiratory rate.	May be an early manifestation of developing complication, e.g., thrombophlebitis, infection, gastrointestinal dysfunction.
Note reports of pain and/or numbness in ulnar area (fourth and fifth digits) of the hand often accompanied by pain/discomfort of the arms and shoulders. Tell the patient that the problem usually resolves with time.	Indicative of a stretch injury of the brachial plexus as a result of the position of the arms during surgery. No specific treatment is currently useful.

119

ACTIONS/INTERVENTIONS

Collaborative

Administer medications as indicated, e.g., propoxyphene and acetaminophen (Darvocet-N), acetaminophen and oxycodone (Tylox).

RATIONALE

Usually provides for adequate control of pain and reduces muscle tension, which improves patient comfort and promotes healing.

NURSING DIAGNOSIS:	ROLE PERFORMANCE, ALTERED
May be related to:	Situational crisis (dependent role)/recuperative process.
	Uncertainty about future.
Possibly evidenced by:	Delay/alteration in physical capacity to resume role.
	Change in usual role or responsibility.
	Change in self/others' perception of role.
DESIRED OUTCOMES/ EVALUATION CRITERIA— PATIENT WILL:	Verbalize realistic perception and acceptance of self in changed role.
	Talk with SO about situation and changes that have occurred.
	Develop realistic plans for adapting to perceived role changes.

ACTIONS/INTERVENTIONS

Independent

Assess patient role in family constellation. Identify concerns about role dysfunction/interruption, e.g., recuperation, health-illness transitions.

Assess level of anxiety, patient's perception of degree of threat to self/life.

Note cultural factors affecting role changes.

Maintain positive attitude toward the patient, providing opportunities for the patient to exercise control as much as possible.

Assist patient/SO to develop strategies for dealing with changes, e.g., shift responsibilities to other family members/friends or neighbors; acquire temporary assistance (homemaker/yardwork); investigate avenues for financial assistance.

Acknowledge reality of grieving process related to role change and help patient to deal realistically with feelings of anger and sadness.

RATIONALE

Helps to know patient responsibilities and how illness affects this role. Dependent role of the patient provokes anxiety and concern about how the patient will be able to manage usual role responsibilities.

Information provides baseline for identifying/individualizing plan of care.

Cultural expectations regarding male/female illness role can determine how patient/SO react to and deal with current situation and may affect future adaptation to perceived changes.

Helps patient to accept changes that are occurring and to begin to realize that control over self is possible.

Planning for changes that may occur/be required promotes sense of control and accomplishment without loss of self-esteem.

Cardiac surgery constitutes a dramatic point in the patient's life, and it will never be the same again. Patient needs to recognize these feelings in order to deal with them and move forward.

NURSING DIAGNOSIS:	BREATHING PATTERN, INEFFECTIVE, HIGH RISK FOR
Risk factors may include:	Inadequate ventilation (pain/muscular weakness). Diminished oxygen-carrying capacity (blood loss).
	Decreased lung expansion (atelectasis or pneumothorax/hemothorax).
Possibly evidenced by:	[Not applicable; presence of signs and symptoms establishes an actual diagnosis.]
DESIRED OUTCOMES/ EVALUATION CRITERIA— PATIENT WILL:	Maintain a normal/effective respiratory pattern free of cyanosis and other signs/symptoms of hypoxia with breath sounds equal bilaterally, lung fields clearing.
	Display complete reexpansion of lungs with absence of pneumothorax/hemothorax.

ACTIONS/INTERVENTIONS	RATIONALE

Independent

Evaluate respiratory rate and depth. Note respiratory effort, e.g., presence of dyspnea, use of accessory muscles, nasal flaring.	Patient responses are variable. Rate and effort may be increased by pain, fear, fever, diminished circulating volume (blood or fluid loss), accumulation of secretions, hypoxia, or gastric distention. Respiratory suppression (decreased rate) can occur from excessive use of narcotic analgesics. Early recognition and treatment of abnormal ventilation may prevent complications.
Auscultate breath sounds. Note areas of diminished/absent breath sounds and presence of adventitious sounds, e.g., crackles or rhonchi.	Breath sounds are often diminished in lung bases for a period of time following surgery due to normally occurring atelectasis. Loss of active breath sounds in an area of previous ventilation may reflect collapse of the lung segment, especially if chest tubes have recently been removed. Crackles or rhonchi may be indicative of fluid accumulation (interstitial edema, pulmonary edema, or infection) or partial airway obstruction (pooling of secretions).
Observe chest excursion. Investigate decreased expansion or lack of symmetry in chest movement.	Air or fluid in the pleural space prevents complete expansion (usually on one side) and requires further assessment of ventilation status.
Observe character of cough and sputum production.	Frequent coughing may simply be throat irritation from operative ET tube placement or can reflect pulmonary congestion. Purulent sputum suggests onset of pulmonary infection.
Inspect skin and mucous membranes for cyanosis.	Cyanosis of lips, nailbeds, or earlobes or general duskiness may indicate a hypoxic condition due to heart failure or pulmonary complications. General pallor (commonly present in immediate postoperative period) may indicate anemia from blood loss/insufficient blood replacement or red blood cell destruction from cardiopulmonary bypass pump.

121

ACTIONS/INTERVENTIONS	RATIONALE
Independent	
Elevate head of bed, place in upright or semi-Fowler's position. Assist with early ambulation/increased time out of bed.	Stimulates respiratory function/lung expansion. Effective in preventing and resolving pulmonary congestion.
Encourage patient participation/responsibility for deep-breathing exercises, use of adjuncts (blow bottles), and coughing, as indicated.	Aids in reexpansion/maintaining patency of small airways especially after removal of chest tubes. Coughing is not necessary unless wheezes/rhonchi are present, indicating retention of secretions.
Reinforce splinting of chest with pillows during deep breathing/coughing.	Reduces incisional tension, promotes maximal lung expansion, and may enhance effectiveness of cough effort.
Explain that coughing/respiratory treatments will not loosen/damage grafts or reopen chest incision.	Provides reassurance that injury will not occur and may enhance cooperation with therapeutic regimen.
Encourage maximal fluid intake within cardiac reserves.	Adequate hydration helps liquefy secretions, facilitating expectoration.
Medicate with analgesic before respiratory treatments, as indicated.	Allows for easier chest movement and reduces discomfort related to incisional pain, facilitating patient cooperation with/effectiveness of respiratory treatments.
Record response to deep-breathing exercises or other respiratory treatment noting breath sounds (before/after treatment), cough/sputum production.	Documents effectiveness of therapy or need for more aggressive interventions.
Investigate/report respiratory distress, diminished/absent breath sounds, tachycardia, severe agitation, drop in BP.	Although not a common complication, hemothorax/pneumothorax may occur following removal of the chest tubes and requires prompt intervention to maintain respiratory function.
Collaborative	
Review chest x-ray reports and laboratory studies (ABGs, hemoglobin) as indicated.	Monitors effectiveness of respiratory therapy and/or documents developing complications. A blood transfusion may be needed if blood loss is the reason for respiratory hypoxemia.
Assist with use of incentive spirometer/blow bottles.	Used to maximize lung inflation, reduce atelectasis, and prevent pulmonary complications.
Administer supplemental oxygen by cannula or mask, as indicated.	Enhances oxygen delivery to the lungs for circulatory uptake, especially in presence of reduced/altered ventilation.
Assist with reinsertion of chest tubes or thoracentesis if indicated.	Reexpands lung by removal of accumulated blood/air and restoration of negative pleural pressure.

NURSING DIAGNOSIS:	**SKIN INTEGRITY, IMPAIRED, ACTUAL**
May be related to:	Surgical incisions, puncture wounds.

Possibly evidenced by:	Disruption of skin surface.
DESIRED OUTCOMES/ EVALUATION CRITERIA— PATIENT WILL:	Demonstrate behaviors/techniques to promote healing, prevent complications.
	Display timely wound healing.

ACTIONS/INTERVENTIONS	RATIONALE
Independent	
Inspect all incisions. Evaluate healing progress. Review expectations for healing with patient.	Healing begins immediately, but complete healing will take time. Chest incision heals first (minimal muscle tissue), but donor site incision (leg) will require more time (more muscle tissue, longer incision, slower circulation). As healing progresses, the incision lines may appear dry with crusty scabs. Underlying tissue may look bruised and feel tense, warm, and lumpy (resolving hematoma).
Suggest wearing soft cotton shirts and loose fitting clothing, cover/pad incisions as indicated, leave incisions open to air as much as possible.	Reduces suture line irritation and pressure from clothing. Leaving incisions open to air promotes healing process and may reduce risk of infection.
Have patient shower in warm water, washing incisions gently. Tell patient to avoid tub baths until approved by physician.	Keeps incision clean, promotes circulation/healing. *Note:* "Climbing" out of tub requires use of arms and pectoral muscles, which can put undue stress on sternotomy.
Support incisions with Steri-strips (as needed) when sutures are removed.	Aids in maintaining approximation of wound edges to promote healing.
Encourage elevation of legs when sitting up in chair.	Promotes circulation, reduces edema to improve tissue healing.
Watch for/report to physician: places in incision that do not heal; reopening of healed incision; any drainage (bloody or purulent); localized area that is swollen with redness, feels increasingly painful, and is hot to touch.	Signs/symptoms indicating failure to heal; development of complications requiring further evaluation/intervention.
Promote adequate nutritional and fluid intake.	Helps to maintain good circulating volume for tissue perfusion and meets cellular energy requirements to facilitate tissue regeneration/healing process.
Collaborative	
Obtain specimen of wound drainage as indicated.	If infection occurs, local and systemic treatments may be required, e.g., peroxide/saline/Betadine soaks, antibiotic therapy.

NURSING DIAGNOSIS:	**KNOWLEDGE DEFICIT [LEARNING NEED], REGARDING CONDITION, POSTOPERATIVE CARE**
May be related to:	Lack of exposure.

	Information misinterpretation.
	Lack of recall.
Possibly evidenced by:	Questions/requests for information.
	Verbalization of problem.
	Statement of misconception.
	Inaccurate follow-through of instructions.
DESIRED OUTCOMES/ EVALUATION CRITERIA— PATIENT WILL:	Participate in learning process.
	Assume responsibility for own learning.
	Begin to look for information/ask questions.
	Verbalize understanding of condition, prognosis, and therapeutic needs.

ACTIONS/INTERVENTIONS

Independent

Reinforce surgeon's explanation of particular surgical procedure, providing diagram as appropriate.

Incorporate this information into discussion about short-/long-term recovery expectations.

Review prescribed exercise program and progress to date. Assist patient/SO to set realistic goals.

Encourage alternating rest periods with activity and light tasks with heavy tasks. Avoid heavy lifting, isometric/strenuous upper-body exercise.

Problem-solve with patient/SO ways to continue progressive activity program during temperature extremes and high wind/pollution days, e.g., walking predetermined distance within own house or local indoor shopping mall/exercise tract.

Schedule rest periods and short naps several times a day.

Reinforce physician's time limitations about lifting, driving, returning to work, and resumption of sexual activity.

Discuss issues concerning resumption of sexual activity, e.g., correlation of stress of sex to other activities;

RATIONALE

Provides individually specific information creating knowledge base for subsequent learning regarding home management.

Length of rehabilitation and prognosis is dependent on type of surgical procedure, preoperative physical condition, and duration of complications.

Individual capabilities and expectations are dependent on type of surgery, underlying cardiac function, and prior physical conditioning.

Prevents excessive fatigue/overexhaustion. *Note:* Strenuous use of arms can place undue stress on sternotomy.

Having a plan will forestall giving up exercise because of interferences such as weather.

Rest and sleep enhance coping abilities, reduce nervousness (common in this phase), and promote healing.

These restrictions are present until after the first postoperative office visit for assessment of sternum healing.

Concerns about sexual activity often go unexpressed, but patients usually desire information about what to expect. In general, patient can safely engage in sex when activity level has advanced to point where patient can climb two flights of stairs (which is about the same amount of energy expenditure).

ACTIONS/INTERVENTIONS	RATIONALE

Independent

Position recommendations;

Patient should avoid positions that restrict breathing (sex increases oxygen demand and consumption). Patient should not support self or partner with arms (breast bone healing, support muscles stretched).

Expectations of sexual performance;

Impotence appears to occur with some regularity in postoperative cardiac surgery patients. Although etiology is unknown, condition usually resolves in time without specific intervention. If situation persists, may require further evaluation.

Appropriate timing, e.g., avoid sex following heavy meal; during periods of emotional distress; when patient is fatigued/exhausted;

Timing of sexual activity may reduce occurrence of complications/angina.

Pharmacologic considerations.

Some patients may require antianginal medications (prophylactically) before sexual activity.

Inflammatory Cardiac Conditions: Pericarditis, Myocarditis, Endocarditis

The following conditions are problems which occur because of invasion of the heart tissues by bacteria or viruses. The most common types are:

Pericarditis: Inflammation of the visceral and parietal pericardium. (May be acute or chronic.)
Myocarditis: Focal or diffuse inflammation of the myocardium.
Endocarditis: Inflammation of the cardiac endothelial lining.

RELATED CONCERNS:

Congestive Heart Failure, p 48
Dysrhythmias, p 94
Psychosocial Aspects of Acute Care, p 899
Valvular Heart Disease, p 102

PATIENT ASSESSMENT DATA BASE

ACTIVITY/REST

May report:	Fatigue, weakness.
May exhibit:	Tachycardia.
	Decreased BP.
	Dyspnea with activity.

CIRCULATION

May report:	History of rheumatic fever, congenital heart disease, MI, cardiac surgery (CABG/valve replacement/prolonged cardiopulmonary bypass).
	Palpitations.
	Fainting spells.
May exhibit:	Tachycardia, dysrhythmias.
	PMI displaced left and inferior (cardiac enlargement).
	Pericardial friction rub (usually intermittent, heard at left sternal border).
	Murmurs of aortic, mitral, tricuspid stenosis/insufficiency; change in preexisting murmurs; papillary muscle dysfunction.
	Gallop rhythm (S_3/S_4 heart sounds). Heart sounds normal in early acute pericarditis.
	Edema, JVD (CHF).
	Petechia (conjunctiva, mucous membranes).
	Splinter hemorrhages (nail beds).
	Osler's nodes (fingers/toes).
	Janeway lesions (palms, soles).

ELIMINATION

May report:	History of kidney disease/renal failure.
	Reduced urine frequency/amount.
May exhibit:	Dark concentrated urine.

PAIN/COMFORT

May report: Pain in anterior chest (mild to severe/sharp) aggravated by inspiration, coughing, swallowing movement, lying down; relieved by sitting up, leaning forward (pericarditis). Not relieved by nitroglycerin.

Chest/back/joint pain (endocarditis).

May exhibit: Distraction behaviors, e.g., restlessness.

RESPIRATION

May report: Shortness of breath; chronic shortness of breath worse at night (myocarditis).

May exhibit: Dyspnea, nocturnal dyspnea.

Cough, inspiratory wheeze.

Tachypnea, crackles, and rhonchi.

Shallow respirations.

SAFETY

May report: History of viral, bacterial, fungal, or parasitic infections (myocarditis); chest trauma; malignant disease/thoracic irradiation; recent dental work; endoscopic examination of GI/GU system.

Compromised immune system, e.g., course of immunosuppressive therapy, SLE, other collagen diseases.

May exhibit: Fever.

TEACHING/LEARNING

May report: Long-term IV therapy or indwelling catheter use or parenteral drug abuse.

Discharge Plan Considerations: **DRG projected mean length of stay: 4.3 days (pericarditis); 5.5 days (myocarditis); 17 days (endocarditis).**

Assistance with food preparation, shopping, transportation, self-care needs, homemaker/home maintenance tasks.

DIAGNOSTIC STUDIES

ECG: May show ischemia, hypertrophy, conduction blocks, dysrhythmias. (ST elevation may occur in most leads.) PR depression, flattened or inverted T waves, low-voltage tracings are common.

Echocardiogram: May reveal pericardial effusion, cardiac hypertrophy, valvular dysfunction, dilatation of chambers.

Cardiac enzymes: CPK may be elevated, but MB isoenzymes are absent.

Angiography: May show valvular stenosis and regurgitation and/or decreased wall motion.

Chest x-ray: May show cardiac enlargement, pulmonary infiltrates.

CBC: May reveal acute/chronic infectious process; anemia.

Blood cultures: Done to isolate causative bacteria, virus, fungus.

ESR: Generally elevated.

ASO titer: Elevated with rheumatic fever (possible precipitator).

ANA titer: Positive with autoimmune diseases, e.g., SLE (possible precipitator).

BUN: May be done to evaluate for uremia (possible precipitator).

Pericardiocentesis: Pericardial fluid may be examined for etiology of infection, such as bacteria, tuberculosis, viral or fungal infections, SLE, rheumatoid disease, malignancy.

NURSING PRIORITIES

1. Relieve pain.
2. Promote rest, provide self-care assistance.
3. Assist in treatment/alleviation of underlying cause.
4. Manage underlying systemic disease/prevent complications.
5. Instruct in disease etiology, treatment, and prevention.

DISCHARGE GOALS

1. Pain alleviated/controlled.
2. Achieves activity level sufficient to meet basic self-care needs.
3. Infection resolved/controlled; fever absent.
4. Hemodynamic stability maintained; free of symptoms of heart failure.
5. Lifestyle changes initiated to prevent recurrence.

NURSING DIAGNOSIS:	PAIN, [ACUTE]
May be related to:	Inflammation of myocardium or pericardium.
	Systemic effects of infection.
	Tissue ischemia (myocardium).
Possibly evidenced by:	Chest pain, radiating to neck/back.
	Joint pain.
	Pain increased by deep inspiration, movement/activity, position.
	Fever, chills.
PATIENT OUTCOMES/ EVALUATION CRITERIA— PATIENT WILL:	Identify methods that provide relief.
	Report pain is relieved/controlled.
	Demonstrate use of relaxation skills and diversional activities as indicated for individual situation.

ACTIONS/INTERVENTIONS	RATIONALE
Independent	
Investigate reports of chest pain, noting onset and aggravating and relieving factors. Note nonverbal clues of discomfort, e.g., lying very still/restlessness, muscle tension, crying.	Pain of pericarditis is typically located substernally and may radiate into neck and back. However, this differs from myocardial ischemia/infarction pain, in that it becomes worse with deep inspiration, movement, or lying down and is relieved by sitting up/leaning forward. *Note:* Chest pain may or may not accompany endocarditis and myocarditis, depending on the presence of ischemia.
Provide quiet environment and comfort measures, e.g., change of position, back rubs, use of heat/cold, emotional support.	These measures can decrease patient's physical and emotional discomfort.

ACTIONS/INTERVENTIONS	RATIONALE
Independent	
Provide appropriate diversional activities.	Redirects attention, provides distraction within individual level of activity.
Collaborative	
Administer medications as indicated:	
Nonsteroidal agents, e.g., indomethacin (Indocin); ASA (aspirin);	May provide relief of pain, reduces inflammatory response.
Antipyretics, e.g., ASA/acetaminophen (Tylenol);	To reduce fever and promote comfort.
Steroids.	May be given for more severe symptoms.
Administer supplemental oxygen as indicated.	Maximizes oxygen available for uptake to reduce myocardial workload and decrease discomfort associated with ischemia.

NURSING DIAGNOSIS:	ACTIVITY INTOLERANCE
May be related to:	Inflammation and degeneration of myocardial muscle cells.
	Restriction of cardiac filling/ventricular contraction, reduced cardiac output.
	Toxins from infecting organism.
Possibly evidenced by:	Reports of weakness/fatigue/dyspnea with activity.
	Changes in vital signs with activity.
	Signs of CHF.
DESIRED OUTCOMES/ EVALUATION CRITERIA— PATIENT WILL:	Report/display measurable increase in activity tolerance.
	Demonstrate a decrease in physiologic signs of intolerance.
	Verbalize understanding of necessary therapeutic restrictions.

ACTIONS/INTERVENTIONS	RATIONALE
Independent	
Assess patient response to activity. Note presence of and changes in reports of weakness, fatigue, and dyspnea associated with activity.	Myocarditis causes inflammation and possible damage to functioning myocardial cells, with resultant CHF. Diminished cardiac filling and output may develop as fluid collects in the pericardial sac when pericarditis is present. Lastly, endocarditis may present with dysfunctional valves, negatively affecting cardiac output.
Monitor heart rate/rhythm, BP, and respiratory rate before/after activity and during as needed.	Helps determine the degree of cardiac and pulmonary decompensation. Decreased BP, tachy-

ACTIONS/INTERVENTIONS

Independent

Maintain bed rest during febrile periods and as indicated.

Plan care with uninterrupted rest/sleep periods.

Assist patient with gradual progressive exercise program as soon as able to be out of bed, noting vital sign response and patient tolerance to increased activity.

Evaluate emotional response to situation/provide support.

Collaborative

Administer supplemental oxygen.

RATIONALE

cardia, dysrhythmias, and tachypnea are indicative of impaired cardiac tolerance to activity.

Promotes resolution of inflammation during acute phase of pericarditis/endocarditis. *Note:* Fever increases oxygen demand and consumption, thereby increasing cardiac workload and reducing activity tolerance.

Provides for balance in demands that activity places on the heart; enhances healing process and emotional coping ability.

As inflammation resolves/underlying condition is treated, patient may be able to resume most desired activities, unless permanent myocardial damage/complications have occurred.

Anxiety will be present because of inflammation/infection and cardiac response (physiologic), as well as the degree of patient's fear and demands on emotional coping skills imposed by a potentially life-threatening illness (psychologic). Encouragement and support will be needed to cope with the frustration of prolonged hospital stay/recovery period.

Increases available oxygen for myocardial uptake to offset increased oxygen consumption that occurs with activity.

NURSING DIAGNOSIS:	CARDIAC OUTPUT, DECREASED, HIGH RISK FOR
Risk factors may include:	Accumulation of fluid within the pericardial sac (pericarditis).
	Valvular stenosis/insufficiency.
	Depressed/constricted ventricular function.
	Degeneration of cardiac muscle (myocarditis).
Possibly evidenced by:	[Not applicable; presence of signs and symptoms establishes an actual diagnosis.]
DESIRED OUTCOMES/ EVALUATION CRITERIA— PATIENT WILL:	Report/display decreased episodes of dyspnea, angina, and dysrhythmias.
	Identify behaviors to reduce cardiac workload.

ACTIONS/INTERVENTIONS	RATIONALE

Independent

Monitor heart rate/cardiac rhythm.

Tachycardia and numerous dysrhythmias can occur as the heart attempts to increase output in response to fever, hypoxia, and acidosis related to ischemia.

Auscultate heart sounds. Note distant/muffled heart tones, murmurs, S_3 and S_4 gallops.

Provides for early detection of developing complications, e.g., CHF, cardiac tamponade.

Encourage bed rest in semi-Fowler's position.

Reduces cardiac workload, maximizes cardiac output.

Provide comfort measures, e.g., back rub and position change, and diversional activities within cardiac tolerance.

Promotes relaxation and redirects attention.

Encourage use of stress management techniques, e.g., guided imagery, breathing exercises.

Behaviors useful to control anxiety, promote relaxation, and reduce cardiac workload.

Investigate rapid pulse, hypotension, narrow pulse pressure, elevated CVP/JVD, changes in heart tones, diminishing level of consciousness.

Clinical manifestations of cardiac tamponade which may occur in pericarditis when accumulation of fluid/exudate within the pericardial sac restricts cardiac filling and output.

Evaluate reports of fatigue, dyspnea, palpitations, continuous chest pain. Note presence of adventitious breath sounds, fever.

Clinical manifestations of CHF that may accompany endocarditis (infection/valve dysfunction) or myocarditis (acute myocardial muscle dysfunction).

Collaborative

Administer supplemental oxygen.

Enhances available oxygen for myocardial function and reduces effects of anaerobic metabolism, which occurs as a result of hypoxia and acidosis.

Administer medications as indicated, e.g., digitalis, diuretics;

May be given to increase myocardial contractility and reduce workload in presence of CHF (myocarditis).

Intravenous antibiotics/antimicrobials.

Given to treat identified pathogen(s) (endocarditis, pericarditis, myocarditis), preventing further cardiac involvement/damage.

Assist with emergency pericardiocentesis.

Procedure may be performed at the bedside to reduce fluid pressure around the heart, which can rapidly restore cardiac output (pericarditis).

Prepare patient for surgery, if indicated.

Valve replacement may be necessary to improve cardiac output (endocarditis). Pericardectomy may be required because of recurrent pericardial fluid accumulation or scar tissue and constriction of cardiac function (pericarditis).

NURSING DIAGNOSIS:	TISSUE PERFUSION, ALTERED, HIGH RISK FOR
Risk factors may include:	Embolization of thrombi/valvular vegetations secondary to endocarditis.

ACTIONS/INTERVENTIONS	RATIONALE
Independent	
Evaluate mental status. Note development of hemiparalysis, aphasia, seizures, vomiting, elevated BP.	Indicators suggesting systemic embolization to brain.
Investigate chest pain, sudden dyspnea accompanied by tachypnea, pleuritic pain, pallor cyanosis.	Arterial emboli, affecting the heart and/or other vital organs, may occur as a result of valvular disease, and/or chronic dysrhythmias. Venous congestion/stasis may lead to thrombus formation in deep veins and embolization to lungs.
Observe extremities for swelling, erythema. Note tenderness/pain, positive Homans' sign.	Prolonged inactivity/bed rest predisposes to venous stasis, increasing risk of developing venous thrombosis.
Observe for hematuria, accompanied by back/ flank pain, oliguria.	Indicative of emboli to kidney(s).
Note reports of pain in upper-left abdomen radiating to left shoulder, local tenderness, abdominal rigidity.	May indicate splenic emboli.
Promote bed rest as appropriate.	May help prevent the formation or migration of emboli in the patient with endocarditis. Prolonged bed rest (often required for patients with endocarditis and myocarditis), however, carries its own risk of development of thromboembolic phenomena.
Encourage active exercises/assist with range of motion as tolerated.	Enhances peripheral circulation and venous return, thereby decreasing risk of thrombus formation.
Collaborative	
Apply/remove antiembolism stockings as indicated.	Use is controversial, but may promote venous circulation and decrease risk of superficial/deep vein thrombus formation.
Administer anticoagulants, e.g., heparin, warfarin (Coumadin).	Heparin may be used prophylactically when the patient requires prolonged bed rest, has sepsis or CHF, and/or before and after valve replacement surgery. *Note:* Heparin is contraindicated in pericarditis and cardiac tamponade. Coumadin is the drug of choice for long-term/discharge therapy after valve replacement, or in presence of peripheral thrombi.

NURSING DIAGNOSIS:	KNOWLEDGE DEFICIT [LEARNING NEED], REGARDING CONDITION/TREATMENT
May be related to:	Lack of information about disease process, ways to prevent recurrence or complications. Need for long-term therapy and follow-up.
Possibly evidenced by:	Requests for information. Failure to improve. Preventable recurrences/complications.
DESIRED OUTCOMES/ EVALUATION CRITERIA— PATIENT WILL:	Verbalize understanding of inflammatory process, treatment needs, and possible complications. Identify/initiate necessary lifestyle or behavior changes to prevent recurrence/development of complications.

ACTIONS/INTERVENTIONS	RATIONALE
Independent	
Explain effects of inflammation on the heart, individualizing for particular patient. Educate concerning symptoms associated with complications/relapse and symptoms to report immediately to health care provider, e.g., fever, increased/unusual chest pain, weight gain, increasing intolerance to activity.	To take responsibility for own health, the patient needs to understand the specific cause, treatment, and expected long-term effects of the particular inflammatory condition, as well as signs/symptoms indicating recurrence/complications.
Instruct patient/SO in dose, purpose, side effects of medications; dietary needs/special considerations; activity allowances/limitations.	Information necessary to promote self-care, enhance compliance with therapeutic regimen, prevent complications.
Review necessity of prolonged antibiotic/antimicrobial therapy.	Lengthy hospital/home IV administration of antibiotics/antimicrobials may be necessary until blood cultures are negative/other blood work indicates absence of infection.
Discuss prophylactic use of antibiotics.	Patients with a history of rheumatic fever are at high risk for recurrences and usually require long-term antibiotic prophylaxis. Patients with valvular problems who do not have a history of rheumatic fever require short-term antibiotic protection for procedures that may cause transient bacteremia. Such procedures include dental procedures, tonsillectomy and/or adenoidectomy; surgical procedures/biopsy of respiratory mucosa; bronchoscopy; incision/drainage of infected tissue; and GU/GI procedures, childbirth.
Identify actions to prevent endocarditis such as:	
Practice good oral hygiene and dental care;	Bacteria commonly found in mouth can enter easily into systemic circulation through the gums.

133

ACTIONS/INTERVENTIONS	RATIONALE
Independent	
Avoid people with current infectious process (especially respiratory);	Development of infections, particularly respiratory streptococcal/pneumococcal or influenza, increase risk of cardiac involvement.
Choose appropriate birth control method (for female patient);	Use of IUDs has been linked to increased risk of pelvic inflammatory processes/infection.
Avoid illicit IV drug use.	Reduces risk of direct access of pathogens to systemic circulation.
Promote practices of general well-being such as good nutritional intake, balance between activity/rest, monitoring of own health status and reporting signs of infection.	Strengthens immune system and resistance to infection.
Obtain immunizations, e.g., influenza vaccines, as indicated.	Reduces risk of acquiring severe infections that can lead to cardiac infections.
Identify support person(s)/resources available postdischarge to meet self-care/home maintenance needs.	Activity intolerance/limitations may impair patient's ability to perform desired/needed tasks.
Stress importance of regular follow-up medical care. Assist patient in making initial appointments.	Understanding reasons for medical supervision and planning for/accepting responsibility for follow-up care reduces risk of recurrence/complications.
Identify predisposing risk factors over which patient may have control, e.g., IV drug use (endocarditis) and problem-solve solutions.	Patient may be motivated by present cardiac problems to seek support to stop drug abuse/detrimental behaviors.

Thrombophlebitis: Deep Vein Thrombosis _____

Thrombophlebitis is a condition in which a clot forms in a vein secondary to inflammation/trauma of the vein wall or because of a partial obstruction of the vein. Clot formation is related to (1) stasis of blood flow, (2) abnormalities in the vessel walls, and (3) alterations in the clotting mechanism.

Thrombophlebitis can affect superficial or deep veins, and while both conditions can cause symptoms, DVT is more serious in terms of potential complications, including pulmonary embolism and postphlebotic syndrome.

RELATED CONCERNS:

Psychosocial Aspects of Acute Care, p 899
Pulmonary Embolism, p 174

PATIENT ASSESSMENT DATA BASE

ACTIVITY/REST

May report:	Occupation which requires sitting or standing for long periods of time.
	Lengthy immobility, (e.g., orthopedic trauma, long hospitalization/bed rest, complicated pregnancy); paralysis/progressive debilitating condition.
	Pain with activity/prolonged standing.
	Fatigue/weakness of affected extremity.
May exhibit:	Generalized or extremity weakness.

CIRCULATION

May report:	History of previous venous thrombosis, preexisting varices.
	Presence of other predisposing factors, e.g., hypertension (pregnancy-induced); diabetes mellitus, MI/valvular heart disease; thrombotic cerebrovascular accident.
May exhibit:	Tachycardia.
	Peripheral pulse diminished in the affected extremity (DVT).
	Varicosities and/or hardened, bumpy/knotty vein (thrombus).
	Skin color/temperature in affected extremity (calf/thigh): pale, cool, edematous (DVT); pinkish red, warm along the course of the vein (superficial).
	Positive Homans' sign (absence does not rule out DVT).

FOOD/FLUID

May exhibit:	Poor skin turgor, dry mucous membranes (dehydration predisposes to hypercoagulability).
	Obesity (predisposes to stasis and pelvic vein pressure).
	Edema of affected extremity (dependent on location of thrombus).

PAIN/COMFORT

May report:	Throbbing, tenderness, aching pain aggravated by standing or movement (affected extremity).
May exhibit:	Guarding of affected extremity.

135

SAFETY

May report: History of direct or indirect injury to extremity or vein (e.g., major trauma/fractures, orthopedic/pelvic surgery, prolonged labor with fetal head pressure on pelvic veins, intravenous therapy).

Presence of malignancy (particularly of the pancreas, lung, GI system).

May exhibit: Fever, chills.

TEACHING/LEARNING

May report: Use of oral contraceptives/estrogens; recent anticoagulant therapy (predisposes to hypercoagulability).

Recurrence/lack of resolution of previous thrombophlebotic episode.

Discharge Plan Considerations: **DRG projected mean length of stay: 7.7 days.**

Assistance with shopping, transportation, and homemaker/maintenance tasks.

Properly fitted antiembolic hose.

DIAGNOSTIC STUDIES

Hematocrit: Hemoconcentration (elevated Hct) potentiates risk of thrombus formation.

Coagulation studies: May reveal hypercoagulability.

Noninvasive vascular studies (Doppler oscillometry, exercise tolerance, impedance plethysmography, and duplex scans): Changes in blood flow and volume identify venous occlusion, vascular damage, and vascular insufficiency.

Trendelenburg test: May demonstrate vessel valve incompetence.

Venography: Radiographically confirms diagnosis through changes in blood flow and/or size of channels.

MRI: May be useful in assessing blood flow turbulence and movement, venous valvular competence.

NURSING PRIORITIES

1. Maintain/enhance tissue perfusion, facilitate resolution of thrombus.
2. Promote optimal comfort.
3. Prevent complications.
4. Provide information about disease process/prognosis and treatment regimen.

DISCHARGE GOALS

1. Tissue perfusion improved in affected limb.
2. Pain/discomfort relieved.
3. Complications prevented/resolved.
4. Disease process/prognosis and therapeutic needs understood.

NURSING DIAGNOSIS:	TISSUE PERFUSION, ALTERED, PERIPHERAL
May be related to:	Decreased blood flow/venous stasis (partial or complete venous obstruction).
Possibly evidenced by:	Tissue edema, pain.
	Diminished peripheral pulses, slow/diminished capillary refill.
	Skin color changes (pallor, erythema).

DESIRED OUTCOMES/ EVALUATION CRITERIA— PATIENT WILL:	Demonstrate improved perfusion as evidenced by peripheral pulses present/equal, skin color and temperature normal, absence of edema.
	Engage in behaviors/actions to enhance tissue perfusion.
	Display increasing tolerance to activity.

ACTIONS/INTERVENTIONS	RATIONALE

Independent

ACTIONS/INTERVENTIONS	RATIONALE
Inspect extremity for skin color and temperature changes, as well as edema (from groin to foot). Note symmetry of calves; measure and record calf circumference. Report proximal progression of inflammatory process, traveling pain.	Symptoms help distinguish between superficial thrombophlebitis and DVT. Redness, heat, tenderness, and localized edema are characteristic of superficial involvement. Pallor and coolness of extremity are characteristic of DVT. Calf-vein involvement of DVT is associated with absence of edema; femoral-vein involvement is associated with mild to moderate edema; iliofemoral-vein thrombosis is characterized by severe edema.
Examine extremity for obviously prominent veins. Palpate (gently) for local tissue tension, stretched skin, knots/bumps along course of vein.	Distention of superficial veins can occur in DVT because of backflow through communicating veins. Evidence of thrombophlebitis in superficial veins may be visible or palpable.
Assess capillary refill and check for Homans' sign.	Diminished capillary refill usually present in DVT. Positive Homans' sign (deep calf pain in affected leg upon dorsiflexion of foot) is not as consistent a clinical manifestation as once thought and may or may not be present.
Promote bed rest during acute phase.	Until treatment is instituted, limitation of activity reduces oxygen and nutrient demands on affected extremity and minimizes the possibility of dislodging thrombus/creating emboli.
Elevate legs when in bed or chair, as indicated. Periodically elevate feet and legs above heart level.	Reduces tissue swelling and rapidly empties superficial and tibial veins, preventing overdistention and thereby increasing venous return. *Note:* Some physicians believe that elevation may potentiate release of thrombus, thus increasing risk of embolization and decreasing circulation to the most distal portion of the extremity.
Initiate active or passive exercises while in bed (e.g., flex/extend/rotate foot periodically). Assist with gradual resumption of ambulation (e.g., walking 10 min/h) as soon as patient is permitted out of bed.	These measures are designed to increase venous return from lower extremities and reduce venous stasis, as well as improve general muscle tone/strength.
Caution patient to avoid crossing legs or hyperflex at knee (seated position with legs dangling, or lying in jackknife position).	Physical restriction of circulation impairs blood flow and increases venous stasis in pelvic, popliteal, and leg vessels, thus increasing swelling and discomfort.
Instruct patient to avoid rubbing/massaging the affected extremity.	This activity potentiates risk of fragmenting/dislodging thrombus, causing embolization and increasing risk of complications.

137

ACTIONS/INTERVENTIONS	RATIONALE

Independent

Encourage deep breathing exercises.	Increases negative pressure in thorax, which assists in emptying large veins.
Increase fluid intake to at least 2000 ml/d, within cardiac tolerance.	Dehydration increases blood viscosity and venous stasis, predisposing to thrombus formation.

Collaborative

Apply warm, moist compresses, or heat cradle to affected extremity if indicated.	May be prescribed to promote vasodilation and venous return and resolution of local edema. Note: May be contraindicated in presence of arterial insufficiency, in which heat can increase cellular oxygen consumption/nutritional needs, furthering imbalance between supply and demand.
Administer anticoagulants, e.g.: Heparin via continuous or intermittent IV, intermittent subcutaneous injections; and/or coumarin derivatives (Coumadin);	Heparin is preferred initially because of its prompt, predictable antagonistic action on thrombin as it is formed and also the removal of activated coagulation factors XII, XI, IX, X (intrinsic pathway), preventing further clot formation. Coumadin has a potent depressant effect on liver formation of prothrombin from vitamin K and impairs formation of Factors VII, IX, X (extrinsic pathway). Coumadin may be used for long-term/postdischarge therapy.
Thrombolytic agents, e.g., streptokinase, urokinase.	May be used for treatment of acute (less than 10 days old) or massive DVT to prevent valvular damage and development of chronic venous insufficiency. Heparin is usually begun several hours after the completion of thrombolytic therapy.
Monitor laboratory studies as indicated: prothrombin time (PT), partial thromboplastin time (PTT), activated partial thromboplastin time (APTT), CBC.	Monitors anticoagulant therapy and presence of risk factors, e.g., hemoconcentration and dehydration, which potentiate clot formation.
Apply/regulate graduated compression stockings, intermittent pneumatic compression, if indicated.	Sequential compression devices may be used to improve blood flow velocity and emptying of vessels by providing artificial muscle-pumping action.
Apply elastic support hose following acute phase. Take care to avoid tourniquet effect.	Properly fitted support hose are useful (once ambulation has begun) to minimize or delay development of postphlebotic syndrome. They must exert a sustained, evenly distributed pressure over entire surface of calves and thighs to reduce the caliber of superficial veins and increase blood flow to deep veins.
Prepare for surgical intervention when indicated.	Thrombectomy (excision of thrombus) is occasionally necessary if inflammation extends proximally or circulation is severely restricted. Multiple/recurrent thrombotic episodes unresponsive to medical treatment (or when anticoagulant therapy is contraindicated) may require insertion of a vena caval screen/umbrella.

NURSING DIAGNOSIS:	PAIN, [ACUTE], [DISCOMFORT]
May be related to:	Diminished arterial circulation and oxygenation of tissues with production/accumulation of lactic acid in tissues.
	Inflammatory process.
Possibly evidenced by:	Reports of pain, tenderness, aching/burning.
	Guarding of affected limb.
	Restlessness, distraction behaviors.
DESIRED OUTCOMES/ EVALUATION CRITERIA— PATIENT WILL:	Report pain/discomfort is alleviated/controlled.
	Verbalize methods that provide relief.
	Display relaxed manner; be able to sleep/rest and engage in desired activity.

ACTIONS/INTERVENTIONS	RATIONALE
Independent	
Assess degree of discomfort/pain. Note guarding of extremity. Palpate leg with caution.	Degree of pain is directly related to extent of circulatory deficit, inflammatory process, degree of hypoxia, and extent of edema associated with thrombus development.
Maintain bed rest during acute phase.	Reduces discomfort associated with muscle contraction and movement.
Elevate affected extremity.	Encourages venous return to facilitate circulation, reducing stasis/edema formation.
Provide foot cradle.	Cradle keeps pressure of bed clothes off the affected leg, thereby reducing pressure discomfort.
Encourage patient to change position frequently.	Decreases/prevents muscle fatigue, helps minimize muscle spasm.
Monitor vital signs, noting elevated temperature.	Elevations in heart rate may indicate increased pain/discomfort or occur in response to fever and inflammatory process. Fever can also increase patient's discomfort.
Investigate reports of sudden and/or sharp chest pain, accompanied by dyspnea, tachycardia, and apprehension.	These signs/symptoms suggest presence of pulmonary emboli as a complication of DVT.
Collaborative	
Administer medications, as indicated:	
Analgesics (narcotic/nonnarcotic);	Relieves pain and decreases muscle tension.
Antipyretics, e.g., acetaminophen.	Reduces fever and inflammation. Note: Risk of bleeding may be increased by concurrent use of drugs that affect platelet function, e.g., ASA and NSAIDs.

139

ACTIONS/INTERVENTIONS

Collaborative

Apply moist heat to extremity, if indicated.

RATIONALE

Causes vasodilation, which increases circulation; relaxes muscles; and may stimulate release of natural endorphins.

NURSING DIAGNOSIS:	KNOWLEDGE DEFICIT [LEARNING NEED], REGARDING CONDITION, TREATMENT PROGRAM
May be related to:	Lack of exposure.
	Misinterpretation of information.
	Unfamiliarity with information resources.
	Lack of recall.
Possibly evidenced by:	Request for information.
	Statement of misconception.
	Inaccurate follow-through of instructions.
	Development of preventable complications.
DESIRED OUTCOMES/ EVALUATION CRITERIA— PATIENT WILL:	Verbalize understanding of disease process, treatment regimen, and limitations.
	Participate in learning process.
	Identify signs/symptoms requiring medical evaluation.
	Correctly perform therapeutic procedure(s) and explain reasons for actions.

ACTIONS/INTERVENTIONS

Independent

Review pathophysiology of condition and signs/symptoms of possible complications, e.g., pulmonary emboli, chronic venous insufficiency, venous stasis ulcers (postphlebotic syndrome).

Explain purpose of activity restrictions and need for balance between activity/rest.

Establish appropriate exercise/activity program.

Problem-solve solutions to predisposing factors that may be present, e.g., employment that requires prolonged standing/sitting; wearing of restrictive clothing (girdles/garters); use of oral con-

RATIONALE

Provides a knowledge base from which patient can make informed choices and understand/identify health care needs.

Rest reduces oxygen and nutrient needs of compromised tissues and decreases risk of fragmentation of thrombosis. Balancing rest with activity prevents exhaustion and further impairment of cellular perfusion.

Aids in developing collateral circulation, enhances venous return, and prevents recurrence.

Actively involves patient in identifying and initiating lifestyle/behavior changes to promote health and prevent recurrence of condition/development of complications.

ACTIONS/INTERVENTIONS	RATIONALE
Independent	
traceptives; obesity, prolonged bed rest/immobility; dehydration.	
Discuss purpose, dosage of anticoagulant. Emphasize importance of taking drug as prescribed.	Promotes patient safety by reducing risk of inadequate therapeutic response/deleterious side effects.
Identify safety precautions, e.g., use of soft toothbrush, electric razor for shaving, gloves for gardening, avoiding sharp objects (including toothpicks), walking barefoot, engaging in rough sports/activities, or forceful blowing of nose.	Reduces the risk of traumatic injury, which potentiates bleeding/clot formation.
Review possible drug interactions and stress need to read ingredient labels of OTC drugs.	Salicylates and excess alcohol decrease prothrombin activity, whereas vitamin K (multivitamins, bananas, green leafy vegetables) increases prothrombin activity. Barbiturates increase metabolism of coumarin drugs; antibiotics alter intestinal flora and may interfere with vitamin K synthesis.
Identify untoward anticoagulant effects requiring medical attention, e.g., bleeding from mucous membranes (nose, gums), continued oozing from cuts/punctures, severe bruising after minimal trauma, development of petechiae.	Early detection of deleterious effects of therapy (prolongation of clotting time) allows for timely intervention and may prevent serious complications.
Stress importance of medical follow-up/laboratory testing.	Understanding that close supervision of anticoagulant therapy is necessary (therapeutic dosage range is narrow and complications may be deadly) promotes patient participation.
Encourage wearing of medical-alert identification bracelet/tag, as indicated.	Alerts emergency health care givers to use of anticoagulants.
Review purpose and demonstrate correct application/removal of antiembolic hose.	Understanding may enhance cooperation with prescribed therapy and prevent improper/ineffective use.
Instruct in meticulous skin care of lower extremities, e.g., prevent/promptly treat breaks in skin and report development of lesions/ulcers or changes in skin color.	Chronic venous congestion/postphlebotic syndrome may develop (especially in presence of severe vascular involvement and/or recurrent episodes) potentiating risk of stasis ulcers/infection.

Raynaud's Disease _____

Raynaud's phenomenon may be either primary or secondary. About 65% of patient's with Raynaud's have the more benign *primary* disease. This form has no known cause, no underlying or associated medical problems, and affects mostly women between the ages of 15 and 40. *Secondary* Raynaud's is potentially more serious, and may stem from one or more activities (e.g., tasks that subject worker's hands to increased wear and tear), medications, or underlying disease that act on the blood vessels in some way (e.g., scleroderma, SLE, rheumatoid arthritis). This syndrome more commonly occurs in men or in women over 40 years of age.

(Note: Not usually treated in hospital. Individual may be hospitalized for other medical/surgical needs.)

RELATED CONCERNS:

Psychosocial Aspects of Acute Care, p 899
Rheumatoid Arthritis, p 875

PATIENT ASSESSMENT DATA BASE

CIRCULATION

May report:	History of hypertension (vasospasm effects).
	Color changes of affected parts on exposure to cold (onset in early adulthood).
May exhibit:	Skin color on fingers/affected parts (dependent on phase at time of observation) may appear dead white (blanching), then cyanotic, then hyperemic (red). Late/progressive signs: skin is white or discolored, shiny, taut, smooth.
	Pulses: Radial and ulnar may be normal (early) or absent (late).
	Nail clubbing/deformities may occur (late).
	Ulcerations and/or areas of gangrene (rare).

EGO INTEGRITY

May report:	Stress and strong emotional reactions (precipitator).

NEUROSENSORY

May report:	Paresthesia, numbness in fingers.
	Recurrent migraine headaches (vasospasm/hormonal effect).
May exhibit:	Awkwardness/loss of fine motor coordination.

PAIN/COMFORT

May report:	Throbbing pain during rubor phase of color change (vasodilation). Sensitivity to pressure on affected part.
May exhibit:	Guarding, restlessness, self-focus.

RESPIRATION

May report:	Use of tobacco.

SAFETY

May report:	Occupation which involves use of vibratory tools or requires frequent squeezing/repetitive movements, e.g., mechanics, farmers, typists, pianists, jackhammer/chainsaw operators (precipitator).

| May exhibit: | Lesions/areas of gangrene on fingertips from the size of a pin to those involving the entire fingertip (very advanced). |

SEXUALITY

| May report: | Correlation of attacks with menses/menopause (hormonal effect). |

TEACHING/LEARNING

| May report: | Other member(s) of family affected with vascular disease, e.g., hypertension, migraine headaches, or Raynaud's disease. |
| Discharge Plan Considerations: | **DRG projected mean length of stay: 4.4 days.** Alteration in medications, change in occupation. Assistance with some homemaker/maintenance tasks (e.g., defrosting refrigerator, shoveling snow). |

DIAGNOSTIC STUDIES

Diagnosis is generally clinical, but studies may be done to rule out chronic arterial occlusive or connective tissue disease.

Allen test: May show occlusion of radial or ulnar pulse proximal to wrist during attack.

Peripheral pulses: Doppler evaluation usually normal but may be reduced or absent during an attack.

Thermogram: Measures and plots areas of temperature changes in tissues showing loss of circulation.

Digital plethysmography: Abnormal perfusion pulse contour and pressure during attacks.

Peripheral arteriography: May be done to visualize small peripheral arteries/rule out arteriovascular disease.

NURSING PRIORITIES

1. Minimize/eliminate ischemic attacks.
2. Support patient responsibility in prevention of complications.
3. Provide information about disease process/prognosis and treatment.

DISCHARGE GOALS

1. Frequency/severity of attacks decreasing.
2. Complications prevented/minimized.
3. Stress reduction techniques used appropriately.
4. Disease progression and therapeutic regimen understood.

NURSING DIAGNOSIS:	PAIN, [ACUTE]/CHRONIC
May be related to:	Vasospasm/altered perfusion of affected tissues. Ischemia/destruction of tissues.
Possibly evidenced by:	Verbal complaints. Guarding of affected parts. Self-focusing. Restlessness.

143

ACTIONS/INTERVENTIONS	RATIONALE
Independent	
Note characteristics of pain and paresthesia.	Changes in severity/duration may indicate progression of disease process/development of complications.
Discuss with patient how and why pain is produced.	Knowledge of pain-producing mechanism allows patient to intervene more effectively to minimize occurrences.
Assist patient to identify precipitating factors or situations, e.g., smoking, exposure to cold and problem-solve solutions.	Vasoconstriction is to be limited as it may lead to tissue damage and gangrene.
Encourage use of stress management techniques, diversional activities.	Promotes relaxation/focusing attention to help in breaking the stress/anxiety/stress cycle, which can worsen vasoconstrictive response and increase pain.
Immerse affected part in warm water.	This method of rewarming encourages vasodilation, stopping vasospasm.
Provide warm room, free of drafts, e.g., block air conditioner vent, keep hallway door closed as indicated.	Eliminates environmental factors that may precipitate an attack.
Monitor effects of medications and treatment.	Individual responses to prescribed therapies may not be adequate to control disease or may produce untoward side effects, indicating need for change in regimen.
Collaborative	
Administer medications as indicated. (Refer to ND: Tissue Perfusion, altered: Peripheral, below.)	Use of vasodilators/antihypertensives may relieve vasospasm and reduce pain.
Prepare for surgical intervention if indicated.	Sympathectomy is sometimes performed when relief of severe symptoms is not obtained by other methods. However, surgical relief is often temporary with symptoms returning within 6 months. This option should be considered when patient has progressive ulceration.

NURSING DIAGNOSIS:	**TISSUE PERFUSION, ALTERED: PERIPHERAL**
May be related to:	Interruption of arterial blood flow.
Possibly evidenced by:	Coolness of affected areas during attack.

Intermittent color changes of tissue, e.g., blanching, cyanosis, reactive hyperemia.

Decreased sensation.

Slow healing of lesions.

Development of ulcerations/gangrene (rare).

DESIRED OUTCOMES/ EVALUATION CRITERIA— PATIENT WILL:

Report/display decreased frequency/severity of vasospastic attacks with healing/absence of lesions.

Identify/initiate appropriate lifestyle and behavior changes to enhance circulation.

ACTIONS/INTERVENTIONS	RATIONALE
Independent	
Observe skin color of affected parts.	Typical skin color changes occur in phases with intermittent blanching (result of sudden vasospasm); cyanosis (ischemia); and rubor (vasodilation/reactive hyperemia). During color changes, affected parts are first cold and numb, then throbbing, with tingling sensations and swelling.
Note diminshed pulses; delayed capillary refill; trophic skin changes (discoloration, shiny/taut); clubbing of nails.	These changes indicate progressive/chronic process.
Evaluate sensation in affected parts, e.g., sharp/dull, hot/cold.	Sensation is often diminished during attack or chronically in advanced disease.
Protect from injury, e.g., refrain from activities using sharp implements, requiring fine motor function, or involving heat/cold (drinking coffee/testing water for bath).	Lack of awareness when sensation is diminished can lead to situations in which the affected parts are damaged.
Inspect and assess skin for ulcerations, lesions, gangrenous areas.	Lesions can occur from pinpoint size to those involving an entire fingertip and may result in infection/serious tissue damage/loss.
Encourage proper nutrition, vitamins.	A well-balanced diet, including adequate protein and hydration, is necessary for proper healing and tissue regeneration.
Collaborative	
Administer medications as indicated:	Individual drugs or combinations may be used, but effectiveness varies and use may be outweighed by presence of undesired side effects.
Vasodilators, e.g., cyclandelate (Cyclospamol), tolazoline (Priscoline); antihypertensives, e.g., methyldopa (Aldomet), reserpine (Serpasil), phenoxybenzamine (Dibenzyline), prazosin (Minipress);	Although site/mechanism of action varies, intended results are reduction of vasoconstriction, relaxation of vasospasm, and a more even blood flow/narrowing of pulse pressure.

ACTIONS/INTERVENTIONS

Collaborative

Calcium channel blockers, e.g., verapamil (Calan).

Obtain specimen of lesion drainage for culture and sensitivity.

Refer to resources providing instruction in biofeedback.

RATIONALE

These drugs used primarily in persons with severe disease or when signs of tissue damage occur. These medications have significant side effects, especially orthostatic hypertension, which may preclude their use.

Lesions may become secondarily infected, further damaging tissues and preventing healing. C&S identifies specific organism and the antibiotic most useful in treating the organism.

May help patient to voluntarily increase the temperature in the fingers by controlling the autonomic nervous system.

NURSING DIAGNOSIS:	**KNOWLEDGE DEFICIT [LEARNING NEED], REGARDING NATURE OF CONDITION, THERAPEUTIC NEEDS**
May be related to:	Lack of knowledge/unfamiliarity with information resources. Misconceptions/misunderstanding.
Possibly evidenced by:	Request for information. Recurrence of attacks.
DESIRED OUTCOMES/ EVALUATION CRITERIA— PATIENT WILL:	Verbalize understanding of need for protection from cold. Demonstrate understanding of medical regimen and symptoms to report to physician. Display lifestyle/behavior changes to reduce occurrence of attacks.

ACTIONS/INTERVENTIONS

Independent

Encourage avoidance of exposure to cold. Educate about the use of extra protection from cold, e.g., warm environment; adequate clothing, (mittens, hats, chemical- or battery-powered hand warmer or socks, warm boots); avoid direct contact with cold objects when possible.

Keep environmental temperature at/above 70°F, eliminate drafts.

Discuss possible move to warmer climate, change of occupation, as indicated.

RATIONALE

Cold exposure is major precipitator of vasoconstriction. Warm clothing and environment help prevent vasoconstriction of digits by keeping the entire body warm. *Note:* Mittens are preferred, because gloves allow cold to surround and absorb heat from each finger.

Reduces risk of precipitating attack.

May be necessary if severe vasospasm attacks continue or ischemic tissue changes occur that cannot be controlled by other means.

ACTIONS/INTERVENTIONS	RATIONALE
Independent	
Stress importance of cessation of smoking. Provide information on local clinics/support groups.	Smoking causes vasoconstriction, which may precipitate/potentiate attacks. Patient usually requires support to accomplish elimination of this activity.
Assist patient in designing methods to avoid or modify stressful episodes. Discuss relaxation techniques.	Stress reduction can limit catecholamine release by the sympathetic nervous system, thereby limiting/aborting the vasoconstriction response.
Stress importance of daily inspection and proper skin-care practices.	Maintaining integrity/health of compromised tissues may prevent progression/development of complications, e.g., lesions, infection, necrosis.
Prevent trauma to distal parts (hands, feet). Carefully trim nails. Advise patient to stop activity/protect affected part when spasm occurs.	Reduces risks of injury from sharp objects such as knives/needles and from burns when sensitivity is diminished.
Discuss and provide information about how to terminate attacks, e.g., immersion of affected part in warm water.	Attack may subside spontaneously or be terminated by slow rewarming (encourages vasodilation). Information can reduce anxiety when patient takes measures to reduce pain.
Discuss purpose, dosage, side effects of medications.	Information necessary for patient to follow through with therapeutic regimen and evaluate effectiveness.
Recommend avoiding use of β-blockers, e.g., propanolol (Inderal).	Contraindicated because they worsen vasospasm.
Investigate water therapy for circulatory conditioning e.g., soaking hands in warm water 3–6 times every other day indoors, then progressing to exposing body to cold while hands are submerged in warm water.	An experimental technique used to "retrain" body response to cold, which has met with success in some trials.

Bibliography

General References

Bellak, JP and Bamford, PA: Nursing Assessment: A Multidimensional Approach. Jones & Bartlett, Boston, 1987.
Berkow, R (ed): The Merck Manual, ed 15. Merck Sharp & Dohme Research Laboratories, Rahway, NJ, 1987.
Cella, JH and Watson, J: Nurse's Manual of Laboratory Tests. FA Davis, Philadelphia, 1989.
Condon, RE and Nyhus, LM (eds): Manual of Surgical Therapeutics, ed 7. Little, Brown & Co, Boston, 1988.
Deglin, JH and Vallerand, AH: Davis's Drug Guide for Nurses, ed 3. FA Davis, Philadelphia, 1992.
Diseases and Disorders Handbook, ed 3. Springhouse, Springhouse, PA, 1989.
Doenges, ME and Moorhouse, MF: Nurse's Pocket Guide: Nursing Diagnoses with Interventions, ed 3. FA Davis, Philadelphia, 1991.
Dunagan, WC and Ridner, ML (eds): Manual of Medical Therapeutics, ed 26. Little, Brown & Co, Boston, 1989.
Fischbach, F: A Manual of Laboratory and Diagnostic Tests, ed 4. JB Lippincott, Philadelphia, 1992.
Guyton, AC: Textbook of Medical Physiology, ed 8. WB Saunders, Philadelphia, 1991.
Kuhn, MM: Pharmacotherapeutics: A Nursing Process Approach, ed 2, FA Davis, 1991.
Professional Guide to Diseases, ed 3. Springhouse, Springhouse, PA, 1989.
Suddarth, DS (ed): The Lippincott Manual of Nursing Practice, ed 5. JB Lippincott, Philadelphia, 1991.
Thomas, CL (ed): Taber's Cyclopedic Medical Dictionary, ed 16. FA Davis, Philadelphia, 1989.
Thompson, JM, McFarland, GK, Hirsh, JE, et al: Mosby's Manual of Clinical Nursing, ed 2. CV Mosby, St Louis, 1989.

Books

Daily, E and Schroeder, J: Hemodynamic Monitoring of the Patient with Acute Myocardial Infarct, ed 4. CV Mosby, 1989.
Wilson, et al (eds): Harrison's Principles of Internal Medicine, ed 12. McGraw Hill, New York,1991.

Articles

Assessing cardiac emergencies. Nursing90 20(8):50, 1990.
Barbier, CC: PTCA: Treating the tough cases. RN 54(2):38, 1991.
Bennet, WI (ed): Sounding out clots. Harvard Medical School Health Letter 15(3):2, 1990.
Braun, AE: Drugs that dissolve clots. RN June 1991, p 52.
Calloway, CK: Zeroing in on chest pain. Nursing90 20:44, 1990.
Cerrato, PL: Hypertension: The role of diet and lifestyle. RN 53(12):46, 1990.
Culligan, M, Todd, B, and Liehr, P: Preventing graftleg complications in CABG patients. Nursing90 20(6):59, 1990.
Drug challenge. Nursing90 20(7):93, 1990.
Drug News: Risk of recurrent MI, stroke is less likely with warfarin. RN 53(11):141, 1990.
Ellstrom, K: What's causing your patient's respiratory distress? Nursing90 20(11):57, 1990.
Ferry, D and Nash, DT: Hypertension: The nurses' role. RN 53(11):54, 1990.
Finesilver, C and Metzler, DJ: Right ventricular infarction: The critically different MI. AJN 21(4):32, 1991.
Gehring, PE: Perfecting the art of vascular assessment. RN 55(1):40, 1992.
Gleeson, B: After myocardial infarction: How to teach a patient in denial. Nursing91 21(5):48, 1991.
Gleeson, B: Loosening the grip of anginal pain. Nursing91 21:33, 1991.
Green, E: Solving the puzzle of chest pain. AJN 22:32, 1992.
Hospital drug quiz. Nursing90 20(2):101, 1990.
Hospital drug quiz. Nursing92 22(2):86, 1992.
Miller, KM: When your patient has an implanted defibrillator. RN 53(6):32, 1990.
Owen, A: Keeping pace with temporary pacemakers. Nursing91 21(4):58, 1991.
Rafalowski, M: Cardiac valve replacement: The homograft. Focus on Critical Care 17(2):112, 1990.
Rodgers, ML: Pericarditis, a different kind of heart disease. Nursing90 20(2):52, 1990.
Rodman, MJ: Hypertension: Step-care management. RN 54(2):24, 1991.
Saul, L: Arrhythmia mimics. AJN 21(3):40, 1991.
Snowberger, P: Sinus arrhythmia. RN 55(1):50, 1992.
Solomon, J: Managing a failing heart. RN 54(8):46, 1991.
Stephenson, J: Raynauds phenomenon: The cold facts. Harvard Medical School Health Letter 17(3):1, 1992.
Teplitz, L: Action Stat! Hypertensive crisis. Nursing90 20(4):33, 1990.
Thompson, VL: Chest pain: Your response to a classic warning. RN 52(4):32, 1989.
Wilson, S: Action Stat! Complications of thrombolytic therapy. Nursing91 21(1):41, 1991.

CHAPTER 5

RESPIRATORY

Chronic Obstructive Pulmonary Disease (COPD) _____

All respiratory diseases characterized by chronic obstruction to airflow fall under the broad classification of COPD. Within that broad category the primary cause of the obstruction may vary, e.g., airway inflammation, mucous plugging, narrowed airway lumina, or airway destruction.

Asthma: Characterized by reversible constriction of bronchial smooth muscle, hypersecretion of mucous, and mucosal inflammation and edema. Precipitating factors include allergens, emotional upheaval, cold weather, exercise, chemicals, medications, and infections.

Chronic bronchitis: Widespread inflammation of airways with narrowing or blocking of airways and increased production of mucoid sputum, leading to ventilation-perfusion mismatch and marked cyanosis.

Emphysema: Most severe form of COPD characterized by recurrent inflammation which damages and eventually destroys alveolar walls creating large blebs or bullae (air spaces) and collapsed bronchioles upon expiration (air-trapping).

Note: Chronic bronchitis and emphysema coexist in many patients and are the two diseases most commonly seen in hospitalized COPD patients. Both diseases are characterized by chronic airflow limitation. Chronic bronchitis and emphysema are usually irreversible, although some effects can be mediated.

RELATED CONCERNS:

Congestive Heart Failure, p 48
Pneumonia, p 162
Psychosocial Aspects of Acute Care, p 899
Ventilatory Assistance (Mechanical), p 226

PATIENT ASSESSMENT DATA BASE

ACTIVITY/REST

May report:	Fatigue, exhaustion, malaise.
	Inability to perform basic ADLs because of breathlessness.
	Inability to sleep, need to sleep sitting up.
	Dyspnea at rest or in response to activity or exercise.

May exhibit:	Fatigue.
	Restlessness, insomnia.
	General debilitation/loss of muscle mass.

CIRCULATION

May report:	Swelling of lower extremities.
May exhibit:	Elevated BP.
	Elevated heart rate/severe tachycardia, dysrhythmias.
	Distended neck veins (advanced disease).
	Dependent edema, may not be related to heart disease.
	Faint heart sounds (due to increased AP chest diameter).
	Skin color/mucous membranes: Normal or bluish/cyanotic; clubbing of nails and peripheral cyanosis.
	Pallor can indicate anemia.

EGO INTEGRITY

May report:	Increased stress factors.
	Changes in lifestyle.
May exhibit:	Anxious, fearful, irritable behavior.

FOOD/FLUID

May report:	Nausea/vomiting.
	Poor appetite/anorexia (emphysema).
	Inability to eat because of respiratory distress.
	Persistent weight loss (emphysema), weight gain may reflect edema (bronchitis).
May exhibit:	Poor skin turgor.
	Dependent edema.
	Diaphoresis.
	Weight loss, decreased muscle mass/subcutaneous fat (emphysema).
	Abdominal palpation may reveal hepatomegaly (bronchitis).

HYGIENE

May report:	Decreased ability/increased need for assistance with ADLs.
May exhibit:	Poor hygiene, body odor.

RESPIRATION

May report:	Shortness of breath (insidious onset with dyspnea predominant symptom in emphysema) especially on exertion; seasonal or episodic occurrence of breathlessness (asthma); sensation of chest tightness, inability to breathe (asthma).
	Chronic "air hunger."
	Persistent cough with sputum production on most days (particularly upon arising), for a minimum of 3 consecutive months each year for at least 2 years. Sputum production (gray, white, or yellow) may be copious (chronic bronchitis).
	Intermittent cough episodes, usually nonproductive in early stages although may become productive (emphysema).

History of recurrent pneumonia, long-term exposure to chemical pollution/respiratory irritants (e.g., cigarette smoke) or occupation dust/fumes (e.g., cotton hemp, asbestos, coal dust, sawdust).

Familial and hereditary factors, i.e., deficiency of alpha$_1$-antitrypsin (emphysema).

Use of oxygen at night or continuously.

May exhibit: Respirations: Usually rapid, may be shallow; prolonged expiratory phase with grunting, pursed-lip breathing (emphysema).

Assumption of 3-point ("tripod") position for breathing (especially with acute exacerbation of chronic bronchitis).

Use of accessory muscles for respiration, e.g., elevated shoulder girdle, retraction of supraclavicular fossae, flaring of nares.

Chest: May appear hyperinflated with increased AP diameter (barrel-shaped); minimal diaphragmatic movement.

Breath sounds: May be faint with expiratory wheezes (emphysema); scattered, fine, or coarse moist crackles (bronchitis); rhonchi, wheezing throughout lung fields on expiration and possibly during inspiration progressing to diminished or absent breath sounds (asthma).

Percussion: Hyperresonant over lung fields (e.g., air-trapping with emphysema); dull over lung fields (e.g., consolidation, fluid, mucus).

Difficulty speaking sentences or more than 4 or 5 words at one time.

Color: Pallor with cyanosis of lips, nailbeds; overall duskiness; ruddy color (chronic bronchitis, "blue bloaters"). Patients with moderate emphysema are often called "pink puffers" because of normal skin color despite abnormal gas exchange and rapid respiratory rate.

Clubbing of the fingers (emphysema).

SAFETY:

May report: History of allergic reactions or sensitivity to substances/environmental factors.

Recent/recurrent infections.

Flushing/perspiration (asthma).

SEXUALITY

May report: Decreased libido.

SOCIAL INTERACTION

May report: Dependent relationship(s).

Lack of support systems.

Insufficient support from/to partner/SO.

Prolonged disease or disability progression.

May exhibit: Inability to converse/maintain voice because of respiratory distress.

Limited physical mobility.

Neglectful relationships with other family members.

TEACHING/LEARNING

May report: Use/misuse of respiratory drugs.

Difficulty stopping smoking.

Regular use of alcohol.

Failure to improve.

151

Discharge Plan Considerations:

DRG projected mean length of stay: 5.9 days.

Assistance with shopping, transportation, self-care needs, homemaker/home maintenance tasks.

Changes in medication/therapeutic treatments.

DIAGNOSTIC STUDIES

Chest x-ray: May reveal hyperinflation of lungs; flattened diaphragm; increased retrosternal air space; decreased vascular markings/bullae (emphysema); increased bronchovascular markings (bronchitis); normal findings during periods of remission (asthma).

Pulmonary function tests: Done to determine cause of dyspnea, to determine whether functional abnormality is obstructive or restrictive, to estimate degree of dysfunction and to evaluate effects of therapy, e.g., bronchodilators.

TLC: Increased in advanced bronchitis and occasionally in asthma; decreased in emphysema.

Inspiratory capacity: Reduced in emphysema.

Residual volume: Increased in emphysema, chronic bronchitis, and asthma.

FEV_1/FVC: Ratio of forced expiratory volume to forced vital capacity is decreased in bronchitis and asthma.

ABGs: Estimates progression of chronic disease process, e.g., most often PaO_2 is decreased, and $PaCO_2$ is normal or increased (chronic bronchitis and emphysema) but is often decreased in asthma; pH normal or acidotic, mild respiratory alkalosis secondary to hyperventilation (moderate emphysema or asthma).

Bronchogram: Can show cylindrical dilation of bronchi on inspiration; bronchial collapse on forced expiration (emphysema); enlarged mucous ducts seen in bronchitis.

CBC and differential: Increased hemoglobin (advanced emphysema), increased eosinophils (asthma).

Blood chemistry: alpha 1-antitrypsin done to verify deficiency and a diagnosis of primary emphysema.

Sputum: Culture to determine presence of infection, identify pathogen; cytologic examination to rule out underlying malignancy or allergic disorder.

ECG: Right axis deviation, peaked P-waves (severe asthma); atrial dysrhythmias (bronchitis), tall, peaked P-waves in leads II, III, AVF (bronchitis, emphysema); vertical QRS axis (emphysema).

Exercise ECG, stress test: Helps in assessing degree of pulmonary dysfunction, evaluating effectiveness of bronchodilator therapy, planning/evaluating exercise program.

NURSING PRIORITIES

1. Maintain airway patency.
2. Assist with measures to facilitate gas exchange.
3. Enhance nutritional intake.
4. Prevent complications, slow progression of condition.
5. Provide information about disease process/prognosis and treatment regimen.

DISCHARGE GOALS

1. Ventilation/oxygenation adequate to meet self-care needs.
2. Nutritional intake meeting caloric needs.
3. Infection free.
4. Disease process/prognosis and therapeutic regimen understood.

NURSING DIAGNOSIS:	AIRWAY CLEARANCE, INEFFECTIVE
May be related to:	Bronchospasm.

	Increased production of secretions, retained secretions, thick, viscous secretions.
	Decreased energy/fatigue.
Possibly evidenced by:	Statement of difficulty breathing.
	Changes in depth/rate of respirations, use of accessory muscles.
	Abnormal breath sounds, e.g., wheezes, rhonchi, crackles.
	Cough (persistent), with/without sputum production.
DESIRED OUTCOMES/ EVALUATION CRITERIA— PATIENT WILL:	Maintain patent airway with breath sounds clear/clearing.
	Demonstrate behaviors to improve airway clearance, e.g., cough effectively and expectorate secretions.

ACTIONS/INTERVENTIONS

Independent

Auscultate breath sounds. Note adventitious breath sounds, e.g., wheezes, crackles, rhonchi.

Assess/monitor respiratory rate. Note inspiratory/expiratory ratio.

Note presence/degree of dyspnea, e.g., reports of "air hunger," restlessness, anxiety, respiratory distress, use of accessory muscles.

Assist the patient to assume.position of comfort, e.g., elevate head of bed, sitting on edge of bed.

Keep environmental pollution to a minimum, e.g., dust, smoke, and feather pillows according to individual situation.

Encourage/assist with abdominal or pursed-lip breathing exercises.

Observe characteristics of cough, e.g., persistent, hacking, moist. Assist with measures to improve effectiveness of cough effort.

RATIONALE

Some degree of bronchospasm is present with obstructions in airway and may/may not be manifested in adventitious breath sounds, e.g., scattered, moist crackles (bronchitis); faint sounds, with expiratory wheezes (emphysema); or absent breath sounds (severe asthma).

Tachypnea is usually present in some degree and may be pronounced on admission or during stress/concurrent acute infectious process. Respirations may be shallow and rapid with prolonged expiration in comparison to inspiration.

Respiratory dysfunction is variable dependent on stage of chronic process in addition to acute process that precipitated hospitalization, e.g., infection, allergic reaction.

Elevation of the head of the bed facilitates respiratory function by use of gravity. However, the patient in severe distress will seek the position that most eases breathing. Supporting arms/legs with table, pillows, and so on helps reduce muscle fatigue and can aid chest expansion.

Precipitators of allergic type of respiratory reactions that can trigger onset of acute episode.

Provides the patient with some means to cope with and control dyspnea and reduce air-trapping.

Cough can be persistent but ineffective, especially if the patient is elderly, acutely ill, or debilitated. Coughing is most effective in an upright or in a head-down position after chest percussion.

153

ACTIONS/INTERVENTIONS	RATIONALE
Independent	
Increase fluid intake to 3000 ml/d *within cardiac tolerance.* Provide warm/tepid liquids. Recommend intake of fluids between, instead of during, meals.	Hydration helps decrease the viscosity of secretions, facilitating expectoration. Using warm liquids may decrease bronchospasm. Fluids during meals can increase gastric distention and pressure on the diaphragm.
Collaborative	
Administer medications as indicated:	
Bronchodilators: e.g., β-agonists: epinephrine (Adrenalin, Vaponefrin); albuterol (Proventil, Ventolin); terbutaline (Brethine, Brethaire); isoetharine (Bronkosol, Bronkometer);	Relaxes smooth muscles and reduces local congestion, reducing airway spasm, wheezing, and mucous production. Medications may be oral, injected, or inhaled.
xanthines, e.g., aminophylline, oxtriphylline (Choledyl); theophylline (Bronkodyl, Theo-Dur);	Decreases mucosal edema and smooth muscle spasm (bronchospasm) by indirectly increasing cyclic AMP. May also reduce muscle fatigue/respiratory failure by increasing diaphragmatic contractility. Although theophylline has been the cornerstone of therapy, use of theophylline may be of little or no benefit in presence of adequate β-agonist regimen. However, it may sustain bronchodilation as effect of β-agonist diminishes between doses. Recent research suggests theophylline use may correlate with reduced frequency of hospitalization.
cromolyn (Intal), flunisolide (Aerobid);	Decreases local airway inflammation and edema by inhibiting effects of histamine and other mediators.
Oral, IV, and inhaled steroids: methylprednisolone (Medrol); dexamethasone (Decadral); antihistamines, e.g., beclomethasone (Vanceril, Beclonent); triamcinolone (Azmacort);	Corticosteroids may be used to prevent allergic reactions/inhibit release of histamine, reducing severity and frequency of airway spasm, respiratory inflammation, and dyspnea.
Antimicrobials;	Various antimicrobials may be indicated for control of respiratory infection/pneumonia. Note: Even in the absence of pneumonia, therapy may enhance airflow and improve outcome.
Analgesics, cough suppressants/antitussives, e.g., codeine, dextromethorphan products (Benylin DM, Comtrex, Novahistine).	Persistent, exhausting cough may need to be suppressed to conserve energy and permit the patient to rest.
Provide supplemental humidification, e.g., ultrasonic nebulizer, aerosol room humidifier.	Humidity reduces viscosity of secretions facilitating expectoration and may help reduce/prevent formation of thick mucous plug in bronchioles.
Assist with respiratory treatments, e.g., IPPB, chest physiotherapy.	Postural drainage and percussion are an important part of the treatment for removal of excessive/sticky secretions and improved ventilation of bottom lung segments. *Note:* May aggravate bronchospasms in asthmatics.
Monitor/graph serial ABGs, pulse oximetry, chest x-ray.	Establishes baseline for monitoring progression/regression of disease process and complications.

NURSING DIAGNOSIS:	GAS EXCHANGE, IMPAIRED
May be related to:	Altered oxygen supply (obstruction of airways by secretions, bronchospasm; air-trapping).
	Alveoli destruction.
Possibly evidenced by:	Dyspnea.
	Confusion, restlessness.
	Inability to move secretions.
	Abnormal ABG values (hypoxia and hypercapnia).
	Changes in vital signs.
	Reduced tolerance for activity.
DESIRED OUTCOMES/ EVALUATION CRITERIA— PATIENT WILL:	Demonstrate improved ventilation and adequate oxygenation of tissues by ABGs within patient's normal range and free of symptoms of respiratory distress.
	Participate in treatment regimen within level of ability/situation.

ACTIONS/INTERVENTIONS	RATIONALE
Independent	
Assess respiratory rate, depth. Note use of accessory muscles, pursed-lip breathing, inability to speak/converse.	Useful in evaluating the degree of respiratory distress, and/or chronicity of the disease process.
Elevate head of bed, assist patient to assume position to ease work of breathing. Encourage deep-slow or pursed-lip breathing as individually needed/tolerated.	Oxygen delivery may be improved by upright position and breathing exercises to decrease airway collapse, dyspnea, and work of breathing.
Assess/routinely monitor skin and mucous membrane color.	Cyanosis may be peripheral (noted in nailbeds) or central (noted around lips/or earlobes). Duskiness and central cyanosis would indicate advanced hypoxemia.
Encourage expectoration of sputum; suction when indicated.	Thick, tenacious, copious secretions are a major source of impaired gas exchange in small airways. Deep suctioning may be required when cough is ineffective for expectoration of secretions.
Auscultate breath sounds, noting areas of decreased airflow and/or adventitious sounds.	Breath sounds may be faint because of decreased airflow or areas of consolidation. Presence of wheezes may indicate bronchospasm/retained secretions. Scattered moist crackles may indicate interstitial fluid/cardiac decompensation.
Palpate for fremitus.	Decrease of vibratory tremors suggests fluid collection or air-trapping.

155

ACTIONS/INTERVENTIONS	RATIONALE

Independent

Monitor level of consciousness/mental status. Investigate changes.

Restlessness and anxiety are common manifestations of hypoxia. Worsening ABGs accompanied by confusion/somnolence are indicative of cerebral dysfunction due to hypoxemia.

Evaluate level of activity tolerance. Provide calm, quiet environment. Limit patient's activity or encourage bed/chair rest during acute phase. Have patient resume activity gradually and increase as individually tolerated.

During severe/acute/refractory respiratory distress the patient may be totally unable to perform basic self-care activities because of hypoxemia and dyspnea. Rest interspersed with care activities remains an important part of treatment regimen. However, an exercise program is aimed at increasing endurance and strength without causing severe dyspnea, and can enhance sense of well-being.

Monitor vital signs and cardiac rhythm.

Tachycardia, dysrhythmias, and changes in BP can reflect effect of systemic hypoxemia on cardiac function.

Collaborative

Monitor/graph serial ABGs and pulse oximetry.

$PaCO_2$ usually elevated (bronchitis, emphysema) and PaO_2 is generally decreased, so that hypoxia is present in a lesser or greater degree. Note: A "normal" or increased $PaCO_2$ signals impending respiratory failure for asthmatics.

Administer supplemental oxygen judiciously as indicated by ABG results and patient tolerance.

May correct/prevent worsening of hypoxia. Note: Chronic emphysema, patient's respiratory drive is determined by the CO_2 level and may be eliminated by excess elevation of PaO_2.

Administer CNS depressant (e.g., antianxiety, sedative, or narcotic) with caution.

May be used to control anxiety/restlessness which increases oxygen consumption/demand, exacerbating dyspnea. Must be monitored closely as respiratory failure can occur.

Assist with intubation, institution/maintenance of mechanical ventilation, and transfer to critical care area dependent on patient directives.

Development of/impending respiratory failure requires prompt life-saving measures.

NURSING DIAGNOSIS:	NUTRITION, ALTERED, LESS THAN BODY REQUIREMENTS
May be related to:	Dyspnea.
	Fatigue.
	Medication side effects.
	Sputum production.
	Anorexia, nausea/vomiting.
Possibly evidenced by:	Weight loss.

Loss of muscle mass, poor muscle tone.

Fatigue.

Reported altered taste sensation.

Aversion to eating, lack of interest in food.

DESIRED OUTCOMES/ EVALUATION CRITERIA— PATIENT WILL:

Display progressive weight gain toward goal as appropriate.

Demonstrate behaviors/lifestyle changes to regain and/or maintain appropriate weight.

ACTIONS/INTERVENTIONS	RATIONALE

Independent

Assess dietary habits, recent food intake. Note degree of difficulty with eating. Evaluate weight and body size (mass).

The patient in acute respiratory distress is often anorectic because of dyspnea, sputum production, medications. In addition, many COPD patients habitually eat poorly, even though respiratory insufficiency creates a hypermetabolic state with increased caloric needs. As a result, patient often is admitted with some degree of malnutrition. People who have emphysema are often thin with wasted musculature.

Auscultate bowel sounds.

Diminished/hypoactive bowel sounds may reflect decreased gastric motility and constipation (common complication) related to limited fluid intake, poor food choices, decreased activity, and hypoxemia.

Give frequent oral care, remove expectorated secretions promptly, provide specific container for disposal of secretions and tissues.

Noxious tastes, smells, and sights are prime deterrents to appetite and can produce nausea and vomiting with increased respiratory difficulty.

Encourage a rest period of 1 hour before and after meals. Provide frequent small feedings.

Helps to reduce fatigue during mealtime and provides opportunity to increase total caloric intake.

Avoid gas-producing foods and carbonated beverages.

Can produce abdominal distention, which hampers abdominal breathing and diaphragmatic movement, and can increase dyspnea.

Avoid very hot or very cold foods.

Extremes in temperature can precipitate/aggravate coughing spasms.

Weigh as indicated.

Useful in determining caloric needs, setting weight goal, and evaluating adequacy of nutritional plan. *Note:* Weight loss may continue initially, despite adequate intake, as edema is resolving.

Collaborative

Consult dietician/nutritional support team to provide easily digested, nutritionally balanced meals by appropriate means, e.g., oral, supplemental/ tube feedings, parenteral nutrition. (Refer to CP: Total Nutritional Support, p 1039)

Method of feeding and caloric requirements is based on individual situation/needs to provide maximal nutrients with minimal patient effort/ energy expenditure.

ACTIONS/INTERVENTIONS

Collaborative

Review laboratory studies, e.g., serum albumin, transferrin, amino acid profile, iron, nitrogen balance studies, glucose, liver function studies, electrolytes. Administer vitamins/minerals/electrolytes as indicated.

Administer supplemental oxygen during meals, as indicated.

RATIONALE

Evaluates/treats deficits and monitors effectiveness of nutritional therapy.

Decreases dyspnea and increases energy for eating enhancing intake.

NURSING DIAGNOSIS:	INFECTION, HIGH RISK FOR
Risk factors may include:	Inadequate primary defenses (decreased ciliary action, stasis of secretions).
	Inadequate acquired immunity (tissue destruction, increased environmental exposure).
	Chronic disease process.
	Malnutrition.
Possibly evidenced by:	[Not applicable; presence of signs and symptoms establishes an actual diagnosis.]
DESIRED OUTCOMES/ EVALUATION CRITERIA— PATIENT WILL:	Verbalize understanding of individual causative/risk factors.
	Identify interventions to prevent/reduce risk of infection.
	Demonstrate techniques, lifestyle changes to promote safe environment.

ACTIONS/INTERVENTIONS

Independent

Monitor temperature.

Review importance of breathing exercises, effective cough, frequent position changes, and adequate fluid intake.

Observe color, character, odor of sputum.

Demonstrate and assist the patient in disposal of tissues and sputum. Stress proper handwashing (nurse and patient), and use gloves when handling/disposing of tissues, sputum containers.

Monitor visitors; provide masks as indicated.

RATIONALE

Fever may be present because of infection and/or dehydration.

These activities promote mobilization and expectoration of secretions to reduce risk of developing pulmonary infection.

Odorous, yellow, or greenish secretions suggest the presence of pulmonary infection.

Prevents spread of fluid-borne pathogens.

Reduces potential for exposure to infectious illnesses, (e.g., URI).

ACTIONS/INTERVENTIONS

Independent

Encourage balance between activity and rest.

Discuss need for adequate nutritional intake.

Collaborative

Obtain sputum specimen by deep coughing or suctioning for Gram stain, culture/sensitivity.

Administer antimicrobials as indicated.

RATIONALE

Reduces oxygen consumption/demand imbalance and improves patient's resistance to infection, promoting healing.

Malnutrition can affect general well-being and lower resistance to infection.

Done to identify causative organism and susceptibility to various antimicrobials.

May be given for specific organisms identified by culture and sensitivity, or be given prophylactically because of high risk.

NURSING DIAGNOSIS:	**KNOWLEDGE DEFICIT [LEARNING NEED], REGARDING CONDITION, TREATMENT**
May be related to:	Lack of information/unfamiliarity with information resources.
	Information misinterpretation.
	Lack of recall/cognitive limitation.
Possibly evidenced by:	Request for information.
	Statement of concerns/misconception.
	Inaccurate follow-through of instructions.
	Development of preventable complications.
DESIRED OUTCOMES/ EVALUATION CRITERIA— PATIENT WILL:	Verbalize understanding of condition/disease process and treatment.
	Identify relationship of current signs/symptoms to the disease process and correlate these with causative factors.
	Initiate necessary lifestyle changes and participate in treatment regimen.

ACTIONS/INTERVENTIONS

Independent

Explain/reinforce explanations of individual disease process. Encourage patient/SO to ask questions.

Instruct/reinforce rationale for breathing exercises, coughing effectively, and general conditioning exercises.

RATIONALE

Decreases anxiety and can lead to improved participation in treatment plan.

Pursed-lip and abdominal/diaphragmatic breathing exercises strengthen muscles of respiration, help minimize collapse of small airways, and pro-

ACTIONS/INTERVENTIONS	RATIONALE
Independent	
	vide the individual with means to control dyspnea. General conditioning exercises increase activity tolerance, muscle strength, and sense of well-being.
Discuss respiratory medications, side effects, adverse reactions.	These patients are frequently on several respiratory drugs at once that have similar side effects and potential drug interactions. It is important that the patient understand the difference between nuisance side effects (medication continued), and untoward or adverse side effects (medication possibly discontinued/changed).
Demonstrate technique for using a metered-dose inhaler (MDI), such as how to hold it, taking 2–5 minutes between puffs, cleaning the inhaler.	Proper administration of drug enhances delivery and effectiveness.
Devise system for recording prescribed intermittent drug/inhaler usage.	Reduces risk of improper use/overdosage of prn medications, especially during acute exacerbations, when cognition may be impaired.
Recommend avoidance of sedative antianxiety agents unless specifically prescribed/approved by physician treating respiratory condition.	Although the patient may be nervous and feel the need for sedatives, these can depress respiratory drive and protective cough mechanisms.
Stress importance of oral care/dental hygiene.	Decreases bacterial growth in the mouth, which can lead to pulmonary infections.
Discuss importance of avoiding people with active respiratory infections. Stress need for routine influenza/pneumococcal vaccinations.	Decreases exposure to and incidence of acquired acute upper respiratory infections.
Discuss individual factors that may aggravate condition, e.g., excessively dry air, wind, environmental temperature extremes, pollen, tobacco smoke, aerosol sprays, air pollution. Encourage patient/SO to explore ways to control these factors in and around the home.	These environmental factors can induce/aggravate bronchial irritation leading to increased secretion production and airway blockage.
Review the harmful effects of smoking and advise cessation of smoking by patient and/or SO.	Cessation of smoking may slow/halt progression of COPD. However, even when patient wants to stop smoking, support groups and medical monitoring may be needed. *Note:* Research studies indicate that "side-stream" or "second hand" smoke can be as detrimental as actually smoking.
Provide information about activity limitations and alternating activities with rest periods to prevent fatigue; ways to conserve energy during activities (e.g., pulling instead of pushing, sitting instead of standing while performing tasks); use of pursed-lip breathing, sidelying position, and possible need for supplemental oxygen during sexual activity.	Having this knowledge can enable patient to make informed choices/decisions to reduce dyspnea, maximize activity level, perform most desired activities, and prevent complications.
Discuss importance of medical follow-up care, periodic chest x-rays, sputum cultures.	Monitoring disease process allows for alterations in therapeutic regimen to meet changing needs and may help prevent complications.

ACTIONS/INTERVENTIONS	RATIONALE
Independent	
Review oxygen requirements/dosage for patient who is discharged on supplemental oxygen.	Reduces risk of misuse (too little/too much) and resultant complications.
Instruct patient/SO in safe use of oxygen and refer to supplier as indicated.	Promotes environmental/physical safety.
Refer to/encourage participation in support groups, e.g., American Lung Association, public health department.	These patients and their SOs may experience anxiety, depression, and other reactions as they deal with a chronic disease that has an impact on their desired lifestyle. Support groups and/or home visits may be desired or needed to provide assistance, emotional support, and respite care.
Refer for evaluation of home care if indicated. Provide a detailed care plan and baseline physical assessment to home care nurse as needed on discharge from acute care.	Provides for continuity of care. May help reduce frequency of rehospitalization.

Pneumonia: Microbial _____

Pneumonia is an inflammation of the lung parenchyma, usually associated with the filling of the alveoli with fluid. Likely causes include various infectious agents, chemical irritants, and radiation therapy. This care plan deals with bacterial and viral pneumonias, e.g., pneumococcal pneumonia, pneumocystis carinni, haemophilus influenza, mycoplasma, Gram-negative.

RELATED CONCERNS:

Adult Respiratory Distress Syndrome (ARDS), p 217
AIDS, p 850
Chronic Obstructive Pulmonary Disease, p 149
Inflammatory Cardiac Conditions, p 126
Intracranial Infections, p 307
Psychosocial Aspects of Acute Care, p 899
Sepsis/Septicemia, p 887
Surgical Intervention, p 918

PATIENT ASSESSMENT DATA BASE

ACTIVITY/REST

May report:	Fatigue, weakness.
	Insomnia.
May exhibit:	Lethargy.
	Decreased tolerance to activity.

CIRCULATION

May report:	History of recent/chronic CHF.
May exhibit:	Tachycardia.
	Flushed appearance or pallor.

EGO INTEGRITY

May report:	Multiple stressors, financial concerns.

FOOD/FLUID

May report:	Loss of appetite, nausea/vomiting.
	History of diabetes mellitus.
May exhibit:	Distended abdomen.
	Hyperactive bowel sounds.
	Dry skin with poor turgor.
	Cachectic appearance (malnutrition).

NEUROSENSORY

May report:	Frontal headache (influenza).
May exhibit:	Changes in mentation (confusion, somnolence).

PAIN/COMFORT

May report: Headache.

Chest pain (pleuritic), aggravated by cough; substernal chest pain (influenza).

Myalgia, arthralgia.

May exhibit: Splinting/guarding over affected area (patient commonly lies on affected side to restrict movement).

RESPIRATION

May report: History of recurrent/chronic URI, COPD, cigarette smoking.

Tachypnea, progressive dyspnea; shallow grunting respirations, use of accessory muscles, nasal flaring.

Cough: Dry hacking (initially) progressing to productive cough.

May exhibit: Sputum: Pink, rusty, or purulent.

Percussion: Dull over consolidated areas.

Fremitus: Tactile and vocal gradually increases with consolidation.

Pleural friction rub.

Breath sounds: Diminished or absent over involved area, or bronchial breath sounds over area(s) of consolidation. Coarse inspiratory crackles.
Color: Pallor or cyanosis of lips/nailbeds.

SAFETY

May report: History of altered immune system: i.e., SLE, AIDS, steroid or chemotherapy use, institutionalization, general debilitation.

Fever (e.g., 102–104° F).

May exhibit: Diaphoresis.

Shaking/recurrent chills.

Rash may be noted in cases of rubeola or varicella.

TEACHING/LEARNING

May report: History of recent surgery; chronic alcohol use.

Discharge Plan Considerations: **DRG projected mean length of stay: 6.8 days.**

Assistance with self-care, homemaker tasks.

Oxygen may be needed, if predisposing condition exists.

DIAGNOSTIC STUDIES

Chest x-ray: Identifies structural distribution (e.g., lobar, bronchial); may also reveal multiple abscesses/infiltrates, empyema (staphylococcus); scattered or localized infiltration (bacterial); or diffuse/extensive nodular infiltrates (more often viral). In mycoplasmal pneumonia, chest x-ray may be clear.

ABGs/pulse oximetry: Abnormalities may be present, depending on extent of lung involvement and underlying lung disease.

Gram stain/cultures of sputum and blood: May be obtained by needle biopsy, transtracheal aspiration, fiberoptic bronchoscopy, or open lung biopsy to recover causative organism. More than 1 type of organism may be present; common bacteria include Diplococcus pneumoniae, Staphylococcus aureus, A-hemolytic streptococcus, Hemophilus influenzae; CMV. Note: Sputum cultures may not identify all offending organisms. Blood cultures may show transient bacteriemia.

CBC: Leukocytosis usually present, although a low WBC may be present in viral infection, immunosuppressed conditions such as AIDS, overwhelming bacterial pneumonia.

Serologic studies, e.g., viral or Legionella titers, cold agglutinins: Assist in differential diagnosis of specific organism.

ESR: Increased.

Lung function studies: Volumes may be decreased (congestion and alveolar collapse); airway pressure may be increased and compliance decreased. Shunting will be present (hypoxemia).

Electrolytes: Sodium and chloride may be low.

Bilirubin: May be increased.

Percutaneous aspiration/open biopsy of lung tissues: May reveal typical intranuclear and cytoplasmic inclusions (CMV); characteristic giant cells (rubeola).

NURSING PRIORITIES

1. Maintain/improve respiratory function.
2. Prevent complications.
3. Support recuperative process.
4. Provide information about disease process/prognosis and treatment.

DISCHARGE GOALS

1. Ventilation and oxygenation adequate for individual needs.
2. Complications prevented/minimized.
3. Disease process/prognosis and therapeutic regimen understood.
4. Lifestyle changes identified/initiated to prevent recurrence.

NURSING DIAGNOSIS:	**AIRWAY CLEARANCE, INEFFECTIVE**
May be related to:	Tracheal bronchial inflammation, edema formation, increased sputum production.
	Pleuritic pain.
	Decreased energy, fatigue.
Possibly evidenced by:	Changes in rate, depth of respirations.
	Abnormal breath sounds, use of accessory muscles.
	Dyspnea, cyanosis.
	Cough, effective or ineffective; with/without sputum production.
DESIRED OUTCOMES/ EVALUATION CRITERIA— PATIENT WILL:	Identify/display behaviors to achieve airway clearance.
	Demonstrate patent airway with breath sounds clearing, absence of dyspnea, cyanosis.

ACTIONS/INTERVENTIONS	RATIONALE
Independent	
Assess rate/depth of respirations and chest movement.	Tachypnea, shallow respirations, and asymmetric chest movement are frequently present because of

ACTIONS/INTERVENTIONS	RATIONALE
Independent	
	discomfort of moving chest wall and/or fluid in lung.
Auscultate lung fields, noting areas of decreased/absent airflow and adventitious breath sounds, e.g., crackles, wheezes.	Decreased airflow occurs in areas consolidated with fluid. Bronchial breath sounds (normal over bronchus) can also occur in consolidated areas. Crackles, rhonchi, and wheezes are heard on inspiration and/or expiration in response to fluid accumulation, thick secretions, and airway spasm/obstruction.
Elevate head of bed, change position frequently.	Lowers diaphragm, promoting chest expansion, aeration of lung segments, mobilization and expectoration of secretions.
Assist patient with frequent deep-breathing exercises. Demonstrate/help patient learn to perform coughing, e.g., splinting chest and effective coughing while in upright position.	Deep breathing facilitates maximum expansion of the lungs/smaller airways. Coughing is a natural self-cleaning mechanism, assisting the cilia to maintain patent airways. Splinting reduces chest discomfort, and an upright position favors deeper, more forceful cough effort.
Suction as indicated.	Stimulates cough or mechanically clears airway in patient who is unable to do so because of ineffective cough or decreased level of consciousness.
Force fluids to at least 2500 ml/d (unless contraindicated). Offer warm, rather than cold, fluids.	Fluids (especially warm liquids) aid in mobilization and expectoration of secretions.
Collaborative	
Assist with/monitor effects of nebulizer treatments and other respiratory physiotherapy, e.g., incentive spirometer, IPPB, blow bottles, percussion, postural drainage. Perform treatments between meals and limit fluids when appropriate.	Facilitates liquefaction and removal of secretions. Postural drainage may not be effective in interstitial pneumonias or those causing alveolar exudate/destruction. Coordination of treatments/schedules and oral intake reduces likelihood of vomiting with coughing, expectorations.
Administer medications as indicated: mucolytics, expectorants, bronchodilators, analgesics.	Aids in reduction of bronchospasm as well as mobilization of secretions. Analgesics are given to improve cough effort by reducing discomfort but should be used cautiously, as they can decrease cough effort/depress respirations.
Provide supplemental fluids, e.g., IV, humidified oxygen, and room humidification.	Fluids are required to replace losses (including insensible) and aid in mobilization of secretions.
Monitor serial chest x-rays, ABGs, pulse oximetry readings. (Refer to ND: Gas Exchange, Impaired, p 166.)	Follows progress and effects of disease process and facilitates necessary alterations in therapy.
Assist with bronchoscopy/thoracentesis, if indicated.	Occasionally needed to remove mucous plugs, drain purulent secretions, and/or prevent atelectasis.

NURSING DIAGNOSIS:	GAS EXCHANGE, IMPAIRED
May be related to:	Alveolar-capillary membrane changes (inflammatory effects).
	Altered oxygen-carrying capacity of blood (fever, shifting oxyhemoglobin curve).
	Altered delivery of oxygen (hypoventilation).
Possibly evidenced by:	Dyspnea, cyanosis.
	Tachycardia.
	Restlessness/changes in mentation.
	Hypoxia.
DESIRED OUTCOMES/ EVALUATION CRITERIA— PATIENT WILL:	Demonstrate improved ventilation and oxygenation of tissues by ABGs within patient's normal range and absence of symptoms of respiratory distress.
	Participate in actions to maximize oxygenation.

ACTIONS/INTERVENTIONS	RATIONALE
Independent	
Assess respiratory rate, depth, and ease.	Manifestations of respiratory distress are dependent on/and indicative of the degree of lung involvement and underlying general health status.
Observe color of skin, mucous membranes, and nail beds, noting presence of peripheral cyanosis (nail beds), or central cyanosis (circumoral).	Cyanosis of nail beds may represent vasoconstriction or the body response to fever/chills. However, cyanosis of earlobes, mucous membranes, and skin around the mouth ("warm membranes"), is indicative of systemic hypoxemia.
Assess mental status.	Restlessness, irritation, confusion, and somnolence may reflect hypoxemia/decreased cerebral oxygenation.
Monitor heart rate/rhythm.	Tachycardia usually present as a result of fever/dehydration but may represent a response to hypoxemia.
Monitor body temperature, as indicated. Assist with comfort measures to reduce fever and chills, e.g., addition/removal of bedcovers, comfortable room temperature, tepid or cool water sponges.	High fever (common in bacterial pneumonia and influenza) greatly increases metabolic demands and oxygen consumption and alters cellular oxygenation.
Maintain bed rest. Encourage use of relaxation techniques and diversional activities.	Prevents overexhaustion and reduces oxygen consumption/demands to facilitate resolution of infection.
Elevate head and encourage frequent position changes, deep breathing, and effective coughing.	These measures promote maximal inspiration, enhance expectoration of secretions to improve ventilation. (Refer to ND: Airway Clearance, ineffective, p 164.)

ACTIONS/INTERVENTIONS

Independent

Assess level of anxiety. Encourage verbalization of concerns/feelings. Answer questions honestly. Visit frequently, arrange for SO/visitors to stay with patient as indicated.

Observe for deterioration in condition, noting hypotension, copious amounts of pink/bloody sputum, pallor, cyanosis, change in level of consciousness, severe dyspnea, restlessness.

Prepare for/transfer to critical care setting if indicated.

Collaborative

Administer oxygen therapy by appropriate means, e.g., nasal prongs, mask, Venturi mask.

Monitor ABGs, pulse oximetry.

RATIONALE

Anxiety is a manifestation of psychologic concerns as well as physiologic response to hypoxia. Providing reassurance and enhancing sense of security can reduce the psychologic component, thereby decreasing oxygen demand and adverse physiologic response.

Shock and pulmonary edema are the most common causes of death in pneumonia and require immediate medical intervention.

Intubation and mechanical ventilation may be required in the event of severe respiratory insufficiency.

The purpose of oxygen therapy is to maintain PaO_2 above 60 mm Hg. Oxygen is administered by the method that provides appropriate delivery within the patient's tolerance.

Follows progress of disease process and facilitates alterations in pulmonary therapy.

NURSING DIAGNOSIS:	INFECTION, HIGH RISK FOR [SPREAD]
Risk factors may include:	Inadequate primary defenses (decreased ciliary action, stasis of respiratory secretions).
	Inadequate secondary defenses (presence of existing infection, immunosuppression) chronic disease, malnutrition.
Possibly evidenced by:	[Not applicable; presence of signs and symptoms establishes an actual diagnosis.]
DESIRED OUTCOMES/ EVALUATION CRITERIA— PATIENT WILL:	Achieve timely resolution of current infection without complications.
	Identify interventions to prevent/reduce risk of infection.

ACTIONS/INTERVENTIONS

Independent

Monitor vital signs closely, especially during initiation of therapy.

Instruct patient concerning the disposition of secretions (e.g., raising and expectoration versus swallowing) and reporting changes in color, amount, odor of secretions.

RATIONALE

During this period of time, potentially fatal complications (hypotension/shock) may develop.

Although patient may find expectoration offensive and attempt to limit or avoid it, it is essential that sputum be disposed of in a safe manner. Changes in characteristics of sputum reflect resolu-

ACTIONS/INTERVENTIONS

Independent

Demonstrate/encourage good handwashing technique.

Change position frequently and provide good pulmonary toilet.

Limit visitors as indicated.

Institute isolation precautions as individually appropriate.

Encourage adequate rest balanced with moderate activity. Promote adequate nutritional intake.

Monitor effectiveness of antimicrobial therapy.

Investigate sudden changes/deterioration in condition, such as increasing chest pain, extra heart sounds, altered sensorium, recurring fever, changes in sputum characteristics.

Collaborative

Administer antimicrobials as indicated by results of sputum/blood cultures: e.g., penicillins, erythromycin, tetracycline, amikacin; cephalosporins: amantadine.

RATIONALE

tion of pneumonia or development of secondary infection.

Effective means of reducing spread/acquisition of infection.

Promotes expectoration, clearing of infection.

Reduces likelihood of exposure to other infectious pathogens.

Dependent on type of infection, response to antibiotics, patient's general health, and development of complications, isolation techniques may be desired to prevent spread/protect patient from other infectious processes.

Facilitates healing process and enhances natural resistance.

Signs of improvement in condition should occur within 24–48 hours.

Delayed recovery or increase in severity of symptoms suggest resistance to antibiotics or secondary infection. Complications affecting any/all organ systems include lung abscess/empyema, bacteremia, pericarditis/endocarditis, meningitis/encephalitis, and superinfections.

These drugs are used to combat most of the microbial pneumonias. Combinations of antiviral and antifungal agents may be used when the pneumonia is a result of mixed organisms.

NURSING DIAGNOSIS:	ACTIVITY INTOLERANCE
May be related to:	Imbalance between oxygen supply and demand.
	General weakness.
	Exhaustion associated with interruption in usual sleep pattern due to discomfort, excessive coughing, and dyspnea.
Possibly evidenced by:	Verbal reports of weakness, fatigue, exhaustion.
	Exertional dyspnea, tachypnea.
	Tachycardia in response to activity.
	Development/worsening of pallor/cyanosis.
DESIRED OUTCOMES/ EVALUATION CRITERIA— PATIENT WILL:	Report/demonstrate a measurable increase in tolerance to activity with absence of dyspnea, excessive fatigue, and vital signs within patient's normal range.

ACTIONS/INTERVENTIONS

Independent

Evaluate patient's response to activity. Note reports of dyspnea, increased weakness/fatigue, and changes in vital signs during and after activities.

Provide a quiet environment and limit visitors during acute phase as indicated. Encourage use of stress management and diversional activities as appropriate.

Explain importance of rest in treatment plan and necessity for balancing activities with rest.

Assist the patient to assume comfortable position for rest and/or sleep.

Assist with self-care activities as necessary. Provide for progressive increase in activities during recovery phase.

RATIONALE

Establishes patient's capabilities/needs and facilitates choice of interventions.

Reduces stress and excess stimulation, promoting rest.

Bed rest is maintained during acute phase to decrease metabolic demands, conserving energy for healing. Activity restrictions thereafter are determined by individual patient response to activity and resolution of respiratory insufficiency.

Patient may be comfortable with head of bed elevated, sleeping in a chair, or resting forward on overbed table with pillow support.

Minimizes exhaustion and helps to balance oxygen supply and demand.

NURSING DIAGNOSIS: PAIN [ACUTE]

May be related to:
Inflammation of lung parenchyma.
Cellular reactions to circulating toxins.
Persistent coughing.

Possibly evidenced by:
Pleuritic chest pain.
Headache, muscle/joint pain.
Guarding of affected area.
Distraction behaviors, restlessness.

DESIRED OUTCOMES/ EVALUATION CRITERIA— PATIENT WILL:
Verbalize relief/control of pain.
Demonstrate relaxed manner, resting/sleeping, and engaging in activity appropriately.

ACTIONS/INTERVENTIONS

Independent

Determine pain characteristics, e.g., sharp, constant, stabbing. Investigate changes in character/location/intensity of pain.

Monitor vital signs.

RATIONALE

Chest pain, usually present to some degree with pneumonia, may also herald the onset of complications of pneumonia such as pericarditis and endocarditis.

Changes in heart rate or BP may indicate that the patient is experiencing pain, especially when other reasons for changes in vital signs have been ruled out.

ACTIONS/INTERVENTIONS

Independent

Provide comfort measures, e.g., back rubs, change of position, quiet music/conversation, relaxation/breathing exercises.

Offer frequent oral hygiene.

Instruct and assist patient in chest splinting techniques during coughing episodes. (Refer to ND: Airway Clearance, ineffective, p 152.)

Collaborative

Administer analgesics and antitussives as indicated.

RATIONALE

Nonanalgesic measures administered with a gentle touch can alleviate discomfort and augment therapeutic effects of analgesics.

Mouth breathing and oxygen therapy can irritate and dry out mucous membranes, potentiating general discomfort.

Aids in control of chest discomfort while enhancing effectiveness of cough effort.

These medications may be used to suppress nonproductive/paroxysmal cough or reduce excess mucous, enhancing general comfort/rest.

NURSING DIAGNOSIS:	NUTRITION, LESS THAN BODY REQUIREMENTS, HIGH RISK FOR
Risk factors may include:	Increased metabolic needs secondary to fever and infectious process.
	Anorexia associated with bacterial toxins, the odor and taste of sputum, and certain aerosol treatments.
	Abdominal distention/gas associated with swallowing air during dyspneic episodes.
Possibly evidenced by:	[Not applicable; presence of signs and symptoms establishes an actual diagnosis.]
DESIRED OUTCOMES/ EVALUATION CRITERIA— PATIENT WILL:	Demonstrate increased appetite. Maintain/regain desired body weight.

ACTIONS/INTERVENTIONS

Independent

Identify factors that are contributing to nausea/vomiting, e.g., copious sputum, aerosol treatments, severe dyspnea, pain.

Provide covered container for sputum and remove at frequent intervals. Provide/assist with oral hygiene after emesis, after aerosol and postural drainage treatments, and before meals.

Schedule respiratory treatments at least 1 hour before meals.

Auscultate for bowel sounds. Observe/palpate for abdominal distention.

RATIONALE

Choice of interventions is dependent on the underlying cause of the problem.

Eliminates noxious sights, tastes, smells from the patient environment and can reduce nausea.

Reduces effects of nausea associated with these treatments.

Bowel sounds may be diminished/absent if the infectious process is severe/prolonged. Abdominal distention may occur as a result of air swallowing

ACTIONS/INTERVENTIONS

Independent

Provide small, frequent meals, including dry foods (toast, crackers) and/or foods that are appealing to patient.

Evaluate general nutritional state, obtain baseline weight.

RATIONALE

or reflect the influence of bacterial toxins on the GI tract.

These measures may enhance intake even though appetite may be slow to return.

Presence of chronic conditions (such as COPD or alcoholism) or financial limitations can contribute to malnutrition, lowered resistance to infection, and/or delayed response to therapy.

NURSING DIAGNOSIS:	FLUID VOLUME DEFICIT, HIGH RISK FOR
Risk factors may include:	Excessive fluid loss (fever, profuse diaphoresis, mouth breathing/hyperventilation, vomiting).
	Decreased oral intake.
Possibly evidenced by:	[Not applicable; presence of signs and symptoms establishes an actual diagnosis.]
DESIRED OUTCOMES/ EVALUATION CRITERIA— PATIENT WILL:	Demonstrate fluid balance evidenced by individually appropriate parameters, e.g., moist mucous membranes, good skin turgor, prompt capillary refill, stable vital signs.

ACTIONS/INTERVENTIONS

Independent

Assess vital sign changes, e.g., increased temperature/prolonged fever, tachycardia, orthostatic hypotension.

Assess skin turgor, moisture of mucous membranes (lips, tongue).

Note reports of nausea/vomiting.

Monitor intake and output, noting color, character of urine. Calculate fluid balance. Be aware of insensible losses. Weigh as indicated.

Force fluids to at least 2500 ml/d or as individually appropriate.

Collaborative

Administer medications as indicated, e.g., antipyretics, antiemetics.

Provide supplemental IV fluids as necessary.

RATIONALE

Elevated temperature/prolonged fever increases metabolic rate and fluid loss through evaporation. Orthostatic BP changes and increasing tachycardia may indicate systemic fluid deficit.

Indirect indicators of adequacy of fluid volume, although oral mucous membranes may be dry because of mouth-breathing and supplemental oxygen.

Presence of these symptoms reduces oral intake.

Provides information about adequacy of fluid volume and replacement needs.

Meets basic fluid needs, reducing risk of dehydration.

Useful in reducing fluid losses.

In presence of reduced intake/excessive loss, use of parenteral route may correct/prevent deficiency.

171

NURSING DIAGNOSIS:	KNOWLEDGE DEFICIT [LEARNING NEED], REGARDING CONDITION AND TREATMENT NEEDS
May be related to:	Lack of exposure.
	Misinterpretation of information.
	Altered recall.
Possibly evidenced by:	Requests for information.
	Statement of misconception.
	Failure to improve/recurrence.
DESIRED OUTCOMES/ EVALUATION CRITERIA— PATIENT WILL:	Verbalize understanding of condition, disease process, and treatment.
	Initiate necessary lifestyle changes and participate in treatment program.

ACTIONS/INTERVENTIONS	RATIONALE
Independent	
Review normal lung function, pathology of condition.	Promotes understanding of current situation and importance of cooperating with treatment regimen.
Discuss debilitating aspects of disease, length of convalescence, and recovery expectations. Identify self-care and homemaker needs/resources.	Information can enhance coping and help reduce anxiety and excessive concern. Respiratory symptoms may be slow to resolve, and fatigue and weakness can persist for an extended period. These factors may be associated with depression and the need for various forms of support and assistance.
Provide information in written as well as verbal form.	Fatigue and depression can affect ability to assimilate information/follow medical regimen.
Stress importance of continuing effective coughing/deep-breathing exercises.	During initial 6–8 weeks after discharge, patient is at greatest risk for recurrence of pneumonia.
Emphasize necessity for continuing antibiotic therapy for prescribed period.	Early discontinuation of antibiotics may result in failure to completely resolve infectious process.
Review importance of cessation of smoking.	Smoking destroys tracheobronchial ciliary action, irritates bronchial mucosa, and inhibits alveolar macrophages, compromising body's natural defense against infection.
Outline steps to enhance general health and well-being, e.g., balanced rest and activity, well-rounded diet, avoidance of crowds during cold/flu season and persons with upper-respiratory infections.	Increases natural defenses/immunity, limits exposure to pathogens.
Stress importance of continuing medical follow-up and obtaining vaccinations/immunizations as appropriate.	May prevent recurrence of pneumonia and/or related complications.

ACTIONS/INTERVENTIONS	RATIONALE
Independent	
Identify signs/symptoms requiring notification of health care provider, e.g., increasing dyspnea, chest pain, prolonged fatigue, weight loss, fever/chills, persistence of productive cough, changes in mentation.	Prompt evaluation and timely intervention may prevent/minimize complications.

Pulmonary Embolism (PE)

Although PE is a relatively common complication among hospitalized patients, it is often not diagnosed. Even with a massive PE, one that blocks at least 50% of a pulmonary artery, signs and symptoms are not clear-cut. Because PE is so elusive and calls for a quick response, it is crucial to take steps to prevent its occurrence.

RELATED CONCERNS:

Psychosocial Aspects of Acute Care, p 899
Thrombophlebitis: Deep Vein Thrombosis, p 135

PATIENT ASSESSMENT DATA BASE

ACTIVITY/REST

May report:	Fatigue and/or weakness.
	Prolonged bed rest/immobility.
May exhibit:	Exertional dyspnea.
	Abnormal heart rate or BP response to activity.
	Sleep disturbances.

CIRCULATION

May report:	History of vein wall injury, such as surgery or trauma to iliac and pelvic veins, varicose veins, sepsis, burns; recent/current invasive procedures, e.g., central lines, hemodynamic monitoring; coagulation problems, e.g., polycythemia, autoimmune hemolytic anemia, sickle cell disease, transmural/subendocardial/RV myocardial infarction, heart failure.
	Palpitations/irregular pulse.
May exhibit:	Tachycardia.
	Dysrhythmias, e.g., chronic atrial fibrillation.
	Extra heart sounds, i.e., S_3 or S_4.
	Murmur of valvular insufficiency.
	Hypotension.
	Pulses may be normal, weak/thready (shock), or full/bounding (polycythemia vera).
	JVD.
	Extremities: Signs of thrombophlebitis, e.g., phlebotic veins, tense muscle tissue, shiny skin, edema; increased skin temperature.

EGO INTEGRITY

May report:	Apprehension, feelings of impending doom.
	Fear of death.
May exhibit:	Restlessness, trembling, panic behavior.
	Facial tension.
	Increased perspiration.

FOOD/FLUID

May report:	Nausea.
May exhibit:	Leg edema.

174

NEUROSENSORY

May report:
Difficulty in concentrating, altered memory/thinking ability.
Fainting.

May exhibit:
Altered attention span.
Disorientation.
Changes in remote/recent/immediate memory.
Lethargy/stupor.

PAIN/COMFORT

May report:
Chest pain.
Discomfort in extremities (if thrombophlebitis is present).

May exhibit:
Self-focusing/narrowed focus.
Distraction behaviors, facial grimacing, moaning, restlessness.
Splinting of the chest.

RESPIRATION

May report:
History of chronic lung disease.
"Air hunger"/dyspnea.
Cough, pink/bloody/brown sputum.

May exhibit:
Tachypnea.
Dyspnea, gasping/shallow respirations.
Decreased breath sounds; crackles, wheezes; pleural friction rub (if pulmonary infarction has occurred).
Cough (hacking/dry or productive of bloody sputum).

SAFETY

May report:
History of cancer, systemic infection, fractures/trauma to lower extremities, burns.

May exhibit:
Low grade fever.

SEXUALITY

May report:
Current pregnancy, recent delivery.

TEACHING/LEARNING

May report:
Use of oral contraceptives, recent discontinuation of anticoagulants.

Discharge Plan Considerations:
DRG projected mean length of stay: 8.8 days.
Alteration of medication regimen.
Assistance with self-care, homemaker/maintenance tasks.

DIAGNOSTIC STUDIES

Lung scan (ventilation/perfusion scan): May reveal pattern of abnormal perfusion in areas of ventilation (ventilation/perfusion mismatch) or absence of both ventilation and perfusion (confirms diagnosis of PE).

Pulmonary angiography: Most specific study for PE. Presence of a filling defect or artery "cutoff" with no distal blood flow confirms diagnosis.

Chest x-ray: Frequently normal (especially in subacute PE), but may demonstrate shadow of a clot, abrupt vessel cutoff, diaphragmatic elevation on affected side, pleural effusion, infiltrates/consolidation.

ABGs: May show decreased PaO_2, $PaCO_2$ (hypoxemia/hypocarbia) and elevated pH (respiratory alkalosis) especially if pulmonary obstruction is severe.

CBC: May reveal elevated Hct (hemoconcentration); increased RBCs (polycythemia).

ECG: May be normal or demonstrate changes indicative of right ventricular strain, e.g., changes in T waves/ST segment, axis deviation/right bundle branch block. Tachycardia and dysrhythmias (new onset of atrial fibrillation) frequently present.

NURSING PRIORITIES

1. Restore/maintain adequate oxygenation/ventilation.
2. Minimize/prevent complications.
3. Relieve anxiety and pain.
4. Provide information about disease process and treatment.

DISCHARGE GOALS

1. Respiratory function adequate for individual needs.
2. Complications minimized/prevented.
3. Anxiety reduced, pain controlled.
4. Disease process, therapy needs, prevention of complications/recurrence understood.

NURSING DIAGNOSIS:	BREATHING PATTERN, INEFFECTIVE
May be related to:	Tracheobronchial obstruction by blood clot, copious secretions, or active bleeding.
	Decreased lung expansion.
	Inflammatory process.
Possibly evidenced by:	Changes in depth and/or rate of respiration.
	Dyspnea/use of accessory muscles of respiration.
	Altered chest excursion.
	Abnormal breath sounds, e.g., crackles, wheezes.
	Cough, with or without sputum production.
DESIRED OUTCOMES/ EVALUATION CRITERIA— PATIENT WILL:	Demonstrate effective respiratory pattern with rate and depth within patient's normal range and lungs clear/clearing.
	Participate in activities/behaviors to enhance respiratory function.

ACTIONS/INTERVENTIONS	RATIONALE
Independent	
Assess respiratory rate, depth, and chest expansion. Note respiratory effort, including use of accessory muscles/nasal flaring.	Rate is usually increased. Dyspnea ("air hunger") and increased work of breathing is present (may be first or only sign in subacute PE). Depth of res-

ACTIONS/INTERVENTIONS	RATIONALE
Independent	
	pirations varies depending on degree of respiratory failure. Chest expansion may be limited due to atelectasis and/or pleuritic chest pain.
Auscultate breath sounds and note presence of adventitious sounds, such as crackles, wheezes, pleural rub.	Breath sounds may be decreased/absent if airway obstruction is secondary to bleeding, clotting, or small airway collapse (atelectasis). Rhonchi and wheezing also accompany airway obstruction/respiratory failure.
Elevate head of bed and assist with frequent changes of position. Get patient out of bed and ambulate as soon as able.	Upright position favors lung expansion and facilitates respiratory effort. Turning and ambulation enhances aeration of different lung segments, thereby improving gas diffusion.
Observe cough pattern and character of secretions.	Alveolar congestion may produce a dry/irritated cough. Bloody sputum may be the result of tissue destruction (pulmonary infarction) or excessive anticoagulation.
Encourage/assist patient in deep-breathing and coughing exercises. Suction orally or nasotracheally if indicated.	May have increased/copious secretions which impair ventilation and add to the discomfort of breathing effort.
Assist patient to deal with fear/anxiety that may be present. (Refer to ND: Fear/Anxiety [Specify Level], p 180.)	Feelings of fear and severe anxiety are associated with inability to breathe/development of hypoxemia and may actually increase oxygen consumption/demand.
Collaborative	
Administer supplemental oxygen.	Maximizes respiratory effort and may reduce work of breathing.
Provide supplemental humidification, e.g., ultrasonic nebulizers.	Delivers moisture to mucous membranes and helps liquefy secretions to facilitate airway clearance.
Assist with chest physiotherapy (e.g., postural drainage and percussion of nonaffected area, blow bottles/incentive spirometer).	Facilitates deeper respiratory effort and promotes drainage of secretions from lung segments into bronchi, where they may more readily be removed by coughing/suctioning.
Prepare for/assist with bronchoscopy.	Occasionally useful to remove blood clots and clear airways.

NURSING DIAGNOSIS:	GAS EXCHANGE, IMPAIRED
May be related to:	Altered blood flow to alveoli or to major portions of the lung.
	Alveolar-capillary membrane changes (atelectasis, airway/alveolar collapse, pulmonary edema/effusion, excessive secretions/active bleeding).

177

Possibly evidenced by:	Profound dyspnea, restlessness, apprehension, somnolence, cyanosis.
	Changes in ABGs/pulse oximetry, e.g., hypoxemia and hypercapnia.
DESIRED OUTCOMES/ EVALUATION CRITERIA— PATIENT WILL:	Demonstrate adequate ventilation/oxygenation by ABGs within patient's normal range.
	Report/display resolution/absence of symptoms of respiratory distress.

ACTIONS/INTERVENTIONS	RATIONALE

Independent

Note respiratory rate and depth, use of accessory muscles, pursed-lip breathing.	Tachypnea and dyspnea accompany pulmonary obstruction. More severe respiratory failure accompanies moderate to severe loss of functional lung units.
Auscultate lungs for areas of decreased/absent breath sounds and the presence of adventitious sounds, e.g., crackles.	Nonventilated areas may be identified by absence of breath sounds. Crackles occur in fluid-filled tissues/airways or may reflect cardiac decompensation.
Observe for generalized duskiness and cyanosis in "warm tissues" such as earlobes, lips, tongue, and buccal membranes.	Indicative of systemic hypoxemia.
Institute measures to restore/maintain patent airways, e.g., coughing, suctioning. (Refer to ND: Breathing Pattern, ineffective, p 176.)	Plugged/collapsed airways reduce number of functional alveoli, negatively affecting gas exchange.
Elevate head of bed as patient requires/tolerates.	Promotes maximal chest expansion, making it easier to breathe, which enhances physiologic/psychologic comfort.
Monitor vital signs.	Tachycardia, tachypnea, and changes in BP occur with advancing hypoxemia and acidosis.
Assess level of consciousness/mentation changes.	Systemic hypoxemia may be reflected first by restlessness and irritability, then by progressively decreased mentation.
Assess activity tolerance, e.g., complaints of weakness/fatigue during any exertion, or vital sign changes. Encourage rest periods and limit activities to patient tolerance.	Hypoxemia reduces ability to participate in activity without profound dyspnea, tachycardia, dysrhythmias, and possible hypotension. These parameters assist in determining patient response to resumed activities and ability to participate in self-care.

Collaborative

Monitor serial ABGs/pulse oximetry.	Hypoxemia is present in varying degrees, depending on the amount of airway obstruction, prior cardiopulmonary function, and presence/absence of shock. Respiratory alkalosis and metabolic acidosis can also occur.

ACTIONS/INTERVENTIONS	RATIONALE
Collaborative	
Administer oxygen by appropriate method.	Maximizes available oxygen for gas exchange. Oxygen is usually administered by nasal cannula in partial pulmonary obstruction. *Note:* If the obstruction is large or hypoxemia does not respond to supplemental oxygenation it may be necessary to move patient to critical care area for intubation and mechanical ventilation.

NURSING DIAGNOSIS:	**TISSUE PERFUSION, ALTERED, CARDIOPULMONARY, [ACTUAL], AND PERIPHERAL, HIGH RISK FOR**
May be related to:	Interruption of blood flow (arterial/venous).
	Exchange problems at alveolar level or at tissue level (acidotic shifting of the oxyhemoglobin curve).
Possibly evidenced by:	Cardiopulmonary: Ventilation/perfusion mismatch.
	Dyspnea.
	Central cyanosis.
	Peripheral: [Not applicable; presence of signs and symptoms establishes an actual diagnosis.]
DESIRED OUTCOMES/ EVALUATION CRITERIA— PATIENT WILL:	Demonstrate increased perfusion as individually appropriate, e.g., usual/normal mental status, cardiac rhythm/rate and peripheral pulses within normal limits, absence of central/peripheral cyanosis, warm/dry skin, urine output, and specific gravity within normal limits.

ACTIONS/INTERVENTIONS	RATIONALE
Independent	
Auscultate heart rate and rhythm. Note development of extra heart sounds.	Tachycardia is present as a result of hypoxemia and a compensatory effort to increase blood flow and tissue perfusion. Rhythm alterations are related to hypoxemia, electrolyte imbalance, and/or increased right heart strain. Extra heart sounds, i.e., S_3, S_4, may be noted as cardiac workload increases/decompensation occurs.
Observe for changes in mental status.	Restlessness, confusion, disorientation, and/or sensory/motor changes may indicate impaired blood flow, hypoxia, or cerebral vascular accident (CVA) as a result of systemic emboli.
Observe color and temperature of skin/mucous membranes.	Pallor or cyanosis of the skin, nail beds, lips/buccal membranes; or cool, mottled skin are indicative of peripheral vasoconstriction (shock) and/or impaired systemic blood flow.

179

ACTIONS/INTERVENTIONS	RATIONALE
Independent	
Measure urine output and note specific gravity.	Progressing shock/reduced cardiac output leads to decreased kidney perfusion, manifested by decreased urine output with normal or increased specific gravity.
Evaluate extremities for presence/absence/quality of pulses. Note calf tenderness/swelling.	PE is frequently precipitated by thrombus arising from deep veins (pelvis or legs). Signs/symptoms may or may not be readily apparent.
Elevate legs/feet when in bed/chair. Encourage patient to exercise legs by flexing/extending feet at the ankles. Avoid use of knee gatch and sitting or standing for long periods of time. Apply/demonstrate how to apply and remove elastic stockings if used.	These measures are intended to reduce venous stasis in the legs and pooling of blood in the pelvic veins to reduce risk of thrombus formation.
Collaborative	
Administer fluids (IV/PO) as indicated.	Increased fluids may be required to reduce hyperviscosity of blood (potentiates thrombus formation) or to support circulating volume/tissue perfusion.
Monitor diagnostic/laboratory studies, e.g., ECG, electrolytes, BUN/Cr, ABGs, PTT, and PT.	Evaluates changes in organ function and monitors effects of heparin and Coumadin, which may require alterations in dosage.
Administer medications as indicated:	
Heparin (intermittent or continuous IV infusion);	Heparin prevents further thrombus formation by preventing clot propagation. Continuous infusion is preferred to prevent peak and ebb levels from increasing coagulation imbalances. Heparin dosage is gradually reduced during addition of oral anticoagulant for long-term therapy.
Warfarin sodium (Coumadin);	Oral agent used for long-term therapy after initial anticoagulation is achieved.
Thrombolytic agents, e.g., streptokinase (Kabikinase, Streptase); urokinase (Abbokinase, Breakinase); alteplase (t-PA, Activase).	Usually indicated in massive pulmonary obstruction when the patient is seriously hemodynamically threatened. *Note:* These patients will probably be initially cared for/transferred to the critical care setting.
Prepare for surgical intervention if indicated.	Vena caval ligation or insertion of an intracaval umbrella may be useful for patients who experience recurrent emboli despite adequate anticoagulation, when anticoagulation is contraindicated, or when septic emboli arising from below the renal veins do not respond to treatment.

NURSING DIAGNOSIS:	**FEAR/ANXIETY [SPECIFY LEVEL]**
May be related to:	Severe dyspnea/inability to breathe normally.
	Perceived threat of death.

Threat to/change in health status.

Physiologic response to hypoxemia/acidosis.

Concern regarding unknown outcome of situation.

Possibly evidenced by:

Restlessness, irritability.

Withdrawal or attack behavior.

Sympathetic stimulation, e.g., cardiovascular excitation pupil dilation, sweating, vomiting, diarrhea.

Crying, voice quivering.

DESIRED OUTCOMES/ EVALUATION CRITERIA— PATIENT WILL:

Report fear/anxiety relieved or reduced to manageable level.

Appear relaxed and resting/sleeping appropriately.

ACTIONS/INTERVENTIONS	RATIONALE
Independent	
Note degree of anxiety and fear. Inform patient/SO that feelings are normal and encourage expression of feelings.	Understanding that feelings (which are based on stressful situation plus an oxygen imbalance that is being treated) are normal may help the patient regain some feeling of control over emotions.
Explain disease process and procedures within level of patient's ability to understand and handle the information. Review current situation and measures being taken to remedy the problems.	Allays anxiety related to the unknown and reduces fears concerning personal safety. In the early phases of the illness, explanations need to be short and repeated frequently because the patient will have a reduced attention span.
Stay with the patient or make arrangements for someone else to be there during acute attack.	Helpful in reducing anxiety associated with perceived abandonment in presence of severe dyspnea/feelings of impending doom.
Provide comfort measures, e.g., back rub, position changes.	Aids in reducing stress and redirecting attention to enhance relaxation and coping abilities.
Assist the patient to identify helpful behaviors, e.g., assuming position of comfort, focused breathing, relaxation techniques.	Gives patient measure of control to reduce anxiety and muscle tension.
Support patient/SO in dealing with the realities of the situation, especially in planning for long recovery period. Involve patient in planning and participating in care.	Coping mechanisms and participation in treatment regimen may be enhanced as patient learns to deal with the outcomes of the illness and regains some sense of control.
Develop activity program within limits of physical ability.	Provides a healthy outlet for energy generated by feelings.
Be alert for out-of-control behavior or escalating cardiopulmonary dysfunction, e.g., worsening dyspnea and tachycardia.	Development of incapacitating anxiety requires further evaluation and possible intervention with anti-anxiety medications.

181

ACTIONS/INTERVENTIONS	RATIONALE
Independent	
Stress importance of adhering to prescribed medication schedule.	Anticoagulation may be required for 6 weeks–6 months following initial episode. Taking the medication at the same time each day in the prescribed amount will help maintain serum anticoagulation levels within the narrow therapeutic range.
Caution patient to be alert for bleeding from mucous membranes (nose and gums), severe bruising after minimal trauma, development of petechiae, continued oozing from cuts or punctures.	Signs of excessive prolongation of clotting time, which may indicate need for reduction or cessation of anticoagulant therapy.
Identify appropriate safety factors, e.g., use of electric instead of regular razor; gentle brushing of teeth and gums; avoiding forceful blowing of nose and scratching/rubbing of skin.	Enables the patient to avoid trauma-induced bleeding.
Discuss importance of reporting for scheduled follow-up laboratory monitoring and physician's visits.	Medical supervision is important as anticoagulant therapy may be altered/discontinued, depending on information obtained.
Recommend avoiding inactivity, e.g., sitting or standing for periods longer than 1 hour; wearing constricting clothing: proper wearing/removal of elastic stockings as prescribed.	Reduces venous pooling and risk of thrombus formation.
Discuss reasons for informing dentists and other care givers of anticoagulation and avoiding use of new medications (including OTC) without prior clearance by health care provider.	May need to postpone procedures or alter anticoagulant therapy to reduce risk of hemorrhage. Drugs such as antacids, antihistamines, and vitamin C can decrease the effect of Coumadin. Alcohol, antibiotics, and ibuprofen can increase the effect of Coumadin.
Encourage patient to wear a medical alert identification bracelet/tag.	Alerts emergency personnel that patient is taking anticoagulants.

ACTIONS/INTERVENTIONS	RATIONALE

Independent

Discuss and provide a written list of signs/symptoms to report to the physician, e.g., severe dyspnea, tachypnea and chest pain, excessive fatigue, unexplained weight gain,dependent edema, chest tightness;

Precautions are particularly relevant to those patients who have forced immobility, have recurrent thrombophlebitis, or have a history of recurrent pulmonary emboli. Note: Patients surviving severe/multiple PE have increased risk of development of right-sided cardiac failure.

Palpitations;

Pulmonary embolus can precipitate dysrhythmias such as atrial fibrillation/flutter.

Calf pain/swelling.

Thrombophlebitis can occur or recur and precipitate PE.

Lung Cancer: Surgical Intervention (Postoperative Care) _____

Lung cancer usually develops within the wall or epithelium of the bronchial tree. The most common types are squamous cell carcinoma, oat cell carcinoma, adenocarcinoma, and large-cell carcinoma. Prognosis is generally poor, varying with the type of cancer and extent of involvement at time of diagnosis. Lung cancer is largely preventable, as 80% of lung cancer patient's are smokers.

Treatment options can include combinations of surgery, radiation, and chemotherapy. Surgery is the primary treatment for Stage I, Stage II, or selected Stage III carcinomas, if the tumor is resectable.

Surgical procedures for operable tumors of the lung include:

1. Pneumonectomy (removal of an entire lung), performed for lesions originating in the mainstem bronchus or lobar bronchus
2. Lobectomy (removal of one lobe), preferred for peripheral carcinoma localized in a lobe
3. Segmental resection, performed when lesion is small and well contained within one segment

RELATED CONCERNS:

Cancer, p 1014
Hemothorax/Pneumothorax, p 195
Psychosocial Aspects of Acute Care, p 899
Radical Neck surgery, p 202
Surgical Interventions, p 918

PATIENT ASSESSMENT DATA BASE (PREOPERATIVE)

Findings are dependent on type, duration of cancer, and extent of metastasis.

ACTIVITY/REST

May report:	Fatigue, inability to maintain usual routine, dyspnea with activity.
May exhibit:	Lassitude (usually in advanced stage).

CIRCULATION

May exhibit:	JVD (vena cava obstruction).
	Heart sounds: Pericardial rub (indicating effusion).
	Tachycardia/dysrhythmias.
	Clubbing of fingers.

EGO INTEGRITY

May report:	Scared feelings, fear of outcome of surgery.
	Denial of severity of condition/potential for malignancy.
May exhibit:	Restlessness, insomnia, repetitive questioning.

ELIMINATION

May report:	Intermittent diarrhea (hormonal imbalance, small-cell carcinoma).
	Increased frequency/amount of urine (hormonal imbalance, epidermoid tumor).

FOOD/FLUID

May report:	Weight loss, poor appetite, decreased food intake.

Difficulty swallowing.

Thirst/increased fluid intake.

May exhibit: Thin, emaciated or wasted appearance (late stages).

Edema of face/neck, chest, back (vena caval obstruction); facial/periorbital edema (hormonal imbalance, small cell carcinoma).

Glucose in urine (hormonal imbalance, epidermoid tumor).

PAIN/COMFORT

May report: Chest pain (not usually present in early stages and not always in advanced stages) which may/may not be affected by position change.

Shoulder/arm pain (particularly with large cell or adenocarcinoma).

Bone/joint pain: Cartilage erosion secondary to increased growth hormones (large cell or adenocarcinoma).

Intermittent abdominal pain.

RESPIRATION

May report: Mild cough or change in usual cough pattern and/or sputum production.

Shortness of breath.

Occupational exposure to pollutants, industrial dusts (e.g., asbestos, iron oxides, coal dust), radioactive material.

Hoarseness, vocal cord paralysis.

History of smoking.

May exhibit: Dyspnea, aggravated by exertion.

Increased tactile fremitus (indicating consolidation).

Brief crackles/wheezes on inspiration or expiration (impaired airflow).

Persistent crackles/wheezes; tracheal shift (space-occupying lesion).

Hemoptysis.

SAFETY

May exhibit: Fever may be present (large cell or adenocarcinoma).

Bruising, discoloration of skin (hormonal imbalance, small cell carcinoma).

SEXUALITY

May exhibit: Gynecomastia (neoplastic hormonal changes, large cell carcinoma).

Amenorrhea/impotence (hormonal imbalance, small cell carcinoma).

TEACHING/LEARNING

May report: Familial risk factors: Cancer (especially lung), tuberculosis.

Failure to improve.

Discharge Plan Considerations: **DRG projected mean length of stay: 11.7 days.**

Assistance with transportation, medications, treatments, self-care, homemaker/maintenance tasks.

DIAGNOSTIC STUDIES

Chest x-ray (PA and lateral), chest tomography: Outlines shape, size and location of lesion. May reveal mass of air in hilar region, pleural effusion, atelectasis, erosion of ribs or vertebrae.

185

Cytologic examinations (sputum, pleural, or lymph node): Performed to assess presence/stage of carcinoma.

Fiberoptic bronchoscopy: Allows for visualization, regional washings, and cytologic brushing of lesions (large percent of bronchogenic carcinomas may be visualized).

Biopsy: May be performed on scalene nodes, hilar lymph nodes, or pleura to establish diagnosis.

Mediastinoscopy: Used for staging of carcinoma.

Radioisotope scans: May be done on lungs, liver, brain, bones, and distant organs for evidence of metastasis.

Pulmonary function studies and ABGs: May be done to assess lung capacity to meet postoperative ventilatory needs.

Skin tests, absolute lymphocyte counts: May be done to evaluate for immunocompetence (common in lung cancers).

Bone scan; CT scan of brain, liver; gallium scan of liver, spleen, bone: To detect metastasis.

NURSING PRIORITIES

1. Maintain/improve respiratory function.
2. Control/alleviate pain.
3. Support efforts to cope with diagnosis/situation.
4. Provide information about disease process/prognosis and therapeutic regimen.

DISCHARGE GOALS

1. Oxygenation/ventilation adequate to meet individual activity needs.
2. Pain controlled.
3. Anxiety/fear decreased to manageable level.
4. Free of preventable complications.
5. Disease process/prognosis and planned therapies understood.

NURSING DIAGNOSIS:	GAS EXCHANGE, IMPAIRED
May be related to:	Removal of lung tissue.
	Altered oxygen supply (hypoventilation).
	Decreased oxygen-carrying capacity of blood (blood loss).
Possibly evidenced by:	Dyspnea.
	Restlessness/changes in mentation.
	Hypoxemia and hypercapnea.
	Cyanosis.
DESIRED OUTCOMES/ EVALUATION CRITERIA— PATIENT WILL:	Demonstrate improved ventilation and adequate oxygenation of tissues by ABGs within patient's normal range.
	Be free of symptoms of respiratory distress.

ACTIONS/INTERVENTIONS	RATIONALE

Independent

Note respiratory rate, depth, and ease of respirations. Observe for use of accessory muscles, pursed-lip breathing, changes in skin/mucous membrane color, e.g., pallor, cyanosis.	Respirations may be increased as a result of pain or as an initial compensatory mechanism to accommodate for loss of lung tissue. However, increased work of breathing and cyanosis may indicate increasing oxygen consumption and energy expenditures and/or reduced respiratory reserve, e.g., elderly patient or extensive chronic obstructive lung disease.
Auscultate lungs for air movement and abnormal breath sounds.	Consolidation and lack of air movement on operative side is normal in the pneumonectomy patient. However, the lobectomy patient should demonstrate normal airflow in remaining lobes.
Investigate restlessness and changes in mentation/level of consciousness.	May indicate increased hypoxia or complications such as mediastinal shift in pneumonectomy patient when accompanied by tachypnea, tachycardia, and tracheal deviation.
Maintain patent airway by positioning, suctioning, use of adjuncts.	Airway obstruction impedes ventilation, impairing gas exchange. (Refer to ND: Airway Clearance, ineffective, p 188.)
Reposition frequently, placing patient in sitting positions as well as supine to side positions.	Maximizes lung expansion and drainage of secretions.
Avoid positioning the patient with a pneumonectomy on the operative side with the remaining lung dependent.	This position reduces lung expansion and decreases perfusion to the "good" lung and could foster the development of a tension pneumothorax secondary to a mediastinal shift and accumulation of fluid in the remaining lung.
Encourage/assist with deep-breathing exercises and pursed-lip breathing as appropriate.	Promotes maximal ventilation and oxygenation and reduces/prevents atelectasis.
Maintain patency of chest drainage system for lobectomy, segmental/wedge resection patient.	Drains fluid from pleural cavity to promote reexpansion of remaining lung segments.
Note changes in amount/type of chest tube drainage.	Bloody drainage should decrease in amount and change to a more serous composition as recovery progresses. A sudden increase in amount of bloody drainage or return to frank bleeding suggests thoracic bleeding/hemothorax; sudden cessation suggests blockage of tube, requiring further evaluation and intervention.
Observe presence/degree of bubbling in water-seal chamber.	Air leaks immediately postoperative are not uncommon, especially following lobectomy or segmental resection. However, this should diminish as healing progresses. Prolonged or new leaks require evaluation to identify problems in the patient versus the drainage system.
Assess patient response to activity. Encourage rest periods/limit activities to patient tolerance.	Increased oxygen consumption/demand and stress of surgery can result in increased dyspnea and changes in vital signs with activity. However, early mobilization is desired to help prevent pulmonary complications and to obtain and maintain

ACTIONS/INTERVENTIONS	RATIONALE
Independent	
	respiratory and circulatory efficiency. Adequate rest balanced with activity can prevent respiratory compromise.
Note development of fever.	Fever within the first 24 hours after surgery is frequently due to atelectasis. Temperature elevation within the 5th to 10th postoperative day usually indicates an infection, e.g., wound or systemic.
Collaborative	
Administer supplemental oxygen, via nasal cannula, partial rebreathing mask, or high humidity face mask, as indicated.	Maximizes available oxygen, especially while ventilation is reduced from anesthetic depression or pain, as well as during period of compensatory physiologic shift of circulation to remaining functional alveolar units.
Assist with/encourage use of incentive spirometer or blow bottles.	Prevents/reduces atelectasis and promotes reexpansion of small airways.
Monitor/graph ABGs, pulse oximetry readings. Note Hb levels.	Decreasing PaO_2 or increasing $PaCO_2$ may indicate need for ventilatory support. Significant blood loss can result in decreased oxygen-carrying capacity, reducing PaO_2.

NURSING DIAGNOSIS:	AIRWAY CLEARANCE, INEFFECTIVE
May be related to:	Increased amount/viscosity of secretions.
	Restricted chest movement/pain.
	Fatigue/weakness.
Possibly evidenced by:	Changes in rate/depth of respiration.
	Abnormal breath sounds.
	Ineffective cough.
	Dyspnea.
DESIRED OUTCOMES/ EVALUATION CRITERIA— PATIENT WILL:	Demonstrate patent airway, with fluid secretions easily expectorated, clear breath sounds, and noiseless respirations.

ACTIONS/INTERVENTIONS	RATIONALE
Independent	
Auscultate chest for character of breath sounds and presence of secretions.	Noisy respirations, rhonchi, and wheezes are indicative of retained secretions and/or airway obstruction.
Assist patient with/instruct in effective deep breathing and coughing with upright position (sitting) and splinting of incision.	Upright position favors maximal lung expansion, and splinting improves force of cough effort to mobilize and remove secretions. Splinting may be

ACTIONS/INTERVENTIONS	RATIONALE
Independent	
	done by nurse (placing hands anteriorly and posteriorly over chest wall) and by patient (with pillows) as strength improves.
Observe amount and character of sputum/aspirated secretions. Investigate changes as indicated.	Increased amounts of colorless (or blood-streaked)/watery secretions are normal initially and should decrease as recovery progresses. Presence of thick/tenacious, bloody, or purulent sputum suggests development of secondary problems (e.g., dehydration, pulmonary edema, local hemorrhage, or infection) requiring correction/treatment.
Suction if cough is weak or rhonchi not cleared by cough effort. Avoid deep endotracheal/nasotracheal suctioning in pneumonectomy patient if possible.	"Routine" suctioning increases risk of hypoxemia and mucosal damage. Deep tracheal suctioning is generally contraindicated following pneumonectomy to reduce the risk of rupture of the bronchial stump suture line. If suctioning is unavoidable, it should be done gently only to induce effective coughing.
Encourage oral fluid intake (at least 2500 ml/d) within cardiac tolerance.	Adequate hydration aids in keeping secretions loose/enhances expectoration.
Assess for pain/discomfort and medicate on a routine basis and prior to breathing exercises.	Encourages the patient to move, cough more effectively, and breathe more deeply to prevent respiratory insufficiency.
Collaborative	
Provide/assist with IPPB, incentive spirometer, blow bottles, postural drainage/percussion as indicated.	Improves pulmonary expansion/ventilation and facilitates removal of secretions. *Note:* Postural drainage may be contraindicated in some patients and in every event must be performed cautiously to prevent respiratory embarrassment and incisional discomfort.
Use humidified oxygen/ultrasonic nebulizer. Provide additional fluids via IV as indicated.	Providing maximal hydration helps loosen/liquefy secretions to promote expectoration. Impaired oral intake necessitates IV supplementation to maintain hydration.
Administer bronchodilators, expectorants, and/or analgesics, as indicated.	Relieves bronchospasm to improve airflow. Expectorants increase mucous production to liquefy and reduce viscosity of secretions, facilitating removal. Alleviation of chest discomfort promotes cooperation with breathing exercises and enhances effectiveness of respiratory therapies.

NURSING DIAGNOSIS:	**PAIN [ACUTE]**
May be related to:	Surgical incision, tissue trauma, and disruption of intercostal nerves.
	Presence of chest tube(s).
	Cancer invasion of pleura, chest wall.

Possibly evidenced by:	Verbal reports of discomfort.
	Guarding of affected area.
	Distraction behaviors, e.g., restlessness.
	Narrowed focus (withdrawal).
	Changes in BP, heart/respiratory rate.
DESIRED OUTCOMES/ EVALUATION CRITERIA— PATIENT WILL:	Report pain relieved/controlled.
	Appear relaxed and sleep/rest appropriately.
	Participate in desired/needed activities.

ACTIONS/INTERVENTIONS	RATIONALE

Independent

Ask patient about pain. Determine pain characteristics, e.g., continuous, aching, stabbing, burning. Have patient rate intensity on a 0–10 scale.	Helpful in evaluating cancer-related pain symptoms, which may involve viscera, nerve, or bone tissue. Use of rating scale aids patient in assessing level of pain and provides tool for evaluating effectiveness of analgesics, enhancing patient control of pain.
Assess patient's verbal and nonverbal pain cues.	Discrepancy between verbal/nonverbal cues may provide clues to degree of pain, need for/effectiveness of interventions.
Note possible pathophysiologic and psychologic causes of pain.	A posterolateral incision is more uncomfortable for the patient than an anterolateral incision. The presence of chest tubes can greatly increase discomfort. In addition, fear, distress, anxiety, and grief over confirmed diagnosis of cancer can impair ability to cope.
Evaluate effectiveness of drug regimen. Encourage sufficient medication to control pain; change medication or time span as appropriate.	Pain perception and pain relief is subjective and thus pain management is best left to the patient's discretion. If the patient is unable to provide input, the nurse should observe physiologic and nonverbal signs of pain and administer medications on a regular basis.
Encourage verbalization of feelings about the pain.	Fears/concerns can increase muscle tension and lower threshold of pain perception. (Refer to ND: Fear/Anxiety [Specify Level], p 191.)
Provide comfort measures, e.g., frequent changes of position, back rubs, support with pillows. Encourage use of relaxation techniques, e.g., visualization, guided imagery, and appropriate diversional activities.	Promotes relaxation and redirects attention. Relieves discomfort and augments therapeutic effects of analgesia.
Schedule rest periods, provide quiet environment.	Decreases fatigue and conserves energy, enhancing coping abilities.
Assist with self-care activities, breathing/arm exercises, and ambulation.	Prevents undue fatigue and incisional strain. Encouragement and physical assistance/support may be needed for some time before the patient is

ACTIONS/INTERVENTIONS

Collaborative

Administer analgesics routinely as indicated, especially 45–60 minutes before respiratory treatments/deep-breathing/coughing exercises. Assist with PCA or analgesia through epidural catheter.

RATIONALE

able or confident enough to perform these activities because of pain or fear of pain.

Maintaining a more constant drug level avoids "peak" periods of pain, aids in muscle healing, and improves respiratory function and emotional comfort/coping.

NURSING DIAGNOSIS:	FEAR/ANXIETY [SPECIFY LEVEL]
May be related to:	Situational crises.
	Threat to/change in health status.
	Perceived threat of death.
Possibly evidenced by:	Withdrawal.
	Apprehension.
	Anger.
	Increased pain, sympathetic stimulation.
	Expressions of denial, shock, guilt, insomnia.
DESIRED OUTCOMES/ EVALUATION CRITERIA— PATIENT WILL:	Acknowledge and discuss fears/concerns.
	Demonstrate appropriate range of feelings and appear relaxed/resting appropriately.
	Verbalize accurate knowledge of situation.
	Report beginning use of individually appropriate coping strategies.

ACTIONS/INTERVENTIONS

Independent

Evaluate patient/SO level of understanding of diagnosis.

Acknowledge reality of patient's fears/concerns and encourage expression of feelings.

Provide opportunity for questions and answer them honestly. Be sure that patient and care providers have the same understanding of terms used.

RATIONALE

Patient and SO are hearing and assimilating new information that includes changes in self-image and lifestyle. Understanding perceptions of those involved sets the tone for individualizing care and provides information necessary for choosing appropriate interventions.

Support may enable the patient to begin exploring/dealing with the reality of cancer and its treatment. Patient may need time to identify feelings and even more time to begin to express them.

Establishes trust and reduces misperceptions/misinterpretation of information.

ACTIONS/INTERVENTIONS

Independent

Accept, but do not reinforce, patient's denial of the situation.

Note comments/behaviors indicative of beginning acceptance and/or use of effective strategies to deal with situation.

Involve patient/SO in care planning. Provide time to prepare for events/treatments.

Provide for patient's physical comfort.

RATIONALE

If extreme denial or anxiety is interfering with progress of recovery, the issues facing the patient need to be explained and resolutions explored.

Fear/anxiety will diminish as patient begins to accept/positively deal with reality. Indicator of patient's readiness to accept responsibility for participation in recovery and to "resume life".

May help restore some feeling of control/independence to patient who feels powerless in dealing with diagnosis and treatment.

It is difficult to deal with emotional issues when experiencing extreme/persistent physical discomfort.

NURSING DIAGNOSIS:	KNOWLEDGE DEFICIT [LEARNING NEED] REGARDING CONDITION, TREATMENT, PROGNOSIS
May be related to:	Lack of exposure, unfamiliarity with information/resources. Information misinterpretation. Lack of recall.
Possibly evidenced by:	Statements of concern. Request for information. Inadequate follow-through of instruction. Inappropriate or exaggerated behaviors, e.g., hysterical, hostile, agitated, apathetic.
DESIRED OUTCOMES/ EVALUATION CRITERIA— PATIENT WILL:	Verbalize understanding of ramifications of diagnosis, treatment regimen. Correctly perform necessary procedures and explain reasons for the actions. Participate in learning process. Initiate necessary lifestyle changes.

ACTIONS/INTERVENTIONS

Independent

Discuss diagnosis, current/planned therapies and expected outcomes.

RATIONALE

Provides individually specific information, creating knowledge base for subsequent learning regarding home management. Radiation or chemotherapy may follow surgical intervention and information is essential to enable the patient/SO to make informed decisions.

ACTIONS/INTERVENTIONS	RATIONALE
Independent	
Reinforce surgeon's explanation of particular surgical procedure providing diagram as appropriate. Incorporate this information into discussion about short-/long-term recovery expectations.	Length of rehabilitation and prognosis is dependent on type of surgical procedure, preoperative physical condition, and duration/degree of complications.
Discuss necessity of planning for follow-up care prior to discharge.	Follow-up assessment of respiratory status and general health is imperative to assure optimal recovery. Also provides opportunity to readdress concerns/questions at a less stressful time.
Identify signs/symptoms requiring medical evaluations, e.g., changes in appearance of incision, development of respiratory difficulty, fever, increased chest pain, changes in appearance of sputum.	Early detection and timely intervention may prevent/minimize complications.
Help patient determine activity tolerance and set goals.	Weakness and fatigue should lessen as lung(s) heal and respiratory function improves during recovery period, especially if cancer was completely removed. If cancer is advanced, it is emotionally helpful for the patient to be able to set realistic activity goals to achieve optimal independence.
Evaluate availability/adequacy of support system(s) and necessity for assistance in self-care/home management.	General weakness and activity limitations may reduce individual's ability to meet own needs.
Recommend alternating rest periods with activity and light tasks with heavy tasks. Stress avoidance of heavy lifting, isometric/strenuous upper-body exercise. Reinforce physician's time limitations about lifting.	Generalized weakness and fatigue are usual in the early recovery period but should diminish as respiratory function improves and healing progresses. Rest and sleep enhance coping abilities, reduce nervousness (common in this phase), and promote healing. *Note:* Strenuous use of arms can place undue stress on incision because chest muscles may be weaker than normal for 3–6 months following surgery.
Recommend stopping any activity that causes undue fatigue or increased shortness of breath.	Exhaustion aggravates respiratory insufficiency.
Encourage inspection of incisions. Review expectations for healing with patient.	Healing begins immediately, but complete healing will take time. As healing progresses, incision lines may appear dry, with crusty scabs. Underlying tissue may look bruised and feel tense, warm, and lumpy (resolving hematoma).
Instruct patient/SO to watch for/report places in incision that do not heal or reopening of healed incision, any drainage (bloody or purulent), localized area of swelling with redness, increased pain, hot to touch.	Signs/symptoms indicating failure to heal, development of complications requiring further medical evaluation/intervention.
Suggest wearing soft cotton shirts and loose fitting clothing, cover/pad incision as indicated, leave incision open to air as much as possible.	Reduces suture line irritation and pressure from clothing. Leaving incisions open to air promotes healing process and may reduce risk of infection.
Shower in warm water, washing incision gently. Avoid tub baths until approved by physician.	Keeps incision clean, promotes circulation/healing. *Note:* "Climbing" out of tub requires use of arms and pectoral muscles, which can put undue stress on incision.

193

ACTIONS/INTERVENTIONS	RATIONALE
Independent	
Support incision with Steri-strips as needed when sutures/staples are removed.	Aids in maintaining approximation of wound edges to promote healing.
Instruct in/provide rationale for arm/shoulder exercises. Have patient/SO demonstrate exercises. Encourage following graded increase in number/intensity of routine repetitions.	Simple arm circles and lifting arms over the head or out to the affected side are initiated on the 1st or 2nd postoperative day to restore normal range of motion of shoulder and to prevent ankylosis of the affected shoulder.
Stress importance of avoiding exposure to smoke, air pollution, and contact with individuals with upper-respiratory infections.	Protects lung(s) from irritation and reduces risk of infection.
Review nutritional/fluid needs. Suggest increasing protein and use of high-calorie snacks as appropriate.	Meeting cellular energy requirements and maintaining good circulating volume for tissue perfusion facilitates tissue regeneration/healing process.
Identify individually appropriate community resources, e.g., American Cancer Society, Visiting Nurse Association, social services.	Agencies such as these offer a broad range of services that can be tailored to provide support and meet individual needs.

Hemothorax/Pneumothorax _____

The lung may collapse partially/completely due to collection of air (pneumothorax), blood (hemothorax), or other fluid (pleural effusion) in the pleural/potential space. The intrathoracic pressure changes induced by increased pleural space volumes reduce lung capacity, causing respiratory distress and gas exchange problems, and producing tension on mediastinal structures that can impede cardiac and systemic circulation. Pneumothorax may be traumatic (open or closed) or spontaneous.

RELATED CONCERNS:

Cardiac Surgery, p 113
Chronic Obstructive Pulmonary Disease, p 149
Psychosocial Aspects of Acute Care, p 899
Pulmonary Tuberculosis, p 241
Ventilatory Assistance (Mechanical), p 226

PATIENT ASSESSMENT DATA BASE

Findings vary, depending on the amount of air and/or fluid accumulation, rate of accumulation, and underlying lung function.

ACTIVITY/REST

May Report: Dyspnea with activity or even at rest.

CIRCULATION

May exhibit: Tachycardia.

Irregular rate/dysrhythmias.

S_3 or S_4/gallop heart rhythm (heart failure secondary to effusion).

Apical pulse (PMI) displaced in presence of mediastinal shift (with tension pneumothorax).

Hamman's sign (crunching sound correlating with heart beat, reflecting air in mediastinum).

BP: hypertension/hypotension.

JVD.

EGO INTEGRITY

May exhibit: Apprehension, irritability.

FOOD/FLUID

May exhibit: Recent placement of central venous IV/pressure line.

PAIN/COMFORT

**May report
(dependent on the
size/area involved):** Unilateral chest pain, aggravated by breathing, coughing.

Sudden onset of symptoms while coughing or straining (spontaneous pneumothorax).

Sharp, stabbing pain aggravated by deep breathing, possibly radiating to neck, shoulders, abdomen (pleural effusion).

May exhibit: Guarding affected area.

Distraction behaviors.

Facial grimacing.

195

RESPIRATION

May report: Difficulty breathing, "air hunger."

Coughing (may be presenting symptom).

History of recent chest surgery/trauma; chronic lung disease, lung inflammation/infection (empyema/effusion); diffuse interstitial disease (sarcoidosis); malignancies, (e.g., obstructive tumor).

Previous spontaneous pneumothorax; spontaneous rupture of emphysematous bulla, subpleural bleb (COPD).

May exhibit: Respirations: Increased rate/tachypnea.

Increased work of breathing, use of accessory muscles in chest, neck; intercostal retractions, forced abdominal expiration.

Breath sounds decreased or absent (involved site).

Fremitus decreased (involved site).

Chest percussion: Hyperresonance over air-filled area (pneumothorax); dullness over fluid-filled area (hemothorax).

Chest observation and palpation: Unequal (paradoxic) chest movement (if trauma, flail); reduced thoracic excursion (affected side).

Skin: Pallor, cyanosis, diaphoresis, subcutaneous crepitation (air in tissues on palpation).

Mentation: Anxiety, restlessness, confusion, stupor.

Use of positive pressure mechanical ventilation/PEEP therapy.

SAFETY

May report: Recent chest trauma.

Radiation/chemotherapy for malignancy.

TEACHING/LEARNING

May report History of familial risk factors: Tuberculosis, cancer.

Recent intrathoracic surgery/lung biopsy.

Evidence of failure to improve.

Discharge Plan Considerations: **DRG projected length of stay: 7.2 days.**

Assistance with self-care, homemaker/maintenance tasks.

DIAGNOSTIC STUDIES

Chest x-ray: Reveals air and/or fluid accumulation in the pleural space; may show shift of mediastinal structures (heart).

ABGs: Variable dependent on degree of compromised lung function, altered breathing mechanics, and ability to compensate. $PaCO_2$ occasionally elevated. PaO_2 may be normal or decreased; oxygen saturation usually decreased.

Thoracentesis: Reveals blood/serosanguinous fluid (hemothorax).

Hb: May be decreased, indicating blood loss.

NURSING PRIORITIES

1. Promote/maintain lung reexpansion for adequate oxygenation/ventilation.
2. Minimize/prevent complications.
3. Reduce discomfort/pain.
4. Provide information about disease process, treatment regimen, and prognosis.

DISCHARGE GOALS

1. Adequate ventilation/oxygenation maintained.
2. Complications prevented/resolved.
3. Pain absent/controlled.
4. Disease process/prognosis and therapy needs understood.

NURSING DIAGNOSIS:	BREATHING PATTERN, INEFFECTIVE
May be related to:	Decreased lung expansion (air/fluid accumulation).
	Musculoskeletal impairment.
	Pain/anxiety.
	Inflammatory process.
Possibly evidenced by:	Dyspnea, tachypnea.
	Changes in depth/equality of respirations.
	Use of accessory muscles, nasal flaring.
	Altered chest excursion.
	Cyanosis, abnormal ABGs.
DESIRED OUTCOMES/ EVALUATION CRITERIA— PATIENT WILL:	Establish a normal/effective respiratory pattern with ABGs within patient's normal range.
	Be free of cyanosis and other signs/symptoms of hypoxia.

ACTIONS/INTERVENTIONS

Independent

Identify etiology/precipitating factors, e.g., spontaneous collapse, trauma, malignancy, infection, complication of mechanical ventilation.

Evaluate respiratory function, noting rapid/shallow respirations, dyspnea, complaints of "air hunger," development of cyanosis, changes in vital signs.

Monitor for synchronous respiratory pattern when using mechanical ventilator. Note changes in airway pressures.

Auscultate breath sounds.

RATIONALE

Understanding the cause of lung collapse is necessary for proper chest tube placement and choice of other therapeutic measures.

Respiratory distress and changes in vital signs may occur as a result of physiologic stress and pain or may indicate development of shock due to hypoxia/hemorrhage.

Difficulty breathing "with" ventilator and/or increasing airway pressures suggests worsening of condition/development of complications (e.g., spontaneous rupture of a bleb, creating a new pneumothorax).

Breath sounds may be diminished or absent in a lobe, lung segment, or entire lung field (unilateral). Atelectatic area will have no breath sounds, and partially collapsed areas have decreased sounds.

197

ACTIONS/INTERVENTIONS	RATIONALE
Independent	
	Evaluation also establishes areas of good air exchange and provides a baseline to evaluate resolution of pneumothorax.
Note chest excursion and position of trachea.	Chest excursion is unequal until lung reexpands. Trachea deviates away from affected side with tension pneumothorax.
Assess fremitus.	Voice and tactile fremitus (vibration) is reduced in fluid-filled/consolidated tissue.
Assist patient with splinting painful area when coughing, deep breathing.	Supporting chest and abdominal muscles makes coughing more effective/less traumatic.
Maintain position of comfort, usually with head of bed elevated. Turn to affected side. Encourage patient to sit up as much as possible.	Promotes maximal inspiration; enhances lung expansion and ventilation in unaffected side.
Maintain a calm attitude, assisting patient to "take control" by the use of slower/deeper respirations.	Assists the patient to deal with the physiologic effects of hypoxia, which may be manifested as anxiety and/or fear.
Once chest tube is inserted:	
Check suction control chamber for correct amount of suction (by water level, wall/table regulator at correct setting);	Maintains prescribed intrapleural negativity, which promotes optimum lung expansion and/or fluid drainage.
Check fluid level in water-seal chamber/bottle; maintain at prescribed level;	Water in a sealed chamber serves as a barrier that prevents atmospheric air from entering the pleural space should the suction source be disconnected and aids in evaluating whether the chest drainage system is functioning appropriately.
Observe water-seal chamber bubbling;	Bubbling during expiration reflects venting of pneumothorax (desired action). Bubbling usually decreases as the lung expands or may occur only during expiration or coughing as the pleural space diminishes. Absence of bubbling may indicate complete lung reexpansion (normal) or represent complications, e.g., obstruction in the tube.
Evaluate for abnormal/continuous water-seal chamber bubbling;	With suction applied, this indicates a persistent air leak that may be from a large pneumothorax at the chest insertion site (patient-centered), or chest drainage unit (system-centered).
Determine location of air leak (patient- or system-centered) by clamping thoracic catheter just distal to exit from chest;	If bubbling stops when catheter is clamped at insertion site, leak is patient-centered (at insertion site or within the patient).
Place petrolatum gauze and/or other appropriate material around the insertion as indicated;	Usually corrects insertion site air leak.
Clamp tubing in stepwise fashion downward toward drainage unit if air leak continues;	Isolates location of a system-centered air leak.
Seal drainage tubing connection sites securely with lengthwise tape or bands according to established policy.	Prevents/corrects air leaks at connector sites.

ACTIONS/INTERVENTIONS	RATIONALE

Independent

Monitor water-seal chamber "tidaling." Note whether change is transient or permanent.

The water-seal chamber serves as an intrapleural manometer (gauges intrapleural pressure); therefore, fluctuation (tidaling) reflects pressure differences between inspiration and expiration. Tidaling of 2–6 cm during inspiration is normal, and may increase briefly during coughing episodes. Continuation of excessive tidal fluctuations may indicate airway obstruction exists or presence of a large pneumothorax.

Position drainage system tubing for optimal function, e.g., coil extra tubing on bed, making sure tubing is not kinked or hanging below entrance to drainage container. Drain accumulated fluid as necessary.

Improper position, kinking, or accumulation of clots/fluid in the tubing changes the desired negative pressure and impedes air/fluid evacuation.

Note character/amount of chest tube drainage.

Useful in evaluating resolution of condition/development of complication or hemorrhage requiring prompt intervention. Note: Some drainage systems are equipped with an auto-transfusion device which allows for salvage of shed blood.

Evaluate need for tube stripping ("milking").

Although it is unlikely that serous or serosanguinous drainage will obstruct tubes, stripping may be necessary to assure/maintain drainage in the presence of fresh bleeding/large blood clots or purulent exudate (empyema).

Strip tubes carefully per protocol, in a manner which minimizes excess negative pressure.

Stripping is usually uncomfortable for the patient because of the change in intrathoracic pressure, which may induce coughing or chest discomfort. Vigorous stripping can create very high intrathoracic suction pressure, which can be injurious (e.g., invagination of tissue into catheter eyelets, collapse of tissues around the catheter, and/or bleeding from rupture of small blood vessels).

If thoracic catheter is disconnected/dislodged:

Observe for signs of respiratory distress. Reconnect thoracic catheter to tubing/suction, if possible, using clean technique. If the catheter is dislodged from the chest, cover insertion site immediately with petrolatum dressing and apply firm pressure. Notify physician at once.

Pneumothorax may recur requiring prompt intervention to prevent fatal pulmonary and circulatory impairment.

After thoracic catheter is removed:

Cover insertion site with sterile occlusive dressing. Observe for signs/symptoms which may indicate recurrence of pneumothorax, e.g., shortness of breath, reports of pain. Inspect insertion site, note character of drainage.

Early detection of developing complication is essential, e.g., recurrence of pneumothorax, presence of infection.

Collaborative

Review serial chest x-rays.

Monitors progress of resolving hemothorax/pneumothorax and reexpansion of lung. Identifies

ACTIONS/INTERVENTIONS

Collaborative

Monitor/graph serial ABGs and pulse oximetry. Review vital capacity/tidal volume measurements.

Administer supplemental oxygen via cannula/mask as indicated.

RATIONALE

malposition of endotracheal tube affecting lung inflation.

Assesses status of gas exchange and ventilation, need for continuation or alterations in therapy.

Aids in reducing work of breathing; promotes relief of respiratory distress and cyanosis associated with hypoxemia.

NURSING DIAGNOSIS:	TRAUMA/SUFFOCATION, HIGH RISK FOR
Risk factors may include:	Concurrent disease/injury process.
	Dependence on external device (chest drainage system).
	Lack of safety education/precautions.
Possibly evidenced by:	[Not applicable; presence of signs and symptoms establishes an actual diagnosis.]
DESIRED OUTCOMES/ EVALUATION CRITERIA— PATIENT WILL:	Recognize need for/seek assistance to prevent complications.
	<u>Caregiver will:</u> Correct/avoid environmental and physical hazards.

ACTIONS/INTERVENTIONS

Independent

Review with patient purpose/function of chest drainage unit, taking note of safety features.

Anchor thoracic catheter to chest wall and provide extra length of tubing before turning or moving patient:

Secure tubing connection sites;

Pad banding sites with gauze/tape.

Secure drainage unit to patient's bed or on stand/cart placed in low-traffic area.

Provide safe transportation if patient is sent off unit for diagnostic purposes. Before transporting: check water-seal chamber for correct fluid level, presence/absence of bubbling; presence/degree/timing of tidaling. Ascertain whether or not chest tube can be clamped or disconnected from suction source.

Monitor thoracic insertion site, noting condition of skin, presence/characteristics of drainage from

RATIONALE

Information on how system works provides reassurance, reducing patient anxiety.

Prevents thoracic catheter dislodgment or tubing disconnection and reduces pain/discomfort associated with pulling or jarring of tubing.

Prevents tubing disconnection.

Protects skin from irritation/pressure.

Maintains upright position and reduces risk of accidental tipping/breaking of unit.

Promotes continuation of optimal evacuation of fluid/air during transport. If patient is draining large amounts of chest fluid or air, tube should not be clamped or suction interrupted because of risk of reaccumulation of fluid/air, compromising respiratory status.

Provides for early recognition and treatment of developing skin/tissue erosion or infection.

ACTIONS/INTERVENTIONS

Independent

around the catheter. Change/reapply sterile occlusive dressing as needed.

Instruct patient to refrain from lying/pulling on tubing.

Identify changes/situations that should be reported to caregivers, e.g., change in sound of bubbling, sudden "air hunger" and chest pain, disconnection of equipment.

Observe for signs of respiratory distress if thoracic catheter is disconnected/dislodged. (Refer to ND: Breathing Pattern, ineffective, p 197.)

RATIONALE

Reduces risk of obstructing drainage/inadvertently disconnecting tubing.

Timely intervention may prevent serious complications.

Pneumothorax may recur/worsen, compromising respiratory function and requiring emergency intervention.

NURSING DIAGNOSIS:	KNOWLEDGE DEFICIT [LEARNING NEED] REGARDING CONDITION, TREATMENT REGIMEN
May be related to:	Lack of exposure to information.
Possibly evidenced by:	Expressions of concern, request for information. Recurrence of problem.
DESIRED OUTCOMES/ EVALUATION CRITERIA— PATIENT WILL:	Verbalize understanding of cause of problem (when known). Identify signs/symptoms requiring medical follow-up. Follow treatment regimen and demonstrate lifestyle changes if necessary to prevent recurrence.

ACTIONS/INTERVENTIONS

Independent

Review pathology of individual problem.

Identify likelihood for recurrence/long-term complications.

Review signs/symptoms requiring immediate medical evaluation, e.g., sudden chest pain, dyspnea/air hunger, progressive respiratory distress.

Review significance of good health practices, e.g., adequate nutrition, rest, exercise.

RATIONALE

Information reduces fear of unknown. Provides knowledge base for understanding underlying dynamics of condition and significance of therapeutic interventions.

Certain underlying lung diseases such as severe COPD and malignancies may increase incidence of recurrence. In otherwise healthy patients who suffered a spontaneous pneumothorax, incidence of recurrence is 10%–50%. Those who have a second spontaneous episode are at high risk for a third incident (60%).

Recurrence of pneumothorax/hemothorax requires medical intervention to prevent/reduce potential complications.

Maintenance of general well-being promotes healing and may prevent/limit recurrences.

201

Radical Neck Surgery: Laryngectomy (Postoperative Care) ____

Head and neck cancer refers to a malignancy that lies above the clavicle but excludes the brain, spinal cord, axial skeleton, and vertebrae. Head and neck cancer accounts for 5.5% of all malignant disease. The majority of the laryngeal neoplasms (95%) are squamous cell carcinomas that arise from the oral cavity. When cancer is limited to the vocal cords (intrinsic) spread may be slow. When the cancer involves the epiglottis (extrinsic) metastases is more common. Current treatment choices include surgery, radiation, and chemotherapy. Carbon dioxide laser may be used for early stage disease. This plan of care focuses on nursing care of the patient undergoing radical surgery of the neck including laryngectomy.

Partial Laryngectomy: Tumors that are limited to only 1 vocal cord are removed and a temporary tracheotomy performed to maintain the airway. After recovery from surgery, the patient's voice will be hoarse.

Hemilaryngectomy: When there is a possibility the cancer includes 1 true and 1 false vocal cord, they are removed along with an arytenoid cartilage and half of the thyroid cartilage. Temporary tracheotomy is performed, and the patient's voice will be hoarse after surgery.

Supraglottic Laryngectomy: When the tumor is located in the epiglottis or false vocal cords, radical neck dissection is done and tracheotomy performed. The patient's voice remains intact; however, swallowing is more difficult because the epiglottis has been removed.

Total Laryngectomy: Advanced cancers that involve a large portion of the larynx require removal of the entire larynx, the hyoid bone, the cricoid cartilage, 2 or 3 tracheal rings, and the strap muscles connected to the larynx. A permanent opening is created in the neck for the trachea, and a laryngectomy tube inserted to keep the stoma open. The lower portion of the posterior pharynx is removed when the tumor extends beyond the epiglottis with the remaining portion sutured to the esophagus after a nasogastric tube is inserted. The patient must breathe through a permanent tracheostomy, with normal speech no longer possible. Swallowing is not a problem because there is no connection between the esophagus and trachea.

RELATED CONCERNS:

Cancer, p 1014
Psychosocial Aspects of Acute Care, p 899
Surgical Intervention, p 918
Total Nutritional Support, p 1039

PATIENT ASSESSMENT DATA BASE

Preoperative data presented here is dependent on specific type/location of cancer process and underlying complications.

EGO INTEGRITY

May report: Feelings of fear about loss of voice, dying, occurrence/recurrence of cancer.

Concern about how surgery will affect family relationships, ability to work, and finances.

May exhibit: Anxiety, depression, anger, and withdrawal.

Denial.

FOOD/FLUID

May report: Difficulty swallowing.

May exhibit: Difficulty swallowing; chokes easily.

Swelling, ulcerations, masses may be noted dependent on location of cancer.

Oral inflammation/drainage, poor dental hygiene.

Leukoplakia, erythroplasia of oral cavity.
Halitosis.
Swelling of tongue.
Altered gag reflex and facial paralysis.

HYGIENE

May exhibit: Neglect of dental hygiene.
Need for assistance in basic care.

NEUROSENSORY

May report: Diplopia (double vision).
Deafness.
Tingling, paresthesia of facial muscles.

May exhibit: Hemiparalysis of face (parotid and submandibular involvement). Persistent hoarseness or loss of voice (dominant and earliest symptom of intrinsic laryngeal cancer).
Difficulty swallowing.
Conduction deafness.
Disruption of mucous membranes.

PAIN/COMFORT

May report: Chronic sore throat, "lump in throat."
Referred pain to ear, facial pain (late stage, probably metastatic).
Pain/burning sensation with swallowing (especially with hot liquids or citrus juices), local pain in oropharynx.
Postoperative: Sore throat or mouth (pain is not usually reported as severe following head and neck surgery, as compared with pain noted prior to surgery).

May exhibit: Guarding behaviors.
Restlessness.
Facial mask of pain.
Alteration in muscle tone.

RESPIRATION

May report: History of smoking/chewing tobacco.
Occupation working with hardwood sawdust, toxic chemicals/fumes, heavy metals.
History of voice overuse, e.g., professional singer or auctioneer.
History of chronic lung disease.
Cough with/without sputum.
Bloody nasal drainage.

May exhibit: Blood-tinged sputum, hemoptysis.
Dyspnea (late).

SAFETY

May report: Excessive sun exposure over a period of years or radiation.
Visual/hearing changes.

May exhibit:	Masses/enlarged nodes.

SOCIAL INTERACTION

May report:	Lack of family/support system (may be result of age group or behaviors, e.g., alcoholism).
	Concerns about ability to communicate, engage in social interactions.
May exhibit:	Persistent hoarseness, change in voice pitch.
	Muffled/garbled speech, reluctance to speak.
	Hesitancy/reluctance of significant others to provide care/be involved in rehabilitation.

TEACHING/LEARNING

May report:	Nonhealing of oral lesions.
	Concurrent use of alcohol/history of alcohol abuse.
Discharge Plan Considerations:	**DRG projected mean length of stay: 7.4 days.**
	Assistance with wound care, treatments, supplies; transportation, shopping; food preparation; self-care, homemaker/maintenance tasks.

DIAGNOSTIC STUDIES

Direct laryngoscopy, laryngeal tomography and biopsy: Are the most reliable diagnostic indicator.

Laryngography: May be performed with contrast to study blood vessels and lymph nodes.

Pulmonary function studies, bone scans, or other organ scans: May be indicated if distant metastasis is suspected.

Chest x-ray: Done to establish baseline lung status and/or identify metastases.

CBC: May reveal anemia, which is a common problem.

Immunologic surveys: May be done for patients receiving chemotherapy/immunotherapy.

Biochemical profile: Changes may occur in organ function as a result of cancer, metastasis, and therapies.

ABGs/pulse oximetry: May be done to establish baseline/monitor status of lungs (ventilation).

NURSING PRIORITIES

1. Maintain patent airway, adequate ventilation.
2. Assist patient in developing alternate communication methods.
3. Restore/maintain skin integrity.
4. Reestablish/maintain adequate nutrition.
5. Provide emotional support for acceptance of altered body image.
6. Provide information about disease process/prognosis and treatment.

DISCHARGE GOALS

1. Ventilation/oxygenation adequate for individual needs.
2. Communicating effectively.
3. Complications prevented/minimized.
4. Beginning to cope with change in body image.
5. Disease process/prognosis and therapeutic regimen understood.

NURSING DIAGNOSIS:	AIRWAY CLEARANCE, INEFFECTIVE
May be related to:	Partial/total removal of the glottis, altering ability to breathe, cough, and swallow.
	Temporary or permanent change to neck breathing (dependent on patent stoma).
	Edema formation (surgical manipulation and lymphatic accumulation).
	Copious and thick secretions.
Possibly evidenced by:	Dyspnea/difficulty breathing.
	Changes in rate/depth of respiration.
	Use of accessory respiratory muscles.
	Abnormal breath sounds.
	Cyanosis.
DESIRED OUTCOMES/ EVALUATION CRITERIA— PATIENT WILL:	Maintain patent airway with breath sounds clear/clearing.
	Expectorate/clear secretion and be free of aspiration.
	Demonstrate behaviors to improve/maintain airway clearance within level of ability/situation.

ACTIONS/INTERVENTIONS

Independent

Monitor respiratory rate/depth; note ease of breathing. Auscultate breath sounds. Investigate restlessness, dyspnea, development of cyanosis.

Elevate head of bed 30–45 degrees.

Encourage swallowing, if patient is able.

Encourage effective coughing and deep breathing.

Suction laryngectomy/tracheostomy tube, oral and nasal cavities. Note amount, color, and consistency of secretions.

RATIONALE

Changes in respirations, use of accessory muscles, and/or presence of rhonchi/wheezes suggests retention of secretions. Airway obstruction (even partial) can lead to ineffective breathing patterns and impaired gas exchange resulting in complications, e.g., pneumonia, respiratory arrest.

Facilitates drainage of secretions, work of breathing, and lung expansion.

Prevents pooling of oral secretions reducing risk of aspiration. *Note:* Swallowing is impaired when the epiglottis is removed and/or significant postoperative edema and pain are present.

Mobilizes secretions to clear airway and helps prevent respiratory complications.

Prevents secretions from obstructing airway, especially when swallowing ability is impaired and patient cannot blow nose. Changes in character of secretions may indicate developing problems (e.g., dehydration, infection) and need for further evaluation/treatment.

205

ACTIONS/INTERVENTIONS

Independent

Demonstrate and encourage patient to begin self-suction procedures as soon as possible. Educate patient in "clean" techniques.

Maintain proper position of laryngectomy/tracheostomy tube. Check/adjust ties as indicated.

Observe tissue surrounding tube for bleeding. Change patient's position to check for pooling of blood behind neck or on posterior dressings.

Change tube/inner cannula as indicated. Instruct patient in cleaning procedures.

Collaborative

Provide supplemental humidification, e.g., compressed air/oxygen mist collar, room humidifier, increased fluid intake.

Monitor serial ABGs/pulse oximetry; chest x-ray.

RATIONALE

Assists patient to exercise some control in postoperative care and prevention of complications. Reduces anxiety associated with difficulty in breathing or inability to handle secretions when alone.

As edema develops/subsides, tube can be displaced compromising airway. Ties should be snug but not constrictive to surrounding tissue or major blood vessels.

Small amount of oozing may be present. However, continued bleeding or sudden eruption of uncontrolled hemorrhage presents a sudden and very real possibility of airway obstruction/suffocation.

Prevents accumulation of secretions and thick mucous plugs from obstructing airway. Note: This is a common cause of respiratory distress/arrest in later postoperative period.

Normal physiologic (nose/nasal passages) means of filtering/humidifying air are bypassed. Supplemental humidity decreases mucous crusting and facilitates coughing/suctioning of secretions through stoma.

Pooling of secretions/presence of atelectasis may lead to pneumonia requiring more aggressive therapeutic measures.

NURSING DIAGNOSIS:	COMMUNICATION, IMPAIRED, VERBAL
May be related to:	Anatomic deficit (removal of vocal cords).
	Physical barrier (tracheostomy tube).
	Required voice rest.
Possibly evidenced by:	Inability to speak.
	Change in vocal characteristics.
DESIRED OUTCOMES/ EVALUATION CRITERIA— PATIENT WILL:	Communicate needs in an effective manner.
	Identify/plan for appropriate alternate speech methods posthealing.

ACTIONS/INTERVENTIONS

Independent

Review preoperative instructions/discussion of why speech and breathing are altered, using anatomic drawings or models to assist in explanations.

RATIONALE

Reinforces teaching at a time when fear of surviving surgery is past.

206

ACTIONS/INTERVENTIONS	RATIONALE

Independent

Determine whether patient has other communication impairment, e.g., hearing, vision, literacy.

Presence of other problems will influence plan for alternate communication.

Provide immediate and continual means to summon nurse, e.g., call light/bell. Let the patient know the summons will be answered immediately. Stop by to check on patient periodically without being summoned. Post notice at central answering system/nursing station that patient is unable to speak.

Patient needs assurance that nurse is vigilant and will respond to summons. Trust and self-esteem are fostered when the nurse cares enough to come at times other than when called by the patient.

Prearrange signals for obtaining immediate help.

May decease patient's anxiety about inability to speak.

Provide alternate means of communication appropriate to patient need, e.g., pad and pencil, magic slate, alphabet/picture board, sign language. Consider placement of IV.

Permits patient to "express" needs/concerns. Note: IV positioned in hand/wrist may limit ability to write or sign.

Allow sufficient time for communication.

Loss of speech and stress of alternate communication can cause frustration and block expression, especially when caregivers seem "too busy" or preoccupied.

Provide nonverbal communication, e.g., touching and physical presence. Anticipate needs.

Communicates concern and meets need for contact with others. Touch is believed to generate complex biochemical events with possible release of endorphins contributing to reduction of anxiety.

Encourage ongoing communication with "outside world," e.g., newspapers, television, radio, calendar, clock.

Maintains contact with "normal lifestyle" and continued communication through other avenues.

Refer to loss of speech as temporary after a partial laryngectomy and/or depending on availability of voice prosthetics.

Provides encouragement and hope for future with the thought that alternate means of communication and speech are available and possible.

Caution patient to not use voice until physician gives permission.

Promotes healing of vocal cord and limits potential for permanent cord dysfunction.

Arrange for meeting with other persons who have experienced this procedure, as appropriate.

Provides role model, enhancing motivation for problem solving and learning new ways to communicate.

Collaborative

Consult with appropriate health team members/therapists/rehabilitation agency (e.g., speech pathologist, social services, laryngectomee clubs) for hospital-based rehabilitation as well as community resources, such as Lost Chord/NewVoice Club, International Association of Laryngectomees, American Cancer Society.

Ability to use alternate voice and speech methods (e.g., electrolarynx, 1-way valved voice prosthesis, esophageal speech) varies greatly, dependent on extent of surgical procedures, patient's age, emotional state, and motivation to return to an active life. Rehabilitation time may be lengthy and require a number of agencies/resources to facilitate/support learning process.

NURSING DIAGNOSIS:	SKIN/TISSUE INTEGRITY, IMPAIRED
May be related to:	Surgical removal of tissues/grafting.

	Radiation or chemotherapeutic agents.
	Altered circulation/reduced blood supply.
	Compromised nutritional status.
	Edema formation.
	Pooling/continuous drainage of secretions (oral, lymph, or chyle).
Possibly evidenced by:	Disruption of skin/tissue surface.
	Destruction of skin/tissue layers.
DESIRED OUTCOMES/ EVALUATION CRITERIA— PATIENT WILL:	Display timely wound healing without complications.
	Demonstrate techniques to promote healing/prevent complications.

ACTIONS/INTERVENTIONS

Independent

Assess skin color/temperature and capillary refill in operative and skin graft areas.

Keep head of bed elevated 30–45 degrees. Monitor facial edema (usually peaks by 3rd–5th postoperative day).

Protect skin flaps and suture lines from tension or pressure. Provide pillows/rolls and instruct patient to support head/neck during activity.

Monitor bloody drainage from surgical sites, suture lines, drains. Measure drainage from hemovac (if used).

Note/report any milky-appearing drainage.

Change dressings as indicated when used.

Cleanse incisions with sterile saline and peroxide (mixed 1:1) after dressings have been removed.

RATIONALE

Skin should be pink or similar to color of surrounding skin. Skin graft flaps should be pink and warm and should blanch (when gentle finger pressure is applied), with return of color within seconds. Cyanosis and slow refill may indicate venous congestion, which can lead to tissue ischemia/necrosis.

Minimizes postoperative tissue congestion and edema related to excision of lymph channels.

Pressure from tubings and tracheostomy tapes or tension on suture lines can alter circulation/cause tissue injury.

Bloody drainage usually declines steadily after first 24 hours. Steady oozing or frank bleeding indicates problem requiring medical attention.

Milky drainage may indicate thoracic lymph duct leakage (can result in depletion of body fluids and electrolytes). Such a leak may heal spontaneously or require surgical closure.

Damp dressings increase risk of tissue damage/infection. Note: Pressure dressings are not used over skin flaps, because blood supply is easily compromised.

Prevents crust formation, which can trap purulent drainage, destroy skin edges, and increase size of wound. Peroxide is not used full strength, because it may cauterize wound edges and impair healing.

ACTIONS/INTERVENTIONS	RATIONALE
Independent	
Monitor donor site if graft performed; check dressings as indicated.	Donor site may be adjacent to operative site or a distant site (e.g., thigh). Pressure dressings are usually removed within 24–48 hours and wound left open to air to promote healing.
Cleanse thoroughly around stoma and neck tubes (if in place) avoiding soap or alcohol. Show patient how to do self-stoma/tube care with clean water and peroxide, using cloth, not tissue or cotton.	Keeping area cleansed promotes healing and comfort. Soap and other drying agents can lead to stomal irritation and possible inflammation. Materials other than cloth may leave fibers in stoma that can irritate or be inhaled into lungs.
Monitor all sites for signs of wound infection, e.g., unusual redness, increasing edema, pain, exudates, and temperature elevation.	Impedes healing, which may already be slow because of changes induced by cancer, cancer therapies, and/or malnutrition.
Collaborative	
Administer oral, IV, and topical antibiotics as indicated.	Prevents/controls infection.
Cover donor sites with petroleum gauze or moisture-impermeable dressing.	Nonadherent dressing covers exposed sensory nerve endings and protects site from contamination.

NURSING DIAGNOSIS:	ORAL MUCOUS MEMBRANES, ALTERED
May be related to:	Dehydration/absence of oral intake.
	Poor/inadequate oral hygiene.
	Pathologic condition (oral cancer).
	Mechanical trauma (oral surgery).
	Decreased saliva production secondary to radiation (common) or surgical procedure (rare).
	Difficulty swallowing and pooling/drooling.
	Nutritional deficits.
Possibly evidenced by:	Xerostomia (dry mouth), oral discomfort.
	Thick/mucoid saliva, decreased saliva production.
	Dry, crusted, coated tongue; inflamed lips.
	Absent teeth/gums, poor dental health, halitosis.
DESIRED OUTCOMES/ EVALUATION CRITERIA— PATIENT WILL:	Report/demonstrate a decrease in symptoms.
	Identify specific interventions to promote healthy oral mucosa.
	Demonstrate techniques to restore/maintain mucosal integrity.

ACTIONS/INTERVENTIONS	RATIONALE
Independent	
Inspect oral cavity and note changes in:	
Saliva;	Damage to salivary glands may decrease production of saliva, resulting in dry mouth. Pooling and drooling of saliva may occur because of compromised swallowing capability or pain in throat and mouth.
Tongue;	Surgery may have included partial resection of tongue, soft palate, and pharynx. This patient will have decreased sensation and movement of tongue, with difficulty swallowing and increased risk of aspiration of secretions, as well as potential for hemorrhage.
Lips;	Surgery may have removed part of lip resulting in uncontrollable drooling.
Teeth and gums;	Teeth may not be intact (surgical) or may be in poor condition because of malnutrition, chemical therapies, and neglect. Gums may also be surgically altered or inflamed because of poor hygiene, long history of smoking/chewing tobacco, or chemical therapies.
Mucous membranes.	May be excessively dry, ulcerated, erythematous, edematous.
Suction oral cavity gently/frequently. Have patient perform self-suctioning when possible or use gauze wick to drain secretions.	Saliva contains digestive enzymes which may be erosive to exposed tissues. Since drooling may be constant, patient can promote own comfort and enhance oral hygiene.
Show patient how to brush inside of mouth, palate, tongue, and teeth frequently.	Reduces bacteria and risk of infection, promotes tissue healing and comfort.
Apply lubrication to lips; provide oral irrigations as indicated.	Counteracts drying effects of therapeutic measures; negates erosive nature of secretions.

NURSING DIAGNOSIS:	PAIN, ACUTE
May be related to:	Surgical incisions.
	Tissue swelling.
	Presence of nasogastric/orogastric feeding tube.
Possibly evidenced by:	Discomfort in surgical areas/pain with swallowing.
	Facial mask of pain.
	Distraction behaviors, restlessness.
	Guarding behavior.

DESIRED OUTCOMES/ EVALUATION CRITERIA— PATIENT WILL:	Report/indicate pain is relieved/controlled. Demonstrate relief of pain/discomfort by reduced tension and relaxed manner, sleeping/resting appropriately.

ACTIONS/INTERVENTIONS	RATIONALE
Independent	
Support head and neck with pillows. Show patient how to support neck during activity.	Muscle weakness results from muscle and nerve resection in the structures of the neck and/or shoulders. Lack of support aggravates discomfort and may result in injury to suture areas.
Provide comfort measures (e.g., back rub, position change) and diversional activities (e.g., television, visiting, reading).	Promotes relaxation and helps the patient refocus attention on something besides self/discomfort. May reduce analgesic dosage needs/frequency.
Encourage patient to expectorate saliva or to suction mouth gently if unable to swallow.	Swallowing causes muscle activity that may be painful because of edema/strain on suture lines.
Investigate changes in characteristics of pain. Check mouth, throat suture lines for fresh trauma.	May reflect developing complications requiring further evaluation/intervention. Tissues are inflamed and congested and may be easily traumatized by suction catheter, feeding tube, and so on.
Note nonverbal indicators and autonomic responses to pain. Evaluate effects of analgesics.	Aids in determining presence of pain, need for/effectiveness of medication.
Medicate before activity/treatments as indicated.	May enhance cooperation and participation in therapeutic regimen.
Schedule care activities to balance with adequate periods of sleep/rest.	Prevents fatigue/exhaustion and may enhance coping with stress/discomfort.
Recommend use of stress management behaviors, e.g., relaxation techniques, guided imagery.	Promotes sense of well-being, may reduce analgesic needs and enhance healing.
Collaborative	
Provide oral irrigations, anesthetic sprays, and gargles. Instruct patient in self-irrigations.	Improves comfort, promotes healing, and reduces halitosis. *Note:* Commercial mouth-washes containing alcohol or phenol are to be avoided because of their drying effect.
Administer analgesics, e.g., codeine, ASA, and Darvon, as indicated.	Degree of pain is related to extent and psychologic impact of surgery as well as general body condition. Studies appear to support the idea that many patients experience less pain after head and neck surgery than prior to surgery.

NURSING DIAGNOSIS:	**NUTRITION, ALTERED, LESS THAN BODY REQUIREMENTS**
May be related to:	Temporary or permanent alteration in mode of food intake. Altered feedback mechanisms of desire to eat, taste, and

smell because of surgical/structural changes, radiation or chemotherapy.

Possibly evidenced by:	Inadequate food intake, perceived inability to ingest food.
	Aversion to eating, lack of interest in food.
	Reported altered taste sensation.
	Weight loss.
	Weakness of muscles required for swallowing or mastication.
DESIRED OUTCOMES/ EVALUATION CRITERIA— PATIENT WILL:	Indicate understanding of importance of nutrition to healing process and general well-being.
	Make dietary choices to meet nutrient needs within individual situation.
	Demonstrate progressive weight gain toward goal, with normalization of laboratory values and timely healing of tissues/incisions.

ACTIONS/INTERVENTIONS	RATIONALE
Independent	
Auscultate bowel sounds.	Feedings are begun only after bowel sounds are restored postoperatively.
Maintain feeding tube, e.g., check for tube placement: flush with warm water as indicated.	Tube is inserted in surgery and usually sutured in place. Initially the tube may be attached to suction to reduce nausea and/or vomiting. Flushing aids in maintaining patency of tube.
Monitor intake and weigh as indicated. Show patient how to monitor and record weight on a scheduled basis.	Provides information regarding nutritional needs and effectiveness of therapy.
Instruct patient/SO in self-feeding techniques, e.g., bulb syringe, bag and funnel method, and blending soft foods if the patient is to go home with a feeding tube. Make sure patient and SO are able to perform this procedure prior to discharge and that appropriate food and equipment are available at home.	Helps promote nutritional success and preserves dignity in the adult who is now forced to be dependent on others for very basic needs in the social setting of meals.
Begin with small feedings and advance as tolerated. Note signs of gastric fullness, regurgitation, diarrhea.	Content of feeding may result in GI intolerance, requiring change in rate or type of formula.
Provide supplemental water by feeding tube or orally if patient can swallow.	Keeps patient hydrated to offset insensible losses and drainage from surgical areas. Meets free water needs associated with enteral feeding.
Encourage patient when relearning swallowing; e.g., maintain quiet environment, have suction equipment on standby, and demonstrate appropriate breathing techniques.	Helps patient to deal with the frustration and safety concerns involved with swallowing. Provides reassurance that measures are available to prevent/ limit aspiration.

ACTIONS/INTERVENTIONS	RATIONALE

Independent

Resume oral feedings when feasible. Stay with patient during meals the first few days.

Oral feedings can usually resume after suture lines are healed (8–10 days) unless further reconstruction is required or patient will be going home with feeding tube. The patient may experience pain or difficulty with chewing and swallowing initially and may require suctioning during meals, in addition to support and encouragement.

Develop and encourage a pleasant environment for meals.

Promotes socialization and maximizes patient comfort when eating difficulties cause embarrassment.

Help patient/SO develop nutritionally balanced home meal plans.

Promotes understanding of individual needs and significance of nutrition in healing and recovery process.

Collaborative

Consult with dietician/nutritional support team as indicated. Incorporate and reinforce dietitian's teaching.

Useful in identifying individual nutritional needs to promote healing and tissue regeneration. Discharge teaching and follow-up by the dietitian may be needed to evaluate patient needs for diet/equipment modifications and meal planning in the home setting.

Provide nutritionally balanced diet (e.g., semisolid/soft foods) or tube feedings (e.g., blended soft food or commercial preparations) as indicated.

Variations can be made to add or limit certain factors, such as fat and sugar, or to provide a food that the patient prefers.

Monitor laboratory studies, e.g., BUN, glucose, liver function, protein, electrolytes.

Indicators of utilization of nutrients as well as organ function.

NURSING DIAGNOSIS:	**BODY IMAGE, DISTURBANCE IN/ROLE PERFORMANCE, ALTERED**
May be related to:	Loss of voice.
	Changes in anatomic contour of face and neck (disfigurement and/or severe functional impairment).
	Presence of chronic illness.
Possibly evidenced by:	Report of fear of rejection by/reaction of others.
	Negative feelings about body change.
	Refusal to verify actual change or preoccupation with change/loss, not looking at self in mirror.
	Change in social involvement.
	Discomfort in social situations.
	Change in self/others' perception of role.
	Anxiety, depression, lack of eye contact.

	Failure of family members to adapt to change or deal with experience constructively.
DESIRED OUTCOMES/ EVALUATION CRITERIA— PATIENT WILL:	Identify feelings and methods for coping with negative perception of self.
	Demonstrate initial adaptation to body changes as evidenced by participating in self-care activities and positive interactions with others.
	Communicate with SO about changes in role that have occurred.
	Begin to develop plans for altered lifestyle.
	Participate in team efforts toward rehabilitation.

ACTIONS/INTERVENTIONS	RATIONALE
Independent	
Discuss meaning of loss/change with patient, identifying perceptions of current situation/future expectations.	Aids in identifying/defining the problem(s) to focus attention and interventions constructively.
Note nonverbal body language, negative attitudes/self-talk. Assess for self-destructive/suicidal behavior.	May indicate depression/despair, need for further assessment/more intense intervention.
Note emotional reactions, e.g., grieving, depression, anger. Allow patient to progress at own rate.	The patient may experience immediate depression after surgery or react with shock and denial. Acceptance of changes cannot be forced, and the grieving process needs time for resolution.
Maintain calm, reassuring manner. Acknowledge and accept expression of feelings of grief, hostility.	May help allay patient's fears of dying, suffocation, inability to communicate, or mutilation. Patient and SO need to feel supported and know that all feelings are appropriate for the type of experience they are going through.
Allow/but do not participate in patient's use of denial, e.g., when patient is reluctant to participate in self-care (e.g., suctioning stoma). Provide care in a nonjudgmental manner.	Denial may be the most helpful defense for the patient in the beginning, permitting the individual to begin to deal with difficult adjustment slowly.
Set limits on maladaptive behaviors, assisting patient to identify positive behaviors that will aid recovery.	Acting-out can result in lowered self-esteem and impede adjustment to new self-image.
Encourage SO to treat patient normally and not as an invalid.	Distortions of body image may be unconsciously reinforced.
Alert staff that facial expressions and other nonverbal behaviors need to convey acceptance and not revulsion.	This patient is very sensitive to nonverbal communication and may make negative assumptions about others' body language.
Encourage identification of anticipated personal/ work conflicts that may arise.	Expressions of concern bring problems into the open where they can be examined/dealt with.

ACTIONS/INTERVENTIONS

Independent

Recognize behavior indicative of overconcern with future lifestyle/relationship functioning.

Encourage patient to deal with situation in small steps.

Provide positive reinforcement for efforts/progress made.

Encourage patient/SO to communicate feelings to each other.

Collaborative

Refer patient/SO to supportive resources, e.g., psychotherapy, social worker, family counseling, pastoral care.

RATIONALE

Ruminating about anticipated losses/reactions of others is nonproductive and is a block to problem solving.

May feel overwhelmed/have difficulty coping with larger picture but can manage 1 piece at a time.

Encourages patient to feel a sense of movement toward recovery.

All those involved may have difficulty in this area (because of the loss of voice function and/or disfigurement) but need to understand that they may gain courage and help from one another.

A multifaceted approach is required to assist patient toward rehabilitation and wellness. Families need assistance in understanding the processes that the patient is going through and to help them with their own emotions. The goal is to enable them to guard against the tendency to withdraw from/isolate the patient from social contact.

NURSING DIAGNOSIS:	KNOWLEDGE DEFICIT [LEARNING NEED], REGARDING CONDITION AND TREATMENT
May be related to:	Lack of information.
	Misinterpretation of information.
	Lack of recall.
	Poor assimilation of material presented.
	Lack of interest in learning.
Possibly evidenced by:	Indications of concern/request for information.
	Inaccurate follow-through of instructions.
	Inappropriate or exaggerated behaviors, e.g., hostile, agitated, apathetic.
DESIRED OUTCOMES/ EVALUATION CRITERIA— PATIENT WILL:	Indicate basic understanding of disease process, surgical intervention, prognosis, treatment needs.
	Demonstrate ability to provide safe care.
	Use resources (rehabilitation team members) appropriately.
	Identify symptoms requiring medical evaluation/intervention.
	Develop plan for/schedule follow-up appointments.

ACTIONS/INTERVENTIONS	RATIONALE

Independent

Ascertain amount of preoperative preparation and retention of information. Assess level of anxiety related to diagnosis and surgery.

Information can provide clues to patient's postoperative reactions. Anxiety may have interfered with understanding of information given before surgery.

Provide/repeat explanations at patient's level of acceptance. Discuss inaccuracies in perception of disease process and therapies with patient and SO.

Overwhelming stressors are present and may be coupled with limited knowledge. Misconceptions are inevitable, but failure to explore and correct them can result in the patient's failing to progress toward health.

Provide written directions for the patient/SO to read and have available for future reference.

Reinforces proper information and may be used as a home reference.

Educate the patient and SO about basic information regarding stoma, e.g.:

Tub baths instead of showers (initially), shampoo by leaning forward, no swimming or water sports;

Prevents water from entering airway/stoma.

Cover stoma with bib/natural fiber scarf (e.g., cotton or silk);

Prevents dust and particles from being inhaled.

Cover stoma when coughing or sneezing;

Normal airways are bypassed, and mucus will exit from stoma.

Reinforce necessity of not smoking.

Necessary to preserve lung function. Note: Patient may need extra support and encouragement to understand that quality of life can be improved by cessation of smoking.

Discuss importance of reporting to caregiver/physician immediately such symptoms as stoma narrowing, presence of "lump" in throat, dysphagia, or bleeding.

May be signs of tracheal stenosis, recurrent cancer, or carotid erosion.

Develop a means of emergency communication at home.

Permits patient to summon assistance when needed.

Recommend wearing medical alert identification tag/bracelet. Encourage family members to become CPR-certified if they are interested/able to do so.

Provides for appropriate care if the patient becomes unconscious or suffers a cardiopulmonary arrest.

Collaborative

Give careful attention to the provision of needed rehabilitative measures, e.g., temporary/permanent prosthesis, dental care, speech therapy, surgical reconstruction, vocational/sexual/marital counseling, financial assistance.

These services can contribute to patient's well-being and have a positive effect on patient's quality of life.

Adult Respiratory Distress Syndrome (ARDS) (Preacute/Postacute Care)

ARDS is a condition of parenchymal lung dysfunction characterized by (1) a major antecedent event, (2) exclusion of cardiogenic causes of pulmonary edema, (3) presence of tachypnea and hypoxia and, (4) patchy infiltrates on chest x-ray.

ARDS (also called shock lung) is the result of pulmonary insult/injury in previously healthy lungs. This syndrome affects approximately 150,000 to 200,000 patients per year, with a mortality rate of 65% for all patients in whom ARDS develops. The predominant risk factor is sepsis. Other predisposing conditions include major trauma, DIC, blood transfusions, aspiration, near-drowning, smoke or chemical inhalation, toxic metabolic disorders, pancreatitis, eclampsia, and drug overdose. Acute care is typically managed in the critical care setting with intubation and mechanical ventilation.

RELATED CONCERNS:

Burns, p 820
Chronic Obstructive Pulmonary Disease, p 149
Hemothorax/Pneumothorax, p 195
Pneumonia, p 162
Psychosocial Aspects of Acute Care, p 899
Ventilatory Assistance (Mechanical), p 226

PATIENT ASSESSMENT DATA BASE

An initial insult is usually followed by a latent period when pulmonary function appears normal (e.g., 12–24 hours following trauma/shock or 5–10 days after onset of sepsis) but gradually deteriorates by stages into respiratory failure. Physical findings vary, depending on the stage at which the diagnosis is made. Early signs are often missed, because many abnormal findings are not evident until later stages.

ACTIVITY/REST

May report:	Lack of energy/fatigue.
	Insomnia.

CIRCULATION

May report:	History of recent cardiac surgery/cardiopulmonary bypass, embolic phenomena (blood, air, fat).
May exhibit:	BP: May be normal or elevated initially (progressing hypoxemia); hypotension occurs in later stages (shock) or may be a precipitating factor as in eclampsia.
	Heart rate: Tachycardia usually present.
	Heart sounds: Normal in early stages; S_2 (pulmonic component) may develop.
	Dysrhythmias can occur, but ECG is frequently normal.
	Skin and mucous membranes: May be pale, cool. Cyanosis usually develops (late stages).

EGO INTEGRITY

May report:	Apprehension, feelings of impending doom.
May exhibit:	Restlessness, agitation, trembling, irritability, changes in mentation, or obtundation.

FOOD/FLUID

May report: Loss of appetite, nausea.

May exhibit: Edema formation/changes in weight.

Loss of/diminished bowel sounds.

NEUROSENSORY

May report/exhibit: Current head trauma.

Mental sluggishness, motor dysfunction.

RESPIRATION

May report: Current aspiration/near-drowning, smoke/gas inhalation, diffuse pulmonary infections.

Sudden or gradual onset of breathing difficulty, "air hunger."

May exhibit: Respirations: Rapid, shallow, grunting.

Increased work of breathing; use of accessory muscles of respiration, e.g., intercostal or substernal retractions, nasal flaring, despite high oxygen concentration.

Breath sounds: May be normal initially. Crackles, rhonchi, and bronchial breath sounds may develop.

Chest percussion: Dull over consolidated areas.

Decreased or unequal chest expansion.

Increased fremitus (vibratory tremors in chest wall noted with palpation).

Thin, frothy sputum.

Pallor or cyanosis.

Decreased mentation, confusion.

SAFETY

May report: Current history of orthopedic trauma/fractures, sepsis, blood transfusions, anaphylactic episode.

SEXUALITY

May report/exhibit: Current/recent pregnancy with development of complications of eclampsia.

TEACHING/LEARNING

May report: Current drug ingestion/overdose.

Discharge Plan Considerations: **DRG projected mean length of stay: 6.0 days.**

Dependent on residual effects/pulmonary damage, may require assistance with transportation, shopping, self-care, homemaker/maintenance tasks.

DIAGNOSTIC STUDIES

Chest x-ray: Unremarkable in initial stages or may reveal minimal patchy, scattered infiltrates located centrally in the perihilar region of the lungs. In later stages, diffuse bilateral interstitial and alveolar infiltrates become evident and may involve all lung lobes. These infiltrates are often described as "ground-glass" appearance or "whiteouts." Heart size is normal (differentiates from cardiogenic pulmonary edema).

ABGs: Serial comparisons show progressing hypoxemia (decreasing PaO_2 despite increased concentrations of inspired oxygen). Hypocapnia (decreased level of CO_2 may be present in initial stages due to com-

218

pensatory hyperventilation. Hypercapnia ($PaCO_2$ greater than 50) reflects ventilatory failure. Respiratory alkalosis (pH greater than 7.45) may occur in early stages, but respiratory acidosis occurs in later stages due to increased deadspace and decreased alveolar ventilation. Metabolic acidosis may also occur in later stages due to rising blood lactate levels, resulting from anaerobic metabolism.

Pulmonary function tests: Lung compliance and lung volumes are decreased, especially FRC. Increased deadspace (V_d/V_t) is produced by areas where vasoconstriction and microemboli have occurred.

Shunt measurement (Qs/Qt): Measures pulmonary blood flow versus systemic blood flow, which provides a clinical measurement of intrapulmonary shunting. Right-to-left shunt is increased.

Alveolar-arterial gradient (A-a gradient): Provides a comparison of the oxygen tension within alveoli and arterial blood. A-a gradient is increased.

Lactic acid level: Elevated

NURSING PRIORITIES

1. Promote/maintain optimal respiratory function and oxygenation.
2. Minimize/prevent complications.
3. Maintain adequate nutrition for healing/respiratory function.
4. Provide for emotional support of patient and family.
5. Provide information about disease process, prognosis, and treatment needs.

DISCHARGE GOALS

1. Breathing spontaneously with appropriate lung tidal volumes.
2. Breath sounds clear/clearing.
3. Free of preventable complications.
4. Dealing realistically with current situation.
5. Disease process, prognosis, and individual therapeutic regimen understood.

NURSING DIAGNOSIS:	AIRWAY CLEARANCE, INEFFECTIVE
May be related to:	Loss of airway cilia function (hypoperfusion). Increased amount/viscosity of pulmonary secretions. Increased airway resistance (interstitial edema).
Possibly evidenced by:	Reports of dyspnea. Changes in depth/rate of respiration, use of accessory muscles for breathing. Cough (effective or ineffective) with/without sputum production. Anxiety/restlessness.
DESIRED OUTCOMES/ EVALUATION CRITERIA— PATIENT WILL:	Verbalize/demonstrate relief from dyspnea. Maintain patent airway with breath sounds clear/absence of rhonchi. Expectorate secretions without difficulty. Demonstrate behaviors to improve/maintain airway clearance.

ACTIONS/INTERVENTIONS	RATIONALE
Independent	
Note changes in respiratory effort and patterns of breathing.	Use of intercostal/abdominal/neck muscles and flaring of nares reflects increased respiratory effort.
Observe for decreased chest wall expansion and presence of/increase in fremitus	Chest expansion may be limited or unequal due to accumulation of fluid, edema, and secretions in sections/lobes. Lung consolidation and fluid-filled areas may increase fremitus.
Note characteristics of breath sounds. (Refer to ND: Gas Exchange, impaired, p 221)	Breath sounds reflect air flow through the tracheo-bronchial tree and are affected by the presence of fluid, mucus, or other obstruction to air flow. Wheezes may be evidence of bronchoconstriction or airway narrowing due to edema. Rhonchi may clear with cough and reflect the collection of mucus in the airway.
Note characteristics of cough (e.g., persistent, effective/ineffective) as well as production and characteristics of sputum.	Cough characteristics may change depending on the cause/etiology of the respiratory failure. Sputum, if present, may be copious, thick/viscous, bloody, and/or purulent.
Maintain proper body/head positioning and use airway adjuncts as needed.	Facilitates maintenance of patent upper airways when patient airway may be compromised, e.g., altered levels of consciousness, sedation, and maxillofacial trauma.
Assist with coughing/deep-breathing exercises, position changes and suctioning, as indicated.	Pooled secretions impair ventilation and predispose to the development of atelectasis and pulmonary infections.
Increase oral intake if possible.	In the absence of heart failure or pulmonary edema and if the patient is not intubated, an increased oral fluid intake may liquefy secretions/enhance expectoration.
Collaborative	
Administer humidified oxygen, IV fluids; provide room humidity as appropriate.	Humidity loosens and mobilizes secretions and promotes the transport of oxygen.
Provide aerosol therapy, ultrasonic nebulization.	Treatments are designed to forcefully deliver oxygen/bronchodilation/humidity to alveoli and to mobilize secretions.
Assist with/administer chest physiotherapy, e.g., postural drainage; chest percussion/vibration, as indicated.	Enhances drainage/elimination of lung secretions into central bronchi, where they may more readily be coughed or suctioned out. Promotes efficient use of respiratory muscles and helps reexpand alveoli.
Administer bronchodilators, e.g., aminophylline, albuterol (Proventil); isoetharine (Bronkosol) and mucolytic agents, e.g., acetylcysteine (Mucomyst); guaifenesin (Robitussin).	Medications are given to relieve bronchospasm, reduce viscosity of secretions, improve ventilation, and facilitate removal of secretions.
Monitor for adverse side effects of medications, e.g., tachycardia, hypertension, tremor, insomnia.	May require alteration of dose/drug choice.

NURSING DIAGNOSIS:	GAS EXCHANGE, IMPAIRED
May be related to:	Accumulation of protein and fluid in interstitial/alveolar spaces.
	Alveolar hypoventilation.
	Loss of surfactant causing alveolar collapse.
Possibly evidenced by:	Tachypnea, use of accessory muscles, cyanosis.
	Changes in ABGs, A-a gradient, and shunt measurement.
	Ventilation/perfusion mismatching with increased dead-space and intrapulmonary shunting.
DESIRED OUTCOMES/ EVALUATION CRITERIA— PATIENT WILL:	Demonstrate improved ventilation and adequate oxygenation by ABGs within normal range and free of symptoms of respiratory distress.
	Participate in treatment regimen within ability/situation.

ACTIONS/INTERVENTIONS	RATIONALE
Independent	
Assess respiratory status frequently, noting increased respiratory rate/effort or change in breathing pattern.	Tachypnea is a compensatory mechanism for hypoxemia, and increased respiratory effort may reflect the degree of hypoxemia.
Note presence/absence of breath sounds and the presence of adventitious sounds, e.g., crackles, wheezes.	Breath sounds may be muffled, unequal, or absent in affected areas. Crackles are evidence of increased fluid in tissue spaces as a result of increased alveolar-capillary membrane permeability. Wheezes may be evidence of bronchoconstriction and/or airway narrowing due to mucus/edema.
Assess for presence of cyanosis.	Usually a significant drop in oxygenation (desaturation of 5 g of hemoglobin) occurs before cyanosis appears. Central cyanosis of "warm organs," e.g., tongue, lips, and earlobes, is most indicative of systemic hypoxemia. Peripheral cyanosis of nail beds/extremities is associated with vasoconstriction.
Observe for drowsiness, apathy, inattentiveness, restlessness, confusion, somnolence.	May reflect progressing hypoxemia and/or acidosis.
Auscultate heart rate and rhythm.	Hypoxemia can cause irritability of the myocardium, producing a variety of dysrhythmias.
Provide for rest periods and a quiet environment.	Conserves patient's energy, reducing oxygen requirements.
Demonstrate/encourage the use of pursed-lip breathing if indicated.	May be especially helpful for patients who are recovering from prolonged/severe illness, resulting in lung parenchymal destruction.

221

ACTIONS/INTERVENTIONS	RATIONALE
Collaborative	
Administer humidified oxygen by CPAP mask as indicated.	Maximizes available oxygen for exchange, by continuous positive airway pressure.
Assist with/provide IPPB treatments.	Promotes full expansion of lungs to improve oxygenation and to administer nebulized medications into respiratory passages. Intubation and ventilatory support are suggested when the PaO_2 is less than 60 mm Hg and does not respond to increased inspired oxygen (FIO_2).
Review serial chest x-rays.	Shows progression or resolution of pulmonary congestion.
Monitor/graph serial ABGs/pulse oximetry.	Reflects ventilation/oxygenation and acid/base status. Used as a basis for evaluating effectiveness of therapies or indicator of need for changes in therapy.
Administer medications as indicated, e.g., steroids, antibiotics, bronchodilators, expectorants.	Treatment for ARDS is largely supportive or is designed to correct the underlying cause of ARDS and to prevent progression and potentially fatal complications of hypoxemia. Steroids may be of benefit in reducing inflammation and promoting surfactant production. Bronchodilators/expectorants promote airway clearance. Antibiotics may be indicated in presence of pulmonary infections/sepsis to treat causative pathogen.

NURSING DIAGNOSIS:	FLUID VOLUME DEFICIT, HIGH RISK FOR
Risk factors may include:	Use of diuretics.
	Compartmental fluid shifts.
Possibly evidenced by:	[Not applicable; presence of signs and symptoms establishes an actual diagnosis.]
DESIRED OUTCOMES/ EVALUATION CRITERIA— PATIENT WILL:	Demonstrate normal fluid volume as evidenced by BP, heart rate, weight, and urine output within patient's normal limits.

ACTIONS/INTERVENTIONS	RATIONALE
Independent	
Monitor vital signs, e.g., BP, heart rate, pulses (equality and volume).	Volume depletion/fluid shifts may increase heart rate, lower BP, and diminish volume of pulses.
Note changes in mentation, skin turgor, hydration of mucous membranes, and character of sputum.	Decreased cardiac output affects cerebral perfusion/function. Fluid deficit can also be identified by decreased skin turgor, dry mucous membranes, and thick viscous secretions.

ACTIONS/INTERVENTIONS	RATIONALE
Independent	
Measure/calculate intake, output, and fluid balance. Note insensible losses.	Provides information about general fluid status. Sequential negative fluid balances may indicate developing deficit.
Weigh daily.	Rapid changes suggest alterations in total body water.
Collaborative	
Administer IV fluids under close observation/with control devices as indicated.	Restores/maintains circulatory volume and osmotic pressure. Note: Despite fluid deficits, fluid administration may result in increased pulmonary congestion, negatively affecting respiratory function.
Monitor/replace electrolytes as indicated.	Electrolytes, especially potassium and sodium may be depleted as a result of diuretic therapy.

NURSING DIAGNOSIS:	**ANXIETY/FEAR (SPECIFY LEVEL)**
May be related to:	Situational crisis.
	Threat to/change in health status; fear of death.
	Physiologic factors (effects of hypoxemia).
Possibly evidenced by:	Expressed concern regarding changes in life events.
	Increased tension and helplessness.
	Apprehension, fear, restlessness.
DESIRED OUTCOMES/ EVALUATION CRITERIA— PATIENT WILL:	Verbalize awareness of feelings of anxiety and healthy ways to deal with them.
	Acknowledge and discuss fears.
	Appear relaxed and report anxiety is reduced to a manageable level.
	Demonstrate problem solving and effective use of resources.

ACTIONS/INTERVENTIONS	RATIONALE
Independent	
Observe for increasing respiratory failure, agitation, restlessness, emotional lability.	Worsening hypoxemia can cause or exacerbate anxiety.
Maintain quiet environment with minimal stimulation. Schedule care and procedures to provide periods of uninterrupted rest.	Reduces anxiety by promoting relaxation and energy conservation.
Demonstrate/assist with relaxation techniques, meditation, guided imaging.	Provides opportunity for patient to manage own anxiety and feel sense of control.

223

ACTIONS/INTERVENTIONS	RATIONALE
Independent	
Identify patient's perception of the threat represented by the situation.	Helps with recognition of extent of anxiety/fear and identification of measures that may be helpful for the individual.
Encourage patient to acknowledge and express feelings.	Initial step in managing feelings is identification and expression. Encourages acceptance of situation and own ability to handle.
Acknowledge reality of stress without denial or reassurance that everything will be all right. Provide information about measures being taken to correct/alleviate condition.	Helps patient to accept what is happening and can reduce level of anxiety/fear of the unknown. False reassurance is not helpful, because neither nurse nor patient knows the final outcome.
Identify techniques patient has used previously to cope with anxiety.	Focuses attention on skills patient already possesses, promoting sense of control.
Assist SO to respond in a positive manner to patient/situation.	Promotes reduction of anxiety to see others remaining calm. Because anxiety is contagious, if SO/staff exhibit their anxiety the patient's coping abilities can be adversely affected.
Collaborative	
Administer sedatives as indicated and monitor for adverse effects.	May be needed to help manage anxiety and promote rest. However, side effects such as respiratory depression may limit or contraindicate use.

NURSING DIAGNOSIS:	KNOWLEDGE DEFICIT [LEARNING NEED], REGARDING CONDITION, THERAPY NEEDS
May be related to:	Lack of information.
	Misinterpretation of information.
	Lack of recall.
Possibly evidenced by:	Request for information.
	Statement of concerns.
DESIRED OUTCOMES/ EVALUATION CRITERIA— PATIENT WILL:	Explain relationship between disease process and therapy.
	Describe/verbalize dietary, medication, and activity regimen.
	Correctly identify signs and symptoms requiring medical attention.
	Formulate plan for follow-up care.

ACTIONS/INTERVENTIONS	RATIONALE
Independent	
Pace learning sessions to meet patient's needs. Give information in clear/concise ways.	Recovery from respiratory compromise/failure may severely hamper the patient's attention span, con-

ACTIONS/INTERVENTIONS

Independent

Assess potential for cooperation with home-treatment regimen. Include SO in sessions as indicated.

Provide information concerning the cause/onset of disease process to patient/SO.

Instruct in preventive measures, if needed. Discuss avoidance of overexertion and importance of maintaining regular rest periods. Avoiding chilling/cold environment and persons with infections.

Provide verbal and written information concerning medications, e.g., purpose, side effects, route, dose, schedules.

Review nutritional counseling regarding meal plans; need for high calorie meals on frequent basis.

Provide guidelines for activity.

Demonstrate adaptive breathing techniques and ways to reduce energy expenditures during ADLs.

Discuss follow-up care, e.g., doctor visits, diagnostic pulmonary function tests, and signs/symptoms requiring evaluation/interventions.

Assist in formulating plan to meet individual needs postdischarge. Identify/refer to appropriate resources, e.g., visiting nurse, home health agency, Meals-on-Wheels, Amblicab.

RATIONALE

centration, and energy for accepting new information/tasks. The SO especially needs to be involved when disease process is severe or chances for recovery limited.

ARDS is a complication of other processes, not a primary diagnosis. Patient/SO are often confused by its development in a previously "healthy" respiratory system.

Lowered resistance persists for a period of time following recovery. Control/avoidance of exposure to environmental factors, such as smoke/fumes, allergic reactions, or infections may be required to avoid further complications.

Providing instruction for safe medication use enables patient to appropriately follow through with medical regimen.

Patient with severe respiratory problems usually has weight loss and anorexia while needing increased nutrients for healing.

Patient should avoid overfatigue and intersperse rest periods with activity to increase strength/stamina and prevent excessive oxygen consumption/demand.

Weakened condition may make it difficult for the patient to manage even simple actions.

Understanding reason and need for follow-up care as well as what constitutes a need for medical attention promotes patient participation and may enhance cooperation with medical regimen.

Permits return to home while providing necessary support during period of recuperation/adjustment.

Ventilatory Assistance (Mechanical)

More and more patients on ventilators are being transferred from ICU to medical-surgical units with problems such as (1) neuromuscular deficits, e.g., quadriplegia with phrenic nerve injury or high C-spine injuries, Guillian-Barre, and ALS; (2) COPD with respiratory atrophy and malnutrition (inability to wean); and (3) restrictive conditions of chest or lungs, e.g., kyphoscoliosis, interstitial fibrosis.

The expectation is that the majority of patients will be weaned prior to discharge. That is the focus of this plan of care. However, it is known that some patients are unsuccessful at weaning or are not candidates for weaning. For those patients, portions of this plan of care would need to be modified.

Volume-cycled ventilators are the primary choice for long-term ventilation of patients whose permanent changes in lung compliance and resistance require increased pressure to provide adequate ventilation (e.g., COPD).

Pressure-cycled ventilators are desirable for patients with relatively normal lung compliance who cannot initiate or sustain respiration because of muscular/phrenic nerve involvement (e.g., quadriplegics).

RELATED CONCERNS:

Adult Respiratory Distress Syndrome, p 217
Cardiac Surgery, p 113
Chronic Obstructive Pulmonary Disease, p 149
Guillian-Barré Syndrome, p 358
Hemothorax/Pneumothorax, p 195
Psychosocial Aspects of Acute Care, p 899
Spinal Cord Injury, p 337
Total Nutritional Support, p 1039

PATIENT ASSESSMENT DATA BASE

Data gathered are dependent on the underlying pathophysiology and/or reason for ventilatory support. Refer to the appropriate plan of care.

Discharge Plan Considerations: **DRG projected mean length of stay: 9.7 days.**
If ventilator-dependent, may require changes in physical layout of home, acquisition of equipment/supplies, provision of a backup power source, instruction of SO/caregivers, provision for continuation of plan of care, assistance with transportation, and coordination of resources/support systems.

DIAGNOSTIC STUDIES

Pulmonary function studies: Determine the ability of the lungs to exchange oxygen and carbon dioxide and include but are not limited to the following:

ABGs: Assesses status of oxygenation and ventilation and acid-base balance.

Vital capacity (VC): Is reduced in restrictive chest or lung conditions; is normal or increased in COPD; normal to decreased in neuromuscular diseases (Guillian-Barré); decreased in conditions limiting thoracic movement (kyphoscoliosis).

Forced vital capacity (FVC): (measured by spirometry): Reduced in restrictive conditions, reduced in asthma, normal to reduced in COPD.

Tidal volume (V_T): May be decreased in both restrictive and obstructive processes.

Negative inspiratory force (NIF): Can be substituted for vital capacity to help determine whether the patient can initiate a breath.

Minute ventilation (V_E): Measures volume of air inhaled and exhaled in 1 minute of normal breathing. This reflects muscle endurance and is a major determinant of work of breathing.

Inspiratory pressure (Pi$_{max}$): Measures respiratory muscle strength (less than -20 cm H_2O is considered insufficient for weaning).

Forced expiratory volume (FEV): Usually decreased in chronic obstructive lung diseases.

Flow-volume (F-V) Loops: Abnormal loops are indicative of large and small airway obstructive disease and restrictive diseases, when far advanced.

Chest x-ray: Monitors resolution/progression of underlying condition (e.g., ARDS) or complications (e.g., atelectasis, pneumonia).

Nutritional assessment: Done to identify nutritional and electrolyte imbalances which might interfere with successful weaning.

NURSING PRIORITIES

1. Promote adequate ventilation and oxygenation.
2. Prevent complications.
3. Provide emotional support for patient/SO.
4. Provide information about disease process/prognosis and treatment needs.

DISCHARGE GOALS

1. Respiratory function adequate to meet individual needs.
2. Complications prevented/minimized.
3. Effective means of communication established.
4. Disease process/prognosis and therapeutic regimen understood (including home ventilatory support if indicated).

NURSING DIAGNOSIS:	BREATHING PATTERN, INEFFECTIVE/ SPONTANEOUS VENTILATION, INABILITY TO SUSTAIN
May be related to:	Respiratory center depression.
	Respiratory muscle weakness/paralysis.
	Noncompliant lung tissue (decreased lung expansion).
	Alteration of patient's usual O_2/CO_2 ratio.
Possibly evidenced by:	Changes in rate and depth of respirations.
	Dyspnea/increased work of breathing, use of accessory muscles.
	Reduced vital capacity/total lung volume.
	Tachypnea/bradypnea or cessation of respirations when off the ventilator.
	Cyanosis.
	Decreased PO_2 and SaO_2; increased PCO_2.
	Increased restlessness, apprehension, and metabolic rate.

ACTIONS/INTERVENTIONS	RATIONALE

Independent

Investigate etiology of respiratory failure.	Understanding the underlying cause of the patient's particular ventilatory problem is essential to the care of the patient, e.g., decisions about future patient capabilities/ventilation needs and most appropriate type of ventilatory support.
Observe overall breathing pattern. Note respiratory rate, distinguishing between spontaneous respirations and ventilator breaths.	Patients on ventilator can experience hyperventilation/hypoventilation, dyspnea/"air hunger," and attempt to correct deficiency by overbreathing.
Auscultate chest periodically, noting presence/absence and equality of breath sounds, adventitious breath sounds, as well as symmetry of chest movement.	Provides information regarding airflow through the tracheobronchial tree and the presence/absence of fluid, mucous obstruction. *Note:* Frequent crackles or rhonchi that do not clear with coughing/suctioning may indicate developing complications (atelectasis, pneumonia, acute bronchospasm, pulmonary edema). Changes in chest symmetry may indicate improper placement of endotracheal tube, development of barotrauma.
Count patient's respirations for 1 full minute and compare to desired/ventilator set rate.	Respirations vary depending on problem requiring ventilatory assistance, e.g., patient may be totally ventilator dependent, or be able to take breath(s) on own between ventilator-delivered breaths. Rapid patient respirations can produce respiratory alkalosis and/or prevent desired volume from being delivered by ventilator. Slow patient respirations/hypoventilation increases $PaCO_2$ levels and may cause acidosis.
Verify that patient's respirations are in phase with the ventilator.	Adjustments may be required in tidal volume, respiratory rate, and/or deadspace of the ventilator or the patient may need sedation to synchronize respirations and reduce work of breathing/energy expenditure.
Elevate head of bed or place in orthopedic chair if possible.	Elevation of the patient's head or getting out of bed while still on the ventilator is both physically and psychologically beneficial.
Inflate tracheal/endotracheal tube cuff properly using minimal leak/occlusive technique. Check cuff	The cuff must be properly inflated to ensure adequate ventilation/delivery of desired tidal volume.

ACTIONS/INTERVENTIONS	RATIONALE

Independent

inflation every 4–8 hours and whenever cuff is deflated/reinflated.

Note: In long-term patients, the cuff may be deflated most of the time or a noncuffed tracheostomy tube used.

Check tubing for obstruction, e.g., kinking or accumulation of water. Drain tubing as indicated, avoiding draining toward the patient or back into the reservoir;

Kinks in tubing prevent adequate volume delivery and increase airway pressure. Water prevents proper gas distribution and predisposes to bacterial growth.

Check ventilator alarms for proper functioning. Do not turn off alarms, even for suctioning. Remove from ventilator and ventilate manually if source of ventilator alarm cannot be quickly identified and rectified. Ascertain that alarms can be heard in the nurses' station.

Ventilators have a series of visual and audible alarms, e.g., oxygen, low/high pressure, I:E ratio. Turning off/failure to reset alarms places patient at risk for unobserved ventilator failure or respiratory distress/arrest.

Keep resuscitation bag at bedside and ventilate manually whenever indicated.

Provides/restores adequate ventilation when patient or equipment problems require that the patient be temporarily removed from the ventilator.

Assist patient in "taking control" of breathing if weaning is attempted/ventilatory support is interrupted during procedure/activity.

Coaching the patient to take slower, deeper breaths, practice abdominal/pursed-lip breathing, assume position of comfort, and use relaxation techniques, can be helpful in maximizing respiratory function.

Collaborative

Assess ventilator settings routinely and readjust as indicated:

Controls/settings are adjusted according to patient's primary disease and results of diagnostic testing in order to maintain parameters within appropriate limits.

Observe oxygen concentration percentage (FIO_2); Verify that oxygen line is in proper outlet/tank; monitor in-line oxygen analyzer or perform periodic oxygen analysis;

FIO_2 is adjusted to maintain an acceptable oxygen percentage and saturation for patient's condition (may be 21% to 100%). Because machine dials are not always accurate, an oxygen analyzer may be used to ascertain that patient is receiving the desired concentration of oxygen.

Assess tidal volume (10–15 ml/kg). Verify proper function of spirometer, bellows or computer readout of delivered volume. Note alterations from desired volume delivery;

Monitors amount of air inspired and expired. Changes may indicate alteration in lung compliance or leakage through machine/around tube cuff (if used).

Note airway pressure;

Airway pressure should remain relatively constant. Increased pressure alarm reading reflects (1) increased airway resistance as may occur with bronchospasm; (2) retained secretions; and/or (3) decreased lung compliance as may occur with obstruction of the ET tube, development of atelectasis, ARDS, pulmonary edema, worsening COPD, or pneumothorax. Low airway pressure alarms may be triggered by pathophysiological conditions causing hypoventilation, e.g., disconnection from ventilator, low ET cuff pressure, ET displaced above the vocal cords, patient is "over-breathing" or out of phase with the ventilator.

229

ACTIONS/INTERVENTIONS

Collaborative

Monitor inspiratory and expiratory (I:E) ratio;

Check sigh rate intervals (usually 1½ to 2 times tidal volume);

Note inspired humidity and temperature.

RATIONALE

Expiratory phase is usually twice the length of the inspiratory rate, but may be longer to compensate for air-trapping to improve gas exchange in the COPD patient.

Sighing promotes maximal ventilation of alveoli to prevent/reduce atelectasis, and enhances movement of secretions.

Usual warming and humidifying function of nasopharynx is bypassed with intubation. Dehydration can dry up normal pulmonary fluids, cause secretions to thicken, and increase risk of infection. Temperature should be maintained at about body temperature to reduce risk of damage to cilia and hyperthermia reactions.

NURSING DIAGNOSIS:	**AIRWAY CLEARANCE, INEFFECTIVE**
May be related to:	Foreign body (artificial airway) in the trachea. Inability to cough/ineffective cough.
Possibly evidenced by:	Changes in rate or depth of respiration. Cyanosis. Abnormal breath sounds. Anxiety/restlessness.
DESIRED OUTCOMES/ EVALUATION CRITERIA— PATIENT WILL:	Maintain patent airway with breath sounds clear and aspiration prevented. <u>Caregiver will:</u> Identify potential complications and initiate appropriate actions.

ACTIONS/INTERVENTIONS

Independent

Assess airway patency.

Evaluate chest movement and auscultate for bilateral breath sounds.

RATIONALE

Obstruction may be caused by accumulation of secretions, mucous plugs, hemorrhage, bronchospasm, and/or problems with the position of tracheostomy/endotracheal tubes.

Symmetrical chest movement with breath sounds throughout lung fields indicates proper tube placement/unobstructed airflow. Lower airway obstruction (e.g., pneumonia/atelectasis) produces changes in breath sounds such as rhonchi, wheezing.

ACTIONS/INTERVENTIONS

Independent

Monitor endotracheal tube placement. Note lip line marking and compare with desired placement. Secure tube carefully with tape or tube holder. Obtain assistance when retaping or repositioning tube.

Note excessive coughing, increased dyspnea, high pressure alarm sounding on ventilator, visible secretions in endotracheal/tracheostomy tube, increased rhonchi.

Suction as needed, limiting duration of suction to 15 seconds or less. Choose appropriate suction catheter. Instill sterile normal saline, if indicated. Hyperventilate with bag before suctioning, using 100% oxygen if appropriate.

Instruct patient in coughing techniques during suctioning, e.g., splinting, timing of breathing, and "quad cough" as indicated.

Reposition/turn periodically.

Encourage/provide fluids within individual capability.

Collaborative

Provide chest physiotherapy as indicated, e.g., postural drainage, percussion.

Administer IV and aerosol bronchodilators as indicated, e.g., aminophylline, metaproterenol sulfate (Alupent); idoetharine hydrochloride (Bronkosol).

Assist with fiberoptic bronchoscopy, if indicated.

RATIONALE

The endotracheal tube may slip into the right main-stem bronchus, thereby obstructing airflow to the left lung and putting patient at risk for a tension pneumothorax.

The intubated patient usually has an ineffective cough reflex, or the patient may have neuromuscular or neurosensory impairment, altering ability to cough. These patients are dependent on alternate means such as suctioning to remove secretions.

Suctioning should not be *routine,* and duration should be limited to reduce hazard of hypoxia. Suction catheter diameter should be less than 50% of the internal diameter of the endotracheal/tracheostomy tube for prevention of hypoxia. Hyperventilation with bag or ventilator sigh on 100% oxygen may be desired to reduce atelectasis and to reduce accidental hypoxia.

Enhances effectiveness of cough effort and secretion clearing.

Promotes drainage of secretions and ventilation to all lung segments, reducing risk of atelectasis.

Helps liquefy secretions, enhancing expectoration.

Promotes ventilation of all lung segments and aids drainage of secretions.

Promotes ventilation and removal of secretions by relaxation of smooth muscle/bronchospasm.

May be performed to remove secretions/mucous plugs.

NURSING DIAGNOSIS:	COMMUNICATION, IMPAIRED, VERBAL
May be related to:	Physical barrier, e.g., endotracheal/tracheostomy tube. Neuromuscular weakness/paralysis.
Possibly evidenced by:	Inability to speak.
DESIRED OUTCOMES/ EVALUATION CRITERIA— PATIENT WILL:	Establish method of communication in which needs can be understood.

RESPIRATORY: Ventilatory Assistance (Mechanical)

231

ACTIONS/INTERVENTIONS	RATIONALE

Independent

Assess patient's ability to communicate by alternate means.

Reasons for long-term ventilatory support are various; patient may be alert and be adept at writing (e.g., chronic COPD with inability to be weaned) or may be lethargic, comatose, or paralyzed. Method of communicating with patient is therefore highly individualized.

Establish means of communication, e.g., maintain eye contact; ask yes/no questions; provide magic slate, paper/pencil, picture/alphabet board; use sign language as appropriate; validate meaning of attempted communications.

Eye contact assures patient of interest in communicating; if patient is able to move head, blink eyes, or is comfortable with simple gestures, a great deal can be done with yes/no questions. Pointing to letter boards or writing is often tiring to patients, who can then become frustrated with the effort needed to attempt conversations. Use of picture boards that express a concept or routine needs may simplify communication. Family members/other caregivers may be able to assist/interpret needs.

Consider form of communication when placing IV.

IV positioned in hand/wrist may limit ability to write or sign.

Place call light/bell within reach, making certain patient is alert and physically capable of using it. Answer call light/bell immediately. Anticipate needs. Tell patient that nurse is immediately available should assistance be required.

Ventilator-dependent patient may be better able to relax, feel safe (not abandoned), and breathe with the ventilator knowing that nurse is vigilant and needs will be met.

Place note at central call station informing staff that patient is unable to speak.

Alerts all staff members to respond to the patient at the bedside instead of over the intercom.

Encourage family/SO to talk with patient, providing information about family and daily happenings.

SO may feel self-conscious in one-sided conversation, but knowledge that he or she is assisting patient to regain/maintain contact with reality as well as enabling patient to feel part of family unit can reduce feelings of awkwardness.

Collaborative

Evaluate need for/appropriateness of talking tracheostomy tubes.

Patients with adequate cognitive/muscular skills may have the ability to manipulate talking tracheostomy tube.

NURSING DIAGNOSIS:	ANXIETY/FEAR [SPECIFY LEVEL]
May be related to:	Situational crises; threat to self-concept.
	Threat of death/dependency on mechanical support.
	Change in health/socioeconomic/role functioning.
	Interpersonal transmission/contagion.
Possibly evidenced by:	Increased muscle/facial tension.
	Insomnia; restlessness.

Hypervigilance.

Feelings of inadequacy.

Fearfulness, uncertainty, apprehension.

Focus on self/negative self-talk.

Expressed concern regarding changes in life events.

DESIRED OUTCOMES/ EVALUATION CRITERIA— PATIENT WILL:

Verbalize/communicate awareness of feelings and healthy ways to deal with them.

Demonstrate problem-solving skills/behaviors to cope with current situation.

Report anxiety/fear is reduced to manageable level.

Appear relaxed and sleeping/resting appropriately.

ACTIONS/INTERVENTIONS	RATIONALE
Independent	
Identify patient's perception of threat represented by situation.	Defines scope of individual problem and influences choice of interventions.
Observe/monitor physical responses, e.g., restlessness, changes in vital signs, repetitive movements. Note congruency of verbal/nonverbal communication.	Useful in evaluating extent/degree of concerns, especially when compared with "verbal" comments.
Encourage patient/SO to acknowledge and express fears.	Provides opportunity for dealing with concerns, clarifies reality of fears, and reduces anxiety to a more manageable level.
Acknowledge the anxiety and fear of the situation. Avoid meaningless reassurance that everything will be all right.	Validates the reality of the situation without minimizing the emotional impact. Provides opportunity for the patient/SO to accept and begin to deal with what has happened, reducing anxiety.
Identify/review with patient/SO the safety precautions being taken, e.g., backup power and oxygen supplies, emergency equipment at hand for suction. Discuss/review the meanings of alarm system.	Provides reassurance to help allay unnecessary anxiety, reduce concerns of the unknown and preplan for response in emergency situation.
Note reactions of SO. Provide opportunity for discussion of personal feelings/concerns and future expectations.	Family members have individual responses to what is happening, and their anxiety may be communicated to the patient, intensifying these emotions.
Identify previous coping strengths of patient/SO and current areas of control/ability.	Focuses attention on own capabilities, increasing sense of control.
Demonstrate/encourage use of relaxation techniques, e.g., focused breathing, guided imagery, progressive relaxation.	Provides active management of situation to reduce feelings of helplessness.

233

ACTIONS/INTERVENTIONS

Independent

Provide/encourage sedentary diversional activities within individual capabilities, e.g., handicrafts, writing, television.

Collaborative

Refer to support groups and therapy as needed.

RATIONALE

Although handicapped by dependence on ventilator, activities that are normal/desired by the individual should be encouraged to enhance quality of life.

May be necessary to provide additional assistance if patient/SO is not managing anxiety or when patient is "identified with the machine."

NURSING DIAGNOSIS:	ORAL MUCOUS MEMBRANES, ALTERED, HIGH RISK FOR
Risk factors may include:	Inability to swallow oral fluids.
	Presence of tube in mouth.
	Lack of or decreased salivation.
	Ineffective oral hygiene.
Possibly evidenced by:	[Not applicable; presence of signs and symptoms establishes an actual diagnosis.]
DESIRED OUTCOMES/ EVALUATION CRITERIA— PATIENT WILL:	Report/demonstrate a decrease in symptoms.
	Caregiver will: Identify specific interventions to promote healthy oral mucosa as appropriate.

ACTIONS/INTERVENTIONS

Independent

Routinely inspect oral cavity, teeth, gums for sores, lesions, bleeding.

Administer mouth care routinely and as needed, especially in the patient with an oral intubation tube, e.g., cleanse mouth with water, saline, or preferred mouth-wash. Brush teeth with soft toothbrush, Waterpik, or moistened swab.

Change position of endotracheal tube/airway on a regular/prn schedule as appropriate.

Apply lip balm; administer oral lubricant solution.

RATIONALE

Early identification of problems provides opportunity for appropriate intervention/preventive measures.

Prevents drying/ulceration of mucous membranes and reduces medium for bacterial growth. Promotes comfort.

Reduces risk of lip and oral mucous membrane ulceration.

Maintains moisture, prevents drying.

NURSING DIAGNOSIS:	NUTRITION, ALTERED, LESS THAN BODY REQUIREMENTS
May be related to:	Altered ability to ingest and properly digest food.
	Increased metabolic demands.

Possibly evidenced by:	Weight loss.
	Aversion to eating.
	Reported altered taste sensation.
	Poor muscle tone.
	Sore, inflamed buccal cavity.
	Absence of/hyperactive bowel sounds.
DESIRED OUTCOMES/ EVALUATION CRITERIA— PATIENT WILL:	Indicate understanding of individual dietary needs.
	Demonstrate progressive weight gain toward goal with normalization of laboratory values.

ACTIONS/INTERVENTIONS	RATIONALE
Independent	
Evaluate ability to eat.	Patient with a tracheostomy tube may be able to eat, but patients with endotracheal tubes must be tube fed or parenterally nourished.
Observe/monitor for generalized muscle wasting, loss of subcutaneous fat.	These symptoms are indicative of depletion of muscle energy and can reduce respiratory muscle function.
Weigh as indicated.	Significant and recent weight loss (7%–10% body weight) and poor nutritional intake provide clues regarding catabolism, muscle glycogen stores, and ventilatory drive sensitivity.
Document oral intake if/when resumed. Offer foods that patient enjoys.	Appetite is usually poor and intake of essential nutrients may be reduced. Offering favorite foods can enhance oral intake.
Provide small frequent feedings of soft/easily digested foods if able to swallow.	Prevents excessive fatigue, enhances intake, and reduces risk of gastric distress.
Encourage/administer fluid intake of at least 2500 ml/d within cardiac tolerance.	Prevents dehydration that can be exacerbated by increased insensible losses (e.g., ventilator/intubation) and reduces risk of constipation.
Assess GI function: Presence/quality of bowel sounds; note changes in abdominal girth, nausea/vomiting. Observe/document changes in bowel movements, e.g., diarrhea/constipation: Test all stools for occult blood.	A functioning GI system is essential for the proper utilization of enteral feedings. Mechanically ventilated patients are at risk of developing abdominal distention (trapped air or ileus) and gastric bleeding (stress ulcers).
Collaborative	
Adjust diet to meet respiratory needs as indicated.	High carbohydrates, protein, and calories may be desired/needed during ventilation to improve respiratory muscle function. Carbohydrates may be reduced and fat somewhat increased just prior to weaning attempts to prevent excessive CO_2 production and reduced respiratory drive.
Monitor laboratory studies as indicated, e.g., serum, transferrin, BUN/Cr, glucose.	Provides information about adequacy of nutritional support/need for change.

NURSING DIAGNOSIS:	INFECTION, HIGH RISK FOR
Risk factors may include:	Inadequate primary defenses (traumatized lung tissue, decreased ciliary action, stasis of body fluids).
	Inadequate secondary defenses (immunosuppression).
	Chronic disease, malnutrition.
	Invasive procedure (intubation).
Possibly evidenced by:	[Not applicable; presence of signs and symptoms establishes an actual diagnosis.]
DESIRED OUTCOMES/ EVALUATION CRITERIA—	Indicate understanding of individual risk factors.
	Identify interventions to prevent/reduce risk of infection.
	Demonstrate techniques to promote safe environment.

ACTIONS/INTERVENTIONS	RATIONALE

Independent

Note risk factors for occurrence of infection.	Intubation, prolonged mechanical ventilation, general debilitation, malnutrition, age, and invasive procedures are factors which potentiate patient's risk of acquiring infection and prolonging recovery. Awareness of individual risk factors provides opportunity to limit effects.
Observe color/odor/characteristics of sputum. Note drainage around tracheostomy tube.	Yellow/green, purulent odorous sputum is indicative of infection; thick, tenacious sputum suggests dehydration.
Reduce nosocomial risk factors via proper handwashing by all caregivers, maintaining sterile suction techniques.	These factors may be the simplest but are the most important keys to prevention of hospital-acquired infection.
Encourage deep breathing, coughing, and frequent position changes.	Maximizes lung expansion and mobilization of secretions to prevent/reduce atelectasis and accumulation of sticky, thick secretions.
Auscultate breath sounds.	Presence of rhonchi/wheezes suggests retained secretions requiring expectoration/suctioning.
Monitor/screen visitors. Avoid contact with persons with upper-respiratory infection.	Individual is already compromised and is at increased risk for development of infections.
Instruct patient in proper secretion disposal, e.g., tissues, soiled tracheostomy dressings.	Reduces transmission of fluid-borne organisms.
Provide respiratory isolation when indicated.	Dependent on specific diagnosis the patient may require protection from others or must prevent transmission of infection to others (e.g., tuberculosis).
Maintain adequate hydration and nutrition. Encourage fluids to 2500 ml/d within cardiac tolerance.	Helps improve general resistance to disease and reduces risk of infection from static secretions.

ACTIONS/INTERVENTIONS

Independent

Encourage self-care/activities to limit of tolerance. Assist with graded exercise program.

Collaborative

Obtain sputum cultures as indicated.

Administer antimicrobials as indicated.

RATIONALE

Improves general well-being and muscle strength and may stimulate immune system recovery.

May be needed to identify pathogens and appropriate antimicrobials.

1 or more agents may be used dependent on identified pathogen(s) if infection does occur.

NURSING DIAGNOSIS:	VENTILATORY WEANING RESPONSE, DYSFUNCTIONAL (DVWR), HIGH RISK FOR,
Risk factors may include:	Sleep disturbance.
	Limited/insufficient energy stores.
	Pain or discomfort.
	Patient perceived inability to wean, decreased motivation.
	Adverse environment (e.g., inadequate monitoring/support).
	History of extended weaning.
Possibly evidenced by:	[Not applicable; presence of signs and symptoms establishes an actual diagnosis.]
DESIRED OUTCOMES/ EVALUATION CRITERIA— PATIENT WILL:	Actively participate in the weaning process.
	Reestablish independent respiration with ABGs within patient's normal range and free of signs of respiratory failure.
	Demonstrate increased tolerance for activity/participate in self-care within level of ability.

ACTIONS/INTERVENTIONS

Independent

Assess physical factors involved in weaning, e.g.:

Stable heart rate/rhythm, BP, and clear breath sounds;

Fever;

Nutritional status and muscle strength.

RATIONALE

The heart will have to work harder to meet increased energy needs associated with weaning. Physician may defer weaning if tachycardia, pulmonary crackles, and hypertension are present.

Increase of 1°F of body temperature raises metabolic rate and oxygen demands by 7%.

Weaning is hard work. Patient must not only be able to withstand the stress of weaning but also must have the stamina to breathe spontaneously for extended periods.

ACTIONS/INTERVENTIONS	RATIONALE
Independent	
Determine psychologic readiness.	Weaning provokes anxiety for the patient regarding concerns about ability to breathe on own and long-term need of ventilator.
Explain weaning techniques, e.g., T piece, SIMV, CPAP, pressure support. Discuss individual plan and expectations.	Assists patient to prepare for weaning process, helps limit fear of unknown, promotes cooperation, and enhances likelihood of a successful outcome.
Provide undisturbed rest/sleep periods. Avoid stressful procedures/situations or nonessential activities.	Maximizes energy for weaning process; limits fatigue and oxygen consumption.
Evaluate/document patient's progress. Note restlessness; changes in BP, heart rate, respiratory rate; use of accessory muscles; discoordinated breathing with ventilator; increased concentration on breathing (mild); patient's concerns about possible machine malfunction; inability to cooperate/respond to coaching; color changes.	Indicators that patient may require slower opportunity to stabilize or may need to stop program.
Recognize/provide encouragement for patient's efforts.	Positive feedback provides reassurance and support for continuation of weaning process.
Monitor response to activity.	Excessive oxygen consumption/demand increases the possibility of failure.
Collaborative	
Consult with dietitian, nutritional support team for adjustments of composition of diet.	Reduction of carbohydrates/fats may be required to prevent excessive production of CO_2 which could alter respiratory drive.
Monitor CBC, serum albumin and prealbumin, transferrin, total iron-binding capacity, and electrolytes (especially potassium, calcium, and phosphorus).	Verifies that nutrition is adequate to meet energy requirements for weaning.
Review chest x-ray and ABGs.	Chest x-rays should show clear lungs or marked improvement in pulmonary congestion or infiltrates. ABGs should document satisfactory oxygenation on an FIO_2 of 40% or less.

NURSING DIAGNOSIS:	KNOWLEDGE DEFICIT [LEARNING NEED] REGARDING CONDITION, PROGNOSIS AND THERAPY NEEDS
May be related to:	Lack of exposure/recall.
	Misinterpretation of information.
	Unfamiliarity with information resources.
	Stress of situational crisis.
Possibly evidenced by:	Questions about care, request for information.
	Reluctance to learn new skills.

	Inaccurate follow-through of instruction.
	Development of preventable complications.
DESIRED OUTCOMES/ EVALUATION CRITERIA— PATIENT/SO/CAREGIVER WILL:	Participate in learning process.
	Exhibit increased interest, shown by verbal/nonverbal cues.
	Assume responsibility for own learning and begin to look for information and to ask questions.
	Indicate understanding of mechanical ventilation therapy.
	Demonstrate behaviors/new skills to meet individual needs/prevent complications.

ACTIONS/INTERVENTIONS	RATIONALE
Independent	
Determine ability and willingness to learn.	Physical condition may preclude patient involvement in care before and after discharge. SO/caregiver may feel inadequate and afraid of machinery and have reservations about ability to learn or deal with overall situation.
Discuss specific condition requiring ventilatory support, what measures are being tried for weaning, short- and long-term goals of treatment.	Provides knowledge base to aid patient/SO in making informed decisions. Weaning efforts may continue for several weeks (extended period of time). Dependence is evidenced by repeatedly increased PCO_2, and/or decline in PaO_2 during weaning attempts, presence of dypsnea, anxiety, tachycardia, perspiration, cyanosis.
Encourage patient/SO to evaluate impact of ventilatory dependence on their lifestyle and what changes they are willing or unwilling to make. Problem-solve solutions to issues raised.	Quality of life must be resolved by the ventilator-dependent patient and caregivers who need to understand that home ventilatory support is a 24-hour job that will affect everyone.
Promote participation in self-care/diversional activities and socialization as appropriate.	Refocuses attention back toward more normal life activities, increases endurance, and helps to prevent depersonalization.
Review issues of general well-being: role of nutrition; assistance with feeding/meal preparation; graded exercise/specific restrictions; rest periods alternated with activity.	Enhances recuperation and assures that individual needs will be met.
Recommend SO/caregivers learn CPR.	Provides sense of security about ability to handle emergency situations that might arise until help can be obtained.
Schedule team conference. Establish in-hospital training for caregivers if patient is to be discharged home on ventilator.	Team approach is needed to coordinate patient's care and teaching program to meet individual needs.

239

ACTIONS/INTERVENTIONS	RATIONALE
Independent	
Instruct caregiver and patient in handwashing techniques, use of sterile technique for suctioning, tracheostomy/stoma care, and chest physiotherapy.	Reduces risk of infection and promotes optimal respiratory function.
Provide both demonstration and "hands on" sessions as well as written material about specific type of ventilator to be used, function, and care of equipment.	Enhances familiarity, reducing anxiety and promoting confidence in implementation of new tasks/skills.
Discuss what/when to report to the health care provider, e.g., signs of respiratory distress, infection.	Helps to reduce general anxiety while promoting timely/appropriate evaluation and intervention to prevent complications.
Ascertain that all needed equipment is in place and that safety concerns have been addressed, e.g., alternate power source (generator, batteries); backup equipment; patient call/alarm system.	Predischarge preparations can ease the transfer process. Planning for potential problems increases sense of security for patient/SO.
Contact community-hospital-based services.	Suppliers of home equipment, physical therapy; emergency power providers; social services; financial assistance aid in procuring equipment and facilitating transition to home.
Refer to vocational/occupational therapist.	Some ventilator-dependent patients are able to resume vocations either while on the ventilator or during the day (while ventilator-dependent at night).

Pulmonary Tuberculosis (TB) _____

TB is on the rise today although many still believe it to be a problem of the past. Although most frequently seen as a pulmonary disease, TB may be extrapulmonary (16%) and affect organs and tissues other than the lungs. Incidence is higher among men, nonwhites, and the foreign-born. In addition, persons at highest risk include those who may have been exposed to the bacillus in the past and those who are debilitated or have lowered immunity because of chronic conditions, such as AIDs, cancer, advanced age, malnutrition, and so on. Most patients are treated as outpatients, but may be hospitalized for diagnostic evaluation/initiation of therapy, adverse drug reactions, or severe illness/debilitation.

RELATED CONCERNS:

Long-Term Care, p 938
Pneumonia, p 162
Psychosocial Aspects of Acute Care, p 899

PATIENT ASSESSMENT DATA BASE

Data are dependent on stage of disease and degree of involvement.

ACTIVITY/REST

May report:	Generalized weakness and fatigue.
	Shortness of breath with exertion.
	Difficulty sleeping with evening or night fever, chills and/or sweats.
	Nightmares.
May exhibit:	Tachycardia, tachypnea/dyspnea on exertion.
	Muscle wasting, pain, and stiffness (advanced stages).

EGO INTEGRITY

May report:	Recent/long-standing stress factors.
	Financial concerns, poverty.
	Feelings of helplessness/hopelessness.
	Cultural/ethnic populations: Native American or recent immigration from Central America, Southeast Asia, Indian subcontinent.
May exhibit:	Denial (especially during early stages).
	Anxiety, apprehension, irritability.

FOOD/FLUID

May report:	Loss of appetite.
	Indigestion.
	Weight loss.
May exhibit:	Poor skin turgor, dry/flaky skin.
	Muscle wasting/loss of subcutaneous fat.

PAIN/COMFORT

May report:	Chest pain aggravated by recurrent cough.
May exhibit:	Guarding of affected area.
	Distraction behaviors, restlessness.

RESPIRATION

May report: Cough, productive or nonproductive.

Shortness of breath.

History of tuberculosis/exposure to infected individual.

May exhibit: Increased respiratory rate (extensive disease or fibrosis of the lung parenchyma and pleura).

Asymmetry in respiratory excursion (pleural effusion).

Dullness to percussion and decreased fremitus (pleural fluid or pleural thickening). Breath sounds; diminished/absent bilaterally or unilaterally (pleural effusion/pneumothorax). Tubular breath sounds and/or whispered pectoriloquies over large lesions. Crackles may be noted over apex of lungs during quick inspiration after a short cough (posttussic crackles).

Sputum characteristics: Green/purulent, yellowish mucoid, or blood-tinged.

Tracheal deviation (bronchogenic spread).

Inattention, marked irritability, change in mentation (advanced stages).

SAFETY

May report: Presence of immunosuppressed conditions, e.g., AIDS, cancer.

Positive HIV test.

May exhibit: Low-grade fever or acute febrile illness.

SOCIAL INTERACTION

May report: Feelings of isolation/rejection because of communicable disease.

Change in usual patterns of responsibility/change in physical capacity to resume role.

TEACHING/LEARNING

May report: Familial history of TB.

General debilitation/poor health status.

Failure to improve/reactivation of TB.

Nonparticipation in therapy.

Discharge Plan Considerations: DRG projected mean length of stay: 6.8 days.

May require assistance with/alteration in drug therapy and assistance in self-care and homemaker/maintenance tasks.

DIAGNOSTIC STUDIES

Sputum culture: Positive for *Mycobacterium tuberculosis* in the active stage of the disease.

Ziehl-Neelsen (Acid-fast stain applied to a smear of body fluid): Positive for acid-fast bacilli.

Skin tests (PPD, Mantoux, tine, Vollmer patch): A positive reaction (area of induration 10 mm or greater, occurring 48–72 hours after interdermal injection of the antigen) indicates past infection and the presence of antibodies but is not necessarily indicative of active disease. A significant reaction in a patient who is clinically ill means that active TB cannot be dismissed as a diagnostic possibility. A significant reaction in healthy persons usually signifies healed TB or an infection caused by a different mycobacterium.

ELISA/Western Blot: May reveal presence of HIV.

Chest x-ray: May show small infiltrations of early lesions in the upper-lung field, calcium deposits of healed primary lesions, or fluid of an effusion. Changes indicating more advanced TB may include cavitation, fibrous areas.

Histologic or tissue cultures (including gastric washings; urine and CSF, skin biopsy): Positive for Mycobacterium tuberculosis.

Needle biopsy of lung tissue: Positive for granulomas of TB; presence of giant cells indicating necrosis.

Electrolytes: May be abnormal depending on the location and severity of infection; e.g., hyponatremia caused by abnormal water retention may be found in extensive chronic pulmonary TB.

ABGs: May be abnormal depending on location, severity and residual damage to the lungs.

Pulmonary function studies: Decreased vital capacity, increased dead space, increased ratio of residual air to total lung capacity, and decreased oxygen saturation are secondary to parenchymal infiltration/fibrosis, loss of lung tissue, and pleural disease (extensive chronic pulmonary TB).

NURSING PRIORITIES

1. Achieve/maintain adequate ventilation/oxygenation.
2. Prevent spread of infection.
3. Support behaviors/tasks to maintain health.
4. Promote effective coping strategies.
5. Provide information about disease process/prognosis and treatment needs.

DISCHARGE GOALS

1. Respiratory function adequate to meet individual need.
2. Complications prevented.
3. Lifestyle/behavior changes adopted to prevent spread of infection.
4. Disease process/prognosis and therapeutic regimen understood.

NURSING DIAGNOSIS:	INFECTION, HIGH RISK FOR, [SPREAD/REACTIVATION]
Risk factors may include:	Inadequate primary defenses, decreased ciliary action/stasis of secretions.
	Tissue destruction/extension of infection.
	Lowered resistance/suppressed inflammatory process.
	Malnutrition.
	Environmental exposure.
	Insufficient knowledge to avoid exposure to pathogens.
Possibly evidenced by:	[Not applicable; presence of signs and symptoms establishes an actual diagnosis.]
DESIRED OUTCOMES/ EVALUATION CRITERIA— PATIENT WILL:	Identify interventions to prevent/reduce risk of spread of infection.
	Demonstrate techniques/initiate lifestyle changes to promote safe environment.

ACTIONS/INTERVENTIONS	RATIONALE

Independent

Review pathology of disease (active/inactive phases; dissemination of infection through bronchi to adjacent tissues or via bloodstream/lymphatic system) and potential spread of infection via airborne droplet during coughing, sneezing, spitting, talking, laughing, singing.

Helps patient realize/accept necessity of adhering to medication regimen to prevent reactivation/complication. Understanding of how the disease is passed and awareness of transmission possibilities help patient/SO to take steps to prevent infection of others.

Identify others at risk, e.g., household members, close associates/friends.

Those exposed may require a course of drug therapy to prevent spread/development of infection.

Instruct patient to cough/sneeze and expectorate into tissue and to refrain from spitting. Review proper disposal of tissue and good handwashing techniques. Encourage return demonstration.

Behaviors necessary to prevent spread of infection.

Review necessity of temporary infection control measures, e.g., mask or respiratory isolation.

May help to reduce the patient's sense of isolation and remove the social stigma associated with communicable diseases.

Monitor temperature as indicated.

Febrile reactions are an indicator of continuing presence of infection.

Identify individual risk factors for reactivation of tuberculosis, e.g., lowered resistance (alcoholism, malnutrition/intestinal bypass surgery); use of immunosuppression drugs/corticosteroids; presence of diabetes mellitus, cancer; postpartum.

Knowledge about these factors helps patient to alter lifestyle and avoid/reduce incidence of exacerbation.

Stress importance of uninterrupted drug therapy.

Contagious period may last only 2–3 days after initiation of chemotherapy, but in presence of cavitation or moderately advanced disease, risk of spread of infection may continue up to 3 months.

Review importance of follow-up and periodic reculturing of sputum for the duration of therapy.

Aids in monitoring the effects and effectiveness of medications and the patient's response to therapy.

Encourage selection/ingestion of well-balanced meals. Provide frequent small "snacks" in place of large meals as appropriate.

Presence of anorexia and/or preexisting malnutrition lower resistance to infectious process and impair healing. Small snacks may enhance overall intake.

Collaborative

Administer antiinfective agents as indicated, e.g.:

Primary drugs: Isoniazid (INH); ethambutal (Myambutol); rifampin (RMP/Rifadin);

A combination of antiinfective agents is used, e.g., 2 primary drugs or a primary plus a secondary drug. INH is usually drug of choice for infected patient and those at risk for developing TB. Short-course chemotherapy of INH and rifampin (for 9 months) with ethambutal (for first 2 months) may be sufficient treatment of uncomplicated pulmonary TB. Ethambutol should be given if CNS or disseminated disease is present or if INH resistance is suspected. Extended therapy (up to 24 months) is indicated for reactivation cases, extrapulmonary reactivated TB, or in the presence of other medical problems, e.g., diabetes mellitus or silicosis. Prophylaxis with INH for 12 months should be considered in HIV positive patients with positive PPD.

ACTIONS/INTERVENTIONS

Collaborative

Pyrazinamide (PZA/Aldinamide); para-amino salicylic (PAS); cycloserine (Seromycin); streptomycin (Strycin).

Monitor laboratory studies, e.g., sputum smear results;

AST/ALT.

Notify local health department.

RATIONALE

These "secondary" drugs may be required when infection is resistant to or intolerant of primary drugs.

Patient who has three consecutive negative sputum smears (takes 3 to 5 months), is adhering to drug regimen, and is asymptomatic will be classified a nontransmitter.

Adverse effects of drug therapy include hepatitis.

Helpful in identifying contacts reducing spread of infection.

NURSING DIAGNOSIS:	AIRWAY CLEARANCE, INEFFECTIVE
May be related to:	Thick, viscous, or bloody secretions.
	Fatigue, poor cough effort.
	Tracheal/pharyngeal edema.
Possibly evidenced by:	Abnormal respiratory rate, rhythm, depth.
	Abnormal breath sounds (rhonchi, wheezes), stridor.
	Dyspnea.
DESIRED OUTCOMES/ EVALUATION CRITERIA— PATIENT WILL:	Maintain patent airway.
	Expectorate secretions without assistance.
	Demonstrate behaviors to improve/maintain airway clearance.
	Participate in treatment regimen, within the level of ability/situation.
	Identify potential complications and initiate appropriate actions.

ACTIONS/INTERVENTIONS

Independent

Assess respiratory function, e.g., breath sounds, rate, rhythm and depth and use of accessory muscles.

Note ability to expectorate mucous/cough effectively; document character, amount of sputum, presence of hemoptysis.

RATIONALE

Diminished breath sounds may reflect atelectasis. Rhonchi, wheezes indicate accumulation of secretions/inability to clear airways that may lead to use of accessory muscles and increased work of breathing.

Expectoration may be difficult when secretions are very thick (i.e., effect of the infection and/or inadequate hydration). Blood-tinged or frankly bloody

245

ACTIONS/INTERVENTIONS	RATIONALE
Independent	
	sputum results from tissue breakdown (cavitation) in the lungs or bronchial ulceration and may require further evaluation/intervention.
Place patient in semi- or high-Fowler's position. Assist patient with coughing and deep-breathing exercises.	Positioning helps maximize lung expansion and decreases respiratory effort. Maximal ventilation may open atelectic areas and promote movement of secretions into larger airways for expectoration.
Clear secretions from mouth and trachea; suction as necessary.	Prevents obstruction/aspiration. Suctioning may be necessary if patient is unable to expectorate secretions.
Maintain fluid intake of at least 2500 ml/d unless contraindicated.	High fluid intake helps to thin secretions, making them easier to expectorate.
Collaborative	
Humidify inspired air/oxygen.	Prevents drying of mucous membranes; helps to thin secretions.
Administer medications as indicated:	
Mucolytic agents, e.g., acetylcysteine (Mucomyst);	Mucolytic agents reduce the thickness and stickiness of pulmonary secretions to facilitate clearance.
Bronchodilators, e.g., oxtriphylline (Choledyl); theophylline (Theo-Dur);	Bronchodilators increase lumen size of the tracheobronchial tree, thus decreasing resistance to airflow.
Corticosteroids (Prednisone).	May be useful in presence of extensive involvement with profound hypoxemia and when inflammatory response is life-threatening.
Be prepared for/assist with emergency intubation.	Intubation may be necessary in rare cases of bronchogenic TB accompanied by laryngeal edema or acute pulmonary bleeding.

NURSING DIAGNOSIS:	**GAS EXCHANGE, IMPAIRED, HIGH RISK FOR**
Risk factors may include:	Decrease in effective lung surface, atelectasis.
	Destruction of alveolar-capillary membrane.
	Thick, viscous secretions.
	Bronchial edema.
Possibly evidenced by:	[Not applicable; presence of signs and symptoms establishes an actual diagnosis.]
DESIRED OUTCOMES/ EVALUATION CRITERIA— PATIENT WILL:	Report absence of/decreased dyspnea.
	Demonstrate improved ventilation and adequate oxygenation of tissues by ABGs within patient's normal ranges.
	Be free of symptoms of respiratory distress.

ACTIONS/INTERVENTIONS	RATIONALE
Independent	
Assess for dyspnea, tachypnea, abnormal/diminished breath sounds, increased respiratory effort, limited chest wall expansion, and fatigue.	Pulmonary TB can cause a wide range of effects in the lungs ranging from a small patch of bronchopneumonia to diffuse intense inflammation, caseous necrosis, pleural effusion, and extensive fibrosis. Respiratory effects can range from mild dyspnea to profound respiratory distress.
Evaluate change in level of consciousness. Note cyanosis and/or change in skin color, including mucous membranes and nail beds.	Accumulation of secretions/airway compromise can impair oxygenation of vital organs and tissues. (Refer to ND: Airway Clearance, ineffective, p 245.)
Demonstrate/encourage pursed-lip breathing during exhalation, especially for patients with fibrosis or parenchymal destruction.	Creates resistance against outflowing air, to prevent collapse/narrowing of the airways, thereby helping to distribute air throughout the lungs and relieve/reduce shortness of breath.
Promote bed rest/activity restriction and assist with self-care activities as necessary.	Reducing oxygen consumption/demand during periods of respiratory compromise may reduce severity of symptoms.
Collaborative	
Monitor serial ABGs/pulse oximetry.	Decreased oxygen content (PaO_2), and/or saturation or increased $PaCO_2$ indicates need for intervention/change in therapeutic regimen.
Provide supplemental oxygen as appropriate.	Aids in correcting the hypoxemia that may occur secondary to decreased ventilation/diminished alveolar lung surface.

NURSING DIAGNOSIS:	**NUTRITION, ALTERED, LESS THAN BODY REQUIREMENTS**
May be related to:	Fatigue.
	Frequent cough/sputum production; dyspnea.
	Anorexia.
	Insufficient financial resources.
Possibly evidenced by:	Weight 10%–20% below ideal for frame and height.
	Reported lack of interest in food, altered taste sensation.
	Poor muscle tone.
DESIRED OUTCOMES/ EVALUATION CRITERIA— PATIENT WILL:	Demonstrate progressive weight gain toward goal with normalization of laboratory values and free of signs of malnutrition.
	Initiate behaviors/lifestyle changes to regain and/or to maintain appropriate weight.

247

ACTIONS/INTERVENTIONS	RATIONALE
Independent	
Document patient's nutritional status on admission, noting skin turgor, current weight and degree of weight loss, integrity of oral mucosa, ability/inability to swallow, presence of bowel tones, history of nausea/vomiting or diarrhea.	Useful in defining degree/extent of problem and appropriate choice of interventions.
Ascertain patient's usual dietary pattern, likes/dislikes.	Helpful in identifying specific needs/strengths. Consideration of individual preferences may improve dietary intake.
Monitor intake/output and weight periodically.	Useful in measuring effectiveness of nutritional and fluid support.
Investigate anorexia, nausea, and vomiting and note possible correlation to medications. Monitor frequency, volume, consistency of stools.	May affect dietary choices and identify areas for problem solving to enhance intake/utilization of nutrients.
Encourage and provide for frequent rest periods.	Helps to conserve energy especially when metabolic requirements are increased with fever.
Provide oral care before and after respiratory treatments.	Reduces bad taste left from sputum or medications used for respiratory treatments that can stimulate the vomiting center.
Encourage small, frequent meals with foods high in protein and carbohydrates.	Maximizes nutrient intake without undue fatigue/energy expenditure from eating large meals and reduces gastric irritation.
Encourage SO to bring foods from home and to share meals with patient unless contraindicated.	Creates a more normal social environment during meal time and helps meet personal, cultural preferences.
Collaborative	
Refer to dietitian for adjustments in dietary composition.	Provides assistance in planning a diet with nutrients adequate to meet patient's metabolic requirements and dietary preferences.
Consult with respiratory therapy to schedule treatments 1–2 hours before/after meals.	May help to reduce the incidence of nausea and vomiting associated with medications or the effects of respiratory treatments on a full stomach.
Monitor laboratory studies, e.g., BUN, serum protein, and albumin.	Low values reflect malnutrition and indicate need for intervention/change in therapeutic regimen.
Administer antipyretics as appropriate.	Fever increases metabolic needs and therefore calorie consumption.

NURSING DIAGNOSIS:	**KNOWLEDGE DEFICIT [LEARNING NEED], REGARDING CONDITION, TREATMENT REGIMEN, AND PREVENTION**
May be related to:	Lack of exposure to/misinterpretation of information.
	Cognitive limitations.
	Inaccurate/incomplete information presented.

Possibly evidenced by:	Request for information.
	Expressed misconceptions about health status.
	Lack of or inaccurate follow-through of instructions/behaviors.
	Expressing or exhibiting feelings of being overwhelmed.
DESIRED OUTCOMES/ EVALUATION CRITERIA— PATIENT WILL:	Verbalize understanding of disease process/prognosis and treatment needs.
	Initiate behaviors/lifestyle changes to improve general well-being and reduce risk of reactivation of TB.
	Identify symptoms requiring evaluation/intervention.
	Describe a plan for receiving adequate follow-up care.

ACTIONS/INTERVENTIONS

Independent

Assess patient's ability to learn, e.g., level of fear, concern, fatigue, participation level, best environment in which patient can learn, how much content, best media, who should be included.

Identify symptoms that should be reported to health care provider, e.g., hemoptysis, chest pain, fever, difficulty breathing, hearing loss, vertigo.

Emphasize the importance of maintaining high-protein and carbohydrate diet and adequate fluid intake. (Refer to ND: Nutrition, Altered, less than body requirements, p 247.)

Provide instruction and specific written information for the patient to refer to, e.g., schedule for medications.

Explain medication dosage, frequency of administration, expected action, and the reason for prolonged treatment. Review potential interactions with other drugs/substances.

Review potential side effects of treatment (e.g., dryness of mouth, constipation, visual disturbances, headache, orthostatic hypertension) and problem-solve solutions.

Stress need to abstain from alcohol while on INH.

Refer for eye examination after starting and then monthly while taking ethambutal.

Encourage patient/SO to verbalize fears/concerns. Answer questions factually. Note prolonged use of denial.

RATIONALE

Learning is dependent on emotional and physical readiness and is achieved at an individual pace.

May indicate progression or reactivation of disease or side effects of medications requiring further evaluation.

Meeting metabolic needs helps to minimize fatigue and promote recovery. Fluids aid in liquefying/expectorating of secretions.

Written information relieves the patient of the burden of having to remember large amounts of information. Repetition strengthens learning.

Enhances cooperation with therapeutic regimen and may prevent discontinuation of medication as patient's condition improves.

May prevent/reduce discomfort associated with therapy and enhance cooperation with regimen.

Combination of INH and alcohol has been linked with increased incidence of hepatitis.

Major side effect is reduced visual acuity; initial sign may be decreased ability to perceive green.

Provides opportunity to correct misconceptions/alleviate anxiety. Inadequate finances/prolonged denial may affect coping with/managing the tasks necessary to regain/maintain health.

249

ACTIONS/INTERVENTIONS	RATIONALE

Independent

Evaluate job-related risk factors, e.g., working in foundry/rock quarry, sandblasting.

Excessive exposure to silicone dust enhances risk of silicosis, which may negatively affect respiratory function/bronchitis.

Encourage abstaining from smoking.

Although smoking does not stimulate recurrence of TB, it does increase the likelihood of respiratory dysfunction/bronchitis.

Review how TB is transmitted (e.g., primarily by inhalation of airborne organisms but may also spread through stools or urine if infection is present in these systems) and hazards of reactivation.

Knowledge may reduce risk of transmission/reactivation. Complications associated with reactivation include cavitation, abscess formation, destructive emphysema, spontaneous pneumothorax, diffuse interstitial fibrosis, serous effusion, empyema, bronchiectasis, hemoptysis, GI ulceration, bronchopleural fistula, tuberculous laryngitis, and miliary spread.

Bibliography

General References

Bellak, JP and Bamford, PA: Nursing Assessment: A Multidimensional Approach. Jones & Bartlett, Boston, 1987.
Berkow, R (ed): The Merck Manual, ed 15. Merck Sharp & Dohme Research Laboratories, Rahway, NJ, 1987.
Cella, JH and Watson, J: Nurse's Manual of Laboratory Tests. FA Davis, Philadelphia, 1989.
Condon, RE and Nyhus, LM (eds): Manual of Surgical Therapeutics, ed 7. Little, Brown & Co, Boston, 1988.
Deglin, JH and Vallerand, AH: Davis's Drug Guide for Nurses, ed 3. FA Davis, Philadelphia, 1992.
Diseases and Disorders Handbook, ed 3. Springhouse, Springhouse, PA, 1989.
Doenges, ME and Moorhouse, MF: Nurse's Pocket Guide: Nursing Diagnoses with Interventions, ed 3. FA Davis, Philadelphia, 1991.
Dunagan, WC and Ridner, ML (eds): Manual of Medical Therapeutics, ed 26. Little, Brown & Co, Boston, 1989.
Fischbach, F: A Manual of Laboratory and Diagnostic Tests, ed 4. JB Lippincott, Philadelphia, 1992.
Guyton, AC: Textbook of Medical Physiology, ed 8. WB Saunders, Philadelphia, 1991.
Kuhn, MM: Pharmacotherapeutics: A Nursing Process Approach, ed 2. FA Davis, Philadelphia, 1991.
Professional Guide to Diseases, ed 3. Springhouse, Springhouse, PA, 1989.
Suddarth, DS (ed): The Lippincott Manual of Nursing Practice, ed 5. JB Lippincott, Philadelphia, 1991.
Thomas, CL (ed): Taber's Cyclopedic Medical Dictionary, ed 16. FA Davis, Philadelphia, 1989.
Thompson, JM, McFarland, GK, Hirsh, JE, et al: Mosby's Manual of Clinical Nursing, ed 2. CV Mosby, St Louis, 1989.

Articles

Anderson, S: ABGs: Six easy steps to interpreting blood gases. AJN 90(8):42, 1990.
Bella, LA: Steroidphobia and the pulmonary patient. AJN 92(2):26, 1992.
Carroll, P: What's new in chest tube management. RN 54(5):34, 1991.
Carroll, P: Nursing the thoracotomy patient. RN 55(6):34, 1992.
Caruthers, DD: Infectious pneumonia in the elderly. AJN 20(2):56, 1990.
Case, SC and Sabo, CE: Adult respiratory distress syndrome: A deadly complication of trauma. Focus on Critical Care 19(2):116, 1992.
Cuzzell, JZ and Rodriquez, LA: How to use a bag-valve-mask devise for artificial ventilation. AJN 89(7):932, 1989.
Ellstrom, K: What's causing your patient's respiratory distress? Nursing90 November: 57, 1990.
Ferland, PA: Are you ready for ventilator patients? Nursing91 21(1):42, 1991.
Geissler, A: Tuberculosis in Colorado Springs: Then and now. University of Phoenix, March 1991 (unpublished).
Grandstom, D: A better way to deliver long-term oxygen therapy. RN 52(9):58, 1989.
Handerhan, B and Allegrezza, N: Getting your patient off a ventilator. RN 52(12):60, 1989.
Holcomb, SS: Pulmonary embolism: Preventing a disaster. RN 54(9):52, 1991.
Janson-Bjerklie, S: Status asthmaticus. AJN 90(9):52, 1990.
Jess, LW: Chronic bronchitis and emphysema: Airing the differences. Nursing92 22(3):34, 1992.

Jess: LW: When your patient has asthma. Nursing92 22(4):48, 1992.

Jordan, K: Chest trauma: How to detect and react to serious trouble. Nursing90 20(9):34, 1990.

Lindell, KO and Mazzocco, MC: Breaking bronchospasm's grip with MDIs. AJN 20(3):35, 1990.

Madsen, LA: Tuberculosis today. RN 53(3):44, 1990.

Matthews, PJ, Matthews, LM, and Mitchell, RR: Airway monitoring and ventilation: What the future holds. Nursing92 22(2):48, 1992.

Mueller, R: Cancer pain: Which drugs for which patients. RN 55(5):38, 1992.

Sawyer, DL and Bruya, MA: Care of the patient having radical neck surgery or permanent laryngectomy: A nursing diagnostic approach. Focus on Critical Care 17(2):167, 1990.

Stiesmeyer, JK: What triggers a ventilator alarm? AJN 91(10):60, 1991.

Thompson, KS, Caddick, K, Mathie, J, et al: Building a critical path for ventilator dependency. AJN 91(7):28, 1991.

Yeaw, EM: How position affects oxygenation: Good lung down? AJN 92(3):27, 1992.

Young, NA and Gorzeman, J: Managing pneumothorax and hemothorax. Nursing91 21(4):56, 1991.

CHAPTER 6

NEUROLOGIC

Headache _____

Headaches may be the most common of all pains experienced by people. They are usually a symptom of an underlying disorder and may occur with or without the presence of organic disease.

Migraine: Cause unknown. However, thought to result from intracranial blood vessel spasms. Similar periodic episodes can occur over an extended period. More frequently seen in teenage and early adult women. May be associated with history of asthma or allergies. May be familial.

Cluster: Thought to be vascular. However, histamine seems to play a role. More common in adolescents and adult men.

Muscle tension: Sustained muscle contractions around scalp, face, neck, upper body; possible cranial artery vasodilation. Occurs in adults with increased incidence in females.

Temporal arteritis: Thought to result from an autoimmune mechanism in patients over 50 years of age.

Other types include: Meningeal, brain tumor, sinus, and posttraumatic.

RELATED CONCERNS:

Cerebrovascular Accident/Stroke, p 290
Craniocerebral Trauma, p 271
Intracranial Infections, p 307
Psychosocial Aspects of Acute Care, p 899

PATIENT ASSESSMENT DATA BASE

Findings are dependent on type/cause of headache. A thorough history may be necessary to differentiate diagnoses.

ACTIVITY/REST

May report: Fatigue, overwork, malaise.

Limitations imposed by condition.

Eye strain, difficulty reading, weakness.

Insomnia, early morning awakening with pain.

Aggravation of headache by changes in posture, exertion, or weather.

CIRCULATION

May report: History of hypertension.

May exhibit: Hypertension.

Vascular pulsation, e.g., temporal area.

Pallor, facial flushing.

EGO INTEGRITY

May report: Specific emotional/environmental stress factors.

Feelings of helplessness, hopelessness, powerlessness, depression.

May exhibit: Apprehension, anxiety, irritability (during headache).

Repression/defense mechanisms (chronic headaches).

FOOD/FLUID

May report: Intake of foods high in vasoactive substances: e.g., caffeine, chocolate, onions, cheese, alcohol, wine, avocados, MSG, sausages, hot dogs, lunch meats, tomatoes, fatty foods, oranges (migraine).

Nausea/vomiting, anorexia (during headache).

Weight loss.

NEUROSENSORY

May report: Dizziness, disorientation (during headache), inability to concentrate.

History of seizures, recent head injury, trauma, stroke, intracranial infection, craniotomy.

Aura: Visual, olfactory, tinnitus.

Visual changes, sensitivity to bright lights/loud noises.

Epistaxis.

Paresthesias, progressive weakness/temporary one-sided paralysis.

May exhibit: Changes in speech pattern/thought processes.

Irritability, excitability.

Decreased deep tendon reflexes.

Papilledema.

PAIN/COMFORT

May report: Characteristics of pain dependent on type of headache, e.g.:

Migraine: May be generalized or unilateral, throbbing quality. May begin around one eye and/or spread to both.

Cluster: Paroxysmal, abrupt, nonthrobbing, unilateral, intense. Involves eye, temple, neck, face. Nasal stuffiness, fluid accumulation under eyes, rhinorrhea, facial flushing. Usually lasts 30–90 minutes. Periods of remission occur.

Muscle tension: Gradual onset, bilateral, pressure, nonthrobbing, intermittent, moderate, fronto-occipital, feeling of tightness/stiffness, aching. May be unrelieved for extended periods.

Meningeal: Severe, generalized, constant pain. May radiate down the neck.

Brain tumor: Pain is intense, steady, generalized, or intermittent, frequently awakens patient. May be localized, positional.

Temporal arteritis: Unilateral or bilateral pain over the temporal area, usually unremitting, throbbing, severe, aching, burning.

Posttraumatic: May be severe and is usually chronic, continuous or intermittent, localized or generalized, variable in intensity, worsened by emotional disturbances, position changes.

Sinus: Gradual onset. Morning headache is worse. Pain is dull, and the pressure positionally aggravated; may be severe, frontal, or occur on one side of face.

Unsuccessful attempts at self-medication with OTC or prescription drugs.

May exhibit: Facial mask of pain, flushing, pallor.

Narrowed focus.

Self-focus.

Distraction behaviors/emotional responses, e.g., crying, restlessness.

Tense musculature in neck area, nuchal rigidity.

SAFETY

May report: History of allergies/allergic reactions.

May exhibit: Fever (meningeal headache).

Gait disturbances, paresthesia, paralysis.

Purulent nasal drainage (sinus headache).

SOCIAL INTERACTION

May report: Changes in role responsibilities/social interaction related to illness.

TEACHING/LEARNING

May report: Family history of hypertension, migraines, stroke, mental illness.

Use of alcohol/other drugs, including caffeine, oral contraceptives, menopausal hormones.

Discharge Plan Considerations: **DRG projected mean length of stay: 3.5 days.**

May require alteration of medication/treatments. Assistance with homemaker tasks during pain episode.

DIAGNOSTIC STUDIES

Skull x-rays: Detects fractures, deviation of structures.

Sinus x-rays: Confirms diagnosis of sinusitis and identifies structural problems, jaw malformations (TMJ).

Visual tests: Acuity, visual fields, refraction assists in making differential diagnosis.

CT scans:

Brain: Detects intracranial masses, ventricular shifts, or intracranial hemorrhage.
Sinus: Detects presence of infection in sphenoidal and ethmoidal areas.

MRI: Detects lesions/tissue abnormalities; provides information about biochemistry, physiology, anatomic structures.

Echoencephalography: Documents displacement of brain structure due to trauma, cerebrovascular accident, or space-occupying lesion.

Electroencephalography: Records brain activity during various activities, headache episode.

Cerebral arteriography: Identifies/substantiates vascular lesions (aneurysm, malformations, space-occupying lesions).

CBC: Leukocytosis is suggestive of infection; presence of anemia may stimulate migraine.

Sedimentation rate: May be normal, ruling out temporal arteritis; elevated in presence of inflammation.

Electrolytes: Imbalance, hypercalcemia may stimulate migraine.

Lumbar puncture: To evaluate/document increased CSF pressure, presence of abnormal cells, blood, infection.

NURSING PRIORITIES

1. Enhance patient comfort.
2. Assist in the detection/elimination of underlying condition.
3. Develop strategies to decrease frequency and duration of headaches.
4. Provide information about cause/treatment/prevention and complications.

DISCHARGE GOALS

1. Pain alleviated/managed.
2. Lifestyle changes/behaviors initiated to control/prevent recurrence.
3. Disease condition/process, therapeutic needs understood.

NURSING DIAGNOSIS:	**PAIN, [ACUTE]/CHRONIC**
May be related to:	Stress and tension.
	Nerve irritation/pressure.
	Vasospasm.
	Increased intracranial pressure.
Possibly evidenced by:	Verbal reports of pain, possibly affected by other factors, e.g., position changes.
	Facial mask of pain, pallor.
	Guarding/distraction behaviors, restlessness.
	Self-focusing; narrowed focus.
	Changes in sleep patterns, insomnia.
	Preoccupation with pain.
	Autonomic responses.
DESIRED OUTCOMES/ EVALUATION CRITERIA— PATIENT WILL:	Report pain relieved/controlled.
	Demonstrate/use behaviors to reduce recurrence.

ACTIONS/INTERVENTIONS	RATIONALE
Independent	
Ascertain duration of problem/episodes, who has been consulted, and what drugs and/or therapies have been used.	Expedites choice of appropriate interventions. Helps identify actions that may have been overlooked/not tried or have failed to help in past episodes.

255

ACTIONS/INTERVENTIONS	RATIONALE

Independent

Investigate reports of pain; note intensity (0–10 scale), characteristics (e.g., dull, throbbing, constant), location, duration, aggravating and relieving factors.	Pain is a subjective experience and must be described by the patient. Identification of pain characteristics and associated factors are essential to choosing appropriate interventions and evaluating effectiveness of therapy.
Note specific probable pathophysiology, e.g., brain/meningeal/sinus infection, cervical spine injury, hypertension, trauma.	Understanding of underlying condition aids in choosing appropriate interventions.
Observe nonverbal pain cues, e.g., facial expressions, body position, restlessness, crying, withdrawal, diaphoresis, changes in heart/respiratory rate, BP.	Indirect indicators of the presence/degree of pain being experienced. Headaches may be both acute and chronic, so physiologic manifestations may or may not be present.
Assess/correlate emotional/physical components of individual situation.	Factors that affect presence/perception of pain.
Evaluate pain behavior.	May be exaggerated because patient's perception of pain is not believed or because patient believes SO/caregivers are discounting reports of pain.
Note effects of pain, e.g., loss of interest in life, decreased activity, weight loss.	Pain may be interfering with life to a serious extent and may lead to development of depression.
Assess degree of personal maladjustment of the patient, such as isolationism.	Patient may be withdrawing from involvement with others/activities because of pain.
Determine issues of secondary gain for the patient/SO, e.g., insurance, mate/family.	These issues need to be recognized/dealt with to help patient recover/cope with condition.
Discuss the physiologic dynamics of tension/anxiety with patient/SO.	Knowledge about how these factors influence headache can help with management.
Instruct patient to report pain as soon as it begins.	Prompt recognition promotes early intervention and may reduce severity of attack.
Place in darkened room as indicated.	May be sensitive to light (photosensitivity), which can intensify attack.
Encourage rest in quiet room.	Decreases excessive stimulation, which may aggravate headache.
Apply cold compresses to head.	Promotes comfort by decreasing vasodilation.
Apply moist/dry heat to head, neck, shoulders as appropriate.	Increases circulation to muscles, promoting relaxation, easing tension.
Massage head/neck/shoulder area if patient can tolerate touch.	Relieves tension and promotes relaxation of muscles.
Use therapeutic touch, visualization, biofeedback, self-hypnosis, and other stress reduction and relaxation techniques.	Provides the patient with some control over pain and/or may alter the pain-sensing mechanism and pain perception.
Encourage patient to use positive affirmations: "I am healing, I am relaxed, I love this life." Ask patient to be aware of internal-external dialogue and say "Stop," or "Cancel" when negative thoughts develop.	Negative thinking can increase tension, increasing pain and disability of headache, making situation more intolerable. Recognition of negative messages and use of positive self-talk can reduce tension, decreasing pain of headache.

ACTIONS/INTERVENTIONS	RATIONALE

Independent

Observe for nausea/vomiting. Provide ice chips, carbonated beverages, crackers as indicated.

Often accompanies severe headache. Measures may promote comfort. *Note:* Beverages containing caffeine may be given with ergot preparations to relieve migraine headaches.

Collaborative

Administer medications as indicated:

Analgesics, e.g., ASA, acetaminophen (Tylenol);

Primary treatments of common tension headaches, are only occasionally useful for vascular headaches.

Mild muscle relaxants, e.g., diazepam (Valium);

Used for general relaxation, sedation, and prevention of migraines.

Nonsteroidal anti-inflammatory agents, e.g., ibuprofen (Motrin); meclofenamate (Meclomen);

Used for anti-inflammatory, analgesic and antipyretic effect.

Narcotics, e.g., Demerol/codeine;

May be required at times to abort severe headache. Regular use should be restricted/avoided.

Prednisone;

Effective treatment for most episodes of cluster headaches.

Vasoactive agents, e.g., Ergot preparations (Cafergot, Wigraine); methysergide maleate (Sansert); Clonidine (Catapres);

Cranial vasoconstrictive agents are useful for reducing frequency and intensity of migraine/cluster headaches. *Note:* Ergot preparations must be given at onset of headache attack.

β-blockers, e.g., propanalol (Inderal); verapamil (Calan); atenolol (Tenormin);

Used to decrease frequency of recurrent vascular/cluster headaches.

Antidepressants, e.g., amitriptyline (Elavil), MAO inhibitors, e.g., isocarboxazid (Marplan); doxepin (Sinequan); nortriptyline (Pamelor);

Useful in treating refractory migraines and alleviating depression, reduces vascular/muscular tension and helps patient cope with situation.

Adrenergic agents: isometheptene mucate (Midrin);

Reduces pain by constricting dilated cranial and cerebral arterioles, providing mild sedation, and by raising pain threshold.

Antiemetics (Tigan);

Reduces discomfort of associated symptoms of nausea and vomiting.

Antibiotics.

Used when brain or sinus infection is present.

Refer for biofeedback, relaxation techniques, physical therapy.

These techniques are useful for reduction of muscle tension and stress, which may be contributing to headache.

Provide information regarding the use of acupressure/acupuncture as appropriate.

Pressure over the unilateral common carotid decreases blood flow to the brain, resulting in lessening of the pain.

Administer supplemental oxygen as indicated.

Shortens the headache attack by 60%–70% in some patients by decreasing hypoxia associated with vascular spasm/constriction.

Assist with/prepare for application of TENS unit.

This device offers a measure of autocontrol by interfering with/blocking the transmission of painful stimuli.

ACTIONS/INTERVENTIONS

RATIONALE

Collaborative

Refer to outpatient headache/pain clinic as indicated.

Ongoing team approach to chronic pain control, which may include counseling, highly structured relaxation sessions, exercise, and medications. May be helpful when other relief measures have failed.

NURSING DIAGNOSIS:	COPING, INDIVIDUAL, INEFFECTIVE, HIGH RISK FOR
Risk factors may include:	Situational crisis.
	Personal vulnerability.
	Inadequate support systems.
	Work overload/no vacations.
	Inadequate relaxation.
	Inadequate coping methods.
	Severe pain, overwhelming threat to self.
Possibly evidenced by:	[Not applicable; presence of signs and symptoms establishes an actual diagnosis.]
DESIRED OUTCOMES/ EVALUATION CRITERIA— PATIENT WILL:	Identify ineffective coping behaviors and consequences.
	Verbalize awareness of own coping abilities.
	Assess the current situation accurately.
	Demonstrate lifestyle changes necessary/appropriate to situation.

ACTIONS/INTERVENTIONS

RATIONALE

Independent

Assess current functional capacity.

Pain of headache (acute or chronic process) can interfere with coping ability.

Discuss usual coping methods, e.g., alcohol intake, smoking habits, eating patterns, physical and mental relaxation strategies.

Maladaptive behaviors may be used to cope with constant pain or may be contributors to continued pain.

Treat the patient with courtesy and respect. Take advantage of teachable moments.

Meets psychologic needs, enhancing self-esteem and promoting opportunities for learning new ways to cope with situation.

Assist patient in dealing with change in concept of body image.

Patient may view self as a person "who has headaches," and beginning to see self as *well* entails seeing self as "one who does not have headaches."

Encourage expression of feelings and discussion of how headaches interfere with work and enjoyment of life.

Enables patient to recognize feelings in relation to pain. Patient may be frustrated with occurrence of headache/treatments and adjustments that need to be made in lifestyle.

ACTIONS/INTERVENTIONS	RATIONALE

Independent

Ascertain impact of illness on sexual needs.

Chronic headache interferes with many aspects of the individual's life, and patient may not broach subject unless asked.

Provide information about cause of headache, treatment, and expected course.

Understanding this information can help the patient make informed choices, learn to cope with events, and gain a sense of control over situation enhancing self-esteem.

Collaborative

Refer for counseling and/or family therapy or assertiveness training classes as indicated.

May need additional help to solve associated problems that are interfering with progress toward wellness.

NURSING DIAGNOSIS: **KNOWLEDGE DEFICIT [LEARNING NEED] REGARDING CONDITION AND TREATMENT NEEDS**

May be related to:

Lack of exposure/lack of recall.

Unfamiliarity with information.

Cognitive limitation.

Possibly evidenced by:

Request for information.

Statement of misconception.

Inappropriate, exaggerated behavior, e.g., hysterical, hostile, agitated, apathetic.

Development of preventable complications.

Inaccurate follow-through of instructions.

DESIRED OUTCOMES/ EVALUATION CRITERIA— PATIENT WILL:

Verbalize understanding of condition and treatment.

Identify relationship of signs/symptoms to condition.

Initiate appropriate lifestyle/behavior changes.

Identify stress situations and specific methods to deal with them.

ACTIONS/INTERVENTIONS	RATIONALE

Independent

Discuss individual etiology of headache when known.

Influences choice of treatment and progress for recovery.

Assist patient in identifying possible precipitating factors, e.g., emotional stressors, temperature extremes, food/environmental allergies.

Avoiding/limiting these factors can often prevent recurrence or frequency of attacks.

Discuss medication regimen/side effects. Review need to reduce/alter medications as indicated.

These patients may become drug-dependent and ignore other forms of therapy.

ACTIONS/INTERVENTIONS	RATIONALE
Independent	
Instruct patient/SO in activity/exercise program, dietary considerations, and physical comfort measures, e.g., massage.	When done correctly, exercise can alleviate pain by increasing endorphin levels in the brain and patient's pain threshold. Dietary restrictions of vasoactive substances will decrease the frequency of headaches. Massage therapy is important in improving circulation to relax muscle tension.
Discuss importance of good body mechanics/posture.	Decreases strain on the muscles of the neck and shoulder areas and can provide overall relief of body tension.
Encourage patient/SO to take time for relaxation and fun.	Overzealous sense of duty can lead to neglect of own well-being, adding to stress and contributing to headache.
Encourage use of right-brain activities, love, and laughter.	Releases body's natural painkillers (endorphins) helping patient to reduce pain of headache.
Encourage use of subliminal music with positive affirmations.	Bypasses logical part of the brain, promoting relaxation.
Encourage patient to keep log of headaches and associated factors/precipitators.	Provides opportunity to identify/control factors that may precipitate a headache.
Provide written information/guidelines.	Resource for the patient to refer to when in doubt about a certain exercise, diet, drug effect/interaction, or side effect.
Identify and discuss potential hazards of unproven and/or nonmedical therapies/remedies.	Patients can become discouraged with lack of relief from standard treatments and may seek other sources that not only do not provide relief but may even be harmful.

Seizure Disorders/Epilepsy

Seizures (convulsions) are the result of uncontrolled electrical discharges from the nerve cells of the cerebral cortex, characterized by sudden, brief attacks of altered consciousness, motor activity, and/or sensory phenomena.

The phases of seizure activity are prodromal, aura, ictal, and postictal. The prodromal phase involves mood or behavior changes that may precede seizure by hours/days. The aura is a premonition of impending seizure activity and may be visual, auditory, or gustatory. The ictal stage is seizure activity, usually musculoskeletal. The postictal stage is a period of confusion/somnolence/irritability that occurs after the seizure.

The main causes for seizures can be divided into six categories:

Drugs: Poisons, alcohol, overdoses of prescription/nonprescription drugs. Drugs are the leading cause of seizures.

Chemical imbalances: Hyperkalemia, hypoglycemia, and acidosis.

Fever: The most frequent cause in young children.

Cerebral pathology: Resulting from head injury, trauma, infections, increased intracranial pressure.

Eclampsia: Prenatal hypertension/toxemia of pregnancy.

Idiopathic: Unknown origin.

RELATED CONCERNS:

Cerebrovascular Accident/Stroke, p 290
Craniocerebral Trauma, p 271
Intracranial Infections, p 307
Psychosocial Aspects of Acute Care, p 899
Substance Dependence, p 1000

PATIENT ASSESSMENT DATA BASE

ACTIVITY/REST

May report:	Fatigue, general weakness.
	Limitation of activities/occupation imposed by self/SO/health care provider or others.
May exhibit:	Altered muscle tone/strength.
	Involuntary movement/contractions of muscles or muscle groups.

CIRCULATION

May exhibit:	Ictal: Hypertension, increased pulse, cyanosis.
	Postictal: Vital signs normal or may be depressed with decreased pulse and respiration.

EGO INTEGRITY

May report:	Internal/external stressors related to condition and/or treatment.
	Irritability; sense of helplessness/hopelessness.
	Changes in relationships.
May exhibit:	Wide range of emotional responses.

ELIMINATION

May report:	Episodic incontinence.
May exhibit:	Ictal: Increased bladder pressure and sphincter tone.
	Postictal: Muscles relaxed resulting in incontinence (urinary/fecal).

FOOD/FLUID

May report: Food sensitivity nausea/vomiting correlating with seizure activity.

May exhibit: Dental/soft tissue damage (injury during seizure).

Gingival hyperplasia (side effect of long-term Dilantin use).

NEUROSENSORY

May report: History of headaches, recurring seizure activity, fainting, dizziness.

History of head trauma, anoxia, cerebral infections.

Presence of aura (stimulation of visual, auditory, hallucinogenic areas).

Postictal: Weakness, muscle pain, areas of paresthesia/paralysis.

May exhibit: Seizure characteristics:

Prodromal phase: Vague changes in emotional reactivity or affective response preceding aura in some cases and lasting minutes to hours.

Generalized Seizures:

Tonic-clonic (grand mal): Rigidity and jerking posturing, vocalization, loss of consciousness, dilated pupils, stertorous respiration, excessive saliva (froth), fecal/urinary incontinence, and biting of the tongue may occur.

Postictal: Patient sleeps 30 minutes to several hours, then may be weak, confused, and amnesic for the episode with nausea and stiff, sore muscles.

Absence (petit mal): Periods of altered awareness or consciousness (staring, fluttering of eyes) lasting 5–30 seconds, which may occur as much as 100 times a day; minor motor seizures may be akinetic (loss of movement), myoclonic (repetitive motor contractions), or atonic (loss of muscle tone).

Postictal: Amnesia for seizure events, no confusion, able to resume activity.

Partial seizures (complex):

Psychomotor/temporal lobe: Patient generally remains conscious, with reactions such as dream state, staring, wandering, irritability, hallucinations, hostility, or fear. May display involuntary motor symptoms (lip smacking) and behaviors that appear purposeful but are inappropriate (automatism) and include impaired judgment, and on occasion, antisocial acts.

Postictal: Absence of memory for these events, mild to moderate confusion.

Partial seizures (simple):

Focal-motor/Jacksonian: Often preceded by aura, lasts 2–15 minutes. No loss of consciousness (unilateral) or loss of consciousness (bilateral). Convulsive movements and temporary disturbance in part controlled by the brain region involved (e.g., frontal lobe [motor dysfunction]; parietal [numbness, tingling]; occipital [bright, flashing lights]; posterotemporal [difficulty speaking]). Convulsions may march along limb or side of body in orderly progression. If restrained during seizure, patient may exhibit combative and uncooperative behavior.

Status epilepticus:

Continuous seizure activity occurring spontaneously or related to abrupt withdrawal of anticonvulsants and other metabolic phenomena. _Note:_ If absence seizures are the pattern, problem may go undetected for a period of time, as the patient does not lose consciousness.

PAIN/COMFORT

May report: Headache, muscle/back soreness postictally.

Paroxysmal abdominal pain during ictal phase (may occur during some partial/focal seizures without loss of consciousness).

May exhibit: Guarding behavior.

Alteration in muscle tone.

Distraction behavior/restlessness.

RESPIRATION

May exhibit: Ictal: Clenched teeth, cyanosis, decreased or rapid respirations; increased mucous secretions.

Postictal: Apnea.

SAFETY

May report: History of accidental falls/injuries, fractures.

Presence of allergies.

May exhibit: Soft tissue injury/ecchymosis.

Decreased general strength/muscle tone.

SOCIAL INTERACTION

May report: Problems with interpersonal relationships within family/socially.

Limitation/avoidance of social contacts.

TEACHING/LEARNING

May report: Familial history of epilepsy.

Drug (including alcohol) use/misuse.

Increased frequency of episodes/failure to improve.

Discharge Plan Considerations: **DRG projected mean length of stay: 3.5 days.**

May require changes in medications, assistance with some homemaker/maintenance tasks relative to issues of safety and transportation.

DIAGNOSTIC STUDIES

Electrolytes: Imbalances may affect/predispose to seizure activity.

Glucose: Hypoglycemia may precipitate seizure.

BUN: Elevation may potentiate seizure activity or may indicate nephrotoxicity related to medication regimen.

CBC: Aplastic anemia may result from drug therapy.

Serum drug levels: To verify therapeutic range of antiepileptic drugs.

Lumbar puncture: Detects abnormal CSF pressure, signs of infections, bleeding (subarachnoid, subdural hemorrhage) as a cause of seizures.

Skull x-rays: Identifies presence of space-occupying lesions, fractures.

Electroencephalogram (EEG): Locates area of cerebral dysfunction; measures brain activity. Brain waves take on characteristic spikes in each type of seizure activity.

Video-EEG monitoring, 24 hours (video picture obtained at same time as EEG): May identify exact focus of seizure activity (advantage of repeated viewing of event with EEG recording).

CT scan: Identifies localized cerebral lesions, infarcts, hematomas, cerebral edema, trauma, abscesses, tumor; can be done with or without contrast medium.

Positron emission tomography (PET): Demonstrates metabolic alterations, e.g., decreased metabolism of glucose at site of lesion.

MRI: Localizes focal lesions.

Magnetoencephalogram: Maps the electrical impulses/potential of brain for abnormal discharge patterns.

Wada: Determines hemispheric dominance (done as a presurgical evaluation prior to temporal lobectomy).

NURSING PRIORITIES

1. Prevent/control seizure activity.
2. Protect patient from injury.
3. Maintain airway/respiratory function.
4. Promote positive self-esteem.
5. Provide information about disease process, prognosis, and treatment needs.

DISCHARGE GOALS

1. Seizure activity controlled.
2. Complications/injury prevented.
3. Capable/competent self-image displayed.
4. Disease process/prognosis, therapeutic regimen, and limitations understood.

NURSING DIAGNOSIS:	**TRAUMA/SUFFOCATION, HIGH RISK FOR**
Risk factors may include:	Weakness, balancing difficulties.
	Cognitive limitations/altered consciousness.
	Loss of large or small muscle coordination.
	Emotional difficulties.
Possibly evidenced by:	[Not applicable; presence of signs and symptoms establishes an actual diagnosis.]
DESIRED OUTCOMES/ EVALUATION CRITERIA— PATIENT WILL:	Verbalize understanding of factors that contribute to possibility of trauma, and/or suffocation and take steps to correct situation.
	Demonstrate behaviors, lifestyle changes to reduce risk factors and protect self from injury.
	Modify environment as indicated to enhance safety.
	Maintain treatment regimen to control/eliminate seizure activity.
	<u>Care givers will:</u> Identify actions/measures to take when seizure occurs.

ACTIONS/INTERVENTIONS	RATIONALE
Independent	
Explore with patient the various stimuli that may precipitate a seizure.	Alcohol, various drugs, and other stimuli (e.g., loss of sleep, flashing lights, prolonged television viewing) may increase brain activity, thereby increasing the potential for seizure activity.

ACTIONS/INTERVENTIONS	RATIONALE
Independent	
Keep padded side rails up with bed in lowest position.	Minimizes injury should seizures (frequent/generalized) occur while patient is in bed.
Encourage patient to smoke only while supervised.	May cause burns if cigarette is accidentally dropped during aura/seizure activity.
Evaluate need for/provide protective headgear.	Use of helmet may provide added protection for individuals who suffer recurrent/severe seizures.
Use metal thermometer or obtain temperature via ear canal when necessary.	Reduces risk of patient biting and breaking glass thermometer or suffering injury if sudden seizure activity should occur.
Maintain strict bed rest if prodromal signs/aura experienced. Explain necessity for these actions.	Patient may feel restless/need to ambulate or even defecate during aura phase, thereby inadvertently removing self from safe environment and easy observation. Understanding importance of providing for own safety needs may enhance patient cooperation.
Stay with patient during/after seizure.	Promotes patient safety.
Insert plastic airway/bite block or soft roll between teeth (if jaw relaxed). Turn head to side/suction airway as indicated.	Reduces risk of oral trauma but should not be "forced" or inserted when teeth are clenched, because dental and soft tissue damage may result. Also helps maintain airway. *Note:* Wooden tongue blades should not be used, because they may splinter and break in patient's mouth. (Refer to ND: Airway Clearance/Breathing Pattern, ineffective, p 266.)
Cradle head, place on soft area, or assist to floor if out of bed. Do not attempt to restrain.	Gentle guiding of extremities reduces risk of physical injury when patient lacks voluntary muscle control. *Note:* If attempt is made to restrain patient during seizure, erratic movements may increase, and patient may injure self or others.
Document type of seizure activity (e.g., location/duration of motor activity, loss of consciousness, incontinence) and frequency/recurrence.	Helps to localize the cerebral area of involvement.
Perform neurologic/vital sign check after seizure, e.g., level of consciousness, orientation, BP, pulse/respiratory rate.	Documents postictal state and time/completeness of recovery to normal state.
Reorient patient following seizure activity.	Patient may be confused, disoriented, and possibly amnesic after the seizure and need help to regain control and alleviate anxiety.
Allow postictal "automatic" behavior without interfering while providing environmental protection.	May display behavior (of motor or psychic origin) that seems inappropriate/irrelevant for time and place. Attempts to control or prevent activity may result in patient becoming aggressive/combative.
Observe for status epilepticus, e.g., one tonic-clonic seizure after another in rapid succession.	This is a life-threatening emergency that may cause respiratory arrest, severe hypoxia, and/or brain and nerve cell damage. Immediate intervention is required to control seizure activity. *Note:*

265

ACTIONS/INTERVENTIONS	RATIONALE
Independent	
	Although absence seizures may become static, they are not usually life-threatening.
Discuss seizure warning signs (if appropriate) and usual seizure pattern. Teach SO to recognize warning signs and how to care for patient during and after seizure.	Enables patient to protect self from injury and recognize changes that require notification of physician/further intervention. Knowing what to do when seizure occurs can prevent injury/complications and decrease SO's feelings of helplessness.
Collaborative	
Administer medications as indicated:	
AEDs, e.g., phenytoin (Dilantin); primidone (Mysoline); carbamazepine (Tegretol); clonazepam (Klonopin); valproic acid (Depakote);	Antiepileptic drugs raise the seizure threshold by stabilizing nerve cell membranes, reducing the excitability of the neurons, or through direct action on the limbic system, thalamus, and hypothalamus. Goal is for optimal suppression of seizure activity with lowest possible dose of drug and with fewest side effects.
Phenobarbital (Luminal);	Potentiates/enhances effects of AEDs and allows for lower dosage to reduce side effects.
Diazepam (Valium);	May be used alone (or in combination with phenobarbital) as a first-line drug to suppress status seizure activity.
Glucose, thiamine.	May be given to restore metabolic balance if seizure is induced by hypoglycemia or alcohol.
Monitor/document AED drug levels, corresponding side effects, and frequency of seizure activity.	Standard therapeutic level may not be optimal for individual patient if untoward side effects develop or seizures are not controlled.
Monitor CBC, electrolytes, glucose levels.	Identifies factors that aggravate/decrease seizure threshold.
Prepare for surgery/electrode implantation as indicated.	Vagal nerve stimulator, magnetic beam therapy, or other surgical intervention (e.g., temporal lobectomy) may be done for intractable seizures or well-localized epileptogenic lesions when patient is disabled and at high risk for serious injury.

NURSING DIAGNOSIS:	AIRWAY CLEARANCE/BREATHING PATTERN, INEFFECTIVE, HIGH RISK FOR
Risk factors may include:	Neuromuscular impairment.
	Tracheobronchial obstruction.
	Perceptual/cognitive impairment.
Possibly evidenced by:	[Not applicable; presence of signs and symptoms establishes an actual diagnosis.]

DESIRED OUTCOMES/ EVALUATION CRITERIA— PATIENT WILL:	Maintain effective respiratory pattern with airway patent/ aspiration prevented.

ACTIONS/INTERVENTIONS	RATIONALE

Independent

Encourage patient to empty mouth of dentures/foreign objects if aura occurs and to avoid chewing gum/sucking lozenges if seizures occur without warning.	Reduces risk of aspiration/foreign bodies lodging in pharynx.
Place in lying position, flat surface; turn head to side during seizure activity.	Promotes drainage of secretions; prevents tongue from obstructing airway.
Loosen clothing from neck/chest and abdominal areas.	Facilitates breathing/chest expansion.
Insert bite stick/airway or soft roll as indicated.	If inserted prior to tightening of the jaw, these devices may prevent biting of tongue and facilitate suctioning/respiratory support if required. Airway adjunct may be indicated after cessation of seizure activity if patient is unconscious and unable to maintain safe position of tongue.
Suction as needed.	Reduces risk of aspiration/asphyxiation.

Collaborative

Administer supplemental oxygen/hand ventilate as needed postictally.	May reduce cerebral hypoxia resulting from decreased circulation/oxygenation secondary to vascular spasm during seizure. *Note:* Artificial ventilation during general seizure activity is of limited or no benefit as it is not possible to move air in/out of lungs during sustained contraction of respiratory musculature. As seizure abates, respiratory function will return unless a secondary problem exists (e.g., foreign body/aspiration).
Prepare for/assist with intubation, if indicated.	Presence of prolonged apnea postictally may require ventilatory support.

NURSING DIAGNOSIS:	SELF-ESTEEM/PERSONAL IDENTITY, DISTURBANCE
May be related to:	Stigma associated with condition.
	Perception of being out of control.
Possibly evidenced by:	Verbalization about changed lifestyle.
	Fear of rejection; negative feelings about body.
	Change in self-perception of role.
	Change in usual patterns of responsibility.
	Lack of follow-through/nonparticipation in therapy.

ACTIONS/INTERVENTIONS	RATIONALE
Independent	
Discuss feelings about diagnosis, perception of threat to self. Encourage expression of feelings.	Reactions vary among individuals, and previous knowledge/experience with this condition will affect acceptance of therapeutic regimen. Verbalization of fears, anger, and concerns about future implications can help patient begin to accept/deal with situation.
Identify possible/anticipated public reaction to condition. Encourage patient to refrain from concealing problem.	Provides opportunity to problem-solve responses and provides measure of control over situation. Concealment is destructive to self-esteem (potentiates denial), blocking progress in dealing with problem and may actually increase risk of injury/negative response when seizure does occur.
Explore with patient current/past successes and strengths.	Focusing on positive aspects can help to alleviate feelings of guilt/self-consciousness and help patient begin to accept manageability of condition.
Avoid overprotecting patient; encourage activities providing supervision/monitoring when indicated.	Participation in as many experiences as possible can lessen depression about limitations. Observation/supervision needs to be provided for such activities as gymnastics, climbing, and water sports.
Determine attitudes/capabilities of SO. Help him/her realize that his/her feelings are normal; however guilt and blame are not helpful.	Negative expectations from SO may affect patient's sense of competency/self-esteem and interfere with support received from SO, limiting potential for optimal management.
Stress importance of staff/SO to remain calm during seizure.	Anxiety of care givers is contagious and can be conveyed to the patient, increasing/multiplying individual's own negative perceptions of situation/self.
Collaborative	
Refer patient/SO to support group, e.g., Epilepsy Foundation of America and National Association of Epilepsy Centers.	Provides opportunity to gain information, support, and ideas for dealing with problems from others who share similar experiences.
Discuss referral for psychotherapy with patient/SO.	Seizures have a profound effect on personal self-esteem, and patient/SO may feel guilt over perceived limitations and public stigma. Counseling can help overcome feelings of inferiority/self-consciousness.

NURSING DIAGNOSIS:	KNOWLEDGE DEFICIT [LEARNING NEED], REGARDING CONDITION AND TREATMENT REGIMEN
May be related to:	Lack of exposure.
	Information misinterpretation; lack of recall.
	Cognitive limitation.
	Failure to improve.
Possibly evidenced by:	Questions.
	Increased/lack of control of seizure activity.
	Lack of follow-through of drug regimen.
DESIRED OUTCOMES/ EVALUATION CRITERIA— PATIENT WILL:	Verbalize understanding of disorder and various stimuli that may increase/potentiate seizure activity.
	Initiate necessary lifestyle/behavior changes as indicated.
	Adhere to prescribed drug regimen.

ACTIONS/INTERVENTIONS	RATIONALE
Independent	
Review pathology/prognosis of condition and life-long need for treatment as indicated.	Provides opportunity to clarify/dispel misconceptions and present condition as something that is manageable within a normal lifestyle.
Review medication regimen, necessity of taking drugs as ordered, and not discontinuing therapy without physician supervision. Include directions for missed dose.	Lack of cooperation with medication regimen is a leading cause of seizure breakthrough. Patient needs to know risks of status epilepticus resulting from abrupt withdrawal of anticonvulsants. Dependent on drug and frequency, patient may be instructed to take missed dose if remembered within a predetermined time frame.
Recommend taking drugs with meals if appropriate.	May reduce incidence of gastric irritation, nausea/vomiting.
Discuss adverse side effects of particular drugs, e.g., drowsiness, hyperactivity, sleep disturbances, gingival hypertrophy, visual disturbances, nausea/vomiting, rashes, syncope/ataxia, birth defects, aplastic anemia.	May indicate need for change in dosage/choice of drug therapy. Promotes involvement/participation in decision-making process, and awareness of potential long-term effects of drug therapy and provides opportunity to minimize/prevent complications.
Provide information about potential drug interactions and necessity of notifying other health care providers of drug regimen.	Knowledge of anticonvulsant use reduces risk of prescribing drugs that may interact, thus altering seizure threshold or therapeutic effect. E.g., Dilantin potentiates anticoagulant effect of Coumadin, whereas INH and chloromycetin increase the effect of Dilantin.
Encourage patient to wear identification tag/bracelet stating the presence of a seizure disorder.	Expedites treatment and diagnosis in emergency situations.

269

ACTIONS/INTERVENTIONS	RATIONALE
Independent	
Stress need for routine follow-up care/laboratory testing as indicated, e.g., CBC should be monitored biannually and in presence of sore throat/fever.	Therapeutic needs may change and/or serious drug side effects (e.g., agranulocytosis or toxicity) may develop.
Review possible effects of hormonal changes.	Alterations in hormonal levels that occur during menstruation and pregnancy may increase risk of seizures.
Discuss significance of maintaining good general health, e.g., adequate diet, rest, moderate exercise, and avoidance of exhaustion, alcohol, caffeine, and stimulant drugs.	Regularity and moderation in activities may aid in reducing/controlling precipitating factors, enhancing sense of general well-being, and strengthening coping ability and self-esteem.
Review importance of good oral hygiene and regular dental care.	Reduces risk of oral infections and gingival hyperplasia.
Identify necessity/promote acceptance of actual limitations; discuss safety measures concerned with driving, using mechanical equipment, climbing ladders, swimming, hobbies, and so on.	Reduces risk of injury to self or others, especially if seizures occur without warning.
Discuss local laws/restrictions pertaining to persons with epilepsy/seizure disorder. Encourage awareness but not necessarily acceptance of these policies.	Although legal/civil rights of persons with epilepsy have improved during the past decade, restrictions still exist in some states pertaining to obtaining driver's license, sterilization, worker's compensation, and required reportability to state agencies.

Craniocerebral Trauma (Acute Rehabilitative Phase)

Craniocerebral trauma (open and closed) includes skull fractures, concussion, cerebral contusion/laceration, and cerebral hemorrhage (subarachnoid, subdural, epidural, intracerebral, brainstem). *Primary* injury may occur from direct blow to head or be indirect (acceleration/deceleration of brain). *Secondary* brain injury can result from diffuse axonal injury, intracranial hypertension, hypoxemia, hypercapnea, or systemic hypotension.

Consequences range from no apparent neurologic disturbance to a persistent vegetative state or death. Therefore, every head injury must be considered potentially serious.

RELATED CONCERNS:

Cerebrovascular Accident/Stroke, p 290
Headache, p 252
Psychosocial Aspects of Acute Care, p 899
Seizure Disorders/Epilepsy, p 261
Total Nutritional Support, p 1039
Upper Gastrointestinal/Esophageal Bleeding, p 454

PATIENT ASSESSMENT DATA BASE

Data are dependent on type, location, and severity of injury and may be complicated by additional injury to other vital organs.

ACTIVITY/REST

May report:	Weakness, fatigue, clumsiness, loss of balance.
May exhibit:	Altered consciousness, lethargy.
	Hemiparesis, quadriparesis.
	Unsteady gait (ataxia).
	Balance problems.
	Orthopedic injuries (trauma).
	Loss of muscle tone, muscle spasticity.

CIRCULATION

May exhibit:	Normal or altered BP (hypertension).
	Changes in heart rate (bradycardia, tachycardia alternating with bradycardia, other dysrhythmias).

EGO INTEGRITY

May report:	Behavior or personality changes (subtle or dramatic).
May exhibit:	Anxiety, irritability, delirium, agitation, confusion, depression, impulsivity.

ELIMINATION

May exhibit:	Bowel/bladder incontinence or dysfunction.

FOOD/FLUID

May report:	Nausea/vomiting, changes in appetite.
May exhibit:	Vomiting (may be projectile).
	Swallowing problems (coughing, drooling, dysphagia).

NEUROSENSORY

May report: Transient loss of consciousness, amnesia surrounding trauma events.

Vertigo, syncope, tinnitus, hearing loss.

Tingling, numbness in extremity.

Visual changes, e.g., acuity, diplopia, photophobia, loss of part of visual field.

Loss of/changes in senses of taste or smell.

May exhibit: Alteration in consciousness, coma.

Mental status changes (orientation, alertness/responsiveness, attention, concentration, problem solving, emotional affect/behavior, memory).

Pupillary changes (response to light, symmetry), deviation of eyes, inability to follow.

Loss of senses, e.g., taste, smell, hearing.

Facial asymmetry.

Unequal, weak handgrip.

Absent/weak deep tendon reflexes.

Apraxia, hemiparesis, quadriparesis.

Posturing (decorticate, decerebrate); seizure activity.

Heightened sensitivity to touch and movement.

Loss of sensation to parts of body.

Difficulty in understanding self/limbs in relation to environment (proprioception).

PAIN/COMFORT

May report: Headache of variable intensity and location (usually long lasting).

May exhibit: Facial grimacing, withdrawal response to painful stimuli, restlessness, moaning.

RESPIRATION

May exhibit: Changes in breathing patterns (e.g., periods of apnea alternating with hyperventilation).

Noisy respirations, stridor, choking.

Rhonchi, wheezes (possible aspiration).

SAFETY

May report: Current trauma/accidental injuries.

May exhibit: Fractures/dislocations.

Impaired vision.

Skin: Head/facial lacerations, abrasions, discoloration, e.g., raccoon eyes, Battles' sign around ears (trauma signs).

Drainage from ears/nose (CSF).

Impaired cognition.

Range of motion impairment, loss of muscle tone, general strength; paralysis.

Fever, altered body temperature regulation.

SOCIAL INTERACTION

May exhibit: Expressive or receptive aphasia, unintelligible speech, repetitive speech, dysarthria, anomia.

TEACHING/LEARNING

May report: Use of alcohol/other drugs.

Discharge Plan Considerations: **DRG projected mean length of stay: 12 days.**
May require assistance with self-care, ambulation, transportation, food preparation, shopping, treatments, medications, homemaker/maintenance tasks; change in physical layout of home or placement in living facility other than home.

DIAGNOSTIC STUDIES

CT scan (with/without contrast): Identifies space-occupying lesions, hemorrhage; determines ventricular size, brain tissue shift. Note: Serial study may be required as ischemic injury/infarct may not be detected for 24–72 hours postinjury.

MRI: Uses similar to those of CT scan with or without use of radioactive contrast.

Cerebral angiography: Demonstrates cerebral circulatory anomalies, e.g., brain tissue shifts secondary to edema, hemorrhage, trauma.

Serial EEG: May reveal presence or development of pathologic waves.

X-rays: Detect changes in bony structure (fractures), shifts of midline structures (bleeding/edema), bone fragments.

BAER: Determines levels of cortical and brainstem function.

PET: Detects changes in metabolic activity in the brain.

CSF, lumbar puncture: May be diagnostic for suspected subarachnoid hemorrhage.

ABGs: Determines presence of ventilation or oxygenation problems that may exacerbate/increase intracranial pressure.

Serum chemistry/electrolytes: May reveal imbalances that contribute to increased intracranial pressure (IICP)/changes in mentation.

Toxicology screen: Detects drugs which may be responsible for/potentiate loss of consciousness.

Serum anticonvulsant levels: May be done to ensure that therapeutic level is adequate to prevent seizure activity.

NURSING PRIORITIES

1. Maximize cerebral perfusion/function.
2. Prevent/minimize complications.
3. Promote optimal functioning/return to preinjury level.
4. Support coping process and family recovery.
5. Provide information about disease process/prognosis, treatment plan, and resources.

DISCHARGE GOALS

1. Cerebral function improved; neurologic deficits resolving/stabilized.
2. Complications prevented or minimized.
3. ADL needs met by self or with assistance of other(s).
4. Family acknowledging reality of situation and involved in recovery program.
5. Disease process/prognosis and treatment regimen understood and available resources identified.

NURSING DIAGNOSIS:	TISSUE PERFUSION, ALTERED, CEREBRAL
May be related to:	Interruption of blood flow by space-occupying lesions (hemorrhage, hematoma); cerebral edema (localized or

generalized response to injury, metabolic alterations, drug/alcohol overdose); decreased systemic BP/hypoxia (hypovolemia, cardiac dysrhythmias).

Possibly evidenced by:	Altered level of consciousness; memory loss.
	Changes in motor/sensory responses, restlessness.
	Changes in vital signs.
DESIRED OUTCOMES/ EVALUATION CRITERIA— PATIENT WILL:	Maintain usual/improved level of consciousness, cognition, and motor/sensory function.
	Demonstrate stable vital signs and absence of signs of increased ICP.

ACTIONS/INTERVENTIONS	RATIONALE
Independent	
Determine factors related to individual situation/ cause for coma/decreased cerebral perfusion and potential for IICP.	Influences choice of interventions. Deterioration in neurologic signs/symptoms or failure to improve after initial insult may require that the patient be transferred to critical care for monitoring of intracranial pressure and/or surgical intervention.
Monitor/document neurologic status frequently and compare with baseline, e.g., Glasgow Coma Scale;	Assesses trends in LOC and potential for IICP and is useful in determining location, extent, and progression/resolution of CNS damage.
Evaluate eye opening, e.g., spontaneous (awake), opens only to painful stimuli, keeps eyes closed (coma);	Determines arousal ability/level of consciousness.
Assess verbal response; note whether patient is alert, oriented to person, place, time or is confused; uses inappropriate words/phrases that make little sense;	Measures appropriateness of speech and content of consciousness. If minimal damage has occurred in the cerebral cortex, the patient may be aroused by verbal stimuli but may appear drowsy or uncooperative. More extensive damage to the cerebral cortex may be displayed by slow response to commands, lapsing into sleep when not stimulated, disorientation, and stupor. Damage to midbrain, pons, and medulla are manifested by lack of appropriate responses to stimuli.
Assess motor response to simple commands, noting purposeful (obeys command, attempts to push stimulus away) and nonpurposeful (posturing) movement. Note limb movement and document right and left sides separately.	Measures overall awareness and ability to respond to external stimuli and best indicates state of consciousness in the patient whose eyes are closed because of trauma or who is aphasic. Consciousness and involuntary movement are integrated if the patient can both grasp and release the tester's hand or hold up 2 fingers on command. Purposeful movement can include grimacing or withdrawing from painful stimuli or movements that the patient desires, e.g., sitting up. Other movements (posturing and abnormal flexion of extremities) usually indicate diffuse cortical

ACTIONS/INTERVENTIONS

Independent

Monitor vital signs, e.g.:

BP, noting onset of/continuing systolic hypertension and widening pulse pressure; observe for hypotension in multiple trauma patient;

Heart rate/rhythm, noting bradycardia, alternating bradycardia/tachycardia, other dysrhythmias;

Respirations, noting patterns and rhythm, e.g., periods of apnea after hyperventilation, Cheyne Stokes breathing.

Evaluate pupils, noting size, shape, equality, light reactivity.

Assess for changes in vision, e.g., double vision (diplopia) blurred vision, alterations in visual field, depth perception.

Assess position/movement of eyes, noting whether in midposition or deviated to side or downward. Note loss of doll's eyes (oculocephalic reflex).

Note presence/absence of reflexes (e.g., blink, cough, gag, Babinski).

Monitor temperature and regulate environmental temperature as indicated. Limit use of blankets;

RATIONALE

damage. Absence of spontaneous movement on one side of the body indicates damage to the motor tracts in the opposite cerebral hemisphere.

Normally, autoregulation maintains constant cerebral blood flow despite fluctuations in systemic BP. Loss of autoregulation may follow local or diffuse cerebral vascular damage. Elevating systolic BP accompanied by decreasing diastolic BP (widening pulse pressure) is an ominous sign of IICP when accompanied by decreased level of consciousness. Hypovolemia/hypotension (associated with multiple trauma) may also result in cerebral ischemia/damage.

Changes in rate (most often bradycardia) and dysrhythmias may develop, reflecting brainstem pressure/injury in the absence of underlying cardiac disease.

Irregularities can suggest location of cerebral insult/increasing ICP and need for further intervention including possible respiratory support. (Refer to ND: Breathing Pattern, ineffective, high risk for, p 277.)

Pupil reactions are regulated by the oculomotor (III) cranial nerve and are useful in determining if the brainstem is intact. Pupil size/equality is determined by balance between parasympathetic and sympathetic enervation. Response to light reflects combined function of optic (II) and oculomotor (III) cranial nerves.

Visual alterations, which can result from microscopic damage to the brain, have consequent safety concerns and influence choice of interventions.

Position and movement of eyes help localize area of brain involvement. An early sign of increased ICP is impaired abduction of eyes, indicating pressure/injury to the fifth cranial nerve. Loss of doll's eyes indicates deterioration in brainstem function and poor prognosis.

Alterations in reflexes reflect injury at level of midbrain or brainstem and have direct implications for patient safety. Loss of blink reflex suggests damage to the pons and medulla. Absence of cough and gag reflexes reflect damage to medulla. Presence of Babinski reflex indicates injury along pyramidal pathways in the brain.

Fever may reflect damage to hypothalamus. Increased metabolic needs and oxygen consump-

ACTIONS/INTERVENTIONS	RATIONALE
Independent	
administer tepid sponge bath in presence of fever. Wrap extremities in blankets when hypothermia blanket is used.	tion occur (especially with fever and shivering), which can further increase ICP.
Monitor intake and output. Weigh as indicated. Note skin turgor, status of mucous membranes.	Useful indicators of total body water, which is an integral part of tissue perfusion. Cerebral trauma/ischemia can result in diabetes insipidus (DI) or SIADH. Alterations may lead to hypovolemia or vascular engorgement, either of which can negatively affect cerebral pressure.
Maintain head/neck in midline or neutral position, support with small towel rolls and pillows. Avoid placing head on large pillows.	Turning head to one side compresses the jugular veins and inhibits cerebral venous drainage, thereby increasing ICP.
Provide rest periods between care activities and limit duration of procedures.	Continual activity can increase ICP by producing a cumulative stimulant effect.
Decrease extraneous stimuli and provide comfort measures, e.g., back massage, quiet environment, soft voice, gentle touch.	Provides calming effect, reduces adverse physiologic response, and promotes rest to maintain/ lower ICP.
Help patient avoid/limit coughing, vomiting, straining at stool/bearing down when possible.	These activities increase intrathoracic and intra-abdominal pressures, which can increase ICP.
Avoid/limit use of restraints.	Mechanical restraints may enhance fight response, increasing ICP. *Note:* Cautious use may be indicated to prevent injury to patient.
Encourage SO to talk to patient.	Familiar voices of family/SO appear to have a relaxing effect on many comatose patients, which can reduce ICP.
Investigate increasing restlessness, moaning, guarding behaviors.	These nonverbal cues may indicate increasing ICP or reflect presence of pain when patient is unable to verbalize complaints. Unrelieved pain can in turn aggravate/potentiate IICP.
Palpate for bladder distention, maintain patency of urinary drainage if used. Monitor for constipation.	May trigger autonomic responses potentiating elevation of ICP.
Observe for seizure activity and protect patient from injury.	Seizures can occur as a result of cerebral irritation, hypoxia, or IICP, and seizures can further elevate ICP, compounding cerebral damage.
Assess for nuchal rigidity, twitching, increased restlessness, irritability, onset of seizure activity.	Indicative of meningeal irritation, which may occur due to interruption of dura, and/or development of infection during acute or recovery period of brain injury.
Collaborative	
Elevate head of bed 15–45 degrees as tolerated/ indicated.	Promotes venous drainage from head, thereby reducing cerebral congestion and edema/risk of IICP.
Restrict fluid intake as indicated. Administer IV fluids with control device.	Fluid restriction may be needed to reduce cerebral edema; minimize fluctuations in vascular load, BP, and ICP.
Administer supplemental oxygen as indicated.	Reduces hypoxemia, which may increase cerebral vasodilation and blood volume, elevating ICP.

ACTIONS/INTERVENTIONS	RATIONALE
Collaborative	
Monitor ABGs/pulse oximetry.	Determines respiratory sufficiency (presence of hypoxia/acidosis) and indicates therapy needs.
Administer medications as indicated:	
Diuretics, e.g., mannitol (Osmitrol); furosemide (Lasix);	Diuretics may be used in acute phase to draw water from brain cells, reducing cerebral edema and ICP.
Steroids, e.g., dexamethasone (Decadron); methylprednisolone (Medrol);	Decreases inflammation, reducing tissue edema.
Anticonvulsant, e.g., phenytoin (Dilantin);	Drug of choice for treatment and prevention of seizure activity.
Chlorpromazine (Thorazine);	Useful in treating posturing and shivering, which can increase ICP. *Note:* This drug can lower the seizure threshold or precipitate Dilantin toxicity.
Mild analgesics, e.g., codeine;	May be indicated to relieve pain and its negative effect on ICP but should be used with caution to prevent respiratory embarrassment.
Sedatives, e.g., diphenhydramine (Benadryl);	May be used to control restlessness, agitation.
Antipyretics, e.g., acetaminophen (Tylenol).	Reduces/controls fever and its deleterious effect on cerebral metabolism/oxygen needs.
Prepare for surgical intervention, if indicated.	Craniotomy or trephination ("burr" holes) may be done to remove bone fragments, elevate depressed fractures, evacuate hematoma, control hemorrhage, and debride necrotic tissue.

NURSING DIAGNOSIS:	BREATHING PATTERN, INEFFECTIVE, HIGH RISK FOR
Risk factors may include:	Neuromuscular impairment (injury to respiratory center of brain).
	Perception or cognitive impairment.
	Tracheobronchial obstruction.
Possibly evidenced by:	[Not applicable; presence of signs and symptoms establishes an actual diagnosis.]
DESIRED OUTCOMES/ EVALUATION CRITERIA— PATIENT WILL:	Maintain a normal/effective respiratory pattern, free of cyanosis, with ABGs within patient's normal range.

ACTIONS/INTERVENTIONS	RATIONALE
Independent	
Monitor rate, rhythm, depth of respiration. Note breathing irregularities.	Changes may indicate onset of pulmonary complications (common following brain injury) or indicate location/extent of brain involvement. Slow respiration, periods of apnea may indicate need for mechanical ventilation.

ACTIONS/INTERVENTIONS	RATIONALE

Independent

Note competence of gag/swallow reflexes and patient's ability to protect own airway. Insert airway adjunct as indicated.	Ability to mobilize or clear secretions is important to airway maintenance. Loss of swallow or cough reflex may indicate need for artificial airway/intubation. *Note:* Soft nasopharyngeal airways may be preferred to prevent stimulation of the gag reflex by hard oropharyngeal airway, which can lead to excessive coughing and increased ICP.
Elevate head of bed as permitted, position on sides as indicated.	Facilitates lung expansion/ventilation and reduces risk of airway obstruction by tongue.
Encourage deep breathing if patient is conscious.	Prevents/reduces atelectasis.
Suction with extreme caution, no longer than 10–15 seconds. Note character, color, odor of secretions.	Suctioning is usually required if patient is comatose or is immobile and unable to clear own airway. Deep tracheal suctioning should be done with caution, because it can cause or aggravate hypoxia, which produces vasoconstriction, adversely affecting cerebral perfusion.
Auscultate breath sounds, noting areas of hypoventilation and presence of adventitious sounds (crackles, rhonchi, wheezes).	Identifies pulmonary problems such as atelectasis, congestion, airway obstruction, which may jeopardize cerebral oxygenation and/or indicate onset of pulmonary infection (common complication of head injury).
Monitor use of respiratory depressant drugs, e.g., sedatives.	Can increase respiratory embarrassment/complications.

Collaborative

Monitor/graph serial ABGs, pulse oximetry.	Determines respiratory sufficiency, acid-base balance, and therapy needs.
Review chest x-rays.	Reveals ventilatory state and signs of developing complications (e.g., atelectasis, pneumonia).
Administer supplemental oxygen.	Maximizes arterial oxygenation and aids in prevention of hypoxia. If respiratory center is depressed, mechanical ventilation may be required.
Assist with chest physiotherapy when indicated.	Although contraindicated in patient with acute IICP, these measures are often necessary in acute rehabilitation phase to mobilize and clear lung fields and reduce atelectasis/pulmonary complications.

NURSING DIAGNOSIS:	SENSORY-PERCEPTUAL ALTERATION, SPECIFY
May be related to:	Altered sensory reception, transmission and/or integration (neurologic trauma or deficit).
Possibly evidenced by:	Disorientation to time, place, persons.
	Change in usual response to stimuli.
	Motor incoordination, alterations in posture, inability to tell position of body parts (proprioception).

Altered communication patterns.

Visual and auditory distortions.

Poor concentration, altered thought processes/bizarre thinking.

Exaggerated emotional responses, change in behavior pattern.

DESIRED OUTCOMES/ EVALUATION CRITERIA— PATIENT WILL:

Regain/maintain usual level of consciousness and perceptual functioning.

Acknowledge changes in ability and presence of residual involvement.

Demonstrate behaviors/lifestyle changes to compensate for/overcome deficits.

ACTIONS/INTERVENTIONS	RATIONALE
Independent	
Evaluate/continually monitor changes in orientation, ability to speak, mood/affect, sensorium, thought process.	Upper cerebral functions are often the first to be affected by altered circulation, oxygenation. Damage may occur at time of initial injury or develop sometime afterward because of swelling or bleeding. Motor, perceptual, cognitive, and personality changes may develop and persist, with gradual normalization of responses or remain permanently to some degree.
Assess sensory awareness, e.g., response to touch, hot/cold, dull/sharp, and awareness of motion and location of body parts. Note problems with vision, other senses.	Information is essential to patient safety. All sensory systems may be affected with changes involving an increase or decrease in sensitivity or loss of sensation/ability to perceive and respond appropriately to stimuli.
Observe behavioral responses, e.g., hostility, crying, inappropriate affect, agitation, hallucinations. (Refer to ND: Thought Processes, altered, p 280.)	Individual responses may be variable but commonalities, such as emotional lability, lowered frustration level, apathy, and impulsiveness exist during recovery from brain injury. Documentation of behavior provides information needed for development of structured rehabilitation.
Document specific changes in abilities, e.g., focusing/tracking with both eyes, following simple verbal instructions, answering "yes" or "no" to questions, feeding self with dominant hand.	Helps localize areas of cerebral dysfunction and identifies signs of progress toward improved neurologic function.
Eliminate extraneous noise/stimuli as necessary.	Reduces anxiety, exaggerated emotional responses/confusion associated with sensory overload.
Speak in calm, quiet voice. Use short, simple sentences. Maintain eye contact.	Patient may have limited attention span/understanding during acute and recovery stages, and these measures can help patient to attend to communication.

ACTIONS/INTERVENTIONS	RATIONALE

Independent

Ascertain/validate patient's perceptions, provide feedback. Reorient patient frequently to environment, staff, and procedures, especially if vision is impaired.

Assists patient to separate reality from altered perceptions. Cognitive dysfunction and/or visual deficits can potentiate disorientation and anxiety.

Provide meaningful stimulation: verbal (talk to patient); olfactory (e.g., oil of clove, coffee); tactile (touch, hand holding); and auditory (tapes, television, radio, visitors). Avoid physical or emotional isolation of patient.

Carefully selected sensory input may be useful for coma stimulation as well as during cognitive retraining.

Provide structured environment, including therapies, activities. Write out schedule for patient (if appropriate) and refer to regularly.

Promotes consistency and reassurance, reducing anxiety associated with the unknown. Promotes sense of control/cognitive retraining.

Schedule adequate rest/uninterrupted sleep periods.

Reduces fatigue, prevents exhaustion, provides for REM sleep (absence of which can aggravate sensory-perceptual deficits).

Use day/night lighting.

Provides for normal sense of passage of time and sleep/wake pattern.

Allow adequate time for communication and performance of activities.

Reduces frustration associated with altered abilities/delayed response pattern.

Provide patient safety, e.g., padded side rails, assistance with ambulation, protection from hot/sharp objects. Note perceptual deficit on chart and at bedside.

Agitation, impaired judgment, poor balance, and sensory deficits increase risk of patient injury.

Identify alternate ways of dealing with perceptual deficits, e.g., arrange bed, personal articles, food to take advantage of functional vision; describe where affected body parts are located.

Enables patient to progress toward independence, enhancing sense of control, while compensating for neurologic deficits.

Collaborative

Refer to physical, occupational, speech, and cognitive therapists.

Interdisciplinary approach can create an integrated treatment plan based on the individual's unique combination of abilities/disabilities with focus on evaluation and functional improvement in physical, cognitive, and perceptual skills.

NURSING DIAGNOSIS:	THOUGHT PROCESSES, ALTERED
May be related to:	Physiologic changes; psychologic conflicts.
Possibly evidenced by:	Memory deficit/changes in remote, recent, immediate memory.
	Distractibility, altered attention span/concentration.
	Disorientation to time, place, person, circumstances, and events.

	Impaired ability to make decisions, problem-solve, reason, abstract, or conceptualize. Personality changes; inappropriate social behavior.
DESIRED OUTCOMES/ EVALUATION CRITERIA— PATIENT WILL:	Maintain/regain usual mentation and reality orientation. Recognize changes in thinking/behavior. Participate in therapeutic regimen/cognitive retraining.

ACTIONS/INTERVENTIONS

Independent

Assess attention span, distractibility. Note level of anxiety.

Confer with SO to compare past behaviors/preinjury personality with current responses.

Maintain consistency in staff assigned to patient as much as possible.

Present reality concisely and briefly, avoid challenging illogical thinking.

Explain procedures and reinforce explanations given by others. Provide information about disease process in relationship to symptoms.

Review necessity of recurrent neurologic evaluations.

Reduce provocative stimuli, negative criticism, arguments, and confrontations.

Listen with regard to patient's verbalizations in spite of speech pattern/content.

Promote socialization within individual limitations.

RATIONALE

Attention span/ability to attend/concentrate may be severely shortened, which both causes and potentiates anxiety, affecting thought processes.

Recovery from head injury includes a phase of agitation, angry responses, and disordered thought sequences/conversation. Presence of hallucinations or alteration in interpretation of stimuli may have been present independent of current condition, or be part of developing sequelae of brain injury. *Note:* SOs often have difficulty accepting and dealing with patient's aberrant behavior and may require assistance in coping with situation.

Provides patient with feelings of stability and control of situation.

Patient may be totally unaware of injury (amnesic) or of extent of injury, and therefore deny reality of injury. Structured reality orientation can reduce defensive reactions.

Loss of internal structure (changes in memory, reasoning, and ability to conceptualize) as well as fear of the unknown affect processing and retention of information, compounding anxiety, confusion, and disorientation.

Understanding that assessments are done frequently to prevent/limit complications and do not necessarily reflect seriousness of patient's condition may help reduce anxiety.

Reduces risk of triggering fight/flight response. Severely brain-injured patient may become violent or physically/verbally abusive.

Conveys interest and worth to individual, enhancing self-esteem and encouraging continued efforts.

Reinforcement of positive behaviors (e.g., appropriate interaction with others) may be helpful in relearning internal structure.

281

ACTIONS/INTERVENTIONS	RATIONALE

Independent

Encourage SO to provide current news/family happenings, and so on.

Promotes maintenance of contact with usual events, enhancing reality orientation and normalization of thinking.

Instruct in relaxation techniques. Provide diversional activities.

Can help refocus attention and reduce anxiety to manageable levels.

Maintain realistic expectations of patient's ability to control own behavior, comprehend, remember information.

It is important to maintain an expectation of the ability to improve and progress to a higher level of functioning to maintain hope and promote continued work of rehabilitation.

Avoid leaving patient alone when agitated, frightened.

Anxiety can lead to loss of control and escalate to panic. Support may provide calming effect, reducing anxiety and risk of injury.

Implement measures to control emotional outbursts/aggressive behavior if needed; e.g., tell patient to "stop," speak in a calm voice, remove from the situation, provide distraction. May need restraint for brief periods of time.

Patient may need help/external control to protect self or others from harm until internal control is regained. Restraints (physical holding, mechanical, pharmacologic) should be used judiciously to avoid escalating violent, irrational behavior.

Inform patient/SO that intellectual function, behavior, and emotional functioning will gradually improve but that some effects may persist for months or even be permanent.

Most brain-injured patients have problems with concentration and memory and may think more slowly; have difficulty problem solving. Recovery may be complete, or residual effects may remain.

Collaborative

Coordinate/participate in cognitive retraining or rehabilitation program as indicated.

Assists with learning methods to compensate for disruption of cognitive skills and addresses problems in concentration, memory, judgment, sequencing, and problem solving.

Refer to support groups, e.g., Brain Injury Association, social services, VNA, and counseling/therapy as needed.

Additional assistance may be helpful in supporting/sustaining recovery efforts.

NURSING DIAGNOSIS:	**PHYSICAL MOBILITY, IMPAIRED**
May be related to:	Perceptual or cognitive impairment.
	Decreased strength/endurance.
	Restrictive therapies/safety precautions, e.g., bed rest, immobilization.
Possibly evidenced by:	Inability to purposefully move within the physical environment, including bed mobility, transfer, ambulation.
	Impaired coordination, limited range of motion, decreased muscle strength/control.
DESIRED OUTCOMES/ EVALUATION CRITERIA— PATIENT WILL:	Regain/maintain optimal position of function, as evidenced by absence of contractures, footdrop.

Maintain/increase strength and function of affected and/or compensatory body part(s).

Demonstrate techniques/behaviors that enable resumption of activities.

Maintain skin integrity, bladder and bowel function.

ACTIONS/INTERVENTIONS

Independent

Review functional ability and reasons for impairment.

Assess degree of immobility, using a scale to rate dependence (0–4).

Position patient to avoid pressure damage. Turn at regular intervals, and make small position changes between turns.

Maintain functional body alignment, e.g., hips, feet, hands. Monitor for proper placement of devices and/or signs of pressure from devices.

Support head and trunk, arms and shoulders, feet and legs when patient is in wheelchair/recliner. Pad chair seat with foam or water-filled cushion, and assist patient to shift weight at frequent intervals.

Provide/assist with range of motion exercises.

Instruct/assist patient with exercise program and use of mobility aids. Increase activity and participation in self-care as tolerated.

Provide meticulous skin care, massaging with emollients and removing wet linen/clothing, keeping bedding free of wrinkles.

Provide eye care, artificial tears; patch eyes as indicated.

RATIONALE

Identifies probable functional impairments and influences choice of interventions.

The patient may be completely independent (0) or require minimal assistance/equipment (1); moderate assistance/supervision/teaching (2); extensive assistance/equipment, and devices (3); or be completely dependent on caregivers (4). Persons in all categories are at risk for injury, but those in categories 2–4 are at greatest risk for hazards associated with immobility.

Regular turning more normally distributes body weight and promotes circulation to all areas. If paralysis or limited cognition is present, patient should be repositioned frequently and positioned on affected side for only brief periods.

Use of high-top tennis shoes, "space boots," and T-bar sheepskin devices can help prevent footdrop. Handsplints are variable and designed to prevent hand deformities and promote optimal function. Use of pillows, bedrolls, and sandbags can help prevent abnormal hip rotation.

Maintains comfortable, safe, and functional posture and prevents/reduces risk of coccyx skin breakdown.

Maintains mobility and function of joints/functional alignment of extremities and reduces venous stasis.

Lengthy convalescence often follows brain injury, and physical reconditioning is an essential part of the program. Involving patient in planning and performing activities is important to promote patient cooperation/sustain program.

Promotes circulation and skin elasticity and reduces risk of skin excoriation.

Protects delicate tissues from drying. Patient may require eye patches during sleep to protect eyes from trauma if unable to keep eyes closed.

ACTIONS/INTERVENTIONS	RATIONALE

Independent

Monitor urinary output. Note color and odor of urine. Assist with bladder retraining when appropriate.

Indwelling catheter used during the acute phase of injury may be needed for an extended period of time before bladder retraining is possible. Once the catheter is removed, several methods of continence control may be tried, e.g., intermittent catheterization (for residual and complete emptying); external catheter; planned intervals on commode; incontinence pads.

Provide fluids within individual tolerance (e.g., neurologic and cardiac), including cranberry juice, as indicated.

Once past the acute phase of head injury and if patient has no other contraindicating factors, forcing fluids will decrease risk of urinary tract infections/stone formation as well as provide other positive effects such as normal stool consistency and optimal skin turgor.

Monitor bowel elimination and provide for/assist with a regular bowel routine. Check for impacted stool; use digital stimulation as indicated. Sit patient upright on commode or stool at regular intervals. Add fiber/bulk/fruit juice to diet as appropriate.

A regular bowel routine requires simple but diligent measures to prevent complications. Stimulation of the internal rectal sphincter will stimulate bowel to empty automatically if stool is soft enough to do so. Upright position aids evacuation.

Inspect for localized tenderness, redness, skin warmth, muscle tension, and/or ropy veins in calves of legs. Observe for sudden dyspnea, tachypnea, fever, respiratory distress, chest pain.

Patient is at risk for development of DVT and PE (especially after trauma), requiring prompt medical evaluation/intervention to prevent serious complications.

Provide air/water mattress, kinetic therapy as appropriate.

Equalizes tissue pressure, enhances circulation, and helps reduce venous stasis to decrease risk of tissue injury.

NURSING DIAGNOSIS:	INFECTION, HIGH RISK FOR
Risk factors may include:	Traumatized tissues, broken skin, invasive procedures.
	Decreased ciliary action, stasis of body fluids.
	Nutritional deficits.
	Suppressed inflammatory response (steroid use).
	Altered integrity of closed system (CSF leak).
Possibly evidenced by:	[Not applicable; presence of signs and symptoms establishes an actual diagnosis.]
DESIRED OUTCOMES/ EVALUATION CRITERIA— PATIENT WILL:	Maintain normothermia, free of signs of infection.
	Achieve timely wound healing when present.

ACTIONS/INTERVENTIONS	RATIONALE
Independent	
Provide meticulous/aseptic care, maintain good handwashing techniques.	First-line defense against nosocomial infections.
Observe areas of impaired skin integrity (e.g., wounds, suture lines, invasive line insertion sites), noting drainage characteristics and presence of inflammation.	Early identification of developing infection permits prompt intervention and prevention of further complications.
Monitor temperature routinely. Note presence of chills, diaphoresis, changes in mentation.	May indicate developing sepsis requiring further evaluation/intervention.
Encourage deep breathing, aggressive pulmonary toilet. Observe sputum characteristics.	Enhances mobilization and clearing of pulmonary secretions to reduce risk of pneumonia, atelectasis. *Note:* Postural drainage should be used with caution if risk of IICP exists.
Provide perineal care. Maintain integrity of closed urinary drainage system if used. Encourage adequate fluid intake.	Reduces potential for bacterial growth/ascending infection.
Observe color/clarity of urine. Note presence of foul odor.	Indicators of developing urinary tract infection requiring prompt intervention.
Screen/restrict access of visitors or caregivers with upper respiratory infections.	Reduces exposure of "compromised host."
Collaborative	
Administer antibiotics as indicated.	Prophylactic therapy may be used in the presence of trauma, CSF leak, or after surgical procedures to reduce risk of nosocomial infections.
Obtain specimens as indicated.	Culture/sensitivity, Gram stain may be done to verify presence of infection and identify causative organism and appropriate treatment choices.

NURSING DIAGNOSIS:	NUTRITION, ALTERED, LESS THAN BODY REQUIREMENTS, HIGH RISK FOR
Risk factors may include:	Altered ability to ingest nutrients (decreased level of consciousness). Weakness of muscles required for chewing, swallowing. Hypermetabolic state.
Possibly evidenced by:	[Not applicable; presence of signs and symptoms establishes an actual diagnosis.]
DESIRED OUTCOMES/ EVALUATION CRITERIA— PATIENT WILL:	Demonstrate maintenance of/progressive weight gain toward goal. Experience no signs of malnutrition, with laboratory values within normal range.

ACTIONS/INTERVENTIONS	RATIONALE

Independent

Assess ability to chew, swallow, cough, handle secretions.	These factors determine choice of feeding as patient must be protected from aspiration.
Auscultate bowel sounds, noting decreased/absent or hyperactive sounds.	GI functioning is usually preserved in brain-injured patients, so bowel sounds help in determining response to feeding or development of complications, e.g., ileus.
Weigh as indicated.	Evaluates effectiveness or need for changes in nutritional therapy.
Provide for feeding safety, e.g., elevate head of bed while eating or during tube feeding.	Reduces risk of regurgitation and/or aspiration.
Divide feedings into small amounts and give frequently.	Enhances digestion and patient's tolerance of nutrients and can improve patient cooperation in eating.
Promote pleasant, relaxing environment, including socialization during meals. Encourage SO to bring in food that patient enjoys.	Although the recovering patient may require assistance with feeding and/or use of assistive devices, meal time socialization with SO or friends can improve intake and normalize the life function of eating.
Check stools, gastric aspirant, vomitus for blood.	Acute/subacute bleeding may occur (Cushing's ulcer) requiring intervention and alternate method of providing nutrition.

Collaborative

Consult with dietitian/nutritional support team.	Effective resource for identifying caloric/nutrient needs dependent on age, body size, desired weight, concurrent conditions (trauma, cardiac/metabolic problems).
Monitor laboratory studies, e.g., serum albumin, transferrin, amino acid profile, iron, BUN, nitrogen balance studies, glucose, AST/ALT, electrolytes.	Identifies nutritional deficiencies, organ function, and response to nutritional therapy.
Administer feedings by appropriate means, e.g., tube feeding, oral feedings with soft foods and thick liquids.	Choice of route is dependent on patient needs/capabilities. Tube feedings (nasogastric, gastric) may be required initially. If the patient is able to swallow, soft foods or semiliquid foods may be more easily managed without aspiration.
Involve speech/occupational/physical therapists when mechanical problem exists, e.g., impaired swallow reflexes, wired jaws, contractures of hands, paralysis.	Individual strategies/devices may be needed to improve ability to eat.

NURSING DIAGNOSIS	FAMILY PROCESS, ALTERED
May be related to:	Situational transition and crisis.
	Uncertainty about outcomes/expectations.

Possibly evidenced by:	Difficulty adapting to change or dealing with traumatic experience constructively.
	Family not meeting needs of its members.
	Difficulty accepting or receiving help appropriately.
	Inability to express or to accept feelings of members.
DESIRED OUTCOMES/ EVALUATION CRITERIA— PATIENT WILL:	Begin to express feelings freely and appropriately.
	Identify internal and external resources to deal with the situation.
	Direct energies in a purposeful manner to plan for resolution of crisis.
	Encourage and allow injured member to progress toward independence.

ACTIONS/INTERVENTIONS	RATIONALE
Independent	
Note components of family unit, availability/involvement of support systems.	Defines family resources and identifies areas of need.
Encourage expression of concerns about seriousness of condition, possibility of death, or incapacity.	Verbalization of fears gets concerns out in the open and can decrease anxiety and enhance coping with reality.
Listen for expressions of helplessness/hopelessness	Joy of survival of victim is replaced by grief/anger at "loss" and necessity of dealing with "new person that family does not know and may not even like." Prolongation of these feelings may result in depression.
Encourage expression of/acknowledge feelings. Do not deny or reassure patient/SO that everything will be all right.	Because it is not possible to predict the outcome, it is more helpful to assist the person to deal with feelings about what is happening instead of giving false reassurance.
Reinforce previous explanations about extent of injury, treatment plan, and prognosis. Provide accurate information at current level of understanding/ability to accept.	Patient/SO are unable to absorb/recall all information, and blocking can occur because of emotional trauma. As time goes by, reinforcement of information can help reduce misconceptions, fear about the unknown/future expectations.
Stress importance of continuous open dialogue between family members.	Provides opportunity to get feelings out in the open. Recognition and awareness promotes resolution of guilt, anger.
Evaluate/discuss family goals and expectations.	Family may believe that if patient is going to live, rehabilitation will bring about a cure. Despite accurate information, expectations may be unrealistic. Also, patient's early recovery may be rapid, then plateau, resulting in disappointment/frustration.

ACTIONS/INTERVENTIONS	RATIONALE
Independent	
Identify individual roles and anticipated/perceived changes.	Responsibilities/roles may have to be partially or completely assumed by others, which can further complicate family coping.
Assess energy direction, e.g., whether efforts at resolution/problem solving are purposeful or scattered.	May need assistance to focus energies in an effective way/enhance coping.
Identify and encourage use of previously successful coping behaviors.	Focuses on strengths and reaffirms individual's ability to deal with current crisis.
Demonstrate and encourage use of stress management skills, e.g., relaxation techniques, breathing exercises, visualization.	Helps redirect attention toward revitalizing self to enhance coping ability.
Help family recognize needs of all members.	Attention may be so focused on injured member that other members feel isolated/abandoned, which can compromise family growth and unity.
Support family grieving for "loss" of member. Acknowledge normality of wide range of feelings and ongoing nature of process.	Although grief may never be fully resolved and family may vacillate among various stages, understanding that this is typical may help members accept/cope with the situation.
Collaborative	
Include family in rehabilitation team meetings and care planning/placement decisions.	Facilitates communication, enables family to be an integral part of the rehabilitation, and provides sense of control.
Identify community resources, e.g., VNA, homemaker service, day care facility, legal/financial counselor.	Provides assistance with problems that may arise because of altered role function.
Refer to family therapy, support groups.	Cognitive/personality changes are usually very difficult for family to deal with. Decreased impulse control, emotional lability, inappropriate sexual or aggressive/violent behavior can disrupt family and result in abandonment/divorce, and so on. Trained therapists and peer role models may assist family to deal with feelings/reality of situation and provide support for decisions that are made.

NURSING DIAGNOSIS:	**KNOWLEDGE DEFICIT [LEARNING NEED] REGARDING CONDITION AND TREATMENT NEEDS**
May be related to:	Lack of exposure, unfamiliarity with information/resources.
	Lack of recall/cognitive limitation.
Possibly evidenced by:	Request for information, statement of misconception.
	Inaccurate follow-through of instructions.

DESIRED OUTCOMES/ EVALUATION CRITERIA— PATIENT WILL:	Participate in learning process.
	Verbalize understanding of condition, treatment regimen, potential complications.
	Initiate necessary lifestyle changes and/or involvement in rehabilitation program.
	Correctly perform necessary procedures.

ACTIONS/INTERVENTIONS	RATIONALE
Independent	
Evaluate capabilities and readiness to learn of both patient and SO.	Permits presentation of material based on individual needs. *Note:* Patient may not be emotionally/ mentally capable of assimilating information.
Review information regarding injury process and aftereffects.	Aids in establishing realistic expectations and promotes understanding of current situation and needs.
Review/reinforce current therapeutic regimen. Identify ways of continuing program after discharge.	Recommended activities, limitations, medication/ therapy needs have been established on the basis of a coordinated interdisciplinary approach, and follow-through is essential to progression of recovery/prevention of complications.
Discuss plans for meeting self-care needs.	Varying levels of assistance may be required/need to be planned based on individual situation.
Provide written instructions and schedules for activity, medication, important facts.	Provides visual reinforcement and reference source after discharge.
Identify signs/symptoms of individual risks, e.g., delayed CSF leak, posttraumatic seizures.	Recognizing developing problems provides opportunity for prompt evaluation and intervention to prevent serious complications.
Discuss with patient/SO development of symptoms, such as reexperiencing traumatic event (flashbacks, intrusive thoughts, repetitive dreams/ nightmares); psychic/emotional numbness; changes in lifestyle, including adoption of self-destructive behaviors.	May indicate occurrence/exacerbation of posttrauma response, which can occur months to years after injury, requiring further evaluation and supportive interventions.
Identify community resources, e.g., head injury support groups, social services, rehabilitation facilities, outpatient programs, VNA.	May be needed to provide assistance with physical care, home management, adjustment to lifestyle changes, as well as emotional and financial concerns.
Refer/reinforce importance of follow-up care by rehabilitation team, e.g., physical/occupational/ speech/vocational therapists, cognitive retrainers.	Diligent work (often for several years with these providers) may eventually overcome residual neurologic deficits and enable patient to resume desired/productive lifestyle.

Cerebrovascular Accident/Stroke _____

Cerebrovascular disease refers to any functional or structural abnormality of the brain caused by a pathologic condition of the cerebral vessels or of the entire cerebral vascular system. This pathology causes either hemorrhage from a tear in the vessel wall or impairs the cerebral circulation by a partial or complete occlusion of the vessel lumen with transient or permanent effects.

RELATED CONCERNS:

Craniocerebral Trauma, p 271
Psychosocial Aspects of Acute Care, p 899
Seizure Disorders, p 261
Total Nutritional Support, p 1039

PATIENT ASSESSMENT DATA BASE

Data collected will be determined by location, severity, and duration of pathology.

ACTIVITY/REST

May report: Difficulties with activity due to weakness, loss of sensation, or paralysis (hemiplegia).

Tiring easily; difficulty resting (pain or muscle twitchings).

May exhibit: Altered muscle tone (flaccid or spastic); paralysis (hemiplegia); generalized weakness.

Visual disturbances.

Altered level of consciousness.

CIRCULATORY

May report: History of postural hypotension, cardiac disease (e.g., MI, rheumatic/valvular heart disease, CHF, bacterial endocarditis), polycythemia.

May exhibit: Arterial hypertension (frequently found unless the CVA is due to embolism or vascular malformation).

Pulse: Rate may vary (preexisting heart conditions, medications, effect of stroke on vasomotor center).

Dysrhythmias, ECG changes.

Bruit in carotid, femoral, and iliac arteries or abdominal aorta.

EGO INTEGRITY

May report: Feelings of helplessness, hopelessness.

May exhibit: Emotional lability and inappropriate response to anger, sadness, happiness.

Difficulty expressing self.

ELIMINATION

May exhibit: Change in voiding patterns, e.g., incontinence, anuria.

Distended abdomen (overdistended bladder); absent bowel sounds (paralytic ileus).

FOOD/FLUID

May report:
Lack of appetite.

Nausea/vomiting during acute event (increased IICP).

Loss of sensation in tongue, cheek, and throat; dysphagia.

History of diabetes, elevated serum lipids.

May exhibit:
Mastication/swallowing problems (palatal and pharyngeal reflex involvement).

Obesity (risk factor).

NEUROSENSORY

May report:
Dizziness/syncope (before CVA/transient during TIA).

Headaches: Severe with intracerebral or subarachnoid hemorrhage.

Tingling/numbness/weakness (commonly reported during TIAs, found in varying degrees in other types of stroke); involved side seems "dead."

Visual deficits, e.g., blurred vision, partial loss of vision (monocular blindness), double vision (diplopia), or other disturbances in visual fields.

Touch: Sensory loss on contralateral side (opposite side) in extremities and sometimes in ipsilateral side (same side) of face.

Disturbance in senses of taste, smell.

May exhibit:
Mental status/LOC: Coma usually present in the initial stages of hemorrhagic disturbances; consciousness is usually preserved when the etiology is thrombotic in nature; altered behavior (e.g., lethargy, apathy, combativeness); altered cognitive function (e.g., memory, problem-solving, sequencing).

Extremities: Weakness/paralysis (contralateral with all kinds of stroke), unequal hand grasp; diminished deep tendon reflexes (contralateral).

Facial paralysis or paresis (ipsilateral).

Aphasia: Defect or loss of language function may be expressive (difficulty producing speech); receptive (difficulty comprehending speech); or global (combination of the two).

Loss of ability to recognize or appreciate import of visual, auditory, tactile stimuli (agnosia), e.g., altered body image awareness, neglect or denial of contralateral side of body, disturbances in perception.

Loss of ability to execute purposeful motor acts despite physical ability and willingness to do so (apraxia).

Pupil size/reaction: Inequality; dilated and fixed pupil on the ipsilateral side (hemorrhage/herniation).

Nuchal rigidity (common in hemorrhagic etiology). Seizures (common in hemorrhagic etiology).

PAIN/COMFORT

May report:
Headache of varying intensity (carotid artery involvement).

May exhibit:
Guarding/distraction behaviors, restlessness, muscle/facial tension.

RESPIRATION

May report:
Smoking (risk factor).

May exhibit:
Inability to swallow/cough/protect airway.

Labored and/or irregular respirations.

Noisy respirations/rhonchi (aspiration of secretions).

SAFETY

May exhibit: Motor/sensory: Problems with vision.

Changes in perception of body spatial orientation (right CVA).

Difficulty seeing objects on left side (RCVA).

Being unaware of affected side.

Inability to recognize familiar objects, colors, words, faces.

Diminished response to heat and cold/altered body temperature regulation.

Swallowing difficulty, inability to meet own nutritional needs.

Impaired judgment, little concern for safety, impatience/lack of insight (RCVA).

SOCIAL INTERACTION

May exhibit: Speech problems, inability to communicate.

TEACHING/LEARNING

May report: Family history of hypertension, strokes; African heritage (risk factor).

Use of oral contraceptives, alcohol abuse (risk factor).

Discharge Plan Considerations: **DRG projected mean length of stay: 7.3 days.**

May require medication regimen/therapeutic treatments.

Assistance with transportation, shopping, food preparation, self-care and home-maker/maintenance tasks.

Changes in physical layout of home; transition placement before return to home setting.

DIAGNOSTIC STUDIES

Cerebral angiography: Helps determine specific cause of stroke, e.g., hemorrhage or obstructed artery, pinpoints site of occlusion or rupture.

CT scan: Demonstrates edema, hematomas, ischemia, and infarctions. *Note:* May not immediately reveal all changes.

Lumbar puncture: Normal pressure and usually clear in cerebral thrombosis, embolism, and TIA. Pressure elevation and grossly bloody fluid suggests subarachnoid and intracerebral hemorrhage. Total protein level may be elevated in cases of thrombosis due to inflammatory process.

MRI: Shows areas of infarction, hemorrhage, arteriovenous malformations.

Doppler ultrasonography: Identifies arteriovenous disease, e.g., problems with carotid system (blood flow/presence of atherosclerotic plaques).

EEG: Identifies problems based on brain waves and may demonstrate specific areas of lesions.

X-rays (skull): May show shift of pineal gland to the opposite side from an expanding mass; calcifications of the internal carotid may be visible in cerebral thrombosis; partial calcification of walls of an aneurysm may be noted in subarachnoid hemorrhage.

NURSING PRIORITIES

1. Promote adequate cerebral perfusion and oxygenation.
2. Prevent/minimize complications and permanent disabilities.
3. Assist patient to gain independence in ADLs.

4. Support coping process and integration of changes into self-concept.
5. Provide information about disease process/prognosis and treatment/rehabilitation needs.

DISCHARGE GOALS

1. Cerebral function improved, neurologic deficits resolving/stabilized.
2. Complications prevented or minimized.
3. ADL needs met by self or with assistance of other(s).
4. Coping with situation in positive manner, planning for the future.
5. Disease process/prognosis, and therapeutic regimen understood.

NURSING DIAGNOSIS:	TISSUE PERFUSION, ALTERED, CEREBRAL
May be related to:	Interruption of blood flow: occlusive disorder, hemorrhage; cerebral vasospasm, cerebral edema.
Possibly evidenced by:	Altered level of consciousness; memory loss.
	Changes in motor/sensory responses; restlessness.
	Sensory, language, intellectual, and emotional deficits.
	Changes in vital signs.
DESIRED OUTCOMES/ EVALUATION CRITERIA— PATIENT WILL:	Maintain usual/improved level of consciousness, cognition, and motor/sensory function.
	Demonstrate stable vital signs and absence of signs of increased ICP.
	Displays no further deterioration/recurrence of deficits.

ACTIONS/INTERVENTIONS	RATIONALE
Independent	
Determine factors related to individual situation/cause for coma/decreased cerebral perfusion, and potential for increased ICP.	Influences choice of interventions. Deterioration in neurologic signs/symptoms or failure to improve after initial insult may require surgical intervention and/or that the patient be transferred to critical care area for monitoring of ICP.
Monitor/document neurologic status frequently and compare with baseline. (Refer to CP: Craniocerebral Trauma, ND: Tissue Perfusion, altered, cerebral, p. 273, for complete neurologic evaluation.)	Assesses trends in LOC and potential for increased ICP and is useful in determining location, extent, and progression/resolution of CNS damage. May also reveal presence of TIA, which may warn of impending thrombotic CVA.
Monitor vital signs, i.e. note: Hypertension/hypotension, compare BP readings in both arms;	Variations may occur because of cerebral pressure/injury in vasomotor area of the brain. Hypertension or postural hypotension may have been a precipitating factor. Hypotension may occur because of shock (circulatory collapse). Increased ICP may occur (tissue edema, clot formation). Subclavian artery blockage may be revealed by difference in pressure readings between arms.

293

ACTIONS/INTERVENTIONS	RATIONALE
Independent	
Heart rate and rhythm; auscultate for murmurs;	Changes in rate, especially bradycardia, can occur because of the brain damage. Dysrhythmias and murmurs may reflect cardiac disease, which may have precipitated CVA (e.g., stroke after MI or from valve dysfunction).
Respiration, noting patterns and rhythm, e.g., periods of apnea after hyperventilation, Cheyne-Stokes breathing.	Irregularities can suggest location of cerebral insult/increasing ICP and need for further intervention, including possible respiratory support. (Refer to CP: Craniocerebral Trauma, ND: Breathing Pattern, ineffective, high risk for, p 277.)
Evaluate pupils, noting size, shape, equality, light reactivity.	Pupil reactions are regulated by the oculomotor (III) cranial nerve and are useful in determining whether the brainstem is intact. Pupil size/equality is determined by balance between parasympathetic and sympathetic enervation. Response to light reflects combined function of the optic (II) and oculomotor (III) cranial nerves.
Document changes in vision, e.g., reports of blurred vision, alterations in visual field/depth perception.	Specific visual alterations reflect area of brain involved, indicate safety concerns, and influence choice of interventions.
Assess higher functions, including speech, if patient is alert. (Refer to ND: Communication, impaired: verbal, p 297.)	Changes in cognition and speech content are an indicator of location/degree of cerebral involvement and may indicate deterioration/increased ICP.
Position with head slightly elevated and in neutral position.	Reduces arterial pressure by promoting venous drainage and may improve cerebral circulation/perfusion.
Maintain bed rest; provide quiet environment; restrict visitors/activities as indicated. Provide rest periods between care activities, limit duration of procedures.	Continual stimulation/activity can increase ICP. Absolute rest and quiet may be needed to prevent rebleeding in the case of hemorrhage.
Prevent straining at stool, holding breath.	Valsalva maneuver increases ICP and potentiates risk of rebleeding.
Assess for nuchal rigidity, twitching, increased restlessness, irritability, onset of seizure activity.	Indicative of meningeal irritation, especially in hemorrhagic disorders. Seizures may reflect increased ICP/cerebral injury, requiring further evaluation and intervention.
Collaborative	
Administer supplemental oxygen as indicated.	Reduces hypoxemia, which can cause cerebral vasodilation and increase pressure/edema formation.
Administer medications as indicated:	
Anticoagulants, e.g., warfarin sodium (Coumadin); heparin, antiplatelet agents (ASA); dipyridamole (Persantine);	May be used to improve cerebral blood flow and prevent further clotting when embolus/thrombosis is the problem. Contraindicated in hypertensive patients because of increased risk of hemorrhage.

ACTIONS/INTERVENTIONS	RATIONALE
Collaborative	
Antifibrolytics, e.g., aminocaproic acid (Amicar);	Used with caution in hemorrhagic disorder to prevent lysis of formed clots and subsequent rebleeding.
Antihypertensives;	Preexisting/chronic hypertension requires cautious treatment, because aggressive management increases the risk of extension of tissue damage. Transient hypertension often occurs during acute stroke and resolves often without therapeutic intervention.
Peripheral vasodilators, e.g., cyclandelate (Cyclospasmol); papaverine (Pavabid/Vasospan); isoxsuprine (Vasodilan);	Used to improve collateral circulation or decrease vasospasm.
Steroids, dexamethasone (Decadron);	Use is controversial in control of cerebral edema.
Phenytoin (Dilantin), phenobarbital;	May be used to control seizures and/or for sedative action. *Note:* Phenobarbital enhances action of antiepileptics.
Stool softeners.	Prevents straining during bowel movement and corresponding increase of ICP.
Prepare for surgery, endarterectomy, microvascular bypass.	May be necessary to resolve situation.
Monitor laboratory studies as indicated, e.g., prothrombin/PTT time, Dilantin level.	Provides information about drug effectiveness/therapeutic level.

NURSING DIAGNOSIS:	**PHYSICAL MOBILITY, IMPAIRED**
May be related to:	Neuromuscular involvement: weakness, paresthesia; flaccid/hypotonic paralysis (initially); spastic paralysis.
	Perceptual/cognitive impairment.
Possibly evidenced by:	Inability to purposefully move within the physical environment; impaired coordination; limited range of motion; decreased muscle strength/control.
DESIRED OUTCOMES/ EVALUATION CRITERIA— PATIENT WILL:	Maintain optimal position of function as evidenced by absence of contractures, footdrop.
	Maintain/increase strength and function of affected or compensatory body part.
	Demonstrate techniques/behaviors that enable resumption of activities.
	Maintain skin integrity.

295

ACTIONS/INTERVENTIONS	RATIONALE
Independent	
Assess functional ability/extent of impairment initially and on a regular basis. Classify according to 0–4 scale. (Refer to CP: Craniocerebral Trauma, ND: Physical Mobility, impaired, p 282.)	Identifies strengths/deficiencies and may provide information regarding recovery. Assists in choice of interventions, because different techniques are used for flaccid and spastic paralysis.
Change positions at least every 2 hours (supine, sidelying) and possibly more often if placed on affected side.	Reduces risk of tissue ischemia/injury. Affected side has poorer circulation and reduced sensation and is more predisposed to skin breakdown/decubitus.
Position in prone position once or twice a day if patient can tolerate.	Helps maintain functional hip extension; however, may increase anxiety, especially about ability to breathe.
Begin active/passive range of motion to all extremities (including splinted) on admission. Encourage exercises such as quadriceps/gluteal exercise, squeezing rubber ball, extension of fingers and legs/feet.	Minimizes muscle atrophy, promotes circulation, helps prevent contractures. Reduces risk of hypercalciuria and osteoporosis if underlying problem is hemorrhage. *Note:* Excessive/imprudent stimulation can predispose to rebleeding.
Prop extremities in functional position, use footboard during the period of flaccid paralysis. Maintain neutral position of head.	Prevents contractures/footdrop and facilitates use when/if function returns. Flaccid paralysis may interfere with ability to support head, whereas spastic paralysis may lead to deviation of head to one side.
Use arm sling when patient in upright position, as indicated.	During flaccid paralysis, use of sling may reduce risk of shoulder subluxation and shoulder-hand syndrome.
Evaluate use of/need for positional aids and/or splints during spastic paralysis:	Flexion contractures occur because flexor muscles are stronger than extensors.
Place pillow under axilla to abduct arm;	Prevents adduction of shoulder and flexion of elbow.
Elevate arm and hand;	Promotes venous return and helps prevent edema formation.
Place hard hand-rolls in the palm with fingers and thumb opposed;	Hard cones decrease the stimulation of finger flexion, maintaining finger and thumb in a functional position.
Place knee and hip in extended position;	Maintains functional position.
Maintain leg in neutral position with a trochanter roll;	Prevents external hip rotation.
Discontinue use of footboard, when appropriate.	Continued use (after change from flaccid to spastic paralysis) can cause excessive pressure on the ball of the foot, enhance spasticity, and actually increase plantar flexion.
Assist to develop sitting balance (e.g., raise head of bed; assist to sit on edge of bed, having patient use the strong arm to support body weight and strong leg to move affected leg; increase sitting time) and standing balance (e.g., put flat walking shoes on patient; support patient's lower back with	Aids in retraining neuronal pathways, enhancing proprioception and motor response.

ACTIONS/INTERVENTIONS	RATIONALE

Independent

hands while positioning own knees outside patient's knees; assist in using parallel bars/walkers).

Observe affected side for color, edema, or other signs of compromised circulation.

Edematous tissue is more easily traumatized and heals more slowly.

Inspect skin, particularly over bony prominences, regularly. Gently massage any reddened areas and provide aids such as sheepskin pads as necessary.

Pressure points over bony prominences are most at risk for decreased perfusion/ischemia. Circulatory stimulation and padding helps prevent skin breakdown and decubitus development.

Get up in chair as soon as vital signs are stable except following cerebral hemorrhage.

Helps stabilize BP (restores vasomotor tone), promotes maintenance of extremities in a functional position and emptying of bladder/kidneys, reducing risk of urinary stones and infections from stasis.

Pad chair seat with foam or waterfilled cushion and assist patient to shift weight at frequent intervals.

Prevents/reduces coccyx pressure/skin breakdown.

Set goals with patient/SO for participation in activities/exercise and position changes.

Promotes sense of expectation of progress/improvement and provides some sense of control/independence.

Encourage patient to assist with movement and exercises using unaffected extremity to support/move weaker side.

May respond as if affected side is no longer part of body and need encouragement and active training to "reincorporate" it as a part of own body.

Collaborative

Provide egg crate mattress, water bed, flotation device, or specialized beds (e.g., kinetic) as indicated.

Promotes even weight distribution decreasing pressure on bony points and helping to prevent skin breakdown/decubitus formation. Specialized beds help with positioning the extremely obese patient, enhances circulation, and reduces venous stasis to decrease risk of tissue injury and complications such as orthostatic pneumonia.

Consult with physical therapist regarding active, resistive exercises and patient ambulation.

Individualized program can be developed to meet particular needs/deal with deficits in balance, coordination, strength.

Assist with electrical stimulation, e.g., TENS unit as indicated.

May assist with muscle restrengthening and increase voluntary muscle control.

Administer muscle relaxants, antispasmodics as indicated, e.g., baclofen, dantrolene.

May be required to relieve spasticity in affected extremities.

NURSING DIAGNOSIS:	COMMUNICATION, IMPAIRED, VERBAL, AND/OR [WRITTEN]
May be related to:	Impaired cerebral circulation; neuromuscular impairment, loss of facial/oral muscle tone/control; generalized weakness/fatigue.
Possibly evidenced by:	Impaired articulation; does not/cannot speak (dysarthria).

297

	Inability to modulate speech, find and name words, identify objects; inability to comprehend written/spoken language.
	Inability to produce written communication.
DESIRED OUTCOMES/ EVALUATION CRITERIA— PATIENT WILL:	Indicate an understanding of the communication problems.
	Establish method of communication in which needs can be expressed.
	Use resources appropriately.

ACTIONS/INTERVENTIONS	RATIONALE
Independent	
Assess type/degree of dysfunction: e.g., patient does not seem to understand words or has trouble speaking or making self understood;	Helps determine area and degree of brain involvement and difficulty patient has with any or all steps of the communication process. Patient may have trouble understanding spoken words (receptive aphasia/damage to Wernicke's speech area); speaking words correctly (expressive aphasia/ damage to Broca's speech areas); or experience damage to both areas.
Differentiate aphasia from dysarthria;	Choice of interventions is dependent on type of impairment. Aphasia is a defect in using and interpreting symbols of language and may involve sensory and/or motor components, e.g., inability to comprehend written/spoken words or write, make signs, speak. A dysarthric person can understand, read, and write language but has difficulty forming/pronouncing words due to weakness and paralysis of oral musculature.
Listen for errors in conversation and provide feedback;	Patient may lose ability to monitor verbal output and be unaware that communication is not sensible. Feedback helps patient realize why caregivers are not understanding/responding appropriately and provides opportunity to clarify content/meaning.
Ask patient to follow simple commands (e.g., "Shut your eyes," "Point to the door"), repeat simple words/sentences;	Tests for receptive aphasia.
Point to objects and ask patient to name them;	Tests for expressive aphasia; e.g., patient may recognize item but not be able to name it.
Have patient produce simple sounds, e.g., "Sh," "Cat";	Identifies dysarthria as motor components of speech (tongue, lip movement, breath control) can affect articulation and may/may not be accompanied by expressive aphasia.
Ask the patient to write name and/or a short sentence. If unable to write, have patient read a short sentence.	Tests for writing disability (agraphia) and deficits in reading comprehension (alexia), which are also part of receptive and expressive aphasia.

ACTIONS/INTERVENTIONS	RATIONALE
Independent	
Post notice at nurses' station and patient's room about speech impairment. Provide special call bell if necessary.	Allays anxiety related to inability to communicate and fear that needs will not be met promptly. Call bell that is activated by minimal pressure is useful when patient is unable to use regular call system.
Provide alternative methods of communication, e.g., writing or felt board, pictures. Provide visual clues (gestures, pictures, "needs" list, demonstration).	Provides for communication of needs/desires based on individual situation/underlying deficit.
Anticipate and provide for patient's needs.	Helpful in decreasing frustration when dependent on others and unable to communicate desires.
Talk directly to patient, speaking slowly and distinctly. Use yes/no questions to begin with, progressing in complexity as patient responds.	Reduces confusion/anxiety at having to process and respond to large amount of information at one time. As retraining progresses, advancing complexity of communication stimulates memory and further enhances word/idea association.
Speak in normal tones and avoid talking too fast. Give patient ample time to respond. Talk without pressing for a response.	Patient is not necessarily hearing impaired, and raising voice may anger patient/cause irritation. Forcing responses can result in frustration and may cause patient to resort to "automatic" speech, e.g., garbled speech, obscenities.
Encourage SO/visitors to persist in efforts to communicate with patient, e.g., reading mail, discussing family happenings.	Reduces patient's social isolation and promotes establishment of effective communication.
Discuss familiar topics, e.g., job, family, hobbies.	Promotes meaningful conversation and provides opportunity to practice skills.
Respect patient's preinjury capabilities; avoid "speaking down" to patient or making patronizing remarks.	Enables patient to feel esteemed, because intellectual abilities often remain intact.
Collaborative	
Consult with/refer to speech therapist.	Assesses individual verbal capabilities and sensory, motor, and cognitive functioning to identify deficits/therapy needs.

NURSING DIAGNOSIS:	SENSORY-PERCEPTUAL ALTERATION
May be related to:	Altered sensory reception, transmission, integration (neurologic trauma or deficit).
	Psychologic stress (narrowed perceptual fields caused by anxiety).
Possibly evidenced by:	Disorientation to time, place, persons.
	Change in behavior pattern/usual response to stimuli; exaggerated emotional responses.
	Poor concentration, altered thought processes/bizarre thinking.

	Reported/measured change in *sensory acuity:* hypoparesthesia; altered *sense of taste/smell.*
	Inability to tell position of body parts (proprioception).
	Inability to recognize/attach meaning to objects (visual agnosia).
	Altered communication patterns.
	Motor incoordination.
DESIRED OUTCOMES/ EVALUATION CRITERIA— PATIENT WILL:	Regain/maintain usual level of consciousness and perceptual functioning.
	Acknowledge changes in ability and presence of residual involvement.
	Demonstrate behaviors to compensate for/overcome deficits.

ACTIONS/INTERVENTIONS	RATIONALE
Independent	
Review pathology of individual condition.	Awareness of type/area of involvement aids in assessing for/anticipating specific deficits and planning care.
Evaluate for visual deficits. Note loss of visual field, changes in depth perception (horizontal/vertical planes), presence of diplopia (double vision).	Presence of visual disorders can negatively affect patient's ability to perceive environment and relearn motor skills and increases risk of accident/injury.
Approach patient from visually intact side. Leave light on; position objects to take advantage of intact visual fields. Patch affected eye if indicated.	Provides for recognition of the presence of persons/objects; may help with depth perception problems; prevents patient from being startled. Patching may decrease the sensory confusion of double vision.
Simplify environment, remove excess equipment/ furniture.	Decreases/limits amount of visual stimuli that may confuse interpretation of environment; reduces risk of accidental injury.
Assess sensory awareness, e.g., differentiation of hot/cold, dull/sharp; position of body parts/muscle, joint sense.	Diminished sensory awareness and impairment of kinesthetic sense negatively affects balance/positioning and appropriateness of movement, which interferes with ambulation, increasing risk of trauma.
Stimulate sense of touch; e.g., give patient objects to touch, grasp. Have patient practice touching walls/other boundaries.	Aids in retraining sensory pathways to integrate reception and interpretation of stimuli. Helps patient orient self spatially and strengthens use of affected side.
Protect from temperature extremes; assess environment for hazards. Recommend testing warm water with unaffected hand.	Promotes patient safety, reducing risk of injury.
Note inattention to body parts, segments of envi-	Presence of agnosia (loss of comprehension of au-

ACTIONS/INTERVENTIONS	RATIONALE

Independent

ronment; lack of recognition of familiar objects/persons.

ditory, visual, or other sensations, although sensory sphere is intact) may lead to/result in unilateral neglect, inability to recognize environmental cues/meaning of commonplace objects, considerable self-care deficits, and disorientation or bizarre behavior.

Encourage patient to watch feet when appropriate and consciously position body parts. Make the patient aware of all neglected body parts, e.g., sensory stimulation to affected side, exercises that bring affected side across midline, reminding person to dress/care for affected ("blind") side.

Use of visual and tactile stimuli assists in reintegration of affected side and allows patient to experience forgotten sensations of normal movement patterns.

Observe behavioral responses, e.g., hostility, crying, inappropriate affect, agitation, hallucination. (Refer to CP: Craniocerebral Trauma, ND: Thought Processes, altered, p 280.)

Individual responses are variable, but commonalities such as emotional lability, lowered frustration threshold, apathy, and impulsiveness may exist, complicating care.

Eliminate extraneous noise/stimuli as necessary.

Reduces anxiety and exaggerated emotional responses/confusion associated with sensory overload.

Speak in calm, quiet voice, using short sentences. Maintain eye contact.

Patient may have limited attention span or problems with comprehension. These measures can help patient to attend to communication.

Ascertain/validate patient's perceptions. Reorient patient frequently to environment, staff, procedures.

Assists patient to identify inconsistencies in reception and integration of stimuli and may reduce perceptual distortion of reality.

NURSING DIAGNOSIS:	SELF-CARE DEFICIT: [SPECIFY]
May be related to:	Neuromuscular impairment, decreased strength and endurance, loss of muscle control/coordination.
	Perceptual/cognitive impairment.
	Pain/discomfort.
	Depression.
Possibly evidenced by:	Impaired ability to perform ADLs, e.g., inability to bring food from receptacle to mouth; inability to wash body part(s), regulate temperature of water; impaired ability to put on/take off clothing; difficulty completing toileting tasks.
DESIRED OUTCOMES/ EVALUATION CRITERIA— PATIENT WILL:	Demonstrate techniques/lifestyle changes to meet self-care needs.
	Perform self-care activities within level of own ability.
	Identify personal/community resources that can provide assistance as needed.

ACTIONS/INTERVENTIONS	RATIONALE

Independent

Assess abilities and level of deficit (0–4 scale) for performing ADLs.

Aids in anticipating/planning for meeting individual needs.

Avoid doing things for the patient that the patient can do, but provide assistance as necessary.

These patients may become fearful and dependent, and although assistance is helpful in preventing frustration, it is important for the patient to do as much as possible for self to maintain self-esteem and promote recovery.

Be aware of impulsive behavior/actions suggestive of impaired judgment.

May indicate need for additional interventions and supervision to promote patient safety.

Maintain a supportive, firm attitude. Allow patient sufficient time to accomplish tasks.

Patients will need empathy but need to know caregivers will be consistent in their assistance.

Provide positive feedback for efforts/accomplishments.

Enhances sense of self-worth, promotes independence, and encourages patient to continue endeavors.

Create plan for visual deficits that are present, e.g.:

Place food and utensils on the tray related to the patient's unaffected side;

Patient will be able to see to eat the food.

Situate the bed so that the patient's unaffected side is facing the room with the affected side to the wall;

Will be able to see when getting in/out of bed, observe anyone who comes into the room.

Position furniture against wall/out of travel path.

Provides for safety when patient is able to move around the room reducing risk of tripping/falling over furniture.

Use self-help devices, e.g., knife-fork combinations, long-handled brushes, extensions for picking things up from floor; toilet riser, shower chair.

Enables patient to manage for self, enhancing independence and self-esteem.

Assess patient's ability to communicate the need to void and/or ability to use urinal, bedpan. Take patient to the bathroom at frequent/periodic intervals for voiding if appropriate.

May have neurogenic bladder, be inattentive, or be unable to communicate needs in acute recovery phase, but usually able to regain independent control of this function as recovery progresses.

Identify previous bowel habits and reestablish normal regimen. Increase bulk in diet; encourage fluid intake, increased activity.

Assists in development of retraining program (independence) and aids in preventing constipation and impaction (long-term effects).

Collaborative

Administer suppositories and stool softeners.

May be necessary at first to aid in establishing regular bowel function.

Consult with physical/occupational therapist.

Provides expert assistance for developing a therapy plan and identifying special equipment needs.

NURSING DIAGNOSIS: SELF-ESTEEM, DISTURBANCE, [SPECIFY]

May be related to: Biophysical, psychosocial, cognitive perceptual changes.

Possibly evidenced by:	Actual change in structure and/or function.
	Change in usual patterns of responsibility/physical capacity to resume role.
	Verbal/nonverbal response to actual or perceived change.
	Negative feelings about body, feelings of helplessness/hopelessness.
	Focus on past strength, function, or appearance.
	Preoccupation with change or loss.
	Not touching/looking at involved body part.
DESIRED OUTCOMES/ EVALUATION CRITERIA— PATIENT WILL:	Talk/communicate with SO about situation and changes that have occurred.
	Verbalize acceptance of self in situation.
	Recognize and incorporate change into self-concept in accurate manner without negating self-esteem.

ACTIONS/INTERVENTIONS	RATIONALE
Independent	
Assess extent of altered perception and related degree of disability.	Determination of individual factors aids in developing plan of care/choice of interventions.
Identify meaning of the loss/dysfunction/change to the patient.	Some patients accept and manage altered function effectively with little adjustment, while others have considerable difficulty recognizing and adjusting to deficits.
Encourage patient to express feelings including hostility or anger.	Demonstrates acceptance of/assists patient to recognize and begin to deal with these feelings.
Note whether patient refers to affected side as "it" or denies affected side and says it is "dead."	Suggests rejection of body part/negative feelings about body image and abilities, indicating need for intervention and emotional support.
Acknowledge statement of feelings about betrayal of body; remain matter-of-fact about reality that patient can still use unaffected side and learn to control affected side. Use words (e.g., weak, affected, right-left) that incorporate that side as part of the whole body.	Helps patient to see that the nurse accepts both sides as part of the whole individual. Allows patient to feel hopeful and begin to accept current situation.
Emphasize small gains either in recovery of function or independence.	Consolidates gains, helps reduce feelings of anger and helplessness, and conveys sense of progress.
Assist and encourage good grooming and make-up habits.	Helps enhance sense of self-esteem and control over one area of life.
Encourage SO to allow patient to do as much as possible for self.	Reestablishes sense of independence and fosters self-worth and enhances rehabilitation process. *Note:* This may be very difficult and frustrating for the SO/caregiver depending on degree of disability and time required for patient to complete activity.

ACTIONS/INTERVENTIONS	RATIONALE

Independent

Support behaviors/efforts such as increased interest/participation in rehabilitation activities.

Suggests possible adaptation to changes and understanding about own role in future lifestyle.

Reinforce use of adaptive devices, e.g., cane, walker, button/zipper hook, leg bag for catheter, and so on.

Increases independence, reduces reliance on others for meeting physical needs, and enables patient to be more socially active.

Monitor for sleep disturbance, increased difficulty concentrating, statements of inability to cope, lethargy, withdrawal.

May indicate onset of depression (common after effect of stroke), which may require further evaluation and intervention.

Collaborative

Refer for neuropsychologic evaluation and/or counseling if indicated.

May facilitate adaptation to role changes that are necessary for a sense of feeling/being a productive person.

NURSING DIAGNOSIS:	SWALLOWING, IMPAIRED, HIGH RISK FOR
Risk factors may include:	Neuromuscular/perceptual impairment.
Possibly evidenced by:	[Not applicable; presence of signs and symptoms establishes an actual diagnosis.]
DESIRED OUTCOMES/ EVALUATION CRITERIA— PATIENT WILL:	Demonstrate feeding methods appropriate to individual situation with aspiration prevented. Maintain desired body weight.

ACTIONS/INTERVENTIONS	RATIONALE

Independent

Review individual pathology/ability to swallow, noting extent of paralysis, facial, tongue involvement, ability to protect airway. Weigh periodically as indicated.

Nutritional interventions/choice of feeding route is determined by these factors.

Promote effective swallowing, e.g.:

Assist patient with head control/support;

Counteracts hyperextension, aiding in prevention of aspiration and enhancing ability to swallow.

Place patient in upright position during and after feeding;

Uses gravity to facilitate swallowing and reduces risk of aspiration.

Stimulate lips to close or manually open mouth by light pressure on lips/under chin, if needed;

Aids in sensory retraining and promotes muscular control.

Place food in unaffected side of mouth;

Provides sensory stimulation (including taste), which may trigger swallowing efforts and enhance intake.

ACTIONS/INTERVENTIONS	RATIONALE

Independent

Touch parts of the cheek with tongue blade/apply ice to weak tongue;

Can improve tongue movement and control (necessary for swallowing) and inhibits tongue protrusion.

Feed slowly in quiet environment;

Enables patient to concentrate on mechanics of eating without external distraction.

Begin oral feedings with semiliquid, soft foods when patient can swallow water. Select/assist patient to select foods that require little or no chewing, are easy to swallow, e.g., custard, applesauce, eggs, soft finger foods;

Soft foods/thick fluids are easier to control in mouth, reducing risk of choking/aspiration.

Encourage use of drinking straw for liquids;

Strengthens facial and swallowing muscles and reduces risk of choking.

Encourage SO to bring favorite foods.

Stimulates feeding efforts and may enhance swallowing/intake.

Maintain accurate I&O; record calorie count.

If swallowing efforts are not sufficient to meet fluid/nutrition needs, alternate methods of feeding must be pursued.

Encourage participation in exercise/activity program.

May increase release of endorphins in the brain, promoting a sense of general well-being and increasing appetite.

Collaborative

Administer IV fluids and/or tube feedings.

May be necessary for fluid replacement and nutrition if patient is unable to take anything orally.

NURSING DIAGNOSIS:	**KNOWLEDGE DEFICIT [LEARNING NEED], REGARDING CONDITION AND TREATMENT**
May be related to:	Lack of exposure.
	Cognitive limitation, information misinterpretation, lack of recall.
	Unfamiliarity with information resources.
Possibly evidenced by:	Request for information.
	Statement of misconception.
	Inaccurate follow-through of instructions.
	Development of preventable complications.
DESIRED OUTCOMES/ EVALUATION CRITERIA— PATIENT WILL:	Participate in learning process.
	Verbalize understanding of condition/prognosis and therapeutic regimen.
	Initiate necessary lifestyle changes.

ACTIONS/INTERVENTIONS	RATIONALE
Independent	
Evaluate type/degree of sensory-perceptual involvement.	Deficits affect the choice of teaching methods and content/complexity of instruction.
Discuss specific pathology and individual potentials.	Aids in establishing realistic expectations and promotes understanding of current situation and needs.
Review current restrictions/limitations and discuss planned/potential resumption of activities (including sexual relations).	Promotes understanding, provides hope for future, and creates expectation of resumption of more "normal" life.
Review/reinforce current therapeutic regimen. Identify ways of continuing program after discharge.	Recommended activities, limitations, and medication/therapy needs are established on the basis of a coordinated interdisciplinary approach. Follow-through is essential to progression of recovery/prevention of complications.
Discuss plans for meeting self-care needs.	Varying levels of assistance may be required/need to be planned for based on individual situation.
Provide written instructions and schedules for activity, medication, important facts.	Provides visual reinforcement and reference source after discharge.
Encourage patient to refer to lists/written communications or notes instead of depending on memory.	Provides aids to support memory and promotes improvement in cognitive skills.
Suggest patient reduce/limit environmental stimuli, especially during cognitive activities.	Multiple/concomitant stimuli may aggravate alteration of thought processes.
Recommend patient seek assistance in problem-solving process and validate decisions, as indicated.	Some patients (especially those with right CVA) may display impaired judgment and impulsive behavior, compromising ability to make sound decisions.
Identify individual risk factors (e.g., hypertension, obesity, smoking, atherosclerosis, use of oral contraceptives) and necessary lifestyle changes.	Promotes general well-being and may reduce risk of recurrence.
Identify signs/symptoms requiring further follow-up, e.g., changes/decline in visual, motor, sensory functions; alteration in mentation or behavioral responses; severe headache.	Prompt evaluation and intervention reduces risk of complications/further loss of function.
Refer to discharge planner/home care supervisor, visiting nurse.	Home environment may require evaluation and modifications to meet individual needs.
Identify community resources, e.g., stroke support clubs, senior services, Meals-on-Wheels, adult day care/respite program, and VNA.	Enhances coping abilities and promotes home management and adjustment to impairments.
Refer to/reinforce importance of follow-up care by rehabilitation team, e.g., physical/occupational/speech/vocational therapists.	Diligent work may eventually overcome/minimize residual deficits.

Intracranial Infections: Meningitis, Encephalitis, Brain Abscess

Intracranial infections can involve brain tissue (encephalitis) or the coverings of the brain and spinal column (meningitis) or be an accumulation of free or encapsulated pus within the brain (abscess). The causative agent can be bacterial, viral, or fungal, and sequelae can range from complete recovery to residual neurologic deficits to death.

RELATED CONCERNS:

Congestive Heart Failure, p 48
Craniocerebral Trauma, p 271
Headache, p 252
Inflammatory Cardiac Conditions, p 126
Psychosocial Aspects of Acute Care, p 899
Seizure Disorders/Epilepsy, p 261
Sepsis/Septicemia, p 887

PATIENT ASSESSMENT DATA BASE

ACTIVITY/REST

May report: Malaise.
Limitations imposed by condition.

May exhibit: Ataxia, gait problems, palsies, involuntary movement.
Generalized weakness, limited range of motion.
Hypotonia.

CIRCULATION

May report: History of underlying cardiopathology, e.g., infective endocarditis, some congenital heart diseases (brain abscess).

May exhibit: BP elevation, decreased pulse, and widening pulse pressure (correlates with increased ICP and effects on the vasomotor center).
Tachycardia, dysrhythmias (acute episode), e.g., sinus dysrhythmia (meningitis).

ELIMINATION

May exhibit: Incontinence and/or retention.

FOOD/FLUID

May report: Loss of appetite.
Difficulty swallowing (acute episode).

May exhibit: Anorexia; vomiting.
Poor skin turgor, dry mucous membranes.

HYGIENE

May exhibit: Dependence for all self-care needs (acute phase).

NEUROSENSORY

May report: Headaches (may be first symptom and is usually severe).
Paresthesia, itching, tingling along course of involved nerve, loss of sensation (damage to cranial nerves).

307

Hyperalgesia/increased sensitivity to pain (meningitis).

Seizure activity (bacterial meningitis or brain abscesses).

Disturbances in vision, e.g., diplopia (initial phase of any of the infections).

Photophobia (meningitis).

Deafness (meningitis or encephalitis) or may be hypersensitive to noise.

Olfactory/gustatory hallucinations.

May exhibit: Mental status/LOC: Altered LOC (lethargy to mild confusion to coma); delusions and hallucinations/organic psychosis (encephalitis).

Memory loss, lack of judgment (can be initial symptoms of developing communicating hydrocephalus following bacterial meningitis).

Aphasia/difficulty communicating.

Eyes (pupil size/reaction): Inequality of size or response to light (increased ICP).

Nystagmus (continuous movement of eyeballs).

Ptosis (drooping of the eyelid).

Facial characteristics: Changes in motor or sensory function (V or VII cranial nerve involvement).

Generalized or focal seizures (abscesses), temporal lobe seizures.

Muscle hypotonia/flaccid paralysis (acute phase meningitis) or tetanic spasms with arching of back and extremities (severe meningitis), spasticity (encephalitis).

Hemiparesis or hemiplegia on occasion (encephalitis/meningitis).

Positive Brudzinski's sign and/or a positive Kernig's sign indicative of meningeal irritation (acute phase).

Nuchal rigidity (meningeal irritation).

Deep tendon reflexes: Altered/accentuated, positive Babinski.

Abdominal reflexes diminished/absent; absence of cremasteric reflex in male (meningitis).

PAIN/COMFORT

May report: Headaches (severe throbbing, frontal) may be worsened by straining; stiff neck/back; pain with ocular movement; photosensitivity; aches; sore throat.

May exhibit: Guarding.

Distraction behaviors/restlessness.

Crying/moaning.

RESPIRATION

May report: History of lung or sinus infection (brain abscess).

May exhibit: Increased work of breathing (initial episode).

Changes in mentation (lethargy to coma) and restlessness.

SAFETY

May report: History of upper respiratory/other infections including mastoiditis, middle ear, sinus, dental abscess; pelvic, abdominal, or skin infections; recent lumbar puncture, surgery, skull fracture/head injury; sickle cell anemia.

Recent immunizations; exposure to meningitis; exposure to measles, mumps, chickenpox, herpes simplex, mononucleosis; animal bites; foreign travel.

Visual/hearing impairment.

May exhibit:	Temperature elevation, diaphoresis, chills.
	Petechial rashes, generalized purpura, subcutaneous bleeding.
	Generalized weakness; flaccid or spastic muscle tone; paralysis or paresis. Impaired sensation.

TEACHING/LEARNING

May report:	History of drug use (brain abscess).
	Drug hypersensitivity (nonbacterial meningitis).
	Previous illness/concurrent medical problems, e.g., chronic condition/general debility, alcoholism, diabetes mellitus, splenectomy, implantation of ventricular shunt.
Discharge Plan Considerations:	**DRG projected mean length of stay: 8.4 days.**
	May require assistance in all areas, including self-care and homemaker/maintenance tasks.

DIAGNOSTIC STUDIES

Lumbar puncture analysis of CSF:

Bacterial meningitis: Pressure elevated, fluid cloudy/milky, increased white cell count and protein; decreased to normal glucose; smear and culture shows presence and type of bacteria.

Viral meningitis: Pressure varies, fluid usually clear, increased white cells; usually normal protein and glucose; Gram stain shows no bacteria, virus cultured only with special procedures.

Encephalitis: Slight increase in pressure unless ICP elevated and then a marked elevation in cerebrospinal pressure, fluid usually clear, increased white cells, slightly elevated protein, normal glucose.

Brain abscess: Elevated pressure, elevated WBC count and protein, and normal glucose. *Note:* LP may be contraindicated as cerebral herniation can occur when ICP is lowered.

Serum glucose: Elevated (meningitis).

Serum LDH: Elevated (bacterial meningitis).

Serum WBC: Marked elevation with increased neutrophils (bacterial infection).

Serum electrolytes: Abnormal.

ESR: Elevated (meningitis).

Blood/nose/throat/urine cultures: May indicate area of "seeding" of infection or indicate type of infectious agent.

MRI/CT scan: May help localize lesion, visualize ventricle size/displacement; rule out cerebral hematoma, hemorrhage, or tumor.

EEG: May show focal or generalized slowing (encephalitis) or increased voltage (abscess).

Chest, skull, and sinus x-rays: May indicate infection or source of intracranial infection.

Carotid arteriography: Locates temporal lobe abscess, posterior study locates cerebellar abscess.

NURSING PRIORITIES

1. Maximize cerebral function and tissue perfusion.
2. Prevent complications/injury.
3. Alleviate anxiety/provide emotional support to patient/SO.
4. Reduce/minimize pain.
5. Provide information about disease process/prognosis and treatment needs.

DISCHARGE GOALS

1. Infectious process(es) resolving/absent.
2. Complications/injury prevented or minimized.
3. Discomfort relieved/controlled.
4. ADL needs met by self or with assistance of other(s).
5. Disease process/prognosis and therapeutic regimen understood.

NURSING DIAGNOSIS:	INFECTION, HIGH RISK FOR, [SPREAD]
Risk factors may include:	Hematogenous dissemination of pathogen.
	Stasis of body fluids.
	Suppressed inflammatory response (medication-induced).
	Exposure of others to pathogens.
Possibly evidenced by:	[Not applicable; presence of signs and symptoms establishes an actual diagnosis.]
DESIRED OUTCOMES/ EVALUATION CRITERIA— PATIENT WILL:	Achieve timely healing, with no evidence of endogenous spread of infection or involvement of others.

ACTIONS/INTERVENTIONS	RATIONALE
Independent	
Provide isolation precautions as indicated.	During early stage of meningococcal meningitis or some encephalitis infections, isolation may be required until organism is known/sufficient doses of antibiotic have been administered to reduce risk of spread to others.
Maintain aseptic techniques and good handwashing by patient/visitors/staff. Monitor and limit visitors/staff as appropriate.	Reduces patient's risk of acquiring secondary infection. Controls spread of infectious agents, prevents exposure to infectious individuals (e.g., those with upper respiratory infection).
Monitor temperature regularly. Note persistence of clinical signs of infectious process.	Drug therapy is usually continued for 5 days after temperature returns to normal and clinical signs clear. Continuation of symptoms may indicate development of acute meningococcemia, which can last weeks/months, or sepsis/hematogenous dissemination of pathogens.
Investigate reports of chest pain, development of irregular pulse/dysrhythmias, or persistent fever.	Secondary infection such as myocarditis/pericarditis may develop requiring further intervention.
Auscultate breath sounds. Monitor respiratory rate and effort.	Presence of rhonchi/wheezes, tachypnea, and increased work of breathing may reflect accumulation of secretions with risk of respiratory infection.
Reposition/turn frequently and encourage deep breathing.	Mobilizes secretions and promotes expectoration, reducing risk of respiratory complications.

ACTIONS/INTERVENTIONS	RATIONALE

Independent

Note urine characteristics, e.g., color, clarity, odor.

Urine stasis, dehydration, and general debility increases risk of bladder/kidney infection/onset of sepsis.

Identify contacts at risk for development of cerebral infectious process and encourage them to seek medical attention.

Those with intimate respiratory contact may require antimicrobial prophylactic therapy to prevent spread of infection.

Collaborative

Administer IV/intrathecal antimicrobial therapy as indicated, e.g., penicillin G (Biotic-T); ampicillin (Amcill); chloramphenicol (Chloromycetin); gentamycin (Garamycin); amphotericin B (Fungizone);

Choice of drug is dependent on type of infection and individual sensitivity. *Note:* Intrathecal administration may be indicated for Gram-negative bacilli, fungi, amoebae.

  vidarabine (Vira-A).

Useful for treatment of herpes simplex encephalitis.

Prepare for surgical intervention, as indicated.

May require drainage of encapsulated brain abscess or removal of infected ventricular shunt to prevent rupture/control spread of infection.

NURSING DIAGNOSIS:	TISSUE PERFUSION, ALTERED: CEREBRAL, HIGH RISK FOR
Risk factors may include:	Cerebral edema altering/interrupting cerebral arterial/venous blood flow.
	Hypovolemia.
	Exchange problems at cellular level (acidosis).
Possibly evidenced by:	[Not applicable; presence of signs and symptoms establishes an actual diagnosis.]
DESIRED OUTCOMES/ EVALUATION CRITERIA— PATIENT WILL:	Maintain usual/improved level of consciousness and motor/sensory function.
	Demonstrate stable vital signs.
	Report absence of/diminished severity of headache.
	Demonstrate improved cognition and absence of signs of increased ICP.

ACTIONS/INTERVENTIONS	RATIONALE

Refer to CP: Craniocerebral Trauma, ND: Tissue Perfusion, p 273, for a more in-depth discussion.

Independent

Maintain bed rest with head flat and monitor vital signs as indicated after lumbar puncture.

Alteration of CSF pressure may potentiate risk of brainstem herniation, requiring immediate medical intervention.

ACTIONS/INTERVENTIONS	RATIONALE
Independent	
Monitor/document neurologic status frequently and compare with baseline, such as Glasgow Coma Scale.	Assesses trends in LOC and potential for IICP and is useful in determining location, extent, and progression/resolution of CNS damage.
Assess for nuchal rigidity, twitching, increased restlessness, irritability, onset of seizure activity.	Indicative of meningeal irritation and may occur in acute and recovery period of brain injury.
Monitor vital signs, e.g.: BP noting onset of/continuing systolic hypertension and widening pulse pressure;	Normally, autoregulation maintains constant cerebral blood flow despite fluctuations in systemic BP. Loss of autoregulation may follow local or diffuse cerebral vascular damage, resulting in IICP. This phenomenon may be manifested by elevated systolic BP accompanied by decreasing diastolic BP (widening pulse pressure).
Heart rate/rhythm;	Changes in rate (most often bradycardia) and dysrhythmias may develop, reflecting brainstem pressure/injury in the absence of underlying cardiac disease.
Respirations, noting patterns and rhythm, e.g., periods of apnea after hyperventilation, Cheyne-Stokes breathing.	Type of respiratory pattern suggests severity of IICP/area of cerebral involvement and may indicate need for intubation with ventilatory support.
Monitor temperature and regulate environmental temperature as indicated. Limit use of blankets; administer tepid sponge bath in presence of fever. Wrap extremities in blankets when hypothermia blanket is used.	Fever is usually due to inflammatory process but may be complicated by damage to hypothalamus. Increased metabolic needs and oxygen consumption occur (especially with shivering), which can increase ICP.
Monitor intake and output. Note urine characteristics, skin turgor, status of mucous membranes.	Hyperthermia increases insensible losses and increases risk of dehydration, especially if level of consciousness/presence of nausea reduces oral intake. *Note:* SIADH release may occur, potentiating fluid retention with edema formation and decreased urinary output.
Help patient avoid/limit coughing, vomiting, straining at stool/bearing down. Encourage patient to exhale during turning/movement in bed.	These activities increase intrathoracic and intra-abdominal pressures, which can increase ICP. Exhaling during repositioning can prevent Valsalva effect.
Provide comfort measures, e.g., back massage, quiet environment, soft voice, gentle touch.	Promotes rest and decreases excessive sensory stimulation.
Provide rest periods between care activities and limit duration of procedures.	Prevents excessive fatigue/exhaustion. Continual activity can increase ICP by producing a cumulative stimulant.
Encourage SO to talk to patient if appropriate.	Hearing familiar voices of family/SO appears to have a relaxing effect on many patients and may reduce ICP.
Collaborative	
Elevate head of bed 15–45 degrees as tolerated/indicated. Keep head in neutral position.	Promotes venous drainage from head, thereby decreasing ICP.

ACTIONS/INTERVENTIONS

Collaborative

Administer IV fluids with control device. Restrict fluid intake and administer hypertonic/electrolyte solutions as indicated.

Monitor ABGs. Provide supplemental oxygen as indicated.

Use hypothermia blanket.

Administer medications as indicated, e.g.:

Steroids: dexamethasone (Decadron); methylprednisolone (Medrol);

Chlorpromazine (Thorazine);

Acetaminophen (Tylenol), rectally or orally.

RATIONALE

Minimizes fluctuations in vascular load and ICP. Fluid restriction may be needed to lower total body water and thereby reduce cerebral edema, especially in presence of SIADH.

Development of acidosis may inhibit release of oxygen at cellular level, worsening cerebral ischemia.

Aids in control/stabilization of extreme temperature elevation, reducing metabolic demands/risk of seizures and promoting patient safety.

May reduce capillary permeability to limit cerebral edema formation; may also reduce risk of rebound phenomena when mannitol is used.

Drug of choice in treating posturing and shivering, which can increase ICP. *Note:* This drug can lower the seizure threshold or precipitate Dilantin toxicity.

Reduces cellular metabolic/oxygen consumption and risk of seizure activity.

NURSING DIAGNOSIS:	TRAUMA, HIGH RISK FOR
Risk factors may include:	Irritation of cerebral cortex predisposing to neural discharge and generalized seizure activity.
	Involvement of localized area (focal seizure).
	Generalized weakness, paralysis, paresthesia.
	Ataxia, vertigo.
Possibly evidenced by:	[Not applicable; presence of signs and symptoms establishes an actual diagnosis.]
DESIRED OUTCOMES/ EVALUATION CRITERIA— PATIENT WILL:	Experience no seizures/concomitant or other injury.

ACTIONS/INTERVENTIONS

Independent

Monitor for twitching of hands, feet, and mouth or other facial muscles.

RATIONALE

Reflects generalized CNS irritability, requiring prompt evaluation and possible intervention to prevent complications.

ACTIONS/INTERVENTIONS

Independent

Provide for patient safety by padding side rails, keeping side rails up, and having a plastic airway or soft roll and suction machine available.

Maintain bed rest during acute phase. Ambulate with assistance as condition improves.

Collaborative

Administer medications as indicated, e.g., phenytoin (Dilantin); diazepam (Valium); phenobarbital (Luminal).

RATIONALE

Protects the patient if seizure occurs. *Note:* Insert oral airway/roll only if jaw relaxed; if inserted when teeth are clenched, dental and soft tissue damage may result.

Reduces risk of falls/injury when vertigo, syncope, ataxia are present.

Indicated for treatment and prevention of seizure activity. *Note:* Phenobarbital may cause respiratory depression and sedation and mask the signs/symptoms of increasing ICP.

NURSING DIAGNOSIS	PAIN, [ACUTE]
May be related to:	Biologic injuring agents, presence of infectious/inflammatory process, circulating toxins.
Possibly evidenced by:	Reports of headache, photophobia, muscle pain/backache.
	Distraction behaviors: crying, moaning, restlessness.
	Guarding behaviors, assumption of a characteristic position.
	Muscular tension; facial mask of pain, pallor.
	Changes in vital signs.
DESIRED OUTCOMES/ EVALUATION CRITERIA— PATIENT WILL:	Report pain is relieved/controlled.
	Display relaxed posture and be able to sleep/rest appropriately.

ACTIONS/INTERVENTIONS

Independent

Provide quiet environment; darken room as indicated.

Promote bed rest, assist with necessary self-care activities.

Place ice bag to head, cool cloth over eyes.

Support assumption of position of comfort, e.g., curled up with head slightly extended in meningitis.

RATIONALE

Reduces reaction to external stimuli/sensitivity to light and promotes rest/relaxation.

Reduces movement that may increase pain.

Promotes vasoconstriction; numbs sensory reception, thereby reducing pain.

Reduces meningeal irritation, resultant discomfort.

ACTIONS/INTERVENTIONS	RATIONALE
Independent	
Provide gentle active/passive range of motion and massage to neck/shoulder muscles.	May help relax tension of muscles, promoting reduction of pain/discomfort.
Use moist heat for neck/back pain if afebrile.	Promotes muscle relaxation and reduces aches/discomfort.
Collaborative	
Administer analgesics, e.g., acetaminophen, codeine.	May be needed to relieve severe pain. Note: Narcotics may be contraindicated as they impact the accuracy of the neurologic assessment.

NURSING DIAGNOSIS:	**PHYSICAL MOBILITY, IMPAIRED**
May be related to:	Neuromuscular impairment, decreased strength/endurance.
	Perceptual/cognitive impairment.
	Pain/discomfort.
	Restrictive therapies (bed rest).
Possibly evidenced by:	Reluctance to attempt movement.
	Impaired coordination and decreased muscle strength/control.
	Limited range of motion.
	Inability to purposefully move within the physical environment
DESIRED OUTCOMES/ EVALUATION CRITERIA— PATIENT WILL:	Regain/maintain optimal position of function as evidenced by absence of contractures, footdrop.
	Maintain/increase general strength and function.
	Maintain skin integrity, bladder and bowel function.

Refer to CP: Craniocerebral Trauma, ND: Physical Mobility, impaired, p 282.

NURSING DIAGNOSIS:	**SENSORY-PERCEPTUAL ALTERATION [SPECIFY]**
May be related to:	Altered sensory reception, transmission, or integration.
Possibly evidenced by:	Photosensitivity.
	Paresthesia, hyperalgesia.
	Change in usual response to stimuli.

	Poor concentration, irritability, restlessness, disorientation.
	Exaggerated emotional responses.
DESIRED OUTCOMES/ EVALUATION CRITERIA— PATIENT WILL:	Regain usual level of consciousness and perceptual functioning.
	Acknowledge changes in ability and presence of residual involvement.
	Demonstrate behaviors/lifestyle changes to compensate for/overcome deficits.

(Refer to CP: Craniocerebral Trauma, ND: Sensory-Perceptual alteration, specify, p 278).

NURSING DIAGNOSIS:	**ANXIETY (SPECIFY)/FEAR**
May be related to:	Situational crisis; interpersonal transmission and contagion.
	Threat of death/change in health status (involvement of brain).
	Separation from support system (hospitalization).
Possibly evidenced by:	Increased tension/helplessness.
	Apprehension/uncertainty of outcome, focus on self.
	Sympathetic stimulation.
	Restlessness.
DESIRED OUTCOMES/ EVALUATION CRITERIA— PATIENT WILL:	Acknowledge and discuss fears.
	Verbalize accurate knowledge of the situation.
	Appear relaxed and report anxiety is reduced to a manageable level.

ACTIONS/INTERVENTIONS	RATIONALE
Independent	
Assess patient's mentation and level of anxiety of patient/SO. Note both verbal and nonverbal cues.	Altered LOC may affect expression of fears but does not negate their presence. Degree of anxiety will affect how information is received by the individual.
Provide explanation of relationship between disease process and symptoms.	Promotes understanding, lessens fear of unknown, and may help reduce anxiety.
Answer questions honestly and give information about favorable prognosis.	Important to the establishment of trust as the diagnosis of meningitis may be frightening, and honesty and accurate information can provide reassurance.

ACTIONS/INTERVENTIONS	RATIONALE
Independent	
Explain and prepare for procedures beforehand.	May alleviate apprehension especially when testing involves the brain.
Allow time to verbalize thoughts and fears.	Brings fears out into the open, where they can be addressed.
Involve patient/SO in care, daily planning, decision-making as much as possible.	Increases feeling of control and encourages independence.
Support planning for realistic lifestyle after illness within limitations but fully using capabilities.	Promotes sense of hope/expectation of recovery.
Explore sources of support: SO, clergy, professional counselor.	Provides reassurance that needed assistance is available to enhance/support coping.
Let SO/patient know that uncharacteristic/inappropriate behavior is related to cerebral involvement and is usually self-limiting.	Bizarre behaviors, as may be seen with temporal lobe involvement in herpes encephalitis, can be very frightening, escalating anxiety and potentiating sense of helplessness/loss of control.
Protect patient's privacy if seizure activity occurs.	Consideration of the patient's need for privacy preserves and conveys a sense of dignity and self-worth, protecting the patient from embarrassment.
Provide explanation to patient/SO; unless permanent damage to the cerebrum occurs, seizure activity will likely subside as the patient recovers.	Seizure activity may be equated with the stigma of epilepsy, and an explanation of what is happening in relationship to the current illness may reduce anxiety, promote understanding of the condition.

NURSING DIAGNOSIS:	**KNOWLEDGE DEFICIT [LEARNING NEED] REGARDING CAUSE OF INFECTION AND TREATMENT NEEDS**
May be related to:	Lack of exposure.
	Information misinterpretation.
	Lack of recall, cognitive limitation.
Possibly evidenced by:	Questions, statement of misconception.
	Request for information.
	Inaccurate follow-through of instruction.
	Inappropriate or exaggerated behaviors (hostile, agitated, apathetic).
DESIRED OUTCOMES/ EVALUATION CRITERIA— PATIENT WILL:	Verbalize understanding of condition/disease process and treatment.
	Correctly perform necessary procedures and explain reasons for the actions.

ACTIONS/INTERVENTIONS	RATIONALE
Independent	
Provide information in short/brief segments.	Decreased attention span may reduce ability to process and retain information.
Discuss anticipated length of convalescence.	Recovery may take several weeks to months, and accurate information about expectations will help patient to cope with enforced inactivity/deal with continued discomfort.
Provide information about need for high protein/carbohydrate diet that should be offered in small/frequent meals.	Promotes healing process. Frequent eating of small amounts of food uses less energy, reduces gastric irritation, and may enhance total intake.
Instruct in progressive range of motion exercises, using warm bath to promote muscle relaxation.	Assists in regaining muscle strength/function.
Discuss importance of adequate rest, scheduling rest periods balanced with activities. Advance activity level as tolerated.	Fatigue often persists beyond usual expectations of patient/SO. Extra rest is needed to help in healing process and enhance coping abilities.
Promote development of diversional activities.	Prevents boredom and helps to maintain sense of purpose in life during recuperation period.
Review medication regimen and stress consulting health care provider before taking other medications/OTC drugs.	Completion of scheduled drug program is necessary for complete resolution of infectious process. Other medications/OTC drugs may be incompatible with prescribed medication regimen.
Discuss prevention of disease as appropriate, e.g., obtaining appropriate vaccinations, swimming only in chlorinated water, obtaining environmental control of mosquitoes, preventing/treating infections.	Acute viral meningitis is often due to such viruses as mumps and herpes. A variety of encephalitic diseases are transmitted by the bite of infective mosquitoes.
Review signs/symptoms requiring physician notification, e.g., nausea/vomiting, recurrence of headache, problems with balance, or changes in mentation.	Prompt evaluation and intervention may prevent relapse/development of complications.
Stress importance of routine reevaluation and outpatient therapies.	Necessary to note progress/resolution of residual symptoms and need for continuation/changes in therapy and to determine functional and neurologic deficits.
Identify community resources/supports.	Presence of functional and/or neurologic deficits will require adaptations by patient/SO/family.

Herniated Nucleus Pulposus (Ruptured Intervertebral Disk) ___

A herniated disk (HNP) is a major cause of severe, chronic, and recurrent back pain. Herniation, either complete or partial, of the nuclear material in the vertebral areas of L4–L5, L5–S1, or C5–C6, C6–C7 is most common and may be the result of trauma or degenerative changes associated with the aging process.

RELATED CONCERNS:

Disk Surgery, p 327
Psychosocial Aspects of Acute Care, p 899

PATIENT ASSESSMENT DATA BASE

Data are dependent on site, severity, whether acute/chronic, effects of surrounding structures, and amount of nerve root compression.

ACTIVITY/REST

May report:	History of occupation requiring heavy lifting, sitting, driving for long periods.
	Need to sleep on bedboard/firm mattress.
	Decreased range of motion of extremities on one side.
	Inability to perform usual/desired activities.
May exhibit:	Atrophy of muscles on the affected side.
	Gait disturbances.

ELIMINATION

May report:	Constipation, difficulty in defecation.
	Urinary incontinence/retention.

EGO INTEGRITY

May report:	Fear of paralysis.
	Financial, employment concerns.
May exhibit:	Anxiety, depression, withdrawal from family/SO.

NEUROSENSORY

May report:	Tingling, numbness, weakness, of arm/leg.
May exhibit:	Decreased deep tendon reflexes; muscle weakness, hypotonia.
	Tenderness/spasm of paravertebral muscles.
	Decreased pain perception (sensory).

PAIN/COMFORT

May report:	Pain knifelike, aggravated by coughing, sneezing, bending, lifting, defecation, straight leg raising or neck flexion; unremitting pain or intermittent episodes of more severe pain; radiation to leg, buttocks area (lumbar) or shoulder; occiput with stiff neck (cervical).
	Heard "snapping" sound at time of initial pain/trauma or felt "back giving way."
	Limited mobility/forward bending.

May exhibit:	Stance: Leans away from affected area.
	Altered gait, walking with a limp, elevated hip on affected side.
	Pain on palpation.

SAFETY

May report:	History of previous back problems.

TEACHING/LEARNING

May report:	Lifestyle: Sedentary or overactive.
Discharge Plan Considerations:	**DRG projected mean length of stay: 10.8 days.**
	May require assistance with transportation, self-care, and homemaker/maintenance tasks.

DIAGNOSTIC STUDIES

Spinal x-rays: May show degenerative changes in spine/intervertebral space or rule out other suspected pathology, e.g., tumors, osteomyelitis.

Electromyography: May localize lesion to level of particular spinal nerve root involved.

Epidural venogram: May be done for cases where myelogram accuracy is limited.

Lumbar puncture: Rules out other related conditions, infection, presence of blood.

LeSeque's sign (straight leg raise test): Supports initial diagnosis of herniated disk when posterior leg pain is present.

CT scan: May reveal spinal canal narrowing, disk protrusion.

MRI: Noninvasive study reveals changes in bone and soft tissues and can validate disk herniation.

Myelogram: May be normal or show "narrowing" of disk space, specific location and size of herniation.

NURSING PRIORITIES

1. Reduce spinal stress, muscle spasm, and pain.
2. Promote optimal functioning.
3. Support patient/SO in rehabilitation process.
4. Provide information concerning condition/prognosis and treatment needs.

DISCHARGE GOALS

1. Pain relieved/controlled.
2. Motor function/sensation restored to optimal level.
3. Proper lifting, posture, exercises demonstrated.
4. Disease/injury process, prognosis, and therapeutic regimen understood.

NURSING DIAGNOSIS:	**PAIN, [ACUTE]/CHRONIC**
May be related to:	Physical injury agents: nerve compression, muscle spasm.
Possibly evidenced by:	Reports of back pain, stiff neck.
	Walking with a limp, inability to walk.
	Guarding behavior, leans toward affected side when standing.
	Decreased tolerance for activity.

Preoccupation with pain, self-narrowed focus.

Altered muscle tone.

Facial mask of pain.

Distraction.

Autonomic responses (when pain is acute).

Changes in sleep patterns.

Physical/social withdrawal.

DESIRED OUTCOMES/ EVALUATION CRITERIA— PATIENT WILL:

Report pain is relieved/controlled.

Verbalize methods that provide relief.

Demonstrate use of therapeutic interventions (e.g., relaxation skills, behavior modification) to relieve pain.

ACTIONS/INTERVENTIONS	RATIONALE
Independent	
Assess reports of pain, noting location, duration, precipitating/aggravating factors. Ask patient to rate on scale of 0–10.	Helps determine choice of interventions and provides basis for comparison and evaluation of therapy.
Maintain bed rest during acute phase. Place patient in semi-Fowler's with spine, hips, knees flexed; supine with/without head elevated 10–30 degrees; or lateral position.	Bed rest in position of comfort allows for decrease of muscle spasm, reduces stress on structures, and facilitates reduction of disk protrusion.
Logroll for position change.	Reduces flexion, twisting, and strain on back.
Assist with application of brace/corset.	Useful during acute phase of ruptured disk to provide support and limit flexion/twisting. Prolonged use can increase muscle weakness and cause further degeneration.
Limit activity during acute phase as indicated.	Decreases forces of gravity and motion, which can relieve muscle spasms and reduce edema and stress on structures around affected disk.
Place needed items, call bell within easy reach.	Reduces risk of straining to reach.
Instruct in relaxation/visualization techniques.	Refocuses attention, aids in reducing muscle tension and promotes healing.
Instruct in/encourage proper body mechanics/ body posture.	Alleviates stress on muscles and prevents further injury.
Provide opportunities to talk/listen to concerns.	Ventilation of worries can help to decrease stress factors present in illness/hospitalization. Provides opportunity to give information/correct misinformation.
Collaborative	
Provide orthopedic bed or place board under mattress.	Provides support and reduces spinal flexion, decreasing spasms.

ACTIONS/INTERVENTIONS	RATIONALE
Collaborative	
Administer medications as indicated:	
Muscle relaxants, e.g., diazepam (Valium); carisoprodol (Soma); methcarbamol (Robaxin);	Relaxes muscles, decreasing pain.
NSAIDs, e.g., ibuprofen (Motrin, Advil); diflurisal (Dolobid); Ketoproten (Orudis); meclofenamate (Meclomen);	Decreases edema and pressure on nerve root(s). *Note:* Epidural or facet joint injection of anti-inflammatory drugs may be tried if other interventions fail to alleviate pain.
Analgesics, e.g., acetaminophen (Tylenol) with codeine; meperidine (Demerol); Hydrocodone (Vicodin); butorphanol (Stadol).	May be required for relief of moderate to severe pain.
Apply physical supports, e.g., lumbar braces, cervical collar.	Support of structures decreases muscle stress/spasms and reduces pain.
Maintain traction if indicated.	Removes weight bearing from affected disk area, increasing intravertebral separation and allowing disk bulge to move away from nerve root.
Consult with physical therapist.	Individual stretching/exercise program can relieve muscle spasm and strengthen back, extensor, abdominal, and quadriceps muscles to increase support to lumbar area.
Apply/monitor use of cold or moist hot packs, diathermy, ultrasound.	Increases circulation to affected muscles, promotes relief of spasms, and enhances patient's relaxation.
Instruct in postmyelogram procedures when appropriate, e.g., force fluids and lie flat or at 30-degree elevation, as indicated for specific number of hours.	Decreases risk of postprocedure headache/spinal fluid leak.
Assist with/prepare for application of TENS.	Decreases stimuli by blocking pain transmission.
Refer to pain clinic.	Coordinated team efforts may include physical as well as psychologic therapy to deal with all aspects of chronic pain and allow patient to increase activity and productivity.

NURSING DIAGNOSIS:	PHYSICAL MOBILITY, IMPAIRED
May be related to:	Pain and discomfort, muscle spasms.
	Restrictive therapies, e.g., bed rest, traction.
	Neuromuscular impairment.
Possibly evidenced by:	Reports of pain on movement.
	Reluctance to attempt/difficulty with purposeful movement.
	Impaired coordination, limited range of motion, decreased muscle strength.

NEUROLOGIC: Herniated Nucleus Pulposus (Ruptured Intervertebral Disk)

DESIRED OUTCOMES/ EVALUATION CRITERIA— PATIENT WILL:	Verbalize understanding of situation/risk factors and individual treatment regimen.
	Demonstrate techniques/behaviors that enable resumption of activities.
	Maintain or increase strength and function of affected and/or compensatory body part.

ACTIONS/INTERVENTIONS	RATIONALE

Independent

Provide for safety measures as indicated by individual situation.	Dependent on area of involvement/type of procedure, imprudent activity increases chance of spinal injury. (Refer to CP: Disk Surgery, ND: Trauma [Spinal], high risk for, p 328.)
Note emotional/behavioral responses to immobility. Provide diversional activities.	Forced immobility may heighten restlessness, irritability. Diversional activity aids in refocusing attention and promotes coping with limitations.
Follow activity/procedures with rest periods. Encourage participation in ADLs within individual limitations.	Enhances healing and builds muscle strength and endurance. Patient participation promotes independence and sense of control.
Provide/assist with passive and active range of motion exercises.	Strengthens abdominal muscles and flexors of spine; promotes good body mechanics.
Encourage lower leg/ankle exercises. Evaluate for edema, erythema of lower extremities, presence of Homans' sign.	Stimulates venous circulation/return decreasing venous stasis and possible thrombus formation.
Assist with activity/progressive ambulation.	Activity limitation is dependent on individual situation but usually progresses slowly according to tolerance.
Demonstrate use of adjunctive devices, e.g., walker, cane.	Provides stability and support to compensate for altered muscle tone/strength and balance.
Provide good skin care; massage pressure points after each position change. Check skin under brace periodically.	Reduces risk of skin irritation/breakdown.

Collaborative

Administer medication for pain approximately 30 minutes prior to turning patient/ambulation, as indicated.	Anticipation of pain can increase muscle tension. Medication can relax patient; enhance comfort and cooperation during activity.
Apply antiembolism stockings as indicated.	Promotes venous return.

NURSING DIAGNOSIS:	ANXIETY [SPECIFY LEVEL]/COPING, INDIVIDUAL, INEFFECTIVE [CHRONIC]
May be related to:	Situational crisis.
	Threat to/change in health status, socioeconomic status, role functioning.

	Recurrent disorder with continuing pain.
	Inadequate relaxation, little or no exercise.
	Inadequate coping methods.
Possibly evidenced by:	Apprehension, uncertainty, helplessness.
	Expressed concerns regarding changes in life events.
	Verbalization of inability to cope.
	Muscular tension, general irritability, restlessness; insomnia/fatigue.
	Inability to meet role expectations.
DESIRED OUTCOMES/ EVALUATION CRITERIA— PATIENT WILL:	Appear relaxed and report anxiety is reduced to a manageable level.
	Identify ineffective coping behaviors and consequences.
	Assess the current situation accurately.
	Demonstrate problem-solving skills.
	Develop plan for necessary lifestyle changes.

ACTIONS/INTERVENTIONS	RATIONALE
Independent	
Assess level of anxiety. Determine how patient has dealt with problems in the past as well as how he/she is coping with current situation.	Aids in identifying strengths and skills that may help patient deal with current situation and/or enable others to provide appropriate assistance.
Provide accurate information and honest answers.	Enables patient to make decisions based on knowledge.
Provide opportunity for expression of concerns, e.g., possible paralysis, effect on sexual ability, changes in employment/finances, altered role responsibilities.	Most patients have concerns that need to be expressed and responded to with accurate information to promote coping with situation.
Assess presence of secondary gains that may interfere with the wish to recover and may impede recovery.	The patient may unconsciously experience advantages such as relief from responsibilities; attention, and control of others. These need to be dealt with positively to promote recovery.
Note behaviors of SO that promote "sick role" for the patient.	SO may unconsciously enable patient to remain dependent by doing things that patient should do for self.
Collaborative	
Refer to community support groups, social services, financial/vocational counselor, marriage therapy/psychotherapy.	Provides support for adapting to changes and provides resources to deal with problems.

NURSING DIAGNOSIS:	KNOWLEDGE DEFICIT [LEARNING NEED] REGARDING CONDITION, PROGNOSIS, AND TREATMENT
May be related to:	Misinformation/lack of knowledge.
	Information misinterpretation, lack of recall.
	Unfamiliarity with information resources.
Possibly evidenced by:	Verbalization of problems.
	Statement of misconception.
	Inaccurate return demonstration.
DESIRED OUTCOMES/ EVALUATION CRITERIA— PATIENT WILL:	Verbalize understanding of condition, prognosis, and treatment.
	Initiate necessary lifestyle changes.
	Participate in treatment regimen.

ACTIONS/INTERVENTIONS	RATIONALE
Independent	
Review disease/injury process and prognosis and activity restrictions/limitations; e.g., avoid riding in car for long periods, refrain from participation in aggressive sports.	Helpful in clarifying and developing understanding and acceptance of necessary lifestyle changes. Full knowledge base provides opportunity for patient to make informed choices. May enhance cooperation with treatment program and achievement of optimal recovery.
Give information about and instruct in proper body mechanics and exercises. Include information about proper posture/body mechanics for standing, sitting, lifting and use of supportive shoes.	Reduces risk of reinjuring back/neck area by using muscles of thighs/buttocks.
Discuss medications and side effects: e.g., some medications cause drowsiness (analgesics, muscle relaxants); others can aggravate ulcer disease (NSAIDs).	Reduces risk of complications/injury.
Recommend use of bedboards/firm mattress, small flat pillow under neck, sleeping on side with knees flexed, avoiding prone position.	May decrease muscle strain through structural support and prevention of hyperextension of spine.
Discuss dietary needs/goals.	High-fiber diet can limit constipation; calorie restrictions promote weight control/reduction, which can decrease pressure on disk.
Avoid prolonged heat application.	Can increase local tissue congestion; decreased sensing of heat can result in thermal injury.
Review use of soft cervical collar.	Maintaining slight flexion of head (allows maximal opening of intervertebral foramina) may be useful for relieving pressure in mild to moderate cervical disk disease. Hyperextension should be avoided.

ACTIONS/INTERVENTIONS

Independent

Encourage regular medical follow-up.

Provide information about what symptoms need to be reported for further evaluation, e.g., sharp pain, loss of sensation/ability to walk.

Review treatment alternatives, e.g.:

Chemonucleolysis;

Surgical interventions.

RATIONALE

Evaluates resolution/progression of degenerative process; monitors development of side effects/ complications of drug therapy; may indicate need for change in therapeutic regimen.

Progression of the process may necessitate further treatment/surgery.

As an alternative to surgery, the enzyme chymopapain may be injected into the disk (dissolves the mucoprotein disk material without effect on surrounding structure). Although many patients experience relief, the procedure is not widely done because of side effects including allergic reaction to the enzyme.

Microdiskectomy may be performed to excise fragments of the disk with a comparatively lower risk than more invasive surgery. Laminectomy with/without spinal fusion may be performed when conservative treatment is ineffective or when neurologic deficits persist.

Disk Surgery

Laminectomy is the excision of a vertebral posterior arch and is commonly performed for injury to the spinal column or to relieve pressure/pain in the presence of an HNP. The procedure may be done with or without fusion of vertebrae.

RELATED CONCERNS:

Psychosocial Aspects of Acute Care, p 899
Surgical Intervention, p 918

PATIENT ASSESSMENT DATA BASE

Refer to CP: Herniated Nucleus Pulposus, p 319.

TEACHING/LEARNING

Discharge Plan Considerations:	**DRG projected mean length of stay: 10.8 days.**
	May require assistance with ADLs, transportation, homemaker/maintenance tasks, vocational counseling, possible changes in layout of home.

DIAGNOSTIC STUDIES

Refer to CP: Herniated Nucleus Pulposus, p 319.

NURSING PRIORITIES

1. Maintain tissue perfusion/neurologic function.
2. Promote comfort and healing.
3. Prevent/minimize complications.
4. Assist with return to normal mobility.
5. Provide information about condition/prognosis, treatment needs and limitations.

DISCHARGE GOALS

1. Neurologic function maintained/improved.
2. Complications prevented.
3. Limited mobility achieved with potential for increasing mobility.
4. Condition/prognosis, therapeutic regimen, and behavior/lifestyle changes are understood.

NURSING DIAGNOSIS:	TISSUE PERFUSION, ALTERED: [SPECIFY]
May be related to:	Diminished/interrupted blood flow (e.g., edema of operative site, hematoma formation.)
	Hypovolemia.
Possibly evidenced by:	Paresthesia; numbness.
	Decreased range of motion, muscle strength.
DESIRED OUTCOMES/ EVALUATION CRITERIA— PATIENT WILL:	Report/demonstrate normal sensations and movement as appropriate.

ACTIONS/INTERVENTIONS	RATIONALE

Independent

Check neurologic signs periodically and compare with baseline. Assess movement/sensation of lower extremities and feet (lumbar) plus hands/arms (cervical).

Although some degree of prior sensory impairment is usually present, deterioration/changes may reflect development/resolution of edema, inflammation of the tissues secondary to damage to motor nerve roots, requiring prompt medical evaluation.

Keep patient flat on back for several hours.

Pressure to operative site reduces risk of hematoma.

Monitor vital signs. Note color, warmth, capillary refill.

Hypotension (especially postural) with corresponding changes in pulse rate may reflect hypovolemia from blood loss, restriction of oral intake, nausea/vomiting.

Monitor intake/output and Hemovac drainage (if used).

Provides information about circulatory status and replacement needs.

Palpate operative site for swelling. Inspect dressing for excess drainage and test for glucose if indicated.

Change in contour of operative site suggests hematoma/edema formation. Inspection may reveal frank bleeding or dura leak of CSF (will test glucose positive), requiring prompt intervention.

Measure Hemovac drainage each shift.

Excessive/prolonged blood loss requires further evaluation to determine appropriate intervention.

Collaborative

Administer IV fluids/blood as indicated.

Fluid replacement is dependent on the degree of hypovolemia and duration of oozing/bleeding/spinal fluid leaking.

Monitor blood counts, e.g., Hb, Hct, and RBC.

Aids in establishing blood replacement needs and monitors effectiveness of therapy.

NURSING DIAGNOSIS:	TRAUMA [SPINAL], HIGH RISK FOR
Risk factors may include:	Temporary weakness of spinal column.
	Balancing difficulties, changes in muscle coordination.
Possibly evidenced by:	[Not applicable; presence of signs and symptoms establishes an actual diagnosis.]
DESIRED OUTCOMES/ EVALUATION CRITERIA— PATIENT WILL:	Maintain proper alignment of spine.
	Recognize need for/seek assistance with activity.

ACTIONS/INTERVENTIONS	RATIONALE

Independent

Post sign at bedside regarding prescribed position.

Reduces risk of inadvertent strain/flexion of operative area.

Provide bedboard/firm mattress.

Aids in stabilizing back.

ACTIONS/INTERVENTIONS	RATIONALE
Independent	
Maintain cervical collar postoperatively with cervical laminectomy procedure.	Decreases muscle spasm and supports the surrounding structures, allowing normal sensory stimulation to occur.
Limit activities when patient has had a spinal fusion.	Movement in the involved vertebral area is eliminated when fusion has been done and recuperation is longer.
Logroll patient from side to side. Have patient fold arms across chest, tighten long back muscles, keeping shoulders and pelvis straight. Use pillows between knees during position change and when on side. Use turning sheet and sufficient personnel when turning, especially on the 1st postoperative day.	Maintains body alignment while turning, preventing twisting motion, which may interfere with healing process.
Assist out of bed: logroll to side of bed, splint back, and raise to sitting position. Avoid prolonged sitting. Move to standing position in single smooth motion.	Avoids twisting and flexing of back while arising from bed/chair, protecting surgical area.
Avoid sudden stretching, twisting, flexing, or jarring of spine.	May cause vertebral collapse, shifting of bone graft, delayed hematoma formation, or subcutaneous wound dehiscence.
Check BP; note reports of dizziness or weakness. Change position slowly.	Presence of postural hypotension may result in fainting/fall and possible injury to surgical site.
Have patient wear firm/flat walking shoes when ambulating.	Reduces risk of falls.
Collaborative	
Apply lumbar brace/cervical collar as appropriate.	May be needed while patient is ambulating to give support to spine and surrounding structures until muscle strength improves. Brace is applied while patient is supine in bed.
Refer to physical therapy. Implement program as outlined.	Strengthening exercises may be indicated during the rehabilitative phase to decrease muscle spasm and strain on the vertebral disk area.

NURSING DIAGNOSIS:	**BREATHING PATTERN, INEFFECTIVE/AIRWAY CLEARANCE, HIGH RISK FOR**
Risk factors may include:	Tracheal/bronchial obstruction/edema. Decreased lung expansion, pain.
Possibly evidenced by:	[Not applicable; presence of signs and symptoms establishes an actual diagnosis.]
DESIRED OUTCOMES/ EVALUATION CRITERIA— PATIENT WILL:	Maintain a normal/effective respiratory pattern free of cyanosis and other signs of hypoxia, with ABGs within patient's normal range.

329

ACTIONS/INTERVENTIONS

Independent

Inspect for edema of face/neck (cervical laminectomy).

Listen for hoarseness.

Auscultate breath sounds, note presence of wheezes/rhonchi.

Assist with cough, turn, and deep breathing.

Collaborative

Administer humidified supplemental oxygen, if indicated.

Monitor/graph ABGs/pulse oximetry.

RATIONALE

Tracheal edema/compression or nerve injury can compromise respiratory function.

May indicate laryngeal nerve injury, which can negatively affect cough (ability to clear airway).

Suggests accumulation of secretions/ineffective airway clearance.

Facilitates movement of secretions and clearing of lungs; reduces risk of respiratory complications (pneumonia).

May be necessary for periods of respiratory distress or evidence of hypoxia.

Monitors effectiveness of breathing pattern/therapy.

NURSING DIAGNOSIS:	PAIN [ACUTE]
May be related to:	Physical agent (surgical manipulation, edema, inflammation).
Possibly evidenced by:	Reports of pain.
	Autonomic responses (diaphoresis, changes in vital signs, pallor).
	Alteration in muscle tone.
	Guarding, distraction behaviors/restlessness.
DESIRED OUTCOMES/ EVALUATION CRITERIA— PATIENT WILL:	Report pain is relieved/controlled.
	Verbalize methods that provide relief.
	Demonstrate use of relaxation skills and diversional activities.

ACTIONS/INTERVENTIONS

Independent

Assess intensity, description, and location/radiation of pain, changes in sensation.

Review expected manifestations/changes in intensity of pain.

RATIONALE

May be mild to severe with radiation to shoulders/occipital area (cervical) or hips/buttocks (lumbar). If bone graft has been taken from the iliac crest, pain may be more severe at the donor site. Numbness/tingling discomfort may reflect return of sensation after nerve root decompression or result from developing edema of compressed nerve/operative site.

Development/resolution of edema and inflammation in the immediate postoperative phase can

ACTIONS/INTERVENTIONS	RATIONALE
Independent	
	affect pressure on various nerves and cause changes in degree of pain (especially 3 days after operation, when muscle spasms/improved nerve root sensation intensify pain).
Allow patient to assume position of comfort if indicated. Use logroll for position change.	Positioning is dictated by physical preference, type of operation (e.g., head of bed may be slightly elevated after cervical laminectomy). Readjustment of position aids in relieving muscle fatigue and discomfort. Logrolling avoids tension in the operative areas and maintains straight spinal alignment.
Provide back rub/massage avoiding operative site.	Relieves/reduces pain by alteration of sensory neurons, muscle relaxation.
Demonstrate/encourage use of relaxation skills, e.g., deep breathing, visualization.	Refocuses attention, reduces muscle tension, promotes sense of well-being, and controls/decreases discomfort.
Provide soft diet, room humidifier; encourage voice rest following cervical laminectomy.	Reduces discomfort associated with sore throat and difficulty swallowing.
Investigate patient reports of return of radicular pain.	Suggests complications (collapsing of disk space, shifting of bone graft or arachnoiditis with adhesions) requiring further medical evaluation and intervention. *Note:* Sciatica and muscle spasms often recur after laminectomy but should resolve within several days or weeks.
Collaborative	
Administer analgesics, as indicated:	Given for pain relief/control.
Narcotics, e.g., morphine, codeine, meperidine (Demerol); oxycodone (Tylox); hydrocondone (Vicodin); acetaminophen (Tylenol) with codeine;	Narcotics are used during the first few postoperative days, then nonnarcotic agents are incorporated as intensity of pain diminishes.
Muscle relaxants, e.g., cyclobenzaprine (Flexeril); diazepam (Valium).	May be used to relieve muscle spasms resulting from intraoperative nerve irritation.
Assist with PCA.	Gives patient control of medication administration (usually narcotics) to achieve a more constant level of comfort, which may enhance healing.
Provide throat sprays/lozenges, viscous xylocaine.	Sore throat may be a major complaint following cervical laminectomy.
Apply TENS unit as needed.	May be used for incisional pain or when nerve involvement continues after discharge.

NURSING DIAGNOSIS:	**PHYSICAL MOBILITY, IMPAIRED**
May be related to:	Neuromuscular impairment.
	Limitations imposed by condition.
	Pain.

Possibly evidenced by:	Impaired coordination, limited range of motion.
	Reluctance to attempt movement.
	Decreased muscle strength/control.
DESIRED OUTCOMES/ EVALUATION CRITERIA— PATIENT WILL:	Demonstrate techniques/behaviors that enable resumption of activities.
	Maintain or increase strength and function of body.
	Verbalize understanding of situation, treatment regimen, and safety measures.

ACTIONS/INTERVENTIONS	RATIONALE
Independent	
Schedule activity/procedures with rest periods. Encourage participation in ADLs within individual limitations.	Enhances healing and builds muscle strength and endurance. Patient participation promotes independence and sense of control.
Provide/assist with passive and active range of motion exercises dependent on surgical procedure.	Strengthens abdominal muscles and flexors of spine; promotes good body mechanics.
Assist with activity/progressive ambulation.	Until healing occurs activity is limited and progressed slowly according to individual tolerance.

(Refer to CP: Herniated Nucleus Pulposus, ND: Physical Mobility, impaired, p 322, for further considerations.)

NURSING DIAGNOSIS:	**CONSTIPATION**
May be related to:	Pain and swelling in surgical area.
	Immobilization, decreased physical activity.
	Altered nerve stimulation, ileus.
	Emotional stress, lack of privacy.
	Changes/restriction of dietary intake.
Possibly evidenced by:	Decreased bowel sounds.
	Increased abdominal girth.
	Reports of abdominal/rectal fullness, nausea.
	Abdominal pain.
	Change in frequency, consistency, and amount of stool.
DESIRED OUTCOMES/ EVALUATION CRITERIA— PATIENT WILL:	Reestablish normal patterns of bowel functioning.
	Pass stool of soft/semiformed consistency without straining.

ACTIONS/INTERVENTIONS	RATIONALE
Independent	
Note abdominal distention and auscultate bowel sounds.	Distention and absence of bowel sounds indicate that bowel is not functioning, possibly due to sudden loss of parasympathetic enervation of the bowel.
Use fracture- or child-size bedpan until allowed out of bed.	Promotes comfort, reduces muscle tension.
Provide privacy.	Promotes psychologic comfort.
Encourage ambulation as able.	Stimulates peristalsis, facilitating passage of flatus.
Collaborative	
Begin progressive diet as tolerated.	Solid foods are not started until bowel sounds have returned/flatus passed and danger of ileus formation has abated.
Provide rectal tube, suppositories, and enemas as needed.	May be necessary to relieve abdominal distention, promote resumption of normal bowel habits.
Administer laxatives, stool softeners as indicated.	Softens stools, promotes normal bowel habits, decreases straining.

NURSING DIAGNOSIS:	URINARY RETENTION, HIGH RISK FOR
Risk factors may include:	Pain and swelling in operative area. Need for remaining flat in bed.
Possibly evidenced by:	[Not applicable; presence of signs and symptoms establishes an actual diagnosis.]
DESIRED OUTCOMES/ EVALUATION CRITERIA— PATIENT WILL:	Empty bladder adequately according to individual need.

ACTIONS/INTERVENTIONS	RATIONALE
Independent	
Observe and record amount/time of voiding.	Determines whether bladder is being emptied and when interventions may be necessary.
Palpate for bladder distention.	May indicate urine retention.
Force fluids.	Maintains kidney function.
Stimulate bladder emptying by running water, pouring warm water over peritoneal area, putting hand in warm water as needed.	Promotes urination by relaxing urinary sphincter.
Collaborative	
Catheterize for bladder residual after voiding when indicated. Insert/maintain indwelling catheter as needed.	Intermittent or continuous catheterization may be necessary for several days postoperatively, until swelling is decreased.

333

NURSING DIAGNOSIS:	KNOWLEDGE DEFICIT [LEARNING NEED], REGARDING CONDITION, PROGNOSIS, AND TREATMENT NEEDS
May be related to:	Lack of exposure.
	Information misinterpretation; lack of recall.
	Unfamiliarity with information resources.
Possibly evidenced by:	Request for information.
	Statement of misconception.
	Inaccurate follow-through of instruction.
DESIRED OUTCOMES/ EVALUATION CRITERIA— PATIENT WILL:	Verbalize understanding of condition, prognosis, and therapeutic regimen.
	Participate in treatment regimen.
	Initiate necessary lifestyle changes.

ACTIONS/INTERVENTIONS	RATIONALE
Independent	
Review particular condition/prognosis.	Individual needs dictate tolerance levels/limitations of activity.
Discuss return to activities, stressing importance of increasing as tolerated.	Although the recuperative period may be lengthy, following prescribed activity program promotes muscle and tissue circulation, healing, and strengthening.
Encourage development of regular exercise program, e.g., walking.	Promotes healing, strengthens abdominal and erector muscles to provide support to the spinal column, and enhances general physical and emotional well-being.
Discuss importance of good posture and avoidance of prolonged standing/sitting. Recommend sitting in straight-backed chair with feet on a footstool or flat on the floor.	Prevents further injuries/stress by maintaining proper alignment of spine.
Stress importance of avoiding activities that increase the flexion of the spine, e.g., climbing stairs, automobile driving/riding, bending at the waist with knees straight, lifting more than 5 lb, engaging in strenuous exercise/sports. Discuss limitations on sexual relations/positions.	Flexing/twisting of the spine aggravates the healing process and increases risk of injury to spinal cord.
Encourage lying-down rest periods, balanced with activity.	Reduces general and spinal fatigue and assists in the healing/recuperative process.
Discuss possibility of unrelieved/renewed pain.	Some pain may continue for several months as activity level increases and scar tissue stretches. Pain relief from surgical procedure could be temporary if other disks have similar amount of degeneration.

ACTIONS/INTERVENTIONS	RATIONALE
Independent	
Discuss use of heat, e.g., warm packs, heating pad, or showers.	Increased circulation to the back/surgical area transports nutrients for healing to the area and resolution of pathogens/exudates out of the area. Decreases muscle spasms that may result from nerve root irritation during healing process.
Discuss judicious use of cold packs before/after stretching activity, if indicated.	May decrease muscle spasm in some instances more effectively than heat.
Avoid tub baths for 3–4 weeks, depending on physician recommendation.	Tub baths increase risk of flexing/twisting of spine as well as danger of falls.
Review dietary/fluid needs.	Should be tailored to reduce risk of constipation and avoid excess weight gain while meeting nutrient needs to facilitate healing.
Review/reinforce incisional care.	Correct care promotes healing, reduces risk of wound infection.
Identify signs/symptoms requiring notification of health care provider, e.g., fever, increased incisional pain, inflammation, wound drainage, decreased sensation/motor activity in extremities.	Prompt evaluation and intervention may prevent complications/permanent injury.
Discuss necessity of follow-up care.	Long-term medical supervision may be needed to manage problems/complications and to reincorporate individual into desired/altered lifestyle and activities.
Review need for/use of immobilization device, as indicated.	Correct application and wearing time is important to gaining the most benefit from the brace.
Assess current lifestyle/job, finances, activities at home and leisure.	Knowledge of current situation allows nurse to highlight areas for possible intervention, such as referral for occupational/vocational testing and counseling.
Listen/communicate with patient regarding alternatives and lifestyle changes. Be sensitive to patient's needs.	Laminectomy and low back pain are a frequent cause of chronic disability. Many patients may have to stop/modify work, creating marital/financial crises. Often the concern that the patient is a malingerer creates further problems in social relationships.
Note overt/covert expressions of concern about sexuality.	Although patient may not ask directly, there may be concerns about the effect of this surgery on not only ability to cope with usual role in the family/community but also ability to perform sexually.
Explore limitations/abilities.	Placing limitations into perspective with abilities allows the patient to understand own situation and exercise choice.
Provide written copy of all instructions.	Useful as a reference after discharge.
Refer to community resources as indicated, e.g., social services, rehabilitation/vocational counseling services.	A team effort can be helpful in providing support during recuperative period.

335

ACTIONS/INTERVENTIONS	RATIONALE
Independent	
Refer for counseling, sex therapy, psychotherapy, as indicated.	Depression is common in illness for which lengthy recuperative time (2–9 months) is expected. Therapy may alleviate further anxiety, assist patient to cope effectively, and enhance healing process. Presence of physical limitations, pain, and depression may negatively impact sexual desire/performance and add additional stress to relationship.

Spinal Cord Injury (Acute Rehabilitative Phase) _____

Spinal cord lesions are classified as complete (total loss of sensation and voluntary motor function) and incomplete (mixed loss of sensation and voluntary motor function).

Physical findings will vary, depending on the level of injury, degree of spinal shock, and phase and degree of recovery:

C1–3: Quadriplegia with total loss of muscular/respiratory function.
C4–5: Quadriplegia with impairment, poor pulmonary capacity, complete dependency for ADLs.
C6–7: Quadriplegia with some arm/hand movement allowing some independence in ADLs.
C7–8: Quadriplegia with limited use of thumb/fingers, increasing independence.
T1–L1: Paraplegia with intact arm function and varying function of intercostal and abdominal muscles.
L1–2 or below: Mixed motor-sensory loss; bowel and bladder dysfunction.

RELATED CONCERNS:

Disk Surgery, p 327
Fractures, p 772
Pneumonia, p 162
Psychosocial Aspects of Acute Care, p 899
Pulmonary Embolism, p 174
Thrombophlebitis, p 135
Total Nutritional Support, p 1039
Upper Gastrointestinal/Esophageal Bleed, p 454
Ventilatory Assistance (Mechanical), p 226

PATIENT ASSESSMENT DATA BASE

ACTIVITY/REST

May exhibit: Paralysis of muscles (flaccid during spinal shock) at/below level of lesion.
Muscle/generalized weakness (cord contusion and compression).

CIRCULATION

May report: Palpitations.
Dizziness with position changes.

May exhibit: Low BP, postural BP changes, bradycardia. Cool, pale extremities.
Absence of perspiration in affected area.

ELIMINATION

May exhibit: Incontinence of bladder and bowel..
Urinary retention.
Abdominal distention; loss of bowel sounds.
Melena, coffee-ground emesis/hematemesis.

EGO INTEGRITY

May report: Denial, disbelief, sadness, anger.
May exhibit: Fear, anxiety, irritability, withdrawal.

FOOD/FLUID

May exhibit: Abdominal distention; loss of bowel sounds (paralytic ileus).

HYGIENE

May exhibit: Variable level of dependence in ADLs.

NEUROSENSORY

May report: Numbness, tingling, burning, twitching of arms/legs.

May exhibit: Flaccid paralysis (spasticity may develop as spinal shock resolves, dependent on area of cord involvement).

Loss of sensation (varying degrees may return after spinal shock resolves).

Loss of muscle/vasomotor tone.

Loss of/asymmetric reflexes, including deep-tendon.

Changes in pupil reaction, ptosis of upper eyelid.

Loss of sweating in affected area.

PAIN/COMFORT

May report: Pain/tenderness in muscles.

Hyperesthesia immediately above level of injury.

May exhibit: Vertebral tenderness, deformity.

RESPIRATION

May report: Shortness of breath, "air hunger", inability to breathe.

May exhibit: Shallow/labored respirations; periods of apnea.

Diminished breath sounds, rhonchi.

Pallor, cyanosis.

SAFETY

May exhibit: Temperature fluctuations (taking on temperature of environment).

SEXUALITY

May report: Expressions of concern about return to normal functioning.

May exhibit: Uncontrolled erection (priapism).

Menstrual irregularities.

TEACHING/LEARNING

Discharge Plan Considerations: **DRG projected mean length of stay: 7.6 days.**

Will require varying degrees of assistance with transportation, shopping, food preparation, self-care, finances, medications/treatment, and homemaker/maintenance tasks.

May require changes in physical layout of home and/or placement in a rehabilitative center.

DIAGNOSTIC STUDIES

Spinal x-rays: Locates level and type of bony injury (fracture, dislocation); determines alignment and reduction after traction or surgery.

CT scan: Locates injury, evaluates structural alterations.

MRI: Identifies spinal cord lesions, edema, and compression.

Myelogram: May be done to visualize spinal column if pathology is unclear or if occlusion of spinal subarachnoid space is suspected (not usually done after penetrating injuries).

Chest x-ray: Demonstrates pulmonary status (e.g., changes in level of diaphragm, atelectasis).

Pulmonary function studies (vital capacity, tidal volume): Measures maximum volume of inspiration and expiration; especially important in patients with low cervical lesions or thoracic lesions with possible phrenic nerve and intercostal muscle involvement.

ABGs: Indicates effectiveness of gas exchange and ventilatory effort.

NURSING PRIORITIES

1. Maximize respiratory function.
2. Prevent further injury to spinal cord.
3. Promote mobility/independence.
4. Prevent or minimize complications.
5. Support psychologic adjustment of patient/SO.
6. Provide information about injury/prognosis, treatment needs and expectations, possible and preventable complications.

DISCHARGE GOALS

1. Ventilatory effort adequate for individual needs.
2. Spinal injury stabilized.
3. Complications prevented/controlled.
4. Self-care needs met by self/with assistance dependent on specific situation.
5. Beginning to cope with current situation and planning for future.
6. Condition/prognosis, therapeutic regimen, and possible complications understood.

NURSING DIAGNOSIS:	BREATHING PATTERN, INEFFECTIVE, HIGH RISK FOR
Risk factors may include:	Impairment of innervation of diaphragm (lesions at or above C–5).
	Complete or mixed loss of intercostal muscle function.
	Reflex abdominal spasms; gastric distension.
Possibly evidenced by:	[Not applicable; presence of signs and symptoms establishes an actual diagnosis.]
DESIRED OUTCOMES/ EVALUATION CRITERIA— PATIENT WILL:	Maintain adequate ventilation as evidenced by absence of respiratory distress and ABGs within acceptable limits.
	Demonstrate appropriate behaviors to support respiratory effort.

ACTIONS/INTERVENTIONS	RATIONALE
Independent	
Maintain patent airway: keep head in neutral position; elevate head of bed slightly if tolerated; use airway adjuncts as indicated.	Patients with high cervical injury and impaired gag/cough reflexes will require assistance in preventing aspiration/maintaining patent airway.

339

ACTIONS/INTERVENTIONS	RATIONALE

Independent

Suction as necessary. Document quality and quantity of secretions.	If cough is ineffective, suctioning may be needed to remove secretions, enhance gas distribution, and reduce risk of respiratory infections. *Note:* "Routine" suctioning increases risk of hypoxia, bradycardia (vagal response), tissue trauma. Therefore, suctioning needs are based on presence of/inability to move secretions.
Assess respiratory function, by asking patient to take a deep breath. Note presence or absence of spontaneous effort and quality of respirations, e.g., labored, using accessory muscles.	C1–C3 injuries result in complete loss of respiratory function. C4–C5 can result in variable loss of respiratory function, depending on phrenic nerve involvement and diaphragmatic function but generally have decreased vital capacity and inspiratory effort. Injuries below C6–C7 have respiratory muscle function preserved; however, weakness/impairment of intercostal muscles may impair effectiveness of cough, sigh, deep-breathing ability.
Auscultate breath sounds. Note areas of absent or decreased breath sounds or development of adventitious sounds (e.g., rhonchi).	Hypoventilation is common and leads to accumulation of secretions, atelectasis, and peneumonia (frequent complications).
Note strength/effectiveness of cough.	Level of injury determines function of intercostal muscles and ability to cough spontaneously/move secretions.
Assist with coughing (as indicated) by placing hands below diaphragm and pushing upward as patient exhales.	"Quad coughing" is performed to add volume to cough and to facilitate expectoration of secretions or to move them high enough to be suctioned out. *Note:* This procedure is usually performed only in stable persons some distance from acute injury.
Observe skin color for developing cyanosis, duskiness.	May reveal impending respiratory failure, need for immediate medical evaluation and intervention.
Assess for abdominal distension and muscle spasm.	Abdominal fullness may impede diaphragmatic excursion, reducing lung expansion and further compromising respiratory function.
Reposition/turn periodically. Avoid/limit prone position when necessary.	Enhances ventilation of all lung segments, mobilizes secretions, reducing risk of complications, e.g., atelectasis and pneumonia. *Note:* Prone position significantly decreases vital capacity, increasing risk of respiratory compromise, failure.
Encourage fluids (at least 2000 ml/d).	Aids in liquefying secretions, promoting mobilization/expectoration.
Monitor/limit visitors as indicated.	General debilitation and respiratory compromise place patient at increased risk for acquiring upper respiratory infections.
Elicit concerns/questions regarding mechanical ventilation devices.	Acknowledges reality of situation.
Provide honest answers.	Future respiratory function/support needs will not be totally known until spinal shock resolves and acute rehabilitative phase is completed. Even though respiratory support may be required, alter-

ACTIONS/INTERVENTIONS

Independent

Assist patient in "taking control" of respirations as indicated. Instruct in and encourage deep breathing, focusing attention on steps of breathing and so on.

Monitor diaphragmatic movement when phrenic pacemaker is implanted.

Collaborative

Measure/graph:

Vital capacity, tidal volume, inspiratory force;

Serial ABGs and/or pulse oximetry.

Administer oxygen by appropriate method, e.g., nasal prongs, mask, intubation/ventilator.

Refer to/consult with respiratory and physical therapists.

Assist with aggressive chest physiotherapy (e.g., chest percussion) and use of respiratory adjuncts (e.g., incentive spirometer, blow bottles).

RATIONALE

native devices/techniques may be used to enhance mobilityand promote independence.

Breathing may no longer be a totally voluntary activity but require conscious effort, depending on level of injury/involvement of respiratory muscles.

Stimulation of phrenic nerve may enhance respiratory effort, decreasing dependency on mechanical ventilator.

Determines level of respiratory muscle function. Serial measurements may be done to predict impending respiratory failure (acute injury) or determine level of function after spinal shock phase and/or while weaning from ventilatory support.

Documents status of ventilation and oxygenation, identifies respiratory problems, e.g., hypoventilation (low PaO_2/elevated $PaCO_2$) and pulmonary complications.

Method is determined by level of injury, degree of respiratory insufficiency, and amount of recovery of respiratory muscle function after spinal shock phase.

Helpful in identifying exercises individually appropriate to stimulate and strengthen respiratory muscles/effort.

Preventing retained secretions is essential to maximize gas diffusion and to reduce risk of pneumonia.

NURSING DIAGNOSIS:	TRAUMA, HIGH RISK FOR, [ADDITIONAL SPINAL INJURY]
Risk factors may include:	Temporary weakness/instability of spinal column.
Possibly evidenced by:	[Not applicable; presence of signs and symptoms establishes an actual diagnosis.]
DESIRED OUTCOMES/ EVALUATION CRITERIA— PATIENT WILL:	Maintain proper alignment of spine without further spinal cord damage.

ACTIONS/INTERVENTIONS	RATIONALE
Independent	
Maintain bed rest and immobilization device(s), e.g., traction, halo, sandbags, hard/soft cervical collars.	Prevents vertebral column instability and aids healing.
Check skeletal traction apparatus to ensure that frames are secure, pulleys aligned, weights hanging free.	Necessary for maintenance of specified traction for reduction and stabilization of vertebral column and prevention of further spinal cord injury.
Check weights for ordered traction pull (usually 10–20 lb).	Weight pull depends on patient's size and amount of reduction needed to maintain vertebral column alignment.
Elevate head of traction frame or bed as indicated.	Creates counterbalance to maintain both patient's position and traction pull.
Reposition at intervals, using adjuncts for turning and support, e.g., turn sheets, foam wedges, blanket rolls, pillows. Use several staff members when turning/logrolling patient. Follow special instructions for traction equipment, kinetic bed, and frames once halo is in place.	Maintains proper spinal column alignment reducing risk of further trauma. *Note:* Grasping the brace/halo vest to turn or reposition patient may cause additional injury.
Collaborative	
Maintain skeletal traction via tongs, calipers, halo/vest, as indicated.	Reduces vertebral fracture/dislocation.
Prepare for surgery, e.g., spinal laminectomy or fusion, if indicated.	Surgery may be indicated for spinal decompression or removal of bony fragments.

NURSING DIAGNOSIS:	PHYSICAL MOBILITY, IMPAIRED
May be related to:	Neuromuscular impairment.
	Immobilization by traction.
Possibly evidenced by:	Inability to purposefully move; paralysis.
	Muscle atrophy; contractures.
DESIRED OUTCOMES/ EVALUATION CRITERIA— PATIENT WILL:	Maintain position of function as evidenced by absence of contractures, footdrop.
	Increase strength of unaffected/compensatory body parts.
	Demonstrate techniques/behaviors that enable resumption of activity.

ACTIONS/INTERVENTIONS	RATIONALE
Independent	
Continually assess motor function (as spinal shock/edema resolves) by requesting that patient perform actions, e.g., shrug shoulders, spread fingers, squeeze/release examiner's hands.	Evaluates status of individual situation (motor-sensory impairment may be mixed and/or not clear) for a specific level of injury affecting type and choice of interventions.

ACTIONS/INTERVENTIONS	RATIONALE

Independent

Provide means to summon help, e.g., special sensitive call light.	Enables patient to have a sense of control and reduces fear of being left alone. *Note:* Quadriplegic on ventilator requires continuous observation in early management.
Perform/assist with full range of motion exercises on all extremities and joints, using slow smooth movements. Hyperextend hips periodically.	Enhances circulation, restores/maintains muscle tone and joint mobility, and prevents disuse contractures and muscle atrophy.
Position arms at 90-degree angle at regular intervals.	Prevents frozen shoulder contractures.
Maintain ankles at 90 degrees with footboard, high-top tennis shoes, and so on. Use trochanter rolls along thighs when in bed.	Prevents footdrop and external rotation of hips.
Elevate lower extremities at intervals when in chair, or raise foot of bed when permitted in individual situation. Assess for edema of feet/ankles.	Loss of vascular tone and "muscle action" results in pooling of blood and venous stasis in the lower abdomen and lower extremities with increased risk of hypotension and thrombus formation.
Plan activities to provide uninterrupted rest periods. Encourage involvement within individual tolerance/ability.	Prevents fatigue, allowing opportunity for maximal efforts/participation by patient.
Measure/monitor BP before and after activity in acute phases or until stable. Change position slowly. Use cardiac bed or tilt table/circoelectric bed as activity level is advanced.	Orthostatic hypotension may occur as a result of venous pooling (secondary to loss of vascular tone). Side-to-side movement or elevation of head can aggravate hypotension and cause syncope.
Reposition periodically even when sitting in chair. Teach patient how to employ weight-shifting techniques.	Reduces pressure areas, promotes peripheral circulation.
Prepare for weight-bearing activities, e.g., use of tilt table for upright position, strengthening/conditioning exercises for unaffected body parts.	Early weight bearing reduces osteoporotic changes in long bones and reduces incidence of urinary infections and kidney stones.
Encourage use of relaxation techniques.	Reduces muscle tension/fatigue, may help limit pain of muscle spasms, spasticity.
Inspect skin daily. Observe for pressure areas, and provide meticulous skin care. Teach patient to inspect skin surfaces and to use a mirror to look at hard-to-see areas.	Altered circulation, loss of sensation, and paralysis potentiate pressure sore formation. This is a lifelong consideration. (Refer to ND: Skin Integrity, impaired, high risk for, p 354.)
Assist with/encourage pulmonary hygiene, e.g., deep breathing, cough, suction. (Refer to ND: Breathing Pattern, ineffective, p 339.)	Immobility/bed rest increases risk of pulmonary infection.
Assess for deep pain, redness, swelling/muscle tension of calf tissues. Record calf and thigh measurements if indicated.	In a high percentage of patients with cervical cord injury, thrombi develop because of altered peripheral circulation, immobilization, and flaccid paralysis.
Investigate sudden onset of dyspnea, cyanosis, and/or other signs of respiratory distress.	Development of pulmonary emboli may be "silent" because pain perception is altered and/or DVT is not readily recognized.

343

ACTIONS/INTERVENTIONS

Collaborative

Place patient in kinetic therapy bed when appropriate.

Apply antiembolic hose/leotard, sequential compression devices (SCD) to legs.

Consult with physical/occupational therapists, rehabilitation team.

Administer muscle relaxants as indicated, e.g., diazepam (Valium); baclofen (Lioresal); cantrolene (Dantrium).

RATIONALE

Effectively immobilizes unstable spinal column, and improves systemic circulation, which is thought to decrease complications associated with immobility.

Limits pooling of blood in lower extremities or abdomen, thus improving vasomotor tone and reducing incidence of thrombus formation and pulmonary emboli.

Helpful in planning and implementing individualized exercise program and identifying/developing assistive devices to maintain function, enhance mobility and independence.

May be useful in limiting or reducing pain associated with spasticity.

NURSING DIAGNOSIS:	**SENSORY-PERCEPTUAL ALTERATION, [SPECIFY]**
May be related to:	Destruction of sensory tracts with altered sensory reception, transmission, and integration.
	Reduced environmental stimuli.
	Psychologic stress (narrowed perceptual fields caused by anxiety).
Possibly evidenced by:	Measured change in sensory acuity, including position of body parts/proprioception.
	Change in usual response to stimuli.
	Motor incoordination.
	Anxiety, disorientation, bizarre thinking.
	Exaggerated emotional responses.
DESIRED OUTCOMES/ EVALUATION CRITERIA— PATIENT WILL:	Recognize sensory impairments.
	Identify behaviors to compensate for deficits.
	Verbalize awareness of sensory needs and potential for deprivation/overload.

ACTIONS/INTERVENTIONS

Independent

Assess/document sensory function or deficit (by means of touch, pinprick, hot/cold, and so on.) progressing from area of deficit to neurologically intact area.

Protect from bodily harm, e.g., falls, positioning of arm or objects, burns.

RATIONALE

Changes may not occur during acute phase, but as spinal shock resolves, changes should be documented by dermatome charts or anatomic land marks, e.g., "2 inches above nipple line."

Patient may not sense pain or be aware of body position.

ACTIONS/INTERVENTIONS

Independent

Assist the patient to recognize and compensate for alterations in sensation.

Explain procedures prior to and during care, identifying the body part involved.

Provide tactile stimulation, touching patient in intact sensory areas, e.g., shoulders, face, head.

Position patient to see surroundings and activities. Provide prism glasses when prone on turning frame. Talk to patient frequently.

Provide diversional activities, e.g., television, radio, music, liberal visitation. Use clocks, calendars, pictures, bulletin boards, and so on. Encourage SO/family to discuss general and personal news.

Provide uninterrupted sleep and rest periods.

Note presence of exaggerated emotional responses, altered thought processes, e.g., disorientation, bizarre thinking.

RATIONALE

May help reduce anxiety of the unknown and prevent injury.

Enhances patient perception of "whole" body.

Touching conveys caring and fulfills a normal physiologic and psychologic need.

Provides sensory input, which may be severely limited, especially when patient is in prone position.

Aids in maintaining reality orientation and provides some sense of normality in daily passage of time.

Reduces sensory overload, enhances orientation and coping abilities, and aids in reestablishing natural sleep patterns.

Indicative of damage to sensory tracts and/or psychologic stress, requiring further assessment and intervention.

NURSING DIAGNOSIS:	PAIN, [ACUTE]
May be related to:	Physical injury.
	Traction apparatus.
Possibly evidenced by:	Hyperesthesia immediately above level of injury.
	Burning pain below level of injury (paraplegia).
	Muscle spasm/spasticity.
	Phantom pain; headaches.
DESIRED OUTCOMES/ EVALUATION CRITERIA— PATIENT WILL:	Report relief of pain/discomfort.
	Identify ways to manage pain.
	Demonstrate use of relaxation skills and diversional activities as individually indicated.

ACTIONS/INTERVENTIONS

Independent

Assess for presence of pain. Help patient identify and quantify pain, e.g., location, type of pain, intensity on scale of 0–10.

RATIONALE

Patient usually reports pain above the level of injury, e.g., chest/back or headache possibly from stabilizer apparatus. After spinal shock phase, patient may report muscle spasms and phantom pain below level of injury.

ACTIONS/INTERVENTIONS

Independent

Evaluate increased irritability, muscle tension, restlessness, unexplained vital sign changes.

Assist patient in identifying precipitating factors.

Provide comfort measures, e.g., position changes, massage, warm/cold packs, as indicated.

Encourage use of relaxation techniques, e.g., guided imagery, visualization, deep-breathing exercises. Provide diversional activities, e.g., television, radio, telephone, unlimited visitors.

Collaborative

Administer medications as indicated: muscle relaxants, e.g., dantrolene (Dantrium); analgesics; antianxiety, e.g., diazepam (Valium).

RATIONALE

Nonverbal cues indicative of pain/discomfort requiring intervention.

Burning pain and muscle spasms can be precipitated/aggravated by multiple factors, e.g., anxiety, tension, external temperature extremes, sitting for long periods, bladder distention.

Alternate measures for pain control are desirable for emotional benefit, in addition to reducing pain medication needs/undesirable effects on respiratory function.

Refocuses attention, promotes sense of control, and may enhance coping abilities.

May be desired to relieve muscle spasm/pain or to alleviate anxiety and promote rest.

NURSING DIAGNOSIS:	GRIEVING, ANTICIPATORY
May be related to:	Perceived/actual loss of physiopsychosocial well-being.
Possibly evidenced by:	Altered communication patterns.
	Expression of distress, choked feelings, e.g., denial, guilt, fear, sadness; altered affect.
	Alterations in sleep patterns.
DESIRED OUTCOMES/ EVALUATION CRITERIA— PATIENT WILL:	Express feelings and begin to progress through recognized stages of grief, focusing on 1 day at a time.

ACTIONS/INTERVENTIONS

Independent

Identify signs of grieving (e.g., shock, denial, anger, depression).

Shock

Note lack of communication or emotional response, absence of questions.

RATIONALE

Patient experiences many emotional reactions to the injury and its actual/potential impact on life. These stages are not static, and the rate at which the patient progresses through them is variable.

Shock is the initial reaction associated with overwhelming injury. Primary concern is to maintain life, and patient may be too ill to express feelings.

ACTIONS/INTERVENTIONS	RATIONALE

Independent

Provide simple, accurate information to patient and SO regarding diagnosis and care. Be honest: do not give false reassurance while providing emotional support.

Patient's awareness of surroundings and activity may be blocked initially, and attention span may be limited. Little is actually known about the final outcome of the patient's injuries during acute phase, and knowledge may add to frustration and grief of family. Therefore, early focus of emotional support may be directed toward SO.

Encourage expressions of sadness, grief, guilt and fear among patient/SO/friends.

Knowledge that these are appropriate feelings that should be expressed may be very supportive to patient/SO.

Incorporate SO into problem solving and planning for patient's care.

Assists in establishing therapeutic relationships. Provides some sense of control of situation of many losses/forced changes and promotes well-being of patient.

Denial

Assist patient/SO to verbalize feelings about situation, avoiding judgment about what is expressed.

Important beginning step to deal with what has happened. Helpful in identifying patient's coping mechanisms.

Note comments indicating that patient expects to walk shortly and/or is making a bargain with God. Do not confront these comments in early phases of rehabilitation.

Patient may not deny entire disability but may deny its permanency. Situation is compounded by actual uncertainty of outcome, and denial may be useful for coping at this time.

Focus on present needs (e.g., range of motion exercises, skin care).

Attention on "here and now" reduces frustration and hopelessness of uncertain future and may make dealing with today's problems more manageable.

Anger

Identify use of manipulative behavior and reactions to caregivers.

Patient may express anger verbally or physically (e.g., spitting, biting). Patient may say that nothing is done right by caregivers/SO or may pit one caregiver against another.

Encourage patient to take control when possible, e.g., establishing care routines, dietary choices, diversional activities.

Helps reduce anger associated with powerlessness and provides patient with some sense of control and expectation of responsibility for own behavior.

Accept expressions of anger and hopelessness. Avoid arguing. Show concern for the patient.

Patient is acknowledged as a worthwhile individual, and nonjudgmental care is provided.

Set limits on acting-out and unacceptable behavior when necessary (e.g., abusive language, sexually aggressive or suggestive behavior).

Although it is important to express negative feelings, patient and staff need to be protected from violence and embarrassment. This phase is traumatic for all involved, and support of family is essential.

Depression

Note loss of interest in living, sleep disturbance, suicidal thoughts, hopelessness. Listen to but do

Phase may last weeks, months, or even years. Acceptance of these feelings and consistent sup-

ACTIONS/INTERVENTIONS

Independent

not confront these expressions. Let patient know nurse is available for support.

Arrange visit by individual similarly affected, as appropriate.

Collaborative

Consult with/refer to psychiatric nurse, social worker, psychiatrist, pastor.

RATIONALE

port during this phase is important to a satisfactory resolution.

Talking with another person who has shared similar feelings/fears, and survived may help patient reach acceptance of reality of condition and deal with perceived/actual losses.

Patient/SO will need assistance to work through feelings of alienation, guilt, and resentment concerning lifestyle and role changes. The family (required to make adaptive changes to a member who may be permanently "different") will benefit from supportive, long-term assistance and/or counseling in coping with these changes and the future. Patient and SO may suffer great spiritual distress, including feelings of guilt, deprivation of peace, and anger at God, which may interfere with resolution of grief process.

NURSING DIAGNOSIS:	SELF-ESTEEM, SITUATIONAL LOW,
May be related to:	Traumatic injury; situational crisis; forced crisis.
Possibly evidenced by:	Verbalization of forced change in lifestyle.
	Fear of rejection/reaction by others.
	Focus on past strength, function, or appearance.
	Negative feelings about body.
	Feelings of helplessness, hopelessness, or powerlessness.
	Actual change in structure and/or function.
	Lack of eye contact.
	Change in physical capacity to resume role.
	Confusion about self, purpose or direction of life.
DESIRED OUTCOMES/ EVALUATION CRITERIA— PATIENT WILL:	Verbalize acceptance of self in situation.
	Recognize and incorporate changes into self-concept in accurate manner without negating self-esteem.
	Develop realistic plans for adapting to new role/role changes.

ACTIONS/INTERVENTIONS	RATIONALE

Independent

Acknowledge difficulty in determining degree of functional incapacity and/or chance of functional improvement.

During acute phase of injury, long-term effects are unknown, which delays the patient's ability to integrate situation into self-concept.

Listen to patient's comments and responses to situation.

Provides clues to view of self, role changes, and needs and is useful for providing information at patient's level of acceptance.

Assess dynamics of patient and SOs (e.g., patient's role in family, cultural factors).

Patient's previous role in family unit is disrupted or altered by injury, adding to difficulty in integrating self-concept. In addition, issues of independence/dependence need to be addressed.

Encourage SO to treat patient as normally as possible (e.g., discussing home situations, family news).

Involving patient in family unit reduces feelings of social isolation, helplessness, and uselessness and provides opportunity for SO to contribute to patient's welfare.

Provide accurate information. Discuss concerns about prognosis and treatment honestly at patient's level of acceptance.

Focus of information should be on present and immediate needs initially and incorporated into long-term rehabilitation goals. Information should be repeated until patient has assimilated or integrated information.

Discuss meaning of loss or change with patient/SO. Assess interactions between patient and SO.

Actual change in body image may be different from that perceived by patient. Distortions may be unconsciously reinforced by SO.

Accept patient, show concern for individual as a person. Encourage patient, identify strengths, give positive reinforcement for progress noted.

Establishes therapeutic atmosphere for patient to begin self-acceptance.

Include patient/SO in care, allowing patient to make decisions and to participate in self-care activities as possible.

Recognizes that patient is still responsible for own life and provides some sense of control over situation. Sets stage for future lifestyle, pattern, and interaction required in daily care. *Note:* Patient may reject all help or may be completely dependent during this phase.

Be alert to sexually oriented jokes/flirting or aggressive behavior. Elicit concerns, fears, feelings about current situation/future expectations.

Anxiety develops as a result of perceived loss/change in masculine/feminine self-image and role. Forced dependency is often devastating especially in light of change in function/appearance.

Be aware of own feelings/reaction to patient's sexual anxiety.

Behavior may be disruptive, creating conflict between patient/staff, further reinforcing negative feelings and possibly eliminating patient's desire to work through situation/participate in rehabilitation.

Arrange visit by similarly affected person if patient desires and/or situation allows.

May be helpful to patient by providing hope for the future/role model.

Collaborative

Refer to counseling/psychotherapy as indicated, e.g., psychiatric nurse/clinical specialist, psychiatrist, social worker, sex therapist.

May need additional assistance to adjust to change in body image/life.

NURSING DIAGNOSIS:	BOWEL INCONTINENCE/CONSTIPATION
May be related to:	Disruption of innervation to bowel and rectum.
	Perceptual impairment.
	Altered dietary and fluid intake.
	Change in activity level.
Possibly evidenced by:	Loss of ability to evacuate bowel voluntarily.
	Constipation.
	Gastric dilatation, ileus.
DESIRED OUTCOMES/ EVALUATION CRITERIA— PATIENT WILL:	Verbalize behaviors/techniques for individual bowel program.
	Reestablish satisfactory bowel elimination pattern.

ACTIONS/INTERVENTIONS	RATIONALE
Independent	
Auscultate bowel sounds, noting location and characteristics.	Bowel sounds may be absent during spinal shock phase. High tinkling sounds may indicate presence of ileus.
Observe for abdominal distention if bowel sounds are decreased or absent.	Loss of peristalsis (related to impaired innervation) paralyzes the bowel, creating ileus and bowel distention. *Note:* Overdistention of the bowel is a precipitator of autonomic dysreflexia once spinal shock subsides. (Refer to ND: Dysreflexia, high risk for, p 352.)
Note complaints of nausea, onset of vomiting. Check vomitus or gastric secretions (if tube in place) and stools for occult blood.	GI bleeding may occur in response to injury (Cushing's ulcer) or as a side effect of certain therapies (steroids or anticoagulants).
Record frequency, characteristics, and amount of stool.	Identifies degree of impairment/dysfunction and level of assistance required.
Recognize signs of/check for presence of impaction, e.g., no formed stool for several days, semiliquid stool, restlessness, increased feelings of fullness in abdomen.	Early intervention is necessary to effectively treat constipation/retained stool and reduce risk of complications.
Establish regular daily bowel program.	This lifelong program is necessary to routinely evacuate the bowel and usually includes digital stimulation, prune juice and/or warm beverage, and use of stool softeners/suppositories at set intervals. Ability to control bowel evacuation is important to the patient's physical independence and social acceptance
Encourage well-balanced diet that includes bulk and roughage as well as increased fluid intake (at least 2000 ml/d), including fruit juices.	Improves consistency of stool for transit through the bowel.

ACTIONS/INTERVENTIONS	RATIONALE

Independent

Observe for incontinence and help patient relate incontinence to change in diet or routine.

Provide meticulous skin care.

Collaborative

Insert/maintain nasogastric tube and attach to suction if appropriate.

Consult with dietitian/nutritional support team.

Insert rectal tube as needed.

Administer medications as indicated:

Stool softeners, laxatives, suppositories, enemas;

Antacids, cimetidine (Tagamet); ranitidine (Zantac).

Patient can eventually achieve fairly normal routine bowel habits, which enhance independence, self-esteem, and socialization.

Loss of sphincter control and innervation in the area potentiates risk of skin irritation/breakdown.

May be used initially to reduce gastric distention and prevent vomiting (reduces risk of aspiration).

Aids in creating dietary plan to meet individual nutritional needs with consideration of state of digestion/bowel function.

Reduces bowel distention, which may precipitate autonomic responses.

Stimulates peristalsis and routine bowel evacuation when necessary.

Reduces or neutralizes gastric acid to prevent gastric irritation or potential for bleeding.

NURSING DIAGNOSIS:	URINARY ELIMINATION: ALTERED PATTERNS
May be related to:	Disruption in bladder innervation. Bladder atony.
Possibly evidenced by:	Bladder distention; incontinence/overflow, retention. Urinary tract infections. Bladder, kidney stone formation. Renal dysfunction.
DESIRED OUTCOMES/ EVALUATION CRITERIA— PATIENT WILL:	Verbalize understanding of condition. Maintain balanced intake/output with clear, odor-free urine. Verbalize/demonstrate behaviors and techniques to prevent retention/urinary infection.

ACTIONS/INTERVENTIONS	RATIONALE

Independent

Assess voiding pattern, e.g., frequency and amount. Compare urine output with fluid intake. Note specific gravity.

Identifies characteristics of bladder function (e.g., effectiveness of bladder emptying, renal function, and fluid balance).

ACTIONS/INTERVENTIONS	RATIONALE
Independent	
Palpate for bladder distention and observe for overflow.	Bladder dysfunction is variable but may include loss of bladder contraction/inability to relax urinary sphincter, resulting in urine retention and reflux incontinence. *Note:* Bladder distention can precipitate autonomic dysreflexia. (Refer to ND: Dysreflexia, high risk for, below.)
Encourage fluid intake (2–4 L/d), including acid ash juices (e.g., cranberry).	Helps maintain renal function, prevents infection and formation of urinary stones. *Note:* Fluid may be restricted for a period during initiation of intermittent catheterization.
Begin bladder retraining per protocol when appropriate, e.g., fluids between certain hours, digital stimulation of trigger area, contraction of abdominal muscles, Credé's maneuver.	Timing and type of bladder program are dependent on type of injury (upper or lower neuron involvement). *Note:* Credé's maneuver should be used with caution because it may precipitate autonomic dysreflexia.
Observe for cloudy or bloody urine, foul odor.	Signs of urinary tract or kidney infection that can potentiate sepsis.
Cleanse perineal area and keep dry. Provide catheter care as appropriate.	Decreases risk of skin irritation/breakdown and development of ascending infection.
Collaborative	
Keep bladder deflated by means of indwelling catheter initially. Begin intermittent catheterization program when appropriate.	Indwelling catheter is used during acute phase for prevention of urinary retention and for monitoring output. Intermittent catheterization may be implemented to reduce complications usually associated with long-term use of indwelling catheters. A suprapubic catheter may also be inserted for long-term management.
Monitor BUN, creatinine, WBC.	Reflects renal function, identifies complications.
Administer medications as indicated, e.g., vitamin C, and/or urinary antiseptics, e.g., methenamine mandelate (Mandelamine).	Maintains acidic environment and discourages bacterial growth.

NURSING DIAGNOSIS:	**DYSREFLEXIA, HIGH RISK FOR**
Risk factors may include:	Altered nerve function (spinal cord injury at T6 and above).
	Bladder/bowel/skin stimulation (tactile, pain, thermal).
Possibly evidenced by:	[Not applicable; presence of signs and symptoms establishes an actual diagnosis.]
DESIRED OUTCOMES/ EVALUATION CRITERIA— PATIENT WILL:	Recognize signs/symptoms of syndrome.
	Identify preventive/corrective measures.
	Experience no episodes of dysreflexia.

ACTIONS/INTERVENTIONS	RATIONALE

Independent

Identify/monitor precipitating risk factors, e.g., bladder/bowel distention or manipulation; bladder spasms, stones, infection; skin/tissue pressure areas, prolonged sitting position; temperature extremes/drafts.

Visceral distention is the most common cause of autonomic dysreflexia, which is considered an emergency. Treatment of acute episode must be carried out immediately (removing stimulus, treating unresolved symptoms), then interventions and rationale must be geared toward prevention.

Observe for signs/symptoms of syndrome, e.g., changes in vital signs, paroxysmal hypertension, tachycardia, or bradycardia, autonomic responses: sweating, flushing above level of lesion, pallor below injury, chills, gooseflesh, nasal stuffiness, diffuse headache. Note associated complaints/symptoms, e.g., chest pains, blurred vision, nausea, metallic taste, Horner's syndrome.

Early detection and immediate intervention is essential to prevent serious consequences/complications.

Stay with patient during episode.

This is a potentially fatal complication. Continuous monitoring/intervention may reduce patient's level of anxiety.

Monitor BP frequently (3–5 minutes) during acute autonomic dysreflexia, and take action to eliminate stimulus. Continue to monitor BP at intervals after symptoms subside.

Aggressive therapy/removal of stimulus may drop BP rapidly resulting in a hypotensive crisis, especially in those patients who routinely have a low BP. In addition, autonomic dysreflexia may recur, particularly if stimulus is not eliminated.

Elevate head of bed to 45-degree angle or place in sitting position.

Lowers BP to prevent intracranial hemorrhage, seizures, or even death. *Note:* Placing quadriplegic in sitting position automatically lowers BP.

Correct/eliminate causative stimulus as able, e.g., bladder, bowel, skin pressure (including loosening tight leg bands/clothing), temperature extremes.

Removing noxious stimulus usually terminates episode and may prevent more serious autonomic dysreflexia, e.g.: in the presence of sunburn, topical anesthetic should be applied. *Note:* Removal of bowel impaction must be delayed until cardiovascular condition is stablized.

Inform patient/SO of warning signals and how to avoid onset of syndrome, e.g., gooseflesh, sweating, piloerection may indicate full bowel; sunburn may precipitate episode.

This lifelong problem can be largely controlled by the avoidance of pressure from overdistention of visceral organs or pressure on the skin.

Collaborative

Administer medications as indicated and monitor response:

Ganglion blockers, e.g., trimethaphan camsylate (Arfonad);

Blocks excessive autonomic nerve transmission.

Atropine sulfate;

Increases heart rate if bradycardia occurs.

Diazoxide (Hyperstat); hydralazine (Apresoline);

Reduces BP if severe/sustained hypertension occurs.

Nifedipine (Procardia);

Sublingual administration may be effective in absence of IV access for Hyperstat.

ACTIONS/INTERVENTIONS	RATIONALE

Independent

Adrenergic blockers, e.g., methysergide maleate (Sansert);	May be used prophylactically if problem persists/recurs frequently.
Antihypertensives, e.g., prazosin (Minipress), phenoxybenzamine (Dibenzyline).	Long-term use may relax bladder neck/enhance bladder emptying, alleviating the most common cause of chronic autonomic dysreflexia.
Obtain urinary culture as indicated.	Presence of infection may trigger autonomic dysreflexia episode.
Apply local anesthetic ointment to rectum; remove impaction if indicated after symptoms subside.	Ointment blocks further autonomic stimulation and eases later removal of impaction without aggravating symptoms.
Prepare patient for pelvic/pudendal nerve block or posterior rhizotomy if indicated.	Procedures may be considered if autonomic dysreflexia does not respond to other therapies.

NURSING DIAGNOSIS:	**SKIN INTEGRITY, IMPAIRED, HIGH RISK FOR**
Risk factors may include:	Altered/inadequate peripheral circulation; sensation.
	Presence of edema; pressure.
	Altered metabolic state.
	Immobility, traction apparatus.
Possibly evidenced by:	[Not applicable; presence of signs and symptoms establishes an actual diagnosis.]
DESIRED OUTCOMES/ EVALUATION CRITERIA— PATIENT WILL:	Identify individual risk factors.
	Verbalize understanding of treatment needs.
	Participate to level of ability to prevent skin breakdown.

ACTIONS/INTERVENTIONS	RATIONALE

Independent

Inspect all skin areas, noting capillary blanching/refill, redness, swelling. Pay particular attention to back of head, skin under halo frame or vest, and folds where skin continuously touches.	Skin is especially prone to breakdown because of changes in peripheral circulation, inability to sense pressure, immobility, altered temperature regulation.
Observe halo and tong insertion sites. Note swelling, redness, drainage. Cleanse routinely and apply antibiotic ointment per protocol.	These sites are prone to inflammation and infection and provide route for pathologic microorganisms to enter cranial cavity.
Massage and lubricate skin with bland lotion/oil. Protect pressure points by use of heel/elbow pads, lamb's wool, foam padding, egg crate mattress. Use skin hardening agents, e.g., tincture of benzoin, Karaya, Sween cream.	Enhances circulation and protects skin surfaces, reducing risk of ulceration. Quadriplegic and paraplegic patients require lifelong protection from decubiti formation, which can cause extensive tissue necrosis and sepsis.

ACTIONS/INTERVENTIONS	RATIONALE

Independent

Reposition frequently whether in bed or in sitting position. Place in prone position periodically.

Improves skin circulation and reduces pressure time on bony prominences.

Wash and dry skin, especially in high moisture areas such as perineum. Take care to avoid wetting lining of brace/halo vest.

Clean, dry skin is less prone to excoriation/breakdown.

Keep bedclothes dry and free of wrinkles, crumbs.

Reduces/prevents skin irritation.

Encourage continuation of regular exercise program.

Stimulates circulation, enhancing cellular nutrition/oxygenation to improve tissue health.

Elevate lower extremities periodically, if tolerated.

Enhances venous return. Reduces edema formation.

Avoid/limit injection of medication below the level of injury.

Reduced circulation and sensation increase risk of delayed absorption, local reaction, and tissue necrosis.

Collaborative

Provide kinetic therapy or alternating-pressure mattress as indicated.

Improves systemic and peripheral circulation and decreases pressure on skin, reducing risk of breakdown.

NURSING DIAGNOSIS:	KNOWLEDGE DEFICIT [LEARNING NEED] REGARDING CONDITION, PROGNOSIS, AND TREATMENT
May be related to:	Lack of exposure.
	Information misinterpretation.
	Unfamiliarity with information resources.
Possibly evidenced by:	Questions; statement of misconception; request for information.
	Inadequate follow-through of instruction.
	Inappropriate or exaggerated behaviors, e.g., hostile, agitated, apathetic.
	Development of preventable complication(s).
DESIRED OUTCOMES/ EVALUATION CRITERIA— PATIENT WILL:	Participate in learning process.
	Verbalize understanding of condition, prognosis, and treatment.
	Correctly perform necessary procedures and explain reasons for the actions.
	Initiate necessary lifestyle changes and participate in treatment regimen.

ACTIONS/INTERVENTIONS	RATIONALE

Independent

Discuss injury process, current prognosis, and future expectations.

Provides common knowledge base necessary for making informed choices and commitment to the therapeutic regimen.

Provide information and demonstrate:

Positioning;

Promotes circulation; reduces tissue pressure and risk of complications.

Use of pillows/supports, splints.

Keeps spine aligned and prevents/limits contractures improving function and independence.

Encourage continued participation in daily exercise/conditioning program and avoidance of fatigue/chills.

Reduces spasticity, risk of thromboemboli (common complication). Increases mobility, muscle strength/tone for improving organ/body function, e.g., squeezing rubber ball, arm exercises enhance upper body strength to increase independence in transfers/wheelchair mobility; tightening/contracting rectum or vaginal muscles improves bladder control; pushing abdomen up, bearing down, contracting abdomen strengthens trunk and improves GI function (paraplegic).

Have SO/caregivers participate in patient care and demonstrate proper procedures, e.g., applications of splints, braces, suctioning, positioning, skin care, transfers, bowel/bladder program, checking temperature of bath water and food.

Allows home caregivers to become adept and more comfortable with the care tasks they are called on to provide and reduces risk of injury/complications.

Recommend applying abdominal binder before arising (quadriplegic) and remind to change position slowly. Use safety belt during bed-to-wheelchair transfers and adequate number of people.

Reduces pooling of blood in abdomen/pelvis, minimizing postural hypotension. Protects the patient from falls and/or injury to caregivers.

Instruct in proper skin care, inspecting all skin areas daily, using adequate padding (foam, silicone gel, water pads) in bed and chair, and keeping skin dry.

Reduces skin irritation, decreasing incidence of decubitus (patient must manage this throughout life).

Discuss necessity of preventing excessive diaphoresis by using tepid bath water, providing comfortable environment (e.g., fans), removing excess clothes.

Reduces skin irritation/possible breakdown.

Review dietary needs including adequate bulk and roughage. Problem solve solutions to alterations in muscular strength/tone and GI function.

Provides adequate nutrition to meet energy needs and promote healing, prevent complications (e.g., constipation, abdominal distention/gas formation).

Review medication regimen. Recommend avoidance of OTC drugs without approval of health care provider.

Enhances patient safety and may improve cooperation with specific regimen.

Discuss ways to identify and manage autonomic dysreflexia.

Patient may be able to recognize signs, but caregivers need to understand how to prevent precipitating factors and know what to do if autonomic dysreflexia occurs. (Refer to ND: Dysreflexia, high risk for, p 352.)

Identify symptoms to report immediately to health care provider, e.g., infection of any kind, especially

Early identification allows for intervention to prevent/minimize complications.

ACTIONS/INTERVENTIONS

Independent

urinary, respiratory; skin breakdown; unresolved autonomic dysreflexia; suspected pregnancy.

Stress importance of continuing with rehabilitation team to achieve specific functional goals as well as long-term monitoring of therapy needs.

Evaluate home layout and make recommendations for necessary changes. Identify equipment/medical supply needs and resources.

Discuss sexual activity and reproductive concerns.

Identify community resources/supports, e.g., health agencies, VNA, financial counselor; service organizations, Spinal Cord Injury Foundation.

Coordinate cooperation among community/rehabilitation resources.

Arrange for transmitter/emergency call system.

Plan for alternate caregivers as needed.

RATIONALE

No matter what the level of injury, individual may ultimately be able to exercise some independence, e.g., manipulate electric wheelchair with mouth stick (C3–C4); be independent for dressing, transfers to bed, car, toilet (C7); total wheelchair independence (C8–T4). Over time, new discoveries continue to impact equipment/therapy needs and patient's potential.

Physical changes may be required to accommodate both patient and support equipment. Prior arrangements facilitate the transfer to the home setting.

Concerns about individual sexuality/resumption of activity is frequently an *unspoken* concern that needs to be addressed. Spinal cord injury affects all areas of sexual functioning. In addition, choice of contraception is impacted by level of spinal cord injury and side effects/adverse complications of specific method. Finally, some female patients may develop autonomic dysreflexia during intercourse or labor/delivery.

Enhances independence, assisting with home management, respite for caregivers.

Various agencies/therapists/individuals in community may be involved in the long-term care and safety of the patient, and coordination can ensure that needs are not overlooked and optimal level of rehabilitation is achieved.

Provides for safety and access to emergency assistance and equipment.

May be needed to provide respite if regular caregivers are ill or other unplanned emergencies arise.

NEUROLOGIC: Spinal Cord Injury (Acute Rehabilitative Phase)

357

Guillain-Barré Syndrome (Acute Polyneuritis) _____

Guillain-Barré is an acute progressively worsening neuromuscular weakness that may lead to complete, but usually temporary paralysis. The initial phase begins with onset of symptoms and usually peaks in 2–3 weeks. When no further deterioration is noted the condition plateaus. The second phase lasts several days to 2 weeks. The recovery phase may last 4–6 months and possibly up to 2 years. Recovery is spontaneous and complete in most patients, although some residual neurologic deficits can persist.

RELATED CONCERNS:

Pneumonia, p 162
Psychosocial Aspects of Acute Care, p 899
Pulmonary Embolism, p 174
Sepsis/Septicemia, p 887
Thrombophlebitis, p 135
Total Nutritional Support, p 1039
Ventilatory Assistance (Mechanical), p 226

PATIENT ASSESSMENT DATA BASE

ACTIVITY/REST

May report:	Symmetrical weakness and paralysis, usually beginning in lower extremities and progressing rapidly upward.
	Tripping, falling.
	Loss of fine motor control of hands.
May exhibit:	Muscle weakness, flaccid paralysis (symmetric).
	Unsteady gait.

CIRCULATION

May exhibit:	Changes in BP (hypertension or hypotension).
	Dysrhythmias, tachycardia/bradycardia.
	Flushing, diaphoresis.

EGO INTEGRITY

May report:	Feelings of anxiety, concern.
May exhibit:	Fear, confusion.

ELIMINATION

May report:	Changes in usual pattern of elimination.
May exhibit:	Weakness of abdominal muscles.
	Loss of anal/bladder sensation and sphincter reflex.

FOOD/FLUID

May report:	Difficulty chewing, swallowing.
May exhibit:	Impaired gag/swallow reflex.

NEUROSENSORY

May report:
Numbness, tingling beginning in toes or fingers and ascending upward (stocking or glove distribution).

Impaired sense of position, vibration, pain, temperature.

Changes in visual acuity.

May exhibit:
Diminished/absent deep tendon reflexes.

Loss of muscle tone, problem with balance.

Facial weakness, eyelid ptosis (cranial nerve involvement).

Loss of ability to speak.

PAIN/COMFORT

May report:
Muscle tenderness; burning, aggravating, aching, pain (especially in shoulders, pelvis, thighs, back, buttocks).

Hypersensitivity to touch.

RESPIRATION

May report:
Difficulty breathing, shortness of breath.

May exhibit:
Shallow respirations, use of accessory muscles, apnea.

Decreased/absent breath sounds.

Reduced vital capacity.

Pallor/cyanosis.

Impaired gag/swallow/cough reflexes.

SAFETY

May report:
Nonspecific viral infection (e.g., upper respiratory infection) approximately 2 weeks prior to onset of symptoms.

History of herpes zoster, cytomegalovirus.

May exhibit:
Fluctuation in body temperature (takes on temperature of the environment).

Decreased muscle strength/tone, paralysis, paresthesia.

SOCIAL INTERACTION

May exhibit:
Loss of ability to speak/communicate.

TEACHING/LEARNING

May report:
Recent illness (upper respiratory infection, gastroenteritis); vaccinations (smallpox, influenza); chronic conditions (lupus erythematosus, Hodgkin's/malignant process); surgery/general anesthesia; trauma.

Discharge Plan Considerations:
DRG projected length of stay: 6 days.

May require assistance with transportation, food preparation, self-care, and homemaker/maintenance tasks. Possible change in layout of home, transfer to rehabilitation setting.

DIAGNOSTIC STUDIES

Serial lumbar puncture: Demonstrates classic phenomenon of normal pressure and normal number of white cells, with elevating protein levels that peak in 4–6 weeks. Because protein elevation may not usually appear in first 4–5 days, serial lumbar punctures may be indicated.

Electromyelography: Results depend on stage and progression of syndrome. Nerve conduction velocity may be slowed. Fibrillations (repetitive firing of the same motor unit) are more common in later stage.

CBC: May reveal leukocytosis during early stage.

Chest x-ray: May demonstrate progressive signs of respiratory involvement, e.g., atelectatic areas, pneumonia.

Pulmonary function studies: May reveal decreased vital capacity, tidal volume, and inspiratory force.

NURSING PRIORITIES

1. Maintain/support respiratory function.
2. Minimize/prevent complications.
3. Provide emotional support to patient/SO.
4. Control/eliminate pain.
5. Provide information about disease process/prognosis and treatment needs.

DISCHARGE GOALS

1. Respiratory function adequate for individual needs.
2. ADL needs met by self or with assistance of others.
3. Complications prevented/controlled.
4. Anxiety/fear reduced to manageable level.
5. Pain minimized/controlled.
6. Disease process/prognosis, therapeutic regimen, and possible complications understood.

NURSING DIAGNOSIS:	BREATHING PATTERN/AIRWAY CLEARANCE, INEFFECTIVE, HIGH RISK FOR
Risk factors may include:	Weakness/paralysis of respiratory muscles. Impaired gag/swallow reflexes.
Possibly evidenced by:	[Not applicable; presence of signs and symptoms establishes an actual diagnosis.]
DESIRED OUTCOMES/ EVALUATION CRITERIA— PATIENT WILL:	Demonstrate adequate ventilation with absence of signs of respiratory distress, breath sounds clear, and ABGs within acceptable limits.

ACTIONS/INTERVENTIONS	RATIONALE
Independent	
Monitor respiratory rate, depth, symmetry. Note increased work of breathing and observe color of skin and mucous membranes.	Increased respiratory distress indicates advancing muscular weakness and/or paralysis, which can result in the need for ventilatory support.
Assess sensation especially noting diminished response at T8 or upper arm/shoulder area.	Decreased sensation often (although not always) precedes motor weakness; e.g., loss at T8 level can affect intercostal muscles, whereas arm/shoulder involvement often precedes respiratory failure.

ACTIONS/INTERVENTIONS	RATIONALE

Independent

Note breathlessness while talking.	Good indicator of interference with respiratory function/diminishing vital capacity.
Auscultate breath sounds, noting absence/development of adventitious sounds, e.g., rhonchi, wheezes.	Increased airway resistance and/or accumulation of secretions will impede gas diffusion and lead to pulmonary complications (e.g., pneumonia).
Elevate head of bed or place patient in supported sitting position.	Enhances lung expansion and cough efforts, decreases work of breathing, and limits risk of aspiration of secretions.
Evaluate gag/swallow/cough reflexes periodically. Suction secretions, noting color and amount of secretions. Keep NPO if necessary.	Once muscles of head and neck are involved, frequent reevaluation of reflexes must be carried out for prevention of aspiration, pulmonary infections, and respiratory failure. Loss of muscle strength and function may result in inability to maintain and/or clear airway.
Investigate reports of dyspnea, chest pain and note increased restlessness.	These patients are at risk for PE (as a result of vascular pooling and immobility), requiring prompt interventions and respiratory support to prevent serious complications/death.
Monitor serial vital capacity, tidal volume, and inspiratory force as indicated.	Detects worsening of muscle paralysis and declining respiratory effort.

Collaborative

Monitor/graph serial ABGs, pulse oximetry.	Determines effectiveness of current ventilation and need for/effectiveness of interventions.
Review chest x-rays.	Reveals changes indicative of pulmonary congestion and/or atelectasis.
Administer supplemental humidified oxygen as indicated, using appropriate route, e.g., cannula, mask, mechanical ventilator.	Treats hypoxemia. Humidity loosens secretions and keeps mucous membranes moist, thereby reducing irritation of airways.
Administer/assist with pulmonary hygiene measures, e.g., breathing exercises/adjuncts, chest percussion, vibration, and postural drainage.	Improves ventilation and reduces atelectasis by mobilizing secretions and enhancing expansion of alveoli.
Provide kinetic therapy bed as indicated.	Continuous movement/position change may be used to enhance circulation and oxygenation of lung segments and to mobilize secretions. This can reduce atelectasis and risk of pulmonary infection and/or emboli.
Prepare for/maintain intubation, mechanical ventilation, as indicated.	10%–20% of patients suffer significant respiratory involvement requiring aggressive interventions/support.
Provide tracheostomy care when present.	May be needed for airway and secretion management. "Talking" tracheostomy may be inserted to facilitate communication, although muscle weakness and copious secretions can limit its effectiveness.

NURSING DIAGNOSIS:	SENSORY-PERCEPTUAL ALTERATION [SPECIFY]
May be related to:	Altered sensory reception, transmission, and/or integration.
	Altered status of sense organs.
	Inability to communicate, speak, or respond.
	Chemical alteration (hypoxia, electrolyte imbalance).
Possibly evidenced by:	Hypoesthesias/hyperesthesias; pain.
	Change in usual response to stimuli.
	Motor incoordination.
	Restlessness, irritability, anxiety.
	Altered communication patterns.
DESIRED OUTCOMES/ EVALUATION CRITERIA— PATIENT WILL:	Verbalize awareness of sensory deficits.
	Maintain usual mentation/orientation.
	Identify interventions to minimize sensory impairments/ complications.

ACTIONS/INTERVENTIONS	RATIONALE
Independent	
Monitor neurologic status periodically (e.g., ability to speak, respond to simple commands and painful stimuli; awareness of hot/cold, dull/sharp). Record serial findings on flow sheets.	Progression and regression of symptoms may vary greatly. Progression is often quite rapid and may peak in a few days/weeks. Onset of recovery usually begins 2–4 weeks after disease progression stops and is much slower. Flow charts are helpful in alerting nurses to impending complications requiring further evaluation/intervention.
Provide alternate means of communication if patient cannot speak, e.g., "blink method," alphabet/picture boards.	If syndrome develops slowly, patient can help establish preferred method of communication. If process is sudden (hours/days), consistent and constant effort on the part of the staff is required to establish effective communication.
Provide safe environment (side rails, protection from thermal injury). Note deficits on chart in room to alert *all* caregivers, e.g., "absence of sensation below. . . ."	Loss of sensation and motor control leaves patient at the mercy of all caregivers, who must maintain a therapeutic environment and prevent injury.
Allow for undisturbed periods of rest and provide diversional activities within patient ability.	Reduces excessive stimuli, which can greatly increase anxiety and diminish coping abilities.
Reorient patient to environment and staff as indicated.	Helps reduce anxiety and is especially helpful if visual deficit is present.
Provide appropriate sensory stimulation, including familiar sounds (music); clocks (time); television (news/entertainment); conversation.	Patient (who is usually conscious) can feel completely isolated as paralysis progresses and during lengthy recovery phase.

ACTIONS/INTERVENTIONS

Independent

Encourage SOs to talk to and touch patient and to keep abreast of family events.

Patch eyes on a rotating basis if ptosis is present.

Collaborative

Refer to multiple resources for assistance, e.g., physical/occupational/speech therapists, pastoral care, social service, rehabilitation departments.

Assist with plasmapheresis as indicated.

Administer medications as indicated, e.g.:

High dose gamma globulin IV;

Corticosteroids.

RATIONALE

Helps SO to feel involved in patient's life (reduces feelings of helplessness/hopelessness) and may reduce patient's anxiety regarding family during separation.

Maintains visual input while decreasing risk of corneal abrasions.

All services/departments coordinate efforts to promote recovery/minimize residual neurologic deficits.

This treatment removes immunoglobulins, complement, fibrinogen, and acute phase proteins, which shorten the duration of illness and respiratory depression for patients classified as "severe" when treatment is begun within 2 weeks.

Research suggests this may enhance antibody response in the presence of severe involvement.

Use is controversial. May improve acute symptoms by suppressing the autoimmune response but not overall outcome.

NURSING DIAGNOSIS:	TISSUE PERFUSION, ALTERED, HIGH RISK FOR
Risk factors may include:	Autonomic nervous system dysfunction, causing vascular pooling with decreased venous return.
	Hypovolemia.
	Interruption of venous blood flow (thrombosis).
Possibly evidenced by:	[Not applicable; presence of signs and symptoms establishes an actual diagnosis.]
DESIRED OUTCOMES/ EVALUATION CRITERIA— PATIENT WILL:	Maintain perfusion with stable vital signs, cardiac dysrhythmias controlled/absent.

ACTIONS/INTERVENTIONS

Independent

Auscultate BP, noting wide fluctuations. Observe for postural hypotension. Exercise care when changing patient's position.

RATIONALE

Changes in BP (severe hypertension/hypotension) occur because of loss of sympathetic outflow to maintain peripheral vascular tone (autonomic dysfunction). Reflexes to adjust BP during position changes (side to side) may be impaired, causing postural hypotension.

ACTIONS/INTERVENTIONS	RATIONALE
Independent	
Monitor heart rate and rhythm. Document dysrhythmias.	Sinus tachycardia/bradycardia may develop because of impaired sympathetic innervation or unopposed vagal stimulation, leading to cardiac arrest. Dysrhythmias can also occur because of hypoxemia, electrolyte imbalance, or reduced cardiac output (secondary to altered vascular tone and venous return).
Monitor body temperature. Provide comfortable environmental temperature, add or remove blankets, use room fans, and so on.	Changes in vasomotor tone create difficulties with temperature regulation (e.g., inability to perspire), and patient may take on temperature of surrounding environment. Warming and cooling should be done with caution to prevent hot or cold injury inasmuch as the patient may have impaired sensation.
Document intake and output.	Relaxation of vascular tone, fluid shifts, and reduced oral intake can decrease circulating volume, negatively affecting BP and urine output.
Change position frequently. Observe skin for signs of irritation. Massage skin over bony prominences. Keep linens dry, wrinkle-free. Wash and dry skin with mild soap, and apply emollients. Provide sheepskin pads as indicated.	Changes in circulation/vascular pooling impair cellular perfusion, increasing risk of tissue ischemia/breakdown.
Elevate foot of bed slightly. Provide passive exercise for ankle/foot. Observe calf for edema, erythema, positive Homans' sign.	Loss of vascular tone and venous stasis increase risk of thrombus formation. *Note:* DVT (which may go unrecognized because the patient cannot sense discomfort) can lead to pulmonary emboli if not detected and promptly treated.
Collaborative	
Administer:	
IV fluids with caution as indicated;	May be needed to correct/prevent hypovolemia/hypotension, but should be used cautiously because patient with impaired vascular tone may be sensitive to even small increases in circulating volume.
Medications: e.g; short-acting antihypertensive drugs;	Occasionally used to alleviate persistent hypertension or mediate autonomic disturbances.
Heparin.	May be used to reduce risk of thrombophlebitis.
Monitor laboratory studies, e.g., CBC or Hb/Hct, serum electrolytes.	Hct is useful in determining hypovolemia/hypervolemia. Hyponatremia may develop, suggesting complication of SIADH.
Provide alternating pressure mattress, kinetic therapy bed, flotation mattress, as indicated.	Enhances circulation and prevents skin complications. *Note:* Kinetic therapy is widely thought to enhance organ perfusion/function and to reduce complications of immobility.
Apply antiembolic stockings or sequential compression devices; remove at scheduled intervals.	Promotes venous return, reduces venous stasis, lessens risk of thrombus formation.

NURSING DIAGNOSIS:	PHYSICAL MOBILITY, IMPAIRED
May be related to:	Neuromuscular impairment.
Possibly evidenced by:	Loss of coordination; partial/complete paralysis.
	Decreased muscle tone/strength.
DESIRED OUTCOMES/ EVALUATION CRITERIA— PATIENT WILL:	Maintain position of function with absence of complications (contractures, decubiti).
	Increase strength and function of affected parts.
	Demonstrate techniques/behaviors that enable resumption of desired activities.

ACTIONS/INTERVENTIONS

Independent

Assess motor strength/functional ability on a scale of 0–5. Perform assessments on a regular basis and compare with baseline.

Position for optimum comfort. Reposition on a regular schedule as individually indicated.

Support extremities and joints with pillows, trochanter rolls, footboards.

Perform passive range of motion exercises. Avoid active exercise during acute phase.

Coordinate care to allow frequent and uninterrupted rest periods.

Encourage activity progression, depending on individual tolerance, e.g., sitting on bedside with support, up in chair, then ambulating as able.

Provide lubrication/artificial tears as needed.

Collaborative

Confer with/refer to physical/occupational therapy.

RATIONALE

Determines progression/regression of syndrome, aiding in establishing goals/patient expectations. *Note:* Quadriplegia (symmetric paralysis) commonly occurs, requiring multiple interventions.

Reduces fatigue, promotes relaxation, decreases risk of skin ischemia/breakdown.

Maintains extremities in functional position; prevents contractures and loss of joint function.

Stimulates circulation, improves muscle tone, and promotes joint mobility. *Note:* Vigorous exercise may exacerbate symptoms, causing physiologic and emotional regression. Also, joints may dislocate as muscles are totally flaccid.

Maximizes energy and prevents undue fatigue.

Overtaxing muscles can increase time needed for remyelination, thereby prolonging recovery time.

Gradual/programmed resumption of activity denotes improvement, promotes normalization of organ function, and has a positive psychologic effect.

Prevents drying of delicate tissues when patient is unable to close/blink eyes appropriately.

Useful in creating individualized muscle strengthening/conditioning exercises and gait training program and identifying assistive devices/braces to maintain mobility and independence in ADLs.

NURSING DIAGNOSIS:	CONSTIPATION/DIARRHEA, HIGH RISK FOR
Risk factors may include:	Neuromuscular impairment (loss of anal sensation and reflexes). Immobility. Changes in dietary/fluid intake.
Possibly evidenced by:	[Not applicable; presence of signs and symptoms establishes an actual diagnosis.]
DESIRED OUTCOMES/ EVALUATION CRITERIA— PATIENT WILL:	Maintain usual pattern of bowel elimination with absence of ileus.

ACTIONS/INTERVENTIONS	RATIONALE
Independent	
Encourage fluid intake of at least 2000 ml/d (if patient able to swallow) in frequent small amounts, including fruit juices (apple, prune).	Promotes softer stool and facilitates elimination.
Provide privacy and upright positioning on bed side commode (if possible) at regularly scheduled times.	Enhances bowel evacuation efforts.
Auscultate bowel sounds, noting presence, absence, or change.	Decreased or absent sounds may indicate onset of ileus owing to loss of intestinal motility and/or electrolyte imbalance. Hyperactive bowel sounds may be noted if diarrhea occurs as a side effect of tube feeding or kinetic therapy.
Note abdominal distention, tenderness. Measure abdominal girth as indicated.	May reflect developing ileus or fecal impaction.
Monitor for nausea, vomiting, cessation of stool.	Rate of progression to complete ileus is variable but can be expected.
Check for rectal impaction in presence of diminished/absent stool or diarrhea.	Gentle manual removal of stool may be necessary, along with other interventions, to stimulate bowel evacuation.
Collaborative	
Administer stool softeners, suppositories, laxatives, or use rectal tube as indicated.	Prevents constipation, reduces abdominal distention, and assists in regulation of bowel function.
Increase dietary intake of fiber and bulk or change rate and type of tube feedings when indicated.	Aids in regulating fecal consistency and reduces complications (diarrhea, constipation).
Insert/maintain nasogastric tube if indicated.	Reduces nausea and vomiting and decompresses abdominal distention associated with loss of peristalsis, presence of ileus.

NURSING DIAGNOSIS:	URINARY RETENTION, HIGH RISK FOR
Risk factors may include:	Neuromuscular impairment (loss of sensation and sphincter reflex). Immobility.
Possibly evidenced by:	[Not applicable; presence of signs and symptoms establishes an actual diagnosis.]
DESIRED OUTCOMES/ EVALUATION CRITERIA— PATIENT WILL:	Demonstrate adequate/timely bladder emptying with absence of urinary retention or infection.

ACTIONS/INTERVENTIONS	RATIONALE
Independent	
Record frequency and amount of voidings.	Provides information for assessment of bladder functioning.
Palpate abdomen for bladder distention.	If sphincter reflex is absent, the bladder will fill and become distended.
Encourage fluid intake (at least 2000 ml/within cardiac tolerance) and include acidifying fruit juices (e.g., cranberry).	Maintains glomerular filtration rate and reduces risk of infection and formation of urinary tract stones.
Perform Credé's maneuver.	Manual pressure on the bladder may facilitate emptying.
Collaborative	
Catheterize for residual urine, as indicated.	Monitors effectiveness of bladder emptying.
Insert/maintain indwelling catheter if necessary.	May be required to correct urinary retention or until resolution of Guillain-Barré syndrome and restoration of bladder control.

NURSING DIAGNOSIS:	NUTRITION, ALTERED: LESS THAN BODY REQUIREMENTS, HIGH RISK FOR
Risk factors may include:	Neuromuscular impairment affecting gag/cough/swallow reflexes and GI function.
Possibly evidenced by:	[Not applicable; presence of signs and symptoms establishes an actual diagnosis.]
DESIRED OUTCOMES/ EVALUATION CRITERIA— PATIENT WILL:	Demonstrate stable weight, normalization of laboratory values, and no signs of malnutrition.

ACTIONS/INTERVENTIONS	RATIONALE

Independent

Assess ability to chew, swallow, cough, on a regular basis.

Muscle weakness and hypoactive/hyperactive reflexes can indicate need for alternative methods of feeding, e.g., tube feeding.

Auscultate bowel sounds, evaluate abdominal distention.

Disturbance of gastric function often occurs because of paralysis/immobility.

Record daily caloric intake.

Identifies nutrient deficiencies and needs.

Note patient's food likes/dislikes and involve in dietary choices. Provide soft/semisolid foods instead of fluids.

Promotes sense of control and may enhance feeding efforts. Soft/semisolid foods reduce the risk of choking/aspiration.

Encourage self-feeding if possible. Allow plenty of time for self-directed efforts. Feed/assist patient as needed.

Degree of loss of motor control affects ability to feed self. Self-esteem and sense of control may be enhanced by self-directed efforts even when very limited.

Encourage SO to participate at mealtime, e.g., feeding and bringing food from home.

Provides socialization time, which may enhance patient's food intake.

Weigh periodically.

Assesses effectiveness of dietary regimen.

Collaborative

Provide high-calorie/high-protein beverages, e.g., eggnog, commercial preparations (Ensure).

Supplemental feedings can increase nutritional intake.

Insert/maintain feeding tube. Administer enteral/parenteral feedings.

May be indicated if patient cannot swallow (or if gag/swallow reflexes are impaired) to assure proper nutrient, caloric, electrolyte, and mineral intake.

NURSING DIAGNOSIS:	ANXIETY [SPECIFY]/FEAR
May be related to:	Situational crisis.
	Threat of death/change in health status.
Possibly evidenced by:	Increased tension, restlessness, helplessness.
	Apprehension, uncertainty, fearfulness.
	Focus on self.
	Sympathetic stimulation.
DESIRED OUTCOMES/ EVALUATION CRITERIA— PATIENT WILL:	Acknowledge and discuss fears.
	Verbalize accurate knowledge of the situation.
	Demonstrate appropriate range of feelings and lessened fear.
	Appear relaxed and report anxiety is reduced to a manageable level.

ACTIONS/INTERVENTIONS

Independent

Place close to nurses' station, check on patient frequently. Reassess ability to use call light regularly.

Provide primary nurse/consistent staff assignment.

Provide alternate means of communication, if necessary.

Discuss body image changes, fears of permanent disability, loss of function, dying, concerns regarding discharge needs/placement.

Provide simple explanations of care; plan care with patient, involving SO.

RATIONALE

Provides reassurance that help is readily available if the patient suddenly becomes incapacitated.

Enhances patient's level of trust and helps to reduce anxiety.

Reduces feelings of helplessness and isolation.

Bringing fears out into the open provides opportunity to assess patient perceptions/information/misinformation and to problem solve ways to deal with situation.

Understanding can enhance cooperation in needed activities. Involving patient/SO in care planning restores some sense of control over life, enhancing self-esteem.

NURSING DIAGNOSIS:	PAIN [ACUTE]
May be related to:	Neuromuscular impairment (paresthesia, dysesthesia).
Possibly evidenced by:	Painful sensations induced by gentle touch on skin. Aching, tenderness of muscles/joints. Altered muscle tone (flaccid, spastic). Guarding behavior.
DESIRED OUTCOMES/ EVALUATION CRITERIA— PATIENT WILL:	Report pain is relieved/controlled. Verbalize methods that provide relief. Demonstrate use of relaxation skills as indicated for individual situation.

ACTIONS/INTERVENTIONS

Independent

Evaluate degree of pain/discomfort using 0–10 scale. Observe for nonverbal cues (e.g., facial mask of pain, withdrawal/crying).

Encourage verbalization of feelings about pain.

Provide heat or cold applications, warm baths, massage, or touch as individually tolerated.

Reposition frequently. Provide support by means of pillows, foam inserts, blankets.

RATIONALE

Encourages patient to "localize/quantify" pain, recognizing changes, improvement.

Reduces feelings of isolation, anger, and anxiety that may enhance pain.

Helps patient gain control over the constant discomfort caused by the paresthesias and decreases muscle stiffness/pain.

Helps alleviate fatigue and muscle tension. Note: Some patients prefer to lie on their backs in a "frog-leg" position.

ACTIONS/INTERVENTIONS	RATIONALE

Independent

Provide passive range of motion exercises.	Decreases joint stiffness.
Instruct in/encourage use of relaxation techniques, e.g., visualization, progressive relaxation exercises, guided imagery, biofeedback.	Redirects focus of attention/perception and enhances coping, which may help alleviate pain.

Collaborative

Administer analgesics as indicated. Avoid use of narcotics.	Useful for alleviating pain when other methods do not help. Narcotics (except codeine, which has a lesser effect) should be avoided when possible because of their respiratory depressant and GI side effects.
Assist with alternate therapies, e.g., ultrasound, diathermy, and use of TENS unit.	Sometimes useful in relieving muscle discomfort.

NURSING DIAGNOSIS:	**KNOWLEDGE DEFICIT [LEARNING NEED] REGARDING CONDITION, PROGNOSIS, AND TREATMENT**
May be related to:	Lack of exposure.
	Information misinterpretation.
	Unfamiliarity with information resources.
	Lack of recall, cognitive limitation.
Possibly evidenced by:	Request for information.
	Statement of misconception.
	Development of preventable complications.
DESIRED OUTCOMES/ EVALUATION CRITERIA— PATIENT WILL:	Participate in learning process.
	Initiate necessary lifestyle changes and participate in rehabilitation efforts as individually able.

ACTIONS/INTERVENTIONS	RATIONALE

Independent

Determine patient's level of knowledge and ability to participate in rehabilitation.	Influences choice of interventions.
Review disease process and prognosis. Provide written literature about the syndrome.	Knowledge base necessary to make informed choices and participate in rehabilitation efforts. Although the syndrome is transient, the residual effects may persist for weeks, months, or longer.
Encourage verbalization, socialization, and independence.	Promotes return to sense of normality and developing a life around present circumstances.
Identify safety measures to meet individual sensorimotor deficits.	Reduces risk of injury/preventable complications.

ACTIONS/INTERVENTIONS

Independent

Work with SO to have necessary equipment in the home before patient is discharged.

Stress importance of avoiding persons with infections, especially upper respiratory.

Instruct and assist patient/SO in learning range of motion and conditioning exercises, transfer techniques, good body mechanics, breathing/speech exercises, use of assistive devices.

Review signs/symptoms requiring medical follow-up, e.g., infectious process (urinary tract infection, upper respiratory infection), urinary retention, constipation.

Discuss need for continued follow-up.

Refer to community resources, e.g., VNA, home health agencies, social services, Guillain-Barré Syndrome Foundation.

RATIONALE

If patient is able to return home, care may be facilitated by assistive devices for mobilization, feeding, and bathing.

Patient is immunosuppressed and at risk for development of infections.

Promotes independence and continued recovery. Process often takes 4–6 months for remyelination and up to 2 years if quadriplegia developed.

Prompt intervention can prevent/minimize complications.

Necessary to monitor improvement, identify treatment needs, and promote optimal recovery. Recovery is usually good, with varying degrees of weakness/atrophy remaining, although ⅓ have permanent residual deficits (hyperreflexia, atrophy, distal muscle weakness, facial paresis).

Support may permit/sustain patient in home setting.

Alzheimer's Disease (Non-Substance-Induced Organic Mental Disorders)

Dementia of the Alzheimer type (DAT) is a specific degenerative process occurring primarily in the cells located at the base of the forebrain which send information to the cerebral cortex and hippocampus. The affected cells first lose their capacity to secrete acetylcholine then degenerate. Once this degeneration begins, there is currently nothing that can be done to revive or replace them. The cause remains unknown, although research is being done in several areas, such as genetics, "slow" viruses, and environmental factors. It is the most common form of dementia characterized by a steady and global decline. In comparison, multi-infarct dementia reflects a pattern of intermittent deterioration in the brain with symptoms that fluctuate, are focal, or progress in a stepwise fashion. Deterioration is thought to occur in response to repeated infarcts of the brain. Nursing management of these patients is essentially the same.

RELATED CONCERNS, DEPENDENT ON PRIMARY REASON FOR HOSPITALIZATION:

Congestive Heart Failure, p 48
Fractures, p 772
Pneumonia, p 162
Psychosocial Aspects of Acute Care, p 899
Surgical Intervention, p 918

PATIENT ASSESSMENT DATA BASE

Note: If history is obtained from SO, individual may be uncomfortable speaking of declining abilities/loss of function in presence of patient. A more frank disclosure of information may be achieved by interviewing SO alone.

ACTIVITY/REST

May report:	Feeling tired.
May exhibit:	Day/night reversal; wakefulness/aimless wandering, disturbance of sleep rhythms.
	Lethargy; decreased interest in usual activities, hobbies; inability to recall what is read/follow plot of television program.
	Impaired motor skills; inability to carry out familiar, purposeful movements.

CIRCULATION

May report:	History of systemic/cerebral vascular disease, hypertension, embolic episode (predisposing factors).

EGO INTEGRITY

May report:	Suspicion or fear of imaginary persons/situations.
	Misperception of environment, misidentification of objects and people, hoarding of objects; belief that misplaced objects are stolen.
	Multiple losses, perceived changes in body image, self-esteem.
May exhibit:	Concealing of inabilities (makes excuses not to perform task; may thumb through a book without reading it).
	Content sitting and watching others.
	Main activity may be hoarding inanimate objects, repetitive motions (fold-unfold-refold linen), hiding articles, or wandering.

Emotional lability: cries easily, laughs inappropriately; variable mood changes (apathy, lethargy, restlessness, short attention span, irritability); sudden angry outbursts (catastrophic reactions).

Strong, depressive overlay; delusions; paranoia.

Clinging to SO.

ELIMINATION

May report: Urgency (may indicate loss of muscle tone).

May exhibit: Incontinence of urine/feces; prone to constipation/impaction with diarrhea.

FOOD/FLUID

May report: History of hypoglycemic episodes (predisposing factor).

Changes in taste, appetite, denial of hunger/need to eat.

Weight loss.

May exhibit: Loss of ability to chew.

Avoidance/refusal to eat (may be trying to conceal lost skills).

Emaciation (advanced stage).

HYGIENE

May report: Need for assistance/dependence on others.

May exhibit: Unkempt/disheveled appearance, body order, poor personal habits.

May forget to go to bathroom, forget steps involved in toileting, or be unable to find the bathroom.

Lack of interest in/forgetting of mealtime; dependence on others for food cooking and preparation at table, feeding, using utensils.

NEUROSENSORY

May report: Denial of symptoms, especially cognitive changes, and/or describe vague, hypochondriacal complaints of fatigue, diarrhea, dizziness, or occasional headache. Insidious decline in cognitive abilities, judgment, recent memory, behavior (as observed by SO).

Loss of proprioception sense (location of body/body parts in space).

History of cerebral/systemic vascular disease, embolic/hypoxic episodes (predisposing factors).

Seizure activity (secondary to the brain damage).

May exhibit: Impaired communication: aphasia and dysphasia; difficulty with finding correct words (especially nouns); repetitive questioning or scattered conversation with substituted meaningless words; fragmented, inaudible speech.

Gradual loss of ability to read or write (fine motor skills).

Neurologic status:

> (May laugh at or feel threatened by these examinations; may change answers during the interview.)
>
> Difficulty in comprehension, abstract thinking.
>
> Usually oriented to person until late in the disease.
>
> Impaired recent memory, intact remote memory (early DAT).
>
> Inability to do simple calculations or repeat names of three objects.

Impaired motor skills with tremors, rigidity, unsteady gait.

Primitive reflexes (e.g., positive snout, suck, palmar).

Hallucinations, delusions, severe depression, mania (advanced stage).

SAFETY

May report: History of serious head injury (may be a predisposing/accelerating factor).

Incidental trauma (falls, burns, and so on).

May exhibit: Ecchymosis; lacerations.

Striking out/violence toward others.

SOCIAL INTERACTION

May report: Forced retirement.

Prior psychosocial factors; individuality and personality influence present altered behavioral patterns.

May exhibit: Loss of social control, inappropriate behavior.

TEACHING/LEARNING

May report: Familial history of DAT (4 times greater than general population).

Use/misuse of medications, OTC drugs, alcohol.

Discharge Plan Considerations: **DRG projected mean length of stay: 6.9 days.** (Determined by the presenting problem/condition [i.e., pneumonia, CHF] as individual's are not usually admitted for DAT.)

May require alteration in medication regimen.

Assistance in all areas; safety concerns; possible changes in physical layout of home; placement out of home.

DIAGNOSTIC STUDIES

While no diagnostic studies are specific for DAT, they are used to rule out reversible problems that may be confused with these dementias.

Antibodies: Abnormally high levels may be found (leading to a theory of an immunologic defect).

CBC, RPR, electrolytes, thyroid studies: May determine and/or eliminate treatable/reversible dysfunctions, e.g., metabolic disease processes, fluid/electrolyte imbalance, neurosyphilis.

B_{12}: May disclose a nutritional deficit.

Dexamethasone suppression test (DST): To rule out treatable depression.

ECG: May be normal; need to rule out cardiac insufficiency.

EEG: May be normal or show some slowing (aids in establishing treatable brain dysfunctions).

Skull x-rays: Usually normal.

Vision/hearing tests: To rule out deficits that may be the cause of/contribute to disorientation, mood swings, altered sensory perceptions (rather than cognitive impairment).

Brain scans, e.g., PET, BEAM, MRI: May show areas of decreased brain metabolism characteristic of DAT.

CT scan: May show widening of ventricles, cortical atrophy.

CSF: Presence of abnormal protein from the brain cells is 90% indicative of DAT.

Alzheimer disease-associated protein (ADAP): Postmortem studies have been positive in more than 80% of DAT patients. Adaptation for live testing is being investigated.

NURSING PRIORITIES

1. Provide safe environment, prevent injury.
2. Promote socially acceptable responses; limit inappropriate behavior.
3. Maximize reality orientation/prevent sensory deprivation/overload.
4. Encourage participation in self-care within individual limitations.
5. Promote coping mechanisms of patient/SO.
6. Support patient/SO in grieving process.
7. Provide information about disease process, prognosis, and resources available for assistance.

DISCHARGE GOALS

1. Adequate supervision/support systems available.
2. Maximal level of independent functioning achieved.
3. Coping skills developed/strengthened and SOs using available resources.
4. Disease process/prognosis and patient expectations/needs understood by SO.

NURSING DIAGNOSIS:	RELOCATION STRESS SYNDROME
May be related to:	Little or no preparation for the transfer to the hospital/long-term care setting.
	Changes in daily routine.
	Sensory impairment, physical deterioration.
	Separation from support systems.
Possibly evidenced by:	Apprehension, irritability, defensiveness, increased confusion, suspiciousness, aggressive behavior.
	Decreased self-assurance, withdrawal.
	Sympathetic stimulation, GI disturbances.
DESIRED OUTCOMES/ EVALUATION CRITERIA— PATIENT WILL:	Adapt to change of environment and alterations in routine.
	Demonstrate appropriate range of feelings and lessened fear.
	Experience no <u>catastrophic</u> event.

ACTIONS/INTERVENTIONS	RATIONALE
Independent	
Place in private room, if appropriate, and incorporate SO into care activities, meal time, and so on.	Hospitalization disrupts patient's routine and can intensify behavioral problems even in the person with cognitive dysfunction. Provides opportunity to control environment and protect others from patient's disruptive behavior. Presence of SO provides reassurance and may reduce sense of isolation.
Determine patient's usual schedule of activities and incorporate into hospital routine as possible.	Consistency provides reassurance and may lessen confusion and enhance cooperation.

375

ACTIONS/INTERVENTIONS

Independent

Identify strengths the individual had previously.

Provide clear, honest information about actions/events.

Note behavior, presence of suspiciousness/paranoia, irritability, defensiveness. Compare with SO's description of customary responses.

Remain calm. Place in quiet environment providing "time out."

Deal with aggressive behavior by imposing calm, firm limits.

Encourage hugging and use of touch unless patient is paranoid or agitated at the moment.

RATIONALE

Facilitates assistance with communication and management of current deficits.

Decreases "surprises." Assists in maintaining trust and orientation. When the patient knows the truth about what is happening, coping may be enhanced.

Increased stress, physical discomfort/pain, and fatigue may temporarily exacerbate mental deterioration (cognitive inaccessibility) and further impair communication (social inaccessibility). This represents a *catastrophic* episode that can escalate into a panic state and violence.

Defuses situation and gives the patient time to regain emotional and behavioral control.

Acceptance can reduce fear and aggressive response.

Provides reassurance, reduces stress, and enhances quality of life.

NURSING DIAGNOSIS:	INJURY/TRAUMA, HIGH RISK FOR
Risk factors may include:	Inability to recognize/identify danger in environment.
	Disorientation, confusion, impaired judgment.
	Weakness, muscular incoordination; seizure activity.
Possibly evidenced by:	[Not applicable; presence of signs and symptoms establishes an actual diagnosis.]
DESIRED OUTCOMES/ EVALUATION CRITERIA— PATIENT WILL:	Experience no injury.
	Caregiver(s) will: recognize potential risks in the environment and identify steps to correct them.

ACTIONS/INTERVENTIONS

Independent

Assess for degree of impairment in ability/competence, presence of impulsive behavior and visual-perceptual deficits. Assist SO to identify risks/potential hazards that may be present.

Eliminate/minimize identified hazards in the environment.

RATIONALE

Identifies potential risks in environment and heightens awareness so caregivers are more alert to dangers. Patient's demonstrating impulsive behavior are at increased risk of injury as they are less able to control their own behavior/actions. Visual-perceptual deficits increase the risk of falls.

A person with cognitive impairment and perceptual disturbances is prone to accidental injury because of the inability to take responsibility for basic safety needs or to evaluate the unforeseen consequences, e.g., may light a stove/cigarette and for-

ACTIONS/INTERVENTIONS

Independent

Distract/redirect patient's attention when behavior is agitated or dangerous, e.g., climbing out of bed.

Provide with an identification bracelet showing name, phone number, and diagnosis. Do not place near access to stairwell or exit.

Dress according to physical environment/individual need.

Monitor for medication side effects, signs of overmedication, e.g., extrapyramidal signs, orthostatic hypotension, visual disturbances, GI upsets.

Avoid continuous use of restraints. Have SO/others stay with patient during periods of acute agitation.

Recommend use of "child proof" locks to secure medications, poisonous substances, tools, sharp

RATIONALE

get it, attempt to eat plastic fruit, misjudge placement of chairs, stairs.

Maintains safety while avoiding a confrontation that could escalate behavior/increase risk of injury.

Facilitates safe return if lost. Because of poor verbal ability and confusion, patient may be unable to state address, phone number, and so on. Patient may wander and be detained by police, appearing confused, irritable; may have violent outbursts and exhibit poor judgment.

The general slowing of metabolic processes results in lowered body heat. The hypothalamus is affected by the disease process, causing person to feel cold. Patient may have seasonal disorientation and may wander out in the cold. *Note:* Leading causes of death are pneumonia/accidents.

Patient may not be able to report signs/symptoms, and drugs can easily build up to toxic levels in the elderly. Dosages/drug choice may need to be altered.

Endangers the individual who succeeds in partial removal of restraints. May increase agitation and potentiate fractures in the elderly (due to reduced calcium in the bones).

As the disease worsens, the patient may fidget with objects/locks (hypermetamorphosis) or put small items in mouth (hyperorality), which potentiates accidental injury/death.

NURSING DIAGNOSIS:	THOUGHT PROCESSES, ALTERED
May be related to:	Irreversible neuronal degeneration.
	Loss of memory.
	Sleep deprivation.
	Psychologic conflicts.
Possibly evidenced by:	Inability to interpret stimuli accurately and evaluate reality.
	Disorientation and difficulty in grasping ideas/commands.
	Paranoia, delusions, confusion/frustration, and changes in behavioral responses.
DESIRED OUTCOMES/ EVALUATION CRITERIA— PATIENT WILL:	Recognize changes in thinking/behavior and causative factors when able.
	Demonstrate a decrease in undesired behaviors, threats, and confusion.

ACTIONS/INTERVENTIONS	RATIONALE
Independent	
Assess degree of cognitive impairment, e.g., changes in orientation to person, place, time; attention span; thinking ability. Talk with SO about changes from usual behavior/length of time problem has existed.	Provides baseline for future evaluation/comparison, and influences choice of interventions. Note: Repeated evaluation of orientation may actually heighten negative responses/patient's level of frustration.
Maintain a pleasant, quiet environment.	Crowds, clutter, and noise generate sensory overload that stresses the impaired neurons.
Approach in a slow, calm manner.	Hurried approaches can startle/threaten the confused patient who misinterprets or feels threatened by imaginary people and/or situations.
Face the individual when conversing.	Arouses attention, particularly in persons with perceptual disturbances.
Address the patient by name.	Names form our self-identity and establish reality and individual recognition. Patient may respond to own name long after failing to recognize SO.
Use lower voice register and speak slowly to patient.	Increases the chance for comprehension. High-pitched, loud tones convey stress/anger, which may trigger memory of previous confrontations and provoke an angry response.
Use short words and simple sentences and give simple (step-by-step) instructions. Repeat as needed.	As the disease progresses, the communication centers in the brain are impaired, hindering the individual's ability to process and comprehend messages.
Pause between phrases or questions. Give hints and use open-ended phrases when possible.	Invites a verbal response and may increase comprehension. Hints stimulate communication and give the person a chance for a positive experience.
Listen with regard despite speech content. Interpret statements, meanings, and words. If possible, supply the correct word.	Conveys interest and worth to the individual. Assisting the patient with word processing aids in decreasing frustration.
Avoid negative criticism, arguments, confrontations (provocative stimuli).	Provocation decreases self-esteem and may be interpreted as a threat that triggers agitation or increases inappropriate behavior.
Use distraction. Talk about real people and real events when patient begins ruminating about false ideas, unless it increases anxiety/agitation.	Rumination serves to promote disorientation. Reality orientation increases patient's sense of reality, self-worth, and personal dignity.
Refrain from forcing activities and communications.	Force decreases cooperation and may increase suspiciousness, delusions.
Use humor with interactions.	Laughter can assist in communication and help reverse emotional lability.
Focus on appropriate behavior. Give positive reinforcement, e.g., a pat on the back, applaud. Use touch judiciously. Respect individual's personal space/response.	Reinforces correctness, appropriate behavior. While touch frequently transcends verbal interchange (conveying warmth, acceptance, and reality), the individual may misinterpret the meaning of touch. Intrusion into personal space may threaten the patient's distorted world.

ACTIONS/INTERVENTIONS	RATIONALE
Independent	
Respect individuality and evaluate specific needs.	Persons experiencing a cognitive decline deserve respect, dignity, and worth as an individual. Patient's past and background are important in maintaining self-concept, planning activities, communicating, and so on.
Allow personal belongings.	Familiarity enhances security and sense of self and decreases feelings of loss/deprivation.
Permit hoarding of safe objects.	Preserves security and counterbalances irrevocable losses.
Create simple, noncompetitive activities paced to the individual's abilities.	Motivates patient in ways that will reinforce usefulness and self-worth and stimulate reality.
Make useful activities out of hoarding and repetitive motions, e.g., collecting junk mail, scrapbook, folding/unfolding linen, bouncing balls, dusting, sweeping floors.	May decrease restlessness and provide option for pleasurable activity.
Assist with finding misplaced items. Label drawers/belongings. Do not challenge patient.	May decrease defensiveness if patient believes he or she is being accused of stealing a misplaced, hoarded, or hidden item. To refute the accusation will not change the belief and may invite anger.
Monitor phone use closely. Post significant phone numbers in prominent place. Secure long-distance numbers.	Can be used as reality orientation, but impaired judgment does not allow for distinguishing long-distance numbers, and makes client easy prey for phone sale pitches.
Evaluate sleep/rest pattern and adequacy. Note lethargy, increasing irritability/confusion, frequent yawning, dark circles under eyes.	Lack of sleep can impair thought processes and coping abilities. (Refer to ND: Sleep Pattern Disturbance, p 381.)
Collaborative	
Administer medications as individually indicated:	
Antipsychotics, e.g., haloperidol (Haldol); thioridazine (Mellaril);	May be used to control agitation, delusions, hallucinations. Mellaril is often preferred because there are fewer extrapyramidal side effects (e.g., dystonia, akathisia); increased confusion; visual problems; and especially gait disturbances. *Note:* Phenathiazines may cause oversedation, excitation, or bizarre reactions.
Vasodilators, e.g., cyclandelate (Cyclospasmol);	May improve mental alertness but requires further research.
Ergoloid mesylates (Hydergine LC);	A metabolic enhancer (increases the brain's ability to metabolize glucose and use oxygen) that has few side effects. Although it does not increase cognition and memory, it may make patient more alert, less anxious/depressed. However, it may be of little value in dementia therapy because there is usually a limited degree of improvement. *Note:* This is an expensive drug, and families need accurate information to make informed therapy decisions and avoid false hopes and disappointment due to lack of dramatic results.

379

ACTIONS/INTERVENTIONS

RATIONALE

Independent

Anxiolytic agents, e.g., diazepam (Valium); lorazepam (Librium); oxazepam (Serax);

More useful in early/mild stages for relief of anxiety. Can increase confusion in the elderly. Note: Serax may be preferred because it is shorter acting.

Thiamine.

Studies are currently underway to verify the usefulness of high doses of thiamine during the early phase of the disease to slow progression of impairment/slightly improve cognition.

NURSING DIAGNOSIS:	SENSORY-PERCEPTUAL ALTERATION: (SPECIFY)
May be related to:	Altered sensory reception, transmission, and/or integration (neurologic disease/deficit).
	Socially restricted environment (homebound/institutionalized).
Possibly evidenced by:	Changes in usual response to stimuli, e.g., spatial disorientation, confusion.
	Exaggerated emotional responses, e.g., anxiety, paranoia, and hallucinations.
	Inability to tell position of body parts.
	Diminished/altered sense of taste.
DESIRED OUTCOMES/ EVALUATION CRITERIA— PATIENT WILL:	Demonstrate improved/appropriate response to stimuli.
	Caregivers will: identify/control external factors that contribute to alterations in sensory-perceptual abilities.

ACTIONS/INTERVENTIONS

RATIONALE

Independent

Assess degree of sensory or perceptual impairment and how it affects the individual, including hearing/visual deficits.

While brain involvement is usually global, a small percentage may exhibit asymmetrical involvement, which may cause the patient to neglect one side of the body (unilateral neglect). Individual may not be able to locate internal cues, recognize hunger/thirst, perceive external pain, or locate body within the environment.

Encourage use of corrective lenses, hearing aids, as appropriate.

May enhance sensory input, limit/reduce misinterpretation of stimuli.

Maintain a reality-oriented relationship and environment. Provide clues (around the clock) to reality orientation with calendars, clocks, notes, cards, signs, music, seasonal hues/color-code rooms, scenic pictures.

Reduces confusion and promotes coping with the frustrating struggles of misperception and being disoriented/confused. Dysfunction in visual/spatial perception interferes with the ability to recognize direction/patterns, and the patient may become lost, even in familiar surroundings. Clues are tangible reminders that aid recognition and may perme-

ACTIONS/INTERVENTIONS	RATIONALE
Independent	
	ate memory gaps and increase independence. *Note:* Pictures of animals/people may be interpreted as intruders by some patients, increasing paranoia and delusions.
Provide quiet, nondistracting environment when indicated, e.g., soft music, plain but colorful wallpaper/paint.	Helps to avoid visual/auditory overload by emphasizing qualities of calmness, consistency. *Note:* Patterned wallpaper may be disturbing to some patients.
Provide touch in a caring way.	May enhance perception of self/body boundaries.
Use sensory games to stimulate reality, e.g., smell Vick's and tell of the time mother used it on you; use spring-fall nature boxes.	Communicates reality through multiple channels.
Indulge in periodic reminiscence (familiar music, historic events, photos, mementos).	Stimulates recollections, awakens memories, aids in the preservation of self/individuality via past accomplishments. Increases feelings of security while easing adaptation to a changed environment.
Provide simple outings, short walks. Monitor activity.	Outings refresh reality and provide pleasurable sensory stimuli, which may reduce suspiciousness/hallucinations caused by feelings of imprisonment. Motor functioning may be decreased, because nerve degeneration results in weakness, decreasing stamina.
Promote balanced physiologic functions, using colorful Nerf/beach balls, arm dancing with music.	Preserves mobility (reducing the potential for bone and muscle atrophy) and provides diversional opportunity for interaction with others.
Involve in activities with others as dictated by invidual situation, e.g., one-to-one visitors, socialization groups at Alzheimer center, occupational therapy.	Provides opportunity for the stimulation of participation with others and may maintain some level of social interaction.

NURSING DIAGNOSIS:	SLEEP PATTERN DISTURBANCE
May be related to:	Sensory impairments.
	Psychologic stress (neurologic impairment).
	Changes in activity pattern.
Possibly evidenced by:	Changes in behavior and performance.
	Disorientation (day/night reversal).
	Irritability.
	Wakefulness/interrupted sleep, increased aimless wandering; inability to identify need/time for sleeping.
	Lethargy, dark circles under eyes, frequent yawning.

DESIRED OUTCOMES/ EVALUATION CRITERIA— PATIENT WILL:	Establish adequate sleep pattern, with wandering reduced.
	Report/appear rested.

ACTIONS/INTERVENTIONS

Independent

Provide for rest/naps, encourage exercise during day, reduce physical/mental activity late in the day.

Avoid use of continuous restraints.

Evaluate level of stress/orientation as day progresses.

Adhere to regular bedtime schedule and rituals. Tell patient that it is time to sleep.

Provide evening snack, warm milk, bath, and back rub.

Reduce fluid intake in the evening. Toilet before retiring.

Provide soft music or "white noise."

Collaborative

Administer medications as indicated for sleep:

    Antidepressants, e.g., amitriptyline (Elavil); doxepin (Senequan); and trazolone (Desyrel);

    Choral hydrate; oxazepam (Serax); triazolam (Halcion).

Avoid use of diphenhydramine (Benadryl).

RATIONALE

While prolonged physical and mental activity results in fatigue, which can increase confusion, programmed activity without overstimulation promotes sleep.

Potentiates sensory deprivation, increases agitation, and restricts rest.

Increasing confusion, disorientation, and uncooperative behaviors (Sundowner's syndrome) may interfere with attaining restful sleep pattern.

Reinforces that it is bedtime and maintains stability of environment. *Note:* Later than normal bedtime may be indicated to allow patient to dissipate excess energy and facilitate falling asleep.

Promotes relaxation and drowsiness.

Decreases need to get up to go to the bathroom/incontinence during the night.

Reduces sensory stimulation by blocking out other environmental sounds that could interfere with restful sleep.

May be effective in treating pseudodementia or depression, improving ability to sleep. However, the anticholinergic properties can induce confusion or worsen cognition, and side effects (e.g., orthostatic hypotension) may limit usefulness.

Used sparingly, low-dose hypnotics may be effective in treating insomnia or Sundowner's syndrome.

Once used for sleep, this drug is now contraindicated because it interferes with the production of acetylcholine, which is already inhibited in the brains of patients with DAT.

NURSING DIAGNOSIS:	SELF-CARE DEFICIT: (SPECIFY)
May be related to:	Cognitive decline; physical limitations.

	Frustration over loss of independence; depression.
Possibly evidenced by:	Impaired ability to perform ADLs, e.g., inability to bring food from receptacle to mouth; inability to wash body part(s), regulate temperature of water; impaired ability to put on/take off clothing; difficulty completing toileting tasks.
DESIRED OUTCOMES/ EVALUATION CRITERIA— PATIENT WILL:	Perform self-care activities within level of own ability. Identify and use personal/community resources that can provide assistance.

ACTIONS/INTERVENTIONS	RATIONALE

Independent

ACTIONS/INTERVENTIONS	RATIONALE
Identify reason for difficulty in dressing/self-care, e.g., physical limitations in motion; apathy/depression; cognitive decline (such as apraxia); or room temperature ("too cold to get dressed").	Underlying cause affects choice of interventions/ strategies. Problem may be minimized by adaptation of clothing or may require consultation from other specialists.
Identify hygienic needs and provide assistance as needed with care of hair/nails/skin, cleaning glasses, brushing teeth.	As the disease progresses, basic hygienic needs may be forgotten. Harm (e.g., infection, gum disease, disheveled appearance) may occur when patient/caregivers become intimidated by grooming problems.
Incorporate usual routine into activity schedule as possible. Wait and/or change the time to approach dressing/hygiene if a problem arises.	Maintaining routine may prevent worsening of confusion and enhance cooperation. Because anger is quickly forgotten, another time or approach may be successful.
Be attentive to nonverbal physiologic symptoms.	Sensory loss and language dysfunction may cause patient to express self-care needs in nonverbal manner, e.g., thirst by panting; need to void by holding self/fidgeting.
Be alert to underlying meaning of verbal statements.	May direct a question to another, such as "Are you cold?" Meaning, "I am cold and need additional clothing."
Supervise but allow as much autonomy as possible.	Eases the frustration over lost independence.
Allot plenty of time to perform tasks.	Tasks which were once easy (e.g., dressing, bathing) are now complicated by decreased motor skills or cognitive and physical change. Time and patience can reduce chaos resulting from trying to hasten this process.
Assist with neat dressing/provide colorful clothes.	Enhances esteem, may diminish sense of loss and convey aliveness.
Offer one item of clothing at a time, in sequential order. Talk through each step 1 at a time.	Simplicity reduces frustration and the potential for rage and despair. Guidance reduces confusion and allows autonomy.
Allow to sleep in shoes/clothing or to wear 2 sets of clothing if patient demands.	Providing no harm is done, altering the "normal" lessens the rebellion and allows rest.

383

NURSING DIAGNOSIS:	NUTRITION, ALTERED: LESS/MORE THAN BODY REQUIREMENTS, HIGH RISK FOR
Risk factors may include:	Sensory changes.
	Impaired judgment and coordination.
	Agitation.
	Forgetfulness, regressed habits, and concealment.
Possibly evidenced by:	[Not applicable; presence of signs and symptoms establishes an actual diagnosis.]
DESIRED OUTCOMES/ EVALUATION CRITERIA— PATIENT WILL:	Ingest nutritionally balanced diet.
	Maintain/regain appropriate weight.

ACTIONS/INTERVENTIONS	RATIONALE
Independent	
Assess SO/patient's knowledge of nutritional needs.	Identifies needs to assist in formulating individual teaching plan. A role reversal situation can occur (e.g., child now cooking for parent, husband taking over "duties" of wife), increasing the need for information.
Determine amount of exercise/pacing patient does.	Nutritional intake may need to be adjusted to meet needs related to individual energy expenditure.
Offer/provide assistance in menu selection.	Patient may be indecisive/overwhelmed by choices or unaware of the need to maintain elemental nutrition.
Provide privacy, when eating habits become an insoluble problem. Accept eating with hands, spills, and whimsical mixtures, e.g., salad dressing in milk or salt and pepper in ice cream. (Note: Avoid separating patient from other people too soon or too frequently.)	Socially unacceptable and embarrassing eating habits develop as the disease progresses. Acceptance preserves esteem; decreases frustration or refusal to eat as a result of anger, frustration. Early separation can result in patient feeling upset and rejected and can actually decrease food intake.
Offer small feedings and/or snacks of 1 or 2 foods around the clock as indicated.	Large feedings may overwhelm the patient, resulting either in complete abstinence or gorging. Small feedings may enhance appropriate intake. Limiting number of foods offered at single time reduces confusion regarding which food to choose.
Provide ample time for eating.	A leisurely approach aids digestion and decreases the chance of anger precipitated by rushing.
Simplify steps of eating, e.g., serve food in courses. Anticipate needs, cut foods, provide soft/finger foods.	Promotes autonomy and independence. Decreases potential frustration/anger over lost abilities.
Place food items in pita bread/paper sack for the patient that paces.	Carrying food may encourage patient to eat.

384

ACTIONS/INTERVENTIONS

Independent

Avoid baby food and excessively hot foods.

Stimulate oral-suck reflex by gentle stroking of the cheeks or stimulating the mouth with a spoon.

Collaborative

Refer to dietitian.

RATIONALE

Baby foods lack adequate nutritional content, fiber, and taste for adults and can add to patient's humiliation. Hot foods may result in mouth burns and/or refusal to eat.

As the disease progresses, the patient may clench teeth and refuse to eat. Stimulating the reflex may increase cooperation/intake.

Assistance may be needed to develop a nutritionally balanced diet individualized to meet patient needs/food preferences.

NURSING DIAGNOSIS:	**CONSTIPATION/INCONTINENCE, [SPECIFY]/ URINARY ELIMINATION, ALTERED PATTERNS**
May be related to:	Disorientation.
	Lost neurologic functioning/muscle tone.
	Inability to locate the bathroom/recognize need.
	Changes in dietary/fluid intake.
Possibly evidenced by:	Inappropriate toileting behaviors.
	Urgency/incontinence/constipation.
DESIRED OUTCOMES/ EVALUATION CRITERIA— PATIENT WILL:	Establish adequate/appropriate pattern of elimination.

ACTIONS/INTERVENTIONS

Independent

Assess prior pattern and compare with current.

Locate bed near a bathroom when possible; make signs for/color code door. Provide adequate lighting, particularly at night.

Take to the toilet at regular intervals. Dictate each step 1 at a time and use positive reinforcement.

Establish bowel/bladder training program. Promote patient participation to level of ability.

Encourage adequate fluid intake during the day (at least 2 L, as appropriate), diet high in fiber, and fruit juices. Limit intake during the late evening and at bedtime.

RATIONALE

Provides information about changes that may require further assessment/intervention.

Promotes orientation/finding bathroom. Incontinence may be attributed to inability to find a toilet.

Adherence to a daily and regular schedule may prevent accidents. Frequently the problem is forgetting what to do, e.g., pushing pants down, position.

Stimulates awareness, enhances regulation of body function, and helps to avoid accidents.

Reduces risk of dehydration/constipation. Restricting intake in evening may reduce frequency/incontinence during the night.

ACTIONS/INTERVENTIONS	RATIONALE

Independent

Avoid a sense of being rushed.	Hurrying may be perceived as intrusion, which leads to anger and lack of cooperation with activity.
Be alert to nonverbal cues, e.g., restlessness, holding self, or picking at clothes.	May signal urgency, inattention to cues, and/or inability to locate bathroom.
Be discreet and respect person's privacy.	Although the patient is confused, a sense of modesty is often retained.
Convey acceptance when incontinence occurs. Change promptly, provide good skin care.	Acceptance is important to decrease the embarrassment and feelings of helplessness that may occur during the changing process. Reduces risk of skin irritation/breakdown.
Monitor appearance/color of urine; note consistency of stool.	Detection of changes provides opportunity to alter interventions to prevent complications or acquire treatment as indicated (e.g., constipation/urinary infection).

Collaborative

Administer stool softeners, Metamucil, glycerin suppository, as indicated.	May be necessary to facilitate/stimulate regular bowel movement.

NURSING DIAGNOSIS:	SEXUAL DYSFUNCTION, HIGH RISK FOR
Risk factors may include:	Confusion, forgetfulness, and disorientation to place or person.
	Altered body function, decrease in habit/control of behavior.
	Lack of intimacy/sexual rejection by SO.
	Lack of privacy.
Possibly evidenced by:	[Not applicable; presence of signs and symptoms establishes an actual diagnosis.]
DESIRED OUTCOMES/ EVALUATION CRITERIA— PATIENT WILL:	Meet sexuality needs in an acceptable manner.
	Experience no episodes of inappropriate behavior.

ACTIONS/INTERVENTIONS	RATIONALE

Independent

Assess individual needs/desires/abilities.	Alternative methods need to be designed for the individual situation to fulfill the need for intimacy and closeness.
Encourage partner to show affection/acceptance.	The cognitively impaired person retains the basic needs for affection, love, acceptance, and sexual expression.

ACTIONS/INTERVENTIONS

Independent

Assure privacy.

Use distraction, as indicated. Remind patient that this is a public area and current behavior is unacceptable.

Provide time to listen/discuss concerns of SO.

RATIONALE

Sexual expression or behavior may differ, and privacy allows sexual expression without embarrassment and/or the objections of others.

Useful tool when there is inappropriate/objectionable behavior, e.g., self-exposure.

May need information and/or counseling about alternatives for sexual activity/aggression.

NURSING DIAGNOSIS:	**FAMILY COPING, INEFFECTIVE: COMPROMISED/ DISABLING**
May be related to:	Disruptive behavior of patient.
	Family grief about their helplessness watching loved one deteriorate.
	Prolonged disease/disability progression that exhausts the supportive capacity of SO.
	Highly ambivalent family relationships.
Possibly evidenced by:	Family becoming embarrassed and socially immobilized.
	Home maintenance becomes extremely difficult and leads to difficult decisions with legal/financial considerations.
DESIRED OUTCOMES/ EVALUATION CRITERIA— PATIENT WILL:	Identify/verbalize resources within themselves to deal with the situation.
	Acknowledge loved one's condition and demonstrate positive coping behaviors in dealing with situation.
	Use outside support systems effectively.

ACTIONS/INTERVENTIONS

Independent

Include all SOs in teaching and planning for home care.

Focus on specific problems as they occur, the "here and now."

Establish priorities.

Be realistic and honest in all matters.

RATIONALE

Can ease the burden of home management and adaptation. Comfortable and familiar lifestyle at home is helpful in preserving the affected individual's need for belonging.

Disease progression follows no set pattern. A premature focus on the possibility of long-term care can impair the ability to cope with present issues.

Helps to create a sense of order and facilitates problem solving.

Decreases stress that surrounds false hopes, e.g., that individual may regain past level of functioning from advertised or unproven medication.

387

ACTIONS/INTERVENTIONS	RATIONALE

Independent

Continually reassess family's ability to care for patient at home.

Behaviors like hoarding, clinging, unjust accusations, angry outbursts, and so on, can precipitate family burnout and interfere with ability to provide effective care.

Help SO/family understand the importance of maintaining psychosocial functioning.

Embarrassing behavior, the demands of care, and so on, may cause psychosocial withdrawal.

Provide time/listen with regard to concerns/anxieties.

SOs require constant support with the multifaceted problems that arise during the course of this illness to ease the process of adaptation and grieving.

Discuss possibility of isolation. Reinforce need for support system.

The belief that a single individual can meet all the needs of the patient increases the potential for physical/mental illness. *Note:* Mortality rate for primary caregivers is actually higher than for the patient with DAT.

Provide positive feedback for efforts.

Reassures individuals that they are doing their best.

Encourage unlimited visitation.

Contact with familiarity forms a base of reality and can provide a reassuring freedom from loneliness. Recurrent contact helps family members realize and accept situation.

Support concerns generated by consideration/decision to place in LTC facility.

Constant care requirements may be more than can be managed by SO. Support is needed for this difficult guilt-producing decision, which may create a financial burden as well.

Collaborative

Refer to local resources, e.g., adult day care, respite care, homemaker services, or a local chapter of Alzheimer's Disease and Related Disorders Association.

Coping with this individual is a full-time, frustrating task. Respite/day care may lighten the burden, reduce potential social isolation, and prevent family burnout. ADRDA provides group support and family teaching and promotes research. Local groups provide a social outlet for sharing grief and promote problem solving with such matters as financial/legal advice, home care, and so on.

NURSING DIAGNOSIS:	GRIEVING, ANTICIPATORY
May be related to:	Patient awareness of something "being wrong" with changes in memory/family reaction, physiopsychosocial well-being.
	Family perception of potential loss of loved one.
Possibly evidenced by:	Expressions of distress/anger at potential loss.
	Choked feelings, crying.
	Alteration in activity level, communication patterns, eating habits, and sleep patterns.

DESIRED OUTCOMES/ EVALUATION CRITERIA— PATIENT WILL:	Express concerns openly.
	Discuss loss and participate in planning for the future.

ACTIONS/INTERVENTIONS	RATIONALE

Independent

Assess degree of deterioration/level of coping.	Information is helpful to understand how much the patient is capable of doing to maintain highest level of independence and to provide encouragement to help individuals deal with losses.
Review past life experiences, role changes, and coping skills.	Opportunity to identify skills that may help individuals cope with grief of current situation more effectively.
Provide open environment for discussion. Use therapeutic communication skills of active listening, acknowledgment, and so on.	Encourages patient/SO to discuss feelings and concerns realistically.
Note statements of despair, hopelessness, "nothing to live for," expressions of anger.	May be indicative of suicidal ideation. Angry behavior may be patient's way of dealing with feelings of despair.
Respect desire not to talk.	May not be ready to deal with grief.
Be honest, do not give false reassurances or dire predictions about the future.	Honesty promotes a trusting relationship. Expressions of gloom, such as "You'll spend the rest of your life in a nursing home" are not helpful. (No one knows what the future holds.)
Discuss with patient/SO ways they can plan together for the future.	Having a part in problem solving/planning can provide a sense of control over anticipated events.
Assist patient/SO to identify positive aspects of the situation.	Ongoing research, possibility of slow progression may offer some hope for the future.
Identify strengths patient/SO sees in self/situation and support systems available.	Recognizing these resources provides opportunity to work through feelings of grief.

Collaborative

Refer to other resources, counseling, clergy, and so on.	May need additional support/assistance to resolve feelings.

NURSING DIAGNOSIS:	HOME MAINTENANCE MANAGEMENT, IMPAIRED/HEALTH MAINTENANCE, ALTERED
May be related to:	Progressively impaired cognitive functioning.
	Complete or partial lack of gross and/or fine motor skills.
	Significant alteration in communication skills.
	Ineffective individual/family coping.
	Insufficient family organization/planning.
	Unfamiliarity with resources; inadequate support systems.

389

Possibly evidenced by:	Overtaxed family members, e.g., exhausted/anxious.
	Household members express difficulty and request help in maintaining home in safe/comfortable fashion.
	Home surroundings appear disorderly/unsafe.
	Reported or observed inability to take responsibility for meeting basic health practices.
	Reported or observed lack of equipment, financial, or other resources; impairment of personal support system.
DESIRED OUTCOMES/ EVALUATION CRITERIA— CAREGIVER WILL:	Identify and correct factors related to difficulty in maintaining a safe environment for the patient.
	Demonstrate appropriate, effective use of resources, e.g., respite care, homemakers, Alzheimer groups.
	Assume responsibility for and adopt lifestyle changes supporting patient health care goals.
	Verbalize ability to cope adequately with existing situation.

ACTIONS/INTERVENTIONS	RATIONALE
Independent	
Evaluate level of cognitive/emotional/physical functioning (level of independence).	Identifies strengths/areas of need and how much responsibility the patient may be expected to assume. (Refer to ND: Self-Care Deficit, p 382.).
Assess environment, noting unsafe factors and ability of patient to care for self.	Determines what changes need to be made to accommodate disabilities. (Refer to ND: Injury/Trauma, high risk for, p 376.)
Assist patient/SO to develop plan for keeping track of/dealing with health needs.	Scheduling can be helpful in managing routine care.
Identify support systems available to patient/SO, e.g., other family members, friends.	Planning and constant care is necessary to maintain patient at home. If family system is unavailable/unaware, patient needs, e.g., nutrition, dental care, eye examinations can be neglected. Primary caregiver may benefit from assistance, e.g., someone to come in and provide relief/respite from constant care.
Evaluate coping abilities, effectiveness, commitment of caregiver(s)/support persons.	Progressive debilitation taxes caregiver(s) and may alter ability to meet patient/own needs. (Refer to ND: Family Coping, ineffective: compromised/disabling, p 387.)
Collaborative	
Identify alternate care sources (such as sitter/day care facility) or senior care services, e.g., Meals on Wheels/respite care.	As patient's condition worsens, SO may need additional help from several sources or may eventually be unable to maintain patient at home.
Refer to supportive services as need indicates.	Medical and social services consultant may be needed to develop ongoing plan/identify resources as needs change.

Multiple Sclerosis

Multiple sclerosis (MS) is the most common of the demyelinating disorders. It is a chronic disorder in which irregular demyelination of both the central and peripheral portions of the nervous system result in varying degrees of motor, sensory, and cognitive dysfunction. MS is characterized by periods of exacerbation, and remission of symptoms and individual prognosis is variable and unpredictable.

RELATED CONCERNS:

Long-Term Care, p 938
Pneumonia, p 162
Psychosocial Aspects of Care, p 899
Sepsis/Septicemia, p 887

PATIENT ASSESSMENT DATA BASE

Degree of symptomatology is dependent on the stage of disease and extent, areas of neuronal involvement.

ACTIVITY/REST

May report: Extreme fatigue/weakness, exaggerated intolerance to activity, needing to rest after even simple activities such as shaving/showering; increased weakness/intolerance to temperature extremes (especially heat, i.e., summer weather, hot tubs).
Numbness, tingling in the extremities.
Sleep disturbances, may awaken early or frequently.

May exhibit: Absence of predictable pattern of symptoms.
Generalized weakness, decreased muscle tone/mass (disuse).
Staggering, dragging of feet, ataxia.

CIRCULATION

May report: Dependent edema (steroid therapy or inactivity).

May exhibit: Blue/mottled, puffy extremities (inactivity).
Capillary fragility (especially on face).

EGO INTEGRITY

May report: Statements reflecting loss of self-esteem/body image.
Expressions of grief.
Anxiety/fear of pain, disability, rejection, pity.
Keeping illness confidential.
Feelings of helplessness, hopelessness.
Personal tragedies (divorce, abandonment by SO/friends).
Difficult time with employment because of excessive fatigue/cognitive dysfunction.

May exhibit: Denial, rejection.
Mood changes, irritability, restlessness, lethargy, euphoria, depression, anger.

391

ELIMINATION

May report: Nocturia.

Incomplete bladder emptying, retention with overflow.

Hesitancy or urgency.

Urinary/bowel incontinence (cerebral/spinal lesions).

Constipation.

Recurrent urinary tract infections.

May exhibit: Loss of sphincter control.

Kidney stone formation, kidney damage.

FOOD/FLUID

May report: Difficulty chewing, swallowing (weak throat muscles).

Problems getting food to mouth (related to intentional tremors of upper extremities).

Frequent hiccups, lasting extended periods.

May exhibit: Difficulty feeding self.

HYGIENE

May report: Difficulty with/dependence in some ADLs.

Use of assistive devices/individual caregiver.

May exhibit: Poor personal habits, disheveled appearance.

NEUROSENSORY

May report: Weakness, paralysis of muscles, numbness, tingling (prickling sensations in parts of the body).

Change in visual acuity (diplopia).

Moving head back and forth while watching television, difficulty driving (distorted visual field), blurred vision.

Memory loss, difficulty with incidental memory, retrieving/recalling, sorting out information (cerebral involvement).

Difficulty making decisions.

Communication difficulties, such as coining words.

Seizures.

May exhibit: Mental status: Mood swings, depression, euphoria, irritability, apathy; lack of judgment; disorientation/confusion; impairment of short-term memory.

Scanning speech, slow hesitant speech, poor articulation.

Partial/total loss of vision in one eye; vision disturbances.

Positional/vibration sense impaired or absent.

Impaired touch/pain sensation.

Facial/trigeminal nerve involvement, nystagmus, diplopia (brainstem involvement).

Loss of motor skills, muscle tone, spastic paresis/total immobility (advanced stages).

Ataxia, loss of coordination, tremors (may be originally misinterpreted as intoxication), intention tremor.

Hyperreflexia, positive Babinski, ankle clonus; absent superficial reflexes (especially abdominal).

PAIN/DISCOMFORT

May report:
Painful spasms, burning pain along nerve path (some patients do not experience normal pain sensations).

Frequency: Varying, may be sporadic/intermittent (possibly once a day) or may be constant.

Duration: Lightninglike, repetitive, intermittent; painful spasms of persistent long-term back pain.

Facial neuralgia (central lesion).

Dull back pain (peripheral lesion).

SAFETY

May report:
Uneasiness around small children or moving objects, fear of falling (loss of position sense).

History of falls/accidental injuries.

Use of ambulation devices.

Vision impairment.

Suicidal ideation.

SEXUALITY

May report:
Relationship stresses.

Impotence/nocturnal erections or ejaculatory difficulties.

Disturbances in sexual functioning (affected by nerve impairment, fatigue, bowel and bladder control problems, and medications).

Enhanced sexual desire.

Problems with positioning.

Genital anesthesia (female).

SOCIAL INTERACTION

May report:
Lack of social activities/involvement.

Withdrawal from interactions with others.

Feelings of isolation (increased divorce rate/loss of friends).

May exhibit:
Speech impairment.

TEACHING/LEARNING

May report:
Use of prescription/OTC medications.

Difficulty retaining information.

Family history of disease (possibly due to common environmental/inherited factors).

Use of "holistic"/natural products/health care practices, "trying out cures."

Discharge Plan Considerations:
DRG projected mean length of stay: 7.1 days.

May require assistance in any or all areas, depending on individual situation.

May eventually need total care/placement in assisted living/long-term care facility.

DIAGNOSTIC STUDIES

MRI: Determines presence of plaques characteristic of MS (along with clinical symptoms, these findings are conclusive).

CT scan: Demonstrates brain lesions, ventricular enlargement or thinning.

Evoked potentials: Visual, brainstem auditory, and somatosensory may be abnormal early in disease process.

Lumbar puncture: CSF may show elevated levels of I_gG and I_gM. Protein level normal or only slightly elevated, oligoclonal bands present on electrophoresis; WBC, slightly elevated; elevated concentration of myelin basic protein may be noted during active demyelination process.

EEG: May be mildly abnormal in some cases.

NURSING PRIORITIES

1. Maintain optimal mobility.
2. Assist with/provide for maintenance of ADLs.
3. Support acceptance of changes in body image/self-esteem and role performance.
4. Provide information about disease process/prognosis, therapeutic needs, and available resources.

DISCHARGE GOALS

1. Remains mobile within limits of individual situation.
2. ADLs are managed by patient/caregivers.
3. Changes in self-concept are acknowledged and being dealt with.
4. Disease process/prognosis, therapeutic regimen are understood and resources identified.

NURSING DIAGNOSIS:	PHYSICAL MOBILITY, IMPAIRED
May be related to:	Neuromuscular impairment, heat/cold intolerance, decreased strength/endurance, fatigue.
	Perceptual/cognitive deficits.
	Pain/discomfort.
	Poor nutrition.
	Sleep disturbances, depression.
	Medication side effects.
Possibly evidenced by:	Statements of concern about ability to perform expected activities.
	Ataxia, paralysis, loss of sensation to limbs.
	Impaired coordination.
	Deconditioned status, decreased muscle strength/control.
DESIRED OUTCOMES/ EVALUATION CRITERIA— PATIENT WILL:	Identify risk factors and individual strengths affecting activity tolerance.
	Identify alternatives to help maintain current activity level.

Participate in conditioning/rehabilitation programs to enhance ability to perform.

Demonstrate techniques/behaviors that enable resumption/continuation of activities.

ACTIONS/INTERVENTIONS	RATIONALE
Independent	
Determine current activity level/physical condition. Assess degree of functional impairment using 0–4 scale.	Provides information to develop plan of care for rehabilitation. *Note:* Motor symptoms are less likely to improve than sensory ones.
Note and accept presence of fatigue.	Studies indicate that the fatigue encountered by patients with MS can be caused by expenditure of minimal energy, is more frequent and severe than "normal" fatigue, has a disproportionate impact on ADLs, has a slower recovery time, and may have no direct relationship between fatigue severity and neurologic status.
Identify/review factors affecting ability to be active, e.g., temperature extremes, inadequate food intake, insomnia, use of medications.	Provides opportunity to problem solve to maintain/improve mobility.
Encourage patient to perform self-care to the maximum of ability as defined by the patient. Do not rush patient.	Promotes independence and sense of control, may decrease feelings of helplessness. (Refer to ND: Self-Care Deficit, p)
Accept when patient is unable to do activities.	Ability can vary from moment to moment. Nonjudgmental acceptance of the patient's evaluation of day-to-day variations in capabilities provides opportunity to promote independence while supporting fluctuations in level of required care.
Evaluate ability to ambulate safely. Provide walking aids, e.g., Canadian canes, braces, walker, wheelchair; review safety considerations.	Walking exercises can improve the safety and efficiency of the patient's gait. Mobility aids can decrease fatigue, enhancing independence and comfort, as well as safety. However, individual may display poor judgment about ability to safely engage in activity.
Plan care with consistent rest periods between activities.	Reduces fatigue, aggravation of muscle weakness.
Reposition frequently when patient is immobile (bed/chairbound). Position/encourage to sleep prone as tolerated.	Reduces continued pressure on same areas, prevents skin breakdown. Minimizes flexor spasms at knees and hips.
Provide massage and active/passive range of motion exercises on a regular schedule. Encourage use of splints/footboards as indicated.	Prevents problems associated with muscle dysfunction and disuse. Helps to maintain muscle tone/strength and joint mobility and decreases risk of loss of calcium from bones.
Encourage stretching exercises and use of cold packs, splints when indicated.	Helps decrease spasticity.

ACTIONS/INTERVENTIONS	RATIONALE
Collaborative	
Consult with physical/occupational therapists.	Useful in developing individual exercise program and identifying devices/equipment needs to relieve spastic muscles, improve motor functioning, prevent/reduce muscular atrophy and contractures. Can also provide structured activities to involve specific areas of deficit (e.g., cognitive, kinesthetic) and therapy (e.g., expressive) to improve sense of self-esteem.
Recommend groups involved in fitness/exercise and/or the Multiple Sclerosis Society.	Can help patient to stay motivated to remain active within the limits of the disability/condition. Group activities need to be selected carefully to meet the patient's need(s) and prevent discouragement or anxiety.
Administer medications as indicated, e.g.:	
Dantrolene (Dantrium);	Muscle relaxant may be used to decrease spasticity; enhance mobility and maintenance of activity. *Note:* Adverse effect may be increased muscle weakness, loss of muscle tone.
Diazepam (Valium); baclofen (Lioresal);	Reduces spasticity by inhibiting spinal cord reflexes. *Note:* Used with caution because may exacerbate general weakness, further reducing mobility.
Steroids, e.g., prednisone (Deltasone); dexamethasone (Decadron); pituitary hormones, (ACTH);	May be used during acute exacerbations to prevent edema at the sclerotic plaques; however, long-term therapy seems to have little effect on progression of symptoms.
Vitamin B;	Supports nerve-cell replication and enhances metabolic functions.
Immunosuppressives, e.g., cyclophosphamide (Cytoxin).	May be tried in effort to slow progression of disease, promote remission.
Assist with alternate therapies, e.g., hyperbaric oxygenation.	Used experimentally (in early stages) to promote remyelinization, although recent results are not promising.

NURSING DIAGNOSIS:	**SELF-CARE DEFICIT: (SPECIFY)**
May be related to:	Neuromuscular/perceptual impairment; intolerance to activity; decreased strength and endurance; motor impairment, tremors.
	Pain, discomfort, fatigue.
	Memory loss.
	Depression.
Possibly evidenced by:	Frustration; inability to perform tasks of self-care.

DESIRED OUTCOMES/ EVALUATION CRITERIA— PATIENT WILL:	Identify individual areas of weakness/needs.
	Demonstrate techniques/lifestyle changes to meet self-care needs.
	Perform self-care activities within level of own ability.
	Identify personal/community resources that provide assistance.

ACTIONS/INTERVENTIONS

Independent

Assist according to degree of disability; allow as much autonomy as possible. Encourage patient input in planning schedule.

Note presence of/accommodate for fatigue.

Allot sufficient time to perform task(s), and display patience when movements are slow.

Anticipate hygienic needs and assist as necessary with care of nails, skin, and hair; mouth care; shaving (use electric razor).

Provide assistive devices/aids as indicated, e.g., shower chair, elevated toilet seat with arm supports.

Problem-solve ways to meet nutritional/fluid needs, e.g., wrap fork handle with tape, cut food, and show patient how to hold cup with both hands.

Collaborative

Consult with occupational therapist.

RATIONALE

Participation in own care can ease the frustration over loss of independence. Patient's quality of life is enhanced when desires/likes are considered in daily activities.

Fatigue encountered by patients with MS can be very debilitating and greatly impact ability to participate in ADLs. The subjective nature of reports of fatigue can be misinterpreted by health care providers and family, leading to conflict and the belief that the patient is "manipulative" when in fact, this is not the case. Patients with MS expend more energy to complete ADLs, increasing the risk of fatigue.

Decreased motor skills/spasticity may interfere with ability to manage even simple activities.

Example by caregiver can set a matter-of-fact tone for acceptance of handling mundane needs that may be embarrassing to patient/repugnant to SO.

Reduces fatigue, enhancing participation in self-care.

Provides for adequate intake and enhances patient's feelings of independence/self-esteem.

Useful in identifying devices/equipment to meet individual's needs, promoting independence and increasing sense of self-worth.

NURSING DIAGNOSIS:	SELF-ESTEEM, DISTURBANCE IN (SPECIFY)
May be related to:	Changes in structure/function.
	Disruption in how patient perceives own body.
	Role reversal; dependence.

Possibly evidenced by:	Confusion about sense of self, purpose, direction in life.
	Denial, withdrawal, anger.
	Negative/self-destructive behavior.
	Use of ineffective coping methods.
	Change in self/other's perception of role/physical capacity to resume role.
DESIRED OUTCOMES/ EVALUATION CRITERIA— PATIENT WILL:	Verbalize realistic view and acceptance of body as it is.
	View self as a capable person.
	Participate in and assume responsibility for meeting own needs.
	Recognize and incorporate changes in self-concept/role without negating self-esteem.
	Develop realistic plans for adapting to role changes.

ACTIONS/INTERVENTIONS	RATIONALE

Independent

Establish/maintain a therapeutic nurse-patient relationship, discussing fears/concerns.	Conveys an attitude of caring and develops a sense of trust between patient and caregiver in which the patient is free to express fears of rejection, loss of previous functioning/appearance, feelings of helplessness, powerlessness about changes that may occur. Promotes a sense of well-being for the patient.
Note withdrawn behaviors/use of denial, or overconcern with body/disease process.	Initially may be a normal protective response, but if prolonged may prevent dealing appropriately with reality and may lead to ineffective coping.
Support use of defense mechanisms, allowing patient to deal with information in own time and way.	Confronting patient with reality of situation may result in increased anxiety and lessened ability to cope with changed self-concept/role.
Acknowledge reality of grieving process related to actual/perceived changes. Help patient deal realistically with feelings of anger and sadness.	Nature of the disease leads to ongoing losses and changes in all aspects of life, blocking resolution of grieving process.
Review information about course of disease, possibility of remissions, prognosis.	When patient learns about disease, and becomes aware that own behavior can significantly affect course/remission, the patient may feel more in control, enhancing sense of self-esteem. Note: Some patients may never have a remission.
Provide accurate verbal and written information about what is happening and discuss with patient/SO.	Helps patient to stay in the "here and now," reduces fear of the unknown, provides reference source for future use.
Explain that labile emotions are not unusual. Problem solve ways to deal with these feelings.	Relieves anxiety and assists with efforts to manage unexpected emotional display.

ACTIONS/INTERVENTIONS	RATIONALE
Independent	
Note presence of depression/impaired thought processes, expressions of suicidal ideation (evaluate on a scale of 1–10).	Adaptation to a long-term, progressively debilitating disease with a fatal outcome is a difficult emotional adjustment. In addition, brain damage may affect adaptation to these life changes. Individual may believe that suicide is the best way to deal with what is happening.
Assess interaction between patient and SO. Note changes in relationship.	SO may unconsciously/consciously reinforce negative attitudes and beliefs of the patient, or issues of secondary gain may interfere with progress and ability to manage situation.
Provide open environment for patient/SO to discuss concerns about sexuality.	Physical and psychologic changes often create stressors within the relationship, affecting usual roles/expectations, further impairing self-concept.
Collaborative	
Consult with occupational therapist/rehabilitation team.	Identifying assistive devices/equipment enhances level of function and participation in ADLs.

NURSING DIAGNOSIS:	**POWERLESSNESS [SPECIFY DEGREE]/HOPELESSNESS**
May be related to:	Illness-related regimen.
	Lifestyle of helplessness.
Possibly evidenced by:	Verbal expressions of having no control or influence over situation.
	Depression over physical deterioration that occurs despite patient compliance with regimen.
	Nonparticipation in care or decision making when opportunities are provided.
	Passivity, decreased verbalization/affect.
	Verbal cues (despondent content, "I can't," sighing).
	Lack of involvement in care/passively allowing care.
DESIRED OUTCOMES/ EVALUATION CRITERIA— PATIENT WILL:	Identify and verbalize feelings.
	Use coping mechanisms to counteract feelings of hopelessness.
	Identify areas over which individual has control.
	Participate/monitor and control own self-care and ADLs within limits of the individual situation.

ACTIONS/INTERVENTIONS	RATIONALE
Independent	
Note behaviors indicative of powerlessness/hopelessness, e.g., statements of despair, "They don't care," "It won't make any difference."	The degree to which the patient believes own situation is hopeless, that he or she is powerless to change what is happening, affects how patient handles life situation.
Acknowledge reality of situation, at the same time expressing hope for the patient.	While the prognosis may be discouraging, remissions may occur; and because the future cannot be predicted, hope for some quality of life should be encouraged.
Determine degree of mastery patient has exhibited in life to the present. Note locus of control, i.e., internal/external.	The patient who has assumed responsibility in life previously will tend to do the same during difficult times of exacerbation of illness. However, if locus of control has been focused outward, patient may blame others and not take control over own circumstances.
Assist patient to identify factors that are under own control, e.g., list things which can or cannot be controlled.	Knowing and accepting what is beyond individual control can reduce helpless/acting out behaviors, promote focusing on areas individual can control.
Encourage patient to assume control over as much of own care as possible.	Even when unable to do much physical care, individual can help to plan care, having a voice in what is/is not desired.
Discuss needs openly with the patient/SO, setting up agreed-on routines for meeting identified needs.	Helps to deal with manipulative behavior, when patient feels powerless and not listened to.
Incorporate patient's daily routine into hospital stay, as possible.	Maintains sense of control/self-determination and independence.
Discuss plans for the future. Suggest visiting alternate care facilities, taking a look at the possibilities for care as condition changes.	When options are considered and plans are made for any eventuality, patient has a sense of control over own circumstances.

NURSING DIAGNOSIS:	COPING, INDIVIDUAL INEFFECTIVE, HIGH RISK FOR
Risk factors may include:	Physiologic changes (cerebral and spinal lesions).
	Psychologic conflicts; anxiety; fear.
	Impaired judgment, short-term memory loss; confusion; unrealistic perceptions/expectations.
	Personal vulnerability; inadequate support systems.
	Multiple life changes.
	Inadequate coping methods.
Possibly evidenced by:	[Not applicable; presence of signs and symptoms establishes an actual diagnosis.]

DESIRED OUTCOMES/ EVALUATION CRITERIA— PATIENT WILL:	Recognize relationship between disease process (cerebral lesions) and emotional responses, changes in thinking/behavior.
	Verbalize awareness of own capabilities/strengths.
	Display effective problem-solving skills.
	Demonstrate behaviors/lifestyle changes to prevent/minimize changes in mentation and maintain reality orientation.

ACTIONS/INTERVENTIONS	RATIONALE

Independent

Assess current functional capacity/limitations; note presence of distorted thinking processes, labile emotions, cognitive dissonance. Note how these affect the individual's coping abilities.

Organic or psychologic effects may cause patient to be easily distracted; display difficulties with concentration; problem solving, dealing with what is happening, being responsible for own care.

Determine patient's understanding of current situation and previous methods of dealing with life's problems.

Provides a clue to how the patient may deal with what is currently happening and helps identify individual resources and need for assistance.

Maintain an honest, reality-oriented relationship.

Reduces confusion and minimizes painful, frustrating struggles associated with adaptation to altered environment/lifestyle.

Encourage verbalization of feelings/fears, accepting what patient says in a nonjudgmental manner. Note statements reflecting powerlessness, inability to cope. (Refer to ND: Powerlessness/Hopelessness, p 399)

May diminish patient's fear, establish trust, and provide an opportunity to identify problems/begin the problem-solving process.

Observe nonverbal communication, e.g., posture, eye contact, movements, gestures, and use of touch. Compare with verbal content and verify meaning with patient as appropriate.

May provide significant information about what the patient is feeling; however, verification is important to ensure accuracy of communication. Discrepancy between feelings and what is being said can interfere with ability to cope, problem solve.

Provide clues for orientation, e.g., calendars, clocks, notecards, organizers/date book.

These serve as tangible reminders that aid recognition and permeate memory gaps and enable patient to cope with situation.

Encourage patient to tape record important information and listen to it periodically.

Repetition will put information in long-term memory, where it is more easily retrieved and can support decision-making/problem-solving process.

Collaborative

Refer to cognitive retraining program.

Improving cognitive abilities can enhance basic thinking skills when attention span is short; ability to process information is impaired; patient is unable to learn new tasks; or insight, judgment, and problem-solving skills are impaired.

Refer to counseling, psychiatric nurse clinical specialist/psychiatrist, as indicated.

May need additional help to resolve issues of self-esteem and regain effective coping skills.

401

NURSING DIAGNOSIS:	FAMILY COPING, INEFFECTIVE: COMPROMISED/ DISABLING
May be related to:	Temporary family disorganization and role changes.
	Situational crisis.
	Patient providing little support in turn for SO.
	Prolonged disease/disability progression that exhausts the supportive capacity of SO.
	SO with chronically unexpressed feelings of guilt, anxiety, hostility, despair.
	Highly ambivalent family relationships.
Possibly evidenced by:	Patient expresses/confirms concern or complaint about SO response to patient's illness.
	SO withdraws or has limited personal communication with patient or displays protective behavior disproportionate to patient's abilities or need for autonomy.
	SO preoccupied with own personal reactions.
	Intolerance, abandonment.
	Neglectful care of the patient.
	Distortion of reality regarding patient's illness.
DESIRED OUTCOMES/ EVALUATION CRITERIA— FAMILY WILL:	Identify/verbalize resources within themselves to deal with the situation.
	Express more realistic understanding and expectations of the patient.
	Interact appropriately with the patient/staff, providing support and assistance as indicated.
	Verbalize knowledge and understanding of disability/disease.

ACTIONS/INTERVENTIONS

Independent

Note length/severity of illness. Determine patient's role in family and how illness has changed the family organization.

Chronic/unresolved illness, accompanied by changes in role performance/responsibility, often exhausts supportive capacity and coping abilities of SO/family.

Evaluate SO's understanding of disease process and expectations for the future.

Inadequate information/misconception regarding disease process and/or unrealistic expectations affect ability to cope with current situation. Note: A particular area of misconception is the fatigue encountered by patients with MS. Family members may view the patient's inability to perform activi-

ACTIONS/INTERVENTIONS

Independent

Assess other factors that are affecting abilities of family members to provide needed support, e.g., own emotional problems, work concerns.

Discuss underlying reasons for patient's behaviors.

Encourage patient/SO to develop and strengthen problem-solving skills to deal with situation.

Encourage free expression of feelings, including frustration, anger, hostility, and hopelessness.

RATIONALE

ties as manipulative behavior rather than an actual physiologic deficit.

Individual members' preoccupation with own needs/concerns can interfere with providing needed care/support for stresses of long-term illness.

Helps SO understand and accept/deal with behaviors that may be triggered by emotional or physical effects of MS.

Family may/may not have handled conflict well before illness and stress of long-term debilitating condition can create additional problems (including unresolved anger).

Individual members may be afraid to express "negative" feelings, believing it will discourage the patient. Free expression promotes awareness and can help with resolution of feelings and problems (especially when done in a caring manner).

NURSING DIAGNOSIS:	URINARY ELIMINATION, ALTERED PATTERNS
May be related to:	Neuromuscular impairment (spinal cord lesions/neurogenic bladder).
Possibly evidenced by:	Incontinence; nocturia. Retention with overflow.
DESIRED OUTCOMES/ EVALUATION CRITERIA— PATIENT WILL:	Verbalize understanding of condition. Demonstrate behaviors/techniques to prevent/minimize infection.

ACTIONS/INTERVENTIONS

Independent

Note reports of frequency, urgency, burning, incontinence, nocturia, size of/force of urinary stream. Palpate bladder after voiding.

Institute bladder training program.

Encourage adequate fluid intake, limiting intake during late evening and at bedtime. Recommend use of cranberry juice/vitamin C.

RATIONALE

Provides information about degree of interference with elimination or may indicate bladder infection. Fullness over bladder following void is indicative of inadequate emptying and requires intervention.

Helps to restore adequate bladder functioning; lessens occurrence of bladder infection.

Sufficient hydration promotes urinary output and aids in preventing infection. Note: When patient is taking sulfa drugs, sufficient fluids are necessary to ensure adequate excretion of drug, reducing risk of cumulative effects.

ACTIONS/INTERVENTIONS	RATIONALE
Independent	
Promote continued mobility.	Decreases risk of developing bladder and urinary tract infection.
Recommend good handwashing/perineal care.	Reduces skin irritation and risk of ascending infection.
Encourage patient to observe for sediment/blood in urine, foul odor, fever.	Indicative of infection requiring further evaluation/treatment.
Collaborative	
Catheterize as indicated.	May be necessary if patient is unable to empty the bladder or retains urine.
Teach self-catheterization.	Helps patient to maintain autonomy and encourages self-care.
Obtain urine culture and sensitivity as indicated.	Colony count over 100,000 indicates presence of infection requiring treatment.
Administer medications as necessary, e.g., antimicrobial agent, nitrofurantoin macrocrystals (Macrodantin).	Bacteriostatic agent that inhibits bacterial growth. Prompt treatment of infection is necessary to prevent serious complications of sepsis/shock.

NURSING DIAGNOSIS:	**KNOWLEDGE DEFICIT [LEARNING NEED] REGARDING CONDITION, PROGNOSIS, AND TREATMENT**
May be related to:	Lack of exposure; information misinterpretation.
	Unfamiliarity with information resources.
	Cognitive limitation, lack of recall.
Possibly evidenced by:	Statement of misconception.
	Request for information.
	Inaccurate follow-through of instruction.
	Inappropriate or exaggerated behaviors (e.g., hysterical, hostile, agitated, apathetic).
DESIRED OUTCOMES/ EVALUATION CRITERIA— PATIENT WILL:	Participate in learning process.
	Assume responsibility for own learning and begin to look for information and to ask questions.
	Verbalize understanding of condition/disease process and treatment.
	Initiate necessary lifestyle changes.
	Participate in prescribed treatment regimen.

ACTIONS/INTERVENTIONS	RATIONALE
Independent	
Evaluate desire/readiness to learn.	Determines amount/level of information to provide patient at any given moment.
Note signs of emotional lability or that patient is in dissociative state (loss of affect, inappropriate emotional responses).	Patient will not process/retain information and will have difficulty learning during this time.
Review disease process/prognosis, effects of climate, emotional stress, overexertion, fatigue.	Clarifies patient/SO understanding of individual situation.
Identify signs/symptoms requiring further evaluation.	Prompt intervention may help limit severity of exacerbation/complications.
Discuss importance of daily routine of rest, exercise, activity, eating, focusing on current capabilities. Instruct in use of appropriate devices to assist with ADLs, e.g., eating utensils, walking aids.	Helps patient to maintain current level of physical independence and may limit fatigue.
Discuss necessity of weight control.	Excess weight can interfere with balance and motor abilities and make care more difficult.
Stress need for stopping exercise/activity just short of fatigue.	Pushing self beyond individual physical limits can result in excessive/prolonged fatigue and discouragement. Patient can become very adept at knowing where this limit is.
Review possible problems that may arise such as decreased perception of heat and pain, susceptibility to skin breakdown, and infections, especially urinary tract infection.	These effects of demyelination and associated complications may compromise patient's safety and/or precipitate an exacerbation of symptoms.
Identify actions that can be taken to avoid injury: e.g., avoid hot baths, inspect skin regularly, take care with transfers and wheelchair/walker mobility, force fluids, and get adequate nutrition. Encourage avoidance of persons with upper respiratory infection.	Review of these factors can help patient take measures to maintain physical state at optimal level/prevent complications.
Discuss/encourage options for enhancing/developing remaining skills, using diversional activities, continuing with usual concerns as able.	Enables patient to maintain "active" quality of life.
Encourage patient to set goals for the future while focusing on the "here and now," what can be done today.	Having a plan for the future helps to retain hope as well as provide opportunity for patient to see that although today is to be lived, one can plan for tomorrow even in the worst of circumstances.
Review specifics of individual medications. Recommend avoidance of OTC drugs.	Reduces likelihood of drug interactions/adverse effects and enhances cooperation with treatment regimen.
Discuss concerns regarding sexual relationships, contraception/reproduction, effects of pregnancy on affected woman. Identify alternate ways to meet individual needs.	Pregnancy may be an issue for the young patient relative to issues of genetic predisposition and/or ability to manage pregnancy or parent offspring. Increased libido is not uncommon and may require adjustments within the existing relationship or in the absence of an acceptable partner. Information about different positions and techniques and/or

ACTIONS/INTERVENTIONS

Independent

RATIONALE

other options for sexual fulfillment (e.g., fondling, cuddling) may enhance personal relationship and feelings of self-worth.

Collaborative

Refer for vocational rehabilitation.

May need assessment of capabilities/job retraining as indicated by individual limitations/disease progression.

Bibliography

General References

Bellak, JP and Bamford, PA: Nursing Assessment: A Multidimensional Approach. Jones & Bartlett, Boston, 1987.
Berkow, R (ed): The Merck Manual, ed 15. Merck Sharp & Dohme Research Laboratories, Rahway, NJ, 1987.
Cella, JH and Watson, J: Nurse's Manual of Laboratory Tests. FA Davis, Philadelphia, 1989.
Condon, RE and Nyhus, LM (eds): Manual of Surgical Therapeutics, ed 7. Little, Brown & Co, Boston, 1988.
Deglin, JH and Vallerand, AH: Davis's Drug Guide for Nurses, ed 3. FA Davis, Philadelphia, 1992.
Diseases and Disorders Handbook, ed 3. Springhouse, Springhouse, PA, 1989.
Doenges, ME and Moorhouse, MF: Nurse's Pocket Guide: Nursing Diagnoses with Interventions, ed 3. FA Davis, Philadelphia, 1991.
Dunagan, WC and Ridner, ML (eds): Manual of Medical Therapeutics, ed 26. Little, Brown & Co, Boston, 1989.
Fischbach, F: A Manual of Laboratory and Diagnostic Tests, ed 4. JB Lippincott, Philadelphia, 1992.
Guyton, AC: Textbook of Medical Physiology, ed 8. WB Saunders, Philadelphia, 1991.
Kuhn, MM: Pharmacotherapeutics: A Nursing Process Approach, ed 2, FA Davis, 1991.
Professional Guide to Diseases, ed 3. Springhouse, Springhouse, PA, 1989.
Suddarth, DS (ed): The Lippincott Manual of Nursing Practice, ed 5. JB Lippincott, Philadelphia, 1991.
Thomas, CL (ed): Taber's Cyclopedic Medical Dictionary, ed 16. FA Davis, Philadelphia, 1989.
Thompson, JM, McFarland, GK, Hirsh, JE, et al: Mosby's Manual of Clinical Nursing, ed 2. CV Mosby, St Louis, 1989.

Books

Acute Pain Management: Operative or Medical Procedures and Trauma: Clinical Practice Guidelines. US Department of Health and Human Services, February 1992.
Barrett, J: Sexuality and Multiple Sclerosis. National Multiple Sclerosis Society, Courtesy of the Multiple Sclerosis Society of Canada, 1992.
Harkulich, JR and Calamita, BA: A Manual for Caregivers of Alzheimer's Disease Clients in Long Term Care. Nursing Home Area Training Centers of Ohio and the Ohio Department of Aging. Ohio, 1988.
Holland, NJ and Madonna, MG: Understanding Bladder Dysfunction in Multiple Sclerosis. National Multiple Sclerosis Society, 1988.
Multiple Sclerosis and Your Emotions. Multiple Sclerosis Clinic, Department of Neurology, University of Utah School of Medicine, Salt Lake City, Utah, 1989.
Waserman, L, et al: Living with Multiple Sclerosis: A Practical Guide. The Massachusetts Chapter of the National Multiple Sclerosis Society, 1988.

Articles

Alzheimer's Research Review, summer 1990, p 1.
Arena, JG, Hannah, SL, Bruno, FM, et al: Electromygraphic biofeedback training for tension headache in the elderly: A prospective study. Biofeedback and Self-Regulation 16(4):379, 1991.
Aumick, JE: Head trauma: Guidelines for care. RN 54(4):27, 1991.
Bagby, G: Advances in anticonvulsant therapy. Headlines, winter 1991, p 2.
Barker, E: Action Stat! Spinal cord injury. Nursing90 20(11):33, 1990.
Basta, S: Pressure sore prevention education with the spinal cord injured. Rehab Nursing 6(1):6, 1991.
Bennett, WI (ed): Aspirin and stroke. Harvard Medical School Health Letter 15(7):1, 1990.
Bennett, WI (ed): Alzheimer's disease: Is it aluminum? Harvard Medical School Health Letter 15(11):1, 1990.
Bennett, WI (ed): Alzheimer's disease: Is there a test? Harvard Medical School Health Letter 16(3):1, 1991.

Bryant, GA: When your patient needs back surgery. RN 55(7):46, 1992.

Cerrato, GE and Rakowski-Reinhardt, AC: Action Stat! Autonomic dysreflexia. Nursing91 21(2): 33, 1991.

Drummond, B: Preventing increased intracranial pressure: Nursing care can make the difference. Focus on Critical Care 17(2):116, 1990.

Dumas, A: Love brings light to a life grown dim. Rocky Mountain News March 1992, p 12–m.

Evans, RL, Griffith, J, Haselkorn, JK, et al: Poststroke family function: An evaluation of the family's role in rehabilitation. Rehab Nursing 17(3):127, 1992.

Finocchiaro, DN and Herzfeld, ST: Understanding autonomic dysreflexia. AJN 90(9):56, 1990.

Hall, GR: This hospital patient has Alzheimer's. AJN 91(10):44, 1991.

Herbsky, EP and Sears, JH: Fatigue in multiple sclerosis: Guidelines for nursing care. Rehab Nursing 17(4):176, 1992.

Kane-Carlsen, PA: Managing patients with TIAs. Nursing92 22(1):34, 1992.

Killam, P: Childhood epilepsy: Myth vs. reality. AJN 92(3):77, 1992.

Misenti, M: Have you ever had a head injury? Headlines March/April 1992, p 12.

Mitiguy, J: New applications of diagnostic techniques: Looking for evidence of mild brain injury. Headlines March/April 1992, p 2.

Morgan, SP: A passage through paralysis. AJN 91(10):70, 1991.

North, B, North, C, and Lee, JL: Living in a halo. AJN 22(4):54, 1992.

Pace, K and Emerich, M: Keeping track of confused patients. Nursing90 June:64, 1990.

Petit, M: Recognizing post-traumatic stress. RN 54(3):56, 1991.

Purath, J: Assessing headache pain. RN 54(10):26, 1991.

Reimer, M: Head-injured patients: How to detect early signs of trouble. Nursing89 19(3):34, 1989.

Ridgeway, G: Demystifying tonic-clonic seizures. Nursing91 21(11):63, 1991.

Saper, JR: Daily chronic headache. Neuro Clin 8(4):891, 1990.

Sherman, DW: Managing an acute head injury. Nursing90 20(4):47, 1990.

Tackenberg, J: Teaching caregivers about Alzheimer's disease. Nursing 92 22(5):75, 1992.

Wilson, HS: Easing life for the Alzheimer's patient. RN 53(12):24, 1990.

White, AA: Oh my aching back. Harvard Medical School Health Letter 15(1):5, 1989.

White, AA: Back pain treatment. Harvard Medical School Health Letter 15(3):4, 1990.

Wolpow, EP: Mild head injury: After the fall. Harvard Health Letter 16(6):1, 1991.

CHAPTER **7**
OPHTHALMOLOGIC

Ocular Disorders _____

CATARACTS (POSTOPERATIVE)

A cataract is a progressively developing opacity of the lens or lens capsule, commonly a result of the aging process that develops in about half of all people over 65. A cataract often occurs bilaterally, but each cataract progresses independently. Surgery is usually done on an outpatient basis; however, an overnight stay may be required due to the presence of other medical conditions.

GLAUCOMA

This condition is the result of inadequate drainage of aqueous humor from the anterior chamber of the eye. Increasing intraocular pressure causes atrophy of the optic nerve and blindness if untreated.

RELATED CONCERNS:

Psychosocial Aspects of Acute Care, p 899
Surgical Intervention, p 918

PATIENT ASSESSMENT DATA BASE

ACTIVITY/REST

May report:	Change in usual activities/hobbies due to altered vision.

FOOD/FLUID

May report:	Nausea/vomiting (acute glaucoma).

NEUROSENSORY

May report:	Visual distortions (blurred/hazy), bright light causing a glare with a gradual loss of peripheral vision, difficulty focusing on close work/adjusting to darkened room (cataracts).
	Cloudy/blurred vision, appearance of halos/rainbows around lights, loss of peripheral vision, photophobia (acute glaucoma).
	Glasses/treatment change does not improve vision.
May exhibit:	Gray or milky white appearance of pupil (cataract).

408

Fixed pupil and red/hard eye with cloudy cornea (glaucoma emergency). Increased tearing.

PAIN/COMFORT

May report: Mild discomfort/tired eyes (chronic glaucoma).

Sudden/persistent severe pain or pressure in and around eye(s), headache (acute glaucoma).

SAFETY

May report: History of hemorrhage, trauma, ocular disease, tumor (glaucoma).

Difficulty seeing, managing activities.

TEACHING/LEARNING

May report: Family history of glaucoma, diabetes, systemic vascular disorders.

History of stress, allergies, vasomotor disturbances (e.g., increased venous pressure), endocrine imbalance, diabetes (glaucoma).

Exposure to radiation; steroid/phenothiazine toxicity.

Discharge Plan Considerations: **DRG projected mean length of stay: 4.2 days.** (Usually done as an outpatient procedure.)

May require assistance with transportation, meal preparation, self-care, home-maker/maintenance tasks.

DIAGNOSTIC STUDIES

Snellen eye chart/telebinocular machine (tests visual acuity and central vision): May be impaired by defects in cornea, lens, aqueous or vitreous humor, refractive error, or disease of the nervous or vascular system supplying the retina or optic pathway.

Visual fields: Reduction may be caused by CVA, pituitary/brain tumor mass, carotid or cerebral artery pathology or glaucoma.

Tonography measurement: Assesses intraocular (IOP) (normal: 12–25 mm Hg).

Gonioscopy measurement: Helps differentiate open angle from angle-closure glaucoma.

Provocative tests: May be useful in establishing presence/type of glaucoma when IOP is normal or only mildly elevated.

Ophthalmoscopy examination: Assesses internal ocular structures, noting optic disk atrophy, papilledema, retinal hemorrhage, and microaneurysms. Dilation and slit-lamp examination confirms diagnosis of cataract.

CBC, sedimentation rate (ESR): Rules out systemic anemia/infection.

ECG, serum cholesterol, and lipid studies: May be done to rule out atherosclerosis, CAD.

Glucose tolerance test/FBS: Determines presence/control of diabetes.

NURSING PRIORITIES

1. Prevent further visual deterioration.
2. Promote adaptation to changes in/reduced visual acuity.
3. Prevent complications.
4. Provide information about disease process/prognosis and treatment needs.

DISCHARGE GOALS

1. Vision maintained at highest possible level.
2. Patient coping with situation in a positive manner.
3. Complications prevented/minimized.
4. Disease process/prognosis and therapeutic regimen understood.

DEGENERATIVE CATARACT (POSTOPERATIVE CARE)

NURSING DIAGNOSIS:	INJURY, HIGH RISK FOR
Risk factors may include:	Increased IOP.
	Intraocular hemorrhage, vitreous loss.
Possibly evidenced by:	[Not applicable; presence of signs and symptoms establishes an actual diagnosis.]
DESIRED OUTCOMES/ EVALUATION CRITERIA— PATIENT WILL:	Verbalize understanding of factors that contribute to possibility of injury.
	Demonstrate behaviors, lifestyle changes to reduce risk factors and to protect self from injury.
	Modify environment as indicated to enhance safety.

ACTIONS/INTERVENTIONS	RATIONALE
Independent	
Discuss postoperative expectations concerning pain, activity restrictions, appearance, eye bandaging.	Can be helpful in allaying fears and enhancing co-operation with necessary restrictions.
Position patient on back, elevate head, or turn to unoperated side as desired.	Rest may be required for only a few minutes to an hour with outpatient surgery or may be required overnight when preexisting conditions/complications are present. Reduces pressure in affected eye, minimizing risk of hemorrhage or suture stress/dehiscence.
Limit activities such as sudden movement of the head, rubbing eyes, bending at the waist.	Reduces stress on operative area/decreases IOP.
Ambulate with assistance; provide bathroom privileges when recovered from anesthesia.	Requires less strain than use of bedpan, which could increase IOP.
Encourage deep breathing, instead of coughing, for pulmonary hygiene.	Coughing increases IOP.
Recommend use of stress management techniques, e.g., guided imagery, visualization, deep-breathing and relaxation exercises.	Promotes relaxation, reduces IOP, and may enhance coping.
Maintain protective eye patch as indicated.	May be used to protect from accidental injury and to reduce eye movement.

ACTIONS/INTERVENTIONS

Independent

Have patient differentiate between discomfort and sudden sharp eye pain. Investigate restlessness, disorientation, disturbance of dressing. Observe for hyphema (bleeding in the eye) by inspecting the eye with a flashlight, as indicated.

Observe for bulging of wound, flat anterior chamber, pear-shaped pupil.

Collaborative

Administer medication as indicated:

Antiemetics, e.g., prochlorperazine (Compazine);

Acetazolamide (Diamox);

Cycloplegics;

Analgesics, e.g., Empirin with codeine, acetaminophen (Tylenol).

RATIONALE

Discomfort is to be expected from the surgical procedure; however, acute pain suggests developing IOP and/or hemorrhage, which may occur due to strain or for no apparent reason (healing tissue is highly vascular, and capillaries are fragile).

Denotes prolapse of iris or wound rupture caused by loosened sutures or pressure on the eye.

Nausea/vomiting can increase IOP, necessitating prompt treatment to prevent ocular injury.

May be given to decrease IOP if elevation occurs; restricts enzymatic action in production of aqueous humor.

May be given to paralyze ciliary muscle to dilate and rest iris after surgery if lens is not implanted.

May be used for mild discomfort to promote rest/prevent restlessness, which may affect IOP. *Note:* Use of aspirin is contraindicated because of increased bleeding tendencies.

NURSING DIAGNOSIS:	INFECTION, HIGH RISK FOR
Risk factors may include:	Invasive procedure (surgical cataract removal).
Possibly evidenced by:	[Not applicable; presence of signs and symptoms establishes an actual diagnosis.]
DESIRED OUTCOMES/ EVALUATION CRITERIA— PATIENT WILL:	Achieve timely wound healing, free of purulent drainage, erythema, and fever. Identify interventions to prevent/reduce risk of infection.

ACTIONS/INTERVENTIONS

Independent

Discuss importance of handwashing before touching/treating eye.

Use/demonstrate proper technique for cleaning eye from inner to outer corner with fresh tissue/cotton ball for each wipe, changing dressings, and inserting contact lens if used.

Stress importance of not touching/rubbing operated eye.

RATIONALE

Diminishes number of bacteria on hands, preventing contamination of operative area.

Aseptic technique reduces risk of spread of bacteria and cross-contamination.

Prevents contamination and disruption of operative site.

ACTIONS/INTERVENTIONS

RATIONALE

Independent

Observe for/discuss signs of developing infection, e.g., redness, lid swelling, purulent drainage. Identify precautions to take if URI occurs.

Eye infection is most likely to develop 2–3 days after procedure and requires prompt intervention. Presence of URI increases risk of cross-contamination.

Collaborative

Administer medications as indicated:

Antibiotics (topical, parenteral, or subconjunctival);

Topical preparations may be used prophylactically, while more aggressive therapy is required if infection develops. *Note:* Steroids may be added to topical antibiotic when patient has IOL implant.

Steroids.

May be used to decrease inflammation.

NURSING DIAGNOSIS:	SENSORY-PERCEPTUAL ALTERATION: VISUAL
May be related to:	Altered sensory reception/status of sense organs.
	Therapeutically restricted environment.
Possibly evidenced by:	Diminished acuity, visual distortions.
	Change in usual response to stimuli.
DESIRED OUTCOMES/ EVALUATION CRITERIA— PATIENT WILL:	Regain visual acuity within limitations of individual situation.
	Recognize sensory impairments and compensate for changes.
	Identify/correct potential hazards in the environment.

ACTIONS/INTERVENTIONS

RATIONALE

Independent

Determine visual acuity, note whether one or both eyes are involved.

Individual needs and choice of interventions will vary because loss of vision is a slow, progressive process. If bilateral, each eye can progress at a different rate, but usually only one eye is corrected per procedure.

Orient patient to surroundings, staff, others in the area.

Provides for increased comfort level and familiarity, reducing anxiety and postoperative disorientation.

Observe for signs of disorientation; keep side rails up until fully recovered from anesthesia.

Waking in an unfamiliar place and having visual limitations may result in confusion in the elderly person. Decreases risk of falling when patient is confused/unfamiliar with size of bed.

Approach from unoperated side, speak and touch often; encourage SO to stay with patient.

Provides appropriate sensory stimulation to offset isolation and reduce confusion.

ACTIONS/INTERVENTIONS

Independent

Caution about dim or blurred vision and irritation of eye, which may occur when using eye drops.

Remind patient using cataract glasses that objects are magnified approximately 25%, peripheral vision is lost, and blind spots may be noted.

Place needed items/position call bell within easy reach on nonoperative side.

RATIONALE

Visual disturbance/irritation may last for 1–2 hours after instillation of eyedrops but gradually decreases with use. *Note:* Local irritation should be reported to physician, but do not stop use of drug in interim.

Changes in acuity and depth perception can cause visual confusion/increase risk of injury until patient learns to compensate.

Allows patient to see objects more easily and facilitates calling for help when needed.

NURSING DIAGNOSIS:	KNOWLEDGE DEFICIT [LEARNING NEED] REGARDING CONDITION, PROGNOSIS, TREATMENT
May be related to:	Unfamiliarity with information resources, information misinterpretation.
	Lack of exposure/recall.
	Cognitive limitation.
Possibly evidenced by:	Questions/statement of misconception.
	Inaccurate follow-through of instruction.
	Development of preventable complications.
DESIRED OUTCOMES/ EVALUATION CRITERIA— PATIENT WILL:	Verbalize understanding of condition/disease process and treatment.
	Correctly perform necessary procedures and explain reasons for the actions.

ACTIONS/INTERVENTIONS

Independent

Review information about individual condition, prognosis, type of procedure/lens.

Stress importance of routine follow-up care. Tell patient to report clouding of vision.

Inform patient to avoid OTC eyedrops.

Discuss possible effects/interactions between eye medications and patient's medical problems, e.g., increase in hypertension, COPD, diabetes. Instruct

–RATIONALE

Enhances understanding and promotes cooperation with postoperative regimen.

Periodic monitoring reduces risk of serious complications. In some patients the posterior capsule may thicken or become hazy within 2 weeks to several years postoperatively, requiring laser therapy to correct visual deficit.

May counteract/interact with prescribed medications.

Use of topical eye medications, e.g., sympathomimetic agents, β-blockers, and anticholinergic agents can cause BP to rise in hypertensive pa-

413

ACTIONS/INTERVENTIONS	RATIONALE

Independent

in proper method of instilling eyedrops to minimize systemic effects.

tients; precipitate dyspnea in patients with COPD; mask the symptoms of a hypoglycemic crisis in insulin-dependent diabetics. Correct application can limit absorption into systemic circulation, minimizing problems such as drug interactions and unwanted/untoward systemic effects.

Instruct patient to avoid reading, squinting; heavy lifting, straining at stool, excessive bending at the waist, blowing nose; use of sprays, dusting powder, smoking (self/others).

Activities that cause eye fatigue/strain, Valsalva maneuver, or increased IOP may compromise surgical results and precipitate hemorrhage. *Note:* Respiratory irritants that cause coughing/sneezing can increase IOP.

Encourage diversional activities such as radio, conversation, television viewing in moderation.

Provides sensory input, maintains sense of normality, passes time more easily when unable to use vision sense fully. *Note:* Moderate watching of television requires less eye movement and is less stressful than reading.

Recommend patient check with doctor about resumption/modification of sexual activities.

May increase IOP, cause accidental injury to eye.

Stress need for wearing protective glasses during day/patching operative eye at night.

Prevents accidental injury to eye and reduces risk of increased IOP due to squinting or position of head.

Suggest patient sleep on back, regulate the intensity of light and wear dark glasses when outside/in bright lighting, shampoo with head slightly tilted back (not forward), cough with mouth/eyes open.

Prevents accidental injury to eye.

Suggest positioning doors so they are completely opened or closed; remove furniture from the travel pathways.

Decreased peripheral vision or altered depth perception may cause patient to walk into partially opened door or trip over furniture.

Encourage adequate intake of fluids, bulk/roughage; use OTC stool softeners, if indicated.

Maintains consistency of stool to avoid straining.

Recommend keeping extra bottle of eyedrops on hand.

Prevents inadvertent discontinuation of medication in the event of loss and so forth.

Identify signs/symptoms requiring prompt medical evaluation, e.g., sharp sudden pain, decreased vision, lid swelling, purulent discharge, redness, watering of eyes, photophobia.

Early intervention can prevent development of serious complications, possible loss of vision.

Glaucoma _____

NURSING DIAGNOSIS:	SENSORY-PERCEPTUAL ALTERATION: VISUAL
May be related to:	Altered sensory reception: altered status of sense organ.
Possibly evidenced by:	Progressive loss of visual field.
DESIRED OUTCOMES/ EVALUATION CRITERIA— PATIENT WILL:	Participate in therapeutic regimen. Maintain current visual field/acuity without further loss.

ACTIONS/INTERVENTIONS

Independent

Ascertain degree/type of visual loss.

Encourage expression of feelings about loss/possibility of loss of vision.

Demonstrate administration of eyedrops, e.g., counting drops, adhering to schedule, not missing doses.

Implement measures to assist patient to manage visual limitations, e.g., reduce clutter, arrange furniture out of travel path; remind to turn head to view subjects; correct for dim light and problems of night vision.

Collaborative

Administer medications as indicated:

Chronic, simple, open-angle type:

Pilocarpine hydrochloride (IsoptoCarpine, Ocusert Pilo, Pilopine HS Gel);

Timolol maleate (Timoptic); betaxalol (Betopic);

Acetazolamide (Diamox);

Narrow angle (angle closure) type:

Myotics (until pupil is constricted);

RATIONALE

Affects patient's future expectations and choice of interventions.

While early intervention may prevent blindness, the patient faces the possibility or may have already experienced partial or complete loss of vision. Although vision loss that has already occurred cannot be restored (even with treatment), further loss can be prevented.

Controls IOP, preventing further loss of vision.

Reduces safety hazards related to changes in visual fields/loss of vision and papillary accommodation to environmental light.

These topical myotic drugs cause pupillary constriction, facilitating the outflow of aqueous humor.

Decreases formation of aqueous humor without changing pupil size, vision, or accommodation. *Note:* Timoptic is contraindicated in the presence of bradycardia or asthma.

Decreases the rate of production of aqueous humor.

Creates contraction of sphincter muscles of the iris, deepens anterior chamber, and dilates vessels of outflow tract during acute attack/prior to surgery.

415

ACTIONS/INTERVENTIONS	RATIONALE
Collaborative	
Carbonic anhydrase inhibitors, e.g., acetazolamide (Diamox);	Decreases secretion of aqueous humor and lowers IOP.
Dipivefrin hydrochloride (Propine);	May be of benefit when patient is unresponsive to other medications. Free of side-effects such as miosis, blurred vision, and night blindness.
hyperosmotic agents, e.g., mannitol (Osmitrol); glycerine.	Used to decrease circulating fluid volume, which will decrease production of aqueous humor if other treatments have not been successful.
Provide sedation, analgesics as necessary.	Acute glaucoma attack is associated with sudden pain, which can precipitate anxiety/agitation, further elevating IOP. *Note:* Medical management may require 4–6 hours before IOP decreases and pain subsides.
Prepare for surgical intervention as indicated:	
Angon laser trabeculoplasty (ALT) or trabeculectomy; Trabeculectomy/trephination;	Filtering operations that create an opening between the anterior chamber and the subjunctival spaces so that aqueous humor can bypass the trabecular mesh block. *Note:* Apradclonidine (Iopidine) eye drops may be used in conjunction with laser therapy to lessen/prevent postprocedure elevations of IOP.
Iridectomy;	Surgical removal of a portion of the iris to facilitate drainage of aqueous humor. Upper iris usually is covered with upper eyelid, and flow of tears washes bacteria downward. *Note:* Bilateral iridectomy is performed because glaucoma usually develops in the other eye.
Malteno valve implantation;	Experimental device used to correct or prevent scarring over/closure of drainage sac created by trabeculectomy.
Cyclodialysis;	Separates ciliary body from the sclera to facilitate outflow of aqueous humor.
Aqueous-venous shunt;	Used in intractable glaucoma.
Diathermy/cryosurgery.	If other treatments fail, destruction of the ciliary body will reduce formation of aqueous humor.

NURSING DIAGNOSIS:	ANXIETY [SPECIFY LEVEL]
May be related to:	Physiologic factors, change in health status; presence of pain; possibility/reality of loss of vision.
	Unmet needs.
	Negative self-talk.
Possibly evidenced by:	Apprehension, uncertainty.
	Expressed concern regarding changes in life events.

DESIRED OUTCOMES/ EVALUATION CRITERIA— PATIENT WILL:	Appear relaxed and report anxiety is reduced to a manageable level.
	Demonstrate problem-solving skills.
	Use resources effectively.

ACTIONS/INTERVENTIONS

Independent

Assess anxiety level, degree of pain experienced/ suddenness of onset of symptoms, and current knowledge of condition.

Provide accurate, honest information. Discuss probability that careful monitoring and treatment can prevent additional visual loss.

Encourage patient to acknowledge concerns and express feelings.

Identify helpful resources/people.

RATIONALE

These factors affect patient perception of threat to self, potentiate the cycle of anxiety, and may interfere with medical attempts to control IOP.

Reduces anxiety related to unknown/future expectations and provides factual basis for making informed choices about treatment.

Provides opportunity for patient to deal with reality of situation, clarify misconceptions, and problem-solve concerns.

Provides reassurance that patient is not alone in dealing with problem.

NURSING DIAGNOSIS:	KNOWLEDGE DEFICIT [LEARNING NEED], REGARDING CONDITION, PROGNOSIS, AND TREATMENT
May be related to:	Lack of exposure/unfamiliarity with resources.
	Lack of recall, information misinterpretation.
Possibly evidenced by:	Questions; statement of misconception.
	Inaccurate follow-through of instruction.
	Development of preventable complications.
DESIRED OUTCOMES/ EVALUATION CRITERIA— PATIENT WILL:	Verbalize understanding of condition, prognosis, and treatment.
	Identify relationship of signs/symptoms to the disease process.
	Correctly perform necessary procedures and explain reasons for the actions.

ACTIONS/INTERVENTIONS

Independent

Discuss necessity of wearing identification, e.g., Medi-Alert bracelet.

RATIONALE

Vital to provide information for caregivers in case of emergency to reduce risk of receiving contraindicated drugs (e.g., atropine).

417

ACTIONS/INTERVENTIONS	RATIONALE
Independent	
Demonstrate proper technique for administration of eye drops. Have patient return demonstration.	Enhances effectiveness of treatment. Provides opportunity for patient to show competence and ask questions.
Review importance of maintaining drug schedule, e.g., eye drops. Discuss medications that should be avoided, e.g., mydriatic drops (atropine/propantheline bromine), overuse of topical steroids.	This disease can be controlled, not cured, and maintaining consistent medication regimen is vital to control. Some drugs cause pupil dilation, increasing IOP and potentiating additional loss of vision.
Identify potential side effects/adverse reactions of treatment, e.g., decreased appetite, nausea/vomiting, diarrhea, fatigue, "drugged" feeling, decreased libido, impotence, cardiac irregularities, syncope, CHF.	Drug side/adverse effects range from uncomfortable to severe/health-threatening. Approximately 50% of patients will develop sensitivity/allergy to parasympathomimetics (e.g., pilocarpine) or anticholinesterase drugs. These problems require medical evaluation and possible change in therapeutic regimen.
Encourage patient to make necessary changes in lifestyle.	A tranquil lifestyle decreases the emotional response to stress, preventing ocular changes that push the iris forward, which may precipitate an acute attack.
Reinforce avoidance of activities, such as heavy lifting/pushing, snow shoveling, wearing tight/constricting clothing.	May increase IOP precipitating acute attack. *Note:* If patient is not experiencing pain, cooperation with drug regimen and acceptance of lifestyle changes are often difficult to sustain.
Discuss dietary considerations, e.g., adequate fluid, bulk/fiber intake.	Measures to maintain consistency of stool to avoid constipation/straining during defecation.
Stress importance of routine checkups.	Important to monitor progression/maintenance of disease to allow for early intervention and prevent further loss of vision.
Advise patient to immediately report severe eye pain, inflammation, increased photophobia, increased lacrimation, changes in visual field/veil-like curtain, blurred vision, flashes of light/particles floating in visual field.	Prompt action may be necessary to prevent further vision loss/other complications, e.g., detached retina.
Recommend family members be examined regularly for signs of glaucoma.	Hereditary tendency of shallow anterior chambers places family members at risk for developing the condition.

Bibliography

General References

Bellak, JP and Bamford, PA: Nursing Assessment: A Multidimensional Approach. Jones & Bartlett, Boston, 1987.

Berkow, R (ed): The Merck Manual, ed 15. Merck Sharp & Dohme Research Laboratories, Rahway, NJ, 1987.

Cella, JH and Watson, J: Nurse's Manual of Laboratory Tests. FA Davis, Philadelphia, 1989.

Condon, RE and Nyhus, LM (eds): Manual of Surgical Therapeutics, ed 7. Little, Brown & Co, Boston, 1988.

Deglin, JH and Vallerand, AH: Davis's Drug Guide for Nurses, ed 3. FA Davis, Philadelphia, 1992.

Diseases and Disorders Handbook, ed 3. Springhouse, Springhouse, PA, 1989.

Doenges, ME and Moorhouse, MF: Nurse's Pocket Guide: Nursing Diagnoses with Interventions, ed 3. FA Davis, Philadelphia, 1991.

Dunagan, WC and Ridner, ML (eds): Manual of Medical Therapeutics, ed 26. Little, Brown & Co, Boston, 1989.
Fischbach, F: A Manual of Laboratory and Diagnostic Tests, ed 4. JB Lippincott, Philadelphia, 1992.
Guyton, AC: Textbook of Medical Physiology, ed 8. WB Saunders, Philadelphia, 1993.
Kuhn, MM: Pharmacotherapeutics: A Nursing Process Approach, ed 2, FA Davis, 1991.
Professional Guide to Diseases, ed 3. Springhouse, Springhouse, PA, 1989.
Suddarth, DS (ed): The Lippincott Manual of Nursing Practice, ed 5. JB Lippincott, Philadelphia, 1991.
Thomas, CL (ed): Taber's Cyclopedic Medical Dictionary, ed 17. FA Davis, Philadelphia, 1993.
Thompson, JM, McFarland, GK, Hirsh, JE et al: Mosby's Manual of Clinical Nursing, ed 2. CV Mosby, St. Louis, 1989.

Articles

Beed, P: Sight restored. Nursing Times 87(30):46, 1991.
Kramer, SG: The triple procedure: Cataract extraction in a different setting. Refractive & Corneal Surgery 7:51, 1991.
Navarro, VB, Tolley, FM, and Alcott, MA: Restoration of sight by corneal transplantation. Crit Care Nurs Q 13(4):72, 1991.
Propine. Allergan pharmaceuticals, Irvine CA, 1991.
Rodman, M: Your guide to the newest drugs. RN 52(3):61, 1989.
Traynor, M: Day case eye surgery. Nursing Times 86(39):54, 1990.
Varma, R, Steinmann, W and Scott, I: Expert agreement in evaluating the optic disc for glaucoma. Ophthalmology 99(2): 215, 1992.

CHAPTER 8

GASTROENTEROLOGY

Eating Disorders: Anorexia Nervosa/Bulimia Nervosa _____

Although these disorders affect women primarily, approximately 5%–10% are men.

Anorexia nervosa is an illness of starvation, brought on by severe disturbance of body image and a morbid fear of obesity.

Bulimia nervosa is an eating disorder (binge-purge syndrome) characterized by extreme overeating and followed by self-induced vomiting. It may include abuse of laxatives and diuretics.

RELATED CONCERNS:

Dysrhythmias, p 94
Fluid and Electrolyte Imbalances, p 1054
Psychosocial Aspects of Acute Care, p 899

PATIENT ASSESSMENT DATA BASE

ACTIVITY/REST

May report:	Disturbed sleep patterns, e.g., early morning insomnia; fatigue.
	Feeling "hyper" and/or anxious.
	Increased activity/participation in high-energy sports.
May exhibit:	Periods of hyperactivity, constant vigorous exercising.

CIRCULATION

May report:	Feeling cold even when room is warm.
May exhibit:	Low BP.
	Tachycardia, bradycardia, dysrhythmias.

EGO INTEGRITY

May report:	Powerlessness/helplessness.
	Distorted (unrealistic) body image—reports self as fat regardless of weight and sees thin body as fat; persistent overconcern with body shape and weight—fears gaining weight.

High self-expectations.

Suppression of anger.

May exhibit: Emotional states of depression, withdrawal, anger, anxiety.

ELIMINATION

May report: Diarrhea/constipation.

Vague abdominal pain and distress, bloating.

Laxative/diuretic use.

FOOD/FLUID

May report: Constant hunger or denial of hunger; normal or exaggerated appetite (rarely vanishes until late in the disorder).

Intense fear of gaining weight; may have prior history of being overweight.

Preoccupation with food, e.g., calorie counting, gourmet cooking.

An unrealistic pleasure in weight loss, while denying self pleasure in other areas.

Refusal to maintain body weight over minimal norm for age/height.

Recurrent episodes of binge eating; a feeling of lack of control over behavior during eating binges. A minimum average of 2 binge eating episodes a week for at least 3 months.

Regularly engaging in either self-induced vomiting or strict dieting or fasting.

May exhibit: Weight loss/maintenance of body weight 15% or more below that expected (anorexia) or weight may be normal or slightly below (bulimia).

No medical illness evident to account for weight loss.

Cachectic appearance; skin may be dry, yellowish/pale, with poor turgor.

Hiding food, cutting food into small pieces, rearranging food on plate.

Irrational thinking about eating, food, and weight.

Binge-purge syndrome (bulimia) independently or as a complication of anorexia.

Peripheral edema.

Swollen salivary glands, sore, inflamed buccal cavity, continuous sore throat.

Vomiting, bloody vomitus (may indicate esophageal tearing, Mallory-Weiss).

Excessive gum chewing.

HYGIENE

May exhibit: Increased hair growth on body (lanugo); hair loss (axillary/pubic).

Hair is dull/not shiny.

Brittle nails.

Signs of erosion of tooth enamel; gums in poor condition.

NEUROSENSORY

May exhibit: Appropriate affect, except in regard to body and eating.

Depressive affect, (may be depressed).

Mental changes (apathy, confusion, memory impairment) brought on by malnutrition/starvation.

Hysterical or obsessive personality style; no other psychiatric illness or evidence of a psychiatric thought disorder present (although a significant number may show evidence of an affective disorder).

PAIN/COMFORT

May report: Headaches.

SAFETY

May exhibit: Decreased body temperature.
Recurrent infectious processes (indicative of depressed immune system).
Eczema/other skin problems.

SOCIAL INTERACTION

May report: Middle-class or upper-class family background.
Passive father/dominant mother, family members closely fused, togetherness prized, personal boundaries not respected.
History of being a quiet, cooperative child.
Problems of control issues in relationships.
Engagement in power struggles.
An emotional crisis of some sort, such as the onset of puberty or a family move.
Altered relationships or problems with relationships (not married, divorced).
Sexual abuse, promiscuity.
Withdrawal from friends/social contacts.
Sense of helplessness.
Shoplifting.

SEXUALITY

May report: Absence of at least three consecutive menstrual cycles.
Denial/loss of sexual interest.

May exhibit: Breast atrophy, amenorrhea.

TEACHING/LEARNING

May report: Family history of higher than normal incidence of depression.
Onset of the illness usually between the ages of 10 and 22.
Health beliefs/practice, e.g., certain foods have "too many" calories, use of "health" foods.
High academic achievement.

Discharge Plan Considerations: **DRG projected mean length of stay: 6.4 days.**
Assistance with maintenance of treatment plan.

DIAGNOSTIC STUDIES

CBC with differential: Determines presence of anemia, leukopenia, lymphocytosis. Blood platelets show significantly less than normal activity by the enzyme monoamine oxidase (thought to be a marker for depression).

Electrolytes: Imbalances may include decreased potassium, sodium, and chloride.

Endocrine studies:

Thyroid function: Thyroxine (T_4) levels usually normal; however, circulating triiodothyronine (T_3) levels may be low.

Pituitary function: TSH response to TRF is abnormal in anorexia nervosa. Propranolol-glucagon stimulation test (studies the response of human GH): depressed level of GH in anorexia nervosa. Gonadotropic hypofunction is noted.

Cortisol metabolism: May be elevated.

DST: (Evaluates hypothalamic-pituitary function) dexamethasone resistance indicates cortisol suppression, suggesting malnutrition and/or depression.

Luteinizing hormone secretions test: Pattern often resembles those of prepubertal girls.

Estrogen: Decreased.

Blood sugar and BMR: May be low.

Other chemistries: AST (SGOT) elevated. Hypercarotenemia, hypoproteinemia, hypocholesterolemia.

MHP 6 levels: Decreased, suggestive of malnutrition/depression.

Urinalysis and renal function: BUN may be elevated; ketones present reflecting starvation; decreased urinary 17-ketosteroids.

ECG: Abnormal with low voltage, T-wave inversion, dysrhythmias.

NURSING PRIORITIES

1. Reestablish adequate/appropriate nutritional intake.
2. Correct fluid and electrolyte imbalance.
3. Assist patient to develop realistic body image/improve self-esteem.
4. Provide support/involve SO, if available, in treatment program.
5. Coordinate total treatment program with other disciplines.
6. Provide information about disease, prognosis, and treatment to patient/SO.

DISCHARGE GOALS

1. Adequate nutrition and fluid intake maintained.
2. Maladaptive coping behaviors and stressors that precipitate anxiety recognized.
3. Adaptive coping strategies and techniques for anxiety reduction and self-control implemented.
4. Self-esteem increased.
5. Disease process, prognosis, and treatment regimen understood.

NURSING DIAGNOSIS:	NUTRITION, ALTERED: LESS THAN BODY REQUIREMENTS
May be related to:	Inadequate food intake; self-induced vomiting.
	Chronic/excessive laxative use.
Possibly evidenced by:	Body weight 15% (or more) below expected, or may be within normal range (bulimia).
	Pale conjunctiva and mucous membranes; poor skin turgor/muscle tone.
	Excessive loss of hair; increased growth of hair on body (lanugo).
	Amenorrhea.
	Electrolyte imbalances.

	Hypothermia.
	Bradycardia; cardiac irregularities; hypotension.
	Edema.
DESIRED OUTCOMES/ EVALUATION CRITERIA— PATIENT WILL:	Verbalize understanding of nutritional needs.
	Establish a dietary pattern with caloric intake adequate to regain/maintain appropriate weight.
	Demonstrate weight gain toward individually expected range.

ACTIONS/INTERVENTIONS

Independent

Establish a minimum weight goal and daily nutritional requirements.

Use a consistent approach. Sit with patient while eating; present and remove food without persuasion and/or comment. Promote pleasant environment and record intake.

Provide smaller meals and supplemental snacks, as appropriate.

Make selective menu available, and allow patient to control choices as much as possible.

Be alert to choices of low-calorie foods/beverages; hoarding food; disposing of food in various places such as pockets or wastebaskets.

Maintain a regular weighing schedule, such as Monday, Wednesday, and Friday before breakfast in same attire, and graph results.

Weigh with back to scale (dependent on program protocols).

Avoid room checks and other control devices whenever possible.

Provide 1-to-1 supervision and have the patient with bulimia remain in the day-room area with no

RATIONALE

Malnutrition is a mood-altering condition leading to depression and agitation and affecting cognitive function/decision making. Improved nutritional status enhances thinking ability, and psychologic work can begin.

Patient detects urgency and may react to pressure. Any comment that might be seen as coercion provides focus on food. When staff responds in a consistent manner, patient can begin to trust staff responses. The single area in which the patient has exercised power and control is food/eating, and he or she may experience guilt or rebellion if forced to eat. Structuring meals and decreasing discussions about food will decrease power struggles with patient and avoid manipulative games.

Gastric dilation may occur if refeeding is too rapid following a period of starvation dieting.

Patient that gains confidence in self and feels in control of environment is more likely to eat preferred foods.

Patient will try to avoid taking in what is viewed as excessive calories and may go to great lengths to avoid eating.

Provides accurate ongoing record of weight loss and/or gain. Also diminishes obsessing about gains and/or losses.

Although some programs prefer patient see the results of the weighing, this can force the issue of trust in patient who usually does not trust others.

Reinforces feelings of powerlessness and are usually not helpful.

Prevents vomiting during/after eating. Patient may desire food and use a binge-purge syndrome to

ACTIONS/INTERVENTIONS	RATIONALE

Independent

bathroom privileges for a specified period (e.g., 2 hours) following eating, if contracting is unsuccessful.

Monitor exercise program and set limits on physical activities. Chart activity/level of work (pacing and so on).

Maintain matter-of-fact, nonjudgmental attitude if giving tube feedings, hyperalimentation, and so on.

Be alert to possibility of patient disconnecting tube and emptying hyperalimentation if used. Check measurements, and tape tubing snugly.

Collaborative

Administer nutritional therapy within a hospital treatment program as indicated.

Involve patient in setting up/carrying out program of behavior modification. Provide reward for weight gain as individually determined; ignore loss.

Provide diet and snacks with substitutions of preferred foods when available.

Administer liquid diet and/or tube feedings/hyperalimentation if needed.

Blenderize and tube feed anything left on the tray after a given period of time if indicated.

Avoid giving laxatives.

Administer medications as indicated:

    Cypropheptadine (Periactin);

---

maintain weight. *Note:* Purging may occur for the first time in a patient as a response to establishment of a weight gain program.

Moderate exercise helps in maintaining muscle tone/weight and combatting depression. However, patient may exercise excessively to burn calories.

Perception of punishment is counterproductive to patient's self-confidence and faith in own ability to control destiny.

Sabotage behavior is common in attempt to prevent weight gain.

Cure of the underlying problem cannot happen without improved nutritional status. Hospitalization provides a controlled environment in which food intake, vomiting/elimination, medications, and activities can be monitored. It also separates the patient from SO (who may be contributing factor) and provides exposure to others with the same problem, creating an atmosphere for sharing.

Provides structured eating situation while allowing patient some control in choices. Behavior modification may be effective in mild cases or for short-term weight gain.

Having a variety of foods available will enable the patient to have a choice of potentially enjoyable foods.

When caloric intake is insufficient to sustain metabolic needs, nutritional support can be used to prevent malnutrition/death while therapy is continuing. High calorie liquid feedings may be given as medication, at preset times separate from meals, as an alternative means of increasing caloric intake.

May be used as part of behavior modification program to provide total intake of needed calories.

Use is counterproductive because they may be used by patient to rid body of food/calories.

A serotonin and histamine antagonist that may be used in high doses to stimulate the appetite, decrease preoccupation with food, and combat depression. Does not appear to have serious side effects, although decreased mental alertness may occur.

ACTIONS/INTERVENTIONS	RATIONALE
Independent	
Tricyclic antidepressants, e.g., amitriptyline (Elavil, Endep);	Lifts depression and stimulates appetite.
Antianxiety agents, e.g., alprazolam (Xanax);	Reduces tension, anxiety/nervousness and may help patient to participate with treatment.
Major tranquilizers, e.g., chlorpromazine (Thorazine).	Promotes weight gain and cooperation with psychotherapeutic program. Major tranquilizers are used only when absolutely necessary, because of extrapyramidal side effects.
Prepare for/assist with ECT if indicated. Help patient understand this is not punishment.	In rare and difficult cases in which malnutrition is severe/life-threatening, a short-term ECT series may enable the patient to begin eating and become accessible to psychotherapy.

NURSING DIAGNOSIS:	**FLUID VOLUME DEFICIT, HIGH RISK FOR/ACTUAL**
May be related to:	Inadequate intake of food and liquids.
	Consistent self-induced vomiting.
	Chronic/excessive laxative/diuretic use.
Possibly evidenced by: (actual)	Dry skin and mucous membranes, decreased skin turgor.
	Increased pulse rate, body temperature, decreased BP.
	Output greater than input (diuretic use); concentrated urine/decreased urine output (dehydration).
	Weakness.
	Change in mental state.
	Hemoconcentration, altered electrolyte balance.
DESIRED OUTCOMES/ EVALUATION CRITERIA—	Maintain/demonstrate improved fluid balance, as evidenced by adequate urine output, stable vital signs, moist mucous membranes, good skin turgor.
	Verbalize understanding of causative factors and behaviors necessary to correct fluid deficit.

ACTIONS/INTERVENTIONS	RATIONALE
Independent	
Monitor vital signs, capillary refill, status of mucous membranes, skin turgor.	Indicators of adequacy of circulating volume. Orthostatic hypotension may occur with risk of falls/injury following sudden changes in position.
Monitor amount and types of fluid intake. Measure urine output accurately.	Patient may abstain from all intake resulting in dehydration or substitute fluids for caloric intake impacting electrolyte balance.

ACTIONS/INTERVENTIONS

Independent

Discuss strategies to stop vomiting and laxative/diuretic use.

Identify actions necessary to regain/maintain optimal fluid balance, e.g., specific fluid intake schedule.

Collaborative

Review electrolyte/renal function test results.

Administer/monitor IV, hyperalimentation;

Potassium supplements, oral or IV as indicated.

RATIONALE

Helping patient deal with the feelings that lead to vomiting and/or laxative/diuretic use will prevent continued fluid loss. *Note:* The patient with bulimia has learned that vomiting provides a release of anxiety.

Involving patient in plan to correct fluid imbalances improves chances for success.

Fluid/electrolyte shifts, decreased renal function can adversely affect patient's recovery/prognosis and may require additional intervention.

Used as an emergency measure to correct fluid/electrolyte imbalance.

May be required to prevent cardiac dysrhythmias.

NURSING DIAGNOSIS:	THOUGHT PROCESSES, ALTERED
May be related to:	Severe malnutrition/electrolyte imbalance.
	Psychologic conflicts, e.g., sense of low self-worth, perceived lack of control.
Possibly evidenced by:	Impaired ability to make decisions, problem-solve.
	Non-reality-based verbalizations.
	Ideas of reference.
	Altered sleep patterns, e.g., may go to bed late (stay up to binge/purge) and get up early.
	Altered attention span/distractibility.
	Perceptual disturbances with failure to recognize hunger; fatigue, anxiety, and depression.
DESIRED OUTCOMES/ EVALUATION CRITERIA— PATIENT WILL:	Verbalize understanding of causative factors and awareness of impairment.
	Demonstrate behaviors to change/prevent malnutrition.
	Display improved ability to make decisions, problem-solve.

ACTIONS/INTERVENTIONS

Independent

Be aware of patient's distorted thinking ability.

RATIONALE

Allows the caregiver to have more realistic expectations of the patient and provide appropriate information and support.

427

ACTIONS/INTERVENTIONS	RATIONALE

Independent

Listen to and do not challenge irrational, illogical thinking. Present reality concisely and briefly.

It is not possible to respond logically when thinking ability is physiologically impaired. The patient needs to hear reality, but challenging leads to distrust and frustration.

Adhere strictly to nutrition regimen.

Improved nutrition is essential to improved brain functioning. (Refer to ND: Nutrition, altered: less than body requirements, p 423.)

Collaborative

Review electrolyte/renal function tests.

Imbalances negatively affect cerebral functioning and may require correction before therapeutic interventions can begin.

NURSING DIAGNOSIS	BODY IMAGE/SELF-ESTEEM CHRONIC LOW
May be related to:	Morbid fear of obesity.
	Perceived loss of control in some aspect of life.
	Unmet dependency needs.
	Personal vulnerability.
	Dysfunctional family system.
	Continual negative evaluation of self.
Possibly evidenced by:	Distorted body image (views self as fat even in the presence of normal body weight or severe emaciation).
	Expresses little concern, uses denial as a defense mechanism, and feels powerless to prevent/make changes.
	Expressions of shame/guilt.
	Overly conforming, dependent on others' opinions.
DESIRED OUTCOMES/ EVALUATION CRITERIA— PATIENT WILL:	Establish a more realistic body image.
	Acknowledge self as an individual.
	Accept responsibility for own actions.

ACTIONS/INTERVENTIONS	RATIONALE

Independent

Establish a therapeutic nurse/patient relationship.

Within a helping relationship, patient can begin to trust and try out new thinking and behaviors.

Promote self-concept without moral judgment.

Patient sees self as weak-willed, even though part of person may feel sense of power and control (e.g., dieting/weight loss).

ACTIONS/INTERVENTIONS	RATIONALE

Independent

Have patient draw picture of self.

Provides opportunity to discuss patient's perception of self/body image and realities of individual situation.

State rules clearly regarding weighing schedule, remaining in sight during medication and eating times, and consequences of not following the rules. Without undue comment, be consistent in carrying out rules.

Consistency is important in establishing trust. As part of the behavior modification program, patient knows risks involved in not following established rules (e.g., decrease in privileges). Failure to follow rules is viewed as the patient's choice and accepted by staff in matter-of-fact manner so as not to provide reinforcement for the undesirable behavior.

Respond (confront) with reality when patient makes unrealistic statements such as "I'm gaining weight; so there's nothing really wrong with me."

Patient may be denying the psychologic aspects of own situation and is often expressing a sense of inadequacy and depression.

Be aware of own reaction to patient's behavior. Avoid arguing.

Feelings of disgust, hostility, and infuriation are not uncommon when caring for these patients. Prognosis often remains poor even with a gain in weight, because other problems may remain. Many patients continue to see themselves as fat, and there is also a high incidence of affective disorders, social phobias, obsessive-compulsive symptoms, drug abuse, and psychosexual dysfunction. Nurse needs to deal with own response/ feelings so they do not interfere with care of patient.

Assist the patient to assume control in areas other than dieting/weight loss, e.g., management of own daily activities, work/leisure choices.

Feelings of personal ineffectiveness, low self-esteem, and perfectionism are often part of the problem. Patient feels helpless to change and requires assistance to problem-solve methods of control in life situations.

Help the patient formulate goals for self (not related to eating) and create a manageable plan to reach those goals, 1 at a time, progressing from simple to more complex.

Patient needs to recognize ability to control other areas in life and may need to learn problem-solving skills to achieve this control. Setting realistic goals fosters success.

Assist patient to confront sexual fears. Provide sex education as necessary.

Major physical/psychologic changes in adolescence can contribute to development of this problem. Feelings of powerlessness and loss of control of feelings (in particular sexual sensations) lead to an unconscious desire to desexualize themselves. Patient often believes that these fears can be overcome by taking control of bodily appearance/ development/function.

Note patient's withdrawal from and/or discomfort in social settings.

May indicate feelings of isolation and fear of rejection/judgment by other's. Avoidance of social situations and contact with others can compound feelings of worthlessness.

Encourage patient to take charge of own life in a more healthful way by making own decisions and accepting self as she or he is at this moment.

Patient often does not know what he or she may want for self. Parents (mother) usually make decisions for patient. Patient may also believe he or

429

ACTIONS/INTERVENTIONS	RATIONALE
Independent	
Encourage acceptance of inadequacies as well as strengths. Let patient know that it is acceptable to be different from family, particularly mother.	she has to be the best in everything and holds self responsible for being perfect. Developing a sense of identity separate from family and maintaining sense of control in other ways besides dieting and weight loss is a desirable goal of therapy/program.
Involve in personal development program, preferably in a group setting. Provide information about proper application of makeup and grooming.	Learning about methods of enhancing personal appearance may be helpful to long-range sense of self-esteem/image. Feedback from others can promote feelings of self-worth.
Suggest disposing of "thin" clothes as weight gain occurs. Recommend consultation with an image consultant.	Provides incentive to at least maintain and not lose weight. Removes visual reminder of thinner self. Positive image enhances sense of self-esteem.
Use interpersonal psychotherapy approach, rather than interpretive therapy.	Interaction between persons is more helpful for the patient to discover feelings/impulses/needs from within own self. Patient has not learned this internal control as a child and may not be able to interpret/attach meaning to behavior.
Encourage patient to express anger and acknowledge when it is verbalized.	Important to know that anger is part of self and as such is acceptable. Expressing anger may need to be taught to patient, because anger is generally considered unacceptable in the family, and therefore patient does not express it.
Assist patient to learn strategies other than eating for dealing with feelings. Have patient keep a diary of feelings, particularly when thinking about food.	Feelings are the underlying issue, and patient often uses food instead of dealing with feelings appropriately. Patient needs to learn to recognize feelings and how to express them clearly.
Assess feelings of helplessness/hopelessness.	Lack of control is a common/underlying problem for this patient and may be accompanied by more serious emotional disorders. *Note:* 54% of patients with anorexia have a history of major affective disorder, and 33% have a history of minor affective disorder.
Be alert to suicidal ideation/behavior.	Intense anxiety/panic about weight gain, depression, hopeless feelings may lead to suicidal attempts, particularly if patient is impulsive.
Collaborative	
Involve in group therapy.	Provides an opportunity to talk about feelings and try out new behaviors.
Refer to occupational/recreational therapy.	Can develop interests and skills to fill time that has been occupied by obsession with eating. Involvement in recreational activities encourages social interactions with others and promotes fun and relaxation.
Refer to therapist trained in dealing with sexuality.	May need professional assistance to deal with sexuality issues and accept self as a sexual adult.

NURSING DIAGNOSIS	SKIN INTEGRITY, IMPAIRED: HIGH RISK FOR/ACTUAL
May be related to:	Altered nutritional/metabolic state; edema.
	Dehydration/cachectic changes (skeletal prominence).
Possibly evidenced by:	Dry/scaly skin with poor turgor.
	Tissue fragility.
	Brittle/dry hair.
	Complaints of itching.
DESIRED OUTCOMES/ EVALUATION CRITERIA:— PATIENT WILL:	Verbalize understanding of causative factors and relief of itching.
	Identify and demonstrate behaviors to maintain soft, supple, intact skin.

ACTIONS/INTERVENTIONS	RATIONALE

Independent

Observe for reddened, blanched, excoriated areas.	These areas are at increased risk of breakdown and require more intense treatment.
Encourage bathing every other day instead of every day.	Frequent baths contribute to dryness of the skin.
Use skin cream twice a day and after bathing.	Lubricates skin and decreases itching.
Massage skin, especially over bony prominences.	Improves circulation to the skin, enhances skin tone.
Discuss importance of frequent position changes, need for remaining active.	Enhances circulation and perfusion to skin by preventing prolonged pressure on tissues.
Stress importance of adequate nutrition/fluid intake. (Refer to ND: Nutrition, altered: less than body requirements, p 423.)	Improved nutrition and hydration will improve skin condition.

NURSING DIAGNOSIS:	FAMILY PROCESS, ALTERED
May be related to:	Issues of control in family.
	Situational/maturational crises.
	History of inadequate coping methods.
Possibly evidenced by:	Dissonance among family members.
	Family developmental tasks not being met.
	Focus on "Identified Patient" (IP).
	Family needs not being met.

	Family member(s) acting as "enablers" for IP.
	Ill-defined family rules, function, and roles.
DESIRED OUTCOMES/ EVALUATION CRITERIA— FAMILY WILL:	Demonstrate individual involvement in problem-solving processes directed at encouraging patient toward independence.
	Express feelings freely and appropriately.
	Demonstrate more autonomous coping behaviors with individual family boundaries more clearly defined.
	Recognize and resolve conflict appropriately with the individuals involved.

ACTIONS/INTERVENTIONS	RATIONALE
Independent	
Identify patterns of interaction. Encourage each family member to speak for self. Do not allow 2 members to discuss a third without that member's participation.	Helpful information for planning interventions. The enmeshed, overinvolved family members often speak for each other and need to learn to be responsible for their own words and actions.
Discourage members from asking for approval from each other. Be alert to verbal or nonverbal checking with others for approval. Acknowledge competent actions of patient.	Each individual needs to develop own internal sense of self-esteem. Individual often is living up to others' (family's) expectations rather than making own choices. Acknowledgment provide recognition of self in positive ways.
Listen with regard when the patient speaks.	Sets an example and provides a sense of competence and self-worth, in that the patient has been heard and attended to.
Encourage individuals not to answer to everything.	Reinforces individualization and return to privacy.
Communicate message of separation, that it is acceptable for family members to be different from each other.	Individuation needs reinforcement. Such a message confronts rigidity and opens options for different behaviors.
Encourage and allow expression of feelings (e.g., crying, anger) by individuals.	Often these families have not allowed free expression of feelings and will need help and permission to learn and accept this.
Prevent intrusion in dyads by other members of the family.	Inappropriate interventions in family subsystems prevent individuals from working out problems successfully.
Reinforce importance of parents as a couple who have rights of their own.	The focus on the child with anorexia is very intense and often is the only area around which the couple interact. The couple needs to explore their own relationship and restore the balance within it to prevent its disintegration.
Prevent patient from intervening in conflicts between parents. Assist parents in identifying and solving their marital differences.	Triangulation occurs in which a parent-child coalition exists. Sometimes the child is openly pressed to ally self with one parent against the other. The symptom (anorexia) is the regulator in the family system, and the parents deny their own conflicts.

ACTIONS/INTERVENTIONS

Independent

Be aware and confront sabotage behavior on the part of family members.

Collaborative

Refer to community resources, such as family therapy groups, parents' groups as indicated; and parent effectiveness classes.

RATIONALE

Feelings of blame, shame, and helplessness may lead to unconscious behavior designed to maintain the status quo.

May help reduce overprotectiveness, support/facilitate the process of dealing with unresolved conflicts and change.

NURSING DIAGNOSIS:	KNOWLEDGE DEFICIT [LEARNING NEED], REGARDING CONDITION, PROGNOSIS, AND TREATMENT NEEDS
May be related to:	Lack of exposure to/unfamiliarity with information about condition.
	Learned maladaptive coping skills.
Possibly evidenced by:	Verbalization of misconception of relationship of current situation and behaviors.
	Preoccupation with extreme fear of obesity and distortion of own body image.
	Refusal to eat; binging and purging.
	Abuse of laxatives and diuretics.
	Excessive exercising.
	Verbalization of need for new information.
	Expressions of desire to learn more adaptive ways of coping with stressors.
DESIRED OUTCOMES/ EVALUATION CRITERIA— PATIENT WILL:	Verbalize awareness of and plan for lifestyle changes to maintain normal weight.
	Identify relationship of signs/symptoms (weight loss, tooth decay) to behaviors of not eating/binge-purging.
	Assume responsibility for own learning.
	Seek out sources/resources to assist with making identified changes.

ACTIONS/INTERVENTIONS

Independent

Determine level of knowledge and readiness to learn.

Note blocks to learning, e.g., physical/intellectual/emotional.

RATIONALE

Learning is easier when it begins where the learner is.

Malnutrition, family problems, drug abuse, affective disorders, and obsessive-compulsive symp-

ACTIONS/INTERVENTIONS

Independent

Review dietary needs, answering questions as indicated. Encourage inclusion of high fiber foods and adequate fluid intake.

Encourage the use of relaxation and other stress-management techniques, e.g., visualization, guided imagery, biofeedback.

Assist with establishing a sensible exercise program. Caution regarding overexercise.

Provide written information for patient/SO(s).

Discuss need for information about sex and sexuality.

Refer to National Association of Anorexia Nervosa and Associated Disorders.

RATIONALE

toms can be blocks to learning requiring resolution before effective learning can occur.

Patient/family may need assistance with planning for new way of eating. Constipation may occur when laxative use is curtailed.

New ways of coping with feelings of anxiety and fear will help patient to manage these feelings in more effective ways, assisting in giving up maladaptive behaviors of not eating/binging-purging.

Exercise can assist with developing a positive body image and combats depression (release of endorphins in the brain enhances sense of well-being). Patient may use excessive exercise as a way of controlling weight.

Helpful as reminder of and reinforcement for learning.

Because avoidance of own sexuality is an issue for this patient, realistic information can be helpful in beginning to deal with self as a sexual being.

May be a helpful source of support and information for patient/SO.

Eating Disorders: Obesity _____

Obesity is defined as an excess accumulation of body fat at least 20% over average weight for age, sex, and height. The general prognosis for achieving and maintaining weight loss is poor. However, the desire for a healthier lifestyle and reduction of risk factors associated with life-threatening illnesses motivates many people toward diets and weight-loss programs.

RELATED CONCERNS:

Cerebrovascular Accident/Stroke, p 290
Cholecystitis with Cholelithiasis, p 523
Cirrhosis of the Liver, p 547
Congestive Heart Failure, p 48
Diabetes Mellitus, p 737
Hypertension, p 34
Myocardial Infarction, p 80
Obesity: Surgical Interventions, p 444
Psychosocial Aspects of Acute Care, p 899
Thrombophlebitis: Deep Vein Thrombosis, p 135

PATIENT ASSESSMENT DATA BASE

ACTIVITY/REST

May report:	Fatigue, constant drowsiness.
	Inability/lack of desire to be active or engage in regular exercise.
	Dyspnea with exertion.
May exhibit:	Increased heart rate/respirations with activity.

CIRCULATION

May exhibit:	Hypertension, edema.

EGO INTEGRITY

May report:	History of cultural/lifestyle factors affecting food choices.
	Weight may/may not be perceived as a problem.
	Eating relieves unpleasant feelings, e.g., loneliness, frustration, boredom.
	Perception of body image as undesirable.
	SO's resistant to weight loss (may sabotage patient's efforts).

FOOD/FLUID

May report:	Normal/excessive ingestion of food.
	Experimentation with numerous types of diets ("yo-yo" dieting) with varied/short-lived results.
	History of recurrent weight loss and gain.
May exhibit:	Weight disproportionate to height.
	Endomorphic body type (soft/round).
	Failure to adjust food intake to diminishing requirements (e.g., change in lifestyle from active to sedentary, aging).

PAIN/COMFORT

May report:	Pain/discomfort on weight-bearing joints or spine.

435

RESPIRATION

May report: Dyspnea.

May exhibit: Cyanosis, respiratory distress (Pickwickian syndrome).

SEXUALITY

May report: Menstrual disturbances, amenorrhea.

TEACHING/LEARNING

May report: Problem may be lifetime or related to life event.

Family history of obesity.

Concomitant health problems may include hypertension, diabetes, gallbladder and cardiovascular disease, hypothyroidism.

Discharge Plan Considerations: **DRG projected mean length of stay: 6.1 days.**

May require support with therapeutic regimen.

DIAGNOSTIC STUDIES

Metabolic/endocrine studies: May reveal abnormalities, e.g., hypothyroidism, hypopituitarism, hypogonadism, Cushing's syndrome (increased insulin levels), hyperglycemia, hyperlipidemia, hyperuricemia, hyperbilirubinemia. It is also suggested that the cause of these disorders may arise out of neuroendocrine abnormalities within the hypothalamus, which result in various chemical disturbances.

Anthropometric measurements: Estimates fat to muscle ratio.

NURSING PRIORITIES

1. Assist patient to identify a workable method of weight control incorporating healthful foods.
2. Promote improved self-concept, including body image, self-esteem.
3. Encourage health practices to provide for weight control throughout life.

DISCHARGE GOALS

1. Healthy patterns for eating and weight control identified.
2. Weight loss toward desired goal established.
3. Positive perception of self verbalized.
4. Plans for future control of weight made.

NURSING DIAGNOSIS:	**NUTRITION, ALTERED: MORE THAN BODY REQUIREMENTS**
May be related to:	Food intake that exceeds body needs.
	Psychosocial factors.
	Socioeconomic status.
Possibly evidenced by:	Weight of 20% or more over optimum body weight; excess body fat by skinfold/other measurements.
	Reported/observed dysfunctional eating patterns, intake more than body requirements.

DESIRED OUTCOMES/ EVALUATION CRITERIA— PATIENT WILL:	Identify inappropriate behaviors and consequences associated with overeating or weight gain. Demonstrate change in eating patterns and involvement in individual exercise program. Display weight loss with optimal maintenance of health.

ACTIONS/INTERVENTIONS	RATIONALE

Independent

ACTIONS/INTERVENTIONS	RATIONALE
Review individual cause for obesity, e.g., organic or nonorganic.	Identifies/influences choice of interventions.
Implement/review daily food diary, e.g., caloric intake, types of food, eating habits.	Provides the opportunity for the individual to focus on/internalize a realistic picture of the amount of food ingested and corresponding eating habits/ feelings. Identifies patterns requiring change and/ or a base on which to tailor the dietary program.
Discuss emotions/events associated with eating.	Helps to identify when patient is eating to satisfy an emotional need, rather than physiologic hunger.
Formulate an eating plan with the patient.	While there is no basis for recommending one diet over another, a good reducing diet should contain foods from all basic food groups with a focus on low-fat intake. It is helpful to keep the plan as similar to patient's usual eating pattern as possible. A plan developed with and agreed to by the patient is more apt to be successful. *Note:* It is important to maintain adequate protein intake to prevent loss of lean muscle mass.
Use knowledge of individual's height, body build, age, gender, and individual patterns of eating, energy, and nutrient requirements.	Standard tables are subject to error when applied to individual situations, and circadian rhythms/ lifestyle patterns need to be considered.
Stress the importance of avoiding fad diets.	Elimination of needed components can lead to metabolic imbalances, e.g., excessive reduction of carbohydrates can lead to fatigue, headache, instability and weakness, metabolic acidosis (ketosis) interfering with effectiveness of weight loss program.
Discuss realistic increment goals for weekly weight loss.	Reasonable weight loss (1–2 lb/wk) results in more lasting effects. Excessive/rapid loss may result in fatigue and irritability and ultimately lead to failure in meeting goals for weight loss. Motivation is more easily sustained by meeting "stair-step" goals.
Weigh periodically as individually indicated, and obtain appropriate body measurements.	Provides information about effectiveness of therapeutic regimen and visual evidence of success of patient's efforts. During hospitalization, for controlled fasting, daily weight may be required. Weekly weight is more appropriate after discharge.
Determine current activity levels and plan progressive exercise program (e.g., walking) tailored to the individual's goals and choice.	Exercise furthers weight loss by reducing appetite, increasing energy, toning muscles, and enhancing sense of well-being and accomplishment. Commit-

437

ACTIONS/INTERVENTIONS

Independent

Develop an appetite reeducation plan with patient.

Stress the importance of avoiding tension at mealtimes and not eating too quickly.

Encourage patient to eat only at a table or designated eating place and to avoid standing while eating.

Discuss restriction of salt intake and diuretic drugs if used.

Collaborative

Consult with dietitian to determine caloric/nutrient requirements for individual weight loss.

Administer medications as indicated:

Appetite-suppressant drugs, e.g., diethylpropion (Tenuate); mazindol (Sanorex);

Hormonal therapy, e.g., thyroid (Euthroid);

Vitamin, mineral supplements.

Maintain fasting regimen and/or stabilization of medical problems, when indicated.

Refer for surgical interventions, e.g., gastric bypass, partitioning, if indicated.

RATIONALE

ment on the part of the patient enables the setting of more realistic goals and adherence to the plan.

Signals of hunger and fullness often are not recognized, have become distorted, or are ignored.

Reducing tension provides a more relaxed eating atmosphere and encourages more leisurely eating patterns. This is important because a period of time is required for the appestat mechanism to know the stomach is full.

Techniques that modify behavior may be helpful in avoiding diet failure.

Water retention may be a problem because of increased fluid intake, as well as the result of fat metabolism.

Individual intake can be calculated by several different formulas, but weight reduction is based on the basal caloric requirement for 24 hours, depending on patient's sex, age, current/desired weight, and length of time estimated to achieve desired weight.

May be used with caution/supervision at the beginning of a weight loss program to support patient during stress of behaviorial/lifestyle changes. They are only effective for a few weeks and may cause problems of addiction in some people.

May be necessary when hypothyroidism is present. When no deficiency is present, replacement therapy is not helpful and may actually be harmful. *Note:* Other hormonal treatments, such as HCG, although widely publicized, have no documented evidence of value.

Obese individuals have large fuel reserves but are often deficient in vitamins and minerals.

Aggressive therapy/support may be necessary to initiate weight loss, although fasting is not generally a treatment of choice. Patient can be monitored more effectively in a controlled setting, to minimize complications such as postural hypotension, anemia, cardiac irregularities, and decreased uric acid excretion with hyperuricemia.

These interventions may be necessary to assist the client lose weight when obesity is life-threatening.

NURSING DIAGNOSIS:	BODY IMAGE/SELF-ESTEEM, DISTURBANCE IN
May be related to:	Biophysical/psychosocial factors such as patient's view of self. (Slimness is valued in this society, and mixed messages are received when thinness is stressed.)
	Family/subculture encouragement of overeating.
	Control, sex, and love issues.
Possibly evidenced by:	Verbalization of negative feelings about body (mental image often does not match physical reality).
	Fear of rejection/reaction by others.
	Feelings of hopelessness/powerlessness.
	Preoccupation with change (attempts to lose weight).
	Lack of follow-through with diet plan.
	Verbalization of powerlessness to change eating habits.
DESIRED OUTCOMES/ EVALUATION CRITERIA— PATIENT WILL:	Verbalize a more realistic self-image.
	Demonstrate some acceptance of self as is rather than an idealized image.
	Acknowledge self as an individual who has responsibility for self.
	Seek information and actively pursue appropriate weight loss.

ACTIONS/INTERVENTIONS	RATIONALE
Independent	
Discuss with the patient view of being fat and what it does for the individual. Be sure to provide privacy during care activities.	Mental image includes our ideal and is usually not up to date. Fat and compulsive eating behaviors may have deep-rooted psychologic implications, e.g., compensating for lack of love and nurturing, or be a defense against intimacy. However, individual usually is sensitive/self-conscious about body.
Have patient recall coping patterns related to food in family of origin and explore how these may affect current situation.	Parents act as role models for the child. Maladaptive coping patterns (overeating) are learned within the family system and are supported through positive reinforcement. Food may be substituted by the parent for affection and love, and eating is associated with a feeling of satisfaction, becoming the primary defense.
Determine relationship history and possibility of sexual abuse.	May contribute to current issues of self-esteem/ patterns of coping.
Determine the patient's motivation for weight loss and assist with goal setting.	The individual may harbor repressed feelings of hostility, which may be expressed inward on the self. Because of a poor self-concept, the person often has difficulty with relationships. *Note:* When

439

ACTIONS/INTERVENTIONS	RATIONALE
Independent	
	losing weight for someone else, the patient is less likely to be successful/maintain weight loss.
Be alert to myths the patient/SO may have about weight and weight loss.	Beliefs about what an ideal body looks like or unconscious motivations can sabotage efforts at weight loss. Some of these include the feminine thought of "If I become thin, men will pursue me or rape me"; the masculine counterpart, "I don't trust myself to stay in control of my sexual feelings"; as well as issues of strength, power, or the "good cook" image.
Assist patient to identify feelings that lead to compulsive eating. Develop strategies for doing something besides eating for dealing with these feelings, e.g., talking with a friend.	Awareness of emotions that lead to overeating can be the first step in behavior change, e.g., people often eat because of depression, anger, and guilt.
Graph weight on a weekly basis.	Provides ongoing visual evidence of weight changes (reality oriented).
Promote open communication avoiding criticism/judgment about patient's behavior.	Supports patient's own responsibility for weight loss; enhances sense of control, and promotes willingness to discuss difficulties/setbacks and problem solve. *Note:* Distrust and accusations of "cheating" on caloric intake are not helpful.
Outline and clearly state responsibilities of patient and nurse.	It is helpful for each individual to understand area of own responsibility in the program so that misunderstandings do not arise.
Be alert to binge-eating and develop strategies for dealing with these episodes, e.g., substituting other actions for eating.	The patient who binges experiences guilt about it, which is also counterproductive, because negative feelings may sabotage further weight loss efforts.
Encourage patient to use imagery to visualize self as desired weight and to practice handling of new behaviors.	Mental rehearsal is very useful to help the patient plan for and deal with anticipated change in self-image or deal with occasions that may arise (family gatherings, special dinners) where confrontations with food will occur.
Provide information about the use of make-up, hairstyles, and ways of dressing to maximize figure assets.	Enhances feelings of self-esteem; promotes improved body image.
Encourage buying clothes as a reward for weight loss instead of food treats.	Properly fitting clothes enhance the body image as small losses are made and the individual feels more positive. Waiting until the desired weight loss is reached can become discouraging.
Suggest the patient dispose of "fat clothes."	Removes the "safety valve" of having clothes available "in case" the weight is regained. Retaining fat clothes can convey the message that the weight loss will not occur/be maintained.
Help staff be aware of and deal with own feelings when caring for this patient.	Judgmental attitudes, feelings of disgust, anger, and weariness can interfere with care/be transmitted to patient, reinforcing negative self-esteem/image.

ACTIONS/INTERVENTIONS	RATIONALE
Collaborative	
Refer to support and/or therapy group.	Support groups can provide companionship, enhance motivation, decrease loneliness and social ostracism, and give practical solutions to common problems. Group therapy can be helpful in dealing with underlying psychologic concerns.

NURSING DIAGNOSIS:	SOCIAL INTERACTION, IMPAIRED
May be related to:	Verbalized or observed discomfort in social situations.
	Self-concept disturbance.
Possibly evidenced by:	Reluctance to participate in social gatherings.
	Verbalization of a sense of discomfort with others.
DESIRED OUTCOMES/ EVALUATION CRITERIA— PATIENT WILL:	Verbalize awareness of feelings that lead to poor social interactions.
	Become involved in achieving positive changes in social behaviors and interpersonal relationships.

ACTIONS/INTERVENTIONS	RATIONALE
Independent	
Review family patterns of relating and social behaviors.	Social interaction is primarily learned within the family of origin. When inadequate patterns are identified, actions for change can be instituted.
Encourage patient to express feelings and perceptions of problems.	Helps to identify and clarify reasons for difficulties in interacting with others, e.g., may feel unloved/unlovable or insecure about sexuality.
Assess patient's use of coping skills and defense mechanisms.	May have coping skills that will be useful in the process of weight loss. Defense mechanisms used to protect the individual may contribute to feelings of aloneness/isolation.
Have patient list behaviors that cause discomfort.	Identifies specific concerns and suggests actions that can be taken to effect change.
Involve in role-playing new ways to deal with identified behaviors/situations.	Practicing these new behaviors enables the individual to become comfortable with them in a safe situation.
Discuss negative self-concepts and self-talk, e.g., "No one wants to be with a fat person," "Who would be interested in talking to me?"	May be impeding positive social interactions.
Encourage use of positive self-talk such as telling oneself "I am OK," or "I can enjoy social activities and do not need to be controlled by what others think or say."	Positive strategies enhance feelings of comfort and support efforts for change.

441

ACTIONS/INTERVENTIONS	RATIONALE

Collaborative

Refer for ongoing family or individual therapy as indicated.

Patient benefits from involvement of SO to provide support and encouragement.

NURSING DIAGNOSIS:	KNOWLEDGE DEFICIT [LEARNING NEED] REGARDING CONDITION, PROGNOSIS, AND TREATMENT NEEDS
May be related to:	Lack of/misinterpretation of information.
	Lack of interest in learning, lack of recall.
	Inaccurate/incomplete information presented.
Possibly evidenced by:	Statements of lack of/request for information about obesity and nutritional requirements.
	Verbalization of problem with weight reduction.
	Inadequate follow-through with previous diet and exercise instruction.
DESIRED OUTCOMES/ EVALUATION CRITERIA— PATIENT WILL:	Assume responsibility for own learning.
	Begin to look for information about nutrition and ways to control weight.
	Verbalize understanding of need for lifestyle changes to maintain/control weight.
	Establish individual goal and plan for attaining that goal.

ACTIONS/INTERVENTIONS	RATIONALE

Independent

Determine level of nutritional knowledge and what patient believes is most urgent need.

Necessary to know what additional information to provide. When patient's views are listened to, trust is enhanced.

Provide information about ways to maintain satisfactory food intake in settings away from home.

"Smart" eating when dining out or when traveling helps individual to manage weight while still enjoying social outlets.

Identify other sources of information, e.g., books, tapes, community classes, groups.

Using different avenues of accessing information will further patient's learning. Involvement with others who are also losing weight can provide support.

Stress necessity of continued follow-up care/counseling, especially when plateaus occur.

As weight is lost, changes in metabolism occur, interfering with further loss by creating a plateau as the body activates a survival mechanism, attempting to prevent "starvation." This requires new strategies and aggressive support to continue weight loss.

ACTIONS/INTERVENTIONS	RATIONALE
Independent	
Reassess caloric requirements every 2–4 weeks.	Changes in weight and exercise may necessitate changes in reducing diet.
Identify alternatives to chosen activity program to accommodate weather, travel, and so on. Discuss use of mechanical devices/equipment for reducing.	Promotes continuation of program. *Note:* Fat loss occurs on a generalized overall basis, and there is no evidence that spot reducing or mechanical devices aid in weight loss in specific areas. However, specific types of exercise or equipment may be useful in *toning* specific body parts.
Discuss necessity of good skin care, especially during summer months.	Prevents skin breakdown in moist skinfolds.
Identify alternative ways to "reward" self/family for accomplishments or to provide solace.	Reduces likelihood of relying on food to deal with feelings.
Encourage involvement in social activities that are not centered around food, e.g., bike ride/nature hike, attending musical event, group sporting activities.	Provides opportunity for pleasure and relaxation without "temptation." Activities/exercise may also use calories to help maintain desired weight.

Obesity: Surgical Interventions (Gastric Partitioning/ Gastroplasty, Gastric Bypass)

A number of surgical treatments for morbid obesity have been tried and discarded because of ineffectiveness or complications. Two procedures now dominate and have advanced beyond the experimental stage. The procedure of choice is vertical-banded gastroplasty. On occasion, gastric bypass may be performed. Weight reduction surgery has been reported to improve several comorbid conditions such as sleep apnea, glucose intolerance and frank diabetes, hypertension, and hyperlipidemia.

Gastroplasty: A small pouch with a restricted outlet is created across stomach just distal to the gastroesophageal junction leaving a small opening through which food passes into stomach.

Gastric bypass: Anastomosis of jejunum to upper portion of stomach, bypassing rest of stomach.

RELATED CONCERNS:

Eating Disorders: Obesity, p 435
Intestinal Surgery, p 500
Peritonitis, p 514
Psychosocial Aspects of Acute Care, p 899
Surgical Intervention, p 918
Thrombophlebitis: Deep Vein Thrombosis, p 135

PATIENT ASSESSMENT DATA BASE

ACTIVITY/REST

May report:	Difficulty sleeping.
	Exertional discomfort, inability to participate in desired activity/sports.

EGO INTEGRITY

May report:	Motivated to lose weight for oneself (or for gratification of others).
	Repressed feelings of hostility toward authority figures.
	History of psychiatric illness/treatment.
May exhibit:	Symptoms of emotional/psychiatric illness.

FOOD/FLUID

May report:	Adequate trials and failure of other treatment approaches.
	Desire to lose weight.
May exhibit:	Weight exceeding ideal body weight by 100% or more (morbid obesity).

TEACHING/LEARNING

May report:	Presence of chronic conditions (hypertension, diabetes, arthritis, sleep apnea, Pickwickian syndrome, infertility).
Discharge Plan Considerations:	**DRG projected mean length of stay: 7.4 days.**
	May require support with therapeutic regimen/weight loss, assistance with self-care, homemaker/maintenance tasks.

DIAGNOSTIC STUDIES

Studies are dependent on individual situations, to rule out underlying disease in addition to preoperative workup including psychiatric evaluation.

NURSING PRIORITIES

1. Support respiratory function.
2. Prevent/minimize complications.
3. Provide appropriate nutritional intake.
4. Provide information regarding surgical procedure, postoperative expectations, and treatment needs.

DISCHARGE GOALS

1. Ventilation and oxygenation adequate for individual needs.
2. Complications prevented/controlled.
3. Nutritional intake modified for specific procedure.
4. Procedure, prognosis, and therapeutic regimen understood.

NURSING DIAGNOSIS:	**BREATHING PATTERNS, INEFFECTIVE**
May be related to:	Decreased lung expansion.
	Pain, anxiety.
	Decreased energy, fatigue.
	Tracheobronchial obstruction.
Possibly evidenced by:	Shortness of breath, dyspnea.
	Tachypnea, respiratory depth changes, reduced vital capacity.
	Wheezes, rhonchi.
	Abnormal ABGs.
DESIRED OUTCOMES/ EVALUATION CRITERIA— PATIENT WILL:	Maintain adequate ventilation.
	Experience no cyanosis or other signs of hypoxia, with ABGs within patient's normal range.

ACTIONS/INTERVENTIONS	RATIONALE
Independent	
Monitor respiratory rate/depth. Auscultate breath sounds. Investigate presence of pallor/cyanosis, increased restlessness, or confusion.	Shallow respirations/effects of anesthesia decrease ventilation, potentiate atelectasis, and may result in hypoxia. *Note:* Many anesthetic agents are fat-soluble, increasing postoperative sedation and respiratory complications.
Elevate head of bed 30 degrees.	Encourages optimal diaphragmatic excursion/lung expansion and minimizes pressure of abdominal contents on the thoracic cavity. *Note:* Kept recumbent, obese patients are at high risk for severe hypoventilation postoperatively.
Encourage deep-breathing exercises. Assist with coughing and splint incision.	Promotes maximal lung expansion and aids in clearing airways, thus reducing risk of atelectasis, pneumonia.

445

ACTIONS/INTERVENTIONS

Independent

Turn periodically and ambulate as early as possible.

Pad side rails and teach patient to use them as armrests.

Use small pillow under head when indicated.

Avoid use of abdominal binders.

Collaborative

Administer supplemental O_2.

Assist in use of IPPB and/or respiratory adjuncts, e.g., incentive spirometer, blow bottles.

Monitor/graph serial ABGs/pulse oximetry when indicated.

RATIONALE

Promotes aeration of all segments of the lung, mobilizing and aiding in expectoration of secretions.

Using the side rail as an armrest allows for greater chest expansion.

Many obese patients have large, thick necks, and use of large, fluffy pillows may obstruct the airway.

Can restrict lung expansion.

Maximizes available O_2 for exchange and reduces work of breathing.

Enhances lung expansion; reduces potential for atelectasis.

Reflects ventilation/oxygenation and acid-base status. Used as a basis for evaluating need for/effectiveness of respiratory therapies.

NURSING DIAGNOSIS:	TISSUE PERFUSION, ALTERED: PERIPHERAL, HIGH RISK FOR
Risk factors may include:	Diminished blood flow, hypovolemia. Immobility/bed rest. Interruption of venous blood flow (thrombosis).
Possibly evidenced by:	[Not applicable; presence of signs and symptoms establishes an actual diagnosis.]
DESIRED OUTCOMES/ EVALUATION CRITERIA— PATIENT WILL:	Maintain perfusion as individually appropriate, e.g., skin warm/dry, peripheral pulses present/strong, vital signs within patient's normal range. Identify causative/risk factors. Demonstrate behaviors to improve/maintain circulation.

ACTIONS/INTERVENTIONS

Independent

Monitor vital signs. Palpate peripheral pulses routinely; evaluate capillary refill and changes in mentation. Note 24-hour fluid balance.

Encourage frequent ROM exercises for legs and ankles.

Assess for Homans' sign, redness, and edema of calf.

RATIONALE

Indicators of circulatory adequacy. (Refer to ND: Fluid Volume Deficit, high risk for, p 447.)

Stimulates circulation in the lower extremities; reduces venous stasis.

Indicators of thrombus formation but may not always be present in obese individual.

ACTIONS/INTERVENTIONS

Independent

Encourage early ambulation; discourage sitting and/or dangling at the bedside.

Provide adequate/appropriate equipment and sufficient staff for handling patient.

Collaborative

Administer heparin therapy, as indicated.

Monitor Hb/Hct and coagulation studies.

RATIONALE

Sitting constricts venous flow, whereas walking encourages venous return.

Helpful in dealing with the bulky patient for moving, bowel care, and ambulating. Reduces risk of traumatic injury.

May be used prophylactically to reduce risk of thrombus formation or to treat thromboemboli.

Provides information about circulatory volume/alterations in coagulation and indicates therapy needs/effectiveness.

NURSING DIAGNOSIS:	FLUID VOLUME DEFICIT, HIGH RISK FOR
Risk factors may include:	Excessive gastric losses: nasogastric suction, diarrhea. Reduced intake.
Possibly evidenced by:	[Not applicable; presence of signs and symptoms establishes an actual diagnosis.]
DESIRED OUTCOMES/ EVALUATION CRITERIA— PATIENT WILL:	Maintain adequate fluid volume with balanced I&O and be free of signs reflecting dehydration.

ACTIONS/INTERVENTIONS

Independent

Assess vital signs, noting changes in BP (postural), tachycardia, fever. Assess skin turgor, capillary refill, and moisture of mucous membranes.

Monitor I&O, noting/measuring diarrhea and NG suction losses.

Evaluate muscle strength/tone. Observe for muscle tremors.

Establish individual needs/replacement schedule.

Encourage increased oral intake when able.

RATIONALE

Indicators of dehydration/hypovolemia, adequacy of current fluid replacement. *Note:* Adequate sized cuff must be used to ensure factual measurement of BP. If cuff is too small, reading will be falsely elevated.

Changes in gastric capacity/intestinal motility and nausea greatly influence intake and fluid needs, increasing risk of dehydration.

Large gastric losses may result in decreased magnesium and calcium, leading to neuromuscular weakness/tetany.

Determined by amount of measured losses/estimated insensible losses and dependent on gastric capacity.

Permits discontinuation of invasive fluid support measures and contributes to return of normal bowel functioning.

447

ACTIONS/INTERVENTIONS

Collaborative

Administer supplemental IV fluids as indicated.

Monitor electrolytes and replace as indicated.

RATIONALE

Replaces fluid losses and restores fluid balance in immediate postoperative phase and/or until patient is able to take sufficient oral fluids.

Use of NG tube, and/or vomiting, onset of diarrhea can deplete electrolytes, affecting organ function.

NURSING DIAGNOSIS:	NUTRITION, ALTERED: LESS THAN BODY REQUIREMENTS, HIGH RISK FOR
Risk factors may include:	Decreased intake, dietary restrictions, early satiety.
	Increased metabolic rate/healing.
	Malabsorption of nutrients/impaired absorption of vitamins.
Possibly evidenced by:	[Not applicable; presence of signs and symptoms establishes an actual diagnosis.]
DESIRED OUTCOMES/ EVALUATION CRITERIA— PATIENT WILL:	Identify individual nutritional needs.
	Demonstrate appropriate weight loss with normalization of laboratory values.
	Display behaviors to maintain adequate nutritional intake.

ACTIONS/INTERVENTIONS

Independent

Establish hourly intake schedule. Instruct in measuring fluids/foods and sipping or eating slowly.

Weigh daily. Establish regular schedule after discharge.

Stress importance of being aware of satiety and stopping intake.

Require that patient sit up to drink/eat.

Determine foods that are gas-forming.

Discuss food preferences with patient and include in pureed diet.

Collaborative

Provide liquid diet, advancing to soft, high in protein and bulk, and low in fat, with liquid supplements as needed.

RATIONALE

After partitioning, gastric capacity is reduced to approximately 50 ml, necessitating frequent/small feedings.

Monitors losses and aids in assessing nutritional needs/effectiveness of therapy.

Overeating may cause nausea/vomiting or damage partitioning.

Reduces possibility of aspiration.

May interfere with appetite/digestion and restrict nutritional intake.

May enhance intake, promote sense of participation/control.

Provides nutrients without exceeding calorie limits *Note:* Liquid diet is usually maintained for 8 weeks after partitioning procedure.

ACTIONS/INTERVENTIONS

Collaborative

Refer to dietitian.

Administer vitamin supplements as well as B$_{12}$ injections, folate, and calcium as indicated.

RATIONALE

May need assistance in planning a diet that meets nutritional needs.

Supplements may be needed to prevent anemia as absorption is impaired. Increased intestinal motility following bypass procedure lowers calcium level and increases absorption of oxalates, which can lead to urinary stone formation.

NURSING DIAGNOSIS:	**SKIN INTEGRITY, IMPAIRED: ACTUAL/HIGH RISK FOR**
May be related to:	Trauma/surgery; difficulty in approximation of suture line of fatty tissue.
	Reduced vascularity, altered circulation.
	Altered nutritional state: obesity.
Possibly evidenced by:	Disruption of skin surface, altered healing.
DESIRED OUTCOMES/ EVALUATION CRITERIA— PATIENT WILL:	Display timely wound healing without complication.
	Demonstrate behaviors to reduce tension on suture line.

ACTIONS/INTERVENTIONS

Independent

Support incision when turning, coughing, deep breathing, and ambulating.

Observe incisions periodically, noting approximation of wound edges, hematoma formation and resolution, bleeding/drainage.

Provide routine incisional care, being careful to keep dressings dry and sterile. Assess patency of drains.

Encourage frequent position change, inspect pressure points, and massage as indicated. Apply transparent skin barrier to elbows/heels.

Provide meticulous skin care; pay particular attention to skin folds.

Provide foam/air mattress or kinetic therapy as indicated.

RATIONALE

Reduces possibility of dehiscence and later incisional hernia.

Influences choice of interventions.

Promotes healing. Accumulation of serosanguinous drainage in subcutaneous layers increases tension on suture line, may delay wound healing, and serves as a medium for bacterial growth.

Reduces pressure on skin, promoting peripheral circulation and reducing risk of skin breakdown. Skin barrier reduces risk of shearing injury.

Moisture or excoriation enhances growth of bacteria that can lead to postoperative infection.

Reduces skin pressure and enhances circulation.

NURSING DIAGNOSIS:	INFECTION, HIGH RISK FOR
Risk factors may include:	Inadequate primary defenses: broken/traumatized tissues, decreased ciliary action, stasis of body fluids. Invasive procedures.
Possibly evidenced by:	[Not applicable; presence of signs and symptoms establishes an actual diagnosis.]
DESIRED OUTCOMES/ EVALUATION CRITERIA— PATIENT WILL:	Achieve timely wound healing free of signs of local or generalized infectious process.

ACTIONS/INTERVENTIONS	RATIONALE
Independent	
Stress proper hand washing technique.	Prevents spread of bacteria, cross-contamination.
Maintain aseptic technique in dressing changes, invasive procedures.	Reduces risk of nosocomial infection.
Inspect surgical incisions/invasive sites for erythema, purulent drainage.	Early detection of developing infection provides for prevention of more serious complications.
Encourage frequent position changes; deep breathing, coughing, use of respiratory adjuncts, e.g., incentive spirometer.	Promotes mobilization of secretions, reducing risk of pneumonia.
Provide routine catheter care/encourage good perineal care.	Prevents ascending bladder infections.
Encourage patient to drink acid-ash juices, such as cranberry.	Maintains urine acidity to retard bacterial growth.
Observe for reports of abdominal pain (especially after 3rd postoperative day), elevated temperature, increased white count.	Suggests possibility of developing peritonitis.
Collaborative	
Apply topical antimicrobials/antibiotics as indicated.	Reduces bacterial or fungal colonization on skin; prevents infection in wound.
Administer IV antibiotics as indicated.	A prophylactic antibiotic regimen is usually standard in these patients to reduce risk of perioperative contamination and/or peritonitis.

NURSING DIAGNOSIS:	DIARRHEA
May be related to:	Rapid transit of food through shortened small intestine. Changes in dietary fiber and bulk. Inflammation, irritation, and malabsorption of bowel.

Possibly evidenced by:	Loose, liquid stools, increased frequency. Increased/hyperactive bowel sounds.
DESIRED OUTCOMES/ EVALUATION CRITERIA— PATIENT WILL:	Verbalize understanding of causative factors and rationale of treatment regimen. Regain near normal bowel function.

ACTIONS/INTERVENTIONS	RATIONALE
Independent	
Observe/record stool frequency, characteristics, and amount.	Diarrhea often develops after resumption of diet.
Encourage diet high in fiber/bulk within dietary limitations, with moderate fluid intake as diet resumes.	Increases consistency of the effluent. Although fluid is necessary for optimal body function, excessive amounts contribute to diarrhea.
Restrict fat intake as indicated.	Low-fat diet reduces risk of steatorrhea and limits laxative effect of decreased fat absorption.
Observe for signs of "dumping syndrome," e.g., instant diarrhea, sweating, nausea, and weakness after eating.	Rapid emptying of food from the stomach may result in gastric distress and alter bowel function.
Assist with frequent perianal care, using ointments as indicated. Provide whirlpool bath.	Anal irritation, excoriation, and pruritus occur because of diarrhea. The patient often cannot reach the area for proper cleansing and may be embarrassed to ask for help.
Collaborative	
Administer medications as indicated, e.g., diphenoxylate with atropine (Lomotil).	May be necessary to control frequency of stools until body readjusts to surgical changes in function.
Monitor serum electrolytes.	Increased gastric losses potentiate the risk of electrolyte imbalance, which can lead to more serious/threatening complications.

NURSING DIAGNOSIS:	**KNOWLEDGE DEFICIT [LEARNING NEED] REGARDING CONDITION, PROGNOSIS, AND TREATMENT NEEDS**
May be related to:	Lack of exposure, unfamiliarity with resources. Information misinterpretation. Lack of recall.
Possibly evidenced by:	Questions, request for information. Statement of misconceptions. Inaccurate follow-through of instructions. Development of preventable complications.

DESIRED OUTCOMES/ EVALUATION CRITERIA— PATIENT WILL:	Verbalize understanding of surgical procedure, potential complications, treatment regimen, and postoperative expectations.
	Initiate necessary lifestyle changes and participate in treatment regimen.

ACTIONS/INTERVENTIONS	RATIONALE

Independent

ACTIONS/INTERVENTIONS	RATIONALE
Review specific surgical procedure and postoperative expectations.	Provides knowledge base on which informed choices can be made and goals formulated. Initial weight loss is rapid with patient often losing half of their total weight loss during the first 6 months. Weight loss then gradually slows over a 2-year period.
Address concerns about altered body size/image.	Anticipation of problems can be helpful in dealing with situations that arise. (Refer to CP: Eating Disorders: Obesity, ND: Body Image/Self-esteem, disturbance in: p 428.) *Note:* Feelings that often occur during more conventional weight loss therapies generally are not encountered in the surgically treated patient.
Review medication regimen, dosage, and side effects.	Knowledge may enhance cooperation with therapeutic regimen and in maintenance of schedule.
Recommend avoidance of alcohol.	May contribute to liver/pancreatic dysfunction.
Discuss responsibility for self-care with patient/SO.	Full cooperation is important for successful outcome after procedure.
Stress importance of regular medical follow-up, including laboratory studies, and discuss possible health problems.	Periodic assessment/evaluation (e.g., over 3–12 months) promotes early recognition/prevention of such complications as liver dysfunction, malnutrition, electrolyte imbalances, and kidney stones, which may develop after bypass.
Encourage progressive exercise/activity program balanced with adequate rest periods.	Promotes weight loss, enhances muscle tone, and minimizes postoperative complications while preventing undue fatigue.
Review proper eating habits, e.g., eat small amounts of food slowly and chew well, sit at table in calm/relaxed environment, eat only at prescribed times, avoid between-meal snacking, do not "make up" skipped feedings.	Focuses attention on eating, increasing awareness of intake and feelings of satiety.
Avoid fluid intake ½ hour before/after meals and use of carbonated beverages.	May cause gastric fullness/gaseous distention, limiting intake.
Identify signs of hypokalemia, e.g., diarrhea, muscle cramps/weakness of lower extremities, weak/irregular pulse, dizziness with position changes.	Increasing dietary intake of potassium (e.g., milk, coffee, potatoes, carrots, bananas, oranges) may correct deficit, preventing serious respiratory/cardiac complications.
Discuss symptoms that may indicate dumping syndrome, e.g., weakness, profuse perspiration,	Generally occurring in early postoperative period (1–3 weeks), syndrome is usually self-limiting but

ACTIONS/INTERVENTIONS	RATIONALE
Independent	
nausea, vomiting, faintness, flushing, and epigastric discomfort or palpitations, occurring during or immediately following meals. Problem solve solutions.	may become chronic and require medical intervention.
Review symptoms requiring medical evaluation, e.g., persistent n/v, abdominal distention, abdominal tenderness, change in pattern of bowel elimination, fever, purulent wound drainage, excessive weight loss or plateauing/weight gain.	Early recognition of developing complications allows for prompt intervention, preventing serious outcome.
Refer to community support groups.	Involvement with others who have dealt with same problems enhances coping; may promote cooperation with therapeutic regimen and long-term positive recovery.

Upper Gastrointestinal/Esophageal Bleeding _____

Bleeding duodenal ulcer is the most frequent cause of massive upper GI hemorrhage, but bleeding may also occur because of gastric ulcers, gastritis, and esophageal varices. Severe vomiting can precipitate gastric bleeding due to a tear of the mucosa at the gastroesophageal junction (Mallory-Weiss syndrome). Stress ulcer can occur owing to severe burns, major trauma/surgery, or severe systemic disease. Esophagitis, esophageal/gastric carcinoma, hiatal hernia, hemophilia, leukemia, and DIC are less common causes of upper GI bleeding.

   Generally, a patient with severe, active bleeding will be admitted directly to the critical care unit; however, a patient may develop GI bleeding on the medical/surgical unit or be admitted there for evaluation/treatment of subacute bleeding.

RELATED CONCERNS:

Cirrhosis of the Liver, p 547
Fluid and Electrolyte Imbalances, p 1054
Psychosocial Aspects of Acute Care, p 899
Renal Failure: Acute, p 618
Subtotal Gastrectomy/Gastric Resection, p 467

PATIENT ASSESSMENT DATA BASE

ACTIVITY/REST

May report:	Weakness, fatigue.
May exhibit:	Tachycardia, tachypnea/hyperventilation (response to activity).

CIRCULATION

May exhibit:	Hypotension (including postural).
	Tachycardia, dysrhythmias (hypovolemia/hypoxemia).
	Weak/thready peripheral pulse.
	Capillary refill slow/delayed (vasoconstriction).
	Skin color: pallor, cyanosis (depending on the amount of blood loss).
	Skin/mucous membrane moisture: diaphoresis (reflecting shock state, acute pain, psychologic response).

EGO INTEGRITY

May report:	Acute or chronic stress factors (financial, relationships, job-related).
	Feelings of helplessness.
May exhibit:	Signs of anxiety, e.g., restlessness, pallor, diaphoresis, narrowed focus, trembling, quivering voice.

ELIMINATION

May report:	History of previous hospitalizations for GI bleeding or related GI problems, e.g., peptic/gastric ulcer, gastritis, gastric surgery, irradiation of gastric area.
	Change in usual bowel patterns/characteristics of stool.
May exhibit:	Abdominal tenderness, distention.
	Bowel sounds: often hyperactive during bleed, hypoactive after bleeding subsides.

Character of stool: diarrhea; dark bloody, tarry, or occasionally bright red stools; frothy, foul-smelling (steatorrhea). Constipation may occur (changes in diet, antacid use).

Urine output: may be decreased, concentrated.

FOOD/FLUID

May report: Anorexia, nausea, vomiting (protracted vomiting suggests pyloric outlet obstruction associated with duodenal ulcer).

Problems swallowing; hiccups.

Heartburn, burping with sour taste, nausea/vomiting.

Food intolerances, e.g., spicy food, chocolate; special diet for preexisting ulcer disease.

Weight loss.

May exhibit: Vomitus: coffee ground or bright red, with or without clots.

Mucous membranes dry, decreased mucous production, poor skin turgor (chronic bleeding).

Urine specific gravity may be elevated.

NEUROSENSORY

May report: Fainting, dizziness/lightheadedness, weakness.

Mental status: level of consciousness may be altered, ranging from slight drowsiness, disorientation/confusion, to stupor and coma (dependent on circulating volume/oxygenation).

PAIN/COMFORT

May report: Pain, described as sharp, dull, burning, gnawing; sudden excruciating pain can accompany perforation.

Vague sensation of discomfort/distress following large meals and relieved by food (acute gastritis).

Left to mid-epigastric pain and/or pain radiating to back occurring 1–2 hours after eating and relieved by antacids (gastric ulcer).

Localized right epigastric pain occurring about 4 hours after meals when stomach is empty and relieved by food or antacids (duodenal ulcers).

Absence of pain (esophageal varices or gastritis).

Precipitating factors: may be foods, smoking, ingestion of alcohol, use of certain drugs (salicylates, reserpine, antibiotics, ibuprofen), psychologic stressors.

May exhibit: Facial grimacing, guarding of affected area, pallor, diaphoresis, narrowed focus.

SAFETY

May report: Drug allergies/sensitivities, e.g., ASA.

May exhibit: Temperature elevation.

Spider angiomas, palmar erythema (reflecting cirrhosis/portal hypertension).

TEACHING/LEARNING

May report: Recent use of prescription/OTC drugs containing ASA, alcohol, steroids. NSAIDs are the leading cause of drug-induced GI bleeding.

Current complaint may reveal admission for related (e.g., anemia) or unrelated (e.g., head trauma) diagnosis; intestinal flu, or severe vomiting episode. Long-standing health problems, e.g., cirrhosis, alcoholism, hepatitis, eating disorders.

Discharge Plan Considerations: **DRG projected mean length of stay: 3.9 days.**

May require changes in therapeutic/medication regimen.

DIAGNOSTIC STUDIES

EGD (esophagogastroduodenoscopy): Key diagnostic test for upper GI bleeding, done to visualize site of bleeding/degree of tissue ulceration/injury.

Barium swallow with x-ray: Done for differential diagnosis of cause/site of lesion.

Gastric analysis: May be done to determine presence of blood, assess secretory activity of gastric mucosa, e.g., increased hydrochloric acid and nocturnal acid formation indicative of duodenal ulcer. Decreased or normal amount suggests gastric ulcer; enormous hypersecretion and acidity may reflect Zollinger-Ellison syndrome.

Angiography: GI vasculature may be reviewed if endoscopy is inconclusive or impractical. Demonstrates collateral circulation and possibly bleeding site.

Stools: Testing for blood will be positive.

Hb/Hct: Decreased levels occur within 6–24 hours after bleeding begins.

WBC: May elevate, reflecting body's response to injury.

BUN: Elevates within 24–48 hours as blood proteins are broken down in the GI tract and kidney filtration is decreased.

Creatinine: Usually not elevated if renal perfusion is maintained.

Ammonia: May be elevated when severe liver dysfunction disrupts the metabolism and proper excretion of urea or when massive whole blood transfusions have been given.

Coagulation profile: Increased platelets and decreased clotting times may be noted, reflecting the body's attempt to restore hemostasis. Severe abnormalities may reveal coagulopathy, e.g., DIC, as cause of bleeding.

ABGs: May reveal initial respiratory alkalosis (compensating for diminished blood flow through lungs). Later, metabolic acidosis develops in response to sluggish liver flow/accumulation of metabolic waste products.

Sodium: May be elevated as a hormonal compensation to conserve body fluid.

Potassium: May initially be depleted because of massive gastric emptying/vomiting or bloody diarrhea. Elevated potassium levels may occur after multiple transfusions of stored blood or with acute renal impairment.

Serum gastrin analysis: Elevated level suggests Zollinger-Ellison syndrome or possible presence of multiple poorly healed ulcers. Normal or low in type B gastritis.

Serum amylase: Elevated with posterior penetration of duodenal ulcer.

Pepsinogen level: Increased by duodenal ulcer; low level suggestive of gastritis.

Serum parietal cell antibodies: Presence suggestive of chronic gastritis.

NURSING PRIORITIES

1. Control hemorrhage.
2. Achieve/maintain hemodynamic stability.
3. Promote stress reduction.
4. Provide information about disease process/prognosis, treatment needs, and potential complications.

DISCHARGE GOALS

1. Hemorrhage curtailed.
2. Hemodynamically stable.
3. Anxiety/fear reduced to manageable level.
4. Disease process/prognosis, therapeutic regimen, and potential complications understood.

NURSING DIAGNOSIS:	FLUID VOLUME DEFICIT, [ACTIVE LOSS]
May be related to:	Hemorrhage.
Possibly evidenced by:	Hypotension, tachycardia, delayed capillary refill.
	Changes in mentation, restlessness.
	Concentrated/decreased urine.
	Pallor, diaphoresis.
	Hemoconcentration.
DESIRED OUTCOMES/ EVALUATION CRITERIA— PATIENT WILL:	Demonstrate improved fluid balance as evidenced by individually adequate urinary output with normal specific gravity, stable vital signs, moist mucous membranes, good skin turgor, prompt capillary refill.

ACTIONS/INTERVENTIONS

Independent

Note characteristics of vomitus and/or drainage.

Monitor vital signs; compare with patient's normal/previous readings. Take BP in sitting, lying, standing position when possible.

Note patient's individual physiologic response to bleeding, e.g., changes in mentation, weakness, restlessness, anxiety; pallor, diaphoresis; tachypnea; temperature elevation.

Measure CVP, if available.

RATIONALE

May be helpful in differentiating cause of gastric distress. Yellow-green bile content implies that the pylorus is open. Fecal content indicates bowel obstruction. Bright red blood signals recent or acute arterial bleeding, perhaps due to gastric ulceration; dark red blood may be old blood (retained in intestine) or venous bleeding from varices. Coffee-ground appearance is suggestive of partially digested blood from slowly oozing area. Undigested food indicates obstruction or gastric tumor.

Changes in BP and pulse may be used for rough estimate of blood loss, (e.g., BP <90 mm Hg, and pulse >110 suggests a 25% decrease in volume or approximately 1000 ml). Postural hypotension reflects a decrease in circulating volume.

Symptomatology may be useful in gauging severity/length of bleeding episode. Worsening of symptoms may reflect continued bleeding or inadequate fluid replacement.

Reflects circulating volume and cardiac response to bleeding and fluid replacement; e.g., CVP values between 5 and 20 cm H_2O usually reflect adequate volume.

ACTIONS/INTERVENTIONS	RATIONALE
Independent	
Monitor I&O, and correlate with weight changes. Measure blood/fluid losses via emesis, gastric suction/lavage, and stools.	Provides guidelines for fluid replacement.
Keep accurate record of subtotals of solutions/ blood during replacement therapy.	Potential exists for overtransfusion of fluids, especially when volume expanders are given before blood transfusions.
Maintain bed rest; prevent vomiting and straining at stool. Schedule activities to provide undisturbed rest periods. Eliminate noxious stimuli.	Activity/vomiting increases intra-abdominal pressure and can predispose to further bleeding.
Elevate head of bed during antacid gavage.	Prevents gastric reflux and aspiration of antacids, which can cause serious pulmonary complications.
Note signs of renewed bleeding after cessation of initial bleeding.	Increased abdominal fullness/distention, nausea or renewed vomiting, and bloody diarrhea may indicate rebleeding.
Observe for secondary bleeding, e.g., nose/gums, oozing from puncture sites, appearance of ecchymotic areas following minimal trauma.	Loss of/inadequate replacement of clotting factors may precipitate development of DIC.
Provide clear/bland fluids when intake resumed. Avoid caffeinated and carbonated beverages.	Caffeine and carbonated beverages stimulate hydrochloric acid production, possibly potentiating rebleeding.
Collaborative	
Administer fluids/blood as indicated:	Fluid replacement is dependent on degree of hypovolemia and duration of bleeding (acute or chronic). Volume expanders (albumin) may be infused until type and cross-match can be completed and blood transfusions begun. Approximately 80%–90% of gastric bleeding is controlled by fluid resuscitation and medical management.
Fresh whole blood/packed red cells;	Fresh whole blood is indicated for acute bleeding (with shock), because stored blood may be deficient in clotting factors. Packed cells may be adequate for stable patients with subacute/chronic bleeding and are required for patients with CHF to prevent fluid overload.
Fresh frozen plasma and/or platelets.	Clotting factors/components are depleted by 2 mechanisms: hemorrhagic loss and the clotting process at the site of bleeding. FFP is an excellent source of clotting factors. Platelet replacement may potentiate formation of platelet plug at injury sites.
Insert/maintain large-bore NG tube in acute bleeding.	Provides avenue for removing irritating gastric secretions, blood, and clots; reduces nausea/ vomiting; and facilitates diagnostic endoscopy. *Note:* Blood remaining in the stomach/intestines will be broken down into ammonia, which can produce a toxic CNS effect, e.g., encephalopathy.

ACTIONS/INTERVENTIONS	RATIONALE

Independent

Perform gastric lavage with cold or room-temperature saline until aspirate is light pink or clear and free of clots. Simultaneous low gastric suctioning with continuous saline infusion through the air port of a salem sump tube may also be used.

Flushes out/breaks up clots and may reduce bleeding by local vasoconstriction. Facilitates visualization by endoscopy to locate bleeding source. *Note:* Research now suggests that iced saline is no more effective than room temperature solution in controlling bleeding, and it may actually damage gastric mucosa as well as lower the patient's core temperature, which could prolong bleeding by inhibiting platelet function.

Administer medications, as indicated:

Cimetidine (Tagamet); ranitidine (Zantac); famotidine (Pepcid); nizatidine (Axid);

Histamine H_2-blockers reduce gastric acid production, increase gastric pH, and reduce irritation to gastric mucosa to aid in healing as well as prevention of lesion formation.

Sucralfate (Carafate);

Antiulcer agent decreases gastric acid secretion and increases the production of protective mucus useful in treating and preventing recurrence of duodenal ulcers. *Note:* Impairs absorption of some drugs, e.g., theophylline, digoxin, phenytoin, tetracycline, amitriptyline.

Omeprazole (Prilosec);

Classified as a substitute benzimidazole, which can completely inhibit acid secretion and has a long duration of action.

Antacids: e.g., Amphojel, Maalox, Mylanta, Riopan;

Antacids (administered orally or by gavage) may be given to maintain gastric pH level at 4.5 or higher to reduce risk of rebleeding. Antacids block the gastric absorption of oral histamine antagonists and therefore should not be administered within 1 hour after oral administration of histamine blockers.

Belladonna; atropine;

Anticholinergics may be used to decrease gastric motility, particularly in peptic ulcer disease after acute bleeding has subsided.

Vasopressin (Pitressin);

Administration of intra-arterial vasocontrictors may be needed in severe, prolonged bleeding (varices).

Vitamin K_1 (AquaMephyton);

Promotes hepatic synthesis of coagulation factors to support clotting. *Note:* Absorption of vitamin K may be decreased by use of sulcralfate.

Phenobarbital;

Mild sedatives may be given to promote rest, reduce intensity of bleeding, and alleviate pain. *Note:* Use with caution to avoid masking signs of developing hypovolemia.

Antiemetics, e.g., metoclopramide (Reglan); prochlorperazine (Compazine);

Alleviates nausea and prevents vomiting.

Supplemental vitamin B_{12};

In diffuse atrophic gastritis, the intrinsic factor necessary for B_{12} absorption from the GI tract is not secreted, and individual may develop pernicious anemia.

ACTIONS/INTERVENTIONS	RATIONALE
Independent	
Antibiotics.	May be used when infection is the cause of chronic gastritis (Campylobacter pylori) or ulcers (Helicobacter pylori). *Note:* Neomycin (Mycifradin) or lactulose (Cephulac) may be used in esophageal varices to block bacterial breakdown of shed blood in the gut to reduce the risk of encephalopathy.
Monitor laboratory studies, e.g.:	
Hb, Hct, RBC count;	Aids in establishing blood replacement needs and monitoring effectiveness of therapy, e.g., 1 U of whole blood should raise Hct 2–3 points. Levels may initially remain stable, due to loss of both plasma and RBCs.
BUN/creatinine levels.	BUN >40 with normal creatinine level indicates major bleeding. BUN should return to patient's normal level approximately 12 hours after bleeding has ceased.
Assist with/prepare for:	
Sclerotherapy;	Injection of an irritating (sclerosing) agent into esophageal varices (to create thrombosis) may be performed to prevent recurrence after initial bleeding is controlled.
Endoscopic variceal ligation (EVL);	This banding technique is used as an effective alternative to sclerotherapy. Active hemorrhage is controlled in a high percentage of patients with fewer complications than with sclerotherapy.
Electrocoagulation or photocoagulation (laser) therapy;	Provides direct coagulation of bleeding sites.
Surgical intervention.	Total/partial gastrectomy, pyloroplasty, and/or vagotomy may be required to control/prevent future gastric bleeding. Shunt procedures (portacaval, splenorenal, mesocaval, or distal splenorenal) may be done to divert blood flow and reduce pressure within esophageal vessels when other measures fail.

NURSING DIAGNOSIS:	TISSUE PERFUSION, ALTERED, HIGH RISK FOR
Risk factors may include:	Hypovolemia.
Possibly evidenced by:	[Not applicable; presence of signs and symptoms establishes an actual diagnosis.]
DESIRED OUTCOMES/ EVALUATION CRITERIA— PATIENT WILL:	Maintain/improve tissue perfusion as evidenced by stabilized vital signs, warm skin, palpable peripheral pulses, ABGs within patient norms, adequate urine output.

ACTIONS/INTERVENTIONS	RATIONALE
Independent	
Investigate changes in level of consciousness, reports of dizziness/headache.	Changes may reflect inadequate cerebral perfusion as a result of reduced arterial blood pressure. *Note:* Changes in sensorium may also reflect elevated ammonia levels/hepatic encephalophathy in patient with liver disease.
Investigate reports of chest pain. Note location, quality, duration, and what relieves pain.	May reflect cardiac ischemia related to decreased perfusion. *Note:* Impaired oxygenation status resulting from blood loss can bring on MI in patient with cardiac disease.
Auscultate apical pulse. Monitor cardiac rate/rhythm if continuous ECG available.	Dysrhythmias and ischemic changes can occur as a result of hypotension, hypoxia, acidosis, electrolyte imbalance, or cooling near the heart if cold saline lavage is used to control bleeding.
Assess skin for coolness, pallor, diaphoresis, delayed capillary refill, and weak, thready peripheral pulses.	Vasoconstriction is a sympathetic response to lowered circulating volume and/or may occur as a side effect of vasopressin administration.
Note urinary output and specific gravity.	Decreased systemic perfusion may cause kidney ischemia/failure manifested by decreased urine output. ATN may develop if hypovolemic state is prolonged.
Note reports of abdominal pain, especially sudden, severe pain or pain radiating to shoulder.	Pain caused by gastric ulcer is often relieved after acute bleeding because of buffering effects of blood. Continued severe or sudden pain may reflect ischemia due to vasoconstrictive therapy; bleeding into biliary tract (hematobilia); or perforation/onset of peritonitis.
Observe skin for pallor, redness. Massage with lotion. Change position frequently.	Compromised peripheral circulation increases risk of skin breakdown.
Collaborative	
Provide supplemental oxygen if indicated.	Treats hypoxemia and lactic acidosis during acute bleed.
Monitor ABGs/pulse oximetry.	Identifies hypoxemia, effectiveness of/need for therapy.
Administer IV fluids as indicated.	Maintains circulating volume and perfusion. Note: Use of Ringer's lactate may be contraindicated in presence of hepatic failure because metabolism of lactate is impaired, and lactic acidosis may develop.

NURSING DIAGNOSIS:	**FEAR/ANXIETY [SPECIFY LEVEL]**
May be related to:	Change in health status, threat of death.
Possibly evidenced by:	Increased tension, restlessness, irritability, fearfulness.
	Trembling, tachycardia, diaphoresis.

461

	Lack of eye contact, focus on self.
	Verbalization of specific concern.
	Withdrawal, panic or attack behavior.
DESIRED OUTCOMES/ EVALUATION CRITERIA— PATIENT WILL:	Discuss fears/concerns recognizing healthy versus unhealthy fears.
	Verbalize appropriate range of feelings.
	Appear relaxed and report anxiety is reduced to a manageable level.
	Demonstrate problem solving and effective use of resources.

ACTIONS/INTERVENTIONS	RATIONALE

Independent

ACTIONS/INTERVENTIONS	RATIONALE
Monitor physiologic responses, e.g., tachypnea, palpitations, dizziness, headache, tingling sensations.	May be indicative of the degree of fear patient is experiencing but may also be related to physical condition/shock state.
Note behavioral clues, e.g., restlessness, irritability, lack of eye contact, combativeness/attack behavior.	Indicators of degree of fear patient is experiencing; e.g., patient may feel out of control of the situation or reach a state of panic.
Encourage verbalization of fear and anxiety; provide feedback.	Establishes a therapeutic relationship. Assists the patient in dealing with feelings and provides opportunity to clarify misconceptions.
Acknowledge that this is a fearful situation and that others have expressed similar fears. Assist patient in expressing feelings by active listening.	When patient is expressing own fear, the validation that these feelings are normal can help patient to feel less isolated.
Provide accurate, concrete information about what is being done, e.g., sensations to expect, usual procedures undertaken.	Involves patient in plan of care and decreases unnecessary anxiety about unknowns.
Provide a calm, restful environment.	Removing patient from outside stressors promotes relaxation, may enhance coping skills.
Encourage SO to stay with patient as able. Respond to call signal promptly. Use touch and eye contact as appropriate.	Helps reduce fear of going through a frightening experience alone.
Provide opportunity for SO to express feelings/concerns. Encourage SO to project positive, realistic attitude.	Helps SO to deal with own anxiety/fears that can be transmitted to the patient. Promotes a supportive attitude that can facilitate recovery.
Demonstrate relaxation techniques, e.g., visualization, deep breathing exercises, guided imagery.	Learning ways to relax can be helpful in reducing fear and anxiety. As the patient with GI bleeding is often a person with type A personality who has difficulty relaxing, learning these skills can be important to recovery and prevention of recurrence.
Help the patient to identify and initiate positive coping behaviors used successfully in the past.	Successful behaviors can be fostered in dealing with current fear, enhancing patient's sense of self-control and providing reassurance.

ACTIONS/INTERVENTIONS

Independent

Encourage and support patient in evaluation of lifestyle.

Collaborative

Administer medications as indicated, e.g.:

Diazepam (Valium); clorazepate (Tranxene); alprazolam (Xanax).

Refer to psychiatric nurse/social services/spiritual advisor.

RATIONALE

Changes may be necessary to avoid recurrence of ulcer condition.

Sedatives/tranquilizers may be used on occasion to reduce anxiety and promote rest, particularly in the ulcer patient.

May need additional assistance during recovery to deal with consequences of emergency situation/adjustments to required/desired changes in lifestyle.

NURSING DIAGNOSIS:	PAIN, [ACUTE]/CHRONIC
May be related to:	Chemical burn of gastric mucosa, oral cavity.
	Physical response, e.g., reflex muscle spasm in the stomach wall.
Possibly evidenced by:	Communication of pain descriptors.
	Abdominal guarding, rigid body posture, facial grimacing.
	Autonomic responses, e.g., changes in vital signs (acute pain).
DESIRED OUTCOMES/ EVALUATION CRITERIA— PATIENT WILL:	Verbalize relief of pain.
	Demonstrate relaxed body posture and be able to sleep/rest appropriately.

ACTIONS/INTERVENTIONS

Independent

Note reports of pain, including location, duration, intensity (0–10 scale).

Review factors that aggravate or alleviate pain.

Note nonverbal pain cues, e.g., restlessness, reluctance to move, abdominal guarding, tachycardia, diaphoresis. Investigate discrepancies between verbal and nonverbal cues.

Provide small, frequent meals as indicated for individual patient.

RATIONALE

Pain is not always present but if present should be compared with patient's previous pain symptoms, which may assist in diagnosis of etiology of bleeding and development of complications.

Helpful in establishing diagnosis and treatment needs.

Nonverbal cues may be both physiologic and psychologic and may be used in conjunction with verbal cues to identify extent/severity of the problem.

Food has an acid neutralizing effect, as well as diluting the gastric contents. Small meals prevent distention and the release of gastrin.

ACTIONS/INTERVENTIONS	RATIONALE
Independent	
Identify and limit foods that create discomfort.	Specific foods that cause distress vary between individuals. Studies indicate pepper is harmful, and coffee (including decaffeinated) can precipitate dyspepsia.
Assist with active/passive ROM exercises.	Reduces joint stiffness, minimizing pain/discomfort.
Provide frequent oral care and comfort measures, e.g., back rub, position change.	Halitosis from stagnant oral secretions is unappetizing and can aggravate nausea. Gingivitis and dental problems may arise.
Collaborative	
Provide and implement prescribed dietary modifications.	Patient may be NPO initially. When oral intake is allowed, food choices will depend on the diagnosis and etiology of the bleeding.
Use regular rather than skim milk, if milk is allowed.	Fat in regular milk may decrease gastric secretions; however, the calcium and protein content (especially in skim milk) increases them.
Administer medications, as indicated, e.g.:	
Analgesics, e.g., morphine sulfate;	May be narcotic of choice to relieve acute/severe pain and reduce peristaltic activity. *Note:* Demerol has been associated with increased incidence of n/v.
Acetaminophen (Tylenol);	Promotes comfort and rest.
Antacids;	Decreases gastric acidity by absorption or by chemical neutralization. Evaluate type of antacid in regard to total health picture, e.g., sodium restriction.
Anticholinergics, e.g., belladonna, atropine.	May be given at bedtime to decrease gastric motility, suppress acid production, delay gastric emptying, and alleviate nocturnal pain associated with gastric ulcer.

NURSING DIAGNOSIS:	**KNOWLEDGE DEFICIT [LEARNING NEED], REGARDING DISEASE PROCESS, PROGNOSIS, AND TREATMENT NEEDS**
May be related to:	Lack of information/recall.
	Unfamiliarity with information resources.
	Information misinterpretation.
Possibly evidenced by:	Verbalization of the problem, request for information, statement of misconceptions.
	Inaccurate follow-through of instructions.
	Development of preventable complications.

DESIRED OUTCOMES/ EVALUATION CRITERIA— PATIENT WILL:	Verbalize understanding of cause of own bleeding episode (if known) and treatment modalities used.
	Begin to discuss own role in preventing recurrence.
	Identify/implement necessary lifestyle changes.
	Participate in treatment regimen.

ACTIONS/INTERVENTIONS	RATIONALE
Independent	
Determine patient perception of cause of bleeding.	Establishes knowledge base and provides some insight into how the teaching plan needs to be constructed for this individual.
Provide/review information regarding etiology of bleeding, cause/effect relationship of lifestyle behaviors, and ways to reduce risk/contributing factors. Encourage questions.	Provides knowledge base on which patient can make informed choices/decisions about future and control of health problems.
Assist patient to identify relationship of food intake and precipitation of/or relief from epigastric pain, including avoidance of gastric irritants, e.g., pepper, caffeine, alcohol, fruit juices, carbonated beverages, smoking, and extremely hot, cold, fatty or spicy foods.	Caffeine and smoking stimulate gastric acidity. Alcohol contributes to erosion of gastric mucosa. Individuals may find that certain foods/fluids increase gastric secretion and pain.
Recommend small, frequent meals/snacks, chewing food slowly, eating at regular time, and avoiding "skipping" meals.	Frequent eating keeps HCl neutralized, dilutes stomach contents to minimize action of acid on gastric mucosa. Small meals prevent gastric overdistention.
Stress importance of reading labels on OTC drugs and avoiding products containing aspirin or switching to enteric-coated aspirin.	Aspirin damages the protective mucosa, permitting gastric erosion, ulceration, and bleeding to occur.
Review significance of signs/symptoms such as coffee-ground emesis, tarry stools, abdominal distention, severe epigastric/abdominal pain radiating to shoulder/back.	Prompt medical evaluation/intervention is required to prevent more serious complications, e.g., perforation, Zollinger-Ellison syndrome.
Support use of stress management techniques, avoidance of emotional stress.	Decreases extrinsic stimulation of HCl, reducing risk of recurrence of bleeding.
Review drug regimen, possible side effects and interaction with other drugs as appropriate.	Helpful to patient's understanding of reason for taking drugs, and what symptoms are important to report to health care provider. *Note:* Aluminum-containing antacids inhibit the intestinal absorption of some drugs affecting scheduling of drug intake.
Encourage patient to inform all health care providers of bleeding history.	May affect drug choices and/or concomitant prescriptions, e.g., misoprostal (Cytotec) can be given with NSAIDs to inhibit gastric acid secretion and reduce risk of gastric irritability/lesions resulting from NSAID therapy.

465

ACTIONS/INTERVENTIONS	RATIONALE
Independent	
Discuss importance of cessation of smoking.	Ulcer healing may be delayed in people who smoke, particularly in those treated with Tagamet. Smoking is also associated with increased risk of peptic ulcer development/recurrence.
Refer to support groups/counseling for lifestyle/behavior changes/reduction of associated risk factors, e.g., substance abuse/stop-smoking clinics.	Alcohol users have a higher incidence of gastritis/esophageal varices, and cigarette smoking is associated with peptic ulcers and delayed healing.

Subtotal Gastrectomy/Gastric Resection _____

Indicated for gastric hemorrhage/intractable ulcers, pyloric obstruction, perforation, cancer.

RELATED CONCERNS:

Cancer, p 1014
Intestinal Surgery, p 500
Pancreatitis, p 561
Peritonitis, p 514
Psychosocial Aspects of Acute Care, p 899
Surgical Intervention, p 918
Total Nutritional Support, p 1039
Upper Gastrointestinal/Esophageal Bleeding, p 454

NURSING PRIORITIES

1. Promote healing and adequate nutritional intake.
2. Prevent complications.
3. Provide information about surgical procedure/prognosis, treatment needs, and concerns.

DISCHARGE GOALS

1. Nutritional intake adequate for individual needs.
2. Complications prevented/minimized.
3. Surgical procedure/prognosis, therapeutic regimen, and long-term needs understood.

(In addition to nursing diagnoses identified in this CP, refer to CP Surgical Intervention, p 918.)

NURSING DIAGNOSIS:	NUTRITION, ALTERED: LESS THAN BODY REQUIREMENTS, HIGH RISK FOR
Risk factors may include:	Restriction of fluids and food.
	Change in digestive process/absorption of nutrients.
Possibly evidenced by:	[Not applicable; presence of signs and symptoms establishes an actual diagnosis.]
DESIRED OUTCOMES/ EVALUATION CRITERIA — PATIENT WILL:	Maintain stable weight/demonstrate progressive weight gain toward goal with normalization of laboratory values.
	Be free of signs of malnutrition.
	Verbalize understanding of functional changes.
	Identify necessary interventions/behaviors to maintain appropriate weight.

ACTIONS/INTERVENTIONS	RATIONALE
Independent	
Maintain patency of NG tube. Do not reposition tube if it becomes dislodged.	Provides rest for GI tract during acute postoperative phase until return of normal function. *Note:* Even though gastric distention may cause stress on the sutures/possible rupture of stump (Billroth II), the tube needs to be repositioned by the physician to prevent injury to the operative area.
Note character and amount of gastric drainage.	Will be bloody for first 12 hours, and then should clear/turn greenish. Continued/recurrent bleeding suggests complications. Decline in output may reflect progression of fluid through the GI tract, suggesting return of function.
Caution the patient to limit the intake of ice chips.	Excessive intake of ice produces nausea and can wash out electrolytes via the NG tube.
Provide oral hygiene on a regular, frequent basis, including petroleum jelly for lips.	Prevents discomfort of dry mouth and cracked lips caused by fluid restriction and the NG tube.
Auscultate for bowel sounds and note passage of flatus.	Peristalsis can be expected to return about the 3rd postoperative day, signaling readiness to resume oral intake.
Monitor tolerance to fluid and food intake, noting abdominal distention, reports of increased pain/cramping, n/v.	Complications of paralytic ileus, obstruction, delayed gastric emptying, and gastric dilatation may occur, possibly requiring reinsertion of NG tube.
Avoid milk (high carbohydrate foods) in the diet.	May trigger dumping syndrome. (Refer to ND; Knowledge Deficit [Learning Need], p 469.)
Note admission weight and compare with subsequent readings.	Provides information about adequacy of dietary intake/determination of nutritional needs.
Collaborative	
Administer IV fluids, hyperalimentation and lipids as indicated.	Meets fluid/nutritional needs until oral intake can be resumed.
Monitor laboratory studies, e.g., Hb/Hct and electrolytes.	Indicators of fluid/nutritional needs and effectiveness of therapy and detects developing complications.
Progress diet as tolerated, advancing from clear liquid to bland diet with several small feedings.	Usually NG tube is clamped for specified periods of time when peristalsis returns, to determine tolerance. After NG tube is removed, intake is advanced gradually to prevent gastric irritation/distention.
Administer medications as indicated:	
Anticholinergics, e.g., atropine, propantheline bromide (Pro-Banthine);	Controls dumping syndrome, enhancing digestion and absorption of nutrients.
Fat-soluble vitamin supplements, including B_{12}, calcium;	Removal of the stomach prevents absorption of B_{12} (due to loss of intrinsic factor) and can lead to pernicious anemia. In addition, rapid emptying of the stomach reduces absorption of calcium.
Iron preparations;	Corrects/prevents iron deficiency anemia.

ACTIONS/INTERVENTIONS

Collaborative

Protein supplements;

Pancreatic enzymes, bile salts;

Medium-chain triglycerides (MCT).

RATIONALE

Additional protein may be helpful for tissue repair and healing.

Enhances digestive process.

Promotes absorption of fats and fat-soluble vitamins to prevent malabsorption problems.

NURSING DIAGNOSIS:	KNOWLEDGE DEFICIT [LEARNING NEED], REGARDING PROCEDURE, PROGNOSIS, AND TREATMENT NEEDS
May be related to:	Lack of exposure/recall. Information misinterpretation. Unfamiliarity with information resources.
Possibly evidenced by:	Questions, statement of misconception. Inaccurate follow-through of instruction. Development of preventable complications.
DESIRED OUTCOMES/ EVALUATION CRITERIA— PATIENT WILL:	Verbalize understanding of procedure, disease process/prognosis, treatment. Correctly perform necessary procedures, explaining reasons for actions.

ACTIONS/INTERVENTIONS

Independent

Review surgical procedure and long-term expectations.

Discuss and identify stress situations and how to avoid them. Investigate job-related issues.

Review dietary needs/regimen (e.g., low carbohydrate, low-fat, high-protein) and importance of maintaining vitamin supplementation.

Discuss the importance of eating small, frequent meals slowly and in a relaxed atmosphere; resting

RATIONALE

Provides knowledge base from which informed choices can be made. Recovery following gastric surgery is often slower than may be anticipated with similar types of surgery. Improved strength and partial normalization of dietary pattern may not be evident for up to 3 months, and full return to usual intake (3 "normal" meals/d) may take up to 12 months. This prolonged convalescence may be difficult for the patient/SO to deal with if he or she has not been prepared.

Can alter gastric motility, interfering with optimal digestion. Note: Patient may require vocational counseling if change in employment is indicated.

May prevent deficiencies and enhance healing and promote cooperation with therapy. Note: Low-fat diet may be required to reduce risk of alkaline reflux gastritis.

These measures can be helpful in avoiding gastric distention/irritation and/or stress on surgical repair,

ACTIONS/INTERVENTIONS	RATIONALE

Independent

after meals; avoiding extremely hot or cold food; restricting high-fiber foods, caffeine, milk products and alcohol, excess sugars and salt; and taking fluids between meals, rather than with food.

dumping syndrome, and reactive hypoglycemia. *Note:* Ice-cold fluids/foods can cause gastric spasms.

Instruct in avoiding certain fibrous foods and discuss the necessity of chewing food well.

Remaining gastric tissue may have reduced ability to digest such foods as citrus skins/seeds, which can collect, forming a mass (phytobezoar formation) that is not excreted.

Recommend foods containing pectin, e.g., citrus fruits, bananas, apples, yellow vegetables, and beans.

Increased intake of these foods may reduce incidence of dumping syndrome.

Identify foods that can cause gastric irritation and increase gastric acid, e.g., chocolate, spicy foods, whole grains, raw vegetables.

Limiting/avoiding these foods reduces risk of gastric bleeding/ulceration in some individuals. *Note:* Ingesting fresh fruits to reduce risk of dumping syndrome should be tempered with adverse effect of gastric irritation.

Identify symptoms that may indicate dumping syndrome, e.g., weakness, profuse perspiration, epigastric fullness, nausea/vomiting, abdominal cramping, faintness, flushing, explosive diarrhea, and palpitations occurring within 15 minutes–1 hour after eating.

Can cause severe discomfort or even shock, and reduces absorption of nutrients. Usually self-limiting (1–3 weeks after surgery) but may become chronic.

Discuss signs of hypoglycemia and corrective interventions, e.g., ingesting of cheese and crackers, orange/grape juice.

Awareness helps patient to take actions to prevent progression of symptoms.

Suggest patient weigh self on a regular basis.

Change in dietary pattern, early satiety, effort of avoiding dumping syndrome may limit intake causing weight loss.

Review medications, purpose, dosage, and schedule as well as possible side effects.

Understanding rationale/therapeutic needs can reduce risk of complications, e.g., anticholinergics/pectin powder may be given to reduce incidence of dumping syndrome; antacids/histamine antagonists reduce gastric irritation.

Caution patient to read labels and avoid products containing ASA, ibuprophen.

Can cause gastric irritation/bleeding.

Discuss reasons and importance of cessation of smoking.

Smoking stimulates gastric acid production and may cause vasoconstriction, compromising mucous membranes and increasing risk of gastric irritation/ulceration.

Identify signs/symptoms requiring medical evaluation, e.g., persistent nausea/vomiting or abdominal fullness, weight loss, diarrhea, foul-smelling fatty or tarry stools, bloody or coffee-ground vomitus/presence of bile, fever. Instruct patient to report changes in pain characteristics.

Prompt recognition and intervention may prevent serious consequences of potential complications such as pancreatitis, peritonitis, and afferent loop syndrome.

Stress importance of regular checkup with health care provider.

Necessary to detect developing complications, e.g., anemia, problems with nutrition, and/or recurrence of disease.

Inflammatory Bowel Disease: Ulcerative Colitis, Regional Enteritis, (Crohn's Disease, Ileocolitis)

Ulcerative colitis (UC) is a chronic condition of unknown cause usually starting in the rectum and distal portions of the colon and possibly spreading upward to involve the sigmoid and descending colon or the entire colon. It is usually intermittent (acute exacerbation with long remissions), but some individuals (30%–40%) have continuous symptoms.

Regional enteritis (Crohn's disease, ileocolitis) may be found in portions of the alimentary tract from the mouth to the anus but is most commonly found in the small intestine (terminal ileum). It is a slowly progressive chronic disease of unknown cause with intermittent acute episodes.

UC and regional enteritis share common symptoms but differ in the degree of severity and complications. Therefore, separate data bases are provided.

RELATED CONCERNS:

Fecal Diversion, p 486
Fluid and Electrolyte Imbalances, p 1054
Intestinal Surgery, p 500
Peritonitis, p 514
Psychosocial Aspects of Acute Care, p 899
Total Nutritional Support, p 1039

PATIENT ASSESSMENT DATA BASE—UC

ACTIVITY/REST

May report:

Weakness, fatigue, malaise, exhaustion.

Insomnia, not sleeping through the night because of diarrhea.

Feeling restless and anxious.

Restriction of activities/work due to effects of disease process.

CIRCULATION

May exhibit:

Tachycardia (response to fever, dehydration, inflammatory process, and pain).

jjBruising, ecchymotic areas (insufficient vitamin K).

BP: hypotension, including postural.

Skin/mucous membranes: poor turgor; dry, cracking of tongue (dehydration/malnutrition).

EGO INTEGRITY

May report:

Anxiety, apprehension, emotional upsets, e.g., feelings of helplessness/hopelessness.

Acute/chronic stress factors, e.g., family/job-related, expense of treatment.

Cultural factor—increased prevalence in Jewish population.

May exhibit:

Withdrawal, narrowed focus, depression.

ELIMINATION

May report:

Stool texture varying from soft-formed to mushy or watery.

Unpredictable, intermittent, frequent, uncontrollable episodes of bloody diarrhea (as many as 20–30 stools/d); sense of urgency/cramping (tenesmus); passing blood/pus/mucus with or without passing feces.

Rectal bleeding.

History of renal stones (dehydration).

May exhibit: Diminished bowel sounds, absence of peristalsis or presence of visible peristalsis.

Hemorrhoids, anal fissures (25%); perianal fistula (more frequently with Crohn's).

Oliguria.

FOOD/FLUID

May report: Anorexia; nausea/vomiting.

Weight loss.

Dietary intolerances/sensitivities, e.g., raw fruits/vegetables, dairy products, fatty foods.

May exhibit: Decreased subcutaneous fat/muscle mass.

Weakness, poor muscle tone and skin turgor.

Mucous membrane pale; sore, inflamed buccal cavity.

HYGIENE

May exhibit: Inability to maintain self-care.

Stomatitis reflecting vitamin deficiency.

Body odor.

PAIN/COMFORT

May report: Pain/tenderness in lower-left quadrant (may be relieved with defecation).

Migratory joint pain, tenderness (arthritis).

Eye pain, photophobia (iritis).

May exhibit: Abdominal tenderness/distention.

SAFETY

May report: History of lupus erythematosus, hemolytic anemia, vasculitis.

Arthritis (worsening of symptoms with exacerbations in bowel disease).

Temperature elevation 104–105° F (acute exacerbation).

Blurred vision.

Allergies to foods/milk products (release of histamine into bowel has an inflammatory effect).

May exhibit: Skin lesions may be present; e.g., erythema nodosum (raised, tender, red, and swollen) on arms, face; pyoderma gangrenosum (purulent pinpoint lesion/boil with a purple border) on trunk, legs, ankles.

Ankylosing spondylitis.

Uveitis, conjunctivitis/iritis.

SEXUALITY

May report: Reduced frequency/avoidance of sexual activity.

SOCIAL INTERACTION

May report: Relationship/role problems related to condition.

Inability to be active socially.

472

TEACHING/LEARNING

May report: Family history of inflammatory bowel disease.

Discharge Plan Considerations: **DRG projected mean length of stay: 7.1 days.**

Assistance with dietary requirements, medication regimen, psychologic support.

DIAGNOSTIC STUDIES

Stool specimens (examinations are used in initial diagnosis and in following disease progression): Mainly composed of mucus, blood, pus, and intestinal organisms, especially *Entamoeba histolytica* (active stage).

Proctosigmoidoscopy: Visualizes ulcerations, edema, hyperemia, and inflammation (result of secondary infection of the mucosa and submucosa). Friability and hemorrhagic areas caused by necrosis and ulceration occur in 85% of these patients.

Cytology and rectal biopsy: Differentiates between infectious process and carcinoma (occurs 10–20 times more often than in general population). Neoplastic changes can be detected, as well as characteristic inflammatory infiltrates called crypt abscesses.

Barium enema: May be performed after visual examination has been done, although rarely done during acute, relapsing stage, because it can exacerbate condition.

Colonoscopy: Identifies adhesions, changes in luminal wall (narrowing/irregularity); rules out bowel obstruction.

CBC: May show hyperchromic anemia (active disease generally present due to blood loss and iron deficiency); leukocytosis may occur, especially in fulminating or complicated cases and in patients on steroid therapy.

Serum iron level: Lowered due to blood loss.

Prothrombin time: Prolonged in severe cases from altered factors VII and X caused by vitamin K deficiency.

ESR: Increased according to severity of disease.

Thrombocytosis: May occur due to inflammatory disease process.

Electrolytes: Decreased potassium and magnesium are common in severe disease.

Albumin level: Decreased because of loss of plasma proteins/disturbed liver function.

Alkaline phosphatase: Increased, along with serum cholesterol and hypoproteinemia, indicating disturbed liver function, (e.g., cholangitis, cirrhosis).

Bone marrow: A generalized depression is common in fulminating types/after a long inflammatory process.

PATIENT ASSESSMENT DATA BASE—REGIONAL ENTERITIS

ACTIVITY/REST

May report: Weakness, fatigue, malaise, exhaustion.

Feeling restless and anxious.

Restriction of activities/work due to effects of disease process.

EGO INTEGRITY

May report: Anxiety, apprehension, emotional upsets, feelings of helplessness/hopelessness.

Acute/chronic stress factors, e.g., family/job-related, expense of treatment.

Cultural factor—increased prevalence in Jewish population, frequency increasing in individuals of Northern European and Anglo-Saxon derivation.

May exhibit: Withdrawal, narrowed focus, depression.

ELIMINATION

May report: Unpredictable, intermittent, frequent, uncontrollable episodes of diarrhea, soft or semiliquid with flatus; foul-smelling and fatty (steatorrhea) stools; melena.

Intermittent constipation.

History of renal stones (increased oxalates in the urine).

May exhibit: Hyperactive bowel sounds with gurgling, splashing sound (borborygmus).

Visible peristalsis.

FOOD/FLUID

May report: Anorexia; n/v.

Weight loss.

Dietary intolerance/sensitivity, e.g., dairy products, fatty foods.

May exhibit: Decreased subcutaneous fat/muscle mass.

Weakness, poor muscle tone and skin turgor.

Mucous membranes pale.

HYGIENE

May exhibit: Inability to maintain self-care.

Body odor.

PAIN/COMFORT

May report: Tender abdomen with cramping pain in lower right quadrant; pain in midlower abdomen (jejunal involvement).

Referred tenderness to periumbilical region.

Migratory joint pain, tenderness (arthritis).

Eye pain, photophobia (iritis).

May exhibit: Abdominal tenderness/distention.

SAFETY

May report: History of arthritis, lupus erythematosus, hemolytic anemia, vasculitis.

Temperature elevation (low-grade fever).

Perianal fissures, anorectal fistula.

Blurred vision.

May exhibit: Skin lesions may be present; erythema nodosum (raised tender, red swelling) on face, arms; pyoderma gangrenosum (purulent pinpoint lesion/boil with a purple border) on trunk, legs, ankles.

Ankylosing spondylitis.

Uveitis, conjunctivitis/iritis.

SOCIAL INTERACTION

May report: Relationship/role problems related to condition. Inability to be active socially.

TEACHING/LEARNING

May report: Family history of inflammatory bowel disease.

Discharge Plan Considerations: **DRG projected mean length of stay: 7.1 days.**

Assistance with dietary requirements, medication regimen, psychologic support.

DIAGNOSTIC STUDIES

Stool examination: Occult blood may be positive (mucosal erosion); steatorrhea and bile salts may be found.

X-rays: Barium swallow may demonstrate luminal narrowing in the terminal ileum, stiffening of the bowel wall, mucosal irritability or ulceration.

Barium enema: Small bowel is nearly always involved, but the rectal area is affected only 50% of the time. Fistulas are frequent and are usually found in the terminal ileum but may be present in segments throughout the GI tract.

Sigmoidoscopic examination: Can demonstrate edematous hyperemic colon mucosa, transverse fissures, or longitudinal ulcers.

Endoscopy: Provides visualization of involved areas.

CBC: Anemia (hypochromic, occasionally macrocytic) may occur due to malnutrition or malabsorption or depressed bone marrow function (chronic inflammatory process); increased WBCs.

ESR: Increased reflecting inflammation.

Albumin/total protein: Decreased.

Cholesterol: Elevated (may have gallstones).

Serum iron-binding folic acid capacity: Decreased due to chronic infection or secondary to blood loss.

Clotting studies: Alterations may occur due to poor vitamin B_{12} absorption.

Electrolytes: Decreased potassium, calcium, and magnesium, with increased sodium.

Urine: Hyperoxaluria (can cause kidney stones).

Urine culture: If *Escherichia coli* organisms are present, suspect fistula formation into the bladder.

NURSING PRIORITIES

1. Control diarrhea/promote optimal bowel function.
2. Minimize/prevent complications.
3. Minimize mental/emotional stress.
4. Provide information about disease process, treatment needs, and long-term aspects/potential complications of recurrent disease.

DISCHARGE GOALS

1. Bowel function stabilized.
2. Complications prevented/controlled.
3. Dealing positively with condition.
4. Disease process/prognosis, therapeutic regimen, and potential complications understood.

NURSING DIAGNOSIS:	DIARRHEA
May be related to:	Inflammation, irritation, or malabsorption of the bowel.
	Presence of toxins.
	Segmental narrowing of the lumen.
Possibly evidenced by:	Increased bowel sounds/peristalsis.
	Frequent, and often severe, watery stools (acute phase).

475

ACTIONS/INTERVENTIONS	RATIONALE

Independent

Observe and record stool frequency, characteristics, amount, and precipitating factors.	Helps differentiate individual disease and assesses severity of episode.
Promote bed rest, provide bedside commode.	Rest decreases intestinal motility as well as reducing the metabolic rate when infection or hemorrhage is a complication. Defecation urges may occur without warning and be uncontrollable, increasing risk of incontinence/falls if facilities are not close at hand.
Remove stool promptly. Provide room deodorizers.	Reduces noxious odors to avoid undue patient embarrassment.
Identify foods and fluids that precipitate diarrhea, e.g., raw vegetables and fruits, whole-grain cereals, condiments, carbonated drinks, milk products.	Avoidance of intestinal irritants promotes intestinal rest.
Restart oral fluid intake gradually. Offer clear liquids hourly; avoid cold fluids.	Provides colon rest by omitting or decreasing the stimulus of foods/fluids. Gradual resumption of liquids may prevent cramping and recurrence of diarrhea; however, cold fluids can increase intestinal motility.
Provide opportunity to vent frustrations related to disease process.	Presence of disease with unknown cause that is difficult to cure and that may require surgical intervention can lead to stress reactions that may aggravate condition.
Observe for fever, tachycardia, lethargy, leukocytosis, decreased serum protein, anxiety, and prostration.	May signify that toxic megacolon or perforation and peritonitis are imminent/have occurred necessitating immediate medical intervention.

Collaborative

Administer medications as indicated:

Anticholinergics, e.g., tincture of belladonna, atropine, diphenoxylate (Lomotil); anodyne suppositories;	Decreases GI motility/propulsion (peristalsis) and diminishes digestive secretions to relieve cramping and diarrhea. *Note:* Use with caution in UC as they may precipitate toxic megacolon.
Sulfasalazine (Azulfidine);	Useful in treating mild/moderate exacerbations. Long-term use may prolong remission. *Note:* Enteric-coated form is preferred.

ACTIONS/INTERVENTIONS	RATIONALE
Collaborative	
Loperamide (Imodium); codeine;	May be required for intense/severe diarrhea. *Note:* Used with caution because toxic dilation may occur.
Mesalamine (Rowasa);	May be given as an enema in place of Azulfidine for patients who are sensitive to sulfa drugs.
Psyllium (Metamucil);	Absorbs water to increase bulk in stools, thereby decreasing diarrhea.
Cholestyramine (Questran);	Binds bile salts, reducing diarrhea that results from excess bile acid.
Steroids, e.g., ACTH, hydrocortisone, prednisolone (Delta-Cortef); prednisone (Deltasone);	Given to decrease inflammatory process. *Note:* Contraindicated in Crohn's disease if intra-abdominal abscesses are suspected.
Azathioprine (Imuran);	Immunosuppressant may be given to block inflammatory response, decrease steroid requirements, promote healing of fistulas. May be given in conjunction with sulfasalazine.
Antacids;	Decreases gastric irritation, preventing inflammation and reducing risk of infection in colitis.
Enema (hydrocortisone), with/without suppository;	Steroid enemas may be given in mild/moderate disease to aid absorption of the drug. May be given with atropine sulfate or belladonna suppository).
Antibiotics.	Treats local suppurative infections.
Assist with/prepare for surgical intervention.	May be necessary if perforation or bowel obstruction occurs or disease is unresponsive to medical treatment.

NURSING DIAGNOSIS:	FLUID VOLUME DEFICIT, HIGH RISK FOR
Risk factors may include:	Excessive losses through normal routes (severe frequent diarrhea, vomiting).
	Hypermetabolic state (inflammation, fever).
	Restricted intake (nausea).
Possibly evidenced by:	[Not applicable; presence of signs and symptoms establishes an actual diagnosis.]
DESIRED OUTCOMES/ EVALUATION CRITERIA— PATIENT WILL:	Maintain adequate fluid volume as evidenced by moist mucous membranes, good skin turgor, and capillary refill; stable vital signs; balanced I&O with urine of normal concentration/amount.

ACTIONS/INTERVENTIONS	RATIONALE
Independent	
Monitor I&O. Note number, character, and amount of stools; estimate insensible fluid losses, e.g., diaphoresis. Measure urine specific gravity; observe for oliguria.	Provides information about overall fluid balance, renal function, and bowel disease control, as well as guidelines for fluid replacement.
Assess vital signs (BP, pulse, temperature).	Hypotension (including postural), tachycardia, fever can indicate response to and/or effect of fluid loss.
Observe for excessively dry skin and mucous membranes, decreased skin turgor, slowed capillary refill.	Indicates excessive fluid loss/resultant dehydration.
Weigh daily.	Indicator of overall fluid and nutritional status.
Maintain oral restrictions, bed rest; avoid exertion.	Colon is placed at rest for healing and to decrease intestinal fluid losses.
Observe for overt bleeding and test stool daily for occult blood.	Inadequate diet and decreased absorption may lead to vitamin K deficiency and defects in coagulation, potentiating risk of hemorrhage.
Note generalized muscle weakness or cardiac dysrhythmias.	Excessive intestinal loss may lead to electrolyte imbalance, e.g., potassium, which is necessary for proper skeletal and cardiac muscle function. Minor alterations in serum levels can result in profound and/or life-threatening symptoms.
Collaborative	
Administer parenteral fluids, blood transfusions as indicated.	Maintenance of bowel rest will require alternate fluid replacement to correct losses/anemia. *Note:* Fluids containing sodium may be restricted in presence of regional enteritis.
Monitor laboratory studies, e.g., electrolytes (especially potassium, magnesium) and ABGs (acid-base balance).	Determines replacement needs and effectiveness of therapy.
Administer medications as indicated:	
Antidiarrheal (Refer to ND: Diarrhea, p 475.);	Reduces fluid losses from intestines.
Antiemetics, e.g., trimethobenzamide (Tigan); hydroxyzine (Vistaril); prochlorperazine (Compazine);	Used to control nausea/vomiting in acute exacerbations.
Antipyretics, e.g., acetaminophen (Tylenol);	Controls fever, reducing insensible losses.
Electrolytes, e.g., potassium supplement (KCl-IV; K-lyte, Slow-K);	Electrolytes are lost in large amounts, especially in pbowel with denuded, ulcerated areas, and diarrhea can also lead to metabolic acidosis through loss of bicarbonate (HCO_3).
Vitamin K (Mephyton).	Stimulates hepatic formation of prothrombin, stabilizing coagulation and reducing risk of hemorrhage.

NURSING DIAGNOSIS:	NUTRITION, ALTERED: LESS THAN BODY REQUIREMENTS
May be related to:	Altered absorption of nutrients. Hypermetabolic state. Medically restricted intake; fear that eating may cause diarrhea.
Possibly evidenced by:	Weight loss; decreased subcutaneous fat/muscle mass; poor muscle tone. Hyperactive bowel sounds; steatorrhea. Pale conjunctiva and mucous membranes. Aversion to eating.
DESIRED OUTCOMES/ EVALUATION CRITERIA— PATIENT WILL:	Demonstrate stable weight or progressive gain toward goal with normalization of laboratory values and absence of signs of malnutrition.

ACTIONS/INTERVENTIONS	RATIONALE
Independent	
Weigh daily.	Provides information about dietary needs/effectiveness of therapy.
Encourage bed rest and/or limited activity during acute phase of illness.	Decreasing metabolic needs aids in preventing caloric depletion and conserves energy.
Recommend rest before meals.	Quiets peristalsis and increases available energy for eating.
Provide oral hygiene.	A clean mouth can enhance the taste of food.
Serve foods in well-ventilated, pleasant surroundings, with unhurried atmosphere, congenial company.	Pleasant environment aids in reducing stress and is more conducive to eating.
Limit foods that might cause abdominal cramping, flatulence (e.g., milk products).	Prevents acute attack/exacerbation of symptoms.
Record intake and changes in symptomatology.	Useful in identifying specific deficiencies and determining GI response to foods.
Promote patient participation in dietary planning as possible.	Provides sense of control for patient and opportunity to select food desired/enjoyed, which may increase intake.
Encourage patient to verbalize feelings concerning resumption of diet.	Hesitation to eat may be result of fear that food will cause exacerbation of symptoms.
Collaborative	
Keep patient NPO as indicated.	Resting the bowel decreases peristalsis and diarrhea, which causes malabsorption/loss of nutrients.

479

ACTIONS/INTERVENTIONS	RATIONALE
Collaborative	
Resume/advance diet as indicated, e.g., clear liquids progressing to bland, low residue; then high-protein, high-calorie, and low-fiber as indicated.	Allows the intestinal tract to readjust to the digestive process. Protein is necessary for tissue healing integrity. Low bulk decreases peristaltic response to meal.
Administer medications as indicated, e.g.:	
Donnatal, barbital sodium with belladonna (Butibel); propanthelene bromide (ProBanthine);	Anticholinergics given 15–30 minutes prior to eating provide relief from cramping pain and diarrhea, decreasing gastric motility and enhancing time for absorption of nutrients.
Iron (Imferon injectable);	Prevents/treats anemia. Oral route for iron supplement is ineffective because of intestinal alterations that severely reduce absorption.
Vitamin B$_{12}$ (Crystimin, Rubisol);	Malabsorption of B$_{12}$ is a result of marked loss of functional ileum. Replacement reverses bone marrow depression caused by prolonged inflammatory process, promoting RBC production/correction of anemia.
Folic acid (Folvite);	Folate deficiency is common in presence of Crohn's disease due to decrease intake/absorption, effect of drug therapy (Azulfidine).
Vitamin C (Ascorbicap).	Promotes tissue healing/regeneration.
Provide TPN, IV therapy as indicated.	This regimen rests the GI tract while providing essential nutrients.

NURSING DIAGNOSIS:	ANXIETY [SPECIFY LEVEL]
May be related to:	Physiologic factors/sympathetic stimulation (inflammatory process).
	Threat to self-concept (perceived or actual).
	Threat to/change in health status, socioeconomic status, role functioning, interaction patterns.
Possibly evidenced by:	Exacerbation of acute stage of disease.
	Increased tension, distress, apprehension.
	Expressed concern regarding changes in life.
	Somatic complaints.
	Focus on self.
DESIRED OUTCOMES/ EVALUATION CRITERIA— PATIENT WILL:	Appear relaxed and report anxiety reduced to a manageable level.
	Verbalize awareness of feelings of anxiety and healthy ways to deal with them.

ACTIONS/INTERVENTIONS	RATIONALE

Independent

Note behavioral clues, e.g., restlessness, irritability, withdrawal, lack of eye contact, demanding behavior.

Indicators of degree of anxiety/stress, e.g., patient may feel out of control at home, work/personal problems. Stress may develop as a result of physical symptoms of condition, as well as reaction of others.

Encourage verbalization of feelings. Provide feedback.

Establishes a therapeutic relationship. Assists the patient/SO in identifying problems causing stress. Patient with severe diarrhea may hesitate to ask for help for fear of becoming a burden to the staff.

Acknowledge that the anxiety and problems are similar to those expressed by others. Active-listen patient's concerns.

Validation that feelings are normal can help to reduce stress/isolation and belief that "I am the only one."

Provide accurate, concrete information about what is being done, e.g., reason for bed rest, restriction of oral intake, and procedures.

Involving patient in plan of care provides sense of control and helps to decrease anxiety.

Provide a calm, restful environment.

Removing patient from outside stressors promotes relaxation; helps to reduce anxiety.

Encourage staff/SO to project caring, concerned attitude.

A supportive manner can help the patient feel less stressed, allowing energy to be directed toward healing/recovery.

Help patient to identify/initiate positive coping behaviors used in the past.

Successful behaviors can be fostered in dealing with current problems/stress, enhancing patient's sense of self-control.

Assist patient to learn new coping mechanisms, e.g., stress management techniques, organizational skills.

Learning new ways to cope can be helpful in reducing stress and anxiety, enhancing disease control.

Collaborative

Administer medications as indicated:

    Sedatives, e.g., barbiturates (Luminal); antianxiety agents, e.g., diazepam (Valium).

May be used to reduce anxiety and to facilitate rest, particularly in the patient with UC.

Refer to clinical specialist psychiatric nurse, social services, spiritual advisor.

May require additional assistance to regain control and cope with acute episodes/exacerbation as well as learning to deal with the chronicity and consequences of the disease and therapeutic regimen.

NURSING DIAGNOSIS:	**PAIN [ACUTE]**
May be related to:	Hyperperistalsis, prolonged diarrhea, skin/tissue irritation, perirectal excoriation, fissures; fistulas.
Possibly evidenced by:	Reports of colicky/cramping abdominal pain/referred pain.
	Guarding/distraction behaviors, restlessness.

	Facial mask of pain.
	Self-focusing.
DESIRED OUTCOMES/ EVALUATION CRITERIA— PATIENT WILL:	Report pain is relieved/controlled.
	Appear relaxed and able to sleep/rest appropriately.

ACTIONS/INTERVENTIONS	RATIONALE
Independent	
Encourage patient to report pain.	May try to tolerate pain, rather than request analgesics.
Assess reports of abdominal cramping or pain, noting location, duration, intensity (0–10 scale). Investigate and report changes in pain characteristics.	Colicky intermittent pain occurs with Crohn's. Predefecation pain frequently occurs in UC with urgency, which may be severe and continuous. Changes in pain characteristics may indicate spread of disease/developing complications, e.g., bladder fistula, perforation, toxic megacolon.
Note nonverbal clues, e.g., restlessness, reluctance to move, abdominal guarding, withdrawal, and depression. Investigate discrepancies between verbal and nonverbal clues.	Body language/nonverbal clues may be both physiologic and psychologic and may be used in conjunction with verbal cues to identify extent/ severity of the problem.
Review factors that aggravate or alleviate pain.	May pinpoint precipitating or aggravating factors (such as stressful events, food intolerance) or identify developing complications.
Permit patient to assume position of comfort, e.g., knees flexed.	Reduces abdominal tension and promotes sense of control.
Provide comfort measures (e.g., back rub, reposition) and diversional activities.	Promotes relaxation, refocuses attention, and may enhance coping abilities.
Cleanse rectal area with mild soap and water/ wipes after each stool and provide skin care, e.g., A&D ointment, Sween ointment, karaya gel, Desitin, petroleum jelly.	Protects skin from bowel acids, preventing excoriation.
Provide sitz bath as appropriate.	Enhances cleanliness and comfort in the presence of perianal irritation/fissures.
Observe for ischiorectal and perianal fistulas.	Fistulas may develop from erosion and weakening of intestinal bowel wall.
Observe/record abdominal distention, increased temperature, decreased BP.	May indicate developing intestinal obstruction from inflammation, edema, and scarring.
Collaborative	
Implement prescribed dietary modifications, e.g., commence with liquids and increase to solid foods as tolerated.	Complete bowel rest can reduce pain, cramping.
Administer medications as indicated:	
Analgesics;	Pain varies from mild to severe and necessitates management to facilitate adequate rest and recovery. *Note:* Opiates should be used with caution, because they may precipitate toxic megacolon.

ACTIONS/INTERVENTIONS	RATIONALE
Collaborative	
Anticholinergics;	Relieves spasms of GI tract and resultant colicky pain.
Anodyne suppositories.	Relaxes rectal muscle, decreasing painful spasms.
Assist with sitz bath as indicated.	Provides local soothing and comfort to irritated rectal area.

NURSING DIAGNOSIS:	COPING, INEFFECTIVE INDIVIDUAL
May be related to:	Multiple stressors, repeated over period of time.
	Unpredictable nature of disease process.
	Personal vulnerability.
	Severe pain.
	Lack of sleep, rest.
	Situational crisis.
	Inadequate coping method; lack of support systems.
Possibly evidenced by:	Verbalization of inability to cope, discouragement, anxiety.
	Preoccupation with physical self, chronic worry, emotional tension, poor self-esteem.
	Depression and dependency.
DESIRED OUTCOMES/ EVALUATION CRITERIA— PATIENT WILL:	Assess the current situation accurately.
	Identify ineffective coping behaviors and consequences.
	Acknowledge own coping abilities.
	Demonstrate necessary lifestyle changes to limit/prevent recurrent episodes.

ACTIONS/INTERVENTIONS	RATIONALE
Independent	
Assess patient/SO understanding and previous methods of dealing with disease process.	Enables the nurse to deal more realistically with current problems. Anxiety and other problems may have interfered with previous health teaching/patient learning.
Determine outside stresses, e.g., family, relationships, social or work environment.	Stress can alter autonomic nervous response and contribute to exacerbation of disease. Even the goal of independence in the dependent patient can be an added stressor.
Provide opportunity for patient to discuss how illness has affected relationship, including sexual concerns.	Stressors of illness affect all areas of life and patient may have difficulty coping with feelings of fatigue/pain in relation to relationship/sexual needs.

483

ACTIONS/INTERVENTIONS	RATIONALE
Independent	
Help patient identify individually effective coping skills.	Use of previously successful behaviors can help patient deal with current situation/plan for future.
Provide emotional support:	
Active-listen in a nonjudgmental manner;	Aids in communication and understanding the patient's view-point. Adds to patient's feelings of self-worth.
Maintain nonjudgmental body language when caring for patient;	Prevents reinforcing patient's feelings of being a burden, e.g., frequent need to empty bedpan.
Assign same staff as much as possible.	Provides a more therapeutic environment and lessens the stress of constant adjustments.
Provide uninterrupted sleep/rest periods.	Exhaustion brought on by the disease tends to magnify problems, interfering with ability to cope.
Encourage use of stress management skills, e.g., relaxation techniques, visualization, guided imagery, deep-breathing exercises.	Refocuses attention, promotes relaxation, and enhances coping abilities.
Collaborative	
Include patient/SO in team conferences to develop individualized program.	Promotes continuity of care and enables patient/SO to feel a part of the plan, giving them a sense of control and increasing cooperation with therapeutic regimen.
Administer medications as indicated: antipsychotics, e.g., thioridazine (Mellaril); antianxiety agents, e.g., lorazepam (Ativan); alprazolam (Xanax).	Aids in psychologic/physical rest. Conserves energy and may strengthen coping abilities.
Refer to resources as indicated, e.g., social worker, psychiatric nurse, spiritual advisor.	Additional support and counseling can assist patient/SO in dealing with specific stress/problem areas.

NURSING DIAGNOSIS:	**KNOWLEDGE DEFICIT [LEARNING NEED] REGARDING CONDITION, PROGNOSIS, AND TREATMENT NEEDS**
May be related to:	Information misinterpretation, lack of recall.
	Unfamiliarity with resources.
Possibly evidenced by:	Questions, request for information, statements of misconceptions.
	Inaccurate follow-through of instructions.
	Development of preventable complications/exacerbations.
DESIRED OUTCOMES/ EVALUATION CRITERIA— PATIENT WILL:	Verbalize understanding of disease processes, treatment.
	Identify stress situations and specific action(s) to deal with them.
	Participate in treatment regimen.
	Initiate necessary lifestyle changes.

ACTIONS/INTERVENTIONS	RATIONALE

Independent

Determine patient's perception of disease process.

Establishes knowledge base and provides some insight into individual learning needs.

Review disease process, cause/effect relationship of factors that precipitate symptoms and identify ways to reduce contributing factors. Encourage questions.

Precipitating/aggravating factors are individual; therefore, the patient needs to be aware of what foods, fluids, and lifestyle factors can precipitate symptoms. Accurate knowledge base provides opportunity for patient to make informed decisions/choices about future and control of chronic disease. Although most patients know about their own disease process, they may have outdated information or misconceptions.

Review medications, purpose, frequency, dosage, and possible side effects.

Promotes understanding and may enhance cooperation with regimen.

Remind patient to observe for side effects if steroids are given on a long-term basis, e.g., ulcers, facial edema, muscle weakness.

Steroids may be used to control inflammation and to effect a remission of the disease; however, drug may lower resistance to infection and cause fluid retention.

Stress importance of skin care, e.g., good hand-washing techniques and perineal skin care.

Reduces spread of bacteria and risk of skin irritation/breakdown, infection.

Recommend cessation of smoking.

Can increase intestinal motility, aggravating symptoms.

Emphasize need for long-term follow-up and periodic reevaluation.

Patients with inflammatory bowel disease are at increased risk for colon/rectal cancer, and regular diagnostic evaluations may be required.

Refer to appropriate community resources, e.g., Public Health Nurse, Ostomy Association, dietitian, support groups, and social services.

Patient may benefit from the services of these agencies in coping with chronicity of the disease and evaluating treatment options.

Fecal Diversions: Postoperative Care of Ileostomy and Colostomy

An ileostomy is an opening in the ileum for the purpose of treating regional and ulcerative colitis and diverting intestinal contents in colon cancer, polyps, and trauma. It is usually permanent.

A colostomy is a diversion of the effluent of the colon, which may be temporary or permanent. Ascending, transverse, and sigmoid colostomies may be performed. Transverse colostomy is usually temporary. A sigmoid colostomy is the most common permanent stoma, usually performed for cancer.

RELATED CONCERNS:

Cancer, p 1014
Fluid and Electrolyte Imbalances, p 1054
Inflammatory Bowel Disease, p 471
Intestinal Surgery, p 500
Psychosocial Aspects of Acute Care, p 899
Surgical Interventions, p 918
Total Nutritional Support, p 1039

PATIENT ASSESSMENT DATA BASE

The data are dependent on the underlying problem, duration, and severity (e.g., obstruction, perforation, inflammation, congenital defects).

TEACHING/LEARNING

Discharge Plan Considerations:	**DRG projected mean length of stay: 9.4 days.** Assistance with dietary concerns, management of ostomy, and acquisition of supplies may be required.

NURSING PRIORITIES

1. Assist patient/SO in psychosocial adjustment.
2. Prevent complications.
3. Support independence in self-care.
4. Provide information about procedure/prognosis, treatment needs, potential complications, and community resources.

DISCHARGE GOALS

1. Adjusting to perceived/actual changes.
2. Complications prevented/minimized.
3. Self-care needs met by self/with assistance dependent on specific situation.
4. Procedure/prognosis, therapeutic regimen, potential complications understood and sources of support identified.

NURSING DIAGNOSIS:	SKIN INTEGRITY, IMPAIRED, HIGH RISK FOR
Risk factors may include:	Absence of sphincter at stoma.
	Character/flow of effluent and flatus from stoma.

	Reaction to product/chemicals; improper fitting of appliance or removal of adhesive.
Possibly evidenced by:	[Not applicable; presence of signs and symptoms establishes an actual diagnosis.]
DESIRED OUTCOMES/ EVALUATION CRITERIA— PATIENT WILL:	Maintain skin integrity. Identify individual risk factors. Demonstrate behaviors/techniques to promote healing/ prevent skin breakdown.

ACTIONS/INTERVENTIONS	RATIONALE
Independent	
Inspect stoma/peristomal skin area with each pouch change. Clean with water and pat dry. Note irritation, bruises (dark, bluish color), rashes.	Monitors healing process/effectiveness of appliances and identifies areas of concern, need for further evaluation/intervention. Maintaining a clean/ dry area helps to prevent skin breakdown. Early identification of stomal necrosis/ischemia or fungal infection (from changes in normal bowel flora) provides for timely interventions to prevent serious complications. Stoma should be red and moist. Ulcerated areas on stoma may be from a pouch opening that is too small or a faceplate that cuts into stoma. In patients with an ileostomy, the effluent is rich in enzymes, increasing the likelihood of skin irritation. In the patient with a colostomy, skin care is not as great a concern, since the enzymes are no longer present in the effluent.
Measure stoma periodically, e.g., each appliance change for first 6 weeks, then once a month for 6 months.	As postoperative edema resolves (during first 6 weeks) size of appliance must be altered to ensure proper fit so that effluent is collected as it flows from the ostomy and contact with the skin is prevented.
Verify that opening on adhesive backing of pouch is at least 1/8 in larger than the base of the stoma with adequate adhesiveness left to apply pouch.	Prevents trauma to the stoma tissue and protects the peristomal skin. Adequate adhesive area is important to maintain a seal. *Note:* Too tight a fit may cause stomal edema or stenosis.
Use a transparent, odor-proof drainable pouch.	A transparent appliance during first 4–6 weeks allows easy observation of stoma without necessity of removing pouch/irritating skin.
Apply effective skin barrier, e.g., stomahesive wafer, karaya gum, Reliaseal (Davol), or similar products.	Protects skin from pouch adhesive, enhances adhesiveness of pouch, and facilitates removal of pouch when necessary. *Note:* Sigmoid colostomy may not require use of a skin barrier once stool becomes formed and elimination is regulated through irrigation.
Empty, irrigate, and cleanse ostomy pouch on a routine basis, using appropriate equipment.	Frequent pouch changes are irritating to the skin and should be avoided. Emptying and rinsing the

ACTIONS/INTERVENTIONS	RATIONALE

Independent

pouch with the proper solution not only removes bacteria and odor-causing stool and flatus but also deodorizes the pouch.

Support surrounding skin when gently removing appliance. Apply adhesive removers as indicated, then wash thoroughly.

Prevents tissue irritation/destruction associated with "pulling" pouch off.

Investigate reports of burning/itching/blistering around stoma.

Indicative of effluent leakage with peristomal irritation, or possibly candida infection, requiring intervention.

Evaluate adhesive product and appliance fit on ongoing basis.

Provides opportunity for problem solving. Determines need for further intervention.

Collaborative

Consult with enterostomal therapist/nurse.

Helpful in choosing products appropriate for patient's particular rehabilitation needs, including type of ostomy, physical/mental status, and financial resources.

Apply corticosteroid aerosol spray and nystatin powder as indicated.

Assists in healing if peristomal irritation persists/fungal infection develops. *Note:* These products can have potent side effects and should be used sparingly.

NURSING DIAGNOSIS:	**BODY IMAGE, DISTURBANCE**
May be related to:	Biophysical: presence of stoma; loss of control of bowel elimination.
	Psychosocial: altered body structure.
	Disease process and associated treatment regimen, e.g., cancer, colitis.
Possibly evidenced by:	Verbalization of change in body image, fear of rejection/reaction of others, and negative feelings about body.
	Actual change in structure and/or function (ostomy).
	Not touching/looking at stoma, refusal to participate in care.
DESIRED OUTCOMES/ EVALUATION CRITERIA— PATIENT WILL:	Verbalize acceptance of self in situation, incorporating change into self-concept without negating self-esteem.
	Demonstrate beginning acceptance by viewing/touching stoma and participating in self-care.
	Verbalize feelings about stoma/illness; begin to deal constructively with situation.

ACTIONS/INTERVENTIONS	RATIONALE

Independent

Ascertain whether counseling was initiated when the possibility and/or necessity of ostomy was first discussed.

Provides information about patient's/SO's level of knowledge about individual situation and process of acceptance.

Encourage patient/SO to verbalize feelings regarding the ostomy. Acknowledge normality of feelings of anger, depression, and grief over loss. Discuss daily "ups and downs" that can occur.

Helps the patient to realize that feelings are not unusual and that feeling guilty about them is not necessary/helpful. Patient needs to recognize feelings before they can be dealt with effectively.

Review reason for surgery and future expectations.

Patient may find it easier to accept/deal with an ostomy done to correct chronic/long-term disease than for traumatic injury, even if ostomy is only temporary. Also, the patient who will be undergoing a second procedure (to convert ostomy to a continent or anal reservoir) may possibly encounter lesser degree of self-image problems because body function eventually will be "more normal".

Note behaviors of withdrawal, increased dependency, manipulation, or noninvolvement in care.

Suggestive of problems in adjustment that may require further evaluation and more extensive therapy.

Provide opportunities for patient/SO to view and touch stoma, using the moment to point out positive signs of healing, normal appearance, and so forth. Remind patient that it will take time to adjust, both physically and emotionally.

Although integration of stoma into body image can take months or even years, looking at the stoma and hearing comments (made in a normal, matter-of-fact manner) can help patient with this acceptance. Touching stoma reassures patient/SO that it is not fragile and that slight movements of stoma actually reflect normal peristalsis.

Provide opportunity for patient to deal with ostomy through participation in self-care.

Independence in self-care helps to improve self-confidence and acceptance of situation.

Plan/schedule care activities with patient.

Promotes sense of control and gives message that patient can handle this, enhancing self-esteem.

Maintain positive approach during care activities, avoiding expressions of disdain or revulsion. Do not take angry expressions personally.

Assists patient/SO to accept body changes and feel all right about self. Anger is most often directed at the situation and lack of control individual has over what has happened (powerlessness), not with the individual caregiver.

Discuss possibility of contacting ostomy visitor, and make arrangements for visit if desired.

Can provide a good support system. Helps to reinforce teaching (shared experiences) and facilitates acceptance of change as patient realizes "life does go on" and can be relatively normal.

NURSING DIAGNOSIS:	PAIN [ACUTE]
May be related to:	Physical factors: e.g., disruption of skin/tissues (incisions/drains).

	Biologic: activity of disease process (cancer, trauma).
	Psychologic factors: e.g., fear, anxiety.
Possibly evidenced by:	Reports of pain, self-focusing.
	Guarding/distraction behaviors, restlessness.
	Autonomic responses, e.g., changes in vital signs.
DESIRED OUTCOMES/ EVALUATION CRITERIA— PATIENT WILL:	Verbalize pain is relieved/controlled.
	Display relief of pain, able to sleep/rest appropriately.
	Demonstrate use of relaxation skills and general comfort measures as indicated for individual situation.

ACTIONS/INTERVENTIONS	RATIONALE

Independent

Assess pain, noting location, characteristics, intensity (0–10 scale).	Helps evaluate degree of discomfort and effectiveness of analgesia or may reveal developing complications; e.g., because abdominal pain usually subsides gradually by the 3rd or 4th postoperative day, continued or increasing pain may reflect delayed healing or peristomal skin irritation. *Note:* Pain in anal area associated with abdominal-perineal resection may persist for months.
Encourage patient to verbalize concerns. Active-listen these concerns, and provide support by acceptance, remaining with patient, and giving appropriate information.	Reduction of anxiety/fear can promote relaxation/comfort.
Provide comfort measures, e.g., mouth care, back rub, repositioning (use proper support measures as needed). Assure patient that position change will not injure stoma.	Prevents drying of oral mucosa and associated discomfort. Reduces muscle tension, promotes relaxation, and may enhance coping abilities.
Encourage use of relaxation techniques, e.g., guided imagery, visualization. Provide diversional activities.	Helps patient to rest more effectively and refocuses attention, thereby reducing pain and discomfort.
Assist with ROM exercises and encourage early ambulation. Avoid prolonged sitting position.	Reduces muscle/joint stiffness. Ambulation returns organs to normal position and promotes return of usual level of functioning. *Note:* Presence of edema, packing, and drains (if perineal resection has been done) increases discomfort and creates a sense of needing to defecate. Ambulation and frequent position changes reduce perineal pressure.
Investigate and report abdominal muscle rigidity, involuntary guarding, and rebound tenderness.	Suggestive of peritoneal inflammation, which requires prompt medical intervention.

Collaborative

Administer medication as indicated, e.g., narcotics, analgesics, PCA.	Relieves pain, enhances comfort, and promotes rest. PCA may be more beneficial, especially following AP repair.

ACTIONS/INTERVENTIONS	RATIONALE

Collaborative

Provide sitz baths.

Relieves local discomfort, reduces edema, and promotes healing of perineal wound.

Apply/monitor effects of TENS unit.

Cutaneous stimulation may be used to block transmission of pain stimulus

---

NURSING DIAGNOSIS:	SKIN/TISSUE INTEGRITY, IMPAIRED: ACTUAL
May be related to:	Invasion of body structure (perineal resection).
	Stasis of secretions/drainage.
	Altered circulation, edema; malnutrition.
Possibly evidenced by:	Disruption of skin/tissue: presence of incision, and sutures, drains.
DESIRED OUTCOMES/ EVALUATION CRITERIA— PATIENT WILL:	Achieve timely wound healing free of signs of infection.

ACTIONS/INTERVENTIONS	RATIONALE

Independent

Observe wounds, note characteristics of drainage.

Postoperative hemorrhage is most likely to occur during first 48 hours, whereas infection may develop at any time. Dependent on type of wound closure (e.g., first or second intention), complete healing may take 6–8 months.

Change dressings as needed using aseptic technique.

Large amounts of serous drainage require that dressings be changed frequently to reduce skin irritation and potential for infection.

Encourage sidelying position with head elevated. Avoid prolonged sitting.

Promotes drainage from perineal wound/drains reducing risk of pooling. Prolonged sitting increases perineal pressure, reducing circulation to wound, and may delay healing.

Collaborative

Irrigate wound as indicated, using normal saline, diluted hydrogen peroxide, or antibiotic solution.

May be required to treat preoperative inflammation/infection or intraoperative contamination.

Provide sitz baths.

Promotes cleanliness and facilitates healing especially after packing is removed (usually day 3–5).

NURSING DIAGNOSIS:	FLUID VOLUME DEFICIT, HIGH RISK FOR
Risk factors may include:	Excessive losses through normal routes, e.g., preoperative emesis and diarrhea.

	Losses through abnormal routes, e.g., NG/intestinal tube, perineal wound drainage tubes.
	High volume ileostomy output.
	Medically restricted intake.
	Altered absorption of fluid, e.g., loss of colon function.
	Hypermetabolic states, e.g., inflammation, healing process.
Possibly evidenced by:	[Not applicable; presence of signs and symptoms establishes an actual diagnosis.]
DESIRED OUTCOMES/ EVALUATION CRITERIA— PATIENT WILL:	Maintain adequate hydration as evidenced by moist mucous membranes, good skin turgor and capillary refill, stable vital signs, and individually appropriate urinary output.

ACTIONS/INTERVENTIONS	RATIONALE
Independent	
Monitor I&O carefully, measure liquid stool. Weigh regularly.	Provides direct indicators of fluid balance. Greatest fluid losses occur with ileostomy, but they generally do not exceed 500–800 ml/d.
Monitor vital signs noting postural hypotension, tachycardia. Evaluate skin turgor, capillary refill, and mucous membranes.	Reflects hydration status/possible need for increased fluid replacement.
Limit intake of ice chips during period of gastric intubation.	Ice chips can stimulate gastric secretions and wash out electrolytes.
Collaborative	
Monitor laboratory results, e.g., Hct and electrolytes.	Detects homeostasis or imbalance and aids in determining replacement needs.
Administer IV fluid and electrolytes as indicated.	May be necessary to maintain adequate tissue perfusion/organ function.

NURSING DIAGNOSIS:	**NUTRITION, ALTERED: LESS THAN BODY REQUIREMENTS, HIGH RISK FOR**
Risk factors may include:	Prolonged anorexia/altered intake preoperatively.
	Hypermetabolic state (preoperative inflammatory disease; healing process).
	Presence of diarrhea/altered absorption.
	Restriction of bulk and residue-containing foods.
Possibly evidenced by:	[Not applicable; presence of signs and symptoms establishes an actual diagnosis.]

DESIRED OUTCOMES/ EVALUATION CRITERIA— PATIENT WILL:	Maintain weight/demonstrate progressive weight gain toward goal with normalization of laboratory values and free of signs of malnutrition.
	Plan diet to meet nutritional needs/limit GI disturbances.

ACTIONS/INTERVENTIONS	RATIONALE
Independent	
Obtain a thorough nutritional assessment.	Identifies deficiencies/needs to aid in choice of interventions.
Auscultate bowel sounds.	Return of intestinal function indicates readiness to resume oral intake.
Resume solid foods slowly.	Reduces incidence of abdominal cramps, nausea.
Identify odor-causing foods (e.g., cabbage, fish, beans) and temporarily restrict from diet. Gradually reintroduce 1 food at a time.	Sensitivity to certain foods is not uncommon following intestinal surgery. Patient can experiment with food several times before determining whether it is creating a problem.
Recommend patient increase use of yogurt and buttermilk.	May help decrease odor formation.
Suggest patient with ileostomy exercise caution in the use of prunes, dates, stewed apricots, strawberries, grapes, bananas, cabbage family, beans, and nuts and avoid cellulose products, e.g., peanuts.	These products increase ileal effluent. Digestion of cellulose requires colon bacteria that are no longer present.
Discuss mechanics of swallowed air as a factor in the formation of flatus and some ways the patient can exercise control.	Drinking through a straw, snoring, anxiety, smoking, ill-fitting dentures, and gulping down food increase the production of flatus. Too much flatus not only necessitates frequent emptying, but can be a causative factor in leakage from too much pressure within the pouch.
Collaborative	
Consult with dietitian.	Helpful in assessing patient's nutritional needs in light of changes in digestion and intestinal function.
Advance diet from liquids to low-residue food when oral intake is resumed.	Low-residue diet may be maintained during first 6–8 weeks to provide adequate time for intestinal healing.
Administer enteral/parenteral feedings when indicated.	In the presence of severe debilitation/intolerance of oral intake, hyperalimentation may be used to supply needed components for healing and prevention of catabolic state.

NURSING DIAGNOSIS:	SLEEP PATTERN DISTURBANCE
May be related to:	External factors: necessity of ostomy care, excessive flatus/ostomy effluent.

	Internal factors: psychologic stress, fear of leakage of pouch/injury to stoma.
Possibly evidenced by:	Verbalizations of interrupted sleep, not feeling well rested.
	Changes in behavior, e.g., irritability, listlessness/lethargy.
DESIRED OUTCOMES/ EVALUATION CRITERIA— PATIENT WILL:	Sleep/rest between disturbances.
	Report increased sense of well-being and feeling rested.

ACTIONS/INTERVENTIONS	RATIONALE
Independent	
Explain necessity to monitor intestinal function in early postoperative period.	Patient is more apt to be tolerant of disturbances by staff if he or she understands the reasons for/importance of care.
Provide adequate pouching system. Empty pouch before retiring and, if necessary, on a preagreed schedule.	Excessive flatus/effluent can occur despite interventions. Emptying on a regular schedule minimizes threat of leakage.
Let patient know that stoma will not be injured when sleeping.	Patient will be able to rest better if feeling secure about stoma and ostomy.
Restrict intake of caffeine-containing foods/fluids.	Caffeine may delay patient's falling asleep and interfere with REM sleep, resulting in patient not feeling well rested.
Support continuation of usual bedtime rituals.	Promotes relaxation and readiness for sleep.
Collaborative	
Determine cause of excessive flatus or effluent, e.g., confer with dietitian regarding restriction of foods if diet-related.	Identification of cause enables institution of corrective measures that may promote sleep/rest.
Administer analgesics, sedatives at bedtime as indicated.	Pain can interfere with patient's ability to fall/remain asleep. Timely medication can enhance rest/sleep during initial postoperative period. *Note:* Pain pathways in the brain lie near the sleep center and may contribute to wakefulness.

NURSING DIAGNOSIS:	CONSTIPATION/DIARRHEA, HIGH RISK FOR
Risk factors may include:	Placement of ostomy in descending or sigmoid colon.
	Inadequate diet/fluid intake.
Possibly evidenced by:	[Not applicable; presence of signs and symptoms establishes an actual diagnosis.]
DESIRED OUTCOMES/ EVALUATION CRITERIA— PATIENT WILL:	Establish an elimination pattern suitable to physical needs and lifestyle with effluent of appropriate amount and consistency.

ACTIONS/INTERVENTIONS	RATIONALE
Independent	
Ascertain patient's previous bowel habits and lifestyle.	Assists in formulation of an effective irrigating schedule for the patient with a colostomy.
Investigate delayed onset/absence of effluent. Auscultate bowel sounds.	Postoperative paralytic/adynamic ileus usually resolves within 48–72 hours and ileostomy should begin draining within 12–24 hours. Delay may indicate persistent ileus or stomal obstruction, which may occur postoperatively because of edema, improperly fitting pouch (too tight), prolapse, or stenosis of the stoma.
Inform the patient with an ileostomy that initially the effluent will be liquid. If constipation occurs, it should be reported to enterostomal nurse or physician.	Although the small intestine eventually begins to take on water-absorbing functions to permit a more semisolid, pasty discharge, constipation may indicate an obstruction. Absence of stool requires emergency medical attention.
Review dietary pattern and amount/type of fluid intake.	Adequate intake of fiber and roughage provides bulk, and fluid is an important factor in determining the consistency of the stool.
Review physiology of the colon and discuss irrigation management of sigmoid ostomy, if appropriate.	This knowledge helps the patient understand individual care needs.
Demonstrate use of irrigation equipment to inject normal saline per protocol until relief is obtained.	Irrigations may be done on a daily basis or prior to special activities. There are differing views on the use of daily irrigations. Many believe cleaning the bowel on a regular basis is helpful. Others believe that this interferes with normal functioning. Most authorities agree that occasional irrigating is useful for emptying the bowel to avoid leakage when special events are planned.
Instruct patient in the use of closed-end pouch or a patch, dressing/Bandaid when irrigation is successful and the sigmoid colostomy effluent becomes more manageable, with stool expelled every 24 hours.	Enables patient to feel more comfortable socially and is less expensive than regular ostomy pouches.
Involve the patient in care of the ostomy on an increasing basis.	Rehabilitation can be facilitated by encouraging patient independence and control.
Collaborative	
Provide TENS unit if indicated.	Electrical stimulation has been used in some patients to stimulate peristalsis and relieve postoperative ileus.

NURSING DIAGNOSIS:	**SEXUAL DYSFUNCTION, HIGH RISK FOR**
Risk factors may include:	Altered body structure/function; radical resection/treatment procedures.
	Vulnerability/psychologic concern about response of SO.

495

	Disruption of sexual response pattern, e.g., erectile difficulty.
Possibly evidenced by:	[Not applicable; presence of signs and symptoms establishes an actual diagnosis.]
DESIRED OUTCOMES/ EVALUATION CRITERIA— PATIENT WILL:	Verbalize understanding of relationship of physical condition to sexual problems.
	Identify satisfying/acceptable sexual practices and explore alternate methods.
	Resume sexual relationship as appropriate.

ACTIONS/INTERVENTIONS	RATIONALE

Independent

Determine the patient/SO sexual relationship prior to the disease and/or surgery and whether they anticipate problems related to presence of ostomy.	Identify future expectations and desires. Mutilation and loss of privacy/control of a bodily function can affect patient's view of personal sexuality. When coupled with the fear of rejection by SO, the desired level of intimacy can be greatly impaired. Sexual needs are very basic, and the patient will be rehabilitated more successfully when a satisfying sexual relationship is continued/developed.
Review with the patient/SO sexual functioning in relation to own situation.	Understanding if nerve damage has altered normal sexual functioning (e.g., erection) helps patient/SO to understand the need for exploring alternate methods of satisfaction.
Reinforce information given by the physician. Encourage questions. Provide additional information as needed.	Reiteration of data previously given assists the patient/SO to hear and process the knowledge again, moving toward acceptance of individual limitations/restrictions and prognosis (e.g., that it may take up to 2 years to regain potency after a radical procedure or that a penile prosthesis may be necessary).
Discuss resumption of sexual activity in approximately 6 weeks after discharge, beginning slowly and progressing (e.g., cuddling/caressing until both partners are comfortable with body image/function changes). Include alternate methods of stimulation as appropriate.	Knowing what to expect in progress of recovery helps patient avoid performance anxiety/reduce risk of "failure." If the couple is willing to try new ideas, this can assist with adjustment and may help to achieve sexual fulfillment.
Encourage dialogue between partners. Suggest wearing pouch cover, T-shirt, or shortie nightgown.	Disguising ostomy appliance may aid in reducing feelings of self-consciousness, embarrassment during sexual activity.
Stress awareness of factors that might be distracting (e.g., unpleasant odors and pouch leakage). Encourage use of sense of humor.	Promotes resolution of solvable problems. Laughter can help individuals to deal more effectively with difficult situation, promote positive sexual experience.
Problem-solve alternative positions for coitus.	Minimizing awkwardness of appliance and physical discomfort can enhance satisfaction.

ACTIONS/INTERVENTIONS

Independent

Discuss/role-play possible interactions or approaches when dealing with new sexual partners.

Provide birth control information as appropriate and stress that impotence does not mean the patient is sterile.

Collaborative

Arrange meeting with an ostomy visitor if appropriate.

Refer to counseling/sex therapy as indicated.

RATIONALE

Rehearsal is helpful in dealing with actual situations when they arise, preventing self-consciousness about "different" body image.

Confusion may exist that can lead to an unwanted pregnancy.

Sharing of how these problems have been resolved by others can be helpful and reduce sense of isolation.

If problems persist longer than several months after surgery, a trained therapist may be required to facilitate communication between patient and SO.

NURSING DIAGNOSIS:	KNOWLEDGE DEFICIT [LEARNING NEED], REGARDING CONDITION, PROGNOSIS, AND TREATMENT NEEDS
May be related to:	Lack of exposure; information misinterpretation; lack of recall. Unfamiliarity with information resources.
Possibly evidenced by:	Questions; statement of misconception/misinformation. Inaccurate follow-through of instruction/performance of ostomy care. Inappropriate or exaggerated behaviors (e.g., hostile, agitated, apathetic, withdrawal).
DESIRED OUTCOMES/ EVALUATION CRITERIA— PATIENT WILL:	Verbalize understanding of condition/disease process, treatment and prognosis. Correctly perform necessary procedures, explain reasons for the action. Initiate necessary lifestyle changes.

ACTIONS/INTERVENTIONS

Independent

Evaluate patient's emotional and physical capabilities.

Review anatomy, physiology, and implications of surgical intervention. Discuss future expectations,

RATIONALE

These factors affect patient's ability to master tasks and willingness to assume responsibility for ostomy care.

Provides knowledge base on which patient can make informed choices and an opportunity to clar-

ACTIONS/INTERVENTIONS	RATIONALE

Independent

including anticipated changes in character of effluent.

ify misconceptions regarding individual situation. (Temporary ileostomy may be converted to ileoanal reservoir at a future date; ileostomy and ascending colostomy cannot be regulated by diet, irrigations, or medications, and so on.)

Include written/picture resources.

Provides references postdischarge to support patient efforts for independence in self-care.

Instruct patient/SO in stomal care. Allot time for return demonstrations and provide positive feedback for efforts.

Promotes positive management and reduces risk of improper ostomy care/development of complications.

Recommend increased fluid intake during warm weather months.

Loss of normal colon function of conserving water and electrolytes can lead to dehydration and constipation.

Discuss possible need to decrease salt intake.

Salt can increase ileal output, potentiating risk of dehydration and increasing frequency of ostomy care needs/patient's inconvenience.

Identify symptoms of electrolyte depletion, e.g., anorexia, abdominal muscle cramps, feelings of faintness or "cold" in arms/legs; general fatigue/weakness, bloating, decreased sensations in arms/legs.

Loss of colon function with altered fluid/electrolyte absorption may result in sodium/potassium deficits requiring dietary correction with foods/fluids high in sodium (e.g., bouillon, Gatorade) or potassium (e.g., orange juice, prunes, tomatoes, bananas, or Gatorade).

Stress importance of chewing food well, adequate intake of fluids with/following meals, and only moderate use of high-fiber foods; avoidance of cellulose.

Reduces risk of bowel obstruction, especially in patient with ileostomy.

Review foods that are/may be a source of flatus (e.g., carbonated drinks, beer, beans, cabbage family, onions, fish, and highly seasoned foods) or odor (e.g., onions, cabbage family, eggs, fish, and beans).

These foods may be restricted or eliminated for better ostomy control, or it may be necessary to empty the pouch more frequently if they are ingested.

Identify foods associated with diarrhea, such as green beans, broccoli, highly seasoned foods.

Promotes better bowel control.

Recommend foods used to manage constipation (e.g., bran, celery, raw fruits), as well as importance of increased fluid intake.

Proper management can prevent/minimize problems of constipation.

Discuss resumption of presurgery level of activity.

Patient should be able to manage same degree of activity as previously enjoyed and in some cases increase activity level.

Talk about the possibility of sleep disturbance, anorexia, loss of interest in usual activities.

"Homecoming depression" may occur, lasting for up to 3 months after surgery, requiring patience/support and ongoing evaluation.

Explain necessity of notifying health care providers and pharmacists of type of ostomy and avoidance of sustained-release medications.

Presence of ostomy may alter rate/extent of absorption of oral medications and increase risk of drug-related complications, e.g., diarrhea/constipation or peristomal excoriation. Liquid, chewable, or injectable forms of medication are preferred for

ACTIONS/INTERVENTIONS	RATIONALE
Independent	patients with ileostomy to maximize absorption of drug.
Counsel patient concerning medication use and problems associated with altered bowel function. Refer to pharmacist for teaching/advice as appropriate.	The patient with an ostomy has 2 key problems, i.e., altered disintegration and absorption of oral drugs and unusual or pronounced adverse effects. Some of the medications, which these patients may respond to differently, include laxatives, salicylates, H_2 receptor antagonists, antibiotics, and diuretics.
Discuss effect of medications on effluent, i.e., changes in color, odor, consistency of stool; need to observe for drug residue indicating incomplete absorption.	Understanding decreases anxiety regarding intestinal function and enhances independence in self-care.
Stress necessity of close monitoring of chronic health conditions requiring routine oral medications.	Monitoring of clinical symptoms and serum blood levels is indicated due to altered drug absorption requiring periodic dosage adjustments.
Identify community resources, e.g., United Ostomy Association, local ostomy support group, enterostomal therapist, VNA, pharmacy/medical supply house.	Continued support after discharge is essential to facilitate the recovery process and patient's independence in care. Enterostomal nurse can be very helpful in solving appliance problems, identifying alternatives to meet individual patient needs.

Intestinal Surgery without Diversion _____

Intestinal surgery may be performed for a number of different conditions, including resection of tumors, diverticuli, polyps, adhesions, regional enteritis. Treatment is concerned with removing the diseased segments when enough tissue is viable to prevent the need for ostomy construction.

RELATED CONCERNS:

Cancer, p 1014
Inflammatory Bowel Disease, p 471
Peritonitis, p 514
Psychosocial Aspects of Acute Care, p 899
Surgical Intervention, p 918
Total Nutritional Support, p 1039

PATIENT ASSESSMENT DATA BASE

The data are dependent on the underlying disease process. Refer to specific CPs where available.

Discharge Plan Considerations: **DRG projected mean length of stay: 6.4 days.**

NURSING PRIORITIES

1. Maintain adequate circulating volume.
2. Control/minimize pain.
3. Prevent complications.
4. Promote proper GI functioning.
5. Provide information about surgical procedure/prognosis, complications, and treatment needs.

DISCHARGE GOALS

1. Fluid intake adequate to maintain circulating volume.
2. Pain relieved/controlled.
3. Complications prevented/minimized.
4. GI function returned, intake adequate to meet nutritional needs.
5. Procedure/prognosis, possible complications, and therapeutic regimen understood.

NURSING DIAGNOSIS:	FLUID VOLUME DEFICIT, HIGH RISK FOR
Risk factors may include:	Excessive losses through normal routes, e.g., vomiting, diarrhea.
	Loss of fluid through abnormal routes, e.g., indwelling drains, NG/intestinal suctioning, hemorrhage.
	Insufficient replacement, fever.
Possibly evidenced by:	[Not applicable; presence of signs and symptoms establishes an actual diagnosis.]
DESIRED OUTCOMES/ EVALUATION CRITERIA— PATIENT WILL:	Maintain adequate hydration as evidenced by moist mucous membranes, good skin turgor and capillary refill, stable vital signs, and individually appropriate urinary output.

ACTIONS/INTERVENTIONS	RATIONALE

Independent

Monitor vital signs frequently, noting increased pulse, postural BP changes, tachypnea, and apprehension. Check dressings and wound frequently during first 24 hours for signs of bright blood or excessive incisional swelling.

Early signs of intestinal hemorrhage and/or hematoma formation, which may cause hypovolemic shock.

Palpate peripheral pulses. Evaluate capillary refill, skin turgor, and status of mucous membranes.

Provides information about general circulating volume and level of hydration.

Note presence of edema.

Edema may occur due to fluid shifts associated with decreased serum albumin/protein levels.

Monitor I&O (include all sources, e.g., emesis, tubes, diarrhea), noting urine output, specific gravity. Calculate 24-hour balance, and weigh daily.

Direct indicators of hydration/organ perfusion and function. Provides guidelines for fluid replacement.

Note presence of/measure abdominal distention.

Fluid shifts from the vascular space reduce circulating volume and impair renal perfusion.

Observe/record quantity, amount, and character of NG drainage. Test pH as indicated. Encourage and assist with frequent changes of position.

Excessive fluid output may cause electrolyte imbalance and metabolic alkalosis with further loss of potassium by the kidneys attempting to compensate. Hyperacidity, as indicated by a pH of less than 5, may identify patients at risk for stress ulcer formation. Repositioning prevents formation of magenstrasse in the stomach, which can channel gastric fluid and air past tip of NG tube into duodenum.

Monitor temperature.

Low-grade fever is common during the first 24–48 hours and can add to fluid losses.

Review cause for surgery and possible effects on fluid balance. Observe for complications, e.g., intestinal obstruction, paralytic ileus, and fistula formation.

Exacerbates fluid and electrolyte losses.

Do guaiac test on stool.

Microscopic/subacute bleeding may not be readily evident.

Collaborative

Maintain patency of NG/intestinal suction. Maintain low, intermittent suction, as indicated.

Promotes bowel decompression to reduce distention/pressure on suture lines and to reduce n/v, which can accompany anesthesia, manipulation of the bowel, or preexisting conditions, e.g., cancer.

Monitor laboratory studies, e.g., Hb/Hct, electrolytes, BUN/Cr.

Provides information about hydration and replacement needs and organ function.

Administer fluids, blood, albumin, electrolytes as indicated.

Maintains circulating volume and electrolyte balance.

NURSING DIAGNOSIS:	PAIN [ACUTE]
May be related to:	Physical agents, e.g., surgical incisions, abdominal distention, presence of NG/intestinal tube.

Possibly evidenced by:	Reports of pain.
	Guarding/distraction behaviors, self-focus.
	Autonomic responses, e.g., changes in BP, pulse, respirations.
DESIRED OUTCOMES/ EVALUATION CRITERIA— PATIENT WILL:	Report pain relieved/controlled.
	Appear relaxed, able to rest/sleep appropriately.

ACTIONS/INTERVENTIONS	RATIONALE
Independent	
Investigate reports of pain, noting location, intensity (0–10 scale), and aggravating/relieving factors. Note nonverbal cues, e.g., muscle guarding, shallow breathing, emotional responses.	Incisional pain can be significant in early postoperative phase, aggravated by movement, coughing, abdominal distention, nausea. Having patient rate own discomfort helps identify appropriate interventions and evaluate effectiveness of analgesia.
Encourage patient to report pain as soon as it begins.	Early intervention in pain control facilitates muscle/tissue healing by reducing muscle tension and improving circulation.
Monitor vital signs.	Autonomic responses can include changes in BP, pulse, and respirations, which should correlate with complaints/relief of pain. Continuation of abnormal vital signs requires further evaluation.
Assess surgical incisions, noting edema; changes in contour of wound (hematoma formation); or inflammation, drying of wound edges.	Bleeding into tissues, swelling, local inflammation, or development of infection can cause increased incisional pain.
Provide comfort measures, e.g., back rub; splinting incision during position changes and coughing/breathing exercises; calm, quiet environment. Encourage use of guided imagery, relaxation techniques. Provide diversional activities.	Provides support (physical, emotional); reduces muscle tension; enhances relaxation; refocuses attention; enhances sense of control and coping abilities.
Give frequent oral care, lubricate lips and nares (when NG tube is present). Tape tube so there is no pressure on the nares.	Irritation of mucous membranes causes patient to swallow more frequently and results in abdominal distention (increased ingestion of air).
Maintain patency of NG/intestinal drainage tubes, irrigating as indicated. Note presence of "gas pain," passage of flatus.	Obstruction of tubes can increase abdominal distention (retention of gas); stress internal suture lines; and greatly increase pain.
Palpate bladder for distention when voiding is delayed. Promote privacy and use nursing measures to promote relaxation when patient is attempting to void. Place in semi-Fowler's or standing position as appropriate.	Psychologic factors and pain may increase muscle tension. Upright position increases intra-abdominal pressure, which may aid in micturition.
Ambulate patient as soon as possible.	Decreases problems that occur because of immobility, e.g., muscle tension, retained flatus.
Recommend breathing through nose instead of mouth.	Reduces air swallowing and resultant distention.

ACTIONS/INTERVENTIONS

Collaborative

Administer analgesics, narcotics as indicated.

Catheterize as necessary.

RATIONALE

Controls/relieves pain to promote rest and enhance cooperation with therapeutic regimen.

Single/multiple straight catheterization or indwelling insertion may be used to empty the bladder until function returns.

NURSING DIAGNOSIS:	INFECTION, HIGH RISK FOR
Risk factors may include:	Inadequate primary defenses, e.g., chronic disease, invasive procedures, malnutrition.
	Opening of the abdominal cavity/bowel with possible contamination, stasis of body fluids, altered peristalsis.
Possibly evidenced by:	[Not applicable; presence of signs and symptoms establishes an actual diagnosis.]
DESIRED OUTCOMES/ EVALUATION CRITERIA— PATIENT WILL:	Achieve timely wound healing; be free of purulent drainage or erythema and fever.

ACTIONS/INTERVENTIONS

Independent

Monitor vital signs, noting temperature elevation.

Observe wound approximation, character of drainage, presence of inflammation.

Monitor respirations, breath sounds. Keep head of bed elevated 35–45 degrees. Assist patient to turn, cough, and deep breathe; assist with incentive spirometer, blow bottles.

Observe for signs/symptoms of peritonitis, e.g., fever, increasing pain, abdominal distention.

Maintain aseptic wound care. Keep dressings dry.

RATIONALE

Evening temperature spike that returns to normal level in the morning is characteristic of infection. Fever of 38°C (100°F) soon after surgery may indicate pulmonary/urinary/wound infection or thrombophlebitis formation. Fever 38.3°C (101°F) of sudden onset and accompanied by chills, fatigue, weakness, tachypnea, tachycardia, and hypotension indicates septic shock. Temperature elevation 4–7 days after surgery is often indicative of wound abscess or fluid leak from anastomosis site.

Development of infection can delay healing.

Pulmonary infections may occur because of respiratory depression (anesthesia, narcotics); ineffective cough (abdominal incision); and abdominal distention (decreased lung expansion).

Although bowel preparation is done before elective surgery, peritonitis can occur when intestine is interrupted, e.g., preoperative rupture; leaking anastomosis (postoperative); or when surgery is an emergency/result of an accidental wound.

Protects patient from cross-contamination during dressing changes. Wet dressings act as a retrograde wick, drawing in external contaminants.

ACTIONS/INTERVENTIONS

Collaborative

Use Montgomery straps to secure dressings, if indicated.

Culture suspicious drainage/secretions; culture both center and outer edges of wound and obtain anaerobic cultures as indicated.

Administer medications as indicated:

Antibiotics, e.g., cefazolin (Ancef).

Do wound irrigations, as needed.

RATIONALE

Frequent removal of tape (especially when drains are present) may cause skin abrasion, which can also become a site of infection.

Multiple organisms may be present in open wounds and after bowel surgery. Anaerobic bacteria, e.g., *Bacteroides fragilis*, can only be detected by anaerobic cultures. Identifying all organisms involved allows for more specific antibiotic therapy.

Given prophylactically and to combat infection.

Combats infection when present.

NURSING DIAGNOSIS:	NUTRITION, ALTERED: LESS THAN BODY REQUIREMENTS, HIGH RISK FOR
Risk factors may include:	Inability to ingest/digest food or absorb sufficient nutrients to meet metabolic demands.
	NPO status; NG/intestinal aspiration.
Possibly evidenced by:	[Not applicable; presence of signs and symptoms establishes an actual diagnosis.]
DESIRED OUTCOMES/ EVALUATION CRITERIA— PATIENT WILL:	Demonstrate maintenance of/progressive weight gain toward goal with normalization of laboratory values and no signs of malnutrition.

ACTIONS/INTERVENTIONS

Independent

Review individual factors that affect ability to ingest/digest food, e.g., NPO status, nausea, paralytic ileus after tube removal.

Weigh as indicated. Record I&O.

Auscultate for bowel sounds; palpate abdomen. Record passage of flatus.

Identify dietary likes/dislikes of patient. Encourage choice of foods high in protein and vitamin C.

Observe for development of diarrhea; "greasy," foul-smelling stools.

RATIONALE

Influences choice of interventions.

Identifies fluid status as well as ascertaining current metabolic needs.

Determines return of peristalsis (usually within 2–4 days).

Increases patient cooperation with dietary regimen. Proteins/vitamin C are prime contributors to tissue maintenance and repair. Malnutrition is a factor in lowered resistance to infection.

Malabsorption syndrome may develop after surgery of small intestine, requiring further evaluation and dietary modifications, e.g., low-fat diet.

ACTIONS/INTERVENTIONS	RATIONALE
Collaborative	
Maintain patency of NG/gastrostomy tube.	Maintains decompression of stomach/bowel; promotes bowel rest/healing.
Administer IV fluids, e.g.:	
Albumin, lipids, electrolytes;	Corrects fluid and electrolyte imbalances. Bowel inflammation, mucosal erosion, infection, or neoplasm may lead to anemia or malabsorption, reducing delivery of nutrients at the cellular level. Restricted diet, gastric/intestinal suction, preoperative bowel preparation may result in electrolyte imbalance, especially sodium and potassium. Loss of plasma; decreased serum albumin (edema, ascites formation, or effusion); and immunodeficiency can prolong wound healing.
Vitamin supplements, with particular attention to vitamin K, parenterally.	Preoperative use of cathartics (bowel preparation) may deplete vitamin supply and/or intestinal problems may have blocked absorption of vitamins. *Note:* Sterilized bowel cannot synthesize vitamin K, decreasing coagulation potential.
Administer medications as indicated:	
Antiemetics, e.g., prochlorperazine (Compazine);	Prevents vomiting.
Antacids and/or histamine inhibitors, e.g., cimetidine (Tagamet).	Neutralizes or decreases acid formation to prevent mucosal erosion and possible ulceration.
Consult with dietitan, nutritional support team. Provide enteral/parenteral TPN as indicated.	Useful in evaluating and establishing individual dietary needs. Many patients present with marked weight loss and are generally debilitated, thus are at greater risk for postoperative complications.
Give liquids, progressing to clear liquid, full diet as tolerated after NG or gastrostomy feeding tube is removed.	Resumption of fluids and diet is essential to return of normal intestinal functioning and promotes adequate nutritional intake.

NURSING DIAGNOSIS:	**SKIN/TISSUE INTEGRITY, IMPAIRED**
May be related to:	External factors: surgical incision, radiation.
	Internal factors: medication, altered nutritional state, altered circulation, immunologic deficit.
	Mechanical factors: pressure, friction.
Possibly evidenced by:	Disruption of integumentary and subcutaneous tissues.
	Invasion of body structures.
DESIRED OUTCOMES/ EVALUATION CRITERIA— PATIENT WILL:	Achieve timely wound healing without complications.

ACTIONS/INTERVENTIONS

Independent

Monitor vital signs frequently noting fever, tachypnea, tachycardia, and apprehension. Check wound frequently for excessive incisional swelling, inflammation, drainage.

Splint incision during coughing and breathing exercises. Apply binder/support for elderly and obese patients if indicated.

Use paper tape/Montgomery straps for dressings as indicated.

Be aware of further risk factors, i.e., malignancies, such as lymphosarcoma and multiple myeloma; radiation therapy of operative site.

If dehiscence occurs:

Maintain calm attitude. Stay with patient. Notify physician;

Keep patient on complete bed rest. Position with knees bent.

If evisceration occurs:

Cover exposed intestines with sterile, moist dressings. Prepare for surgical repair of wound.

Review laboratory values for anemia and decreased serum albumin. Note leukocyte count.

RATIONALE

May be indicative of hematoma formation/developing infection, which contributes to delayed wound healing and increases risk of wound separation/dehiscence.

Minimizes stress/tension on healing wound edges. The aging process and atherosclerosis contribute to diminished circulation to the wound. Fatty tissue is difficult to approximate, and suture line is more easily disrupted.

Frequent dressing changes may result in damage to skin from strong adhesives.

Reduces immunocompetence, thus interfering with wound healing and resistance to infection. Promotes vasculitis and fibrosis in connective tissue, interfering with delivery of oxygen and nutrients necessary for healing.

Stressful situation in which it is extremely important to prevent panic in both the patient and the nurse.

Reduces intra-abdominal tension. May prevent evisceration from occurring.

Prevents drying of mucosal tissue.

Anemia and edema formation can interfere with healing. Steroid therapy and anticancer drugs reduce leukocyte count and suppress capillary formation and fibrogenesis.

NURSING DIAGNOSIS:	CONSTIPATION [SPECIFY]/DIARRHEA
May be related to:	Effects of anesthesia, surgical manipulation.
	Less than adequate dietary intake and bulk.
	Physical inactivity, immobility; inflammation, irritation, malabsorption of bowel.
	Pain, medication effects.
Possibly evidenced by:	Absence of stool (immediately postoperatively); constipation; diarrhea.
DESIRED OUTCOMES/ EVALUATION CRITERIA— PATIENT WILL:	Reestablish normal pattern of bowel functioning.

ACTIONS/INTERVENTIONS

Independent

Auscultate bowel sounds.

Investigate reports of abdominal pain.

Observe bowel movements, noting color, consistency, and amount.

Encourage nonirritating foods/fluids when oral intake is resumed.

Collaborative

Provide stool softener, glycerine suppository as indicated.

RATIONALE

Return of GI function may be delayed by depressant effects of anesthesia, paralytic ileus, intraperitoneal inflammation, medications. Presence of abnormal sounds (e.g., high-pitched tinkling or prolonged growling sounds) suggests development of complications.

May be related to gas distention or developing complications, e.g., ileus.

Indicator of return of GI function, identifies appropriate interventions.

Reduces risk of mucosal irritation/diarrhea.

May be necessary to gently stimulate peristalsis/stool evacuation.

NURSING DIAGNOSIS:	KNOWLEDGE DEFICIT [LEARNING NEED] REGARDING CONDITION, PROGNOSIS, AND TREATMENT NEEDS
May be related to:	Lack of exposure/recall. Information misinterpretation. Unfamiliarity with information resources.
Possibly evidenced by:	Questions; request for information. Statement of misconception. Inaccurate follow-through of instruction.
DESIRED OUTCOMES/ EVALUATION CRITERIA— PATIENT WILL:	Verbalize understanding of disease process and treatment. Identify relationship of signs/symptoms to the disease process and correlate symptoms with causative factors. Correctly perform necessary procedures and explain reasons for actions.

ACTIONS/INTERVENTIONS

Independent

Review surgical procedure and postoperative expectations.

Discuss importance of adequate fluid intake, dietary needs.

RATIONALE

Provides knowledge base on which patient can make informed choices.

Promotes healing and normalization of bowel function.

ACTIONS/INTERVENTIONS	RATIONALE
Independent	
Demonstrate appropriate wound care/dressing change. Encourage showering and use of mild soap to clean wound.	Promotes healing, reduces risk of infection, provides opportunity to observe wound healing.
Review care of gastrostomy tube if patient is to be discharged with one in place:	Promotes independence, enhances self-care abilities.
Mark position of tube at skin level;	Provides baseline to note change in position, slipping in/out of wound.
Demonstrate proper irrigation techniques and care of irrigation set as indicated;	Flushing maintains patency of tube, especially after bolus administration of feedings/medication. Proper care of the irrigation set helps prevent growth of bacteria.
Review skin care need around tube insertion site;	Helps prevent skin breakdown, reduces risk of infection.
Discuss procedure to follow if tube becomes dislodged/position changes.	Timely intervention may prevent untoward complications.
Identify signs/symptoms requiring medical evaluation, e.g., persistent fever, swelling, erythema, or opening of wound edges, changes in characteristics of drainage.	Early recognition of complications and prompt intervention may prevent progression to serious, life-threatening situation.
Review activity limitations/restrictions, e.g., no heavy lifting for 6–8 weeks, avoidance of strenuous exercise/sports.	Reduces risk of incisional strain/trauma, hernia formation.
Encourage progressive advancement of activity as tolerated and balance with adequate rest periods.	Prevents fatigue, stimulates circulation and normalization of organ function, promotes healing.

Appendectomy

Removal of an inflamed appendix may be performed as an outpatient procedure using an endoscopic approach. However, the presence of multiple adhesions, retroperitoneal positioning of the appendix or the likelihood of rupture necessitates an open (traditional) procedure.

RELATED CONCERNS:

Peritonitis, p 514
Psychosocial Aspects of Acute Care, p 899
Surgical Intervention, p 918

PATIENT ASSESSMENT DATA BASE (PREOPERATIVE)

ACTIVITY/REST

May report:	Malaise.

CIRCULATION

May exhibit:	Tachycardia.

ELIMINATION

May report:	Constipation of recent onset.
	Diarrhea (occasional).
May exhibit:	Abdominal distention, tenderness/rebound tenderness, rigidity.
	Decreased or absent bowel sounds.

FOOD/FLUID

May report:	Anorexia.
	Nausea/vomiting.

PAIN/COMFORT

May report:	Abdominal pain around the epigastrium and umbilicus, which becomes increasingly severe and localizes at McBurney's point (halfway between umbilicus and crest of right ileum), aggravated by walking, sneezing, coughing, or deep respiration (sudden cessation of pain suggests perforation or infarction of the appendix).
	Varied reports of pain/vague symptoms (due to location of appendix, e.g., retrocecally or next to ureter).
May exhibit:	Guarding behavior; lying on side or back with knees flexed; increased right lower quadrant (RLQ) pain with extension of right leg/upright position.
	Rebound tenderness on left side suggests peritoneal inflammation.

SAFETY

May exhibit:	Fever (usually low-grade).

RESPIRATION

May exhibit:	Tachypnea; shallow respirations.

TEACHING/LEARNING

May report: History of other conditions associated with abdominal pain, e.g., acute pyelitis, ureteral stone, acute salpingitis, regional ileitis.

May occur at any age.

Discharge Plan Considerations: **DRG projected mean length of stay: 4.2 days.**

May need brief assistance with transportation, home maker tasks.

DIAGNOSTIC STUDIES

WBC: Leukocytosis above 12,000/mm^3, neutrophil count elevated to 75%.

Urinalysis: Normal, but erythrocytes/leukocytes may be present.

Abdominal x-rays: May reveal hardened bit of fecal material in appendix (fecalith), localized ileus.

NURSING PRIORITIES

1. Promote comfort.
2. Prevent complications.
3. Provide information about surgical procedure/prognosis, treatment needs, and potential complications.

DISCHARGE GOALS

1. Complications prevented/minimized.
2. Pain alleviated/controlled.
3. Surgical procedure/prognosis, therapeutic regimen, and possible complications understood.

NURSING DIAGNOSIS:	INFECTION, HIGH RISK FOR
Risk factors may include:	Inadequate primary defenses; perforation/rupture of the appendix; peritonitis; abscess formation.
	Invasive procedures, surgical incision.
Possibly evidenced by:	[Not applicable; presence of signs and symptoms establishes an actual diagnosis.]
DESIRED OUTCOMES/ EVALUATION CRITERIA— PATIENT WILL:	Achieve timely wound healing; free of signs of infection/inflammation, purulent drainage, erythema, and fever.

ACTIONS/INTERVENTIONS	RATIONALE
Independent	
Monitor vital signs. Note onset of fever, chills, diaphoresis, changes in mentation, reports of increasing abdominal pain.	Suggestive of presence of infection/developing sepsis, abscess, peritonitis.
Practice good hand washing and aseptic wound care. Provide pericare.	Reduces risk of spread of bacteria.
Inspect incision and dressings. Note characteristics of drainage from wound/drains (if inserted), presence of erythema.	Provides for early detection of developing infectious process, and/or monitors resolution of preexisting peritonitis.

ACTIONS/INTERVENTIONS	RATIONALE

Independent

Provide accurate, honest information to patient/SO.

Being informed about progress of situation provides emotional support, helping to decrease anxiety.

Collaborative

Obtain drainage specimens if indicated.

Gram stain, culture, and sensitivity are useful in identifying causative organism and choice of therapy.

Administer antibiotics as indicated.

May be given prophylactically or to reduce number of organisms (in preexisting infection) to decrease spread and seeding of the abdominal cavity.

Assist with I&D if indicated.

May be necessary to drain contents of localized abscess.

NURSING DIAGNOSIS:	**FLUID VOLUME DEFICIT, HIGH RISK FOR**
Risk factors may include:	Preoperative vomiting. Postoperative restrictions (e.g., NPO). Hypermetabolic state (e.g., fever, healing process). Inflammation of peritoneum with sequestration of fluid.
Possibly evidenced by:	[Not applicable; presence of signs and symptoms establishes an actual diagnosis.]
DESIRED OUTCOMES/ EVALUATION CRITERIA— PATIENT WILL:	Maintain adequate fluid balance as evidenced by moist mucous membranes, good skin turgor, stable vital signs, and individually adequate urinary output.

ACTIONS/INTERVENTIONS	RATIONALE

Independent

Monitor BP and pulse.

Variations help identify fluctuating intravascular volumes.

Inspect mucous membranes; assess skin turgor and capillary refill.

Indicators of adequacy of peripheral circulation and cellular hydration.

Monitor I&O; note urine color/concentration, specific gravity.

Decreasing output of concentrated urine with increasing specific gravity suggests dehydration/need for increased fluids.

Auscultate bowel sounds. Note passing of flatus, bowel movement.

Indicators of return of peristalsis, readiness to begin oral intake.

Provide clear liquids in small amounts when oral intake is resumed, and progress diet as tolerated.

Reduces risk of gastric irritation/vomiting to minimize fluid loss.

Give frequent mouth care with special attention to protection of the lips.

Dehydration results in drying and painful cracking of the lips and mouth.

ACTIONS/INTERVENTIONS	RATIONALE
Collaborative	
Maintain gastric/intestinal suction.	An NG tube is usually inserted preoperatively and maintained in immediate postoperative phase to decompress the bowel, promote intestinal rest, prevent vomiting.
Administer IV fluids and electrolytes.	The peritoneum reacts to irritation/infection by producing large amounts of fluid that may reduce the circulating blood volume, resulting in hypovolemia. Dehydration and relative electrolyte imbalances may occur.

NURSING DIAGNOSIS:	PAIN, [ACUTE]
May be related to:	Distention of intestinal tissues by inflammation.
	Presence of surgical incision.
Possibly evidenced by:	Reports of pain.
	Facial grimacing, muscle guarding; distraction behaviors.
	Autonomic responses.
DESIRED OUTCOMES/ EVALUATION CRITERIA— PATIENT WILL:	Report pain is relieved/controlled.
	Appear relaxed, able to sleep/rest appropriately.

ACTIONS/INTERVENTIONS	RATIONALE
Independent	
Assess pain, noting location, characteristics, severity (0–10 scale). Investigate and report changes in pain as appropriate.	Useful in monitoring effectiveness of medication, progression of healing. Changes in characteristics of pain may indicate developing abscess/peritonitis, requiring prompt medical evaluation and intervention.
Keep at rest in semi-Fowler's position.	Gravity localizes inflammatory exudate into lower abdomen or pelvis, relieving abdominal tension, which is accentuated by supine position.
Encourage early ambulation.	Promotes normalization of organ function, e.g., stimulates peristalsis and passing of flatus, reducing abdominal discomfort.
Provide diversional activities.	Refocuses attention, promotes relaxation, and may enhance coping abilities.
Collaborative	
Keep NPO/maintain NG suction initially.	Decreases discomfort of early intestinal peristalsis and gastric irritation/vomiting.

ACTIONS/INTERVENTIONS

Collaborative

Administer analgesics as indicated.

Place ice bag on abdomen.

RATIONALE

Relief of pain facilitates cooperation with other therapeutic interventions, e.g., ambulation, pulmonary toilet.

Soothes and relieves pain through desensitization of nerve endings. *Note:* Do not use heat, because it may cause tissue congestion.

NURSING DIAGNOSIS:	**KNOWLEDGE DEFICIT [LEARNING NEED] REGARDING CONDITION, PROGNOSIS, AND TREATMENT NEEDS.**
May be related to:	Lack of exposure/recall; information misinterpretation.
	Unfamiliarity with information resources.
Possibly evidenced by:	Questions; request for information; verbalization of the problem/concerns.
	Statement of misconception.
	Inaccurate follow-through of instruction.
	Development of preventable complications.
DESIRED OUTCOMES/ EVALUATION CRITERIA— PATIENT WILL:	Verbalize understanding of disease process, treatment, and potential complications.
	Participate in treatment regimen.

ACTIONS/INTERVENTIONS

Independent

Review postoperative activity restrictions, e.g., heavy lifting, exercise, sex, sports, driving.

Encourage progressive activities as tolerated with periodic rest periods.

Recommend use of mild laxative/stool softeners as necessary and avoidance of enemas.

Discuss care of incision, including dressing changes, bathing restrictions, and return to physician for suture/staple removal.

Identify symptoms requiring medical evaluation, e.g., increasing pain; edema/erythema of wound; presence of drainage, fever.

RATIONALE

Provides information for patient to plan for return to usual routines without untoward incidence.

Prevents fatigue, promotes healing and feeling of well-being, and facilitates resumption of normal activities.

Assists with return to usual bowel function; prevents undue straining for defecation.

Understanding promotes cooperation with therapeutic regimen, enhancing healing and recovery process.

Prompt intervention reduces risk of serious complications, e.g., delayed wound healing, peritonitis.

Peritonitis

Inflammation of the peritoneal cavity can be primary or secondary, acute or chronic and results from contamination of the peritoneal capacity by either bacteria or chemicals. Primary peritonitis is not associated with an underlying bowel disorder (e.g., cirrhosis with/ascites, urinary system); secondary sources of inflammation are from the GI tract, ovaries/uterus, traumatic injuries or surgical contaminants. Surgical intervention may be curative in localized peritonitis, e.g., appendicitis/appendectomy, ulcer plication, and bowel resection. If peritonitis is diffuse, medical management is necessary before or in place of surgical treatment.

RELATED CONCERNS:

PATIENT ASSESSMENT DATA BASE

ACTIVITY/REST

May report: Weakness.

May exhibit: Difficulty ambulating.

CIRCULATION

May exhibit: Tachycardia, diaphoresis, pallor, hypotension (signs of shock).
Tissue edema.

ELIMINATION

May report: Inability to pass stool or flatus.
Diarrhea (occasionally).

May exhibit: Hiccups; abdominal distention; quiet abdomen.
Decreased urinary output, dark color.
Decreased/absent bowel sounds (ileus); intermittent loud, rushing bowel sounds (obstruction); abdominal rigidity, distention, rebound tenderness. Hyperresonance/tympany (ileus); loss of dullness over liver (free air in abdomen).

FOOD/FLUID

May report: Anorexia, nausea/vomiting; thirst.

May exhibit: Projectile vomiting.
Dry mucous membranes, swollen tongue, poor skin turgor.

PAIN/COMFORT

May report: Sudden, severe abdominal pain, generalized or localized, referred to shoulder, intensified by movement.

May exhibit: Distention, rigidity, rebound tenderness.

Muscle guarding (abdomen); flexion of knees; distraction behaviors; restlessness; self-focus.

RESPIRATION

May exhibit: Shallow respirations, tachypnea.

SAFETY

May report: Fever, chills.

SEXUALITY

May report: History of pelvic organ inflammation (salpingitis); puerperal infection; septic abortion; retroperitoneal abscess.

TEACHING/LEARNING

May report: History of recent trauma with abdominal penetration, e.g., gunshot/stab wound or blunt trauma to the abdomen; bladder perforation/rupture; disease of GI tract, e.g., appendicitis with perforation, gangrenous/ruptured gall bladder, perforated carcinoma of the stomach, perforated gastric/duodenal ulcer, gangrenous obstruction of the bowel, perforation of diverticulum, UC, regional ileitis; strangulated hernia.

Discharge Plan Considerations: **DRG projected length of stay: 5.1 days.**
Assistance with homemaker/maintenance tasks.

DIAGNOSTIC STUDIES

CBC: WBCs elevated, sometimes greater than 20,000. RBC count may be increased, indicating hemoconcentration.

Serum protein/albumin: May be decreased owing to fluid shifts.

Serum amylase: Usually elevated.

Serum electrolytes: Hypokalemia may be present.

ABGs: Respiratory alkalosis and metabolic acidosis may be noted.

Cultures: Causative organism may be identified from blood, exudate/secretions or ascitic fluid.

Abdominal x-ray examination: May reveal gas distention of bowel/ileus. If a perforated viscera is the etiology, free air will be found in the abdomen.

Chest x-ray: May reveal elevation of diaphragm.

Paracentesis: Peritoneal fluid samples may contain blood, pus/exudate, amylase, bile, and creatinine.

NURSING PRIORITIES

1. Control infection.
2. Restore/maintain circulating volume.
3. Promote comfort.
4. Maintain nutrition.
5. Provide information about disease process, possible complications, and treatment needs.

DISCHARGE GOALS

1. Infection resolved.
2. Complications prevented/minimized.
3. Pain relieved.
4. Disease process, potential complications, and therapeutic regimen understood.

NURSING DIAGNOSIS:	INFECTION, HIGH RISK FOR [SEPTICEMIA]
Risk factors may include:	Inadequate primary defenses (broken skin, traumatized tissue, altered peristalsis). Inadequate secondary defenses (immunosuppression). Invasive procedures.
Possibly evidenced by:	[Not applicable; presence of signs and symptoms establishes an actual diagnosis.]
DESIRED OUTCOMES/ EVALUATION CRITERIA— PATIENT WILL:	Achieve timely healing; be free of purulent drainage or erythema; be afebrile. Verbalize understanding of the individual causative/risk factor(s).

ACTIONS/INTERVENTIONS

Independent

Note individual risk factors, e.g., abdominal trauma, acute appendicitis, peritoneal dialysis.

Assess vital signs frequently, noting unresolved or progressing hypotension, decreased pulse pressure, tachycardia, fever, tachypnea.

Note changes in mental status (e.g., confusion, stupor).

Note skin color, temperature, moisture.

Monitor urine output.

Maintain strict aseptic technique in care of abdominal drains, incisions/open wounds, dressings, and invasive sites. Cleanse with Betadine or other appropriate solution.

Observe drainage from wounds/drains.

Maintain sterile technique when catheterizing patient, and provide catheter care/perineal cleansing on a routine basis.

RATIONALE

Influences choice of interventions.

Signs of impending septic shock. Circulating endotoxins eventually produce vasodilation, loss of fluid from circulation, and a low cardiac output state.

Hypoxemia, hypotension, and acidosis can cause deteriorating mental status.

Warm, flushed, dry skin is early sign of septicemia. Later manifestations include cool, clammy pale skin and cyanosis as shock becomes refractory.

Oliguria develops as a result of decreased renal perfusion, circulating toxins effects of antibiotics.

Prevents access or limits spread of infecting organisms/cross-contamination.

Provides information about status of infection.

Prevents access, limits bacterial growth in urinary tract.

516

ACTIONS/INTERVENTIONS	RATIONALE

Independent

Monitor/restrict visitors and staff as appropriate. Provide protective isolation if indicated.

Reduces risk of exposure to/acquisition of secondary infection in immunosuppressed patient.

Collaborative

Obtain specimens/monitor results of serial blood, urine, wound cultures.

Identifies causative microorganisms and helps in assessing effectiveness of antimicrobial regimen.

Assist with peritoneal aspiration, if indicated.

May be done to remove fluid and to identify infecting organisms so appropriate antibiotic therapy can be instituted.

Administer antimicrobials, e.g., gentamicin (Garamycin); amikacin (Amikin); clindamycin (Cleocin); IV/peritoneal lavage.

Therapy is directed at anaerobic bacteria and aerobic Gram-negative bacilli. Lavage may be used to remove necrotic debris and treat inflammation that is poorly localized/diffuse.

Prepare for surgical intervention if indicated.

May be treatment of choice (curative) in acute, localized peritonitis, e.g., to drain localized abscess, remove peritoneal exudates, remove ruptured appendix/gallbladder, plicate perforated ulcer, or resect bowel.

NURSING DIAGNOSIS:	FLUID VOLUME DEFICIT, [ACTIVE LOSS]
May be related to:	Fluid shifts from extracellular, intravascular, and interstitial compartments into intestines and/or peritoneal space.
	Vomiting; NG/intestinal aspiration.
	Fever.
	Medically restricted intake.
Possibly evidenced by:	Dry mucous membranes, poor skin turgor, delayed capillary refill, weak peripheral pulses.
	Diminished urinary output, dark/concentrated urine.
	Hypotension, tachycardia.
DESIRED OUTCOMES/ EVALUATION CRITERIA— PATIENT WILL:	Demonstrate improved fluid balance as evidenced by adequate urinary output with normal specific gravity, stable vital signs, moist mucous membranes, good skin turgor, prompt capillary refill, and weight within acceptable range.

ACTIONS/INTERVENTIONS	RATIONALE

Independent

Monitor vital signs, noting presence of hypotension (including postural changes), tachycardia, tachypnea, fever. Measure CVP if available.

Aids in evaluating degree of fluid deficit/effectiveness of fluid replacement therapy and response to medications.

ACTIONS/INTERVENTIONS	RATIONALE
Independent	
Maintain accurate I&O and correlate with daily weights. Include measured/estimated losses, e.g., gastric suction, drains, dressings, hemovacs, diaphoresis, abdominal girth.	Reflects overall hydration status. Urine output may be diminished owing to hypovolemia and decreased renal perfusion, but weight may still increase, reflecting tissue edema/ascites accumulation. Gastric suction losses may be large, and a great deal of fluid can be sequestered in the bowel and peritoneal space (ascites).
Measure urine specific gravity.	Reflects hydration status and changes in renal function, which may warn of developing acute renal failure in response to hypovolemia, effect of toxins. *Note:* Many antibiotics also have nephrotoxic effects which may further affect kidney function/urine output.
Observe skin/mucous membrane dryness, turgor. Note peripheral/sacral edema.	Hypovolemia, fluid shifts, and nutritional deficits contribute to poor skin turgor, taut edematous tissues.
Eliminate noxious sights/smells from environment. Limit intake of ice chips.	Reduces gastric stimulation and vomiting response. *Note:* Excess use of ice chips during gastric aspiration can increase gastric washout of electrolytes.
Change position frequently, provide frequent skin care, and maintain dry/wrinkle free bedding.	Edematous tissue with compromised circulation is prone to breakdown.
Collaborative	
Monitor laboratory studies, e.g., Hb/Hct, electrolytes, protein, albumin, BUN, Cr.	Provides information about hydration, organ function. Varied alterations with significant consequences to systemic function are possible as a result of fluid shifts, hypovolemia, hypoxemia, circulating toxins, and necrotic tissue products.
Administer plasma/blood, fluids, electrolytes, diuretics as indicated.	Replenishes/maintains circulating volume and electrolyte balance. Colloids (plasma, blood) help move water back into intravascular compartment by increasing osmotic pressure gradient. Diuretics may be used to assist in excretion of toxins and to enhance renal function.
Maintain NPO with nasogastric/intestinal aspiration.	Reduces hyperactivity of bowel and diarrhea losses.

NURSING DIAGNOSIS:	**PAIN [ACUTE]**
May be related to:	Chemical irritation of the parietal peritoneum (toxins).
	Trauma to tissues.
	Accumulation of fluid in abdominal/peritoneal cavity (abdominal distention).

Possibly evidenced by:	Verbalizations of pain.
	Muscle guarding, rebound tenderness.
	Facial mask of pain, self-focus.
	Distraction behavior, autonomic/emotional responses (anxiety).
DESIRED OUTCOMES/ EVALUATION CRITERIA— PATIENT WILL:	Report pain is relieved/controlled.
	Demonstrate use of relaxation skills, other methods to promote comfort.

ACTIONS/INTERVENTIONS	RATIONALE
Independent	
Investigate pain reports, noting location, duration, intensity (0–10 scale), and characteristics (dull, sharp, constant).	Changes in location/intensity are not uncommon but may reflect developing complications. Pain tends to become constant, more intense, and diffuse over the entire abdomen as inflammatory process accelerates; pain may localize if an abscess develops.
Maintain semi-Fowler's position as indicated.	Facilitates fluid/wound drainage by gravity, reducing diaphragmatic irritation/abdominal tension, and thereby reducing pain.
Move patient slowly and deliberately, splinting painful area.	Reduces muscle tension/guarding, which may help minimize pain of movement.
Provide comfort measures, e.g., massage, backrubs, deep breathing, relaxation/visualization exercises.	Promotes relaxation and may enhance patient's coping abilities by refocusing attention.
Provide frequent oral care. Remove noxious environmental stimuli.	Reduces n/v, which can increase intra-abdominal pressure/pain.
Collaborative	
Administer medications as indicated:	
Analgesics, narcotics;	Reduces metabolic rate and intestinal irritation from circulating/local toxins, which aids in pain relief and promotes healing. *Note:* Pain is usually severe and may require narcotic pain control. Analgesics may be withheld during diagnostic process as they can mask signs/symptoms.
Antiemetics, e.g., hydroxyzine (Vistaril);	Reduces n/v, which can increase abdominal pain.
Antipyretics, e.g., acetaminophen (Tylenol).	Reduces discomfort associated with fever/chills.

NURSING DIAGNOSIS:	**NUTRITION, ALTERED: LESS THAN BODY REQUIREMENTS, HIGH RISK FOR**
Risk factors may include:	Nausea/vomiting, intestinal dysfunction.

	Metabolic abnormalities.
	Increased metabolic needs.
Possibly evidenced by:	[Not applicable; presence of signs and symptoms establishes an actual diagnosis.]
DESIRED OUTCOMES/ EVALUATION CRITERIA— PATIENT WILL:	Maintain usual weight and positive nitrogen balance.

ACTIONS/INTERVENTIONS

Independent

Monitor NG tube output. Note presence of vomiting/diarrhea.

Auscultate bowel sounds, noting absent/hyperactive sounds.

Measure abdominal girth.

Weigh regularly.

Assess abdomen frequently for return to softness, reappearance of normal bowel sounds, and passage of flatus.

Collaborative

Monitor BUN, protein, albumin, glucose, nitrogen balance as indicated.

Advance diet as tolerated, e.g., clear liquid to soft.

Administer hyperalimentation (TPN) as indicated.

RATIONALE

Large amounts of gastric aspirant and vomiting/diarrhea suggest bowel obstruction, requiring further evaluation.

Although bowel sounds are frequently absent, inflammation/irritation of the intestine may be accompanied by intestinal hyperactivity, diminished water absorption, and diarrhea.

Provides quantitative evidence of changes in gastric/intestinal distention and/or accumulation of ascites.

Initial losses/gains reflect changes in hydration, but sustained losses suggest nutritional deficit.

Indicates return of normal bowel function and ability to resume oral intake.

Reflects organ function and nutritional status/ needs.

Careful progression of diet when intake is resumed reduces risk of gastric irritation.

Promotes nutrient utilization and positive nitrogen balance in patients who are unable to assimilate nutrients in a normal fashion.

NURSING DIAGNOSIS:	**ANXIETY [SPECIFY]/FEAR**
May be related to:	Situational crisis.
	Threat of death/change in health status.
	Physiologic factors, hypermetabolic state.
Possibly evidenced by:	Increased tension/helplessness.
	Apprehension, uncertainty, worry.

Sense of impending doom.

Sympathetic stimulation; restlessness; focus on self.

| DESIRED OUTCOMES/ EVALUATION CRITERIA— PATIENT WILL: | Verbalize awareness of feelings and healthy ways to deal with them.
Report anxiety is reduced to a manageable level.
Appear relaxed. |
|---|---|

ACTIONS/INTERVENTIONS	RATIONALE

Independent

Evaluate anxiety level, noting patient's verbal and nonverbal response. Encourage free expression of emotions.	Apprehension may be escalated by severe pain, increasingly ill feeling, urgency of diagnostic procedures, and possibility of surgery.
Provide information regarding disease process and anticipated treatment.	Knowing what to expect can reduce anxiety.
Schedule adequate rest and uninterrupted periods for sleep.	Limits fatigue, conserves energy, and can enhance coping ability.

Refer to CP: Psychosocial Aspects of Acute Care, p 899 for additional interventions.

NURSING DIAGNOSIS:	KNOWLEDGE DEFICIT [LEARNING NEED], REGARDING CONDITION, PROGNOSIS, AND TREATMENT NEEDS
May be related to:	Lack of exposure/recall.
Information misinterpretation.
Unfamiliarity with information resources.
Possibly evidenced by:	Questions; request for information.
Statement of misconception.
Inaccurate follow-through of instruction.
DESIRED OUTCOMES/ EVALUATION CRITERIA— PATIENT WILL:	Verbalize understanding of disease process and treatment.
Identify relationship of signs/symptoms to the disease process and correlate symptoms with causative factors.
Correctly perform necessary procedures and explain reasons for actions.

ACTIONS/INTERVENTIONS	RATIONALE

Independent

Review underlying disease process and recovery expectations.	Provides knowledge base on which patient can make informed choices.

521

ACTIONS/INTERVENTIONS	RATIONALE

Independent

Discuss medication regimen, schedule, and possible side effects.

Antibiotics may be continued after discharge, dependent on length of stay.

Recommend gradual resumption of usual activities as tolerated, allowing for adequate rest.

Prevents fatigue, enhances feeling of well-being.

Review activity restrictions/limitations, e.g., avoid heavy lifting, constipation.

Avoids unnecessary increase of intra-abdominal pressure and muscle tension.

Demonstrate aseptic dressing change, wound care.

Reduces risk of contamination. Provides opportunity to evaluate healing process.

Identify signs/symptoms requiring medical evaluation, e.g., recurrent abdominal pain/distention, vomiting, fever, chills, or presence of purulent drainage, swelling/erythema of surgical incision (if present).

Early recognition and treatment of developing complications may prevent more serious illness/injury.

Cholecystitis with Cholelithiasis _____

Cholecystitis is an acute or chronic inflammation of the gallbladder, usually associated with gallstone(s) impacted in the cystic duct, causing distention of the gallbladder. Stones (calculi) are made up of cholesterol, calcium bilirubinate, or a mixture, caused by changes in the bile composition. Gallstones can develop in the common bile duct, the cystic duct, hepatic duct, small bile duct, and pancreatic duct. Crystals can also form in the submucosa of the gallbladder causing widespread inflammation. Acute cholecystitis with cholelithiasis is usually treated by surgery, although several other treatment methods (fragmentation and dissolution of stones) are now being used. This plan of care deals with the acutely ill, hospitalized patient.

RELATED CONCERNS:

Cholecystectomy, p 531
Fluid and Electrolyte Imbalances, p 1054
Psychosocial Aspects of Acute Care, p 899
Total Nutritional Support, p 1039

PATIENT ASSESSMENT DATA BASE

ACTIVITY/REST

May report:	Fatigue.
May exhibit:	Restlessness.

CIRCULATION

May exhibit:	Tachycardia, diaphoresis.

ELIMINATION

May report:	Change in color of urine and stools.
May exhibit:	Abdominal distention.
	Palpable mass in upper right quadrant.
	Dark, concentrated urine.
	Clay-colored stool, steatorrhea.

FOOD/FLUID

May report:	Anorexia, nausea/vomiting.
	Intolerance of fatty and "gas-forming" foods; recurrent regurgitation, heartburn, indigestion, flatulence, bloating (dyspepsia).
	Belching (eructation).
May exhibit:	Obesity; recent weight loss.

PAIN/COMFORT

May report:	Severe upper abdominal pain, may radiate to back or right shoulder.
	Midepigastric colicky pain associated with eating.
	Pain starting suddenly and usually peaking in 30 minutes.
May exhibit:	Rebound tenderness, muscle guarding or rigidity when RUQ is palpated; positive Murphy's sign.

523

RESPIRATION

May exhibit: Increased respiratory rate.

Splinted respiration marked by short, shallow breathing.

SAFETY

May exhibit: Fever, chills.

Jaundice, with dry, itching skin (pruritus).

Bleeding tendencies (vitamin K deficiency).

TEACHING/LEARNING

May report: Familial tendency for gallstones.

Recent pregnancy/delivery; history of DM, inflammatory bowel disease, blood dyscrasias.

Discharge Plan Considerations: **DRG projected mean length of stay: 3.4 days.**

May require support with dietary changes/weight reduction.

DIAGNOSTIC STUDIES

CBC: Moderate leukocytosis (acute).

Serum bilirubin and amylase: Elevated.

Serum liver enzymes—AST (SGOT); ALT (SGPT); LDH: Slight elevation; alkaline phosphatase and 5-nucleotidase: markedly elevated in biliary obstruction.

Prothrombin levels: Reduced when obstruction to the flow of bile into the intestine decreases absorption of vitamin K.

Ultrasound: Reveals calculi, with gallbladder and/or bile duct distention (frequently the initial diagnostic procedure).

Endoscopic retrograde cholangiopancreatography: Visualizes biliary tree by cannulation of the common bile duct through the duodenum.

Percutaneous transhepatic cholangiography: Fluoroscopic imaging distinguishes between gallbladder disease and cancer of the pancreas (when jaundice is present).

Cholecystograms (for chronic cholecystitis): Reveals stones in the biliary system. Note: contraindicated in acute cholecystitis because the patient is too ill to take the dye by mouth.

CT scan: May reveal gallbladder cysts, dilation of bile ducts, and distinguish between obstructive/nonobstructive jaundice.

Liver scan (with radioactive dye): Shows obstruction of the biliary tree.

Abdominal x-ray films (multipositional): Reveal radiopaque (calcified) gallstones, calcification of the wall or enlargement of the gallbladder.

Chest x-ray: Rule out respiratory causes of referred pain.

NURSING PRIORITIES

1. Relieve pain and promote rest.
2. Maintain fluid and electrolyte balance.
3. Prevent complications.
4. Provide information about disease process, prognosis, and treatment needs.

DISCHARGE GOALS

1. Pain relieved.
2. Homeostasis achieved.
3. Complications prevented/minimized.
4. Disease process, prognosis, and therapeutic regimen understood.

NURSING DIAGNOSIS:	PAIN, [ACUTE]
May be related to:	Biologic injuring agents: obstruction/ductal spasm, inflammatory process, tissue ischemia/necrosis.
Possibly evidenced by:	Reports of pain, biliary colic (waves of pain).
	Facial mask of pain; guarding behavior.
	Autonomic responses (changes in BP, pulse).
	Self-focusing; narrowed focus.
DESIRED OUTCOMES/ EVALUATION CRITERIA— PATIENT WILL:	Report pain is relieved/controlled.
	Demonstrate use of relaxation skills and diversional activities as indicated for individual situation.

ACTIONS/INTERVENTIONS

Independent

Observe and document location, severity (0–10 scale), and character of pain (steady, intermittent, colicky).

Note response to medication, and report to physician if pain is not being relieved.

Promote bed rest, allowing patient to assume position of comfort.

Use soft/cotton linens; calamine lotion; oil (Alpha-Keri) bath; cool/moist compresses as indicated.

Control environmental temperature.

Encourage use of relaxation techniques, e.g., guided imagery, visualization, deep-breathing exercises. Provide diversional activities.

Make time to listen to and maintain frequent contact with patient.

RATIONALE

Assists in differentiating cause of pain and provides information about disease progression/resolution, development of complications, and effectiveness of interventions.

Severe pain not relieved by routine measures may indicate developing complications/need for further intervention.

Bed rest in low-Fowler's position reduces intra-abdominal pressure; however, patient will naturally assume least painful position.

Reduces irritation/dryness of the skin and itching sensation.

Cool surroundings aid in minimizing dermal discomfort.

Promotes rest, redirects attention, may enhance coping.

Helpful in alleviating anxiety and refocusing attention, which can relieve pain.

ACTIONS/INTERVENTIONS	RATIONALE
Collaborative	
Maintain NPO status, insert/maintain NG suction as indicated.	Removes gastric secretions that stimulate release of cholecystokinin and gallbladder contractions.
Administer medications as indicated:	
anticholinergics, e.g., atropine, propantheline (Pro-Banthine);	Relieves reflex spasm/smooth muscle contraction and assists with pain management.
sedatives, e.g., phenobarbital;	Promotes rest and relaxes smooth muscle, relieving pain.
narcotics, e.g., meperidine hydrochloride (Demerol); Morphine sulfate;	Given to reduce severe pain. Morphine is used with caution because it may increase spasms of the sphincter of Oddi, although nitroglycerin may be given to reduce morphine-induced spasms if they occur.
monoctanoin (Moctanin);	This medication may be tried after a cholecystectomy for retained stones, or for newly formed large stones in the bile duct. It is a lengthy treatment (1–3 weeks) and is administered via a nasal-biliary tube. A cholangiogram is done periodically to monitor stone dissolution.
Smooth muscle relaxants, e.g., papaverine (Pavabid); nitroglycerin, amyl nitrate;	Relieves ductal spasm.
chenodeoxycholic acid (Chenix); ursodeoxycholic acid (UCDA, Actigall);	These natural bile acids decrease cholesterol synthesis, dissolving gallstones. Success of this treatment depends on the number and size of gallstone (3 or fewer stones under 20 mm in diameter).
antibiotics.	To treat infectious process reducing inflammation.
Prepare for procedures, e.g.:	Choice of procedure is dictated by individual situation.
endoscopic papillotomy (removal of ductal stone);	
extracorporeal shock wave lithotripsy (ESWL);	Shock wave treatment indicated when patient has mild or moderate symptoms, cholesterol stones in gallbladder are 0.5 mm or larger, and there is no biliary tract obstruction. Depending on the machine being used, the patient may sit in a tank of water or lie prone on a water-filled cushion. Treatment takes about 1–2 hours and is 75%–95% successful.
endoscopic sphincterotomy;	Procedure done to widen the mouth of the common bile duct where it empties into the duodenum. This procedure may also include the manual retrieval of stones from the duct by means of a tiny basket or balloon on the end of the endoscope. Stones must be smaller than 15 mm.
surgical intervention.	Cholecystectomy may be indicated due to size of stones and degree of tissue involvement/presence of necrosis.

NURSING DIAGNOSIS:	FLUID VOLUME DEFICIT, HIGH RISK FOR
Risk factors may include:	Excessive losses through gastric suction; vomiting, distention, and gastric hypermotility.
	Medically restricted intake.
	Altered clotting process.
Possibly evidenced by:	[Not applicable; presence of signs and symptoms establishes an actual diagnosis.]
DESIRED OUTCOMES/ EVALUATION CRITERIA— PATIENT WILL:	Demonstrate adequate fluid balance evidenced by stable vital signs, moist mucous membranes, good skin turgor, capillary refill, individually appropriate urinary output, absence of vomiting.

ACTIONS/INTERVENTIONS

Independent

Maintain accurate I&O, noting output less than intake, increased urine specific gravity. Assess skin/mucous membranes, peripheral pulses, and capillary refill.

Monitor for signs/symptoms of increased/continued n/v, abdominal cramps, weakness, twitching, seizures, irregular heart rate, paresthesia, hypoactive or absent bowel sounds, depressed respirations.

Eliminate noxious sights/smells from environment.

Perform frequent oral hygiene with mouthwash; apply lubricants.

Use small gauge needles for injections and apply firm pressure for longer than usual after venipuncture.

Assess for unusual bleeding, e.g., oozing from injection sites, epistaxis, bleeding gums, ecchymosis, petechiae, hematemesis/melena.

Collaborative

Keep patient NPO as necessary.

Insert NG tube, connect to suction, and maintain patency as indicated.

Administer antiemetics, e.g., prochlorperazine (Compazine).

RATIONALE

Provides information about fluid status/circulating volume and replacement needs.

Prolonged vomiting, gastric aspiration, and restricted oral intake can lead to deficits in sodium, potassium, and chloride.

Reduces stimulation of vomiting center.

Decreases dryness of oral mucous membranes; reduces risk of oral bleeding.

Reduces trauma, risk of bleeding/hematoma formation.

Blood prothrombin is reduced and coagulation time prolonged when bile flow is obstructed, increasing risk of bleeding/hemorrhage.

Decreases GI secretions and motility.

Provides rest for GI tract.

Reduces nausea and prevents vomiting.

527

ACTIONS/INTERVENTIONS

Collaborative

Review laboratory studies, e.g., Hb/Hct; electrolytes; ABGs (pH); clotting times.

Administer IV fluids, electrolytes, and vitamin K.

RATIONALE

Aids in evaluating circulating volume, identifies deficits, and influences choice of intervention for replacement/correction.

Maintains circulating volume and corrects imbalances.

NURSING DIAGNOSIS:	NUTRITION, ALTERED: LESS THAN BODY REQUIREMENTS, HIGH RISK FOR
Risk factors may include:	Self-imposed or prescribed dietary restrictions; nausea/vomiting, dyspepsia, pain. Loss of nutrients; impaired fat digestion due to obstruction of bile flow.
Possibly evidenced by:	[Not applicable; presence of signs and symptoms establishes an actual diagnosis.]
DESIRED OUTCOMES/ EVALUATION CRITERIA— PATIENT WILL:	Report relief of nausea/vomiting. Demonstrate progression toward desired weight gain or maintain weight as individually appropriate.

ACTIONS/INTERVENTIONS

Independent

Assess for abdominal distention, frequent belching, guarding, reluctance to move.

Estimate/calculate caloric intake. Keep comments about appetite to a minimum.

Weigh as indicated.

Consult with patient about likes/dislikes, foods that cause distress, and preferred meal schedule.

Provide a pleasant atmosphere at mealtime; remove noxious stimuli.

Provide oral hygiene before meals.

Offer effervescent drinks with meals, if tolerated.

Ambulate and increase activity as tolerated.

RATIONALE

Nonverbal signs of discomfort associated with impaired digestion, gas pain.

Identifies nutritional deficiencies/needs. Focusing on problem creates a negative atmosphere and may interfere with intake.

Monitors effectiveness of dietary plan.

Involving patient in planning enables patient to have a sense of control and encourages eating.

Useful in promoting appetite/reducing nausea.

A clean mouth enhances appetite.

May lessen nausea and relieve gas. *Note:* May be contraindicated if beverage causes gas formation/gastric discomfort.

Helpful in expulsion of flatus, reduction of abdominal distention. Contributes to overall recovery and sense of well-being and decreases possibility of secondary problems related to immobility (e.g., pneumonia, thrombophlebitis).

ACTIONS/INTERVENTIONS

Collaborative

Consult with dietitian/nutritional support team as indicated.

Begin low-fat liquid diet after NG tube is removed.

Advance diet as tolerated, usually low-fat, high fiber. Restrict gas-producing foods (e.g., onions, cabbage, popcorn) and foods/fluids high in fats (e.g., butter, fried foods, nuts).

Administer bile salts, e.g., Bilron; Zanchol; dehydrocholic acid (Decholin), as indicated.

Monitor laboratory studies, e.g., BUN, serum albumin/protein, transferrin levels.

Provide TPN as needed.

RATIONALE

Useful in establishing individual nutritional needs via most appropriate route.

Limiting fat content reduces stimulation of gallbladder and pain associated with incomplete fat digestion and is helpful in preventing recurrence.

Meets nutritional requirements while minimizing stimulation of the gallbladder.

Promotes digestion and absorption of fats, fat-soluble vitamins, cholesterol. Useful in chronic cholecystitis.

Provides information about nutritional deficits/effectiveness of therapy.

Alternate feeding may be required dependent on degree of disability/gallbladder involvement and need for prolonged gastric rest.

NURSING DIAGNOSIS:	KNOWLEDGE DEFICIT [LEARNING NEED] REGARDING CONDITION, PROGNOSIS, AND TREATMENT NEEDS
May be related to:	Lack of knowledge/recall.
	Information misinterpretation.
	Unfamiliarity with information resources.
Possibly evidenced by:	Questions; request for information.
	Statement of misconception.
	Inaccurate follow-through of instruction.
	Development of preventable complications.
DESIRED OUTCOMES/ EVALUATION CRITERIA— PATIENT WILL:	Verbalize understanding of disease process, treatment, prognosis.
	Initiate necessary lifestyle changes and participate in treatment regimen.

ACTIONS/INTERVENTIONS

Independent

Provide explanations of/reasons for test procedures and preparation needed.

Review disease process/prognosis. Discuss hospitalization and prospective treatment as indicated. Encourage questions, expression of concern.

RATIONALE

Information can decrease anxiety, thereby reducing sympathetic stimulation.

Provides knowledge base on which patient can make informed choices. Effective communication and support at this time can diminish anxiety and promote healing.

ACTIONS/INTERVENTIONS	RATIONALE
Independent	
Review drug regimen, possible side effects.	Gallstones often recur, necessitating long-term therapy. Development of diarrhea/cramps during chenodiol therapy may be dose related/correctable. *Note:* Women of childbearing age should be counseled regarding birth control to prevent pregnancy and risk of fetal hepatic damage.
Discuss weight reduction programs if indicated.	Obesity is a risk factor associated with cholecystitis, and weight loss is beneficial in medical management of chronic condition.
Instruct patient to avoid food/fluids high in fats (e.g., whole milk, ice cream, butter, fried foods, nuts, gravies, pork); gas-producers (e.g., cabbage, beans, onions, carbonated beverages); or gastric irritants (e.g., spicy foods, caffeine, citrus).	Prevents/limits recurrence of gallbladder attacks.
Review signs/symptoms requiring medical intervention, e.g., recurrent fever; persistent n/v, or pain; jaundice of skin or eyes, itching; dark urine; clay-colored stools; blood in urine, stools; vomitus; or bleeding from mucous membranes.	Indicative of progression of disease process/development of complications requiring further intervention.
Recommend resting in semi-Fowler's position after meals.	Promotes flow of bile and general relaxation during initial digestive process.
Suggest patient limit gum chewing, sucking on straw/hard candy, or smoking.	Promotes gas formation, which can increase gastric distention/discomfort.
Discuss avoidance of aspirin-containing products, forceful blowing of nose, straining for bowel movement, contact sports. Recommend use of soft toothbrush, electric razor.	Reduces risk of bleeding related to changes in coagulation time, mucosal irritation, and trauma.

Cholecystectomy

Cholecystectomy is the treatment of choice for many patients with multiple/large gallstones either because of acute symptomatology or to prevent recurrence of stones. Cholecystectomy can now be performed by laser through laparoscopic incisions. This procedure is usually done on an outpatient basis. However, in the presence of suspected complications, e.g., empyema, gangrene, or perforation, an in-patient stay and more involved surgical intervention is indicated.

RELATED CONCERNS:

Cholecystitis/Cholelithiasis, p 523
Pancreatitis, p 561
Peritonitis, p 514
Psychosocial Aspects of Acute Care, p 899
Surgical Intervention, p 918

PATIENT ASSESSMENT DATA BASE/DIAGNOSTIC STUDIES

Refer to CP: Cholecystitis with Cholelithiasis, p 523.

TEACHING/LEARNING

Discharge Plan Considerations: **DRG projected mean length of stay: 8.2 days.**
May require assistance with wound care/supplies, homemaker tasks.

NURSING PRIORITIES

1. Promote respiratory function.
2. Prevent complications.
3. Provide information about disease, procedure(s), prognosis, and treatment needs.

DISCHARGE GOALS

1. Ventilation/oxygenation adequate for individual needs.
2. Complications prevented/minimized.
3. Disease process, surgical procedure, prognosis, and therapeutic regimen understood.

NURSING DIAGNOSIS:	BREATHING PATTERN, INEFFECTIVE
May be related to:	Pain.
	Muscular impairment.
	Decreased energy/fatigue.
Possibly evidenced by:	Tachypnea.
	Respiratory depth changes, reduced vital capacity.
	Holding breath; reluctance to cough.
DESIRED OUTCOMES/ EVALUATION CRITERIA— PATIENT WILL:	Establish effective breathing pattern.
	Experience no signs of respiratory compromise/complications.

ACTIONS/INTERVENTIONS	RATIONALE
Independent	
Observe respiratory rate/depth.	Shallow breathing, splinting with respirations, holding breath may result in hypoventilation/atelectasis.
Auscultate breath sounds.	Areas of decreased/absent breath sounds suggest atelectasis, whereas adventitious sounds (wheezes, rhonchi) reflect congestion.
Assist patient to turn, cough, and deep breath periodically. Show patient how to splint incision. Instruct in effective breathing techniques.	Promotes ventilation of all lung segments and mobilization and expectoration of secretions.
Elevate head of bed, maintain low-Fowler's position. Support abdomen when coughing, ambulating.	Facilitates lung expansion. Splinting provides incisional support/decreases muscle tension to promote cooperation with therapeutic regimen.
Collaborative	
Assist with respiratory treatments, e.g., incentive spirometer.	Maximizes expansion of lungs to prevent/resolve atelectasis.
Administer analgesics before breathing treatments/therapeutic activities.	Facilitates more effective coughing, deep breathing, and activity.

NURSING DIAGNOSIS:	FLUID VOLUME DEFICIT, HIGH RISK FOR
Risk factors may include:	Losses from NG aspiration, vomiting.
	Medically restricted intake.
	Altered coagulation, e.g., reduced prothrombin, prolonged coagulation time.
Possibly evidenced by:	[Not applicable; presence of signs and symptoms establishes an actual diagnosis.]
DESIRED OUTCOMES/ EVALUATION CRITERIA— PATIENT WILL:	Display adequate fluid balance as evidenced by stable vital signs, moist mucous membranes, good skin turgor/capillary refill, and individually appropriate urinary output.

ACTIONS/INTERVENTIONS	RATIONALE
Independent	
Monitor I&O, including drainage from NG, T-tube, and wound. Weigh patient periodically.	Provides information about replacement needs and organ function. Initially, 200–500 ml of bile drainage is to be expected, decreasing as more bile enters the intestine. Continuing large amounts of bile drainage may be an indication of obstruction or, occasionally, a biliary fistula.
Monitor vital signs. Assess mucous membranes, skin turgor, peripheral pulses, and capillary refill.	Indicators of adequacy of circulating volume/perfusion.

ACTIONS/INTERVENTIONS	RATIONALE
Independent	
Observe for signs of bleeding, e.g., hematemesis, melena; petechiae, ecchymosis.	Prothrombin is reduced and coagulation time prolonged when bile flow is obstructed, increasing risk of bleeding/hemorrhage.
Use small-gauge needles for injections, and apply firm pressure for longer than usual after venipuncture.	Reduces trauma, risk of bleeding/hematoma.
Have the patient use cotton/sponge swabs and mouthwash instead of a toothbrush.	Avoids trauma and bleeding of the gums.
Collaborative	
Monitor laboratory studies, e.g., Hb/Hct, electrolytes, prothrombin level/clotting time.	Provides information about circulating volume, electrolyte balance, and adequacy of clotting factors.
Administer IV fluids, blood products, as indicated;	Maintains adequate circulating volume and aids in replacement of clotting factors.
Electrolytes;	Corrects imbalances resulting from excessive gastric/wound losses.
vitamin K.	Provides replacement of factors necessary for clotting process.

NURSING DIAGNOSIS:	**SKIN/TISSUE INTEGRITY, IMPAIRED**
May be related to:	Chemical substance (bile), stasis of secretions.
	Altered nutritional state (obesity)/metabolic state.
	Invasion of body structure (T tube).
Possibly evidenced by:	Disruption of skin/subcutaneous tissues.
DESIRED OUTCOMES/ EVALUATION CRITERIA— PATIENT WILL:	Achieve timely wound healing without complications.
	Demonstrate behaviors to promote healing/prevent skin breakdown.

ACTIONS/INTERVENTIONS	RATIONALE
Independent	
Check the T tube and incisional drains; make sure they are free flowing.	T tube may remain in common bile duct for 7–10 days to remove retained stones. Incision site drains are used to remove any accumulated fluid and bile. Correct positioning prevents backup of the bile in the operative area.
Maintain T tube in closed collection system.	Prevents skin irritation and facilitates measurement of output. Reduces risk of contamination.

533

ACTIONS/INTERVENTIONS	RATIONALE
Independent	
Observe the color and character of the drainage. Use a disposable ostomy bag over a stab wound drain.	Initially, drainage may contain blood and blood-stained fluid, normally changing to greenish brown (bile color) after the first several hours. Ostomy appliance may be used to collect heavy drainage for more accurate measurement of output and protection of the skin.
Anchor drainage tube, allowing sufficient tubing to permit free turning, and avoid kinks and twists.	Avoids dislodging tube and/or occlusion of the lumen.
Place patient in low- or semi-Fowler's position.	Facilitates drainage of bile.
Observe for hiccups, abdominal distention, or signs of peritonitis, pancreatitis.	Dislodgment of the T tube can result in diaphragmatic irritation or more serious complications if bile drains into abdomen or pancreatic duct is obstructed.
Change dressings as often as necessary. Clean the skin with soap and water. Use sterile petroleum jelly gauze, zinc oxide, or karaya powder around the incision.	Keeps the skin around the incision clean and provides a barrier to protect skin from excoriation.
Apply Montgomery straps.	Facilitates frequent dressing changes and minimizes skin trauma.
Monitor endoscopic puncture sites (3–5) if endoscopic procedure is done.	These areas may bleed or staples and steristrips may loosen at puncture wound sites.
Observe skin, sclerae, urine for change in color.	Developing jaundice may indicate obstruction of bile flow.
Note color and consistency of stools.	Clay-colored stools result when bile is not present in the intestines.
Investigate reports of increased/unrelenting RUQ pain; development of fever, tachycardia; leakage of bile drainage around tube/from wound.	Signs suggestive of abscess or fistula formation, requiring medical intervention.
Collaborative	
Administer antibiotics as indicated.	Necessary for treatment of abscess/infection.
Clamp the T tube per schedule.	Tests the patency of the common bile duct before tube is removed.
Prepare for surgical interventions as indicated.	I&D or fistulectomy may be required to treat abscess/fistula.
Monitor laboratory studies, e.g., WBC.	Leukocytosis reflects inflammatory process, e.g., abcess formation or development of peritonitis/pancreatitis.

NURSING DIAGNOSIS:	**KNOWLEDGE DEFICIT [LEARNING NEED], REGARDING CONDITION, PROGNOSIS, AND TREATMENT NEEDS**
May be related to:	Lack of exposure; information misinterpretation.

	Unfamiliarity with information resources.
	Lack of recall.
Possibly evidenced by:	Questions; statement of misconception.
	Request for information.
	Inaccurate follow-through of instructions.
DESIRED OUTCOMES/ EVALUATION CRITERIA— PATIENT WILL:	Verbalize understanding of disease process, surgical procedure/prognosis, and treatment.
	Correctly perform necessary procedures and explain reasons for the actions.
	Initiate necessary lifestyle changes and participate in treatment regimen.

ACTIONS/INTERVENTIONS	RATIONALE
Independent	
Review disease process, surgical procedure/prognosis.	Provides knowledge base on which patient can make informed choices.
Demonstrate care of incisions/dressings and drains.	Promotes independence in care and reduces risk of complications (e.g., infection, biliary obstruction).
Recommend periodic drainage of T tube collection bag and recording of output.	Reduces risk of reflux, strain on tube/appliance seal. Provides information about resolution of ductal edema/return of ductal function.
Stress importance of maintaining low-fat diet, eating frequent small meals, gradual reintroduction of foods/fluids containing fats over a 4–6 month period.	During initial 6 months after surgery, low-fat diet limits need for bile and reduces discomfort associated with inadequate digestion of fats.
Discuss use of florantyrone (Sancho) or dehydrocholic acid (Decholin).	Oral replacement of bile salts may be required to facilitate fat absorption.
Avoid alcoholic beverages.	Minimizes risk of pancreatic involvement.
Inform patient that loose stools may occur for several months.	Intestines require time to adjust to stimulus of continuous output of bile.
Advise patient to note and avoid foods that seem to aggravate the diarrhea.	Although dietary changes are not usually necessary, certain restrictions may be helpful; e.g., fats in small amounts are usually tolerated. After a period of adjustment, patient usually will not have problems with most foods.
Identify signs/symptoms requiring notification of physician, e.g., dark urine, jaundiced color of eyes/skin, clay-colored stools, excessive stools, or recurrent heartburn, bloating.	Indicators of obstruction of bile flow/altered digestion, requiring further evaluation and intervention.
Review activity limitations dependent on individual situation.	Resumption of usual activities is normally accomplished within 4–6 weeks.

Hepatitis

Inflammation of the liver can be due to bacterial invasion, injury by physical or chemical agents (nonviral), or viral infections (Hepatitis A, B, C, D, E).

RELATED CONCERNS:

Alcoholism (Acute), p 960
Cirrhosis, p 547
Depressants, p 993
Psychosocial Aspects of Acute Care, p 899
Renal Dialysis, p 646
Stimulants, p 983
Total Nutritional Support, p 1039

PATIENT ASSESSMENT DATA BASE

Data are dependent on the cause and severity of liver involvement/damage.

ACTIVITY/REST

May report: Fatigue, weakness, general malaise.

CIRCULATION

May exhibit: Bradycardia (severe hyperbilirubinemia).
Jaundiced sclera, skin, mucous membranes.

ELIMINATION

May report: Dark urine.
Diarrhea/constipation; clay-colored stools.
Current/recent hemodialysis.

FOOD/FLUID

May report: Loss of appetite (anorexia), weight loss or gain (edema).
Nausea/vomiting.

May exhibit: Ascites.

NEUROSENSORY

May exhibit: Irritability, drowsiness, lethargy, asterixis.

PAIN/COMFORT

May report: Abdominal cramping, RUQ tenderness.
Myalgias, arthralgias; headache.
Itching (pruritus).

May exhibit: Muscle guarding, restlessness.

RESPIRATION

May report: Distaste for/aversion to cigarettes (smokers).

SAFETY

May report: Recent transfusion of blood/blood products.

May exhibit: Fever.

Urticaria, maculopapular lesions, irregular patches of erythema.

Exacerbation of acne.

Spider angiomas, palmar erythema, gynecomastia in men (sometimes present in alcoholic hepatitis).

Splenomegaly, posterior cervical node enlargement.

SEXUALITY

May report: Lifestyle/behaviors increasing risk of exposure (e.g., sexually active homosexual/bisexual male).

TEACHING/LEARNING

May report: History of known/possible exposure to virus, bacteria, or toxins (contaminated food, water, needles, surgical equipment or blood); carriers (symptomatic or asymptomatic); recent surgical procedure with halothane anesthesia; exposure to toxic chemicals (e.g., carbon tetrachloride, vinyl chloride); prescription drug use (e.g., sulfonamides, phenothiazines, isoniazid).

Travel to/immigrants from China, Africa, Southeast Asia, Middle East (Hepatitis B [HB] is endemic in these areas).

Street (IV) drug or alcohol use.

Concurrent diabetes, CHF, malignancy or renal disease.

Recent flulike upper respiratory infection.

Discharge Plan Considerations: **DRG projected mean length of stay: 6.7 days.**

May require assistance with homemaker/maintenance tasks.

DIAGNOSTIC STUDIES

Liver function tests: Abnormal (4–10 times normal values). Note: Of limited value in differentiating viral from nonviral hepatitis.

AST (SGOT)/ALT (SGPT): Initially elevated. May rise 1–2 weeks before jaundice is apparent, then declines.

CBC: RBCs decreased due to decreased life of RBCs (liver enzyme alterations) or result of hemorrhage.

Leukopenia: Thrombocytopenia may be present (splenomegaly).

Differential WBC: Leukocytosis, monocytosis, atypical lymphocytes, and plasma cells.

Alkaline phosphatase: Slight elevation (unless severe cholestasis present).

Stools: Clay-colored, steatorrhea (decreased hepatic function).

Serum albumin: Decreased.

Blood sugar: Transient hyperglycemia/hypoglycemia (altered liver function).

Anti-HAV I_gM: Positive in type A.

HbsAG: May be positive (type B) or negative (type A). Note: May be diagnostic before clinical symptoms occur.

Prothrombin time: May be prolonged (liver dysfunction).

Serum bilirubin: Above 2.5 mg/100 ml. (If above 200 mg/100 ml, poor prognosis is probable due to increased cellular necrosis.)

BSP excretion test: Blood level elevated.

Liver biopsy: Defines diagnosis and extent of necrosis.

537

Liver scan: Aids in estimation of severity of parenchymal damage.

Urinalysis: Elevated bilirubin levels; protein/hematuria may occur.

NURSING PRIORITIES

1. Reduce demands on liver while promoting physical well-being.
2. Prevent complications.
3. Enhance self-concept, acceptance of situation.
4. Provide information about disease process, prognosis, and treatment needs.

DISCHARGE GOALS

1. Meeting basic self-care needs.
2. Complications prevented/minimized.
3. Dealing with reality of current situation.
4. Disease process, prognosis, and therapeutic regimen understood.

NURSING DIAGNOSIS:	ACTIVITY INTOLERANCE
May be related to:	Generalized weakness; decreased strength/endurance; pain.
	Imposed activity restrictions; depression.
Possibly evidenced by:	Reports of fatigue, exertional discomfort.
	Decreased muscle strength.
	Reluctance to attempt movement.
DESIRED OUTCOMES/ EVALUATION CRITERIA— PATIENT WILL:	Verbalize understanding of situation/risk factors and individual treatment regimen.
	Demonstrate techniques/behaviors that enable resumption of activities.
	Report a measurable increase in activity tolerance.

ACTIONS/INTERVENTIONS	RATIONALE
Independent	
Promote bed/chair rest. Provide quiet environment; limit visitors as needed.	Promotes rest and relaxation. Available energy is used for healing. Activity and an upright position are believed to decrease hepatic blood flow, which prevents optimal circulation to the liver cells.
Change position frequently. Provide good skin care.	Promotes optimal respiratory function and minimizes pressure areas to reduce risk of tissue breakdown.
Do necessary tasks quickly and at one time as tolerated.	Allows for extended periods of uninterrupted rest.

ACTIONS/INTERVENTIONS	RATIONALE
Independent	
Increase activity as tolerated, assist with passive/active ROM exercises.	Prolonged bed rest can be debilitating. This can be offset by limited activity alternating with rest periods.
Encourage use of stress management techniques, e.g., progressive relaxation, visualization, guided imagery. Provide appropriate diversional activities, e.g., radio, TV, reading.	Promotes relaxation and conserves energy, redirects attention, and may enhance coping.
Monitor for recurrence of anorexia and liver tenderness/enlargement.	Indicates lack of resolution/exacerbation of the disease, requiring further rest, change in therapeutic regimen.
Collaborative	
Administer antidote or assist with procedures as indicated (e.g.: lavage, catharsis, hyperventilation) dependent on route of exposure.	Removal of causative agent in toxic hepatitis may limit degree of tissue involvement/damage.
Administer medications as indicated: sedatives, antianxiety agents, e.g., diazepam (Valium); lorazepam (Ativan).	Assists in managing required rest. *Note:* Use of barbiturates and tranquilizers, such as Compazine and Thorazine, is contraindicated due to hepatotoxic effects.
Monitor liver enzyme levels.	Aids in determining appropriate levels of activity, as premature increase in activity potentiates risk of relapse.

NURSING DIAGNOSIS:	NUTRITION, ALTERED: LESS THAN BODY REQUIREMENTS
May be related to:	Insufficient intake to meet metabolic demands: anorexia, nausea/vomiting.
	Altered absorption and metabolism of ingested foods: reduced peristalsis (visceral reflexes), bile stasis.
	Increased calorie needs/hypermetabolic state.
Possibly evidenced by:	Aversion to eating/lack of interest in food.
	Altered taste sensation.
	Abdominal pain/cramping.
	Loss of weight; poor muscle tone.
DESIRED OUTCOMES/ EVALUATION CRITERIA— PATIENT WILL:	Initiate behaviors, lifestyle changes to regain/maintain appropriate weight.
	Demonstrate progressive weight gain toward goal with normalization of laboratory values and free of signs of malnutrition.

ACTIONS/INTERVENTIONS	RATIONALE
Independent	
Monitor dietary intake/calorie count. Give several small feedings and offer largest meal at breakfast.	Large meals are difficult to manage when patient is anorexic. Anorexia may also worsen during the day, making intake of food difficult later in the day.
Provide mouth care before meals.	Eliminating unpleasant taste may enhance appetite.
Recommend eating in upright position.	Reduces sensation of abdominal fullness and may enhance intake.
Encourage intake of fruit juices, carbonated beverages, and hard candy throughout the day.	These supply extra calories and may be more easily digested/tolerated when other foods are not.
Collaborative	
Consult with dietitian, nutritional support team to provide diet according to patient's needs, with fat and protein intake as tolerated.	Useful in formulating dietary program to meet individual needs. Fat metabolism varies according to bile production and excretion and may necessitate restriction of fat intake if diarrhea develops. If tolerated, a normal or increased protein intake will help with liver regeneration. Protein restriction may be indicated in severe disease (e.g., fulminating hepatitis) because the accumulation of the end products of protein metabolism can potentiate hepatic encephalopathy.
Monitor blood glucose.	Hyperglycemia/hypoglycemia may develop, necessitating dietary changes/insulin administration.
Administer medications as indicated:	
Antiemetics, e.g., metalopramide (Reglan); trimethobenzamide (Tigan);	Given ½ hour before meals, may reduce nausea and increase food tolerance. *Note:* Compazine is contraindicated in hepatic disease.
Antacids, e.g., Mylanta, Titralac;	Counteracts gastric acidity reducing irritation/risk of bleeding.
Vitamins, e.g., B complex, C, other dietary supplements as indicated;	Corrects deficiencies and aids in the healing process.
Steroid therapy, e.g., Prednisone (Deltasone), alone or in combination with azathioprine (Imuran).	Steroids may be contraindicated as they can increase risk of relapse/development of chronic hepatitis in patients with viral hepatitis. However, anti-inflammatory effect may be useful in chronic active hepatitis (especially idiopathic) to reduce n/v and enable patient to retain food and fluids. Steroids may decrease serum aminotransferase and bilirubin levels, but they do not affect liver necrosis or regeneration. Combination therapy has fewer steroid-related side effects.
Provide supplemental feedings/TPN if needed.	May be necessary to meet caloric requirements if marked deficits are present/symptoms are prolonged.

NURSING DIAGNOSIS:	FLUID VOLUME DEFICIT, HIGH RISK FOR
Risk factors may include:	Excessive losses through vomiting and diarrhea, third-space shift (ascites). Altered clotting process.
Possibly evidenced by:	[Not applicable; presence of signs and symptoms establishes an actual diagnosis.]
DESIRED OUTCOMES/ EVALUATION CRITERIA— PATIENT WILL:	Maintain adequate hydration, as evidenced by stable vital signs, good skin turgor, capillary refill, strong peripheral pulses, and individually appropriate urinary output.

ACTIONS/INTERVENTIONS	RATIONALE
Independent	
Monitor I&O, compare with daily weight. Note enteric losses, e.g., vomiting and diarrhea.	Provides information about replacement needs/effects of therapy. *Note:* Diarrhea may be due to transient flulike response to viral infection and may represent a more serious problem of obstructed portal blood flow with vascular congestion in the GI tract or be the result of medication use (neomycin, lactulose) to decrease serum ammonia levels in the presence of hepatic encephalopathy.
Assess vital signs, peripheral pulses, capillary refill, skin turgor, and mucous membranes.	Indicators of circulating volume/perfusion.
Check for ascites or edema formation. Measure abdominal girth as indicated.	Useful in monitoring progression/resolution of fluid shifts (edema/ascites).
Use small-gauge needles for injections, applying pressure for longer than usual after venipuncture.	Reduces possibility of bleeding into tissues.
Have patient use cotton/sponge swabs and mouthwash instead of toothbrush.	Avoids trauma and bleeding of the gums.
Observe for signs of bleeding, e.g., hematuria/melena, ecchymosis, oozing from gums/puncture sites.	Prothrombin levels are reduced and coagulation times prolonged when vitamin K absorption is altered in GI tract and synthesis of prothrombin is decreased in affected liver.
Collaborative	
Monitor laboratory values, e.g., Hb/Hct, Na+, albumin, and clotting times.	Reflects hydration and identifies sodium retention/protein deficits which may lead to edema formation. Deficits in clotting potentiate risk of bleeding/hemorrhage.
Administer IV fluids (usually glucose), electrolytes;	Provides fluid and electrolyte replacement.
Protein hydrolysates;	Correction of albumin/protein deficits can aid in return of fluid from tissues to the circulatory system.
vitamin K;	Because absorption is altered, supplementation may prevent coagulation problems, which may oc-

541

ACTIONS/INTERVENTIONS

Collaborative

Antacids or H$_2$-receptor antagonists, e.g., cimetadine (Tagamet);

Antidiarrheal agents, e.g., diphenoxylate and atropine (Lomotil);

Fresh frozen plasma.

RATIONALE

cur if clotting factors/prothrombin time is depressed.

Neutralizes/reduces gastric secretions to lower risk of gastric irritation/bleeding.

Reduces fluid/electrolyte loss from GI tract.

May be required to replace clotting factors in the presence of coagulation defects.

NURSING DIAGNOSIS:	SELF-ESTEEM, SITUATIONAL LOW
May be related to:	Annoying/debilitating symptoms, confinement/isolation, length of illness/recovery period.
Possibly evidenced by:	Verbalization of change in lifestyle; fear of rejection/reaction of others, negative feelings about body; feelings of helplessness. Depression; lack of follow-through; self-destructive behavior.
DESIRED OUTCOMES/ EVALUATION CRITERIA— PATIENT WILL:	Identify feelings and methods for coping with negative perception of self. Verbalize acceptance of self in situation, including length of recovery/need for isolation. Acknowledge self as worthwhile; be responsible for self.

ACTIONS/INTERVENTIONS

Independent

Contract with patient regarding time for listening. Encourage discussion of feelings/concerns.

Avoid making moral judgments regarding lifestyle (alcohol use/sexual practices).

Discuss recovery expectations.

RATIONALE

Establishing time enhances trusting relationship. Opportunity to express feelings allows patient to feel more in control of the situation. Verbalization decreases anxiety and depression and facilitates positive coping behaviors. Patient may need to express feelings about being ill; length and cost of illness; possibility of infecting others; and in severe illness, fear of death. May have concerns regarding the stigma of the disease.

Patient may already feel upset/angry, and condemn self; judgments from others will further damage self-esteem.

Recovery period may be prolonged (up to 6 months), potentiating family/situational stress and necessitating need for planning, support, and follow-up.

ACTIONS/INTERVENTIONS

Independent

Assess effect of illness on economic factors of patient/SO.

Offer diversional activities based on energy levels.

Suggest patient wear bright reds or blues/blacks instead of yellows or greens.

Collaborative

Make appropriate referrals for help, as needed, e.g., discharge planners, social services, and/or other community agencies.

RATIONALE

Financial problems may exist because of loss of patient's role functioning in the family/prolonged recovery.

Enables patient to use time and energy in constructive ways that enhance self-esteem and minimize anxiety and depression.

Enhances appearance, because yellow skin tones are intensified by yellow/green colors. Jaundice usually peaks within 1–2 weeks, then gradually resolves over 2–4 weeks.

Can facilitate problem solving and help involved individuals to cope more effectively with situation.

NURSING DIAGNOSIS:	INFECTION, HIGH RISK FOR
Risk factors may include:	Inadequate secondary defenses (e.g., leukopenia, suppressed inflammatory response) and immunosuppression. Malnutrition. Insufficient knowledge to avoid exposure to pathogens.
Possibly evidenced by:	[Not applicable; presence of signs and symptoms establishes an actual diagnosis.]
DESIRED OUTCOMES/ EVALUATION CRITERIA— PATIENT WILL:	Verbalize understanding of individual causative/risk factor(s). Demonstrate techniques; initiate lifestyle changes to avoid reinfection/transmission to others.

ACTIONS/INTERVENTIONS

Independent

Establish isolation techniques for enteric and respiratory infections according to hospital policy; include effective hand washing.

RATIONALE

Prevents transmission of viral disease to others. Thorough hand washing is effective in preventing virus transmission. Type A (infectious) is transmitted by oral-fecal route, contaminated water, and milk and food, especially inadequately cooked shellfish. Type B (serum) is transmitted by contaminated blood/blood products; needle punctures; open wounds; and contact with saliva, urine, stool, and semen. Type C is also transmitted by exposure to blood/blood products. Incidence of both HBV and HCV has increased among hospital personnel and high-risk patients. *Note:* Toxic and al-

543

ACTIONS/INTERVENTIONS	RATIONALE

Independent

	coholic hepatitis are not communicable and do not require special measures/isolation.
Monitor/restrict visitors as indicated.	Patient exposure to infectious processes (especially respiratory) potentiates risk of secondary complications.
Explain isolation procedures to patient/SO.	Understanding of reasons for safeguarding themselves and others can lessen feelings of isolation and stigmatization. Isolation may last 2–3 weeks from onset of illness, depending on type/duration of symptoms.
Give information regarding availability of γ-globulin, ISG, HBIG, hepatitis B vaccine (Recombivax HB, Engerix-B) through health department or family physician.	May be effective in preventing viral hepatitis in those who have been exposed, depending on type of hepatitis and period of incubation.
Administer medications as indicated:	
Antiviral drugs: vidaralune (Vira-A), acyclovir (Zovirax);	Useful in treating chronic active hepatitis.
Interferon alfa-2b (Intron-A);	Effective in treating liver disease related to HCV.
Antibiotics appropriate to causative agents (e.g., Gram-negative, anaerobic bacteria) or secondary process.	Treatment of bacterial hepatitis, or to prevent/limit secondary infections.

NURSING DIAGNOSIS:	SKIN/TISSUE INTEGRITY, IMPAIRED, HIGH RISK FOR
Risk factors may include:	Chemical substance: bile salt accumulation in the tissues.
Possibly evidenced by:	[Not applicable; presence of signs and symptoms establishes an actual diagnosis.]
DESIRED OUTCOMES/ EVALUATION CRITERIA— PATIENT WILL:	Display intact skin/tissues, free of excoriation. Report absence/decrease of pruritus/scratching.

ACTIONS/INTERVENTIONS	RATIONALE

Independent

Use cool showers and baking soda or starch baths. Avoid use of alkaline soaps. Apply calamine lotion as indicated.	Prevents excessive dryness of skin. Provides relief from itching.
Provide diversional activities.	Aids in refocusing attention, reducing tendency to scratch.
Suggest use of knuckles if desire to scratch is uncontrollable. Keep fingernails cut short, apply gloves on comatose patient or during hours of	Reduces potential for dermal injury.

544

ACTIONS/INTERVENTIONS

Independent

sleep. Recommend loose-fitting clothing. Provide soft cotton linens.

Provide a soothing massage at bedtime.

Avoid comments regarding patient's appearance.

Collaborative

Administer medications as indicated:

   Antihistamines, e.g., methdilazine (Tacaryl); diphenhydramine (Benadryl);

   Antilipemics, e.g., cholestyramine (Questran).

RATIONALE

May be helpful in promoting sleep by reducing skin irritation.

Minimizes psychologic stress associated with skin changes.

Relieves itching. *Note:* Use cautiously in severe hepatic disease.

May be used to bind bile acids in the intestine and prevent their absorption. Note side effects of nausea and constipation.

NURSING DIAGNOSIS:	KNOWLEDGE DEFICIT [LEARNING NEED], REGARDING CONDITION, PROGNOSIS, AND TREATMENT NEEDS
May be related to:	Lack of exposure/recall; information misinterpretation. Unfamiliarity with resources.
Possibly evidenced by:	Questions; statement of misconception. Request for information. Inaccurate follow-through of instruction.
DESIRED OUTCOMES/ EVALUATION CRITERIA— PATIENT WILL:	Verbalize understanding of disease process and treatment. Identify relationship of signs/symptoms to the disease and correlate symptoms with causative factors. Initiate necessary lifestyle changes and participate in treat-

---

ACTIONS/INTERVENTIONS

Independent

Assess level of understanding of the disease process, expectations/prognosis, possible treatment options.

Provide specific information regarding prevention/ transmission of disease, e.g., contacts may require

RATIONALE

Identifies areas of lack of knowledge/misinformation and provides opportunity to give additional information as necessary. *Note:* Liver transplantation may be required in the presence of fulminating disease with liver failure.

Needs/recommendations will vary with type of hepatitis (causative agent) and individual situation.

545

ACTIONS/INTERVENTIONS	RATIONALE
Independent	
γ-globulin; personal items should not be shared; strict hand washing and sanitizing of clothes, dishes, and toilet facilities while liver enzymes are elevated. Avoid intimate contact, such as kissing and sexual contact and exposure to infections, especially URI.	
Plan resumption of activity as tolerated with adequate periods of rest. Discuss restriction of heavy lifting, strenuous exercise/ contact sports.	It is not necessary to wait until serum bilirubin levels return to normal to resume activity (may take as long as 2 months), but strenuous activity needs to be limited until the liver returns to normal size. When patient begins to feel better, he or she needs to understand the importance of continued adequate rest in preventing relapse or recurrence. (Relapse occurs in 5%–25% of adults.) Note: Energy level may take up to 3–6 months to return to normal.
Help patient identify diversional activities.	Enjoyable activities will help patient avoid focusing on prolonged convalescence.
Encourage continuation of balanced diet.	Promotes general well-being and enhances energy for healing process/tissue regeneration.
Identify ways to maintain usual bowel function, e.g., adequate intake of fluids/dietary roughage, moderate activity/exercise to tolerance.	Decreased level of activity, changes in food/fluid intake, and slowed bowel motility may result in constipation.
Discuss the side effects and dangers of taking OTC/prescribed drugs (e.g., acetaminophen, aspirin, sulfonamides, some anesthetics) and necessity of notifying future health care providers of diagnosis.	Some drugs are toxic to the liver; many others are metabolized by the liver and should be avoided in severe liver diseases because they may cause cumulative toxic effects/chronic hepatitis.
Discuss restrictions on donating blood.	Prevents spread of infectious disease. Most state laws prevent accepting as donors those who have a history of any type of hepatitis.
Emphasize importance of follow-up physical examination and laboratory evaluation.	Disease process may take several months to resolve. If symptoms persist longer than 6 months, liver biopsy may be required to verify presence of chronic hepatitis.
Review necessity of avoidance of alcohol for a minimum of 6–12 months or longer based on individual tolerance.	Increases hepatic irritation and may interfere with recovery.
Refer to community resources, drug/alcohol treatment program as indicated.	May need additional assistance to withdraw from substance and maintain abstinence to avoid further liver damage.

Cirrhosis of the Liver

Cirrhosis is a chronic disease of the liver characterized by alteration in structure and degenerative changes, impairing cellular function and impeding blood flow through the liver. Causes include malnutrition, inflammation (bacterial or viral), and poisons (e.g., alcohol, carbon tetrachloride, acetaminophen).

RELATED CONCERNS:

Alcoholism (Acute), p 960
Fluid and Electrolyte Imbalances, p 1054
Psychosocial Aspects of Acute Care, p 899
Renal Dialysis, p 646
Renal Failure: Acute, p 618
Total Nutritional Support, p 1039
Upper Gastrointestinal/Esophageal Bleeding, p 454

PATIENT ASSESSMENT DATA BASE

Data are dependent on underlying cause of the condition.

ACTIVITY/REST

May report:	Weakness, fatigue, exhaustion.
May exhibit:	Lethargy.
	Decreased muscle mass/tone.

CIRCULATION

May report:	History of chronic CHF, pericarditis, rheumatic heart disease, cancer (liver malfunction leading to liver failure).
May exhibit:	Hypertension or hypotension (fluid shifts).
	Dysrhythmias, extra heart sounds (S_3, S_4).
	JVD; distended abdominal veins.

ELIMINATION

May report:	Flatulence.
	Diarrhea or constipation; gradual abdominal enlargement.
May exhibit:	Abdominal distention (hepatomegaly, splenomegaly, ascites).
	Decreased/absent bowel sounds.
	Clay-colored stools, melena.
	Dark, concentrated urine.

FOOD/FLUID

May report:	Anorexia, food intolerance/indigestion.
	Nausea/vomiting.
May exhibit:	Weight loss or gain (fluid).
	Tissue wasting.
	Edema generalized in tissues.
	Dry skin, poor turgor.
	Jaundice; spider angiomas.
	Halitosis/fetor hepaticus, bleeding gums.

NEUROSENSORY

May report: SO(s) may report personality changes, depressed mentation.

May exhibit: Changes in mentation, confusion, hallucinations, coma.

Slowed/slurred speech.

Asterixis (hepatic encephalopathy).

PAIN/COMFORT

May report: Abdominal tenderness/RUQ pain.

Pruritus.

Peripheral neuritis.

May exhibit: Guarding/distraction behaviors.

Self-focus.

RESPIRATION

May report: Dyspnea.

May exhibit: Tachypnea, shallow respiration, adventitious breath sounds.

Limited thoracic expansion (ascites).

Hypoxia.

SAFETY

May report: Pruritus.

May exhibit: Fever (more common in alcoholic cirrhosis).

Jaundice, ecchymosis, petechiae.

Spider angiomas/telangiectasis, palmar erythema.

SEXUALITY

May report: Menstrual disorders, impotence.

May exhibit: Testicular atrophy, gynecomastia, loss of hair (chest, underarm, pubic).

TEACHING/LEARNING

May report: History of long-term alcohol use/abuse, alcoholic liver disease.

History of biliary disease, hepatitis, exposure to toxins; liver trauma; upper GI bleeding; episodes of bleeding esophageal varices; use of drugs affecting liver function.

Discharge Plan
Considerations: **DRG projected mean length of stay: 7.2 days.**

May need assistance with homemaker/management tasks.

DIAGNOSTIC STUDIES

Liver scans/biopsy: Detects fatty infiltrates, fibrosis, destruction of hepatic tissues.

Cholecystography/cholangiography: Visualizes bile duct disease, which may be a predisposing factor.

Esophagoscopy: May demonstrate presence of esophageal varices.

Percutaneous transhepatic portography: Visualizes portal venous system circulation.

Serum bilirubin: Elevated because of cellular disruption, inability of liver to conjugate, or biliary obstruction.

548 *AST (SGOT)/ALT (SPGT), LDH:* Increased owing to cellular damage and release of enzymes.

Alkaline phosphatase: Elevated owing to reduced excretion.

Serum albumin: Decreased owing to depressed synthesis.

Globulins (I_gA and I_gG): Increased synthesis.

CBC: Hb/Hct and RBCs may be decreased because of bleeding. RBC destruction and anemia is seen with hypersplenism and iron deficiency. Leukopenia may be present as a result of hypersplenism.

Prothrombin time/PTT: Prolonged (decreased synthesis of prothrombin).

Fibrinogen: Decreased.

BUN: Elevation indicates breakdown of blood/protein.

Serum ammonia: Elevated owing to inability to convert ammonia to urea.

Serum glucose: Hypoglycemia suggests impaired glycogenesis.

Electrolytes: Hypokalemia may reflect increased aldosterone, although various imbalances may occur.

Calcium: May be decreased due to impaired absorption of vitamin D.

Nutrient studies: Deficiency of vitamins A, B_{12}, C, K; folic acid, and iron may be noted.

Urine urobilinogen: May/may not be present. Serves as guide for differentiating liver disease, hemolytic disease, and biliary obstruction.

Fecal urobilinogen: Decreased excretion.

NURSING PRIORITIES

1. Maintain adequate nutrition.
2. Prevent complications.
3. Enhance self-concept, acceptance of situation.
4. Provide information about disease process/prognosis, potential complications, and treatment needs.

DISCHARGE GOALS

1. Nutritional intake adequate for individual needs.
2. Complications prevented/minimized.
3. Dealing with current reality.
4. Disease process, prognosis, potential complications, and therapeutic regimen understood.

NURSING DIAGNOSIS:	NUTRITION, ALTERED: LESS THAN BODY REQUIREMENTS
May be related to:	Inadequate diet; inability to process/digest nutrients.
	Anorexia, n/v, indigestion, early satiety (ascites).
	Abnormal bowel function.
Possibly evidenced by:	Weight loss.
	Changes in bowel sounds and function.
	Poor muscle tone/wasting.
	Imbalances in nutritional studies.
DESIRED OUTCOMES/ EVALUATION CRITERIA— PATIENT WILL:	Demonstrate progressive weight gain toward goal with normalization of laboratory values.
	Experience no further signs of malnutrition.

ACTIONS/INTERVENTIONS	RATIONALE
Independent	
Measure dietary intake by calorie count.	Provides information about intake needs/deficiencies.
Weigh as indicated. Compare changes in fluid status, recent weight history, triceps skin measurement.	It may be difficult to use weight as a direct indicator of nutritional status in view of edema/ascites. Triceps skinfold measurement is useful in assessing changes in muscle mass and subcutaneous fat reserves.
Assist and encourage patient to eat; explain reasons for the type of diet. Feed patient if tiring easily, or have SO assist patient. Consider preferences in food choices.	Proper diet is vital to recovery. Patient may eat better if family is involved and preferred food is included as much as possible.
Encourage patient to eat all meals/supplementary feedings.	Patient may pick at food or eat only a few bites because of loss of interest in food and experience nausea, generalized weakness, malaise.
Serve small, frequent meals.	Poor tolerance to larger meals may be due to increased intra-abdominal pressure/ascites.
Provide salt substitutes if allowed; avoid those containing ammonium.	Salt substitutes enhance the flavor of food and aid in increasing appetite; ammonia potentiates risk of encephalopathy.
Restrict intake of caffeine, gas-producing or spicy and excessively hot or cold foods.	Aids in reducing gastric irritation/diarrhea and abdominal discomfort that may impair oral intake/digestion.
Provide soft foods, avoid roughage if indicated.	Hemorrhage from esophageal varices may occur in advanced cirrhosis.
Provide mouth care frequently and prior to meals.	Patient is prone to sore and/or bleeding gums and bad taste in mouth, which adds to anorexia.
Promote undisturbed rest periods, especially before meals.	Conserving energy reduces metabolic demands on the liver and promotes cellular regeneration.
Recommend cessation of smoking.	Reduces excessive gastric stimulation and risk of irritation/bleeding.
Collaborative	
Monitor laboratory studies, e.g., serum glucose, albumin, total protein, ammonia.	Glucose may be decreased because of impaired glycogenesis, depleted glycogen stores, or inadequate intake. Protein may be low because of impaired metabolism, decreased hepatic synthesis, or loss into peritoneal cavity (ascites). Elevation of ammonia level may require restriction of protein intake to prevent serious complications.
Maintain NPO status when indicated.	Initially, GI rest may be required to reduce demands on the liver and production of GI ammonia/urea.
Consult with dietitian to provide diet that is high in calories and simple carbohydrates, low in fat, and moderate to high in protein; limit sodium and fluid as necessary. Provide liquid supplements as indicated.	High-calorie foods are desired inasmuch as patient intake is usually limited. Carbohydrates supply readily available energy. Fats are poorly absorbed because of liver dysfunction and may contribute to abdominal discomfort. Proteins are

ACTIONS/INTERVENTIONS	RATIONALE
Collaborative	
	needed to improve serum protein levels to reduce edema and to promote liver cell regeneration. *Note:* Protein and foods high in ammonia (e.g., gelatin) are restricted if ammonia level is elevated or if patient has clinical signs of hepatic encephalopathy. In addition, these individuals may tolerate vegetable protein better than meat protein.
Administer tube feedings, hyperalimentation, lipids if indicated.	May be required to supplement diet or to provide nutrients when patient is too nauseated or anorexic to eat or esophageal varices interfere with oral intake.
Administer medications as indicated, e.g.:	
Vitamin supplements, thiamine, iron, folic acid;	Patient is usually vitamin-deficient because of previous poor diet. Also, the injured liver is unable to store vitamins A, B complex, D, and K. An iron and folic acid-deficiency-induced anemia may also exist.
Zinc;	Enhances sense of taste/smell, which may stimulate appetite.
Digestive enzymes, e.g., pancreatin (Viokase);	Promotes digestion of fats and may reduce steatorrhea/diarrhea.
Antiemetics, e.g., trimethobenzamide (Tigan).	Used with caution to reduce n/v and increase oral intake.

NURSING DIAGNOSIS:	**FLUID VOLUME, ALTERED: EXCESS**
May be related to:	Compromised regulatory mechanism (e.g., SIADH, decreased plasma proteins, malnutrition).
	Excess sodium/fluid intake.
Possibly evidenced by:	Edema, anasarca, weight gain.
	Intake greater than output, oliguria, changes in urine specific gravity.
	Dyspnea, adventitious breath sounds, pleural effusion.
	BP changes, including CVP.
	JVD, positive hepatojugular reflex.
	Altered electrolytes.
	Change in mental status.
DESIRED OUTCOMES/ EVALUATION CRITERIA— PATIENT WILL:	Demonstrate stabilized fluid volume, with balanced I&O, stable weight, vital signs within patient's normal range, and absence of edema.

ACTIONS/INTERVENTIONS	RATIONALE

Independent

Measure I&O, noting positive balance (intake in excess of output). Weigh daily, and note gain greater than 0.5 kg/d.

Reflects circulating volume status, developing/resolution of fluid shifts, and response to therapy. Positive balance/weight gain often reflects continuing fluid retention. *Note:* Decreased circulating volume (fluid shifts) may directly affect renal function /urine output, resulting in hepatorenal syndrome.

Monitor BP and CVP. Note JVD/abdominal vein distention.

BP elevations are usually associated with fluid volume excess but may not occur because of fluid shifts out of the vascular space. Distention of external jugular and abdominal veins is associated with vascular congestion.

Assess respiratory status, noting increased respiratory rate, dyspnea.

Indicative of pulmonary congestion/edema.

Auscultate lungs, noting diminished/absent breath sounds and developing adventitious sounds (e.g., crackles).

Increasing pulmonary congestion may result in consolidation, impaired gas exchange, and complications, e.g., pulmonary edema.

Monitor for cardiac dysrhythmias. Auscultate heart sounds, noting development of S_3/S_4 gallop rhythm.

May be caused by CHF, decreased coronary arterial perfusion, and electrolyte imbalance.

Assess degree of peripheral/dependent edema.

Fluids shift into tissues as a result of sodium and water retention, decreased albumin, and increased ADH.

Measure abdominal girth.

Reflects accumulation of fluid (ascites) resulting from loss of plasma proteins/fluid into peritoneal space. *Note:* Excessive fluid accumulation can reduce circulating volume creating a deficit (signs of dehydration).

Encourage bed rest when ascites is present.

May promote recumbency induced diuresis.

Provide frequent mouth care; occasional ice chips (if NPO).

Decreases sensation of thirst.

Collaborative

Monitor serum albumin and electrolytes (particularly potassium and sodium).

Decreased serum albumin affects plasma colloid osmotic pressure, resulting in edema formation. Reduced renal blood flow accompanied by elevated ADH and aldosterone levels and the use of diuretics (to reduce total body water) may cause various electrolyte shifts/imbalances.

Monitor serial chest x-rays.

Vascular congestion, pulmonary edema, and pleural effusions frequently occur.

Restrict sodium and fluids as indicated.

Sodium may be restricted to minimize fluid retention in extravascular spaces. Fluid restriction may be necessary to correct/prevent dilutional hyponatremia.

Administer salt-free albumin/plasma expanders as indicated.

Albumin may be used to increase the colloid osmotic pressure in the vascular compartment

ACTIONS/INTERVENTIONS

Collaborative

Administer medications as indicated:

Diuretics, e.g., spironolactone (Aldactone); furosemide (Lasix);

Potassium;

Positive inotropic drugs and arterial vasodilators.

RATIONALE

(pulling fluid into vascular space), thereby increasing effective circulating volume and decreasing ascitic formation.

Used with caution to control edema and ascites, block effect of aldosterone, and increase water excretion while sparing potassium when conservative therapy with bed rest and sodium restriction do not alleviate problem.

Serum and cellular potassium are usually depleted because of liver disease as well as urinary losses.

Given to increase cardiac output/improve renal blood flow and function, thereby reducing excess fluid.

NURSING DIAGNOSIS:	SKIN INTEGRITY, IMPAIRED, HIGH RISK FOR
Risk factors may include:	Altered circulation/metabolic state. Accumulation of bile salts in skin. Poor skin turgor, skeletal prominence, presence of edema, ascites.
Possibly evidenced by:	[Not applicable; presence of signs and symptoms establishes an actual diagnosis.]
DESIRED OUTCOMES/ EVALUATION CRITERIA— PATIENT WILL:	Maintain skin integrity. Identify individual risk factors and demonstrate behaviors/techniques to prevent skin breakdown.

ACTIONS/INTERVENTIONS

Independent

Inspect skin surfaces/pressure points routinely. Massage bony prominences or areas of continued stress. Use emollient lotions; limit use of soap for bathing.

Reposition on a regular schedule, while in bed/chair: assist with active/passive ROM exercises.

Elevate lower extremities.

Keep linens dry and free of wrinkles.

RATIONALE

Edematous tissues are more prone to breakdown and to the formation of decubiti. Ascites may stretch the skin to the point of tearing in severe cirrhosis.

Repositioning reduces pressure on edematous tissues to improve circulation. Exercises enhance circulation and improve/maintain joint mobility.

Enhances venous return and reduces edema formation in extremities.

Moisture aggravates pruritus and increases risk of skin breakdown.

ACTIONS/INTERVENTIONS

Independent

Clip fingernails short; provide mittens/gloves if indicated.

Provide perineal care following urination and bowel movement.

Use alternating pressure mattress, egg carton mattress, waterbed, sheepskins, as indicated.

Apply calamine lotion, provide baking soda baths. Administer cholestyramine (Questran) if indicated.

RATIONALE

Prevents the patient from inadvertently injuring the skin, especially while sleeping.

Prevents skin excoriation breakdown from bile salts.

Reduces dermal pressure, increases circulation, and diminishes risk of tissue ischemia/breakdown.

May be soothing for itching associated with jaundice, bile salts in skin.

NURSING DIAGNOSIS:	BREATHING PATTERN, INEFFECTIVE, HIGH RISK FOR
Risk factors may include:	Intra-abdominal fluid collection (ascites).
	Decreased lung expansion, accumulated secretions.
	Decreased energy, fatigue.
Possibly evidenced by:	[Not applicable; presence of signs and symptoms establishes an actual diagnosis.]
DESIRED OUTCOMES/ EVALUATION CRITERIA— PATIENT WILL:	Maintain effective respiratory pattern; be free of dyspnea and cyanosis, with ABGs and vital capacity within acceptable range.

ACTIONS/INTERVENTIONS

Independent

Monitor respiratory rate, depth, and effort.

Auscultate breath sounds, noting crackles, wheezes, rhonchi.

Investigate changes in level of consciousness.

Keep head of bed elevated. Position on sides.

Reposition frequently; encourage deep-breathing exercises and coughing.

Monitor temperature. Note presence of chills, increased coughing, changes in color/character of sputum.

RATIONALE

Rapid shallow respirations/dyspnea may be present due to hypoxia and/or fluid accumulation in abdomen.

Indicates developing complications, (e.g., presence of adventitious sounds reflects accumulation of fluid/secretions; absent/diminished sounds suggest atelectasis) increasing risk of infection.

Changes in mentation may reflect hypoxemia and respiratory failure, which often accompany hepatic coma.

Facilitates breathing by reducing pressure on the diaphragm and minimizes risk of aspiration of secretions.

Aids in lung expansion and mobilizing secretions.

Indicative of onset of infection, e.g., pneumonia.

ACTIONS/INTERVENTIONS

Collaborative

Monitor serial ABGs, pulse oximetry, vital capacity measurements, chest x-rays.

Administer supplemental O_2 as indicated.

Assist with respiratory adjuncts, e.g., incentive spirometer, blow bottles.

Prepare for/assist with procedure, e.g:

Paracentesis;

Peritoneovenous shunt.

RATIONALE

Reveals changes in respiratory status, developing pulmonary complications.

May be necessary to treat/prevent hypoxia. If respirations/oxygenation inadequate, mechanical ventilation may be required.

Reduces incidence of atelectasis, enhances mobilization of secretions.

Occasionally done to remove ascites fluid when respiratory embarrassment is not corrected by other measures.

Surgical implant of a catheter to return accumulated fluid in the abdominal cavity to systemic circulation via the vena cava, providing long-term relief of ascites and improvement in respiratory function.

NURSING DIAGNOSIS:	INJURY, HIGH RISK FOR [HEMORRHAGE]
Risk factors may include:	Abnormal blood profile: altered clotting factors (decreased production of prothrombin, fibrinogen, and factors VIII, IX, and X; impaired vitamin K absorption; and release of thromboplastin). Portal hypertension, development of esophageal varices.
Possibly evidenced by:	[Not applicable; presence of signs and symptoms establishes an actual diagnosis.]
DESIRED OUTCOMES/ EVALUATION CRITERIA— PATIENT WILL:	Maintain homeostasis with absence of bleeding. Demonstrate behaviors to reduce risk of bleeding.

ACTIONS/INTERVENTIONS

Independent

Assess for signs/symptoms of GI bleed; e.g., check all secretions for frank or occult blood. Observe color and consistency of stools, NG drainage, or vomitus.

Observe for presence of petechiae, ecchymosis, bleeding from one or more sites.

Monitor pulse, BP, and CVP if available.

RATIONALE

The GI tract (esophagus and rectum) is the most usual source of bleeding due to mucosal fragility and alterations in hemostasis associated with cirrhosis.

Subacute DIC may develop secondary to altered clotting factors.

An increased pulse with decreased BP and CVP can indicate loss of circulating blood volume, requiring further evaluation.

ACTIONS/INTERVENTIONS	RATIONALE
Independent	
Note changes in mentation/level of consciousness.	Changes may indicate decreased cerebral perfusion secondary to hypovolemia, hypoxemia.
Avoid rectal temperature; be gentle with GI tube insertions.	Rectal and esophageal vessels are most vulnerable to rupture.
Encourage use of soft toothbrush, electric razor, avoiding straining for stool, forceful nose blowing, and so forth.	In the presence of clotting factor disturbances, minimal trauma can cause mucosal bleeding.
Use small needles for injections. Apply pressure to small bleeding/venipuncture sites for longer than usual.	Minimizes damage to tissues, reducing risk of bleeding/hematoma.
Avoid use of aspirin-containing products.	Prolongs coagulation, potentiating risk of hemorrhage.
Collaborative	
Monitor Hb/Hct and clotting factors.	Indicators of anemia, active bleeding or impending complications (e.g., DIC).
Administer medications as indicated:	
Supplemental vitamins (e.g., vitamins K, D, and C);	Promotes prothrombin synthesis and coagulation if liver is functional. Vitamin C deficiencies increase susceptibility of GI system to irritation/bleeding.
Stool softeners.	Prevents straining for stool with resultant increase in intra-abdominal pressure and risk of vascular rupture/hemorrhage.
Provide gastric lavage with room temperature/cool saline solution or water as indicated.	Evacuation of blood from GI tract reduces ammonia production and risk of hepatic encephalopathy.
Assist with insertion/maintenance of GI/esophageal tube (e.g., Sengstaken-Blakemore tube).	Temporarily controls bleeding of esophageal varices when control by other means (e.g., lavage) and hemodynamic stability cannot be achieved.
Prepare for surgical procedures, e.g., direct ligation (banding) of varices, esophagogastric resection, splenorenalportacaval anastomosis.	May be needed to control active hemorrhage or to decrease portal and collateral blood vessel pressure to minimize risk of recurrence of bleeding.

NURSING DIAGNOSIS:	THOUGHT PROCESSES, ALTERED, HIGH RISK FOR
Risk factors may include:	Physiologic changes: increased serum ammonia level, inability of liver to detoxify certain enzymes/drugs.
Possibly evidenced by:	[Not applicable; presence of signs and symptoms establishes an actual diagnosis.]
DESIRED OUTCOMES/ EVALUATION CRITERIA— PATIENT WILL:	Maintain usual level of mentation/reality orientation. Demonstrate behaviors/lifestyle changes to prevent/minimize changes in mentation.

ACTIONS/INTERVENTIONS	RATIONALE

Independent

Observe for changes in behavior and mentation, e.g., lethargy, confusion, drowsiness, slowing/slurring of speech, and irritability (may be intermittent). Arouse patient at intervals as indicated.

Ongoing assessment of behavior and mental status is important because of fluctuating nature of impending hepatic coma.

Note development/presence of asterixis, fetor hepaticus, seizure activity.

Suggests elevating serum ammonia levels; increased risk of progression to encephalopathy.

Consult with SO about patient's usual behavior and mentation.

Provides baseline for comparison of current status.

Have patient write name periodically and keep this record for comparison. Report deterioration of ability. Have patient do simple arithmetic computations.

Easy test of neurologic status and muscle coordination.

Reorient to time, place, person as needed.

Assists in maintaining reality orientation, reducing confusion/anxiety.

Maintain a pleasant, quiet environment and approach in a slow, calm manner. Provide uninterrupted rest periods.

Reduces excessive stimulation/sensory overload, promotes relaxation, and may enhance coping.

Provide continuity of care. If possible, assign same nurse over a period of time.

Familiarity provides reassurance, aids in reducing anxiety, and provides a more accurate documentation of subtle changes.

Reduce provocative stimuli, confrontation. Refrain from forcing activities. Assess potential for violent behavior.

Avoids triggering agitated, violent responses; promotes patient safety.

Discuss current situation, future expectation.

Patient/SO may be reassured that intellectual (as well as emotional) function may improve as liver involvement resolves.

Maintain bed rest, assist with self-care activities.

Reduces metabolic demands on liver, prevents fatigue, and promotes healing, lowering risk of ammonia buildup.

Leave side rails up and pad if necessary. Provide close supervision.

Reduces risk of injury when confusion, seizures, or violent behavior occurs.

Investigate temperature elevations. Monitor for signs of infection.

Infection may precipitate hepatic encephalopathy owing to tissue catabolism and release of nitrogen.

Avoid use of narcotics or sedatives, tranquilizers, and limit/restrict use of medications metabolized by the liver.

Certain drugs are toxic to the liver, while other drugs may not be metabolized because of cirrhosis, causing cumulative effects that affect mentation, mask signs of developing encephalopathy, or precipitate coma.

Collaborative

Monitor laboratory studies, e.g., ammonia, electrolytes, pH, BUN, glucose, CBC with differential.

Elevated ammonia levels, hypokalemia, metabolic alkalosis, hypoglycemia, anemia, and infection can precipitate or potentiate development of hepatic coma.

Eliminate or restrict protein in diet. Provide glucose supplements, adequate hydration.

Ammonia (product of the breakdown of protein in the GI tract) is responsible for mental changes in

ACTIONS/INTERVENTIONS

Collaborative

Administer medications as indicated:

  Electrolytes:

  Stool softeners, colonic purges (e.g., magnesium sulfate), enemas, Lactulose;

  Bactericidal agents, e.g., neomycin (Neobiotic); kanamycin (Kantrex).

Administer supplemental O_2.

Assist with procedures as indicated, e.g., dialysis, plasmapheresis, or extracorporeal liver perfusion.

RATIONALE

hepatic encephalopathy. Dietary changes may result in constipation, which also increases bacterial action and formation of ammonia. Glucose provides a source of energy, reducing need for protein catabolism. *Note:* Vegetable protein may be better tolerated than meat sources.

Corrects imbalances and may improve cerebral function/metabolism of ammonia.

Removes protein and blood from intestines. Acidifying the intestine produces diarrhea and decreases production of nitrogenous substances, reducing risk/severity of encephalopathy.

Destroys intestinal bacteria, reducing production of ammonia, to prevent encephalopathy.

Mentation is affected by O_2 concentration and utilization in the brain.

May be used to reduce serum ammonia levels if encephalopathy develops/other measures are not successful.

NURSING DIAGNOSIS:	SELF-ESTEEM/BODY IMAGE, DISTURBANCE IN
May be related to:	Biophysical changes/altered physical appearance.
	Uncertainty of prognosis, changes in role function.
	Personal vulnerability.
	Self-destructive behavior (alcohol-induced disease).
Possibly evidenced by:	Verbalization of change/restriction in lifestyle.
	Fear of rejection or of reaction by others.
	Negative feelings about body/abilities.
	Feelings of helplessness, hopelessness, or powerlessness.
DESIRED OUTCOMES/ EVALUATION CRITERIA— PATIENT WILL:	Verbalize understanding of changes and acceptance of self in the present situation.
	Identify feelings and methods for coping with negative perception of self.

ACTIONS/INTERVENTIONS

Independent

Discuss situation/encourage verbalization of fears/concerns. Explain relationship between nature of disease and symptoms.

RATIONALE

The patient is very sensitive to body changes and may also experience feelings of guilt when cause is related to alcohol (80%) or other drug use.

ACTIONS/INTERVENTIONS

Independent

Support and encourage patient; provide care with a positive, friendly attitude.

Encourage family/SO to verbalize feelings, visit/participate in care.

Assist patient/SO to cope with change in appearance; suggest clothing that does not emphasize altered appearance, e.g., use of red, blue, or black clothing.

Collaborative

Refer to support services, e.g., counselors, psychiatric resources, social service, clergy, and/or alcohol treatment program.

RATIONALE

Caregivers sometimes allow judgmental feelings to affect the care of the patient and need to make every effort to help the patient feel valued as a person.

Family members may feel guilty about the patient's condition and fearful of impending death. They need nonjudgmental emotional support and free access to the patient. Participation in care helps them feel useful and promotes trust between staff, patient, and SO.

Patient may present unattractive appearance due to jaundice, ascites, ecchymotic areas. Providing support can enhance self-esteem and promote patient sense of control.

Increased vulnerability/concerns associated with this illness may require services of additional professional resources.

NURSING DIAGNOSIS:	KNOWLEDGE DEFICIT [LEARNING NEED], REGARDING CONDITION, PROGNOSIS, AND TREATMENT NEEDS
May be related to:	Lack of exposure/recall; information misinterpretation. Unfamiliarity with information resources.
Possibly evidenced by:	Questions; request for information. Statement of misconception. Inaccurate follow-through of instruction. Development of complications.
DESIRED OUTCOMES/ EVALUATION CRITERIA— PATIENT WILL:	Verbalize understanding of disease process/prognosis. Correlate symptoms with causative factors. Initiate necessary lifestyle changes and participate in care.

ACTIONS/INTERVENTIONS

Independent

Review disease process/prognosis and future expectations.

Stress importance of avoiding alcohol. Give information about community services available to aid in alcohol rehabilitation if indicated.

RATIONALE

Provides knowledge base on which patient can make informed choices.

Alcohol is the leading cause in the development of cirrhosis.

ACTIONS/INTERVENTIONS	RATIONALE
Independent	
Inform the patient of altered effects of medications with cirrhosis and the importance of using only drugs prescribed or cleared by a physician who is familiar with patient's history.	Some drugs are hepatotoxic (especially narcotics, sedatives, and hypnotics). In addition, the damaged liver has a decreased ability to metabolize all drugs, potentiating cumulative effect and/or aggravation of bleeding tendencies.
Review procedure for maintaining function of peritoneovenous shunt when present.	Insertion of a Denver shunt requires the patient to periodically pump the chamber to maintain patency of the device. Patients with a LeVeen shunt may wear an abdominal binder and/or engage in Valsalva's maneuver to maintain shunt function.
Assist patient in identifying support person(s).	Because of length of recovery, potential for relapses, and slow convalescence, support systems are extremely important in maintaining behavior modifications.
Emphasize the importance of good nutrition. Recommend avoidance of onions and strong cheeses. Provide written dietary instructions.	Proper dietary maintenance and avoidance of foods high in ammonia aids in remission of symptoms and helps prevent further liver damage. Written instructions will be helpful for patient to refer to at home.
Stress necessity of follow-up care and adherence to therapeutic regimen.	Chronic nature of disease has potential for life-threatening complications. Provides opportunity for evaluation of effectiveness of regimen including patency of shunt if used.
Discuss sodium and salt substitute restrictions and necessity of reading food/OTC drug labels.	Minimizes ascites and edema formation. Overuse of substitutes may result in other electrolyte imbalances. Food, OTC/personal care products (e.g., antacids, some mouthwashes) may contain high sodium content, or alcohol.
Encourage scheduling activities with adequate rest periods.	Adequate rest decreases metabolic demands on the body and increases energy available for tissue regeneration.
Promote diversional activities that are enjoyable to the patient.	Prevents boredom and minimizes anxiety and depression.
Recommend avoidance of persons with infections, especially URI.	Decreased resistance, altered nutritional status, and immune response (e.g., leukopenia may occur with splenomegaly) potentiate risk of infection.
Identify environmental dangers, e.g., carbon tetrachloride-type cleaning agents, exposure to hepatitis.	Can precipitate recurrence.
Instruct patient/SO of signs/symptoms that warrant notification of health care provider, e.g., increased abdominal girth; rapid weight loss/gain; increased peripheral edema; increased dyspnea, fever; blood in stool or urine; excess bleeding of any kind, jaundice.	Prompt reporting of symptoms reduces risk of further hepatic damage and provides opportunity to treat complications before they become life-threatening.
Instruct SO to notify health care providers of any confusion, untidiness, night wandering, tremors, or personality change.	Changes (reflecting deterioration) may be more apparent to SO, although insidious changes may be noted by others with less frequent contact with patient.

Pancreatitis

Pancreatitis is a painful inflammatory condition in which the pancreatic enzymes are prematurely activated resulting in autodigestion of the pancreas. Pancreatitis may be acute or chronic, with symptoms mild to severe.

RELATED CONCERNS:

Adult Respiratory Distress Syndrome (ARDS), p 217
Alcoholism (Acute), p 960
Diabetes Mellitus/Diabetic Ketoacidosis, p 737
Peritonitis, p 514
Psychosocial Aspects of Acute Care, p 899
Renal Failure: Acute, p 618
Sepsis/Septicemia, p 887
Total Nutritional Support, p 1039

PATIENT ASSESSMENT DATA BASE

CIRCULATION

May exhibit:
Hypertension (acute pain); hypotension and tachycardia (hypovolemic shock or toxemia).

Edema, ascites.

Skin pale, cold, mottled with diaphoresis (vasoconstriction/fluid shifts); jaundiced (inflammation/obstruction of common duct); blue-green-brown discoloration around umbilicus (Cullen's sign) from accumulation of blood (hemorrhagic pancreatitis).

EGO INTEGRITY

May exhibit:
Agitation, restlessness, distress, apprehension.

ELIMINATION

May report:
Diarrhea, vomiting.

May exhibit:
Abdominal guarding, distention, and rebound tenderness; rigidity.

Bowel sounds decreased/absent (reduced peristalsis/ileus).

Dark amber or brown, foamy urine (bile).

Frothy, foul-smelling, grayish, greasy, nonformed stool (steatorrhea).

Polyuria (developing DM).

FOOD/FLUID

May report:
Food intolerance, anorexia, persistent vomiting, retching, dry heaves.

Weight loss.

NEUROSENSORY

May exhibit:
Confusion, agitation.

Coarse tremors of extremities (hypocalcemia).

PAIN/COMFORT

May report:
Unrelenting severe deep abdominal pain, usually located in the epigastrium and

periumbilical regions but may radiate to the back. Onset may be sudden and is often associated with heavy drinking or a large meal.

Radiation to chest and back, may increase in supine position.

May exhibit: May curl up with both arms over abdomen.

RESPIRATION

May exhibit: Tachypnea, with/without dyspnea.

Decreased depth of respiration with splinting/guarding actions.

Bibasilar crackles (pleural effusion).

SAFETY

May exhibit: Fever.

SEXUALITY

May exhibit: Current pregnancy (3rd trimester) with shifting of abdominal contents and compression of biliary tract.

TEACHING/LEARNING

May report: Family history of pancreatitis.

History of cholelithiasis with partial or complete common bile duct obstruction; gastritis, duodenal ulcer, duodenitis; diverticulitis; Crohn's disease; recent abdominal surgery (e.g., procedures on the pancreas, biliary tract, stomach, or duodenum), external abdominal trauma.

Excessive alcohol intake.

Use of medications, e.g., antihypertensives, opiates, thiazides, steroids, some antibiotics, estrogens.

Discharge Plan Considerations: **DRG projected mean length of stay: 6.1 days.**

May require assistance with dietary program, homemaker/maintenance tasks.

DIAGNOSTIC STUDIES

CT scan: Determines extent of edema and necrosis.

Ultrasound of abdomen: May be used to identify pancreatic inflammation, abscess, pseudocysts, carcinoma, or obstruction of biliary tract.

Endoscopy: Visualization of pancreatic ducts is useful to diagnose fistulas, obstructive biliary disease, and pancreatic duct strictures/anomalies. Note: This procedure is contraindicated in acute phase.

CT-guided needle aspiration: Done to determine if infection is present.

Abdominal x-rays: May demonstrate dilated loop of small bowel adjacent to pancreas or other intra-abdominal precipitator of pancreatitis, presence of free intraperitoneal air caused by perforation or abscess formation, pancreatic calcification.

Upper GI series: Frequently exhibits evidence of pancreatic enlargement/inflammation.

Serum amylase: Increased due to obstruction of normal outflow of pancreatic enzymes (normal level does not rule out disease).

Urine amylase: Increased within 2–3 days after onset of attack.

Serum lipase: Usually elevates along with amylase, but stays elevated longer.

Serum bilirubin: Increase is common (may be caused by alcoholic liver disease or compression of common bile duct).

Alkaline phosphatase: Usually elevated if pancreatitis is accompanied by biliary disease.

Serum albumin and protein: May be decreased (increased capillary permeability and transudation of fluid into extracellular space).

Serum calcium: Hypocalcemia may appear 2–3 days after onset of illness (usually indicates fat necrosis and may accompany pancreatic necrosis).

Potassium: Hypokalemia may occur because of gastric losses; hyperkalemia may develop secondary to tissue necrosis, acidosis, renal insufficiency.

Triglycerides: Levels may exceed 1700 mg/dL and may be causative agent in acute pancreatitis.

LDH/AST (SGOT): May be elevated up to 15 times normal because of biliary and liver involvement.

CBC: WBC of 10,000–25,000 is present in 80% of patients. Hb may be lowered because of bleeding. Hct is usually elevated (hemoconcentration associated with vomiting or from effusion of fluid into pancreas or retroperitoneal area).

Serum glucose: Transient elevations are common, especially during initial/acute attacks. Sustained hyperglycemia reflects widespread β cell damage and pancreatic necrosis and is a poor prognostic sign.

PTT: Prolonged if coagulopathy develops due to liver involvement and fat necrosis.

Urinalysis: Amylase, myoglobin, hematuria, and proteinuria may be present (glomerular damage).

Stool: Increased fat content (steatorrhea) indicative of insufficient digestion of fats and protein.

NURSING PRIORITIES

1. Control pain and promote comfort.
2. Prevent/treat fluid and electrolyte imbalance.
3. Reduce pancreatic stimulation while maintaining adequate nutrition.
4. Prevent complications.
5. Provide information about disease process/prognosis and treatment needs.

DISCHARGE GOALS

1. Pain relieved/controlled.
2. Hemodynamically stable.
3. Complications prevented/minimized.
4. Disease process/prognosis, potential complications, and therapeutic regimen understood.

NURSING DIAGNOSIS:	PAIN [ACUTE]
May be related to:	Obstruction of pancreatic, biliary ducts.
	Chemical contamination of peritoneal surfaces by pancreatic exudate/autodigestion of pancreas.
	Extension of inflammation to the retroperitoneal nerve plexus.
Possibly evidenced by:	Reports of pain.
	Self-focusing, grimacing, distraction/guarding behaviors.
	Autonomic responses, alteration in muscle tone.
DESIRED OUTCOMES/ EVALUATION CRITERIA— PATIENT WILL:	Report pain is relieved/controlled.
	Follow prescribed therapeutic regimen.
	Demonstrate use of methods that provide relief.

ACTIONS/INTERVENTIONS	RATIONALE
Independent	
Investigate verbal reports of pain, noting specific location and intensity (0–10 scale). Note factors that aggravate and relieve pain.	Pain is often diffuse, severe, and unrelenting in acute or hemorrhagic pancreatitis. Severe pain is often the major symptom in patients with chronic pancreatitis. Isolated pain in the RUQ reflects involvement of the head of the pancreas. Pain in the LUQ suggests involvement of the pancreatic tail. Localized pain may indicate development of pseudocysts or abscesses.
Maintain bed rest during acute attack. Provide quiet, restful environment.	Decreases metabolic rate and GI stimulation/secretions, thereby reducing pancreatic activity.
Promote position of comfort, e.g., on one side with knees flexed, sitting up and leaning forward.	Reduces abdominal pressure/tension, providing some measure of comfort and pain relief. *Note:* Supine position often increases pain.
Provide alternate comfort measures (e.g., back rub); encourage relaxation techniques (e.g., guided imagery, visualization); quiet diversional activities (e.g., TV, radio).	Promotes relaxation and enables patient to refocus attention; may enhance coping.
Keep environment free of food odors.	Sensory stimulation can activate pancreatic enzymes, increasing pain.
Administer analgesics in timely manner (smaller, more frequent doses).	Severe/prolonged pain can aggravate shock and is more difficult to relieve, requiring larger doses of medication, which can mask underlying problems/complications and may contribute to respiratory depression.
Maintain meticulous skin care, especially in presence of draining abdominal wall fistulas.	Pancreatic enzymes can digest the skin and tissues of the abdominal wall, creating a chemical burn.
Collaborative	
Administer medications as indicated:	
Narcotic analgesics, e.g., meperidine (Demerol);	Meperidine is usually effective in relieving pain and may be preferred over morphine, which can display side effect of biliary-pancreatic spasms. Paravertebral block has been used to achieve prolonged pain control. *Note:* Patients who have recurrent or chronic pancreatitis episodes may be difficult to manage because they may become addicted to the narcotics given for pain control.
Sedatives, e.g., diazepam (Valium); antispasmodics, e.g., atropine;	Potentiates action of narcotic to promote rest and to reduce muscular/ductal spasm, thereby reducing metabolic needs, enzyme secretions.
Antacids, e.g., Mylanta, Maalox, Amphogel, Riopan;	Neutralizes gastric acid to reduce production of pancreatic enzymes and to reduce incidence of upper GI bleeding.
Cimetidine (Tagamet); ranitidine (Zantac).	Decreasing secretion of HCl reduces stimulation of the pancreas and associated pain.
Withhold food and fluid as indicated.	Limits/reduces release of pancreatic enzymes and resultant pain.

ACTIONS/INTERVENTIONS

Collaborative

Maintain gastric suction when used.

Prepare for surgical intervention if indicated.

RATIONALE

Prevents accumulation of gastric secretions, which can stimulate pancreatic enzyme activity.

Surgical exploration may be required in presence of intractable pain/complications involving the biliary tract.

NURSING DIAGNOSIS:	FLUID VOLUME DEFICIT, HIGH RISK FOR
Risk factors may include:	Excessive losses: vomiting, gastric suctioning.
	Increase in size of vascular bed (vasodilation, effects of kinins).
	Thirdspace fluid transudation, ascites formation.
	Alteration of clotting process, hemorrhage.
Possibly evidenced by:	[Not applicable; presence of signs and symptoms establishes an actual diagnosis.]
DESIRED OUTCOMES/ EVALUATION CRITERIA— PATIENT WILL:	Maintain adequate hydration as evidenced by stable vital signs, good skin turgor, prompt capillary refill, strong peripheral pulses, and individually appropriate urinary output.

ACTIONS/INTERVENTIONS

Independent

Monitor BP and measure CVP if available.

Measure I&O including vomiting/gastric aspirate, diarrhea. Calculate 24-hour fluid balance.

Note decrease in urine output (less than 400 ml/24 hours).

Record color and character of gastric drainage as well as noting pH and presence of occult blood.

Weigh as indicated. Correlate with calculated fluid balance.

Note poor skin turgor, dry skin/mucous membranes, reports of thirst.

RATIONALE

Fluid sequestration (shifts into thirdspace,) bleeding, and release of vasodilators (kinins) and cardiac depressant factor triggered by pancreatic ischemia may result in profound hypotension. Reduced cardiac output/poor organ perfusion secondary to a hypotensive episode can precipitate widespread systemic complications.

Indicators of replacement needs/effectiveness of therapy.

Oliguria may occur, signaling renal impairment/ ATN, related to increase in renal vascular resistance or reduced/altered renal blood flow.

Risk of gastric bleeding/hemorrhage is high.

Weight loss may suggest hypovolemia; however, edema, fluid retention, and ascites may be reflected by increased or stable weight, even in the presence of muscle wasting.

Further physiologic indicators of dehydration.

ACTIONS/INTERVENTIONS	RATIONALE

Independent

Observe/record peripheral and dependent edema. Measure abdominal girth if ascites present.

Edema/fluid shifts occur as a result of increased vascular permeability, sodium retention, and decreased colloid osmotic pressure in the intravascular compartment. *Note:* Fluid loss (sequestration) of greater than 6 L/48 h is considered a poor prognostic sign.

Investigate changes in sensorium, e.g., confusion, slowed responses.

Changes may be related to hypovolemia, hypoxia, electrolyte imbalance, or impending delirium tremens (in the patient with acute pancreatitis secondary to excessive alcohol intake). Severe pancreatic disease may cause toxic psychosis.

Auscultate heart sounds, note rate and rhythm. Monitor/document rhythm changes.

Cardiac changes/dysrhythmias may reflect hypovolemia and/or electrolyte imbalance, commonly hypokalemia/hypocalcemia. Hyperkalemia may occur related to tissue necrosis, acidosis, and renal insufficiency and may precipitate lethal dysrhythmias if uncorrected. S_3 gallop in conjunction with JVD and crackles suggest heart failure/pulmonary edema. *Note:* Cardiovascular complications are common and include MI, pericarditis, and pericardial effusion with/without tamponade.

Inspect skin for petechiae, hematomas, and unusual wound or venipuncture bleeding. Note hematuria, mucous membrane bleeding, and bloody gastric contents.

DIC may be initiated by release of active pancreatic proteases into the circulation. The most frequently affected organs are the kidneys, skin, and lungs.

Observe/report coarse muscle tremors, twitching, positive Chvostek's or Trousseau's sign.

Symptoms of calcium imbalance. Calcium binds with free fats in the intestine and is lost by secretion in the stool.

Collaborative

Administer fluid replacement as indicated, e.g., saline solutions, albumin, blood/blood products, dextran.

Choice of replacement solution may be less important than rapidity and adequacy of volume restoration. Saline solutions and albumin may be used to promote mobilization of fluid back into vascular space. Low molecular-weight dextran is sometimes used to reduce risk of renal dysfunction and pulmonary edema associated with pancreatitis.

Monitor laboratory studies, e.g., Hb/Hct, protein, albumin, electrolytes, BUN, creatinine, urine osmolality and sodium/potassium, coagulation studies.

Identifies deficits/replacement needs and developing complications, e.g., ATN, DIC.

Replace electrolytes, e.g., sodium, potassium, chloride, calcium as indicated.

Decreased oral intake and excessive losses greatly affect electrolyte/acid base balance, which is necessary to maintain optimal cellular/organ function.

Prepare for/assist with peritoneal lavage, hemoperitoneal dialysis.

Removes toxic chemicals/pancreatic enzymes and allows for more rapid correction of metabolic abnormalities in severe/unresponsive cases of acute pancreatitis.

NURSING DIAGNOSIS:	NUTRITION, ALTERED: LESS THAN BODY REQUIREMENTS
May be related to:	Vomiting, decreased oral intake.
	Prescribed dietary restrictions.
	Loss of digestive enzymes and insulin (related to pancreatic outflow obstruction or necrosis/autodigestion).
Possibly evidenced by:	Reported inadequate food intake.
	Aversion to eating, reported altered taste sensation, lack of interest in food.
	Weight loss.
	Poor muscle tone.
DESIRED OUTCOMES/ EVALUATION CRITERIA— PATIENT WILL:	Demonstrate progressive weight gain toward goal with normalization of laboratory values.
	Experience no signs of malnutrition.
	Demonstrate behaviors, lifestyle changes to regain and/or maintain appropriate weight.

ACTIONS/INTERVENTIONS	RATIONALE
Independent	
Assess abdomen, noting presence/character of bowel sounds, abdominal distention, and reports of nausea.	Gastric distention and intestinal atony are frequently present, resulting in reduced/absent bowel sounds. Return of bowel sounds and relief of symptoms signal readiness for discontinuation of gastric aspiration (NG tube).
Provide frequent oral care.	Decreases vomiting stimulus and inflammation/irritation of dry mucous membranes associated with dehydration and mouth breathing when NG is in place.
Assist patient in selecting food/fluids that meet nutritional needs and restrictions when diet is resumed.	Previous dietary habits may be unsatisfactory in meeting current needs for tissue regeneration and healing. Use of gastric stimulants, e.g., caffeine, alcohol, cigarettes, gas-producing foods or ingestion of large meals may result in excessive stimulation of the pancreas/recurrence of symptoms.
Observe color/consistency/amount of stools. Note frothy consistency/foul odor.	Steatorrhea may develop from incomplete digestion of fats.
Note signs of increased thirst and urination or changes in mentation and visual acuity.	May warn of developing hyperglycemia associated with increased release of glucagon (damage to α cells) or decreased release of insulin (damage to β cells).
Test urine for sugar and acetone.	Early detection of inadequate glucose utilization may prevent development of ketoacidosis.

567

ACTIONS/INTERVENTIONS	RATIONALE
Collaborative	
Maintain NPO status and gastric suctioning in acute phase.	Prevents stimulation and release of pancreatic enzymes (secretin), released when chyme and HCl acid enter the duodenum.
Monitor serum glucose.	Indicator of insulin needs because hyperglycemia is frequently present although not usually in levels high enough to produce ketoacidosis.
Administer hyperalimentation and lipids, if indicated.	IV administration of calories, lipids, and amino acids should be instituted before nutrition/nitrogen depletion is advanced.
Resume oral intake with clear liquids and advance diet slowly to provide high protein, high carbohydrate diet, when indicated.	Oral feedings given too early in the course of illness may exacerbate symptoms. Loss of pancreatic function/reduced insulin production may require initiation of a diabetic diet.
Provide medium-chain triglycerides (e.g., MCT, Portagen).	MCTs provide supplemental calories/nutrients that do not require pancreatic enzymes for digestion/absorption.
Administer medications as indicated:	
Vitamins, e.g., A, D, E, K;	Replacement required as fat metabolism is altered, reducing absorption/storage of fat-soluble vitamins.
Replacement enzymes, e.g., pancreatin (Viokase), pancrelipase (Cotazym);	Used in chronic pancreatitis to correct deficiencies to promote digestion and absorption of nutrients.
Anticholinergics, e.g., methantheline bromide (Banthine);	Thought to reduce pancreatic and gastric secretions with depression of the vagal mechanisms and decrease of motility. The decrease in volume and concentration of enzymes provide rest for the inflamed area. *Note:* These drugs are contraindicated in the presence of shock/paralytic ileus, and current drug studies have not proven their efficiency.
Insulin;	Corrects persistent hyperglycemia caused by injury to β cells and increased release of glucocorticoids. Insulin therapy is usually short-term unless permanent damage to pancreas occurs.

NURSING DIAGNOSIS:	INFECTION, HIGH RISK FOR
Risk factors may include:	Inadequate primary defenses: stasis of body fluids, altered peristalsis, change in pH secretions.
	Immunosuppression.
	Nutritional deficiencies.
	Tissue destruction, chronic disease.

Possibly evidenced by:	[Not applicable; presence of signs and symptoms establishes an actual diagnosis.]
DESIRED OUTCOMES/ EVALUATION CRITERIA— PATIENT WILL:	Achieve timely healing, free of signs of infection. Be afebrile. Participate in activities to reduce risk of infection.

ACTIONS/INTERVENTIONS

Independent

Use strict aseptic technique when changing surgical dressings or working with IV lines, indwelling catheters/tubes, drains. Change soiled dressings promptly.

Stress importance of good hand washing.

Observe rate and characteristics of respirations, breath sounds. Note occurrence of cough and sputum production.

Encourage frequent position changes, deep breathing and coughing. Assist with ambulation as soon as stable.

Observe for signs of infection, e.g.:

Fever and respiratory distress in conjunction with jaundice;

Increased abdominal pain, rigidity/rebound tenderness, diminished/absent bowel sounds;

Increased abdominal pain/tenderness, recurrent fever (greater than 101°F), leukocytosis, hypotension, tachycardia, and chills.

Collaborative

Obtain culture specimens, e.g., blood, wound, urine, sputum, or pancreatic aspirate.

Administer antibiotic therapy as indicated:

cephalosporins, e.g., cefoxitin sodium (Mefoxin); plus aminoglycosides, e.g., gentamicin (Garamycin); tobramycin (Nebcin).

Prepare for surgical intervention as necessary.

RATIONALE

Limits sources of infection, which can lead to sepsis in a compromised patient. *Note:* Studies indicate that infectious complications are responsible for about 80% of deaths associated with pancreatitis.

Reduces risk of cross-contamination.

Fluid accumulation and limited mobility predisposes to respiratory infections and atelectasis. Accumulation of ascites fluid may cause elevated diaphragm and shallow abdominal breathing.

Enhances ventilation of all lung segments and promotes mobilization of secretions.

Cholestatic jaundice and decreased pulmonary function may be first sign of sepsis involving Gram-negative organisms.

Suggestive of peritonitis.

Abscesses can occur 2 or more weeks after the onset of pancreatitis (mortality can exceed 50%) and should be suspected whenever the patient is deteriorating despite supportive measures.

Identifies presence of infection and causative organism.

Broad spectrum antibiotics are generally recommended for sepsis. However, therapy will be based on the specific organisms cultured.

Abscesses may be surgically drained with resection of necrotic tissue. Sump tubes may be inserted for antibiotic irrigation and drainage of pancreatic debris. Pseudocysts (persisting for several weeks) may be drained because of the risk and incidence of infection/rupture.

ACTIONS/INTERVENTIONS	RATIONALE
Independent	
Review specific cause of current episode and prognosis.	Provides knowledge base on which patient can make informed choices.
Discuss other causative/associated factors, e.g., excessive alcohol intake, gallbladder disease, duodenal ulcer, hyperlipoproteinenemias, some drugs (e.g., oral contraceptives, thiazides, Lasix, INH, glucocorticoids, sulfonamides).	Avoidance may help to limit damage and prevent development of a chronic condition.
Explore availability of treatment programs/rehabilitation of chemical dependency if indicated.	Alcohol abuse is currently the most common cause of recurrence of chronic pancreatitis. Other drug usage is increasing as a factor, whether prescribed or illicit. *Note:* Pain of pancreatitis can be severe and prolonged and may lead to narcotic dependence, requiring need for referral to pain clinic.
Stress the importance of follow-up care, and review symptoms that need to be reported immediately to physician, e.g., recurrence of pain, persistent fever, n/v, abdominal distention, frothy/foul-smelling stools, general intolerance of food.	Prolonged recovery period requires close monitoring to prevent recurrence/complications, e.g., infection, pancreatic pseudocysts.
Review importance of initially continuing bland, low-fat diet with frequent small feedings and restricted caffeine, with gradual resumption of a normal diet within individual tolerance.	Understanding the purpose of the diet in maximizing the use of available enzymes while avoiding overstimulation of the pancreas may enhance patient involvement in self-monitoring of dietary needs and responses to foods.

ACTIONS/INTERVENTIONS	RATIONALE

Independent

Instruct in use of pancreatic enzyme replacements and bile salt therapy as indicated, avoiding concomitant ingestion of hot foods/fluids.

If permanent damage has occurred to the pancreas, exocrine deficiencies will occur, requiring long-term replacement. Hot foods/fluids can inactivate enzymes.

Recommend cessation of smoking.

Nicotine stimulates gastric secretions and unnecessary pancreatic activity.

Discuss signs/symptoms of DM, i.e., polydipsia, polyuria, weakness, weight loss.

Damage to the β cells may result in a temporary or permanent alteration of insulin production.

Bibliography

General References

Bellak, JP and Bamford, PA: Nursing Assessment: A Multidimensional Approach. Jones & Bartlett, Boston, 1987.
Berkow, R (ed): The Merck Manual, ed 15. Merck Sharp & Dohme Research Laboratories, Rahway, NJ, 1987.
Cella, JH and Watson, J: Nurse's Manual of Laboratory Tests. FA Davis, Philadelphia, 1989.
Condon, RE and Nyhus, LM, (eds): Manual of Surgical Therapeutics, ed 7. Little, Brown & Co, Boston, 1988.
Deglin, JH and Vallerand, AH: Davis's Drug Guide for Nurses, ed 3. FA Davis, Philadelphia, 1992.
Diseases and Disorders Handbook, ed 3. Springhouse, Springhouse, PA, 1989.
Doenges, ME and Moorhouse, MF: Nurse's Pocket Guide: Nursing Diagnoses with Interventions, ed 3. FA Davis, Philadelphia, 1991.
Dunagan, WC and Ridner, ML (eds): Manual of Medical Therapeutics, ed 26. Little, Brown & Co, Boston, 1989.
Fischbach, F: A Manual of Laboratory and Diagnostic Tests, ed 4. JB Lippincott, Philadelphia, 1992.
Guyton, AC: Textbook of Medical Physiology, ed 8. WB Saunders, Philadelphia, 1991.
Kuhn, MM: Pharmacotherapeutics: A Nursing Process Approach, ed 2, FA Davis, 1991.
Professional Guide to Diseases, ed 3. Springhouse, Springhouse, PA, 1989.
Suddarth, DS (ed): The Lippincott Manual of Nursing Practice, ed 5. JB Lippincott, Philadelphia, 1991.
Thomas, CL (ed): Taber's Cyclopedic Medical Dictionary, ed 16. FA Davis, Philadelphia, 1989.
Thompson, JM, McFarland, GK, Hirsh, JE, et al: Mosby's Manual of Clinical Nursing, ed 2. CV Mosby, St Louis, 1989.

Articles

Alltop, SA: Teaching for discharge: Gastrotomy tubes. RN 51(11):42, 1989.
Benedict, P and Haddad, A: Postop teaching for the colostomy patient. RN 52(3):85, 1989.
Bowden, PR, Glombicki, AP, and Smith, JL: Diagnosis of lower GI bleeding. Hospital Medicine, February 1992, p 50.
Brentin, L and Sick, A: Caring for the morbidly obese. AJN 91(8):40, 1991.
Bryant, GA: When the bowel is blocked. RN 55(1):58, 1992
Cerrato, PL: Would a new diet help your gallstone patient? RN 52(7):59, 1989.
Butler, L: Hepatitis: A nurse's story. RN 55(4):66, 1992.
Champion, M: NSAIDs and the gut: A gloomy picture. Gastroenterology Observer 1991, p 2.
Dalton-Lochner, D and Connor, PA: Beyond ileostomy: Surgery for a normal life. RN 52(7):29, 1989.
Forse, RA, Karam, B, MacLean, LD, et al: Antibiotic prophylaxis for surgery in morbidly obese patients. Surgery 6(4):750, 1989.
Grau, PA: Are you at risk for Hepatitis B? Nursing91 21(3):44, 1991.
Grauwitz, DF: Endoscopic cholecystectomy: The patient-friendly alternative. Nursing90 20(12):58, 1990.
Heeg, JM and Coleman, DA: Hepatitis kills. RN 55(4):60, 1992.
Hoffman, S: Hepatitis, C: Earning its letter. Harvard Medical School Health Letter October 1990, p 3.
Isenberg, JI: Should safety concerns with available ulcer treatment influence drug selection? J Clin Gastroenterol 90(Suppl 2):S48, 1990.
Jordan, PH: Surgery for peptic ulcer disease. Curr Probl Surg April 1991, p 270.
Jeter, KF: Clinical Reviews: Meeting the various needs of the ostomy patient. The Consultant Pharmacist November/December 1986, p 287.
Johnston, JH: Gastrointestinal endoscopy [Editorial]. 30(5):313, 1984.
Jurf, JB, Clements, L, and Lorente, J: Cholecystectomy made easier. AJN 20(12):38, 1990.
Lancaster, S and Stockbridge, J: PV shunts relieve ascites. RN 55(8):58, 1992.

Long, L: Ileostomy care: Overcoming the obstacles. Nursing91 21(10):73, 1991.

Madda, MA: Helping ostomy patients manage medications. Nursing91 21(3):47, 1991.

Martin, FL: When the liver breaks down. RN 55(8):52, 1992.

McCarthy, DM: Clinical drug appraisals: Nisoprostol. Drug Therapy July 1989, p 59.

Pachter, A: Should nurses receive the Hepatitis B vaccine? Nursing88 18(6):51, 1988.

Pasner, D: What's wrong with this stoma? AJN 20(4):46, 1990.

Reveille, RM: Endoscopic Variceal Ligation: Equipment and Technique. University of Colorado Health Sciences Center, Denver, unpublished.

Robinson, M, Mills, RJ, and Euler, AR: Ranitidine prevents duodenal ulcers associated with non-steroidal anti-inflammatory drug therapy. Aliment Pharmacol Therap 91(5):143, 1991.

Rowland, GA, Marks, DA, and Torres, WE: The new gallstone destroyers and dissolvers. AJN 19(11):1473, 1989.

Silverstein, F: Upper GI bleeding. Audio-Digest Gastroenterology 4(9): 1990.

Smith, A: When the pancreas self-destructs. AJN 91(9):38, 1991.

Steiner, JF: Counseling the ostomy patient to overcome medication problems. Home Health Care, 1989.

Sugarman, HJ: Gastric surgery for morbid obesity. Problems in General Surgery 4(2):258, 1987.

Thompson, C: Managing acute pancreatitis. RN 55(3):52, 1992.

Van Neil, J: What's wrong with this peristomal skin? AJN 91(12):44, 1991.

Wardell, TL: Assessing and managing gastric ulcer. Nursing91 21(3):34, 1991.

Willis, DA, Harbit, MD, and Julius, LM: Gallstones: Alternatives to surgery. RN 53(4): 44, 1990.

CHAPTER 9

DISEASES OF THE BLOOD/BLOOD-FORMING ORGANS

Anemias (Iron Deficiency, Pernicious, Aplastic, Hemolytic) _____

Anemia is a symptom of an underlying condition, such as loss of blood components, inadequate elements, or lack of required nutrients for the formation of blood cells, that results in the decreased oxygen-carrying capacity of the blood. There are numerous types of anemias with various causes. The following types of anemia are discussed here: Iron deficiency (ID), the result of inadequate absorption or excessive loss of iron; *pernicious* (PA), the result of a lack of the intrinsic factor essential for the absorption of vitamin B_{12}; *aplastic,* due to failure of bone marrow; and *hemolytic,* due to shortened RBC life span. Nursing care for the anemic patient has a common theme even though the medical treatments vary widely.

RELATED CONCERNS

AIDS, p 850
Burns, p 820
Cancer, p 1014
Cirrhosis, p 547
Congestive Heart Failure, p 48
Intestinal Surgery, p 500
Psychosocial Aspects of Acute Care, p 899
Renal Failure: Acute, p 618
Renal Failure: Chronic, p 632
Rheumatoid Arthritis, p 875
Tuberculosis, p 241
Upper Gastrointestinal/Esophageal Bleeding, p 454

PATIENT ASSESSMENT DATA BASE

ACTIVITY/REST

May report:	Fatigue, weakness, general malaise.
	Loss of productivity; diminished enthusiasm for work.
	Low exercise tolerance.
	Greater need for rest and sleep.
May exhibit:	Tachycardia/tachypnea; dyspnea on exertion or at rest.
	Lethargy, withdrawal, apathy, lassitude, and lack of interest in surroundings.

573

Muscle weakness and decreased strength.

Ataxia, unsteady gait.

Slumping of shoulders, drooping posture, slow walk, and other cues indicative of fatigue.

CIRCULATION

May report:
History of chronic blood loss, e.g., chronic GI bleeding, heavy menses (ID); angina, CHF (due to increased workload of the heart).

History of chronic infective endocarditis.

Palpitations (compensatory tachycardia).

May exhibit:
BP: Increased systolic with stable diastolic and a widened pulse pressure; postural hypotension.

Dysrhythmias: ECG abnormalities, e.g., ST-segment depression and flattening or depression of the T wave; tachycardia.

Throbbing carotid pulsations (compensatory mechanism to provide oxygen/nutrients to cells).

Heart sounds: Systolic murmur (ID).

Extremities (color): Pallor of the skin and mucous membranes (conjunctiva, mouth, pharynx, lips) and nail beds. (Note: In black patients, pallor may appear as a grayish cast); waxy, pale skin (aplastic, PA) or bright lemon yellow (PA).

Sclera: Blue or pearl white (ID).

Capillary refill delayed (diminished blood flow to the periphery and compensatory vasoconstriction).

Nails: Brittle, spoon-shaped (koilonychia) (ID).

Hair: Dry, brittle, thinning; premature graying (PA).

EGO INTEGRITY

May report:
Religious/cultural beliefs affecting treatment choices, e.g., refusal of blood transfusions.

May exhibit:
Depression.

ELIMINATION

May report:
History of pyelonephritis, renal failure.

Flatulence, malabsorption syndrome (ID).

Hematemesis, fresh blood in stool, melena.

Diarrhea or constipation.

Diminished urine output.

May exhibit:
Abdominal distention.

FOOD/FLUID

May report:
Decreased dietary intake, low intake of animal protein/high intake of cereal products (ID).

Mouth or tongue pain, difficulty swallowing (ulcerations in pharynx).

Nausea/vomiting, dyspepsia, anorexia.

Recent weight loss.

Insatiable craving or pica for ice, dirt, cornstarch, paint, clay, and so forth. (ID).

May exhibit:	Beefy red/smooth appearance of tongue (PA; folic acid and vitamin B_{12} deficiencies). Dry, pale mucous membranes. Skin turgor: Poor, with dry, shriveled appearance/loss of elasticity (ID). Stomatitis and glossitis (deficiency states). Lips: cheilitis, i.e., inflammation of the lips with cracking at the corners of the mouth (ID).

HYGIENE

May exhibit:	Debilitated, unkempt appearance.

NEUROSENSORY

May report:	Headaches, fainting, dizziness, vertigo, tinnitus, inability to concentrate. Insomnia, dimness of vision, and spots before eyes. Weakness, poor balance, wobbly legs; paresthesias of hands/feet (PA); claudication. Sensation of being cold.
May exhibit:	Irritability, restlessness, depression, drowsiness, apathy. Mentation: Notable slowing and dullness in response. Ophthalmic: Retinal hemorrhages (aplastic, PA). Epistaxis, bleeding from other orifices (aplastic). Disturbed coordination, ataxia: Decreased vibratory and position sense, positive Romberg's sign, paralysis (PA).

PAIN/COMFORT

May report:	Vague abdominal pains; headache (ID).

RESPIRATION

May report:	History of TB, lung abscesses. Shortness of breath at rest and with activity.
May exhibit:	Tachypnea, orthopnea, and dyspnea.

SAFETY

May report:	History of occupational exposure to chemicals, e.g., benzene, lead, insecticides, phenylbutazone, naphthalene. History of exposure to radiation either as a treatment modality or by accident. History of cancer, cancer therapies. Cold and/or heat intolerance. Previous blood transfusions. Impaired vision. Poor wound healing, frequent infections.
May exhibit:	Low grade fever, chills, night sweats. Generalized lymphadenopathy. Petechiae and ecchymosis (aplastic).

SEXUALITY

May report: Changes in menstrual flow, e.g., menorrhagia or amenorrhea (ID).

Loss of libido (men and women).

Impotence.

May exhibit: Pale cervix and vaginal walls.

TEACHING/LEARNING

May report: Family tendency for anemia (ID/PA).

Past/present use of anticonvulsants, antibiotics, chemotherapeutic agents (bone marrow failure), aspirin, anti-inflammatory drugs, or anticoagulants.

Chronic use of alcohol.

Recent/current episode of active bleeding (ID).

History of liver, renal disease; hematologic problems; celiac or other malabsorption disease; regional enteritis; tapeworm manifestations; polyendocrinopathies; autoimmune problem (e.g., antibodies to parietal cells, intrinsic factor, thyroid and T-cell antibodies).

Prior surgeries, e.g., splenectomy; tumor excision; prosthetic valve replacement; surgical excision of duodenum or gastric resection, partial/total gastrectomy (ID/PA).

History of problems with wound healing or bleeding; chronic infections, (RA), chronic granulomatous disease, or cancer (secondary anemias).

Discharge Plan Considerations: **DRG projected mean length of stay: 4.6 days.**

May require assistance with treatment (injections); self-care activities and/or homemaker/maintenance tasks; changes in dietary plan.

DIAGNOSTIC STUDIES

CBC: Hemoglobin and hematocrit decreased.

Erythrocyte count: Decreased (PA), severely decreased (aplastic); MCV and MCH decreased and microcytic with hypochromic erythrocytes (ID), elevated (PA). Pancytopenia (aplastic).

Reticulocyte count: Varies, e.g., decreased (PA), elevated (bone marrow response to blood loss/hemolysis).

Stained RBC examination: Detects changes in color and shape (may indicate particular type of anemia).

ESR: Elevation indicates presence of inflammatory reaction, e.g., increased RBC destruction or malignant disease.

RBC survival time: Useful in the differential diagnosis of the anemias, e.g., in certain types of anemias, RBCs have shortened life spans.

Erythrocyte fragility test: Decreased (ID).

WBCs: Total cell count as well as specific WBCs (differential) may be increased (hemolytic) or decreased (aplastic).

Platelet count: Decreased (aplastic); elevated (ID); normal or high (hemolytic).

Hemoglobin electrophoresis: Identifies type of hemoglobin structure.

Serum bilirubin (unconjugated): Elevated (PA, hemolytic).

Serum folate and vitamin B$_{12}$: Aids in diagnosing anemias related to deficiencies in intake/absorption.

Serum iron: Absent (ID); high (hemolytic).

Serum TIBC: Increased (ID).

Serum ferritin: Decreased (ID).

Bleeding time: Prolonged (aplastic).

Serum LDH: May be elevated (PA).

Schilling test: Decreased urinary excretion of vitamin B_{12} (PA).

Guaiac: May be positive for occult blood in urine, stools, and gastric contents, reflecting acute/chronic bleeding (ID).

Gastric analysis: Decreased secretions with elevated pH and absence of free hydrochloric acid (PA).

Bone marrow aspiration/biopsy examination: Cells may show changes in number, size and shape, helping to differentiate type of anemia, e.g., increased megaloblasts (PA), fatty marrow with diminished blood cells (aplastic).

Endoscopic and radiographic studies: Checks for bleeding sites; GI bleeding.

NURSING PRIORITIES

1. Enhance tissue perfusion.
2. Provide nutritional/fluid needs.
3. Prevent complications.
4. Provide information about disease process, prognosis, and treatment regimen.

DISCHARGE GOALS

1. ADLs met by self or with assistance of others.
2. Complications prevented/minimized.
3. Disease process/prognosis and therapeutic regimen understood.

NURSING DIAGNOSIS:	TISSUE PERFUSION, ALTERED: (SPECIFY)
May be related to:	Reduction of cellular components necessary for delivery of oxygen/nutrients to the cells.
Possibly evidenced by:	Palpitations, angina.
	Pallor of skin, mucous membranes; dry, brittle nails and hair.
	Cold extremities.
	Decreased urinary output.
	Nausea/vomiting, abdominal distension.
	Changes in BP, delayed capillary refill.
	Inability to concentrate, disorientation.
DESIRED OUTCOMES/ EVALUATION CRITERIA— PATIENT WILL:	Demonstrate adequate perfusion as individually appropriate, e.g., stable vital signs; pinkish mucous membranes, good capillary refill; adequate urine output; usual mentation.

ACTIONS/INTERVENTIONS	RATIONALE
Independent	
Monitor vital signs, assess capillary refill, color of skin/mucous membranes, nail beds.	Provides information about degree/adequacy of tissue perfusion and helps to determine needed interventions.
Elevate head of bed as tolerated.	Enhances lung expansion to maximize oxygenation for cellular uptake. *Note:* May be contraindicated if hypotension is present.
Monitor respiratory effort; auscultate breath sounds noting adventitious sounds.	Presence of dyspnea, crackles may reflect developing CHF due to prolonged cardiac strain/compensatory elevation of cardiac output.
Investigate reports of chest pain, palpitations.	Cellular ischemia affects myocardial tissues/potentiates risk of infarction.
Assess for slowed verbal response, irritability, agitation, impaired memory, confusion.	May indicate impaired cerebral function due to hypoxia or vitamin B_{12} deficiency.
Orient/reorient patient as needed. Write out schedule of activities for patient to refer to. Provide sufficient time for patient to complete thoughts, communication, and activities.	Aids in improving thought processes and ability to perform/maintain needed ADLs.
Note reports of feeling cold. Maintain environmental temperature and body warmth as indicated.	Vasoconstriction (shunting of blood to vital organs) decreases peripheral circulation, impairing tissue perfusion. Patient's comfort/need for warmth must be balanced with need to avoid excessive heat with resultant vasodilation (reduces organ perfusion).
Avoid the use of heating pads or hot water bottles. Measure temperature of bath water with a thermometer.	Thermoreceptors in the dermal tissues may be dulled due to oxygen deprivation.
Collaborative	
Monitor laboratory studies, e.g., Hb/Hct and RBC count, ABGs.	Identifies deficiencies and treatment needs/response to therapy.
Administer whole blood/packed RBCs, blood products as indicated. Monitor closely for transfusion complications.	Increases number of oxygen-carrying cells; corrects deficiencies to reduce risk of hemorrhage.
Administer supplemental oxygen as indicated.	Maximizes oxygen transport to tissues.
Prepare for surgical intervention if indicated.	Bone marrow transplant may be done in presence of bone marrow failure/aplastic anemia.

NURSING DIAGNOSIS:	ACTIVITY INTOLERANCE
May be related to:	Imbalance between oxygen supply (delivery) and demand.
Possibly evidenced by:	Weakness and fatigue.

	Reports of decreased exercise/activity tolerance.
	Greater need for sleep/rest.
	Palpitations, tachycardia, increased BP/respiratory response with minor exertion.
DESIRED OUTCOMES/ EVALUATION CRITERIA— PATIENT WILL:	Report an increase in activity tolerance (including ADLs).
	Demonstrate a decrease in physiologic signs of intolerance, e.g., pulse, respirations, and BP remain within patient's normal range.

ACTIONS/INTERVENTIONS

Independent

Assess patient's ability to perform normal tasks/ADLs, noting reports of weakness, fatigue, and difficulty accomplishing tasks.

Assess for loss of balance/gait disturbance, muscle weakness.

Monitor BP, pulse, respirations, during and after activity. Note adverse responses to increased levels of activity (e.g., increased HR/BP, dysrhythmias, dizziness, dyspnea, tachypnea, and so forth).

Provide quiet atmosphere. Maintain bed rest if indicated. Monitor and limit visitors, phone calls, and repeated unplanned interruptions.

Change patient's position slowly and monitor for dizziness.

Prioritize nursing care schedules to enhance rest. Alternate rest periods with activity periods.

Provide assistance with activities/ambulation as necessary, allowing patient to do as much as possible.

Plan activity progression with patient, including activities that the patient views as essential. Increase activity levels as tolerated.

Use energy-saving techniques, e.g., shower chair, sitting to perform tasks.

Instruct patient to stop activity if palpitations, chest pain, shortness of breath, weakness, or dizziness occur.

RATIONALE

Influences choice of interventions/needed assistance.

May indicate neurologic changes associated with vitamin B_{12} deficiency affecting patient safety/risk of injury.

Cardiopulmonary manifestations result from attempts by the heart and lungs to bring adequate amounts of oxygen to the tissues.

Enhances rest to lower body's oxygen requirements and reduces strain on the heart and lungs.

Postural hypotension or cerebral hypoxia may cause dizziness, fainting, and increased risk of injury.

Maintains energy level and alleviates strain on the cardiac and respiratory systems.

While help may be necessary, self-esteem is enhanced when patient does some things for self.

Promotes gradual return to normal activity level and improved muscle tone/stamina without undue fatigue. Increases self-esteem and sense of control.

Encourages patient to do as much as possible, while conserving limited energy and preventing fatigue.

Excessive cardiopulmonary strain/stress may lead to decompensation/failure.

579

NURSING DIAGNOSIS:	NUTRITION, ALTERED: LESS THAN BODY REQUIREMENTS
May be related to:	Failure to ingest or inability to digest food/absorb nutrients necessary for formation of normal RBCs.
Possibly evidenced by:	Weight loss/weight below normal for age, height, and build.
	Decreased triceps skinfold measurement.
	Changes in gums, oral mucous membranes.
	Decreased tolerance for activity, weakness, and loss of muscle tone.
DESIRED OUTCOMES/ EVALUATION CRITERIA— PATIENT WILL:	Demonstrate progressive weight gain or stable weight, with normalization of laboratory values.
	Experience no signs of malnutrition.
	Demonstrate behaviors, lifestyle changes to regain and/or maintain appropriate weight.

ACTIONS/INTERVENTIONS	RATIONALE
Independent	
Assess nutritional history, including food preferences.	Identifies deficiencies, suggests possible interventions.
Observe and record patient's food intake.	Monitors caloric intake or insufficient quality of food consumption.
Weigh daily.	Monitors weight loss or effectiveness of nutritional interventions.
Provide attractive, appetizing meals in a pleasant atmosphere.	May promote appetite and enhance intake.
Provide small, frequent meals and/or between-meal nourishments.	Eating small meals may reduce fatigue and thus enhance intake, while preventing gastric distension.
Observe and record occurrence of nausea/vomiting, flatus, and other related symptoms.	GI symptoms may reflect effects of anemias (hypoxia) on organs.
Provide and assist with good oral hygiene; before and after meals, use soft-bristled toothbrush for gentle brushing. Provide dilute mouthwash if oral mucosa is ulcerated.	Enhances appetite and oral intake. Diminishes bacterial growth, minimizing possibility of infection. Special mouth-care techniques may be needed if tissue fragile/ulcerated/bleeding and pain is severe.
Collaborative	
Consult with dietitian.	Aids in establishing dietary plan to meet individual needs.
Monitor laboratory studies, e.g., Hb/Hct, BUN, albumin, protein, transferrin, serum iron, B_{12}, folic acid, TIBC, serum electrolytes.	Evaluates effectiveness of treatment regimen, including dietary sources of needed nutrients.

ACTIONS/INTERVENTIONS

Collaborative

Administer medications as indicated, e.g.:

    Vitamin and mineral supplements, e.g, cyanocobalamin (vitamin B_{12}), folic acid (Folvite); ascorbic acid (vitamin C);

    Iron dextran (IM/IV);

    Oral iron supplements, e.g., ferrous sulfate (Feosol); ferrous gluconate (Fergon).

    Hydrochloric acid (HCl);

Antifungal or anesthetic mouthwash if indicated.

Provide bland diet, low in roughage, avoiding hot, spicy, or very acidic foods as indicated.

Provide nutritional supplements, e.g., Ensure, Isocal.

RATIONALE

Replacements needed depend on type of anemia and/or presence of poor oral intake and identified deficiencies.

Administered until estimated deficit is corrected and is reserved for those who cannot absorb or comply with oral iron therapy, or when blood loss is too rapid for oral replacement to be effective.

May be useful in some types of iron deficiency anemias.

Potentiates absorption of vitamin B_{12} during initial weeks of therapy.

May be needed in the presence of stomatitis/glossitis to promote oral tissue healing and facilitate intake.

When oral lesions are present, pain may restrict type of foods patient can tolerate.

Enhances intake of protein and calories.

NURSING DIAGNOSIS:	SKIN INTEGRITY, IMPAIRED, HIGH RISK FOR
Risk factors may include:	Circulatory and neurologic changes (anemia).
	Impaired mobility.
	Nutritional deficits.
Possibly evidenced by:	[Not applicable; presence of signs and symptoms establishes an actual diagnosis.]
DESIRED OUTCOMES/ EVALUATION CRITERIA— PATIENT WILL:	Maintain skin integrity.
	Identify individual risk factors/behaviors to prevent dermal injury.

ACTIONS/INTERVENTIONS

Independent

Assess skin integrity, noting changes in turgor, altered color, local warmth, erythema, excoriation.

Reposition periodically and massage bony surfaces when patient is sedentary or in bed.

Keep skin surfaces dry and clean. Limit use of soap.

RATIONALE

Condition of the skin is affected by circulation, nutrition, and immobility. Tissues may become fragile and prone to infection and breakdown.

Increases circulation to all skin areas limiting tissue ischemia/effects of cellular hypoxia.

Moist, contaminated areas provide excellent media for growth of pathogenic organisms. Soap may dry skin excessively and increase irritation.

ACTIONS/INTERVENTIONS	RATIONALE

Independent

Assist with active or passive ROM exercises.

Promotes circulation to tissues, prevents stasis.

Collaborative

Use protective devices, e.g., sheepskin, egg-crate, alternating air pressure/water mattress, heel/elbow protectors, and pillows as indicated.

Avoids skin breakdown by preventing/reducing pressure against skin surfaces.

NURSING DIAGNOSIS:	CONSTIPATION OR DIARRHEA
May be related to:	Decreased dietary intake; changes in digestive processes.
	Drug therapy side effects.
Possibly evidenced by:	Changes in frequency, characteristics, and amount of stool.
	Nausea/vomiting, decreased appetite.
	Reports of abdominal pain, urgency, cramping.
	Altered bowel sounds.
DESIRED OUTCOMES/ EVALUATION CRITERIA— PATIENT WILL:	Establish/return to normal patterns of bowel functioning.
	Demonstrate changes in behaviors/lifestyle, as necessitated by causative, contributing factors.

ACTIONS/INTERVENTIONS	RATIONALE

Independent

Observe stool color, consistency, frequency, and amount.

Assists in identifying causative/contributing factors and appropriate interventions.

Auscultate bowel sounds.

Bowel sounds are generally increased in diarrhea and decreased in constipation.

Monitor intake and output with specific attention to food/fluid intake.

May identify dehydration, excessive loss of fluids or aid in identifying dietary deficiencies.

Encourage fluid intake of 2500–3000 ml/d within cardiac tolerance.

Assists in improving stool consistency if constipated. Will help to maintain hydration status if diarrhea is present.

Avoid foods that are gas forming.

Decreases gastric distress and abdominal distention.

Assess perianal skin condition frequently, noting changes in skin condition or beginning breakdown. Perform pericare after each BM if diarrhea is present.

Prevents skin excoriation and breakdown.

Collaborative

Consult with dietitian to provide well-balanced diet high in fiber and bulk.

Fiber resists enzymatic digestion and absorbs liquids in its passage along the intestinal tract and thereby produces bulk, which acts as a stimulant to defecation.

ACTIONS/INTERVENTIONS	RATIONALE
Collaborative	
Provide stool softeners, mild stimulants, bulk-forming laxatives, or enemas as indicated. Monitor effectiveness.	Facilitates defecation when constipation is present.
Administer antidiarrheal medications, e.g., diphenoxylate hydrochloride with atropine (Lomotil) and water-absorbing drugs, e.g., Metamucil.	Decreases intestinal motility when diarrhea is present.

NURSING DIAGNOSIS:	**INFECTION, HIGH RISK FOR**
Risk factors may include:	Inadequate secondary defenses, e.g., decreased hemoglobin, leukopenia, or decreased granulocytes (suppressed inflammatory response).
	Inadequate primary defenses, e.g., broken skin, stasis of body fluids; invasive procedures; chronic disease, malnutrition.
Possibly evidenced by:	[Not applicable; presence of signs and symptoms establishes an actual diagnosis.]
DESIRED OUTCOMES/ EVALUATION CRITERIA— PATIENT WILL:	Identify behaviors to prevent/reduce risk of infection.
	Achieve timely wound healing, free of purulent drainage or erythema, and be afebrile.

ACTIONS/INTERVENTIONS	RATIONALE
Independent	
Promote good hand washing by health care givers and patient.	Prevents cross-contamination/bacterial colonization. *Note:* Patient with severe/aplastic anemia may be at risk from normal skin flora.
Maintain strict aseptic techniques with procedures/wound care.	Reduces risk of bacterial colonization/infection.
Provide meticulous skin, oral, and perianal care.	Reduces risk of skin/tissue breakdown and infection.
Encourage frequent position changes/ambulation, coughing, and deep-breathing exercises.	Promotes ventilation of all lung segments and aids in mobilizing secretions to prevent pneumonia.
Promote adequate fluid intake.	Assists in liquefying respiratory secretions to facilitate expectoration and prevent stasis of body fluids (e.g., respiratory and renal).
Monitor/limit visitors. Provide isolation if appropriate. Restrict live plants/cut flowers.	Limits exposure to bacteria/infections. Protective isolation may be required in aplastic anemia, when immune response is most compromised.
Monitor temperature. Note presence of chills and tachycardia with/without fever.	Reflective of inflammatory process/infection requiring evaluation/treatment.
Observe for wound erythema/drainage.	Indicators of local infection. *Note:* Pus formation may be absent if granulocytes are depressed.

583

ACTIONS/INTERVENTIONS

Collaborative

Obtain specimens for culture/sensitivity as indicated.

Administer topical antiseptics; systemic antibiotics.

RATIONALE

Verifies presence of infection, identifies specific pathogen and influences choice of treatment.

May be used prophylactically to reduce colonization or used to treat specific infectious process.

NURSING DIAGNOSIS:	KNOWLEDGE DEFICIT [LEARNING NEED], REGARDING CONDITION, PROGNOSIS, AND TREATMENT NEEDS
May be related to:	Lack of exposure/recall. Information misinterpretation. Unfamiliarity with information resources.
Possibly evidenced by:	Questions; request for information. Statement of misconception. Inaccurate follow-through of instruction. Development of preventable complications.
DESIRED OUTCOMES/ EVALUATION CRITERIA— PATIENT WILL:	Verbalize understanding of the nature of the disease process, diagnostic procedures, and treatment plan. Identify causative factors. Initiate necessary behaviors/lifestyle changes.

ACTIONS/INTERVENTIONS

Independent

Provide information about specific anemia. Discuss the fact that therapy depends on the type and severity of the anemia.

Review purpose and preparations for diagnostic studies.

Explain that blood taken for laboratory studies will not worsen anemia.

Review required diet alterations to meet specific dietary needs (determined by type of anemia/deficiency).

Assess resources (e.g., financial and cooking).

Encourage cessation of smoking.

RATIONALE

Provides knowledge base on which patient can make informed choices. Allays anxiety and may promote cooperation with therapeutic regimen.

Anxiety/fear of the unknown increases stress level, which in turn increases the cardiac workload. Knowledge of what to expect can diminish anxiety.

This is often an unspoken concern that can potentiate patient's anxiety.

Red meat, liver, egg yolks, green leafy vegetables, whole wheat bread, and dried fruits are sources of iron. Green vegetables, whole grains, liver, and citrus fruits are sources of folic acid and vitamin C (enhances absorption of iron).

Inadequate resources may affect ability to purchase/prepare appropriate food items.

Decreases available oxygen and causes vasoconstriction.

ACTIONS/INTERVENTIONS	RATIONALE

Independent

Instruct and demonstrate self-administration of oral iron preparations:

Iron replacement usually takes 3–6 months, whereas vitamin B_{12} injections may be necessary for the rest of the patient's life.

Discuss importance of taking only prescribed dosages;

Overdose of iron medication can be toxic.

Advise taking with meals or immediately after meals;

Iron is best absorbed on an empty stomach. However, iron salts are gastric irritants and may cause dyspepsia, diarrhea, and abdominal discomfort if taken on an empty stomach.

Dilute liquid preparations (preferably with orange juice) and administer through a straw;

Undiluted liquid iron preparations may stain the teeth. Ascorbic acid promotes iron absorption.

Caution that BM may appear greenish black/tarry;

Excretion of excessive iron will change stool color.

Stress importance of good oral hygiene measures.

Certain iron supplements (e.g., Feosol) may leave deposits on teeth and gums.

Instruct patient/SO about parenteral iron administration:

Z-track administration of medication;

Prevents extravasation (leaking) with accompanying pain.

Use separate needles for withdrawing and injecting the medication;

Medication may stain the skin.

Caution regarding possible systemic reaction, (e.g., flushing, vomiting, nausea, myalgia) and discuss importance of reporting symptoms.

Possible side effects of therapy requiring reevaluation of drug choice and dosage.

Discuss increased susceptibility to infections, signs/symptoms requiring medical intervention, e.g., fever, sore throat; erythema/draining wound; cloudy urine, burning with urination.

Decreased leukocyte production potentiates risk of infection. *Note:* Purulent drainage may not form in absence of granulocytes (aplastic).

Identify safety concerns, e.g., avoidance of forceful blowing of nose, contact sports, constipation/straining for stool; use of electric razors, soft toothbrush.

Reduces risk of hemorrhage from fragile tissues.

Review good oral hygiene, necessity for regular dental care.

Effects of anemia (oral lesions) and/or iron supplements increase risk of infection/bacteremia.

Instruct to avoid use of aspirin products.

Increases bleeding tendencies.

Refer to appropriate community resources when indicated, e.g., social services for food stamps, Meals-on-Wheels.

May need assistance with groceries/meal preparation.

Sickle Cell Crisis

Sickle cell anemia is a genetic disease that primarily affects blacks and people of Mediterranean descent. It renders the individual vulnerable to repeated painful crises that can progressively destroy vital organs. These crises are:

Vaso-occlusive/thrombocytic crisis: Related to infection, dehydration, fever, hypoxia, and characterized by multiple infarcts of bones, joints, and other target organs, with tissue pain and necrosis caused by plugs of sickled cells in the microcirculation.

Hypoplastic/aplastic crisis: May be secondary to severe (usually viral) infection or folic acid deficiency, resulting in cessation of production of RBCs and bone marrow.

Hyperhemolytic crisis: Reticulocytes are increased in peripheral blood; and bone marrow is hyperplastic. Characterized by anemia and jaundice (effects of hemolysis).

Sequestration crisis: Massive, sudden erythrostasis with pooling of blood in the viscera (splenomegaly), resulting in hypovolemic shock/possible death. This crisis occurs in patients with intact splenic function.

RELATED CONCERNS

Cerebrovascular Accident/Stroke, p 290
Cholecystitis with Cholelithiasis, p 523
Cirrhosis of the Liver, p 547
Congestive Heart Failure, p 48
Pneumonia, p 162
Psychosocial Aspects of Acute Care, p 899
Pulmonary Embolism, p 174
Seizure Disorders, p 261
Sepsis/Septicemia, p 887

PATIENT ASSESSMENT DATA BASE

ACTIVITY/REST

May report:	Lethargy, fatigue, weakness, general malaise.
	Loss of productivity; decreased exercise tolerance; greater need for sleep and rest.
May exhibit:	Listlessness; severe weakness and increasing pallor (aplastic crisis).
	Gait disturbances (pain, kyphosis, lordosis); inability to walk (pain).
	Poor body posture (slumping of shoulders indicative of fatigue).
	Decreased ROM (swollen, inflamed joints); joint, bone deformities.
	Generalized retarded growth; tower-shaped skull with frontal bossing; disproportionately long arms and legs, short trunk, narrowed shoulders/hips, and long, tapered fingers.

CIRCULATION

May report:	Palpitations or anginal chest pain (concomitant CAD/myocardial ischemia).
	Intermittent claudication.
May exhibit:	Apical pulse: PMI may be displaced to the left (cardiomegaly).
	Tachycardia, dysrhythmias (hypoxia), systolic murmurs.
	BP: widened pulse pressure.
	Generalized symptoms of shock, e.g., hypotension, rapid thready pulse, and shallow respirations (sequestration crisis).
	Peripheral pulses: Throbbing on palpation.
	Bruits (reflects compensatory mechanisms of anemia; may also be auscultated over the spleen due to multiple splenic infarcts).

Capillary refill delayed (anemia or hypovolemia).

Skin color: Pallor or cyanosis of skin, mucous membranes, and conjunctiva. Note: Pallor may appear as yellowish brown color in brown-skinned patients, and as ashen gray in black-skinned patients. Jaundice: Scleral icterus, generalized icteric coloring (excessive RBC hemolysis).

Dry skin/mucous membranes.

Diaphoresis (either sequestration or vaso-occlusive crisis; acute pain or shock).

ELIMINATION

May report: Frequent voiding, voiding in large amounts, nocturia.

May exhibit: RUQ abdominal tenderness, enlargement/distention (hepatomegaly); ascites.

LUQ fullness (enlarged spleen or may be atrophic and nonfunctional from repeated splenic infarcts and fibrosis).

Dilute, pale, straw-colored urine; hematuria or smoky appearance (multiple renal infarcts).

Urine specific gravity decreased (may be fixed with progressive renal disease).

EGO INTEGRITY

May report: Resentment and frustration with disease, fear of rejection from others.

Generalized poor self-esteem/poor self-concept.

Concern regarding being a burden to SOs; financial concerns, possible loss of insurance/benefits; lost time at work/school, fear of genetic transmission of disease.

May exhibit: Anxiety, restlessness, irritability, apprehension, withdrawal, narrowed focus, self-focusing, unresponsiveness to questions, regression; depression, decreased self-esteem. Dependent relationship with whomever can offer security and protection.

FOOD/FLUID

May report: Thirst.
Anorexia, nausea/vomiting.

May exhibit: Height/weight usually in the lower percentiles.
Poor skin turgor with visible tenting (crisis, infection, and dehydration).
Dry skin, mucous membranes.
JVD and general peripheral edema (concomitant CHF).

HYGIENE

May report: Difficulty maintaining ADLs (pain or severe anemia).

May exhibit: Slovenly, unkempt appearance.

NEUROSENSORY

May report: Headaches or dizziness.

Transient visual disturbances (e.g., hemianopsia, nystagmus).

Tingling in the extremities.

Disturbances in pain and position sense.

May exhibit: Mental status: Usually unaffected except in cases of severe sickling (cerebral infarction/intracranial hemorrhage).

Weakness of the mouth, tongue, and facial muscles; aphasia (in cerebral infarction when dominant hemisphere infarcted).

Abnormal reflexes, decreased muscle strength/tone; abnormal involuntary movements; hemiplegia or sudden hemiparesis, quadriplegia.

Ataxia, seizures.

Meningeal irritation (intracranial hemorrhage), e.g., decreasing level of consciousness, nuchal rigidity, focal neurologic deficits, vomiting, severe headache.

PAIN/COMFORT

May report:

Pain as severe, throbbing, gnawing of varied location (localized, migratory, or generalized).

Recurrent, sharp, transient headaches.

Back pain (changes in vertebral column from recurrent infarctions); joint/bone pain accompanied by warmth, tenderness, erythema, and occasional effusions (vaso-occlusive crisis). Note: Deep bone infarctions may have no apparent signs of irritation.

Gallbladder tenderness and pain (excessive accumulation of bilirubin due to increased erythrocyte destruction).

May exhibit:

Sensitivity to palpation over affected areas.

Holding joints in position of comfort; decreased ROM (result of pain and swollen joints).

Maladaptive pain behaviors, e.g., guilt for being ill, denial of any aspect of disease, indulgence in precipitating factors (overwork, strenuous exercise).

RESPIRATION

May report:

Dyspnea on exertion or at rest.

History of repeated pulmonary infections/infarctions, pulmonary fibrosis, pulmonary hypertension or cor pulmonale.

May exhibit:

Acute respiratory distress, e.g., dyspnea, chest pain, and cyanosis (especially in crisis).

Bronchial/bronchovesicular sounds in lung periphery; diminished breath sounds (pulmonary fibrosis).

Crackles, rhonchi, wheezes, diminished breath sounds (CHF).

Increased AP diameter of the chest (barrel chest).

SAFETY

May report:

History of transfusions.

May exhibit:

Low-grade fever.

Impaired vision (sickle retinopathy), decreased visual acuity (temporary/permanent blindness).

Leg ulcers (common in adult patients, especially found on the internal and external malleoli and the medial aspect of the tibia).

Lymphadenopathy.

SEXUALITY

May report:

Loss of libido; amenorrhea; priapism, impotence.

May exhibit:

Delayed sexual maturity.

Pale cervix and vaginal walls (anemia).

588

TEACHING/LEARNING

May report: History of CHF (chronic anemic state); pulmonary hypertension or cor pulmonale (multiple pulmonary infections/infarctions); chronic leg ulcers, delayed healing.

Discharge Plan Considerations: **DRG projected mean length of stay: 4.6 days.**
May need assistance with shopping, transportation, self-care, homemaker/maintenance tasks.

DIAGNOSTIC STUDIES

CBC: Reticulocytosis (count may vary from 30%–50%); leukocytosis (especially in vaso-occlusive crisis), decreased Hb/Hct and total RBCs, thrombocytosis, and a normal to decreased MCV.

Stained RBC examination: Demonstrates partially or completely sickled, crescent-shaped cells, anisocytosis, poikilocytosis, polychromasia, target cells, Howell-Jolly bodies, basophilic stippling, occasional nucleated RBCs (normoblasts).

Sickle-turbidity tube test (Sickledex): Routine screening test that determines the presence of hemoglobin S but does not differentiate between sickle cell anemia and trait.

Hemoglobin electrophoresis: Identifies any abnormal hemoglobin types and differentiates between sickle cell trait and sickle cell anemia. Results may be inaccurate if patient has received a blood transfusion within 3–4 months prior to testing.

ESR: Elevated.

Erythrocyte fragility: Decreased (osmotic fragility or RBC fragility). RBC survival time: Decreased (accelerated breakdown).

ABGs: May reflect decreased PO_2 (defects in gas exchange at the alveolar capillary level); acidosis (hypoxemia and acidic states in vaso-occlusive crisis).

Serum bilirubin (total and indirect): Elevated (increased RBC hemolysis).

Acid phosphatase: Elevated (release of erythrocytic ACP into the serum).

Alkaline phosphatase: Elevated during vaso-occlusive crisis (bone and liver damage).

LDH: Elevated (RBC hemolysis).

Serum potassium and uric acid: Elevated during vaso-occlusive crisis (RBC hemolysis).

Serum iron: May be elevated or normal (increased iron absorption due to excessive RBC destruction).

TIBC: Normal or decreased.

Urine/fecal urobilinogen: Increased (more sensitive indicators of RBC destruction than serum levels).

IVP: May be done to evaluate kidney damage.

Bone radiographs: May demonstrate skeletal changes, e.g., osteoporosis, osteosclerosis, osteomyelitis, or avascular necrosis.

X-rays: May indicate bone thinning, osteoporosis.

NURSING PRIORITIES

1. Promote adequate cellular oxygenation/perfusion.
2. Alleviate pain.
3. Prevent complications.
4. Provide information about disease, process/prognosis, and treatment needs.

DISCHARGE GOALS

1. Oxygenation/perfusion adequate to meet cellular needs.
2. Pain relieved/controlled.
3. Complications prevented/minimized.
4. Disease process, future expectations, potential complications, and therapeutic regimen understood.

589

NURSING DIAGNOSIS:	GAS EXCHANGE, IMPAIRED
May be related to:	Decreased oxygen-carrying capacity of the blood, reduced RBC life span/premature destruction, abnormal RBC structure; sensitivity to low oxygen tension (strenuous exercise, increase in altitude).
	Increased blood viscosity (occlusions created by sickled cells packing together within the capillaries) and pulmonary congestion (impairment of surface phagocytosis).
	Predisposition to bacterial pneumonia, pulmonary infarcts.
Possibly evidenced by:	Dyspnea, use of accessory muscles.
	Restlessness, confusion.
	Tachycardia.
	Cyanosis (hypoxia).
DESIRED OUTCOMES/ EVALUATION CRITERIA— PATIENT WILL:	Demonstrate improved ventilation/oxygenation as evidenced by respiratory rate within normal limits, absence of cyanosis and use of accessory muscles; normal breath sounds.
	Participate in ADLs without weakness and fatigue.
	Display improved pulmonary function tests improved/normal.

ACTIONS/INTERVENTIONS	RATIONALE
Independent	
Monitor respiratory rate/depth, use of accessory muscles, areas of cyanosis.	Indicators of adequacy of respiratory function or degree of compromise, and therapy needs/effectiveness.
Auscultate breath sounds, noting presence/absence, and adventitious sounds.	Development of atelectasis and stasis of secretions can impair gas exchange.
Monitor vital signs; note changes in cardiac rhythm.	Compensatory changes in vital signs and development of dysrhythmias reflect effects of hypoxia on cardiovascular system.
Assess reports of chest pain and increasing fatigue. Observe for signs of increased fever, cough, adventitious breath sounds.	Reflective of developing respiratory infection, which increases the workload of the heart and oxygen demand.
Assist in turning, coughing, and deep breathing.	Promotes optimal chest expansion, mobilization of secretions, and aeration of all lung fields; reduces risk of stasis of secretions/pneumonia.
Assess level of consciousness/mentation regularly.	Brain tissue is very sensitive to decreases in oxygen and may be an early indicator of developing hypoxia.
Assess activity tolerance; limit activities to within patient tolerance or place patient on bed rest. Assist with ADLs and mobility as needed.	Reduction of the metabolic requirements of the body reduces the oxygen requirements/degree of hypoxia.

ACTIONS/INTERVENTIONS	RATIONALE

Independent

Encourage patient to alternate periods of rest and activity. Schedule rest periods as indicated.

Demonstrate and encourage use of relaxation techniques, e.g., guided imagery and visualization.

Promote adequate fluid intake, e.g., 2–3 L/d within cardiac tolerance.

Screen visitors/staff.

Collaborative

Administer supplemental humidified oxygen as indicated.

Monitor laboratory studies, e.g., CBC, cultures, ABGs/pulse oximetry, chest x-ray, pulmonary function tests.

Perform/assist with chest physiotherapy, IPPB, and incentive spirometer.

Administer packed RBCs or exchange transfusions as indicated.

Administer medications as indicated:

Antipyretics, e.g., acetaminophen (Tylenol);

Antibiotics.

Protects from overfatigue, reduces oxygen demands/degree of hypoxia.

Relaxation decreases muscle tension and anxiety and hence the metabolic demand for oxygen.

Sufficient intake is necessary to provide for mobilization of secretions and to prevent hyperviscosity of blood/capillary occlusion.

Protects from potential sources of respiratory infection.

Maximizes oxygen transport to tissues, particularly in presence of pulmonary insults/pneumonia.

Patients are particularly prone to pneumonia, which is potentially fatal due to its hypoxemic effect of increasing sickling.

Done to mobilize secretions and increase aeration of lung fields.

Increases number of oxygen-carrying cells, dilutes the percentage of hemoglobin S (to prevent sickling), improves circulation, and dislodges sickled cells. Packed RBCs are usually used because they are less likely to create circulatory overload. Note: Partial transfusions are sometimes used prophylactically in high-risk individuals, e.g., chronic, severe leg ulcers, preparation for general anesthesia, third trimester of pregnancy.

Maintains normothermia to reduce metabolic oxygen demands without affecting serum pH, which may occur with aspirin.

A broad-spectrum antibiotic is started immediately pending culture results of suspected infections, then may be changed when the specific pathogen is identified.

NURSING DIAGNOSIS:	TISSUE PERFUSION, ALTERED: DECREASED
May be related to:	Vaso-occlusive nature of sickling, inflammatory response.
	AV shunts in both pulmonary and peripheral circulation.
	Myocardial damage from small infarcts, iron deposits, and fibrosis.

Possibly evidenced by:	Changes in vital signs; diminished peripheral pulses/capillary refill; general pallor.
	Decreased mentation, restlessness.
	Angina, palpitations.
	Tingling in extremities, intermittent claudication, bone pain.
	Transient visual disturbances.
	Ulcerations of lower extremities, delayed healing.
DESIRED OUTCOMES/ EVALUATION CRITERIA— PATIENT WILL:	Demonstrate improved tissue perfusion as evidenced by stabilized vital signs, strong/palpable peripheral pulses, adequate urine output, absence of pain; alert and oriented; normal capillary refill; skin warm/dry; nail beds, lips, and ear lobes are natural pale, pink color; absence of paresthesias.

ACTIONS/INTERVENTIONS

Independent

Monitor vital signs carefully. Assess pulses for rate, rhythm, and volume. Note hypotension; rapid, weak, thready pulse; and increased/shallow respirations.

Assess skin for coolness, pallor, cyanosis, diaphoresis, delayed capillary refill.

Note changes in level of consciousness; reports of headaches, dizziness; development of sensory/motor deficits (e.g., hemiparesis or paralysis), seizures.

Maintain adequate fluid intake. (Refer to ND: Fluid Volume Deficit, High Risk For p 593.) Monitor urine output.

Assess lower extremities for skin texture, edema, ulcerations (especially of internal and external malleoli).

Investigate reports of change in character of pain, or development of bone pain, angina, tingling of extremities, eye pain/vision disturbances.

Maintain environmental temperature and body warmth.

Evaluate for developing edema (including genitals in men).

RATIONALE

Sludging and sickling in peripheral vessels may lead to complete or partial obliteration of a vessel with diminished perfusion to surrounding tissues. Sudden massive splenic sequestration of cells can lead to shock.

Changes reflect diminished circulation/hypoxia potentiating capillary occlusion. (Refer to ND: Gas Exchange, Impaired, p 590.)

Changes may reflect diminished perfusion to the CNS due to ischemia or infarction. Stagnant cells must be mobilized immediately to reduce further ischemia/infarction.

Dehydration not only causes hypovolemia but increases sickling and occlusion of capillaries. Decreased renal perfusion/failure may occur due to vascular occlusion.

Reduced peripheral circulation often leads to dermal changes and delayed healing.

Changes may reflect increased sickling of cells/diminished circulation with further involvement of organs, e.g., MI or pulmonary infarction, occlusion of vasculature of the eye.

Prevents vasoconstriction; aids in maintaining circulation and perfusion.

Vaso-occlusion/circulatory stasis may lead to edema of extremities (and priapism in men) potentiating risk of tissue ischemia/necrosis.

ACTIONS/INTERVENTIONS	RATIONALE

Collaborative

Monitor laboratory studies, e.g.:

ABGs, CBC, LDH, AST (SGOT)/ALT (SGPT), CPK, BUN:

Decreased tissue perfusion may lead to gradual infarction of organ tissues such as the brain, liver, spleen, kidney, skeletal muscle, and so forth with consequent release of intracellular enzymes.

Serum electrolytes. Provide replacements as indicated.

Electrolyte losses (especially sodium) are increased during crisis because of fever, diarrhea, vomiting, diaphoresis.

Administer hypo-osmolar solutions (e.g., 0.45 NS) via an infusion pump.

Hydration lowers the hemoglobin S concentration within the RBCs, which decreases the sickling tendency, and also reduces blood viscosity which helps to maintain perfusion. Infusion pump may prevent circulatory overload. *Note:* D5W or LR may cause RBC hemolysis and potentiate thrombus formation.

Administer experimental antisickling agents (e.g., sodium cyanate) or antineoplastic agents, carefully (e.g., hydroxyurea [Hydrea]) observing for possible lethal side effects.

Antisickling agents (currently under investigational use) are aimed at prolonging erythrocyte survival and preventing sickling by affecting cell membrane changes. *Note:* Use of anticoagulants, plasma expanders, nitrates, vasodilators, and alkylating agents have proven essentially unsuccessful in the management of the vaso-occlusive crisis.

Assist with/prepare for surgical diathermy or photocoagulation.

Direct coagulation of bleeding sites in the eye (resulting from vascular stasis/edema) may prevent progression of proliferative changes if initiated early.

Assist/prepare for needle aspiration of blood from corpora cavernosa;

Sickling within the penis can cause sustained erection (priapism) and edema. Removal of sludged sickled cells can improve circulation, decreasing psychologic trauma and risk of necrosis/infection.

Surgical intervention.

Direct incision and ligation of the dorsal arteries of the penis and saphenocavernous shunting may be necessary in severe cases of priapism to prevent tissue necrosis.

NURSING DIAGNOSIS:	FLUID VOLUME DEFICIT, HIGH RISK FOR
Risk factors may include:	Increased fluid needs, e.g., hypermetabolic state/fever, inflammatory processes.
	Renal parenchymal damage/infarctions limiting the kidneys' ability to concentrate urine (hyposthenuria).
	[Not applicable; presence of signs and symptoms establishes an actual diagnosis.]

DISEASES OF THE BLOOD/BLOOD-FORMING ORGANS: Sickle Cell Crisis

593

DESIRED OUTCOMES/ EVALUATION CRITERIA— PATIENT WILL:	Maintain adequate fluid balance as evidenced by individually appropriate urine output with a near-normal specific gravity, stable vital signs, moist mucous membranes, good skin turgor, and prompt capillary refill.

ACTIONS/INTERVENTIONS	RATIONALE
Independent	
Maintain accurate I&O. Weigh daily.	Patient may reduce fluid intake during periods of crisis because of malaise, anorexia, and so on. Dehydration from vomiting, diarrhea, fever, may reduce urine output and precipitate a vaso-occlusive crisis.
Note urine characteristics and specific gravity.	Kidney can lose its ability to concentrate urine, resulting in excessive losses of dilute urine.
Monitor vital signs, comparing with patient's normal/previous readings. Take BP in lying, sitting, and standing positions if possible.	Reduction of circulating blood volume can occur from increased fluid loss resulting in hypotension and tachycardia.
Observe for fever, changes in level of consciousness, poor skin turgor, dryness of skin and mucous membranes, pain.	Symptoms reflective of dehydration/hemoconcentration with consequent vaso-occlusive state.
Monitor vital signs closely during blood transfusions and note presence of dyspnea, crackles, rhonchi, wheezes, JVD, diminished breath sounds, cough, frothy sputum, and cyanosis.	Patient's heart may already be weakened and prone to failure due to chronic demands placed on it by the anemic state. Heart may be unable to tolerate the added fluid volume from transfusions or rapid IV fluid administered to treat crisis/shock.
Collaborative	
Administer fluids as indicated.	Replaces losses/deficits; may reverse renal concentration of RBCs/presence of failure. Fluids must be given immediately (especially in CNS involvement) to decrease hemoconcentration and prevent further infarction.
Monitor laboratory studies, e.g., Hb/Hct, serum and urine electrolytes.	Elevations may indicate hemoconcentration. Kidneys' loss of ability to concentrate urine may result in serum depletions of Na+, K+, and Cl−.

NURSING DIAGNOSIS:	PAIN, [ACUTE]/CHRONIC
May be related to:	Intravascular sickling with localized stasis, occlusion, and infarction/necrosis.
	Activation of pain fibers due to deprivation of oxygen and nutrients, accumulation of noxious metabolites.
Possibly evidenced by:	Localized, migratory, or more generalized pain, described as throbbing, gnawing, or severe and incapacitating, affecting peripheral extremities; bones, joints, back; abdomen; or head (headaches recurrent/transient).

Decreased ROM, guarding of the affected areas.

Facial grimacing, narrowed/self-focus.

DESIRED OUTCOMES/ EVALUATION CRITERIA— PATIENT WILL:

Verbalize relief/control of pain.

Demonstrate relaxed body posture, have freedom of movement, be able to sleep/rest appropriately.

ACTIONS/INTERVENTIONS	RATIONALE

Independent

Assess reports of pain, including location, duration, and intensity (scale of 0–10).

Observe nonverbal pain cues, e.g., gait disturbances, body positioning, reluctance to move, facial expressions, and physiologic manifestations of pain (e.g., elevated BP, tachycardia, increased respiratory rate). Explore discrepancies between verbal and nonverbal cues.

Discuss with the patient/SO what pain relief measures were effective in the past.

Explore alternate pain relief measures, e.g., relaxation techniques, biofeedback, yoga, meditation, progressive relaxation techniques, distraction (e.g., visual auditory, tactile kinesthetic, guided imagery, and breathing techniques).

Provide support for and carefully position affected extremities.

Apply local massage gently to affected areas.

Encourage ROM exercises.

Plan activities during peak analgesic effects.

Maintain adequate fluid intake.

Collaborative

Apply warm, moist compresses to affected joints or other painful areas. Avoid use of ice or cold compresses.

Administer medications as indicated: narcotics, e.g., meperidine (Demerol), morphine; nonnarcotic analgesics, e.g., acetaminophen (Tylenol) or sedatives, e.g., hydroxyzine (Vistaril).

Administer/monitor RBC transfusion.

Sickling of cells potentiates cellular hypoxia and may lead to infarction of tissue/resultant pain.

Pain is very unique to each patient; therefore, one may encounter varying descriptions due to individualized perceptions. Nonverbal cues may aid in evaluation of pain and effectiveness of therapy.

Involves patient/SO in care and allows for identification of remedies that have already been found to relieve pain. Helpful in establishing individualized treatment needs.

May reduce reliance on pharmacologic therapy and enhance patient's sense of control.

Reduces edema, discomfort, and risk of injury, especially if osteomyelitis is present.

Helps to reduce muscle tension.

Prevents joint stiffness and possible contracture formation.

Maximizes movement of joints, enhancing mobility.

Dehydration increases sickling/vaso-occlusion and corresponding pain.

Warmth causes vasodilation and increases circulation to hypoxic areas. Cold causes vasoconstriction and compounds the crisis.

Reduces pain and promotes rest and comfort. *Note:* Tylenol can be used for control of headache, pain, and fever. Aspirin should be avoided because it alters blood pH and can make cells sickle more easily.

Frequency of painful crises may be reduced by routine partial exchange transfusions to maintain population of normal RBCs.

NURSING DIAGNOSIS:	PHYSICAL MOBILITY, IMPAIRED
May be related to:	Multiple/recurrent bone infarctions or infections (weight-bearing bones). Pain/discomfort: Kyphosis of upper back/lordosis of lower back, possible joint effusions. Osteoporosis with fragmentation/collapse of femoral head or vertebra (compression deformities). Bacterial infections (osteomyelitis).
Possibly evidenced by:	Reports of pain. Limited joint ROM, reluctance to move, inability to walk/perform ADLs, guarding of joints, gait disturbances. Generalized weakness, therapeutic restrictions (e.g., bed rest)
DESIRED OUTCOMES/ EVALUATION CRITERIA— PATIENT WILL:	Resume ADLs. Participate in activities with absence of or improvement in gait disturbances, increased joint ROM, and absence of inflammatory signs.

(Refer to CP: Long-Term Care, ND: Physical Mobility, Impaired, p 955.)

NURSING DIAGNOSIS:	SKIN INTEGRITY, IMPAIRED: HIGH RISK FOR
Risk factors may include:	Impaired circulation (venous stasis and vaso-occlusion); altered sensation. Decreased mobility/bed rest.
Possibly evidenced by:	[Not applicable; presence of signs and symptoms establishes an actual diagnosis.]
DESIRED OUTCOMES/ EVALUATION CRITERIA— PATIENT WILL:	Prevent dermal ischemic injury. Participate in behaviors to reduce risk factors/skin breakdown. Observe improvement in wound/lesion healing if present.

ACTIONS/INTERVENTIONS	RATIONALE

Independent

Reposition frequently, even when sitting in chair.	Prevents prolonged tissue pressure where circula-

ACTIONS/INTERVENTIONS	RATIONALE

Independent

Inspect skin/pressure points regularly for redness, provide gentle massage.

tion is already compromised, reducing risk of tissue trauma/ischemia.

Poor circulation may predispose to rapid skin breakdown.

Protect bony prominences with sheepskin, heel/elbow protectors, pillows, as indicated.

Decreases pressure on tissues, preventing skin breakdown.

Keep skin surfaces dry and clean; linens dry/wrinkle-free.

Moist, contaminated areas provide excellent media for growth of pathogenic organisms.

Monitor leg bruises, cuts, bumps closely for ulcer formation.

Potential entry sites for pathogenic organisms. In presence of altered immune system, this increases risk of infection/delayed healing.

Elevate lower extremities when sitting.

Enhances venous return reducing venous stasis/edema formation.

Collaborative

Provide egg-crate, alternating air pressure or water mattresses.

Reduces tissue pressure and aids in maximizing cellular perfusion to prevent dermal injury.

Monitor status of ischemic areas, ulcer. Note distribution, size, depth, character, and drainage. Cleanse with hydrogen peroxide, boric acid, or povidone-iodine (Betadine) solutions as indicated.

Improvement or delayed healing reflects status of tissue perfusion and effectiveness of interventions. *Note:* These patients are at increased risk of serious complications because of lowered resistance to infection, and decreased nutrients for healing.

Prepare for/assist with hyperbaric oxygenation to ulcer sites.

Maximizes oxygen delivery to tissues, enhancing healing.

NURSING DIAGNOSIS: **INFECTION, HIGH RISK FOR**

Risk factors may include: Chronic disease process, tissue destruction, e.g., infarction, fibrosis, loss of spleen (autosplenectomy).

Inadequate primary defenses (broken skin, stasis of body fluids, decreased ciliary action).

Possibly evidenced by: [Not applicable; presence of signs and symptoms establishes an actual diagnosis.]

DESIRED OUTCOMES/ EVALUATION CRITERIA— PATIENT WILL: Verbalize understanding of individual causative/risk factors.

Identify interventions to prevent/reduce risk of infection.

(Refer to CPs: Pneumonia, microbial p 162; Sepsis/Septicemia, p 887; Fractures, ND: Infection, High Risk For, p 785.)

NURSING DIAGNOSIS:	KNOWLEDGE DEFICIT [LEARNING NEED] REGARDING CONDITION, PROGNOSIS, AND TREATMENT NEEDS
May be related to:	Lack of exposure/recall.
	Information misinterpretation.
	Unfamiliarity with resources.
Possibly evidenced by:	Questions; request for information.
	Statement of misconceptions.
	Inaccurate follow-through of instructions; development of preventable complications.
	Verbal/nonverbal cues of anxiety.
DESIRED OUTCOMES/ EVALUATION CRITERIA— PATIENT WILL:	Verbalize understanding of disease process, including symptoms of crisis.
	Initiate necessary behaviors/lifestyle changes to prevent complications.
	Identify need for continued medical follow-up; genetic counseling/family planning services.

ACTIONS/INTERVENTIONS	RATIONALE
Independent	
Review disease process and treatment needs.	Provides knowledge base on which patient can make informed choices.
Assess patient's knowledge of precipitating factors, e.g.:	
Travel to places more than 7000 ft above sea level or flying in unpressurized aircraft;	Decreased oxygen tension present at higher altitudes causes hypoxia and potentiates sickling of cells.
Strenuous physical activity/contact type sports, and extremely warm temperatures;	Increases metabolic demand for oxygen and increases insensible fluid losses (evaporation and perspiration), which may increase blood viscosity and tendency to sickle.
Cold environmental temperatures, failure to dress warmly when engaging in winter activities; wearing tight, restrictive clothing; stressful situations.	Causes peripheral vasoconstriction, which may result in sludging of the circulation, increased sickling, and may precipitate a vaso-occlusive crisis.
Encourage consumption of at least 4–6 qt of fluid daily, during a steady state of the disease. Increase the amount to 6–8 qt during a painful crisis or while engaging in activities that might precipitate dehydration.	Prevents dehydration and consequent hyperviscosity that can potentiate sickling/crisis.
Encourage ROM exercise and regular physical activity with a balance between rest and activity.	Prevents bone demineralization and may reduce risk of fractures. Aids in maintaining level of resistance and decreases oxygen needs.

ACTIONS/INTERVENTIONS	RATIONALE

Independent

Review patient's current diet, reinforcing the importance of diet including liver, green leafy vegetables, citrus fruits, and wheat germ. Provide necessary instruction regarding supplementary vitamins such as folic acid.

Sound nutrition is essential because of increased demands placed on bone marrow (e.g., folate and vitamin B_{12} are used in greater quantities than usual), and folic acid supplements are frequently ordered to prevent aplastic crisis.

Discourage smoking and alcohol consumption; identify community support groups.

Nicotine induces peripheral vasoconstriction and decreases oxygen tension, which may contribute to cellular hypoxia and sickling. Alcohol increases the possibility of dehydration (precipitating sickling). Maintaining these changes in behavior/lifestyle may require prolonged support.

Discuss principles of skin/extremity care and protection from injury. Encourage prompt treatment of cuts, insect bites, sores.

Due to impaired tissue perfusion, especially in the periphery, distal extremities are especially susceptible to altered skin integrity/infection.

Include instructions on care of any leg ulcers that might develop.

Fosters independence and maintenance of self-care at home.

Instruct patient to avoid persons with infections such as URI.

Altered immune response places patient at risk for infections, especially bacterial pneumonia.

Recommend patient avoid cold remedies and decongestants containing ephedrine. Stress the importance of reading labels on OTC drugs and consulting health care provider prior to consuming any drugs.

Those remedies containing vasoconstrictors may decrease peripheral tissue perfusion and cause sludging of sickled cells.

Discuss conditions for which medical attention should be sought, e.g.:

Urine that appears blood tinged or smoky;

Symptoms suggestive of sickling in the renal medulla.

Indigestion, persistent vomiting, diarrhea, high fever, excessive thirst;

Dehydration may trigger a vaso-occlusive crisis.

Severe joint or bone pain;

May signify a vaso-occlusive crisis due to sickling in the bones or spleen (ischemia or infarction) or onset of osteomyelitis.

Severe chest pain, with or without cough;

May reflect angina, impending MI, or pneumonia.

Abdominal pain; gastric distress following meals;

High incidence of gallbladder disease/stone formation.

Fever, swelling, redness, increasing fatigue/pallor, leg ulcers, dizziness, drowsiness.

Suggestive of infections that may precipitate a vaso-occlusive crisis if dehydration develops. *Note:* Severe infections are the most frequent cause of aplastic crisis.

Assist patient to strengthen coping abilities, e.g., deal appropriately with anxiety, get adequate information, use relaxation techniques.

Promotes patient's sense of control, may avert a crisis.

Suggest wearing a medical alert bracelet or carrying a card.

May prevent inappropriate treatment in emergency situation.

ACTIONS/INTERVENTIONS	RATIONALE
Independent	
Discuss genetic implications of the disease. Encourage SO/family members to seek testing to determine presence of hemoglobin S.	Hereditary nature of the disease with the possibility of transmitting the mutation may have a bearing on the decision to have children.
Explore concerns regarding childbearing/family planning and refer to community resources as indicated.	Provides opportunity to correct misconceptions/present information necessary to make informed decisions. Pregnancy can precipitate a vaso-occlusive crisis because the placenta's tortuous blood supply and low oxygen tension potentiates sickling, which in turn can lead to fetal hypoxia.
Encourage patient to have routine follow-ups, e.g.:	
Periodic laboratory studies, e.g., CBC;	Monitors changes in blood components; identifies need for changes in treatment regimen.
Biannual dental examination;	Sound oral hygiene limits opportunity for bacterial invasion/sepsis.
Annual ophthalmologic examination.	May develop sickle retinopathy with either proliferative or nonproliferative ocular changes.
Determine need for vocational/career guidance.	Sedentary career may be necessary because of the decreased oxygen-carrying capacity and diminished exercise tolerance.
Encourage participation in community support groups available to sickle cell patients/SO, such as the National Association for Sickle Cell Anemia, March of Dimes, Public Health/VNA nurse.	Helpful in adjustment to long-term situation; reduces feelings of isolation and enhances problem solving through sharing of common experiences. *Note:* Failure to resolve concerns/deal with situation may require more intensive therapy/psychologic support.

Leukemias

The term leukemia describes a variety of cancers that arise in the blood-forming organs of the body (spleen, lymphatic system, bone marrow). They are differentiated according to the leukocytic system that is involved. The common trait of all leukemias is the unregulated proliferation of WBCs in the bone marrow that replaces the normal elements. There is an apparent abnormality in the hematopoietic stem cell, which results in its inability to differentiate into normal cells. As the normal cells are replaced by leukemic cells, anemia, neutropenia, and thrombocytopenia occur. In adults, the most common of the acute leukemias is acute myelocytic leukemia, which involves neutrophils, a type of granulocyte. The most common of the chronic leukemias is chronic lymphocytic leukemia, which is characterized by an abnormal increase in lymphocytes.

RELATED CONCERNS

Cancer, p 1014
Psychosocial Aspects of Acute Care, p 899

PATIENT ASSESSMENT DATA BASE

The data are dependent on degree/duration of the disease and other organ involvement.

ACTIVITY/REST

May report: Fatigue, malaise, weakness; inability to engage in usual activities.

May exhibit: Muscle wasting.
                     Increased need for sleep, somnolence.

CIRCULATION

May report: Palpitations.

May exhibit: Tachycardia, heart murmurs.
                     Pallor of skin, mucous membranes.
                     Cranial nerve deficits and/or signs of cerebral hemorrhage.

ELIMINATION

May report: Diarrhea; perianal tenderness, pain.
                     Bright red blood on tissue paper, tarry stools.
                     Blood in urine, decreased urine output.

May exhibit: Perianal abscess; hematuria.

EGO INTEGRITY

May report: Feelings of helplessness/hopelessness.

May exhibit: Depression, withdrawal, anxiety, fear, anger, irritability.
                     Mood changes, confusion.

FOOD/FLUID

May report: Loss of appetite, anorexia, vomiting.
                     Change in taste/taste distortions.
                     Weight loss.
                     Pharyngitis, dysphagia.

May exhibit:	Abdominal distention, decreased bowel sounds.
	Splenomegaly, hepatomegaly; jaundice.
	Stomatitis, oral ulcerations.
	Gum hypertrophy (gum infiltration may be indicative of acute monocytic leukemia).

NEUROSENSORY

May report:	Lack of coordination/decreased coordination.
	Mood changes, confusion, disorientation, lack of concentration.
	Dizziness; numbness, tingling, paresthesias.
May exhibit:	Muscle irritability, seizure activity.

PAIN/COMFORT

May report:	Abdominal pain, headaches, bone/joint pain; sternal tenderness, muscle cramping.
May exhibit:	Guarding/distraction behaviors, restlessness; self-focus.

RESPIRATION

May report:	Shortness of breath with minimal exertion.
May exhibit:	Dyspnea, tachypnea.
	Cough.
	Crackles, rhonchi.
	Decreased breath sounds.

SAFETY

May report:	History of recent/recurrent infections; falls.
	Visual disturbances/impairment.
	Spontaneous uncontrollable bleeding with minimal trauma.
May exhibit:	Fever, infections.
	Bruises, purpura, retinal hemorrhages, gum bleeding, or epistaxis.
	Enlarged lymph nodes, spleen, or liver (due to tissue invasion).
	Papilledema and exophthalmos.
	Leukemic infiltrates in the dermis.

SEXUALITY

May report:	Changes in libido.
	Changes in menstrual flow, menorrhagia.
	Impotence.

TEACHING/LEARNING

May report:	History of exposure to chemicals, e.g., benzene, phenylbutazone, and chloramphenicol; excessive levels of ionizing radiation; previous treatment with chemotherapy, especially alkalating agents.
	Chromosomal disorder, e.g., Down syndrome or Franconi's aplastic anemia.

602

Discharge Plan Considerations: **DRG projected mean length of stay: 3.9 days.**

May need assistance with therapy and treatment needs/supplies, shopping, food preparation, self-care activities, homemaker/maintenance tasks, transportation.

DIAGNOSTIC STUDIES

CBC: Indicates a normocytic, normochromic anemia.

Hemoglobin: May be less than 10 g/100 ml.

Reticulocytes: Count is usually low.

Platelet count: May be very low (<50,000/mm).

WBC: May be more than 50,000/cm with increased immature WBCs ("shift to left"). Leukemic blast cells may be present.

PT/PTT: Prolonged.

LDH: May be elevated.

Serum/urine uric acid: May be elevated.

Serum muramidase (a lysozyme): Elevated in acute monocytic and myelomonocytic leukemias.

Serum copper: Elevated.

Serum zinc: Decreased.

Bone marrow biopsy: Abnormal WBCs usually make up 50% or more of the WBCs in the bone marrow. Often 60%–90% of the cells are blast cells, with erythroid precursors, mature cells, and megakaryocytes reduced.

Chest x-ray and lymph node biopsies: May indicate degree of involvement.

NURSING PRIORITIES

1. Prevent infection during acute phases of disease/treatment.
2. Maintain circulating blood volume.
3. Alleviate pain.
4. Promote optimal physical functioning.
5. Provide psychologic support.
6. Provide information about disease process/prognosis and treatment needs.

DISCHARGE GOALS

1. Complications prevented/minimized.
2. Pain relieved/controlled.
3. ADLs met by self or with assistance.
4. Dealing with disease realistically.
5. Disease process/prognosis and therapeutic regimen understood.

(Refer to CP: Cancer, p 1014, for further discussion/expansion of interventions related to cancer care and for patient teaching.)

NURSING DIAGNOSIS:	INFECTION, HIGH RISK FOR
Risk factors may include:	Inadequate secondary defenses: Alterations in mature WBC (low granulocyte and abnormal lymphocyte count), increased number of immature lymphocytes; immunosuppression, bone marrow suppression (effects of therapy/transplant).

	Inadequate primary defenses (stasis of body fluids, traumatized tissue).
	Invasive procedures.
	Malnutrition; chronic disease.
Possibly evidenced by:	[Not applicable; presence of signs and symptoms establishes an actual diagnosis.]
DESIRED OUTCOMES/ EVALUATION CRITERIA— PATIENT WILL:	Identify actions to prevent/reduce risk of infection.
	Demonstrate techniques, lifestyle changes to promote safe environment, achieve timely healing.

ACTIONS/INTERVENTIONS	RATIONALE

Independent

Place in private room. Screen/limit visitors as indicated. Prohibit use of live plants/cut flowers. Restrict fresh fruits and vegetables.	Protects patient from potential sources of pathogens/infection. *Note:* Profound bone marrow suppression, neutropenia, and chemotherapy place the patient at great risk for infection.
Require good hand washing protocol for all personnel and visitors.	Prevents cross-contamination/reduces risk of infection.
Monitor temperature. Note correlation between temperature elevations and chemotherapy treatments. Observe for fever associated with tachycardia, hypotension, subtle mental changes.	Progressive hyperthermia occurs in some types of infections, and fever (unrelated to drugs or blood products) occurs in most leukemia patients. *Note:* Septicemia may occur without fever.
Prevent chilling; force fluids. Administer tepid sponge bath.	Helps reduce fever, which contributes to fluid imbalance, discomfort, and CNS complications.
Encourage frequent turning, deep breathing, coughing.	Prevents stasis of respiratory secretions, reducing risk of atelectasis/pneumonia.
Auscultate breath sounds, noting crackles, rhonchi; inspect secretions for changes in characteristics, e.g., increased sputum production or cloudy, foul-smelling urine with urgency or burning.	Early intervention is essential to prevent sepsis/septicemia in immunosuppressed person.
Handle patient gently. Keep linens dry/wrinkle-free.	Prevents sheet burn/skin excoriation.
Inspect skin for tender, erythematous areas; open wounds. Cleanse skin with antibacterial solutions.	May indicate local infection. *Note:* Open wounds may not produce pus because of insufficient number of granulocytes.
Inspect oral mucous membranes. Provide good oral hygiene. Use a soft toothbrush for frequent mouth care.	The oral cavity is an excellent medium for growth of organisms.
Promote good perianal hygiene. Provide sitz baths, using Betadine or Hibiclens if indicated.	Promotes cleanliness, reducing risk of perianal abscess; enhances circulation and healing.
Provide uninterrupted rest periods.	Conserves energy for healing, cellular regeneration.

ACTIONS/INTERVENTIONS	RATIONALE
Independent	
Encourage increased intake of foods high in protein and fluids.	Enhances antibody formation and prevents dehydration.
Avoid/limit invasive procedures (e.g., venipuncture and injections) as possible.	Break in skin could provide an entry for pathogenic/potentially lethal organisms. Use of tunneled catheter or implanted port can effectively reduce need for invasive procedure and risk of infection. *Note:* Myelosuppression may be cumulative in nature especially when multiple drug therapy (including steroids) is prescribed.
Collaborative	
Monitor laboratory studies, e.g.:	
CBC, noting whether WBC falls or sudden changes occur in neutrophils;	Decreased numbers of normal/mature WBCs can result from the disease process or chemotherapy, compromising the immune response and increasing risk of infection.
Gram stain cultures/sensitivity.	Verifies presence of infections; identifies specific organisms and appropriate therapy.
Review serial chest x-rays.	Indicator of development/resolution of respiratory complications.
Administer medications as indicated, e.g., antibiotics.	May be given prophylactically or to treat specific infection.
Avoid use of aspirin-containing antipyretics.	Aspirin can cause gastric bleeding and further decrease platelet count.
Provide low-bacteria diet, e.g., cooked, processed foods.	Minimizes potential sources of bacterial contamination.

NURSING DIAGNOSIS:	**FLUID VOLUME DEFICIT, HIGH RISK FOR**
Risk factors may include:	Excessive losses, e.g., vomiting, hemorrhage, diarrhea.
	Decreased fluid intake, e.g., nausea, anorexia.
	Increased fluid need, e.g., hypermetabolic state, fever; predisposition for kidney stone formation.
Possibly evidenced by:	[Not applicable; presence of signs and symptoms establishes an actual diagnosis.]
DESIRED OUTCOMES/ EVALUATION CRITERIA— PATIENT WILL:	Demonstrate adequate fluid volume, as evidenced by stable vital signs; palpable pulses; urine output, specific gravity, and pH within normal limits.
	Identify individual risk factors and appropriate interventions.
	Initiate behaviors/lifestyle changes to prevent development of fluid volume deficit.

ACTIONS/INTERVENTIONS	RATIONALE
Independent	
Monitor intake/output. Calculate insensible losses and fluid balance. Note decreased urine in presence of adequate intake. Measure specific gravity and urine pH.	Decreased circulation secondary to destruction of RBCs and their precipitation in the kidney tubules and/or development of kidney stones (related to elevated uric acid levels) may lead to urinary retention or renal failure.
Weigh daily.	Measure of adequacy of fluid replacement as well as kidney function. Continued intake greater than output may indicate renal insult/obstruction.
Monitor BP and heart rate.	Changes may reflect effects of hypovolemia (bleeding/dehydration).
Evaluate skin turgor, capillary refill, and general condition of mucous membranes.	Indirect indicators of fluid status/hydration.
Note presence of nausea, fever.	Affects intake, fluid needs, and route of replacement.
Encourage fluids of up to 3–4 L/d when oral intake is resumed.	Promotes urine flow, prevents uric acid precipitation, and enhances clearance of antineoplastic drugs.
Inspect skin/mucous membranes for petechiae, ecchymotic areas; note bleeding gums, frank or occult blood in stools and urine; oozing from invasive-line sites.	Suppression of bone marrow and platelet production places the patient at risk for spontaneous/uncontrolled bleeding.
Implement measures to prevent tissue injury/bleeding, e.g., gentle brushing of teeth or gums with soft toothbrush, cotton swab, or sponge-tipped applicator; using electric razor and avoiding sharp razors when shaving; avoid forceful nose blowing, and needle sticks when possible; use sustained pressure on oozing puncture sites.	Fragile tissues and altered clotting mechanisms increase the risk of hemorrhage following even minor trauma.
Limit oral care to mouthwash if indicated (a mixture of ¼ tsp baking soda in 4–8 oz water or hydrogen peroxide in water). Avoid mouthwashes with alcohol.	When bleeding is present even gentle brushing may cause more tissue damage. Alcohol has a drying effect and may be painful to irritated tissues.
Provide soft diet.	May help reduce gum irritation.
Collaborative	
Administer IV fluids as indicated.	Maintains fluid/electrolyte balance in the absence of oral intake; reduces risk of renal complications.
Monitor laboratory studies, e.g., platelets, Hb/Hct, clotting.	When the platelet count is less than 20,000/mm (due to proliferation of WBCs and/or bone marrow suppression secondary to antineoplastic drugs), the patient is prone to spontaneous life-threatening bleeding. Decreasing Hb/Hct is indicative of bleeding (may be occult).
Administer RBCs, platelets, clotting factors.	Restores/normalizes RBC count and oxygen-carrying capacity to correct anemia. Used to prevent/treat hemorrhage.

ACTIONS/INTERVENTIONS	RATIONALE

Collaborative

Maintain external central vascular access device (subclavian or tunneled catheter or implanted port).

Administer medications as indicated, e.g.:

Ondansetron (Zofran);

Allopurinol (Zyloprim);

Potassium acetate or citrate, sodium bicarbonate;

Stool softeners.

Eliminates peripheral venipuncture as source of bleeding.

Relieves nausea/vomiting associated with administration of chemotherapy agents.

Although use is controversial, may be given to reduce the chances of nephropathy as a result of uric acid production.

May be used to alkalinize the urine preventing formation of kidney stones.

Helpful in reducing straining at stool with trauma to rectal tissues.

NURSING DIAGNOSIS:	PAIN [ACUTE]
May be related to:	Physical agents, e.g., enlarged organs/lymph nodes, bone marrow packed with leukemic cells.
	Chemical agents, e.g., antileukemic treatments.
	Psychologic manifestations, e.g., anxiety, fear.
Possibly evidenced by:	Reports of pain (bone, nerve, headaches, and so forth.)
	Guarding/distraction behaviors, facial grimacing, alteration in muscle tone.
	Autonomic responses.
DESIRED OUTCOMES/ EVALUATION CRITERIA— PATIENT WILL:	Report pain is relieved/controlled.
	Demonstrate behaviors to manage pain.
	Appear relaxed and able to sleep/rest appropriately.

ACTIONS/INTERVENTIONS	RATIONALE

Independent

Investigate reports of pain. Note changes in degree and site (use scale of 0–10).

Monitor vital signs, note nonverbal cues, e.g., muscle tension, restlessness.

Provide quiet environment and reduce stressful stimuli, e.g., noise, lighting, constant interruptions.

Helpful in assessing need for intervention; may indicate developing complications.

May be useful in evaluating verbal comments and effectiveness of interventions.

Promotes rest and enhances coping abilities.

ACTIONS/INTERVENTIONS	RATIONALE
Independent	
Place in position of comfort and support joints, extremities with pillows/padding.	May decrease associated bone/joint discomfort.
Reposition periodically and provide/assist with gentle ROM exercises.	Improves tissue circulation and joint mobility.
Provide comfort measures (e.g., massage, cool packs), and psychologic support (e.g., encouragement, presence).	Minimizes need for/enhances effects of medication.
Review/promote patient's own comfort interventions, position, physical activity/nonactivity, and so forth.	Successful management of pain requires patient involvement. Use of effective techniques provides positive reinforcement, promotes sense of control, and prepares patient for interventions to be used after discharge.
Evaluate and support patient's coping mechanisms.	Using own learned perceptions/behaviors to manage pain can help the patient to cope more effectively.
Encourage use of stress management techniques, e.g., relaxation/deep-breathing exercises, guided imagery, visualization; Therapeutic Touch.	Facilitates relaxation, augments pharmacologic therapy, and enhances coping abilities.
Assist with/provide diversional, relaxation techniques.	Helps with pain management by redirecting attention.
Collaborative	
Monitor uric acid level.	Rapid turnover and destruction of leukemic cells during chemotherapy elevates uric acid, causing swollen, painful joints.
Administer medications as indicated:	
Analgesics, e.g., acetaminophen (Tylenol);	Given for mild pain not relieved by comfort measures. *Note:* Avoid aspirin-containing products as they may potentiate hemorrhage.
Narcotics, e.g., codeine, meperidine (Demerol), morphine, hydromorphone (Dilaudid);	Used when pain is severe. Use of PCA may be beneficial in preventing peaks and valleys of intermittent administration.
Antianxiety agents, e.g., diazepam (Valium), lorazepam (Ativan).	May be given to enhance the action of analgesics/narcotics.

NURSING DIAGNOSIS:	**ACTIVITY INTOLERANCE**
May be related to:	Generalized weakness; reduced energy stores, increased metabolic rate from massive production of leukocytes.
	Imbalance between oxygen supply and demand (anemia/hypoxia).
	Therapeutic restrictions (isolation/bed rest); effect of drug therapy.

Possibly evidenced by:	Verbal report of fatigue or weakness.
	Exertional discomfort or dyspnea.
	Abnormal heart rate or BP response.
DESIRED OUTCOMES/ EVALUATION CRITERIA— PATIENT WILL:	Report a measurable increase in activity tolerance.
	Participate in ADLs to level of ability.
	Demonstrate a decrease in physiologic signs of intolerance; e.g., pulse, respiration, and BP remain within patient's normal range.

ACTIONS/INTERVENTIONS	RATIONALE
Independent	
Evaluate reports of fatigue, noting inability to participate in activities or ADLs.	Effects of leukemia, anemia, and chemotherapy may be cumulative (especially during acute and active treatment phase), necessitating assistance.
Provide quiet environment and uninterrupted rest periods. Encourage rest periods before meals.	Restores energy needed for activity and cellular regeneration/tissue healing.
Implement energy-saving techniques, e.g., sitting, rather than standing, use of shower chair. Assist with ambulation/other activities as indicated.	Maximizes available energy for self-care tasks.
Schedule meals around chemotherapy. Give oral hygiene before meals and administer antiemetics as indicated.	May enhance intake by reducing nausea. (Refer to CP: Cancer, ND: Nutrition, Altered: Less Than Body Requirements, p 1023.)
Collaborative	
Provide supplemental oxygen.	Maximizes oxygen available for cellular uptake.

NURSING DIAGNOSIS:	**KNOWLEDGE DEFICIT [LEARNING NEED] REGARDING DISEASE, PROGNOSIS, AND TREATMENT NEEDS**
May be related to:	Lack of exposure to resources.
	Information misinterpretation/lack of recall.
Possibly evidenced by:	Verbalization of problem/request for information.
	Statement of misconception.
DESIRED OUTCOMES/ EVALUATION CRITERIA— PATIENT WILL:	Verbalize understanding of condition/disease process and treatment.
	Initiate necessary lifestyle changes.
	Participate in treatment regimen.

ACTIONS/INTERVENTIONS	RATIONALE
Independent	
Review pathology of specific form of leukemia and various treatment options.	Treatments can include various antineoplastic drugs, whole body or liver/spleen radiation, transfusions, and/or bone marrow transplant.
(For additional interventions refer to CP: Cancer, ND: Knowledge Deficit, p 1036.)	

Lymphomas

Malignant lymphomas are cancers of the lymphoid tissue, classified according to four primary features: cell type, degree of differentiation, type of reaction elicited by tumor cells, and growth patterns. If a nodular growth pattern is observed, the term *nodular* is used after the cell type. If no mention of growth pattern is made, the lymphoma is of a *diffuse* type.

HODGKIN'S DISEASE:

The malignant cell of origin for Hodgkin's is not known, but it is thought to be derived from a B-lymphocyte, T-lymphocyte, or macrophage cell line.

Hodgkin's disease is divided into four different categories: lymphocyte-predominant, mixed cellularity, lymphocyte-depleted, and nodular sclerosing. The lymphocyte-predominant and nodular sclerosing types usually have a more favorable prognosis than the other two types. Stages I–IV of Hodgkin's disease range from one lymph node region to involvement of multiple systems in the body. Treatment for Hodgkin's disease includes extensive radiotherapy, a combination of radiotherapy and chemotherapy, or chemotherapy alone. The use of autologous bone marrow transplant with high-dose chemotherapy is under investigation.

NON-HODGKIN'S DISEASE:

Non-Hodgkin's lymphoma is a malignancy of the B-lymphocyte and T-lymphocyte cell systems. Most patients with non-Hodgkin's lymphoma fall into two broad categories related to their clinical features: the nodular, indolent type and the diffuse, aggressive lymphomas. For treatment purposes, they may also be classified as low-, intermediate-, or high-grade lymphomas. Treatment for non-Hodgkin's lymphomas includes radiotherapy or chemotherapy (usually multiple combinations of antineoplastic agents).

RELATED CONCERNS

Anemias, p 573
Cancer, p 1014
Leukemias, p 601
Psychosocial Aspects of Acute Care, p 899
Spinal Cord Injury, p 337

PATIENT ASSESSMENT DATA BASE

ACTIVITY/REST

May report:	Fatigue, weakness, or general malaise.
	Loss of productivity and decreased exercise tolerance.
	Need for more sleep and rest.
May exhibit:	Diminished strength, slumping of the shoulders, slow walk, and other cues indicative of fatigue.
	Night sweats.

CIRCULATION

May report:	Palpitations, angina/chest pain.
May exhibit:	Tachycardia, dysrhythmias.
	Cyanosis of the face and neck (obstruction of venous drainage from enlarged lymph nodes is a rare occurrence).
	Scleral icterus and a generalized icteric coloring related to liver damage and consequent obstruction of bile ducts by enlarged lymph nodes (may be a late sign).
	Pallor (anemia), diaphoresis, night sweats.

EGO INTEGRITY

May report:
Stress factors, e.g., school, job, family.

Fear/anxiety related to diagnosis and possible fear of dying.

Anxiety/fear related to diagnostic testing and treatment modalities (chemotherapy and radiation therapy).

Financial concerns: Hospital costs, treatment expenses, fear of losing job-related benefits due to lost time from work.

Relationship status: Fear and anxiety related to being a burden on the family.

May exhibit:
Varied behaviors, e.g., angry, withdrawn, passive.

ELIMINATION

May report:
Changes in characteristics of urine and/or stool.

History of intestinal obstruction, e.g., intussusception, or malabsorption syndrome (infiltration from retroperitoneal lymph nodes).

May exhibit:
RUQ tenderness and enlargement on palpation (hepatomegaly).

LUQ tenderness and enlargement on palpation (splenomegaly).

Decreased output, dark/concentrated urine, anuria (ureteral obstruction/renal failure).

Bowel and bladder dysfunction (spinal cord compression occurs late).

FOOD/FLUID

May report:
Anorexia/loss of appetite.

Dysphagia (pressure on the esophagus).

Recent unexplained weight loss equivalent to 10% or more of body weight in previous 6 months with no attempt at dieting.

May exhibit:
Swelling of the face, neck, jaw, or right arm (secondary to superior vena cava compression by enlarged lymph nodes).

Extremities: Edema of the lower extremities related to inferior vena cava obstruction from intra-abdominal lymph node enlargement (non-Hodgkin's).

Ascites (inferior vena cava obstruction related to intra-abdominal lymph node enlargement).

NEUROSENSORY

May report:
Nerve pain (neuralgias) reflecting compression of nerve roots by enlarged lymph nodes in the brachial, lumbar, and sacral plexuses.

Muscle weakness, paresthesia.

May exhibit:
Mental status: lethargy, withdrawal, general lack of interest in surroundings. Paraplegia (spinal cord compression from vertebral body, disk involvement with compression/degeneration, or compromised blood supply to the spinal cord).

PAIN/COMFORT

May report:
Tenderness/pain over involved lymph nodes, e.g., in or around the mediastinum; chest pain, back pain (vertebral compression); generalized bone pain (lymphomatous bone involvement).

Immediate pain in involved areas following ingestion of alcohol.

May exhibit:
Self-focusing; guarding behaviors.

RESPIRATION

May report:
Dyspnea on exertion or at rest; chest pain.

May exhibit:
Dyspnea; tachypnea.

Dry, nonproductive cough.

Signs of respiratory distress, e.g., increased respiratory rate and depth, use of accessory muscles, stridor, cyanosis.

Hoarseness/laryngeal paralysis (pressure from enlarged nodes on the laryngeal nerve).

SAFETY

May report:
History of frequent/recurrent infections (abnormalities in cellular immunity predispose the patient to systemic herpes virus infections, TB, toxoplasmosis, or bacterial infections).

History of mononucleosis (higher risk of Hodgkin's disease in patient with high titers of Epstein-Barr virus). History of ulcers/perforation, gastric bleeding.

Waxing and waning pattern of lymph node size.

Cyclical pattern of evening temperature elevations lasting a few days to weeks (Pel-Ebstein fever) followed by alternate afebrile periods; drenching night sweats without chills.

Generalized rash/pruritus.

May exhibit:
Unexplained, persistent fever greater than 38°C (100.4°F) without symptoms of infection.

Asymmetric, painless, yet swollen/enlarged lymph nodes (cervical nodes most commonly involved, left side more than right; then axillary and mediastinal nodes).

Nodes may feel rubbery and hard, discrete and movable.

Tonsilar enlargement.

Generalized pruritus.

Patchy areas of loss of melanin pigmentation (vitiligo).

SEXUALITY

May report:
Concern about fertility/pregnancy (while disease does not affect either, treatment does).

Decreased libido.

TEACHING/LEARNING

May report:
Familial risk factors (higher incidence among families of Hodgkin's patients than that of general population).

Occupational exposure to herbicides (woodworkers/chemists).

Discharge Plan Considerations:
DRG projected mean length of stay: 3.9 days, with surgical intervention, 10.1 days.

May need assistance with medical therapies/supplies, self-care activities and/or homemaker/maintenance tasks, transportation, shopping.

DIAGNOSTIC STUDIES

These diseases are staged according to the microscopic appearance of involved lymph nodes and the extent and severity of the disorder. Accurate staging is most important in deciding on subsequent treatment regimens and prognosis.

Blood studies may vary from completely normal to marked abnormalities. In stage I, few patients have abnormal blood findings.

CBC:

WBC: Variable, may be normal, decreased, or markedly elevated.

Differential WBC: Neutrophilia, monocytosis, basophilia, and eosinophilia may be found. Complete lymphopenia (late symptom).

RBC and Hb/Hct: Decreased.

Erythrocytes:

Stained RBC examination: May demonstrate mild-to-moderate normocytic, normochromic anemia (hypersplenism).

ESR: Elevated during active stages and indicates inflammatory or malignant disease. Useful to monitor patients in remission and to detect early evidence of recurrence of disease.

Erythrocyte osmotic fragility: Increased.

Platelets: Decreased (may be severely depleted; bone marrow replacement by the lymphoma and by hypersplenism).

Coombs' test: Positive reaction (hemolytic anemia) may occur; however, a negative result usually occurs in advanced disease.

Serum iron and TIBC: Decreased.

Serum alkaline phosphatase: Elevation may indicate either liver or bone involvement.

Serum copper: Elevation may be seen in exacerbations.

Serum calcium: May be elevated when bone is involved.

Serum uric acid: Elevated related to increased destruction of nucleoproteins, and liver and kidney involvement.

BUN: May be elevated when kidney involvement is present. Serum creatinine, bilirubin, ASL (SGOT), creatinine clearance, and so forth may be done to detect organ involvement.

Hypergammaglobulinemia is common; *hypogammaglobulinemia* may occur in advanced disease.

Chest x-ray: May reveal mediastinal or hilar adenopathy, nodular infiltrates, or pleural effusions.

X-rays of thoracic, lumbar vertebrae, proximal extremities, pelvis, or areas of bone tenderness: Determine areas of involvement and assist in staging.

IVP: May be done to detect renal involvement or ureteral deviation by involved nodes.

Whole lung tomography or chest CT scan: Done if hilar adenopathy is present. Reveals possible involvement of mediastinal lymph nodes.

Abdominal CT scans: May be done to rule out diseased nodes in the abdomen and pelvis and in organs not accessible by physical examination.

Abdominal ultrasound: Evaluates extent of involvement of retroperitoneal lymph nodes.

Bone scans: Done to detect bone involvement.

Gallium-67 scintigraphy: Proven useful for detecting recurrent nodal disease, especially above the diaphragm.

Bone marrow biopsy: Determines bone marrow involvement. Bone marrow invasion is seen in advanced stages.

Lymph node biopsy: Establishes the diagnosis of Hodgkin's disease based on the presence of the Reed-Sternberg cell.

Mediastinoscopy: May be performed to establish mediastinal node involvement.

Staging laparotomy: May be done to obtain specimens of retroperitoneal nodes, of both lobes of the liver, and/or remove the spleen. (Splenectomy is controversial because it may increase the risk of infection and is currently not usually implemented unless the patient has clinical manifestations of stage IV disease. Laparoscopy sometimes done as an alternative approach to obtain specimens).

NURSING PRIORITIES

1. Provide physical and psychologic support during extensive diagnostic testing and treatment regimen.
2. Prevent complications.
3. Alleviate pain.
4. Provide information about disease process/prognosis and treatment needs.

DISCHARGE GOALS

1. Complications prevented/diminished.
2. Dealing with situation realistically.
3. Pain relieved/controlled.
4. Disease process/prognosis, possible complications, and therapeutic regimen understood.

(Refer to CPs: Cancer, p 1014, Leukemias, p 601, for general nursing diagnoses and interventions.)

NURSING DIAGNOSIS:	BREATHING PATTERN/AIRWAY CLEARANCE, INEFFECTIVE, HIGH RISK FOR
Risk factors may include:	Tracheobronchial obstruction: Enlarged mediastinal nodes and/or airway edema (Hodgkin's and non-Hodgkin's); superior vena cava syndrome (non-Hodgkin's).
Possibly evidenced by:	[Not applicable; presence of signs and symptoms establishes an actual diagnosis.]
DESIRED OUTCOMES/ EVALUATION CRITERIA— PATIENT WILL:	Maintain a normal/effective respiratory pattern, free of dyspnea, cyanosis, or other signs of respiratory distress.

ACTIONS/INTERVENTIONS	RATIONALE
Independent	
Assess/monitor respiratory rate, depth, rhythm. Note reports of dyspnea and/or use of accessory muscles, nasal flaring, altered chest excursion.	Changes (such as tachypnea, dyspnea, use of accessory muscles) may indicate progression of respiratory involvement/compromise requiring prompt intervention.
Place patient in position of comfort, usually with head of bed elevated or sitting upright leaning forward (weight supported on arms), feet dangling.	Maximizes lung expansion, decreases work of breathing, and reduces risk of aspiration.
Reposition and assist with turning periodically.	Promotes aeration of all lung segments and mobilizes secretions.
Instruct in/assist with deep-breathing techniques and/or pursed lip or abdominal diaphragmatic breathing if indicated.	Helps promote gas diffusion and expansion of small airways. Provides patient with some control over respiration, helping to reduce anxiety.
Monitor/evaluate skin color, noting pallor, development of cyanosis (particularly in nail beds, earlobes, and lips).	Proliferation of WBCs can reduce oxygen-carrying capacity of the blood, leading to hypoxemia.

615

ACTIONS/INTERVENTIONS	RATIONALE

Independent

Assess respiratory response to activity. Note reports of dyspnea/"air hunger," increased fatigue. Schedule rest periods between activities.

Decreased cellular oxygenation reduces activity tolerance. Rest reduces oxygen demands and prevents fatigue and dyspnea.

Identify/encourage energy saving techniques, e.g., rest periods before and after meals, use of shower chair, sitting for care.

Aids in reducing fatigue and dyspnea and conserves energy for cellular regeneration and respiratory function.

Promote bed rest and provide care as indicated during acute/prolonged exacerbation.

Worsening respiratory involvement/hypoxia may necessitate cessation of activity to prevent more serious respiratory compromise.

Encourage expression of feelings. Acknowledge reality of situation and normality of feelings.

Anxiety increases oxygen demand and hypoxemia potentiates respiratory distress/cardiac symptoms, which in turn escalates anxiety.

Provide calm, quiet environment.

Promotes relaxation, conserving energy and reducing oxygen demand.

Observe for neck vein distension, headache, dizziness, periorbital/facial edema, dyspnea and stridor.

Non-Hodgkin's patients are at risk for superior vena cava syndrome, which may result in tracheal deviation and airway obstruction, representing an oncologic emergency.

Collaborative

Provide supplemental oxygen.

Maximizes oxygen available for circulatory uptake; aids in reducing hypoxemia.

Monitor laboratory studies, e.g., ABGs, oximetry.

Measures adequacy of respiratory function and effectiveness of therapy.

Assist with respiratory treatments/adjuncts, e.g., IPPB, incentive spirometer.

Promotes maximal aeration of all lung segments, preventing atelectasis.

Administer analgesics and tranquilizers as indicated.

Reducing physiologic responses to pain/anxiety decreases oxygen demands and may limit respiratory compromise.

Assist with intubation and mechanical ventilation.

May be necessary to support respiratory function until airway edema is resolved.

Prepare for emergency radiation therapy when indicated.

Treatment of choice for superior vena cava syndrome.

Bibliography

General References

Bellak, JP and Bamford, PA: Nursing Assessment: A Multidimensional Approach. Jones & Bartlett, Boston, 1987.
Berkow, R (ed): The Merck Manual, ed 15. Merck Sharp & Dohme Research Laboratories, Rahway, NJ, 1987.
Cella, JH and Watson, J: Nurse's Manual of Laboratory Tests. FA Davis, Philadelphia, 1989.
Condon, RE and Nyhus, LM (eds): Manual of Surgical Therapeutics, ed 7. Little, Brown & Co, Boston, 1988.
Deglin, JH, Vallerand, AH, and Russin, MM: Davis's Drug Guide for Nurses, ed 2. FA Davis, Philadelphia, 1991.
Diseases and Disorders Handbook, ed 3. Springhouse Corp, Springhouse, PA, 1989.
Doenges, ME and Moorhouse, MF: Nurse's Pocket Guide: Nursing Diagnoses with Interventions, ed 3. FA Davis, Philadelphia, 1991.
Dunagan, WC and Ridner, ML (eds): Manual of Medical Therapeutics, ed 26. Little, Brown & Co, Boston, 1989.
Fischbach, F: A Manual of Laboratory and Diagnostic Tests, ed 4. JB Lippincott, Philadelphia, 1992.

Guyton, AC: Textbook of Medical Physiology, ed 8. WB Saunders, Philadelphia, 1991.
Kuhn, MM: Pharmacotherapeutics: A Nursing Process Approach, ed 2. FA Davis, Philadelphia, 1991.
Professional Guide to Diseases, ed 3. Springhouse Corp, Springhouse, PA, 1989.
Suddarth, DS (ed): The Lippincott Manual of Nursing Practice, ed 5. JB Lippincott, Philadelphia, 1991.
Thomas, CL (ed): Taber's Cyclopedic Medical Dictionary, ed 16. FA Davis, Philadelphia, 1989.
Thompson, JM, et al: Mosby's Manual of Clinical Nursing, ed 2. CV Mosby, St Louis, 1989.

Books

A Cancer Source Book for Nurses, ed 6. American Cancer Society, Atlanta, 1991.
Adult Acute Myeloid Leukemia. National Cancer Institutes, PDQ Information for Patients. Rocky Mountain Cancer Information Systems. August 1991.
Otto, S: Oncology Nursing. Mosby Yearbook. CV Mosby, St Louis, 1991.
What You Need to Know about Adult Leukemia. NIH Pub No. 91-1572, October 1990.
What You Need to Know about Hodgkin's Disease. NIH Pub No. 92-1555. August, 1991.
What You Need to Know about Non-Hodgkin's Lymphomas. NIH Pub No 92-1567, August 1991.

Articles

Froberg, JH: The anemias: Causes and courses of action, Part I. RN 52(1):24, 1989.
Froberg, JH: The anemias: Causes and courses of action, Part II. RN 52(3):52, 1989.
Froberg, JH: The anemias: Causes and courses of action, Part III. RN 52(5):42, 1989.
Mueller, R: Cancer pain: Which drugs for which patient? RN 55(5):38, 1992.
Meyer, C: New drugs—The class of 1991. AJN 21(12):41, 1991.
Rivers, R and Williamson, N: Sickle cell anemia: Complex disease, nursing challenge. RN 53(6):24, 1990.
Simonson, GM. Caring for patients with acute myelocytic leukemia. AJN 88(3):304, 1988.
Strong, B: The voice from the mattress: How to care more sensitively for your cancer patients. Nursing 92, 22(5):47, 1992.

Renal Failure: Acute _____

Acute renal failure (ARF) can be divided into three major classifications dependent on site:

Prerenal: Interference with renal perfusion (e.g., volume depletion, volume shifts ("third-space" sequestration of fluid), or volume expansion) and manifested by decreased glomerular filtration rate (GFR).

Renal (or intrarenal): Parenchymal changes caused by ischemia or nephrotoxic substances. Acute tubular necrosis (ATN) accounts for 90% of cases of acute oliguria. Destruction of tubular epithelial cells results from (1) ischemia/hypoperfusion (similar to prerenal hypoperfusion except that correction of the causative factor may be followed by continued oliguria for up to 30 days) and/or (2) direct damage from nephrotoxins.

Postrenal: Occurs as the result of an obstruction in the urinary tract anywhere from the tubules to the urethral meatus.

Note: Iatrogenically induced ARF should be considered when other sources have been ruled out. The most common causative factors are administration of potentially nephrotoxic agents.

RELATED CONCERNS

Fluid and Electrolyte Imbalances, p 1054
Psychosocial Aspects of Acute Care, p 899
Renal Dialysis, p 646
Renal Failure: Chronic, p 632
Sepsis/Septicemia, p 887
Total Nutritional Support, p 1039
Upper Gastrointestinal Bleeding, p 454

PATIENT ASSESSMENT DATA BASE

ACTIVITY/REST

May report:	Fatigue, weakness, malaise.
May exhibit:	Muscle weakness, loss of tone.

CIRCULATION

May exhibit:	Hypotension or hypertension (including malignant hypertension, eclampsia/pregnancy-induced hypertension).

Cardiac dysrhythmias.

Weak/thready pulses, orthostatic hypotension (hypovolemia).

JVD, full/bounding pulses (hypervolemia).

Generalized tissue edema (including periorbital area, ankles, sacrum).

Pallor. Bleeding tendencies.

ELIMINATION

May report: Change in usual urination pattern: Increased frequency, polyuria (early failure), or decreased frequency/oliguria (later phase).

Dysuria, hesitancy, urgency, and retention (inflammation/obstruction/infection). Abdominal bloating, diarrhea, or constipation.

History of BPH, stones/calculi.

May exhibit: Change in urinary color, e.g., deep yellow, red, brown, cloudy.

Oliguria (usually 12–21 days); polyuria (2–6 L/d).

FOOD/FLUID

May report: Weight gain (edema), weight loss (dehydration).

Nausea, anorexia, heartburn, vomiting.

Use of diuretics.

May exhibit: Changes in skin turgor/moisture.

Edema (generalized, dependent).

NEUROSENSORY

May report: Headache, blurred vision.

Muscle cramps/twitching; "restless leg" syndrome.

May exhibit: Altered mental state, e.g., decreased attention span, inability to concentrate, loss of memory, confusion, decreasing level of consciousness (azotemia, electrolyte/acid/base imbalance).

Twitching, muscle fasciculations, seizure activity.

PAIN/COMFORT

May report: Flank pain, headache.

May exhibit: Guarding/distraction behaviors, restlessness.

RESPIRATION

May report: Shortness of breath.

May exhibit: Tachypnea, dyspnea, increased rate/depth (Kussmaul's respiration); ammonia breath.

Cough productive of pink-tinged sputum (pulmonary edema).

SAFETY

May report: Recent transfusion reaction.

May exhibit: Fever (sepsis, dehydration).

Petechiae, ecchymotic areas on skin.

Pruritus, dry skin.

619

TEACHING/LEARNING

May report: Family history of polycystic disease, hereditary nephritis, urinary calculus, malignancy.

History of exposure to toxins, e.g., drugs, environmental poisons.

Current/recent use of nephrotoxic drugs, e.g., aminoglycosides, amphotericin B; anesthetics; vasodilators.

Recent diagnostic testing with radiographic contrast media.

Concurrent conditions: Tumors in the urinary tract; Gram-negative sepsis; trauma/crush injuries, hemorrhage, DIC, burns, electrocution injury; autoimmune disorders (e.g., scleroderma, vasculitis), vascular occlusion/surgery, DM, cardiac/liver failure.

Discharge Plan Considerations: **DRG projected mean length of stay: 6.4 days.**

May require alteration/assistance with medications, treatments, supplies; transportation, homemaker/maintenance tasks.

DIAGNOSTIC STUDIES

Urine:

Volume: Usually less than 400 ml/24 h (oliguric phase), which occurs within 24–48 hours after renal insult.

Color: Dirty, brown sediment indicates presence of blood, Hb, myoglobin, porphyrins.

Specific gravity: Less than 1.020 reflects kidney disease, e.g., glomerulonephritis; pyelonephritis with loss of ability to concentrate; fixed at 1.010 reflects severe renal damage.

pH: Greater than 7 found in UTIs, renal tubular necrosis, and chronic renal failure (CRF).

Osmolality: Less than 350 mOsm/kg is indicative of tubular damage, and urine/serum ratio is often 1:1.

Creatinine clearance: May be significantly decreased before BUN and serum creatinine show significant elevation.

Sodium: Usually decreased but may be greater than 40 mEq/L if kidney is not able to resorb sodium.

Bicarbonate: Elevated if metabolic acidosis is present.

RBCs: May be present because of infection, stones, trauma, tumor, or altered GF.

Protein: High-grade proteinuria (3–4+) strongly indicates glomerular damage when RBCs and casts are also present. Low-grade proteinuria (1–2+) and WBCs may be indicative of infection or interstitial nephritis. In ATN, there is usually minimal proteinuria.

Casts: Usually signal renal disease or infection. Cellular casts with brownish pigments and numerous renal tubular epithelial cells are diagnostic of ATN. Red casts suggest acute glomerular nephritis.

Blood:

Hb: Decreased in presence of anemia.

RBCs: Often decreased owing to increased fragility/decreased survival.

pH: Metabolic acidosis (less than 7.2) may develop because of decreased renal ability to excrete hydrogen and end products of metabolism.

BUN/Cr: Usually rise in proportion with ratio of 10:1.

Serum osmolality: Greater than 285 mOsm/kg; often equal to urine.

Potassium: Elevated related to retention as well as cellular shifts (acidosis) or tissue release (red cell hemolysis).

Sodium: Usually increased, but may vary.

pH, calcium, and bicarbonate: Decreased.

Chloride, phosphorus, and magnesium: Increased.

Protein: Decreased serum level may reflect protein loss via urine, fluid shifts, decreased intake, or decreased synthesis owing to lack of essential amino acids.

Radionuclide imaging: May reveal calicectasis, hydronephrosis, narrowing, and delayed filling or emptying as a cause of ARF.

KUB (abdomen): Demonstrates size of kidneys/ureters/bladder, presence of cysts, tumors, and kidney displacement or obstruction (stones).

Retrograde pyelogram: Outlines abnormalities of renal pelvis and ureters.

Renal arteriogram: Assesses renal circulation and identifies extravascularities, masses.

Voiding cystoureterogram: Shows bladder size, reflux into ureters, retention.

Renal ultrasound: Determines kidney size and presence of masses, cysts, obstruction in upper urinary tract.

CT scan: Cross-sectional view of kidney and urinary tract detects presence/extent of disease.

MRI: Provides information about soft tissue.

Excretory urography (intravenous urogram or pyelogram): Radiopaque contrast concentrates in urine and facilitates visualization of kidneys, ureters and bladder.

Endourology: Direct visualization may be done of urethra, bladder, ureters, and kidney to diagnose problems, biopsy, and remove small lesions and/or calculi.

ECG: May be abnormal reflecting electrolyte and acid/base imbalances.

NURSING PRIORITIES

1. Reestablish/maintain fluid and electrolyte balance.
2. Prevent complications.
3. Provide emotional support for patient/SO.
4. Provide information about disease process/prognosis and treatment needs.

DISCHARGE GOALS

1. Homeostasis achieved.
2. Complications prevented/minimized.
3. Dealing realistically with current situation.
4. Disease process/prognosis and therapeutic regimen understood.

NURSING DIAGNOSIS:	**FLUID VOLUME, ALTERED: EXCESS**
May be related to:	Compromised regulatory mechanism (renal failure) with retention of water.
Possibly evidenced by:	Intake greater than output, oliguria; changes in urine specific gravity.
	Venous distention; BP/CVP changes.
	Generalized tissue edema, weight gain.
	Changes in mental status, restlessness.
	Decreased Hb/Hct, altered electrolytes, pulmonary congestion on x-ray.
DESIRED OUTCOMES/ EVALUATION CRITERIA— PATIENT WILL:	Display appropriate urinary output with specific gravity/ laboratory studies near normal; have a stable weight, vital signs within patient's normal range; have absence of edema.

ACTIONS/INTERVENTIONS	RATIONALE
Independent	
Monitor HR, BP, and CVP.	Tachycardia and hypertension can occur because of (1) failure of the kidneys to excrete urine, (2) excessive fluid resuscitation during efforts to treat hypovolemia/hypotension or convert oliguric phase of renal failure, and/or (3) changes in the renin–angiotensin system. *Note:* Invasive monitoring may be needed for assessing intravascular volume, especially in patients with poor cardiac function.
Record accurate I&O. Include "hidden" fluids such as antibiotic additives. Measure GI losses, and estimate insensible losses, e.g., diaphoresis.	Necessary for determining renal function, fluid replacement needs, and reducing risk of fluid overload. *Note:* Hypervolemia occurs in the anuric phase of ARF.
Monitor urine specific gravity.	Measures the kidney's ability to concentrate urine. In intrarenal failure, specific gravity is usually equal to/less than 1.010, indicating loss of ability to concentrate the urine.
Plan oral fluid replacement with patient, within multiple restrictions. Space desired beverages throughout 24 hours. Vary offerings, e.g., hot, cold, frozen.	Helps avoid periods without fluids, minimizing boredom of limited choices and reducing sense of deprivation and thirst.
Weigh daily on same scale with same equipment and clothing.	Daily body weight is best monitor of fluid status. A weight gain of more than 0.5 kg/d suggests fluid retention.
Assess skin, face, dependent areas for edema. Evaluate degree of edema (on scale of +1 to +4).	Edema occurs primarily in dependent tissues of the body, e.g., hands, feet, lumbosacral area. Patient can gain up to 10 lb (4.5 kg) of fluid before pitting edema is detected. Periorbital edema may be a presenting sign of this fluid shift, because these fragile tissues are easily distended by even minimal fluid accumulation.
Auscultate lung and heart sounds.	Fluid overload may lead to pulmonary edema and CHF evidenced by development of adventitious breath sounds, extra heart sounds. (Refer to ND: Cardiac Output, Decreased, high risk for, p 624.)
Assess level of consciousness; investigate changes in mentation, presence of restlessness.	May reflect fluid shifts, accumulation of toxins, acidosis, electrolyte imbalances, or developing hypoxia.
Collaborative	
Correct any reversible cause of ARF, e.g., improve renal perfusion, maximize cardiac output, relieve obstruction via surgery.	May be able to return to normal functioning, preventing or limiting residual effects.
Monitor laboratory studies, e.g.:	
BUN, Cr;	Assesses progression and management of renal dysfunction/failure. Although both values may be increased, creatinine is a better indicator of renal

ACTIONS/INTERVENTIONS	RATIONALE
Collaborative	
	function because it is not affected by hydration, diet, and tissue catabolism.
Urine sodium and creatinine;	In ATN, tubular functional integrity is lost and sodium resorption is impaired, resulting in increased sodium excretion. Urine creatinine is usually decreased as serum creatinine elevates.
Serum sodium;	Hyponatremia may result from fluid overload (dilutional) or inability of kidney to conserve sodium. Hypernatremia indicates deficit of total body water.
Serum potassium;	Lack of renal excretion and/or selective retention of potassium to excrete excess hydrogen ions (corrects acidosis) leads to hyperkalemia.
Hb/Hct;	Decreased values may indicate hemodilution (hypervolemia); however, during prolonged failure, anemia frequently develops as a result of RBC loss/decreased production. Other possible causes (active or occult hemorrhage) should also be evaluated.
Serial chest x-rays.	Increased cardiac size, prominent pulmonary vascular markings, pleural effusion, infiltrates/congestion indicate acute responses to fluid overload, or chronic changes associated with renal and heart failure.
Administer/restrict fluids as indicated.	Fluid management is usually calculated to replace output from all sources plus estimated insensible losses (metabolism, diaphoresis). Prerenal failure (azotemia) is treated with volume replacement and/or vasopressors. The oliguric patient with adequate circulating volume or fluid overload who is unresponsive to fluid restriction and diuretics requires dialysis.
Administer medications as indicated:	
Diuretics, e.g., furosemide (Lasix), mannitol (Osmitrol);	Given early in oliguric phase of ARF in an effort to convert to nonoliguric phase, to flush the tubular lumen of debris, reduce hyperkalemia, and promote adequate urine volume.
Antihypertensives, e.g., clonidine (Catapres); methyldopa (Aldomet); prazosin (Minipress).	May be given to treat hypertension by counteracting effects of decreased renal blood flow, and/or circulating volume overload.
Insert/maintain indwelling catheter, as indicated.	Catheterization excludes lower tract obstruction and provides means of accurate monitoring of urine output during acute phase. However, indwelling catheterization may be contraindicated due to increased risk of infection.
Prepare for dialysis as indicated.	Done to correct volume overload, electrolyte and acid/base imbalances, and to remove toxins.

623

ACTIONS/INTERVENTIONS	RATIONALE
Independent	
Monitor BP and heart rate.	Fluid volume excess, combined with hypertension (often occurs in renal failure) and effects of uremia, increases cardiac workload and can lead to cardiac failure. In ARF, cardiac failure is usually reversible.
Observe ECG or telemetry for changes in rhythm.	Changes in electromechanical function may become evident in response to progressing renal failure/accumulation of toxins and electrolyte imbalance. For example, hyperkalemia is associated with peaked T wave, wide QRS, prolonged PR interval, flattened/absent P wave. Hypokalemia is associated with flat T wave, peaked P wave, and appearance of U waves. Prolonged QT interval may reflect calcium deficit.
Auscultate heart sounds.	Development of S_3/S_4 are indicative of failure. Pericardial friction rub may be only manifestation of uremic pericarditis, requiring prompt intervention/possibly acute dialysis.
Assess color of skin, mucous membranes, and nail beds. Note capillary refill time.	Pallor may reflect vasoconstriction or anemia. Cyanosis may be related to pulmonary congestion and/or cardiac failure.
Note occurrence of slow pulse, hypotension, flushing, nausea/vomiting, and depressed level of consciousness (CNS depression).	Using drugs (e.g., antacids) containing magnesium can result in hypermagnesmia, potentiating neuromuscular dysfunction and risk of respiratory/cardiac arrest.
Investigate reports of muscle cramps, numbness/tingling of fingers, with muscle twitching, hyperreflexia.	Neuromuscular indicators of hypocalcemia, which can also affect cardiac contractility and function.

ACTIONS/INTERVENTIONS	RATIONALE

ACTIONS/INTERVENTIONS

Independent

Maintain bed rest or encourage adequate rest and provide assistance with care and desired activities.

Collaborative

Monitor laboratory studies, e.g.:

Potassium;

Calcium;

Magnesium.

Administer/restrict fluids as indicated (Refer to NDs: Fluid Volume, excess, p 621 and Fluid Volume Deficit, high risk for, p 629.)

Provide supplemental oxygen if indicated.

Administer medications as indicated:

Inotropic agents, e.g., digoxin (Lanoxin);

Calcium gluconate;

Aluminum hydroxide gels (Amphojel, Basalgel);

Glucose/insulin solution;

Sodium bicarbonate or sodium citrate;

Sodium polystyrene sulfonate (Kayexalate) with/without sorbitol.

RATIONALE

Reduces oxygen consumption/cardiac workload.

During oliguric phase, hyperkalemia may develop but shift to hypokalemia in diuretic or recovery phase. Any potassium value associated with ECG changes requires intervention. *Note:* A serum level of 6.5 mEq or greater constitutes a medical emergency.

In addition to its own cardiac effects, calcium deficit enhances the toxic effects of potassium.

Dialysis or calcium administration may be necessary to combat the CNS-depressive effects of an elevated serum magnesium level.

Cardiac output is dependent on circulating volume (affected by both fluid excess and deficit) and myocardial muscle function.

Maximizes available oxygen for myocardial uptake to reduce cardiac workload and cellular hypoxia.

May be used to improve cardiac output by increasing myocardial contractility and stroke volume. Dosage is dependent on renal function and potassium balance to obtain therapeutic effect without toxicity.

Serum calcium is often low but usually does not require specific treatment in ARF. If treatment is required, calcium gluconate may be given to treat hypocalcemia and to offset the effects of hyperkalemia by modifying cardiac irritability.

Increased phosphate levels may occur as a result of failure of GF and require use of phosphate-binding antacids to limit phosphate absorption from the GI tract.

Temporary measure to lower serum potassium by driving potassium into cells when cardiac rhythm is endangered.

May be used to correct acidosis or hyperkalemia (by increasing serum pH) if patient is severely acidotic and not fluid overloaded.

Exchange resin that trades sodium for potassium in the GI tract to lower serum potassium level.

ACTIONS/INTERVENTIONS

Collaborative

Prepare for/assist with dialysis as necessary.

RATIONALE

Sorbitol may be included to cause osmotic diarrhea to help excrete potassium.

May be indicated for persistent dysrhythmias, progressive heart failure unresponsive to other therapies.

NURSING DIAGNOSIS:	NUTRITION, ALTERED: LESS THAN BODY REQUIREMENTS, HIGH RISK FOR
Risk factors may include:	Protein catabolism; dietary restrictions to reduce nitrogenous waste products.
	Increased metabolic needs.
	Anorexia, nausea/vomiting; ulcerations of oral mucosa.
Possibly evidenced by:	[Not applicable; presence of signs and symptoms establishes an actual diagnosis.]
DESIRED OUTCOMES/ EVALUATION CRITERIA— PATIENT WILL:	Maintain/regain weight as indicated by individual situation, free of edema.

ACTIONS/INTERVENTIONS

Independent

Assess/document dietary intake.

Provide frequent, small feedings.

Give patient/SO a list of permitted foods/fluids and encourage involvement in menu choices.

Offer frequent mouth care/rinse with dilute (25%) acetic acid solution; provide gum, hard candy, breath mints between meals.

Weigh daily.

Collaborative

Monitor laboratory studies, e.g., BUN, serum albumin, transferrin, sodium, and potassium.

RATIONALE

Aids in identifying deficiencies and dietary needs. General physical condition, uremic symptoms (e.g., nausea, anorexia, altered taste), and multiple dietary restrictions affect food intake.

Minimizes anorexia and nausea associated with uremic state/diminished peristalsis.

Provides patient with a measure of control within dietary restrictions. Food from home may enhance appetite.

Mucous membranes may become dry and cracked. Mouth care soothes, lubricates, and helps freshen mouth taste, which is often unpleasant owing to uremia and restricted oral intake. Rinsing with acetic acid helps neutralize ammonia formed by conversion of urea.

The fasting/catabolic patient will normally lose 0.2–0.5 kg/d. Changes in excess of 0.5 kg may reflect shifts in fluid balance.

Indicators of nutritional needs, restrictions, and necessity for/effectiveness of therapy.

ACTIONS/INTERVENTIONS	RATIONALE
Collaborative	
Consult with dietitian/nutritional support team.	Determines individual calorie and nutrient needs within the restrictions, and identifies most effective route and product, e.g., oral supplements, tube feedings, hyperalimentation.
Provide high calorie, low/moderate protein diet. Include complex carbohydrates and fat sources to meet caloric needs (avoiding concentrated sugar sources) and essential amino acids.	The amount of needed exogenous protein is less than normal unless the patient is on dialysis. Carbohydrates meet energy needs and limit tissue catabolism, preventing ketoacid formation from protein and fat oxidation. Carbohydrate intolerance mimicking DM may occur in severe renal failure. Essential amino acids improve nitrogen balance and nutritional status.
Restrict potassium, sodium, and phosphorus intake as indicated.	Restriction of these electrolytes may be needed to prevent further renal damage, especially if dialysis is not part of treatment, and/or during recovery phase of ARF.
Administer medications as indicated:	
Iron preparations;	Iron deficiency may occur if protein is restricted, patient is anemic, or GI function is impaired.
Calcium;	Restores normal serum levels to improve cardiac and neuromuscular function, blood clotting, and bone metabolism.
Vitamin D;	Necessary to facilitate absorption of calcium from the GI tract.
B complex vitamins;	Vital as coenzyme in cell growth and actions. Intake is decreased owing to protein restrictions.
Antiemetics, e.g., prochlorperazine (Compazine), trimethobenzamide (Tigan).	Given to relieve n/v and may enhance oral intake.

NURSING DIAGNOSIS:	**FATIGUE**
May be related to:	Decreased metabolic energy production/dietary restrictions, anemia.
	Increased energy requirements, e.g., fever/inflammation, tissue regeneration.
Possibly evidenced by:	Overwhelming lack of energy.
	Inability to maintain usual activities, decreased performance.
	Lethargy, disinterest in surroundings.
DESIRED OUTCOMES/ EVALUATION CRITERIA— PATIENT WILL:	Report improved sense of energy.
	Participate in desired activities.

ACTIONS/INTERVENTIONS	RATIONALE
Independent	
Evaluate reports of fatigue, difficulty accomplishing tasks. Note ability to sleep/rest appropriately.	Determines degree (progression/resolution) of disabling effects.
Assess ability to participate in desired/required activities.	Identifies individual needs and aids in choosing appropriate interventions.
Identify stress/psychologic factors that may be contributory.	May have an accumulative effect (along with physiologic factors) that can be reduced when concerns and fears are acknowledged/addressed.
Plan care with adequate rest periods.	Prevents excessive fatigue and conserves energy for healing, tissue regeneration.
Provide assistance with ADLs and ambulation.	Conserves energy, permits continuation of normal/required activities, provides for patient safety.
Increase level of participation as patient tolerates.	Promotes sense of improvement/enhances well-being, and limits frustration.
Collaborative	
Monitor electrolyte levels, including calcium, magnesium, and potassium.	Imbalances can impair neuromuscular function requiring increased energy expenditure to accomplish tasks and potentiating feelings of fatigue.

NURSING DIAGNOSIS:	INFECTION, HIGH RISK FOR
Risk factors may include:	Depression of immunologic defenses (secondary to uremia).
	Invasive procedures/devices (e.g., urinary catheter).
	Changes in dietary intake/malnutrition.
Possibly evidenced by:	[Not applicable; presence of signs and symptoms establishes an actual diagnosis.]
DESIRED OUTCOMES/ EVALUATION CRITERIA— PATIENT WILL:	Experience no signs/symptoms of infection.

ACTIONS/INTERVENTIONS	RATIONALE
Independent	
Promote good hand washing by patient and staff.	Reduces risk of cross-contamination.
Avoid invasive procedures, instrumentation, and manipulation of indwelling catheters, whenever possible. Use aseptic technique when caring for/manipulating IV/invasive lines. Change site/dressings per protocol. Note edema, purulent drainage.	Limits introduction of bacteria into body. Early detection/treatment of developing infection may prevent sepsis.

ACTIONS/INTERVENTIONS

Independent

Provide routine catheter care and promote meticulous perianal care. Keep urinary drainage system closed and remove indwelling catheter as soon as possible.

Encourage deep breathing, coughing, frequent position changes.

Assess skin integrity. (Refer to CP: Renal Failure: Chronic; ND: Skin Integrity, impaired, high risk for, p 639.)

Monitor vital signs.

Collaborative

Monitor laboratory studies, e.g., WBC with differential.

Obtain specimen(s) for culture and sensitivity and administer appropriate antibiotics as indicated.

RATIONALE

Reduces bacterial colonization and risk of ascending UTI.

Prevents atelectasis and mobilizes secretions to reduce risk of pulmonary infections.

Excoriations from scratching may become secondarily infected.

Fever with increased pulse and respirations is typical of increased metabolic rate resulting from inflammatory process, although sepsis can occur without a febrile response.

Although elevated WBCs may indicate generalized infection, leukocytosis is commonly seen in ARF and may reflect inflammation/injury within the kidney. A shifting of the differential to the left is indicative of infection.

Verification of infection and identification of specific organism aids in choice of the most effective treatment.

NURSING DIAGNOSIS:	FLUID VOLUME DEFICIT, HIGH RISK FOR
Risk factors may include:	Excessive loss of fluid (diuretic phase of ARF, with rising urinary volume and delayed return of tubular reabsorption capabilities.)
Possibly evidenced by:	[Not applicable; presence of signs and symptoms establishes an actual diagnosis.]
DESIRED OUTCOMES/ EVALUATION CRITERIA— PATIENT WILL:	Display I&O near balance; good skin turgor, moist mucous membranes, palpable peripheral pulses, stable weight and vital signs, electrolytes within normal range.

ACTIONS/INTERVENTIONS

Independent

Measure I&O accurately. Weigh daily. Calculate insensible fluid losses.

RATIONALE

Helps estimate fluid replacement needs. Fluid intake should approximate losses through urine, nasogastric/wound drainage, and insensible losses (e.g., diaphoresis and metabolism). *Note:* Some sources believe that fluid replacement should not exceed two thirds of the previous day's output to prevent prolonging the diuresis.

ACTIONS/INTERVENTIONS	RATIONALE
Independent	
Provide allowed fluids throughout 24-hour period.	Diuretic phase of ARF may revert to oliguric phase if fluid intake is not maintained or nocturnal dehydration occurs.
Monitor BP (noting postural changes) and heart rate.	Orthostatic hypotension and tachycardia suggests hypovolemia.
Note signs/symptoms of dehydration, e.g., dry mucous membranes, thirst, dulled sensorium, peripheral vasoconstriction.	In diuretic phase of renal failure, urine output can exceed 3 L/d. Extracellular fluid volume depletion activates the thirst center, and Na depletion causes persistent thirst, unrelieved by drinking water. Continued fluid losses/inadequate replacement may lead to hypovolemic state.
Control environmental temperature; limit bed linens as indicated.	May reduce diaphoresis, which contributes to overall fluid losses.
Collaborative	
Monitor laboratory studies, e.g., sodium.	In nonoliguric ARF or in diuretic phase of ARF, large urine losses may result in sodium wasting while elevated urinary sodium acts osmotically to increase fluid losses. Restriction of sodium may be indicated to break the cycle.

NURSING DIAGNOSIS:	**KNOWLEDGE DEFICIT [LEARNING NEED] REGARDING CONDITION, PROGNOSIS, AND TREATMENT NEEDS**
May be related to:	Lack of exposure/recall.
	Information misinterpretation.
	Unfamiliarity with information resources.
Possibly evidenced by:	Questions/request for information, statement of misconception.
	Inaccurate follow-through of instructions, development of preventable complications.
DESIRED OUTCOMES/ EVALUATION CRITERIA— PATIENT WILL:	Verbalize understanding of condition/disease process, prognosis, and treatment.
	Identify relationship of signs/symptoms to the disease process and correlate symptoms with causative factors.
	Initiate necessary lifestyle changes and participate in treatment regimen.

ACTIONS/INTERVENTIONS	RATIONALE
Independent	
Review disease process, prognosis, and precipitating factors if known.	Provides knowledge base on which patient can make informed choices.
Explain level of renal function after acute episode is over.	Patient may experience residual defects in kidney function which may/may not be permanent.
Discuss renal dialysis or transplantation if these are likely options for the future.	Although these options would have been previously presented by the physician, the patient may now be at a point when decisions must be made and may desire additional input.
Review dietary plan/restrictions. Include fact sheet listing food restrictions.	Adequate nutrition is necessary to promote healing/tissue regeneration while adherence to restrictions may prevent complications.
Encourage patient to observe characteristics of urine and amount/frequency of output.	Changes may reflect alterations in renal function/need for dialysis.
Establish regular schedule for weighing.	Useful tool for monitoring fluid and dietary status/needs.
Review fluid intake/restriction. Remind patient to spread fluids over entire day and to include all fluids (e.g., ice) in daily fluid counts.	Depending on the cause of ARF, patient may need to either restrict or increase intake of fluids.
Discuss activity restriction and gradual resumption of desired activity. Encourage use of energy-saving, relaxation, and diversional techniques.	Patient with severe ARF may need to restrict activity and/or may feel weak for an extended period during lengthy recovery phase, requiring measures to conserve energy and reduce boredom/depression.
Discuss/review medication use. Encourage patient to discuss all medications (including OTC drugs) with physician.	Medications that are concentrated in/excreted by the kidneys can cause toxic cumulative reactions and/or permanent damage to kidneys.
Stress necessity of follow-up care, laboratory studies.	Renal function may be slow to return following acute failure (up to 12 months) and deficits may persist, requiring changes in therapy to avoid recurrence/complications.
Identify symptoms requiring medical intervention, e.g., decreased urinary output, sudden weight gain, presence of edema, lethargy, bleeding, signs of infection; altered mentation.	Prompt evaluation and intervention may prevent serious complications/progression to CRF.

Renal Failure: Chronic _____

Chronic renal failure (CRF) is usually the end result of a gradually progressive loss of kidney function. Causes include chronic glomerulonephritis, chronic infections, vascular diseases (nephrosclerosis), obstructive processes (calculi), collagen diseases (systemic lupus), nephrotoxic agents (aminoglycosides), endocrine diseases (diabetes).

This syndrome progresses through stages and produces major changes in all body systems.

RELATED CONCERNS

Congestive Heart Failure, p 48
Psychosocial Aspects of Acute Care, p 899
Upper Gastrointestinal/Esophageal Bleeding, p 454
    Additional associated nursing diagnoses are found in:
    Renal Dialysis, p 646
    Renal Failure: Acute, p 618

PATIENT ASSESSMENT DATA BASE

ACTIVITY/REST

May report: Extreme fatigue, weakness, malaise.

                  Sleep disturbances (insomnia/restlessness or somnolence).

May exhibit: Muscle weakness, loss of tone, decreased ROM.

CIRCULATION

May report: History of prolonged or severe hypertension.

                  Palpitations; chest pain (angina).

May exhibit: Hypertension; JVD, full/bounding pulses, generalized tissue and pitting edema of feet, legs, hands.

                  Cardiac dysrhythmias.

                  Weak thready pulses, orthostatic hypotension reflects hypovolemia, which is rare in end-stage disease.

                  Pericardial friction rub (response to accumulated wastes).

                  Pallor; bronze-gray, yellow skin.

                  Bleeding tendencies.

EGO INTEGRITY

May report: Stress factors, e.g., financial, relationship, and so on.

                  Feelings of helplessness, hopelessness, powerlessness.

May exhibit: Denial, anxiety, fear, anger, irritability, personality changes.

ELIMINATION

May report: Decreased urinary frequency, oliguria, anuria (advanced failure).

                  Abdominal bloating, diarrhea, or constipation.

May exhibit: Change in urine color, e.g., deep yellow, red, brown, cloudy.

                  Oliguria, may become anuric.

FOOD/FLUID

May report: Rapid weight gain (edema), weight loss (malnutrition).

Anorexia, heartburn, n/v; unpleasant metallic taste in the mouth (ammonia breath).

Use of diuretics.

May exhibit: Abdominal distention/ascites, liver enlargement (end-stage).

Changes in skin turgor/moisture.

Edema (generalized, dependent).

Gum ulcerations, bleeding of gums/tongue.

Muscle wasting, decreased subcutaneous fat, debilitated appearance.

NEUROSENSORY

May report: Headache, blurred vision.

Muscle cramps/twitching; "restless leg" syndrome; burning numbness of soles of feet.

Numbness/tingling and weakness, especially of lower extremities (peripheral neuropathy).

May exhibit: Altered mental state, e.g., decreased attention span, inability to concentrate, loss of memory, confusion, decreasing level of consciousness, stupor, coma.

Diminished DTRs.

Positive Chvostek's and Trousseau's signs.

Twitching, muscle fasciculations, seizure activity.

Thin, brittle nails; thin hair.

PAIN/COMFORT

May report: Flank pain; headache; muscle cramps/leg pain (worse at night).

May exhibit: Guarding/distraction behaviors, restlessness.

RESPIRATION

May report: Shortness of breath; paroxysmal nocturnal dyspnea; cough with/without thick, tenacious sputum.

May exhibit: Tachypnea, dyspnea, increased rate/depth (Kussmaul's respiration).

Cough productive of pink-tinged sputum (pulmonary edema).

SAFETY

May report: Itching skin.

Recent/recurrent infections.

May exhibit: Pruritus.

Fever (sepsis, dehydration); normothermia may actually represent an elevation in the patient who has developed a lower-than-normal body temperature (effect of CRF/depressed immune response).

Petechiae, ecchymotic areas on skin.

Bone fractures; calcium phosphate deposits (metastatic calcifications) in skin, soft tissues, joints; limited joint movement.

SEXUALITY

May report: Decreased libido; amenorrhea; infertility.

SOCIAL INTERACTION

May report: Difficulties imposed by condition, e.g., unable to work, maintain usual role function in family.

TEACHING/LEARNING

May report: Family history of DM (high risk for renal failure), polycystic disease, hereditary nephritis, urinary calculus, malignancy.

History of exposure to toxins, e.g., drugs, environmental poisons.

Current/recent use of nephrotoxic antibiotics.

Discharge Plan Considerations: **DRG projected mean length of stay: 6.4 days.**

May require alteration/assistance with medications, treatments, supplies; transportation, homemaker/maintenance tasks.

DIAGNOSTIC STUDIES

Urine:

Volume: Usually less than 400 ml/24 h (oliguria) or urine is absent (anuria).

Color: Abnormally cloudy urine may be caused from pus, bacteria, fat, colloidal particles, phosphates, or urates. Dirty, brown sediment indicates presence of blood, Hb, myoglobin, porphyrins.

Specific gravity: Less than 1.015 (fixed at 1.010 reflects severe renal damage).

Osmolality: Less than 350 mOsm/kg is indicative of tubular damage, and urine/serum ratio is often 1:1.

Creatinine clearance: May be significantly decreased.

Sodium: Greater than 40 mEq/L because kidney is not able to reabsorb sodium.

Protein: High-grade proteinuria (3–4+) strongly indicates glomerular damage when RBCs and casts are also present.

Blood:

BUN/Cr: Elevated, usually rise in proportion. Creatinine level of 10 mg/dL suggests end stage (may be as low as 5).

CBC: Hct: Decreased in presence of anemia. *Hb:* Usually less than 7–8 g/dL. *RBCs:* Life span decreased owing to erythropoietin deficiency as well as azotemia.

ABGs: pH: Decreased metabolic acidosis (less than 7.2) occurs because of loss of renal ability to excrete hydrogen and ammonia or end products of protein catabolism. Bicarbonate decreased. PCO_2 decreased.

Serum sodium: May be low (if kidney "wastes sodium") or normal (reflecting dilutional state of hypernatremia).

Potassium: Elevated related to retention as well as cellular shifts (acidosis) or tissue release (RBC hemolysis). In end-stage disease, ECG changes may not occur until potassium is 6.5 mEq or greater.

Magnesium/phosphorus: Elevated.

Calcium: Decreased.

Proteins (especially albumin): Decreased serum level may reflect protein loss via urine, fluid shifts, decreased intake, or decreased synthesis owing to lack of essential amino acids.

Serum osmolality: Greater than 285 mOsm/kg; often equal to urine.

KUB x-rays: Demonstrates size of kidneys/ureters/bladder and presence of obstruction (stones).

Retrograde pyelogram: Outlines abnormalities of renal pelvis and ureters.

Renal arteriogram: Assesses renal circulation and identifies extravascularities, masses.

Voiding cystourethrogram: Shows bladder size, reflux into ureters, retention.

Renal ultrasound: Determines kidney size and presence of masses, cysts, obstruction in upper urinary tract.

Renal biopsy: May be done endoscopically to examine tissue cells for histologic diagnosis.

Renal endoscopy, nephroscopy: Done to examine renal pelvis; flush out calculi, hematuria and remove selected tumors.

ECG: May be abnormal reflecting electrolyte and acid/base imbalances.

X-rays of feet, skull, spinal column, and hands: May reveal demineralization, calcifications.

NURSING PRIORITIES

1. Maintain homeostasis.
2. Prevent complications.
3. Provide information about disease process/prognosis and treatment needs.
4. Support adjustment to lifestyle changes.

DISCHARGE GOALS

1. Fluid/electrolyte balance stabilized.
2. Complications prevented/minimized.
3. Disease process/prognosis and therapeutic regimen understood.
4. Dealing realistically with situation; initiating necessary lifestyle changes.

NURSING DIAGNOSIS:	CARDIAC OUTPUT, DECREASED, HIGH RISK FOR
Risk factors may include:	Fluid imbalances affecting circulating volume, myocardial workload, and systemic vascular resistance.
	Alterations in rate, rhythm, cardiac conduction (electrolyte imbalances, hypoxia).
	Accumulation of toxins (urea), soft-tissue calcification (deposition of Ca^{2+} phosphate).
Possibly evidenced by:	[Not applicable; presence of signs and symptoms establishes an actual diagnosis.]
DESIRED OUTCOMES/ EVALUATION CRITERIA— PATIENT WILL:	Maintain cardiac output as evidenced by BP and heart rate within patient's normal range; peripheral pulses strong and equal with prompt capillary refill time.

ACTIONS/INTERVENTIONS	RATIONALE

(In addition to those in CP: Renal Failure: Acute; ND: Cardiac Output, Decreased, high risk for, p 624:)

Independent

Auscultate heart and lung sounds. Evaluate presence of peripheral edema/vascular congestion and reports of dyspnea.	S_3/S_4 heart sounds with muffled tones, tachycardia, irregular heart rate, tachypnea, dyspnea, crackles, wheezes, and edema/jugular distention suggest CHF.

635

ACTIONS/INTERVENTIONS	RATIONALE

Independent

Assess presence/degree of hypertension: monitor BP; note postural changes, e.g., sitting, lying, standing.

Significant hypertension can occur because of disturbances in the renin–angiotensin aldosterone system (caused by renal dysfunction). Although hypertension is common, orthostatic hypotension may occur due to intravascular fluid deficit, response to effects of antihypertensive medications, or uremic pericardial tamponade.

Investigate reports of chest pain, noting location, radiation, severity (0–10 scale), and whether or not it is intensified by deep inspiration and supine position.

While hypertension and chronic CHF may cause MI, approximately half of CRF patients on dialysis develop pericarditis, potentiating risk of pericardial effusion/tamponade.

Evaluate heart sounds (note friction rub), BP, peripheral pulses, capillary refill, vascular congestion, temperature, and sensorium/mentation.

Presence of sudden hypotension, paradoxic pulse, narrow pulse pressure, diminished/absent peripheral pulses, marked jugular distention, pallor, and a rapid mental deterioration indicate tamponade, which is a medical emergency.

Assess activity level, response to activity.

Weakness can be attributed to CHF as well as anemia.

Collaborative

Monitor laboratory studies, e.g.:

Electrolytes (potassium, sodium, calcium, magnesium), BUN;

Imbalances can alter electrical conduction and cardiac function.

Chest x-rays.

Useful in identifying developing cardiac failure or soft-tissue calcification.

Administer antihypertensive drugs, e.g., prazosin (Minipress), captopril (Capoten), clonidine (Catapres), hydralazine (Apresoline).

Reduces systemic vascular resistance and/or renin release to decrease myocardial workload and aid in prevention of CHF and/or MI.

Assist with pericardiocentesis as indicated.

Accumulation of fluid within pericardial sac can compromise cardiac filling and myocardial contractility impairing cardiac output and potentiating risk of cardiac arrest.

Prepare for dialysis.

Reduction of uremic toxins and correction of electrolyte imbalances and fluid overload may limit/prevent cardiac manifestations, including hypertension and pericardial effusion.

NURSING DIAGNOSIS:	INJURY, HIGH RISK FOR, (ABNORMAL BLOOD PROFILE)
Risk factors may include:	Suppressed erythropoietin production/secretion; decreased RBC production and survival; altered clotting factors; increased capillary fragility.
Possibly evidenced by:	[Not applicable; presence of signs and symptoms establishes an actual diagnosis.]

DESIRED OUTCOMES/ EVALUATION CRITERIA— PATIENT WILL:	Experience no signs/symptoms of bleeding/hemorrhage. Maintain/demonstrate improvement in laboratory values.

ACTIONS/INTERVENTIONS

Independent

Note reports of increasing fatigue, weakness. Observe for tachycardia, pallor of skin/mucous membranes, dyspnea, and chest pain. Plan patient activities to avoid fatigue.

Monitor level of consciousness and behavior.

Evaluate response to activity, ability to perform tasks. Assist as needed and develop schedule for rest.

Limit vascular sampling, combine laboratory tests when possible.

Observe for oozing from venipuncture sites, bleeding/ecchymotic areas following slight trauma, petechiae; joint swelling or mucous membrane involvement, e.g., bleeding gums, recurrent epistaxis, hematemesis, melena, and hazy/red urine.

Hematest GI secretions/stool for blood.

Provide soft toothbrush, electric razor; use smallest needle possible and apply prolonged pressure following injections/vascular punctures.

Collaborative

Monitor laboratory studies, e.g.:

   CBC: RBCs, Hb/Hct;

   Platelet count, clotting factors;

   PT level.

Administer fresh blood, packed RBCs as indicated.

RATIONALE

May reflect effects of anemia, and cardiac response necessary to keep cells oxygenated.

Anemia may cause cerebral hypoxia manifested by changes in mentation, orientation, and behavioral responses.

Anemia decreases tissue oxygenation and increases fatigue, which may require intervention, changes in activity, and rest.

Recurrent/excessive blood sampling can worsen anemia.

Bleeding can occur easily because of capillary fragility/altered clotting functions and may worsen anemia.

Stress and hemostatic abnormalities may result in GI hemorrhage.

Reduces risk of bleeding/hematoma formation.

Uremia (e.g., elevated ammonia, urea, other toxins) decreases production of erythropoietin and depresses RBC production and survival time. In chronic renal failure, hemoglobin and hematocrit are usually low but tolerated; e.g., patient may not be symptomatic until Hb is below 7.

Suppression of platelet formation and inadequate levels of factors III and VIII impair clotting and potentiate risk of bleeding. *Note:* Bleeding may become intractable in end-stage disease.

Abnormal prothrombin consumption lowers serum levels and impairs clotting.

May be necessary when patient is symptomatic with anemia. Packed RBCs are usually given when patient is fluid overloaded or being dialyzed. Washed RBCs are used to prevent hyperkalemia associated with stored blood.

637

ACTIONS/INTERVENTIONS

Collaborative

Administer medications, as indicated, e.g.:

Iron preparations, folic acid (Folvite), cyanocobalamin (Betalin);

Cimetidine (Tagamet); ranitidine (Zantac); antacids;

Hemastatics/fibrinolysis inhibitors, e.g., aminocaproic acid (Amicar);

Stool softeners (Colace); bulk laxative (Metamucil).

RATIONALE

Useful in correcting symptomatic anemia related to nutritional/dialysis-induced deficits. *Note:* Iron should not be given with phosphate binders because they may decrease iron absorption.

May be given prophylactically to reduce/neutralize gastric acid and thereby reduce the risk of GI hemorrhage.

Inhibits bleeding that does not subside spontaneously/respond to usual treatment.

Straining to pass hard-formed stool increases likelihood of mucosa/rectal bleed.

NURSING DIAGNOSIS:	THOUGHT PROCESSES, ALTERED
May be related to:	Physiologic changes: accumulation of toxins (e.g., urea, ammonia), metabolic acidosis, hypoxia; electrolyte imbalances, metastatic calcifications in the brain.
Possibly evidenced by:	Disorientation to person, place, time.
	Memory deficit.
	Altered attention span, decreased ability to grasp ideas.
	Impaired ability to make decisions, problem solve.
	Changes in sensorium: somnolence, stupor, coma.
	Changes in behavior: irritability, withdrawal, depression, psychosis.
DESIRED OUTCOMES/ EVALUATION CRITERIA— PATIENT WILL:	Regain usual level of mentation.
	Identify ways to compensate for cognitive impairment/ memory deficits.

ACTIONS/INTERVENTIONS

Independent

Assess extent of impairment in thinking ability, memory, and orientation. Note attention span.

Ascertain from SO, patient's usual level of mentation.

RATIONALE

Uremic syndrome's effect can begin with minor confusion/irritability and progress to altered personality or inability to assimilate information and participate in care. Awareness of changes provides opportunity for evaluation and intervention.

Provides comparison to evaluate progression/resolution of impairment.

ACTIONS/INTERVENTIONS	RATIONALE
Independent	
Provide SO with information about patient's status.	Some improvement in mentation may be expected with restoration of more normal levels of BUN, electrolytes, and serum pH.
Provide quiet/calm environment and judicious use of television, radio, and visitation.	Minimizes environmental stimuli to reduce sensory overload/increased confusion while preventing sensory deprivation.
Reorient to surroundings, person, and so forth. Provide calendars, clocks, outside window.	Provides clues to aid in recognition of reality.
Present reality concisely, briefly, and do not challenge illogical thinking.	Confrontation potentiates defensive reactions and may lead to patient mistrust and heightened denial of reality.
Communicate information/instructions in simple, short sentences. Ask direct, yes/no questions. Repeat explanations as necessary.	May aid in reducing confusion and increases possibility that communications will be understood/remembered.
Establish a regular schedule for expected activities.	Aids in maintaining reality orientation and may reduce fear/confusion.
Promote adequate rest and undisturbed periods for sleep.	Sleep deprivation may further impair cognitive abilities.
Collaborative	
Monitor laboratory studies, e.g., BUN/creatinine, serum electrolytes, glucose level, and ABGs (PO_2, pH).	Correction of elevations/imbalances can have profound effects on cognition/mentation.
Provide supplemental O_2 as indicated.	Correction of hypoxia alone can improve cognition.
Avoid use of barbiturates and opiates.	Drugs normally detoxified in the kidneys will have increased half-life/cumulative effects, worsening confusion.
Prepare for dialysis.	Marked deterioration of thought processes may indicate worsening of azotemia and general condition, requiring prompt intervention to regain homeostasis.

NURSING DIAGNOSIS:	SKIN INTEGRITY, IMPAIRED, HIGH RISK FOR
Risk factors may include:	Altered metabolic state, circulation (anemia with tissue ischemia), and sensation (peripheral neuropathy).
	Alterations in skin turgor (edema/dehydration).
	Reduced activity/immobility.
	Accumulation of toxins in the skin.
Possibly evidenced by:	[Not applicable; presence of signs and symptoms establishes an actual diagnosis.]

ACTIONS/INTERVENTIONS	RATIONALE
Independent	
Inspect skin for changes in color, turgor, vascularity. Note redness, excoriation. Observe for ecchymosis, purpura.	Indicates areas of poor circulation/breakdown that may lead to decubitus formation/infection.
Monitor fluid intake and hydration of skin and mucous membranes.	Detects presence of dehydration or overhydration that affect circulation and tissue integrity at the cellular level.
Inspect dependent areas for edema.	Edematous tissues are more prone to breakdown.
Change position frequently; move patient carefully; pad bony prominences with sheepskin, elbow/heel protectors.	Decreases pressure on edematous, poorly perfused tissues to reduce ischemia. Elevation promotes venous return limiting venous stasis/edema formation.
Provide soothing skin care. Restrict use of soaps. Apply ointments or creams (e.g., lanolin, Aquaphor).	Baking soda, cornstarch baths decrease itching and are less drying than soaps. Lotions and ointments may be desired to relieve dry, cracked skin.
Keep linens dry, wrinkle-free.	Reduces dermal irritation and risk of skin breakdown.
Investigate reports of itching.	Although dialysis has largely eliminated skin problems associated with uremic frost, itching can occur because the skin is an excretory route for waste products, e.g., phosphate crystals (associated with hyperparathyroidism in end-stage disease).
Recommend patient use cool, moist compresses to apply pressure (rather than scratch) pruritic areas. Keep fingernails short; provide gloves during sleep if needed.	Alleviates discomfort and reduces risk of dermal injury.
Suggest wearing loose-fitting cotton garments.	Prevents direct dermal irritation and promotes evaporation of moisture on the skin.
Collaborative	
Provide foam/flotation mattress.	Reduces prolonged pressure on tissues, which can limit cellular perfusion potentiating ischemia/necrosis.

Possibly evidenced by:	[Not applicable; presence of signs and symptoms establishes an actual diagnosis.]
DESIRED OUTCOMES/ EVALUATION CRITERIA— PATIENT WILL:	Maintain integrity of mucous membranes. Identify/initiate specific interventions to promote healthy oral mucosa.

ACTIONS/INTERVENTIONS	RATIONALE
Independent	
Inspect oral cavity; note moistness, character of saliva, presence of inflammation, ulcerations, leukoplakia.	Provides opportunity for prompt intervention and prevention of infection.
Provide fluids throughout 24-hour period within prescribed limit.	Prevents excessive oral dryness from prolonged period without oral intake.
Offer frequent mouth care/rinse with 25% acetic acid solution; provide gum, hard candy, breath mints between meals.	Mucous membranes may become dry and cracked. Mouth care soothes, lubricates, and helps freshen mouth taste, which is often unpleasant owing to uremia and restricted oral intake. Rinsing with acetic acid helps neutralize ammonia formed by conversion of urea.
Encourage good dental hygiene after meals and at bedtime. Recommend avoidance of dental floss.	Reduces bacterial growth and potential for infection. Dental floss may cut gums, potentiating bleeding.
Recommend patient stop smoking and avoid lemon/glycerine products/mouthwash containing alcohol.	These substances are irritating to the mucosa and have a drying effect, potentiating discomfort.
Provide artificial saliva as needed, e.g., Ora-Lube.	Prevents dryness, buffers acids, and promotes comfort.
Collaborative	
Administer medications as indicated, e.g., antihistamines: cyproheptadine (Periactin).	May be given for relief of itching.

NURSING DIAGNOSIS:	**KNOWLEDGE DEFICIT [LEARNING NEED], REGARDING CONDITION, PROGNOSIS, AND TREATMENT NEEDS**
May be related to:	Cognitive limitation. Lack of exposure/recall, information misinterpretation.
Possibly evidenced by:	Questions/request for information, statement of misconception. Inaccurate follow-through of instructions/development of preventable complications.

ACTIONS/INTERVENTIONS	RATIONALE

(In addition to interventions outlined in CP: Renal Failure: Acute; Knowledge Deficit, p 630.)

Independent

ACTIONS/INTERVENTIONS	RATIONALE
Review disease process/prognosis and future expectations.	Provides knowledge base on which patient can make informed choices.
Review dietary restrictions, including phosphorus (e.g., milk products, poultry, corn, peanuts) and magnesium. (e.g., whole grain products, legumes).	Retention of phosphorus stimulates the parathyroid glands to shift calcium from bones (renal osteodystrophy), and accumulation of magnesium can impair neuromuscular function and mentation.
Discuss other nutritional concerns, e.g., regulating protein intake according to level of renal function.	Metabolites that accumulate in blood derive almost entirely from protein catabolism; as renal function declines proteins may be restricted proportionately.
Encourage high calorie intake, especially from carbohydrates.	Spares protein, prevents wasting, and provides energy.
Discuss drug therapy, including use of calcium supplements and phosphate binders, e.g., aluminum hydroxide antacids (Amphogel, Basalgel) and avoidance of magnesium antacids (Mylanta, Maalox, Gelusil).	Prevents serious complications, e.g., reducing phosphate absorption from the GI tract and supplying calcium to maintain normal serum levels, reducing risk of bone demineralization/fractures, tetany. Use of aluminum-containing products should be monitored, however, because accumulation in the bones potentiates osteodystrophy. Magnesium products potentiate risk of hypermagnesemia.
Stress importance of reading all product labels (drugs and food) and not taking medications without prior approval of health care provider.	It is difficult to maintain electrolyte balance when exogenous intake is not factored into dietary restrictions, e.g., hypercalcemia can result from routine supplement use in combination with increased dietary intake of calcium-fortified foods and medications containing calcium.
Review measures to prevent bleeding/hemorrhage, e.g., use of soft toothbrush, electric razor; avoidance of constipation, forceful blowing of nose, strenuous exercise/contact sports.	Reduces risks related to alteration of clotting factors/decreased platelet count.
Instruct in self observation and monitoring of BP, including scheduling rest period before taking BP, using same arm/position.	Incidence of hypertension is increased in CRF, often requiring management with antihypertensive drugs, necessitating close observation of treatment effects, e.g., vascular response to medication.

ACTIONS/INTERVENTIONS	RATIONALE

Independent

Caution against exposure to external temperature extremes, e.g., heating pad/snow.

Peripheral neuropathy may develop, especially in lower extremities (effects of uremia, electrolyte/acid/base imbalances), impairing peripheral sensation and potentiating risk of tissue injury.

Establish routine exercise program, within individual ability; intersperse adequate rest periods with activities.

Aids in maintaining muscle tone and joint flexibility. Reduces risks associated with immobility (including bone demineralization) while preventing fatigue.

Address sexual concerns.

Physiologic effects of uremia/antihypertensive therapy may impair sexual desire/performance.

Identify available resources as indicated. Stress necessity of medical and laboratory follow-up.

Close monitoring of renal function and electrolyte balance is necessary to readjust treatment and/or make decisions about dialysis/transplantation.

Identify signs/symptoms requiring immediate medical evaluation, e.g.:

Low-grade fever, chills, changes in characteristics of urine/sputum, tissue swelling/drainage, oral ulcerations;

Depressed immune system, anemia, malnutrition all contribute to increased risk of infection.

Numbness/tingling of digits, abdominal/muscle cramps, carpopedal spasms;

Uremia and decreased absorption of calcium may lead to peripheral neuropathies.

Joint swelling/tenderness, decreased ROM, reduced muscle strength;

Hyperphosphatemia with corresponding calcium shifts from the bone may result in deposition of the excess calcium phosphate as calcifications in joints and soft tissues. Symptoms of skeletal involvement are often noted before impairment in organ function is evident.

Headaches, blurred vision, periorbital/sacral edema, "red eyes".

Suggestive of development/poor control of hypertension, and/or changes in eyes caused by calcium.

Review strategies to prevent constipation, including stool softeners (Colace) and bulk laxatives (Metamucil) but avoiding magnesium products (Milk of Magnesia).

Reduced fluid intake, changes in dietary pattern, and use of phosphate-binding products often result in constipation that is not responsive to nonmedical interventions. Use of products containing magnesium increases risk of hypermagnesemia.

NURSING DIAGNOSIS:	NONCOMPLIANCE [COMPLIANCE, ALTERED] (SPECIFY)
May be related to:	Patient value system: Health beliefs, cultural influences.
	Changes in mentation; lack of/refusal of support systems/resources.
	Complexities, costs, side effects of therapy.
Possibly evidenced by:	Reported unwillingness to follow therapeutic regimen.

643

	Failure to progress; exacerbation of symptoms; development of complications.
	Denial of the reality of the situation.
DESIRED OUTCOMES/ EVALUATION CRITERIA— PATIENT WILL:	Verbalize accurate knowledge of disease and understanding of therapeutic regimen.
	Participate in the development of goals and treatment plan.
	Make choices at level of readiness based on accurate information.
	Identify/use resources appropriately.

ACTIONS/INTERVENTIONS	RATIONALE
Independent	
Ascertain patient's/SO's perception/understanding of situation and consequences of behavior.	Provides insight into how the patient views own illness and treatment regimen and aids in understanding problems patient is encountering.
Determine value system (health care beliefs and cultural values).	Therapeutic regimen may be incongruent with patient's social/cultural lifestyle and perceived role/responsibilities.
Listen to/Active-listen patient's complaints/comments.	Conveys message of concern, belief in individual's capability to resolve situation in a positive manner.
Identify behaviors indicative of failure to follow treatment program.	May give information about reasons for lack of cooperation and clarifies areas that need problem solving.
Assess level of anxiety, locus of control, feelings of hopelessness/powerlessness.	Severe level of anxiety interferes with patient's ability to cope with situation. Even when patient is internally motivated (internal locus of control), patient tends to become passive/dependent in long-term, debilitating illness.
Determine psychologic meanings of behavior.	Patient may deny reality of physical condition/chronic irreversible disease process; stage of the grieving process may be reflected in angry, acting-out, or withdrawn behavior.
Evaluate support systems/resources used by the patient. Recommend alternatives as appropriate.	Presence of adequate support systems assists patient to handle difficulties of a long-term illness.
Assess attitudes of health care providers toward patient/behavior.	Judgmental approaches may create barriers/power struggles that alienate the patient, reducing likelihood of achieving compromise.
Accept patient's choice/point of view, even if it appears to be self-destructive.	Patient has the right to make own decisions/choices, and acceptance may give a sense of control, which will help patient to look more clearly at consequences of choice.

ACTIONS/INTERVENTIONS	RATIONALE

Independent

Establish graduated goals with patient; modify regimen as necessary/possible.

When patient has participated in setting of goals, a sense of investment encourages cooperation and willingness to adhere to/work with program as established.

Develop a system of self-monitoring, e.g., BP, weight; provide copies of laboratory reports.

Provides a sense of control, enables patient to follow own progress and to make informed choices.

Provide positive feedback for efforts/involvement in therapy.

Promotes sense of self-esteem, encourages continued participation in regimen.

Renal Dialysis

Dialysis is a process that substitutes functionally for impaired renal function by removing excess fluid and/or accumulated endogenous or exogenous toxins. Dialysis is most often used for patients with acute or chronic (end stage) renal disease. The two most common types are hemodialysis and peritoneal dialysis.

RELATED CONCERNS:

Anemias, p 573
Congestive Heart Failure, p 48
Peritonitis, p 514
Psychosocial Aspects of Acute Care, p 899
Sepsis/Septicemia, p 887
Total Nutritional Support, p 1039

PATIENT ASSESSMENT DATA BASE

Refer to CPs: Renal Failure: Acute, p 618; Renal Failure: Chronic, p 632 for assessment information.

Discharge Plan Considerations:	**DRG projected mean length of stay: 2.2 days to initiate therapy. Otherwise, usually done as outpatients.**
	May require assistance with treatment regimen, transportation, ADLs, home-maker/maintenance tasks.

DIAGNOSTIC STUDIES

Procedures and results are variable, depending on cause (e.g., removal of excess fluid or toxins/drugs), degree of renal involvement, and patient considerations (e.g., distance from treatment center, cognition, available support).

NURSING PRIORITIES

1. Promote homeostasis.
2. Maintain comfort.
3. Prevent complications.
4. Support patient independence/self-care.
5. Provide information about disease process/prognosis and treatment needs.

DISCHARGE GOALS

1. Fluid and electrolyte balance maximized.
2. Complications prevented/minimized.
3. Discomfort alleviated.
4. Dealing realistically with current situation; independent within limits of condition.
5. Disease process/prognosis and therapeutic regimen understood.

GENERAL CONSIDERATIONS

This section addresses the general nursing management issues of the patient receiving some form of dialysis.

NURSING DIAGNOSIS:	**NUTRITION, ALTERED: LESS THAN BODY REQUIREMENTS**
May be related to:	GI disturbances (result of uremia); anorexia, n/v and stomatitis.

	Dietary restrictions (bland, tasteless food).
	Loss of protein during dialysis (crosses the semipermeable membrane/peritoneum).
Possibly evidenced by:	Inadequate food intake, aversion to eating, altered taste sensation.
	Poor muscle tone/weakness.
	Sore, inflamed buccal cavity; pale conjunctiva/mucous membranes.
DESIRED OUTCOMES/ EVALUATION CRITERIA— PATIENT WILL:	Demonstrate stable weight/gain toward goal with normalization of laboratory values and no signs of malnutrition.

ACTIONS/INTERVENTIONS	RATIONALE
Independent	
Monitor food/fluid ingested and calculate daily caloric intake.	Identifies nutritional deficits/therapy needs.
Recommend patient keep a food diary, including estimation of ingested amounts of electrolytes (of individual concern, e.g., sodium, potassium, chloride, magnesium), and protein.	Helps patient to realize "big picture" and allows opportunity to alter dietary choices to meet individual desires within identified restriction.
Measure muscle mass via triceps skinfold or similar procedure.	Assesses adequacy of nutrient utilization by measuring changes in fat deposits that may suggest presence/absence of tissue catabolism.
Note presence of nausea/anorexia.	Symptoms accompany accumulation of endogenous toxins that can alter/reduce intake and require intervention.
Encourage patient to participate in menu planning.	May enhance oral intake and promote sense of control/responsibility.
Serve small, frequent meals. Schedule meals according to dialysis needs.	Smaller portions may enhance intake. Type of dialysis influences meal patterns, e.g., patients receiving hemodialysis might not be fed directly before/ during procedure, because this can alter fluid removal; and patients undergoing peritoneal dialysis may be unable to ingest food while abdomen is distended with dialysate.
Promote visits by SO during meals.	Provides diversion and promotes social aspects of eating.
Provide frequent mouth care.	Reduces discomfort of oral stomatitis and undesirable/metallic taste in mouth, which can interfere with food intake.
Collaborative	
Refer to dietitian.	Useful for individualizing dietary program to meet cultural/lifestyle needs enhancing patient cooperation.

647

ACTIONS/INTERVENTIONS	RATIONALE
Collaborative	
Provide a high-carbohydrate diet that includes ordered amount of high-quality protein and essential amino acids with restriction of sodium/potassium as indicated.	Provides sufficient nutrients to improve energy, prevent muscle wasting, promote tissue regeneration/healing, and electrolyte balance.
Administer multivitamins, including ascorbic acid, folic acid, vitamin D, and iron supplements, as indicated.	Replaces vitamins lost because of malnutrition/anemia or during dialysis.
Administer parenteral supplements as indicated.	Hyperalimentation may be needed to enhance renal tubular regeneration/resolution of underlying disease process and to provide nutrients if oral/enteral feeding is contraindicated.
Monitor serum protein/albumin levels.	Indicator of protein needs. *Note:* Peritoneal dialysis is associated with significant protein loss.
Administer antiemetics, e.g., prochlorperazine (Compazine).	Reduces stimulation of the vomiting center.
Insert/maintain nasogastric tube if indicated.	May be necessary when persistent vomiting occurs or when enteric feeding is desired.

NURSING DIAGNOSIS:	PHYSICAL MOBILITY, IMPAIRED
May be related to:	Restrictive therapies, e.g., lengthy dialysis procedure.
	Fear of/real danger of dislodging dialysis lines/catheter.
	Decreased strength/endurance; musculoskeletal impairment.
	Perceptual/cognitive impairment.
Possibly evidenced by:	Reluctance to attempt movement.
	Inability to move within physical environment.
	Decreased muscle mass/tone and strength.
	Impaired coordination.
	Pain, discomfort.
DESIRED OUTCOMES/ EVALUATION CRITERIA— PATIENT WILL:	Maintain optimal mobility/function.
	Display increased strength and be free of associated complications (contractures, decubiti).

ACTIONS/INTERVENTIONS	RATIONALE
Independent	
Assess activity limitations, noting presence/degree of restriction/ability.	Influences choice of interventions.

ACTIONS/INTERVENTIONS	RATIONALE
Independent	
Change position frequently when on bed rest; support affected body parts/joints with pillows, rolls, sheepskin, elbow/heel pads as indicated.	Decreases discomfort, maintains muscle strength/joint mobility, enhances circulation, and prevents skin breakdown.
Provide skin massage. Keep skin clean and dry well. Keep linens dry and wrinkle-free.	Stimulates circulation; prevents skin irritation.
Encourage deep breathing and coughing. Elevate head of bed as allowed. Turn side to side.	Mobilizes secretions, improves lung expansion, and reduces risk of respiratory complications, e.g., atelectasis, pneumonia.
Provide diversion as appropriate to patient's condition, e.g., visitors, radio/television, books.	Decreases boredom; promotes relaxation.
Assist with active/passive ROM exercises.	Maintains joint flexibility, prevents contractures, and aids in reducing muscle tension.
Institute a planned activity program with patient's input.	Increases patient's energy and sense of well-being/control.
Collaborative	
Provide foam/flotation mattress.	Reduces tissue pressure and may enhance circulation, thereby reducing risk of dermal ischemia/breakdown.
Implement exercise program when appropriate.	Studies have shown that regular exercise programs have benefitted end-stage renal disease patients both physically and emotionally, and, in stable patients, has not been shown to have adverse effects.

NURSING DIAGNOSIS:	**SELF-CARE DEFICIT (SPECIFY)**
May be related to:	Perceptual/cognitive impairment (accumulated toxins).
	Intolerance to activity; decreased strength and endurance; pain/discomfort.
Possibly evidenced by:	Reported inability to carry out ADLs.
	Disheveled/unkempt appearance, strong body odor.
DESIRED OUTCOMES/ EVALUATION CRITERIA— PATIENT WILL:	Participate in ADLs within level of own ability/constraints of the illness.

ACTIONS/INTERVENTIONS	RATIONALE
Independent	
Determine patient's ability to participate in self-care activities (scale of 0–4).	Underlying condition will dictate level of deficit/needs.
Provide assistance with activities as necessary.	Meets needs while supporting patient participation and independence.

ACTIONS/INTERVENTIONS

Independent

Encourage/use energy saving techniques, e.g., sitting, not standing; shower chair; doing tasks in small increments.

Schedule activities allowing patient sufficient time to accomplish tasks to fullest extent of ability.

RATIONALE

Conserves energy, reduces fatigue, and enhances patient ability to perform tasks.

Unhurried approach reduces frustration, promotes patient participation, enhancing self-esteem.

NURSING DIAGNOSIS:	CONSTIPATION, HIGH RISK FOR
Risk factors may include:	Decreased fluid intake, altered dietary pattern.
	Reduced intestinal motility, compression of bowel (peritoneal dialysate); electrolyte imbalances; decreased mobility.
Possibly evidenced by:	[Not applicable; presence of signs and symptoms establishes an actual diagnosis.]
DESIRED OUTCOMES/ EVALUATION CRITERIA— PATIENT WILL:	Maintain normal patterns of bowel function.

ACTIONS/INTERVENTIONS

Independent

Auscultate bowel sounds. Note consistency/frequency of BMs, presence of abdominal distention.

Review current medication regimen.

Ascertain usual dietary pattern/food choices.

Add fresh fruits, vegetables, and fiber to diet (within restrictions) when indicated.

Encourage/assist with ambulation when able.

Provide privacy at bedside commode/bathroom.

Collaborative

Administer stool softeners (e.g., Colace), bulk-forming laxatives (e.g., Metamucil) as indicated.

Keep patient NPO; insert NG tube as indicated.

RATIONALE

Decreased bowel sounds, passage of hard-formed/dry stools suggests constipation and requires ongoing intervention to manage.

Side effects of some drugs (e.g., iron products, some antacids) may compound problem.

Although restrictions may be present, thoughtful consideration of menu choices can aid in controlling problem.

Provides bulk, which improves stool consistency.

Activity may stimulate peristalsis, promoting return to normal bowel activity.

Promotes psychologic comfort needed for elimination.

Produces a softer/more easily evacuated stool.

Decompresses stomach when recurrent/unrelieved vomiting occurs. Large gastric output suggests ileus (common early complication of peritoneal dialysis) with accumulation of gas and intestinal fluid that cannot be passed rectally.

NURSING DIAGNOSIS:	THOUGHT PROCESSES, ALTERED
May be related to:	Physiologic changes, e.g., presence of uremic toxins, electrolyte imbalances, hypervolemia/fluid shifts; hyperglycemia (infusion of a dialysate with a high-glucose concentration).
Possibly evidenced by:	Changes in mentation/behavior, e.g., decreased concentration, memory; disorientation; altered sleep patterns; lethargy, confusion, stupor, dementia.
DESIRED OUTCOMES/ EVALUATION CRITERIA— PATIENT WILL:	Regain usual/improved level of mentation. Recognize changes in thinking/behavior and demonstrate behaviors to prevent/minimize changes.

ACTIONS/INTERVENTIONS	RATIONALE
Independent	
Assess for behavioral change/change in level of consciousness, e.g., orientation to time, place, and person.	May indicate level of uremic toxicity, response to or developing complication of dialysis, and requires further assessment/intervention.
Keep explanations simple, reorient frequently. Provide "normal" day/night lighting patterns, clock, calendar.	Improves reality orientation.
Provide a safe environment, restrain as indicated, pad side rails.	Prevents patient trauma and/or inadvertent removal of dialysis lines/catheter.
Drain peritoneal dialysate promptly at end of specified equilibration period.	Prompt outflow will decrease risk of hyperglycemia/hyperosmolar fluid shifts affecting cerebral function.
Investigate reports of headache, associated with onset of nausea/vomiting, confusion/agitation, hypertension, tremors, or seizure activity.	May reflect development of disequilibrium syndrome, which can occur near completion of/following hemodialysis and is thought to be caused by ultrafiltration or by the too rapid removal of urea from the bloodstream not accompanied by equivalent removal from brain tissue. The hypertonic CSF causes a fluid shift into the brain, resulting in cerebral edema.
Monitor changes in speech pattern, development of dementia, myoclonus activity during hemodialysis.	Occasionally, accumulation of aluminum may cause dialysis dementia, progressing to death if untreated.
Collaborative	
Monitor BUN/Cr, serum glucose; alternate/change dialysate concentrations or add insulin as indicated.	Follows progression/resolution of azotemia. Hyperglycemia may develop secondary to glucose crossing peritoneal membrane and entering circulation. May require initiation of insulin therapy.
Obtain aluminum level as indicated.	Elevation may warn of impending cerebral involvement/dialysis dementia.

651

ACTIONS/INTERVENTIONS

Collaborative

Administer medication, as indicated, e.g., phenytoin (Dilantin).

RATIONALE

If disequilibrium syndrome occurs during dialysis, medication may be needed to control seizures in addition to a change in dialysis prescription or discontinuation of therapy.

NURSING DIAGNOSIS:	ANXIETY [SPECIFY LEVEL]/FEAR
May be related to:	Situational crisis, threat to self-concept; change in health status/role functioning, socioeconomic status.
	Threat of death, unknown consequences/outcome.
DESIRED OUTCOMES/ EVALUATION CRITERIA— PATIENT WILL:	Verbalize awareness of feelings and reduction of anxiety/fear to a manageable level.
	Demonstrate problem-solving skills and effective use of resources.
	Appear relaxed, able to rest/sleep appropriately.

ACTIONS/INTERVENTIONS

Independent

Assess level of fear of both patient and SO. Note signs of denial, depression, or narrowed focus of attention.

Explain procedures/care as delivered. Repeat explanations frequently/as needed.

Acknowledge normalcy of feelings in this situation.

Encourage and provide opportunities for patient/SO to ask questions and verbalize concerns.

Encourage SO to participate in care, as indicated.

Acknowledge concerns of patient/SO.

Point out positive indicators of treatment, e.g., improvement in laboratory values, stable BP, lessened fatigue.

RATIONALE

Helps determine the kind of interventions required.

Fear of unknown is lessened by information/knowledge and may enhance acceptance of dialysis. Alteration in thought processes and high levels of anxiety/fear may reduce comprehension, requiring repetition of important information.

Knowing feelings are normal can allay fear that patient is losing control.

Creates feeling of openness and cooperation and provides information that will assist in problem identification/solving.

Involvement promotes sense of sharing, strengthens feelings of usefulness, provides opportunity to acknowledge individual capabilities, and may lessen fear of the unknown.

Prognosis/possibility of need for long-term dialysis and resultant lifestyle changes are a major concern for this patient and those who may be involved in future care.

Promotes sense of success/progress.

NURSING DIAGNOSIS:	BODY IMAGE/SELF-ESTEEM, DISTURBANCE IN
May be related to:	Situational crisis, chronic illness with changes in usual roles.
Possibly evidenced by:	Verbalization of changes in lifestyle; focus on past function, negative feelings about body; feelings of helplessness, powerlessness.
	Extension of body boundary to incorporate environmental objects (e.g., dialysis machine).
	Change in social involvement.
	Overdependence on others for care, not taking responsibility for self-care/lack of follow-through, self-destructive behavior.
DESIRED OUTCOMES/ EVALUATION CRITERIA— PATIENT WILL:	Identify feelings and methods for coping with negative perception of self.
	Verbalize acceptance of self in situation.
	Demonstrate adaptation to changes/events that have occurred, as evidenced by setting realistic goals and active participation in care/life.

ACTIONS/INTERVENTIONS	RATIONALE
Independent	
Assess level of patient's knowledge about condition and treatment, and anxiety related to current situation.	Identifies extent of problem/concern and interventions necessary.
Discuss meaning of loss/change to the patient.	Some patients may view situation as a challenge, though many have difficulty dealing with changes in life/role performance and loss of ability to control own body.
Note withdrawn behavior, ineffective use of denial or behaviors indicative of overconcern with body and its functions.	Indicators of developing difficulty handling stress of what is happening.
Assess use of addictive substances (e.g., alcohol), self-destructive/suicidal behavior.	May reflect dysfunctional coping and attempt to handle problems in an ineffective manner.
Determine stage of grieving. Note signs of severe/prolonged depression.	Identification of stage patient is experiencing provides guide to recognizing and dealing appropriately with behavior. Prolonged depression may indicate need for further intervention.
Acknowledge normalcy of feelings.	Recognition that feelings are to be expected helps patient to accept and deal with them more effectively.
Encourage verbalization of personal and work conflicts that may arise, and Active-listen concerns.	Helps patient to identify problems and problem-solve solutions.

653

ACTIONS/INTERVENTIONS

Independent

Determine patient's role in family constellation and patient's perception of expectation of self and others.

Recommend SO treat patient normally and not as an invalid.

Assist patient to incorporate disease management into lifestyle.

Identify strengths, past successes, previous methods patient has used to deal with life stressors.

Help patient identify areas over which they have some measure of control. Provide opportunity to participate in decision-making process.

Collaborative

Refer to health care/community resources, e.g., support groups, psychiatric nurse specialist, social service, vocational counselor.

RATIONALE

Long-term/permanent illness and disability alter patient's ability to fulfill usual role(s) in family/work setting. Unrealistic expectations can undermine self-esteem and affect outcome of illness.

Conveys expectation that patient is able to manage situation and helps to maintain sense of self-esteem and purpose in life.

Necessities of treatment assume a more normal aspect when they are a part of the daily routine.

Focusing on these reminders of own ability to deal with problems can help patient to deal with current situation.

Provides sense of control over uncontrollable situation, fostering independence.

Provides additional assistance for long-term management of chronic illness/change in lifestyle.

NURSING DIAGNOSIS:	KNOWLEDGE DEFICIT [LEARNING NEED] REGARDING CONDITION, PROGNOSIS, AND TREATMENT NEEDS
May be related to:	Lack of exposure/recall.
	Unfamiliarity with information resources.
	Cognitive limitations.
Possibly evidenced by:	Questions/request for information; statement of misconception.
	Inaccurate follow-through of instruction; development of preventable complications.
DESIRED OUTCOMES/ EVALUATION CRITERIA— PATIENT WILL:	Verbalize understanding of condition and relationship of signs/symptoms of the disease process.
	Correctly perform necessary procedures and explain reasons for actions.

ACTIONS/INTERVENTIONS

Independent

Note level of anxiety/fear and alteration of thought processes.

RATIONALE

These factors directly affect ability to participate/ access and use knowledge. In addition, studies in-

ACTIONS/INTERVENTIONS

Independent

Review particular disease process, procedures, and purpose of dialysis in terms understandable to the patient. Repeat explanations as required.

Acknowledge that certain feelings/patterns of response are normal during course of therapy.

Encourage and provide opportunity for questions.

Stress necessity of reading all product labels (food/beverage and OTC drugs) and not taking medications without prior approval of health care provider.

Discuss significance of maintaining nutritious eating habits; preventing wide fluctuation of fluid/electrolyte balance; avoidance of crowds/people with infectious processes.

Instruct patient/SO in home dialysis as indicated:

Purpose of dialysis;

Operation and maintenance of equipment (including vascular shunt); sources of supplies;

Aseptic/clean technique;

Self-monitoring of effectiveness of procedure;

Management of potential complications;

Contact person.

Instruct patient about Epoetin alpha, when indicated. Have patient/SO demonstrate ability to self-administer and state adverse side effects and health care practices associated with Epoetin alpha therapy.

RATIONALE

dicate that during the dialysis procedure, the patient's cognitive function may be impaired and that patients themselves state that they feel "fuzzy." Therefore, learning may not be optimal during this time.

Providing information at the level of the patient/SO understanding will reduce anxiety and misconceptions about what the patient is experiencing.

Patient/SO may initially be hopeful and positive about the future, but as treatment continues and progress is less dramatic, they can become discouraged/depressed, and conflicts of dependence/independence may develop.

Enhances learning process, promotes informed decision making, and reduces anxiety associated with the unknown.

It is difficult to maintain electrolyte balance when exogenous intake is not factored into dietary restriction, e.g., hypercalcemia can result from routine supplement use in combination with increased dietary intake of calcium-fortified foods and medicines.

Depressed immune system, presence of anemia, invasive procedures, and malnutrition potentiate risk of infection.

Provides knowledge base on which patient can make informed observations/choices.

Information diminishes anxiety of the unknown and provides opportunity for patient to be knowledgeable about own care.

Prevents contamination and reduces risk of infection.

Provides information necessary to evaluate effects of therapy/need for change.

Reduces concerns regarding personal well-being; supports efforts at self-care.

Readily available support person can answer questions, troubleshoot problems, and facilitate timely medical intervention when indicated.

Epogen was recently approved by the Food and Drug Administration for the management of the anemia associated with CRF. The drug is given to increase and maintain RBC production, which can allow the patient to feel better and stronger.

ACTIONS/INTERVENTIONS	RATIONALE
Independent	
	Contraindications may include adverse side effects such as polycythemia/increased clotting, failure to administer correctly or have appropriate follow-up.
Identify health care/community resources, e.g., dialysis support group, social services, mental health clinic.	Knowledge and use of these resources assists patient/SO to manage own care more effectively. Interaction with others in similar situation provides opportunity for discussion of options and in making informed choices, e.g., stopping dialysis, renal transplantation.

(Plan of care continues on next page.)

Renal Dialysis: Peritoneal _____

The peritoneum serves as the semipermeable membrane permitting transfer of nitrogenous wastes/toxins and fluid from the blood into a dialysate solution. Peritoneal dialysis is sometimes preferred because it uses a simpler technique and provides more gradual physiologic changes than hemodialysis.

Manual single bottle method is usually done as an inpatient procedure with short dwell times of only 30–60 minutes and is repeated until desired effects are achieved.

Continuous ambulatory peritoneal dialysis (CAPD) permits the patient to manage procedure at home with bag and gravity flow, using a prolonged dwell time at night and a total of 3–5 cycles daily, 7 days a week.

Continuous cycling peritoneal dialysis (CCPD) mechanically cycles shorter dwell times during night, with a longer dwell time during daylight hours, increasing the patient's independence.

NURSING DIAGNOSIS:	FLUID VOLUME, EXCESS, HIGH RISK FOR
Risk factors may include:	Inadequate osmotic gradient of dialysate.
	Fluid retention (malpositioned or kinked/clotted catheter, bowel distention; peritonitis, scarring of peritoneum).
	Excessive PO/IV intake.
Possibly evidenced by:	[Not applicable; presence of signs and symptoms establishes an actual diagnosis.]
DESIRED OUTCOMES/ EVALUATION CRITERIA— PATIENT WILL:	Demonstrate dialysate outflow exceeding/approximating infusion.
	Experience no rapid weight gain, edema, pulmonary congestion.

ACTIONS/INTERVENTIONS	RATIONALE
Independent	
Maintain a record of inflow/outflow volumes, and cumulative fluid balance.	In most cases, the amount drained should equal or exceed the amount instilled. A positive balance indicates need of further evaluation.
Record serial weights, compare with I&O balance. Weigh patient when abdomen is empty of dialysate (consistent reference point).	Serial body weights are an accurate indicator of fluid volume status. A positive fluid balance with an increase in weight indicates fluid retention.
Assess patency of catheter, noting difficulty in drainage. Note presence of fibrin strings/plugs.	Slowing of flow rate/presence of fibrin suggests partial catheter occlusion requiring further evaluation/intervention.
Check tubing for kinks; note placement of bottles/bags. Anchor catheter so that adequate inflow/outflow is achieved.	Improper functioning of equipment may result in retained fluid in abdomen and insufficient clearance of toxins.
Turn from side to side, elevate the head of the bed, apply gentle pressure to the abdomen.	May enhance outflow of fluid when catheter is malpositioned/obstructed by the omentum.
Note abdominal distention associated with decreased bowel sounds, changes in stool consistency, reports of constipation.	Bowel distention/constipation may impede outflow of effluent. (Refer to ND: Constipation, p 650.)

ACTIONS/INTERVENTIONS

Independent

Monitor BP and pulse, noting hypertension, bounding pulses, neck vein distention, peripheral edema; measure CVP if available.

Evaluate development of tachypnea, dyspnea, increased respiratory effort. Drain dialysate, and notify physician.

Assess for headache, muscle cramps, mental confusion, disorientation.

Collaborative

Alter dialysate regimen as indicated.

Monitor serum sodium.

Add heparin to initial dialysis runs, assist with irrigation of catheter with heparinized saline.

Maintain fluid restriction as indicated.

RATIONALE

Elevations indicate hypervolemia. Assess heart and breath sounds, noting S_3 and/or crackles, rhonchi. Fluid overload may potentiate CHF/pulmonary edema.

Abdominal distention/diaphragmatic compression may cause respiratory distress.

Symptoms suggest hyponatremia or water intoxication.

Changes may be needed in the glucose or sodium concentration to facilitate efficient dialysis.

Hypernatremia may be present, although serum levels may reflect dilutional effect of fluid volume overload.

May be useful in preventing fibrin clot formation, which can obstruct peritoneal catheter.

Fluid restrictions may have to be continued to decrease fluid volume overload.

NURSING DIAGNOSIS:	FLUID VOLUME DEFICIT, HIGH RISK FOR
Risk factors may include:	Use of hypertonic dialysate with excessive removal of fluid from circulating volume.
Possibly evidenced by:	[Not applicable; presence of signs and symptoms establishes an actual diagnosis.]
DESIRED OUTCOMES/ EVALUATION CRITERIA— PATIENT WILL:	Achieve desired alteration in fluid volume and weight with BP electrolyte levels within acceptable range. Experience no symptoms of dehydration.

ACTIONS/INTERVENTIONS

Independent

Maintain record of inflow/outflow volumes and individual/cumulative fluid balance.

Adhere to schedule for draining dialysate from abdomen.

Weigh when abdomen is empty, following initial 6–10 runs, then as indicated.

Monitor BP (lying and sitting) and pulse. Note level of jugular pulsation.

RATIONALE

Provides information about the status of the patient's loss or gain at the end of each exchange.

Prolonged dwell times, especially when 4.5% glucose solution is used, may cause excess fluid loss.

Detects rate of fluid removal by comparison with baseline body weights.

Decreased BP, postural hypotension, and tachycardia are early signs of hypovolemia.

ACTIONS/INTERVENTIONS	RATIONALE

Independent

Note reports of dizziness, nausea, increasing thirst.

May indicate hypovolemia/hyperosmolar syndrome.

Inspect mucous membranes, evaluate skin turgor, peripheral pulses, capillary refill.

Dry mucous membranes, poor skin turgor and diminished pulses/capillary refill are indicators of dehydration and need for increased intake/changes in strength of dialysate.

Collaborative

Monitor laboratory studies as indicated, e.g.:

Serum sodium and glucose levels;

Hypertonic solutions may cause hypernatremia by removing more water than sodium. In addition, dextrose may be absorbed from the dialysate, thereby elevating serum glucose.

Serum potassium levels.

Hypokalemia may occur and can cause cardiac dysrhythmias.

NURSING DIAGNOSIS:	TRAUMA, HIGH RISK FOR
Risk factors may include:	Catheter inserted into peritoneal cavity. Site near the bowel/bladder with potential for perforation during insertion or by manipulation of the catheter.
Possibly evidenced by:	[Not applicable; presence of signs and symptoms establishes an actual diagnosis.]
DESIRED OUTCOMES/ EVALUATION CRITERIA— PATIENT WILL:	Experience no injury to bowel or bladder.

ACTIONS/INTERVENTIONS	RATIONALE

Independent

Have patient empty bladder prior to peritoneal catheter insertion if indwelling catheter not present.

An empty bladder is more distant from insertion site and reduces likelihood of being punctured during catheter insertion.

Anchor catheter/tubing with tape. Stress importance of patient avoiding pulling/pushing on catheter. Restrain hands if indicated

Reduces risk of trauma by manipulation of the catheter.

Note presence of fecal material in dialysate effluent, or strong urge to defecate, accompanied by severe, watery diarrhea.

Suggests bowel perforation with mixing of dialysate and bowel contents.

Note reports of intense urge to void, or large urine output following initiation of dialysis run. Test urine for sugar as indicated.

Suggests bladder perforation with dialysate leaking into bladder. Presence of glucose-containing dialysate in the bladder, will elevate glucose level of urine.

659

ACTIONS/INTERVENTIONS	RATIONALE

Independent

Stop dialysis if there is evidence of bowel/bladder perforation, leaving peritoneal catheter in place.	Prompt action will prevent further injury. Immediate surgical repair may be required. Leaving catheter in place facilitates diagnosing/locating the perforation.

NURSING DIAGNOSIS:	**PAIN, [ACUTE]**
May be related to:	Insertion of catheter through abdominal wall/catheter irritation, improper catheter placement.
	Irritation/infection within the peritoneal cavity.
	Infusion of cold or acidic dialysate, abdominal distention, rapid infusion of dialysate.
Possibly evidenced by:	Reports of pain.
	Self-focusing.
	Guarding/distraction behaviors, restlessness.
DESIRED OUTCOMES/ EVALUATION CRITERIA— PATIENT WILL:	Verbalize decrease of pain/discomfort.
	Demonstrate relaxed posture/facial expression, able to sleep/rest appropriately.

ACTIONS/INTERVENTIONS	RATIONALE

Independent

Investigate patient's reports of pain; note intensity (0–10), location, and precipitating factors.	Assists in identification of source of pain and appropriate interventions.
Explain that initial discomfort usually subsides after the first few exchanges.	Explanation may reduce anxiety, and promote relaxation during procedure.
Monitor for pain that begins during inflow and continues during equilibration phase. Slow infusion rate as indicated.	Pain will occur at these times if acidic dialysate causes chemical irritation of peritoneal membrane.
Note discomfort that is most pronounced near the end of inflow. Instill no more than 2000 ml of solution at a single time.	Likely the result of abdominal distention from dialysate. Amount of infusion may have to be decreased initially.
Note report of pain in area of shoulder blade. Prevent air from entering peritoneal cavity during infusion.	Inadvertent introduction of air into the abdomen irritates the diaphragm and results in referred pain to shoulder blade. This type of discomfort may also be reported during initiation of therapy/during infusions and usually is related to stretching/irritation of the diaphragm with abdominal distention. Smaller exchange volumes may be required until patient adjusts.
Elevate head of bed at intervals. Turn patient from side to side. Provide back care and tissue massage.	Position changes may relieve abdominal and general muscle discomfort.

ACTIONS/INTERVENTIONS

Independent

Warm dialysate to body temperature before infusing.

Monitor for severe/continuous abdominal pain, and temperature elevation (especially after dialysis has been discontinued).

Encourage use of relaxation techniques, e.g., deep-breathing exercises, guided imagery, visualization. Provide diversional activities.

Collaborative

Administer analgesics.

Add sodium hydroxide to dialysate, if indicated.

(RATIONALE

Warming the solution increases the rate of urea removal by dilating peritoneal vessels. Cold dialysate causes vasoconstriction, which can cause discomfort and/or excessively lower the core body temperature, precipitating cardiac arrest.

May indicate developing peritonitis. (Refer to ND: Infection, high risk for, [peritonitis] this page.)

Redirects attention, promotes sense of control.

Relieves pain and discomfort.

Occasionally used to alter pH if patient is not tolerating acidic dialysate.

NURSING DIAGNOSIS:	INFECTION, HIGH RISK FOR, [PERITONITIS]
Risk factors may include:	Contamination of the catheter during insertion, periodic changing of tubings/bottles/bags. Skin contaminants at catheter insertion site. Sterile peritonitis (response to the composition of dialysate).
Possibly evidenced by:	[Not applicable; presence of signs and symptoms establishes an actual diagnosis.]
DESIRED OUTCOMES/ EVALUATION CRITERIA— PATIENT WILL:	Identify interventions to prevent/reduce risk of infection. Experience no signs/symptoms of infection.

ACTIONS/INTERVENTIONS

Independent

Observe meticulous aseptic techniques and wear masks during catheter insertion, dressing changes and whenever the system is opened. Change tubings per protocol.

Change dressings as indicated being careful not to dislodge the catheter. Note character, color, odor of drainage from around insertion site.

RATIONALE

Prevents the introduction of organisms and airborne contamination that may cause infection.

Moist environment promotes bacterial growth. Purulent drainage at insertion site suggests presence of local infection. *Note:* Polyurethane adhesive film (e.g., Blister film) dressings have been found to decrease amount of pressure on catheter and exit site, as well as incidence of site infections.

ACTIONS/INTERVENTIONS

Independent

Observe color and clarity of effluent.

Apply povidene-iodine (Betadine) barrier in distal, clamped portion of catheter when intermittent dialysis therapy used.

Investigate reports of nausea/vomiting; increased/severe abdominal pain, rebound tenderness, fever, and leukocytosis.

Collaborative

Monitor WBC count of effluent.

Obtain specimens of blood, effluent, and/or drainage from insertion site as indicated for culture/sensitivity.

Monitor renal clearance/BUN, Cr.

Administer antibiotics systemically or in dialysate as indicated.

RATIONALE

Cloudy effluent is suggestive of peritoneal infection.

Reduces risk of bacterial entry through catheter between dialysis treatments when catheter is disconnected from closed system.

Signs/symptoms suggesting peritonitis, requiring prompt intervention.

Presence of WBCs initially may reflect normal response to a foreign substance; however, continued/new elevation suggests developing infection.

Identifies types of organism(s) present, choice of interventions.

Choice and dosage of antibiotics will be influenced by renal function.

Treats infection, prevents sepsis.

NURSING DIAGNOSIS	BREATHING PATTERN, INEFFECTIVE, HIGH RISK FOR
Risk factors may include:	Abdominal pressure/restricted diaphragmatic excursion; rapid infusion of dialysate; pain. Inflammatory process (e.g., atelectasis/pneumonia).
Possibly evidenced by:	[Not applicable; presence of signs and symptoms establishes an actual diagnosis.]
DESIRED OUTCOMES/ EVALUATION CRITERIA— PATIENT WILL:	Display an effective respiratory pattern with clear breath sounds, ABGs within patient's normal range. Experience no signs of dyspnea/cyanosis.

ACTIONS/INTERVENTIONS

Independent

Monitor respiratory rate/effort. Reduce infusion rate if dyspnea is present.

Auscultate lungs, noting decreased, absent, or adventitious breath sounds, e.g., crackles/wheezes/rhonchi.

RATIONALE

Tachypnea, dyspnea, shortness of breath, and shallow breathing during dialysis suggests diaphragmatic pressure from distended peritoneal cavity or may indicate developing complications.

Decreased areas of ventilation suggest presence of atelectasis, whereas adventitious sounds may suggest fluid overload, retained secretions, or infection.

ACTIONS/INTERVENTIONS	RATIONALE
Independent	
Note character, amount, and color of secretions.	Patient is susceptible to pulmonary infections as a result of depressed cough reflex and respiratory effort, increased viscosity of secretions, as well as altered immune response and chronic/debilitating disease.
Elevate head of bed. Promote deep-breathing exercises and coughing.	Facilitates chest expansion/ventilation and mobilization of secretions.
Collaborative	
Review ABGs/pulse oximetry and serial chest x-rays.	Changes in PaO_2/$PaCO_2$ and appearance of infiltrates/congestion on chest x-ray suggests developing pulmonary problems.
Administer supplemental O_2 as indicated.	Maximizes oxygen for vascular uptake, preventing/lessening hypoxia.
Administer analgesics as indicated.	Alleviates pain, promotes comfortable breathing, maximal cough effort.

(Plan of care continues on next page.)

Acute Hemodialysis _____

Blood is shunted through an artificial kidney (dialyzer) for removal of toxins/excess fluid and then returned to the venous circulation. Hemodialysis is a faster and more efficient method than peritoneal dialysis for removing urea and other toxic products, but requires permanent AV access.

NURSING DIAGNOSIS:	INJURY, HIGH RISK FOR, LOSS OF VASCULAR ACCESS
Risk factors may include:	Clotting; hemorrhage related to accidental disconnection; infection.
Possibly evidenced by:	[Not applicable; presence of signs and symptoms establishes an actual diagnosis.]
DESIRED OUTCOMES/ EVALUATION CRITERIA— PATIENT WILL:	Maintain patent vascular access.

ACTIONS/INTERVENTIONS	RATIONALE
Independent	
Clotting:	
Monitor internal AV shunt patency at frequent intervals:	
Palpate for distal thrill;	Thrill is caused by turbulence of high-pressure arterial blood flow entering low-pressure venous system and should be palpable above venous exit site.
Auscultate for a bruit;	Bruit is the sound caused by the turbulence of arterial blood entering venous system and should be audible by stethoscope, although may be very faint.
Note color of blood and/or obvious separation of cells and serum;	Change of color from uniform medium red to dark purplish red suggests sluggish blood flow/early clotting. Separation in tubing is indicative of clotting. Very dark reddish-black blood next to clear yellow fluid indicates full clot formation.
Palpate skin around shunt for warmth.	Diminished blood flow will result in "coolness" of shunt.
Notify physician and/or initiate declotting procedure if there is evidence of loss of shunt patency.	Rapid intervention may save access; however, declotting must be done by experienced personnel.
Evaluate reports of pain, numbness/tingling; note extremity swelling distal to access.	May indicate inadequate blood supply.
Avoid trauma to shunt; e.g., handle tubing gently, maintain cannula alignment. Limit activity of extremity. Avoid taking BP or drawing blood samples in shunt extremity. Instruct patient not to sleep or carry packages, books, purse on affected extremity.	Decreases risk of clotting/disconnection.

664

ACTIONS/INTERVENTIONS	RATIONALE

Independent

Hemorrhage:

Attach two cannula clamps to shunt dressing. Have tourniquet available. If cannulas separate, clamp first the arterial then the venous cannula. If tubing comes out of vessel, clamp cannula that is still in place and apply direct pressure to bleeding site. Place tourniquet above site or inflate BP cuff to pressure just above patient's systolic BP.

Prevents massive blood loss if cannula separates or shunt is dislodged while awaiting medical assistance.

Infection:

Assess skin around vascular access, noting redness, swelling, local warmth, exudate, tenderness.

Signs of local infection, which can progress to sepsis if untreated.

Avoid contamination of access site. Use aseptic technique and masks when giving shunt care, applying/changing dressings, and when starting/completing dialysis process.

Prevents introduction of organisms that can cause infection.

Monitor temperature. Note presence of fever, chills, hypotension.

Signs of infection/sepsis requiring prompt medical intervention.

Collaborative

Culture the site/obtain blood samples as indicated.

Determines presence of pathogens.

Administer medications as indicated, e.g.:

Heparin (low-dose);

Infused on arterial side of filter to prevent clotting in the filter without systemic side effects.

Antibiotics (systemic and/or topical).

Prompt treatment of infection may save access, prevent sepsis.

NURSING DIAGNOSIS: **FLUID VOLUME DEFICIT, HIGH RISK FOR**

Risk factors may include: Ultrafiltration.
Fluid restrictions; actual blood loss (systemic heparinization or disconnection of the shunt).

Possibly evidenced by: [Not applicable; presence of signs and symptoms establishes an actual diagnosis.]

DESIRED OUTCOMES/ EVALUATION CRITERIA— PATIENT WILL: Maintain fluid balance as evidenced by stable/appropriate weight and vital signs, good skin turgor, moist mucous membranes, absence of bleeding.

ACTIONS/INTERVENTIONS	RATIONALE

Independent

Measure all sources of I&O. Have patient keep diary.

Aids in evaluating fluid status, especially when compared with weights. *Note:* Urine output is an inaccurate evaluation of renal function in dialysis

665

ACTIONS/INTERVENTIONS	RATIONALE
Independent	
	patients. Some persons have water output with little renal clearance of toxins. Other persons have oliguria or anuria.
Weigh daily before/after dialysis run.	Weight loss over precisely measured time is a measure of ultrafiltration and fluid removal.
Monitor BP, pulse, and hemodynamic pressures if available during dialysis.	Hypotension, tachycardia, falling hemodynamic pressures suggest volume depletion.
Note/ascertain whether diuretics and/or antihypertensives are to be withheld.	Dialysis potentiates hypotensive effects if these drugs have been ingested.
Verify continuity of shunt/access catheter.	Disconnected shunt/open access will permit exsanguination.
Apply external shunt dressing. Permit no puncture of shunt.	Minimizes stress on cannula insertion site to reduce inadvertent dislodgement and bleeding from site.
Place patient in a supine/Trendelenburg's position as necessary.	Maximizes venous return when hypotension occurs.
Assess for oozing or frank bleeding at access site, mucous membranes, incisions/wounds. Hematest/guaiac stools, gastric drainage.	Systemic heparinization during dialysis increases clotting times and places patient at risk for bleeding, especially during the first 4 hours after procedure.
Collaborative	
Monitor laboratory studies as indicated:	
Hb/Hct;	May be reduced because of anemia, hemodilution, or actual blood loss.
Serum electrolytes and pH;	Imbalances may require changes in the dialysate solution or supplemental replacement to achieve balance.
Clotting times, e.g., ACT, PT/PTT, and platelet count.	Use of heparin to prevent clotting in blood lines and hemofilter alters coagulation and potentiates active bleeding.
Administer IV solutions (e.g., normal saline)/volume expanders (e.g., albumin) during dialysis as indicated:	Saline/dextrose solutions, electrolytes, and $NaHCO_3$ may be infused in the venous side of CAV hemofilter when high ultrafiltration rates are used for removal of extracellular fluid and toxic solutes. Volume expanders may be required during/following hemodialysis if sudden/marked hypotension occurs.
Blood/packed RBCs if needed.	Destruction of RBCs (hemolysis) by mechanical dialysis, hemorrhagic losses, decreased RBC production may result in profound/progressive anemia.
Reduce rate of ultrafiltration during dialysis as indicated.	Reduces the amount of water being removed and may correct hypotension/hypovolemia.
Administer protamine sulfate if indicated.	May be needed to return clotting times to normal or if heparin rebound occurs (up to 16 hours after hemodialysis).

NURSING DIAGNOSIS:	FLUID VOLUME, EXCESS, HIGH RISK FOR
Risk factors may include:	Rapid/excessive fluid intake; IV, blood, plasma expanders, saline given to support BP during dialysis.
Possibly evidenced by:	[Not applicable; presence of signs and symptoms establishes an actual diagnosis.]
DESIRED OUTCOMES/ EVALUATION CRITERIA— PATIENT WILL:	Maintain "dry weight" within patient's normal range; free of edema; breath sounds clear and serum sodium levels within normal limits.

ACTIONS/INTERVENTIONS	RATIONALE
Independent	
Measure all sources of I&O. Weigh routinely.	Aids in evaluating fluid status especially when compared with weight. Weight gain between treatments should not exceed 0.5 kg/d.
Monitor BP, pulse.	Hypertension and tachycardia between hemodialysis runs may result from fluid overload and/or heart failure.
Note presence of peripheral/sacral edema, respiratory rales, dyspnea, orthopnea, distended neck veins, ECG changes indicative of ventricular hypertrophy.	Fluid volume excess because of inefficient dialysis or repeated hypervolemia between dialysis treatments may cause/exacerbate heart failure, as indicated by signs/symptoms of respiratory and/or systemic venous congestion.
Note changes in mentation. (Refer to ND: Thought Processes, Altered, p 651.)	Fluid overload/hypervolemia, may potentiate cerebral edema (disequilibrium syndrome).
Collaborative	
Monitor serum sodium levels. Restrict sodium intake as indicated.	High sodium levels are associated with fluid overload, edema, hypertension, and cardiac complications.
Restrict po/IV fluid intake as indicated, spacing allowed fluids through 24-hour period.	The intermittent nature of hemodialysis results in fluid retention/overload between procedures and may require fluid restriction. Spacing fluids helps reduce thirst.

Urinary Diversions/Urostomy (Postoperative Care) _____

Ileal conduit: Ureters are anastomosed to a segment of ileum resected with the blood supply intact (usually 15–20 cm long). The proximal section is closed, and the distal end brought to skin opening to form a stoma (a passageway, not a storage reservoir).

Colonic conduit: This is a similar procedure using a segment of colon.

Ureterostomy: The ureter(s) is brought directly through the abdominal wall to form its own stoma.

Continent diversion: A section of intestine is used to form a pouch inside the patient's abdomen creating a reservoir that the patient periodically drains by inserting a catheter through the stoma, thus negating the need for an external collecting device. In some male patients, with a Kock pouch (reservoir using small intestine), drainage may be achieved through the urethra and penis rather than an abdominal stoma.

RELATED CONCERNS

Peritonitis, p 514
Psychosocial Aspects of Acute Care, p 899

PATIENT ASSESSMENT DATA BASE

Data are dependent on underlying problem, duration, and severity, e.g., malignant bladder tumor, congenital malformations, trauma, chronic infections, or intractable incontinence due to injury/disease of other body systems (e.g., multiple sclerosis). (Refer to appropriate CP.)

TEACHING/LEARNING

Discharge Plan Considerations: **DRG projected mean length of stay: 5.5 days.**
May require assistance with management of ostomy and acquisition of supplies.

DIAGNOSTIC STUDIES

IVP: Visualizes size/location of kidneys and ureters and rules out presence of tumors elsewhere in urinary tract.

Cystoscopy with biopsy: Determines tumor location/degree of malignancy. Ultraviolet cystoscopy outlines bladder lesion.

Bone scan: Determines presence of metastatic disease.

Bilateral pedal lymphangiogram: Determines involvement of pelvic nodes, where bladder tumor easily seeds because of close proximity.

CT scan: Defines size of tumor mass, degree of pelvic spread.

Urine cystoscopy: Detects tumor cells in urine (for determining presence and type of tumor).

Endoscopy: Evaluates intestines for use as conduit.

Conduitogram: Assesses length and emptying ability of the conduit and presence of stricture, obstruction, reflux, angulation, calculi, or tumor (may complicate or contraindicate use as a urinary diversion).

NURSING PRIORITIES

1. Assist patient/SO in physical/psychosocial adjustment.
2. Prevent complications.
3. Support independence in self-care.
4. Provide information about procedure/prognosis, treatment needs, potential complications, and resources.

DISCHARGE GOALS

1. Adjusting to perceived/actual changes.
2. Complications prevented/minimized.

3. Self-care needs met by self/with assistance as necessary.
4. Procedure/prognosis, therapeutic regimen, potential complications understood and sources of support identified.

NURSING DIAGNOSIS:	SKIN INTEGRITY, IMPAIRED, HIGH RISK FOR
Risk factors may include:	Absence of sphincter at stoma [actual].
	Character/flow of urine from stoma.
	Reaction to product/chemicals; improper fitting of appliance or removal of adhesive.
Possibly evidenced by:	[Not applicable; presence of signs and symptoms establishes an actual diagnosis.]
DESIRED OUTCOMES/ EVALUATION CRITERIA— PATIENT WILL:	Maintain skin integrity.
	Identify individual risk factors.
	Demonstrate behaviors/techniques to promote healing/ prevent skin breakdown.

ACTIONS/INTERVENTIONS	RATIONALE
Independent	
Inspect stoma/peristomal skin. Note irritation, bruises (dark, bluish color), rashes, status of sutures.	Monitors healing process/effectiveness of appliances, and identifies areas of concern, need for further evaluation/intervention. Stoma should be pink or reddish, similar to mucous membranes. Color changes may be temporary, but persistent changes may require surgical intervention. Early identification of stomal necrosis/ischemia or fungal infection provides for timely interventions to prevent skin necrosis.
Clean with water and pat dry (or use hair dryer on cool setting).	Maintaining a clean/dry area helps to prevent skin breakdown.
Handle stoma gently to prevent irritation.	Mucosa has good blood supply and bleeds easily with rubbing or trauma.
Measure stoma periodically, e.g., each appliance change for first 6 weeks, then monthly times 6.	As postoperative edema resolves (during first 6 weeks), size of appliance must be altered to ensure proper fit so that urine is collected as it flows from the stoma, and contact with the skin is prevented.
Apply effective sealant barrier, e.g., Skin Prep or similar products.	Protects skin from pouch adhesive, enhances adhesiveness of pouch, and facilitates removal of pouch when necessary.
Make sure opening for adhesive backing of pouch is at least ⅛ in larger than the base of the stoma, with adequate adhesiveness left to apply pouch.	Prevents trauma to the stoma tissue and protects the peristomal skin. Adequate adhesive area is important to maintain a seal. *Note:* Too tight a fit may cause stomal edema or stenosis.

669

ACTIONS/INTERVENTIONS	RATIONALE
Independent	
Use a transparent, odor-proof drainable pouch Keep gauze square/wick over stoma while cleansing area, and have patient cough or strain before applying pouch.	A transparent appliance during first 4–6 weeks allows easy observation of stoma and stents (when used) without necessity of removing pouch and irritating skin. Covering stoma prevents urine from wetting the peristomal area during pouch changes. Coughing empties distal portion of conduit, followed by a brief pause in drainage to facilitate application of pouch.
Avoid use of karaya-type appliances.	Will not protect skin as urine melts karaya.
Apply waterproof tape around pouch edges if desired.	Reinforces anchoring.
Connect collecting pouch to continuous bedside drainage system, when necessary.	May be needed during times when rate of urine formation is increased, e.g., while IV fluids are administered. Weight of the urine can cause pouch to pull loose/leak when pouch becomes more than half full.
Cleanse ostomy pouch on a routine basis, using vinegar solution.	Frequent pouch changes are irritating to the skin and should be avoided. Emptying and rinsing the pouch with vinegar not only removes bacteria but also deodorizes the pouch.
Change pouch every 3–5 days or as needed for leakage. Remove appliance gently while supporting skin. Use adhesive removers as indicated and wash off completely.	Prevents tissue irritation/destruction associated with "pulling" pouch off.
Investigate reports of burning/itching around stoma.	Suggests peristomal irritation or possibly *Candida* infections, both requiring intervention. *Note:* Continuous exposure of skin to urine can cause hyperplasia around stoma, affecting pouch fit and increasing risk of infection.
Evaluate adhesive product and appliance fit on ongoing basis.	Provides opportunity for problem solving. Determines need for further intervention.
Monitor for distention of lower abdomen (with ileal conduit); assess bowel sounds.	Intestinal distention can cause tension on new suture lines with possibility of rupture.
Collaborative	
Consult with enterostomal nurse.	Helpful in problem solving and choosing products appropriate for patient needs, considering stoma characteristics, patient's physical/mental status, and financial resources. In the presence of persistent or recurring problems, the ostomy nurse has a wider range of knowledge and resources.
Apply antifungal spray or powder, as indicated.	Assists in healing if peristomal irritation is caused by fungal infection. *Note:* These products can have potent side effects and should be used sparingly. Creams/ointments are to be avoided, because they interfere with adhesion of the appliance.

NURSING DIAGNOSIS:	BODY IMAGE, DISTURBANCE
May be related to:	Biophysical: Presence of stoma; loss of control of urine elimination.
	Psychosocial: Altered body structure.
	Disease process and associated treatment regimen, e.g., cancer.
Possibly evidenced by:	Verbalization of change in body image, fear of rejection/reaction of others, and negative feelings about body.
	Actual change in structure and/or function (ostomy).
	Not touching/looking at stoma, refusal to participate in care.
DESIRED OUTCOMES/ EVALUATION CRITERIA— PATIENT WILL:	Demonstrate beginning acceptance by viewing/touching stoma and participating in self-care.
	Verbalize feelings about stoma/illness; begin to deal constructively with situation.
	Verbalize acceptance of self in situation, incorporating change into self-concept without negating self-esteem.

ACTIONS/INTERVENTIONS

Independent

Review reason for surgery and future expectations.

Ascertain whether counseling was initiated when the possibility and/or necessity of urinary diversion was first discussed.

Answer all questions concerning urostomy and its function.

Encourage the patient/SO to verbalize feelings. Acknowledge normality of feelings of anger, depression, and grief over loss. Discuss daily "ups and downs" that can occur after discharge.

Note behaviors of withdrawal, increased dependency, manipulation, or noninvolvement in care.

RATIONALE

Patient may find it easier to accept/deal with an ostomy done for chronic/long-term disease (e.g., intractable incontinence, infections) than for traumatic injury.

Provides information about patient's/SO's level of knowledge about individual situation and process of acceptance.

Establishes rapport and conveys interest/concern of caregiver. Provides additional information for patient to consider.

Provides opportunity to deal with issues/misconceptions. Helps the patient/SO to realize that feelings experienced are not unusual and that feeling guilty for them is not necessary/helpful. Patient needs to recognize feelings before they can be dealt with effectively.

Suggestive of problems in adjustment that may require further evaluation and more extensive therapy. May reflect grief response to loss of body part/function and worry over acceptance by others as well as fear of further disability/loss of life from cancer.

671

ACTIONS/INTERVENTIONS

Independent

Provide opportunities for patient/SO to view and touch stoma, using the moment to point out positive signs of healing, normal appearance, and so forth.

Provide opportunity for patient to deal with ostomy through participation in self-care.

Maintain positive approach, during care activities, avoiding expressions of disdain or revulsion. Do not take patient's angry expressions personally.

Plan/schedule care activities with patient.

Discuss possibility of contacting ostomy/urostomy visitor and make arrangements for visit if desired.

Discuss sexual functioning and penile implant, if applicable, and alternate ways for sexual pleasuring. (Refer to ND: Sexual Dysfunction, high risk for, p 676.)

RATIONALE

Although integration of stoma into body image can take months or even years, looking at the stoma and hearing comments (made in a normal, matter-of-fact manner) can help patient with this acceptance. Touching stoma reassures patient/SO that it is not fragile and that slight movements of stoma actually reflect normal peristalsis.

Independence in self-care helps to improve self-esteem.

Assists patient/SO to accept body changes and feel all right about self. Anger is most often directed at the situation and lack of control individual has over what has happened (powerlessness), not the individual care giver.

Promotes sense of control, and gives message that the patient can handle this, enhancing self-esteem.

Can provide a good support system. Helps to reinforce teaching (shared experiences) and facilitates acceptance of change as patient realizes "life does go on" and can be relatively normal.

Patient may experience anticipatory anxiety, fear of failure in relation to sex after surgery, usually because of ignorance, lack of knowledge. Surgery that removes the bladder and prostate (removed with the bladder) may disrupt parasympathetic nerve fibers that control erection in men, although newer techniques are available that may be used in individual cases to preserve these nerves.

NURSING DIAGNOSIS:	PAIN, [ACUTE]
May be related to:	Physical factors, e.g., disruption of skin/tissues (incisions/drains).
	Biologic: Activity of disease process (cancer, trauma).
	Psychologic factors, e.g., fear, anxiety.
Possibly evidenced by:	Reports of pain, self-focusing.
	Guarding/distraction behaviors, restlessness.
	Autonomic responses, e.g., changes in vital signs.
DESIRED OUTCOMES/ EVALUATION CRITERIA— PATIENT WILL:	Verbalize/display relief of pain.
	Demonstrate ability to assist with general comfort measures and able to sleep/rest appropriately.

ACTIONS/INTERVENTIONS	RATIONALE
Independent	
Assess pain, noting location, characteristics, intensity (0–10 scale).	Helps evaluate degree of discomfort and effectiveness of analgesia or may reveal developing complications, e.g., because abdominal pain usually subsides gradually by the third or fourth postoperative day, continued or increasing pain may reflect delayed healing, peristomal skin irritation, infection, intestinal obstruction.
Auscultate bowel sounds; note passage of flatus.	Indicates reestablishment of bowel function. Lack of return of bowel sounds/function within 72 hours may indicate presence of complication, e.g., peritonitis, hypokalemia, mechanical obstruction.
Note urine flow and characteristics.	Decreased flow may reflect urinary retention (due to edema) with increased pressure in upper urinary tract or leakage into peritoneal cavity (failure of anastomosis). Cloudy urine may be normal (presence of mucus) or indicate infectious process.
Encourage patient to verbalize concerns. Active-listen these concerns and provide support by acceptance, remaining with patient and giving appropriate information.	Reduction of anxiety/fear can promote relaxation/comfort.
Provide comfort measures, e.g., back rub, repositioning (using body support measures as needed). Assure patient that position change will not injure stoma.	Reduces muscle tension, promotes relaxation and may enhance coping abilities.
Encourage use of relaxation techniques, e.g., guided imagery, visualization, diversional activities.	Helps patient to rest more effectively and refocuses attention, which may enhance coping ability, reducing pain and discomfort.
Assist with ROM exercises and encourage early ambulation.	Reduces muscle/joint stiffness. Ambulation returns organs to normal position and promotes return of peristalsis/passage of flatus and feelings of general well-being.
Investigate and report abdominal muscle rigidity, involuntary guarding, and rebound tenderness.	Suggestive of peritoneal inflammation, requiring prompt medical intervention.
Collaborative	
Administer medications as indicated, e.g., narcotics, analgesics; PCA.	Relieves pain, enhances comfort, and promotes rest. PCA may be more beneficial than intermittent analgesia, especially following radical resection.
Provide sitz baths, if indicated.	Relieves local discomfort, reduces edema, and promotes healing of perineal wound associated with radical procedure.
Apply/monitor effects of TENS unit.	Cutaneous stimulation may be used to block transmission of pain stimulus.
Maintain patency of NG tube.	Decompresses stomach/intestines; prevents abdominal distention when intestinal function is impaired.

ACTIONS/INTERVENTIONS	RATIONALE

Independent

ACTIONS/INTERVENTIONS	RATIONALE
Empty ostomy pouch when it becomes one third full once IV fluids and continuous pouch drainage have been discontinued.	Reduces risk of urinary reflux and maintains integrity of appliance seal. *Note:* Urinary pouches are available with antireflux valve.
Document urine characteristics, and note whether changes are associated with reports of flank pain.	Cloudy odorous urine indicates infection (possibly pyelonephritis); however, urine normally contains mucus after a conduit procedure.
Test urine pH with Nitrazine paper (use fresh specimen, not from pouch); notify physician if greater than 6.5.	Urine is normally acidic, which discourages bacterial growth/UTIs. *Note:* Presence of alkaline urine also creates favorable environment for stone formation in presence of hypercalciuria.
Report sudden cessation of urethral drainage.	Constant drainage usually subsides within 10 days. However, abrupt cessation may indicate plugging and lead to abscess formation.
Note red rash around stoma.	Rash is most commonly caused by yeast. Urine leakage or allergy to appliance or products may also cause red, irritated areas.
Inspect incision line around stoma. Observe and document wound drainage, signs of incisional inflammation, systemic indicators of sepsis.	Provides baseline reference. Complications may include interrupted anastomosis of intestine/bowel or ureteral conduit, with leakage of bowel contents into abdomen or urine into peritoneal cavity.
Change dressings as indicated when used.	Moist dressings act as a wick to the wound and provide media for bacterial growth.
Assess skin-fold areas in groin, perineum, under arms and breasts.	Use of antibiotics and trapping of moisture in skin-fold areas increases risk of monilial infections.
Monitor vital signs.	Elevation of temperature suggests incisional or UTI and/or respiratory complications.
Auscultate breath sounds.	Patient is at high risk for development of respiratory complications because of length of time under anesthesia. Often this patient is older and may already have a compromised immune system. Also, painful abdominal incisions cause patient to

ACTIONS/INTERVENTIONS	RATIONALE
	breathe more shallowly than normal and to limit coughing. Accumulation of secretions in respiratory system predisposes to atelectasis and infections.

Collaborative

ACTIONS/INTERVENTIONS	RATIONALE
Use pouch with antireflux valve, if available.	Prevents backflow of urine into stoma, reducing risk of infection.
Obtain specimens of exudates, urine, sputum, blood as indicated.	Identifies source of infection/most effective treatment. Infected urine may cause pyelonephritis. *Note:* Urine specimen must be obtained from the conduit because the pouch is considered contaminated.
Administer medications as indicated:	
Cephalosporins, e.g., cefoxitin (Mefoxin), cefazolin (Ancef);	Given to treat identified infection or may be given prophylactically, especially with history of recurrent pyelonephritis.
Antifungal powder;	Used to treat yeast infections around stoma.
Ascorbic acid/vitamin C.	Given to acidify urine, reduce bacterial growth/risk of infection. *Note:* Large doses of vitamin C can impair GI absorption of B_{12}, potentiating pernicious anemia.
Assist with injection of IV methylene blue.	Dye appearing in wound drainage signifies urine leakage into peritoneal cavity and need for surgical repair.

NURSING DIAGNOSIS:	URINARY ELIMINATION: ALTERED
May be related to:	Surgical diversion; tissue trauma, postoperative edema.
Possibly evidenced by:	Loss of continence. Changes in amount, character of urine; urinary retention.
DESIRED OUTCOMES/ EVALUATION CRITERIA— PATIENT WILL:	Display continuous flow of urine, with output adequate for individual situation.

ACTIONS/INTERVENTIONS	RATIONALE

Independent

ACTIONS/INTERVENTIONS	RATIONALE
Assess for presence of stents/ureteral catheters. Label "right" and "left" and observe urine flow through each.	Maintains patency of ureters and assists in healing of anastomosis by keeping it urine free.
Record urinary output; investigate sudden reduction/cessation of urine flow.	Sudden decrease in urine flow may indicate obstruction/dysfunction, (e.g., blockage by edema or mucus) or dehydration. *Note:* Reduced urinary output (not related to hypovolemia) associated with abdominal distention, fever and clear/watery

ACTIONS/INTERVENTIONS	RATIONALE
Independent	
	discharge from incision suggests urinary fistula also requiring prompt intervention.
Observe and record color of urine. Note hematuria, and/or bleeding from stoma.	Urine may be slightly pink, which should clear up in 2–3 days. Rubbing/washing stoma may cause temporary oozing due to vascular nature of tissues. Continued bleeding, frank blood in the pouch, or oozing around the base of stoma requires medical evaluation/intervention.
Position tubing and drainage pouch so that it allows unimpeded flow of urine. Monitor/protect placement of stents.	Blocked drainage allows pressure to build within urinary tract, risking anastomosis leakage and damage to renal parenchyma. *Note:* Stents inserted to maintain patency of ureters during period of postoperative edema may be inadvertently dislodged, compromising urine flow.
Demonstrate self-catheterization techniques and reservoir irrigations as appropriate.	Patients with continent diversions do not require an external collection device. Periodic catheterization empties the internal reservoir. Daily irrigations remove accumulated mucous from the reservoir. *Note:* Patient's with Kock pouches connected to the urethra are instructed to void every 2 hours during the day and every 3 hours during the night. This is done by bearing down and applying hand pressure on the lower abdomen to aid in emptying the reservoir.
Encourage increased fluids and maintain accurate intake.	Maintains hydration and good urine flow.
Monitor vital signs. Assess peripheral pulses, skin turgor, capillary refill, and oral mucosa. Weigh daily.	Indicators of fluid balance. Reflects level of hydration and effectiveness of fluid replacement therapy.
Collaborative	
Administer IV fluids as indicated.	Assists in maintaining hydration/adequate circulating volume and urinary flow.
Monitor electrolytes, ABGs, calcium.	Impaired renal function in patient with intestinal conduit increases risk of severe electrolyte and/or acid/base problems, e.g., hyperchloremic acidosis. Elevated calcium levels increase risk of crystal/stone formation, affecting both urinary flow and tissue integrity.
Prepare for diagnostic testing, procedures as indicated.	Retrograde ileogram may be done to evaluate patency of conduit; nephrostomy tube or stents may be inserted to maintain urine flow until edema/obstruction is resolved.

NURSING DIAGNOSIS:	**SEXUAL DYSFUNCTION, HIGH RISK FOR**
Risk factors may include:	Altered body structure/function; radical resection/treatment procedures.

Vulnerability/psychologic concern about response of SO.

Disruption of sexual response pattern, e.g., erection difficulty.

Possibly evidenced by: [Not applicable; presence of signs and symptoms establishes an actual diagnosis.]

DESIRED OUTCOMES/ EVALUATION CRITERIA— PATIENT WILL: Verbalize understanding of relationship of physical condition to sexual problems.

Identify satisfying/acceptable sexual practices and explore alternate methods.

Resume sexual relationship as appropriate.

ACTIONS/INTERVENTIONS	RATIONALE
Independent	
Ascertain the patient's/SO's sexual relationship prior to the disease and/or surgery. Identify future expectations and desires.	Mutilation and loss of privacy/control of a bodily function can affect patient's view of personal sexuality. When coupled with the fear of rejection by SO, the desired level of intimacy can be greatly impaired. Sexual needs are very basic, and the patient will be rehabilitated more successfully when a satisfying sexual relationship is continued/developed.
Review with the patient/SO anatomy and physiology of sexual functioning in relation to own situation.	Understanding normal physiology helps patient/ SO understand the mechanisms of nerve damage and need for exploring alternative methods of satisfaction.
Reinforce information given by the physician. Encourage questions. Provide additional information as needed.	Reiteration of previously given information assists the patient/SO to hear and process the knowledge again, moving toward acceptance of individual limitations/restrictions and prognosis (e.g., that it may take up to 2 years to regain potency after a radical procedure or that a penile prosthesis may be necessary).
Discuss resumption of sexual activity approximately 6 weeks after discharge, beginning slowly and progressing (e.g., cuddling/caressing until both partners are comfortable with body image/ function changes). Include alternate methods of stimulation as appropriate.	Knowing what to expect in progress of recovery helps patient avoid performance anxiety/reduce risk of "failure." If the couple is willing to try new ideas, this can assist with adjustment and may help to achieve sexual fulfillment.
Encourage dialogue between patient/SO. Suggest wearing pouch cover, T-shirt, or shortie nightgown.	Disguising urostomy appliance may aid in reducing feelings of self-consciousness, embarrassment during sexual activity.
Stress awareness of factors that might be distracting (e.g., unpleasant odors and pouch leakage).	Promotes resolution of solvable problems.
Encourage use of a sense of humor.	Laughter can help individuals to deal more effectively with difficult situation and promote a positive sexual experience.

677

ACTIONS/INTERVENTIONS	RATIONALE

Independent

Problem-solve alternative positions for coitus.	Minimizing awkwardness of appliance and physical discomfort can enhance satisfaction.
Discuss/role play possible interactions or approaches when dealing with new sexual partners.	Rehearsal helps to deal with actual situations when they arise, preventing self-consciousness about "different" body image.
Provide birth control information as appropriate and stress that impotence does not mean the patient is necessarily sterile.	Confusion about impotency and sterility may exist that can lead to an unwanted pregnancy.

Collaborative

Arrange meeting with an ostomy visitor if appropriate.	Sharing of how these problems have been resolved by others can be helpful and reduce sense of isolation.
Refer to counseling/sex therapy as indicated.	If problems persist longer than several months after surgery, a trained therapist may be required to facilitate communication between patient and SO.

NURSING DIAGNOSIS:	**KNOWLEDGE DEFICIT [LEARNING NEED] REGARDING CONDITION, PROGNOSIS, AND TREATMENT NEEDS.**
May be related to:	Lack of exposure/recall; information misinterpretation.
	Unfamiliarity with information resources.
Possibly evidenced by:	Questions; statement of misconception/misinformation.
	Inaccurate follow-through of instruction/performance of urostomy care.
	Inappropriate or exaggerated behaviors (e.g., hostile, agitated, apathetic, withdrawn).
DESIRED OUTCOMES/ EVALUATION CRITERIA— PATIENT WILL:	Verbalize understanding of condition/disease process and treatment and prognosis.
	Correctly perform necessary procedures, explain reasons for the action.
	Initiate necessary lifestyle changes.

ACTIONS/INTERVENTIONS	RATIONALE

Independent

Evaluate patient's emotional and physical capabilities.	These factors affect patient's ability to master tasks and willingness to assume responsibility for ostomy care.
Review anatomy, physiology, and implications of surgical intervention. Discuss future expectations.	Provides knowledge base on which patient can make informed choices and an opportunity to clarify misconceptions regarding individual situation.

ACTIONS/INTERVENTIONS	RATIONALE

Independent

Include written/picture resources.

Provides references postdischarge to support patient efforts for independence in self-care.

Instruct patient/SO in stomal care as appropriate. Allot time for return demonstrations and provide positive feedback for efforts.

Promotes positive management and reduces risk of improper ostomy care.

Assure that stoma and appliance are odorless, nonleaking.

When patient feels confident about urostomy, energy/attention can be focused on other tasks.

Demonstrate padding to absorb urethral drainage; ask patient to report changes in amount, odor, character.

Small amount of leakage may continue for several weeks after prostate surgery with bladder left in place (temporary diversion procedure).

Recommend routine clipping/trimming of hair around stoma to edges of pouch adhesive.

Hair can be pulled out when the pouch is changed causing irritation of hair follicles and increasing risk of local infection.

Encourage patients with Kock pouch to lengthen voiding interval by 1 hour each week unless discomfort noted.

Increases capacity of reservoir to achieve a more normal voiding pattern. Presence of discomfort suggests reservoir is full necessitating prompt emptying.

Instruct patient in a progressive exercise program to include Kegel's exercises and stop/start of urinary stream.

Improves tone of pelvic muscles and the external sphincter to enhance continence when patient voids through penis.

Encourage optimal nutrition.

Promotes wound healing, increases utilization of energy to facilitate tissue repair. Anorexia may be present for several months postoperatively requiring conscious effort to meet nutritional needs.

Discuss use of acid–ash diet (e.g., cranberries, prunes, plums, cereals, rice, peanuts, noodles, cheese, poultry, fish); avoidance of salt substitutes, sodium bicarbonate, and antacids; and cautious use of products containing calcium.

May be useful in acidifying urine to decrease risk of infection and crystal/stone formation. Products containing bicarbonate/calcium potentiate risk of crystal/stone formation affecting both urinary flow and tissue integrity. *Note:* Use of sulfa drugs requires alkaline urine for optimal absorption; so acid–ash diet/vitamin C supplements should be withheld.

Discuss importance of maintaining normal weight.

Changes in weight can affect size of stoma/appliance fit. *Note:* Weight loss of 10–20 lb is not uncommon due to intestinal involvement and anorexia.

Stress necessity of increased fluid intake of at least 2–3 L/d; of cranberry juice or ascorbic acid/vitamin C tablets; avoidance of citrus fruits as indicated.

Maintains urinary output and promotes acidic urine to reduce risk of infection and stone formation. *Note:* Oranges/citrus fruits make urine alkaline and therefore are contraindicated. Large doses of vitamin C can inhibit B_{12} absorption requiring periodic monitoring of B_{12} levels.

Discuss resumption of presurgery level of activity and possibility of sleep disturbance, anorexia, loss of interest in usual activities.

Patient should be able to manage same degree of activity as previously enjoyed and in some cases increase activity level except for contact sports. "Homecoming depression" may occur, lasting for up to 3 months after surgery, requiring patience/support and ongoing evaluation.

ACTIONS/INTERVENTIONS	RATIONALE
Independent	
Encourage regular activity/exercise program.	Immobility/inactivity increases urinary stasis and calcium shift out of bones, potentiating risk of stone formation and resultant urinary obstruction, infection.
Identify signs/symptoms requiring medical evaluation, e.g., changes in character, amount and flow of urine, unusual drainage from wound; fatigue/muscle weakness, anorexia, abdominal distention, confusion.	Early detection and prompt intervention of developing problems such as UTI, stricture, intestinal fistula may prevent more serious complications. Urinary electrolytes (especially chloride) are resorbed in the intestinal conduit, which leads to compensatory bicarbonate loss, lowered serum pH (metabolic acidosis), and potassium deficit.
Stress importance of follow-up appointments.	Monitors healing, disease process; provides opportunity for discussion of appliance fitting problems, generalized health, and adaptation to condition. *Note:* Extensive surgery requires prolonged recuperation for regaining strength and endurance.
Identify community resources, e.g., United Ostomy Association, and local ostomy support group, enterostomal therapist, VNA, pharmacy/medical supply house.	Continued support after discharge is essential to facilitate the recovery process and patient's independence in care. Enterostomal nurse can be very helpful in solving appliance problems and identifying alternatives to meet individual patient needs.

Benign Prostatic Hyperplasia _____

Progressive enlargement of the prostate gland (commonly seen in men older than age 50) causing varying degrees of urethral obstruction and restriction of urinary flow.

RELATED CONCERNS

Prostatectomy, p 689
Psychosocial Aspects of Acute Care, p 899
Renal Failure: Acute, p 618

PATIENT ASSESSMENT DATA BASE

CIRCULATION

May exhibit:	Elevated BP (renal effects of advanced enlargement).

ELIMINATION

May report:	Decreased force/caliber of urinary stream; dribbling.
	Hesitancy in initiating voiding.
	Inability to empty bladder completely; urgency and frequency of urination.
	Nocturia, dysuria, hematuria.
	Sitting to void.
	Recurrent UTIs, history of calculi (urinary stasis).
	Constipation (protrusion of prostate into rectum).
May exhibit:	Firm mass in lower abdomen (distended bladder), bladder tenderness.
	Inguinal hernia; hemorrhoids (result of increased abdominal pressure required to empty bladder against resistance).

FOOD/FLUID

May report:	Anorexia; nausea, vomiting.
	Recent weight loss.

PAIN/COMFORT

May report:	Suprapubic, flank, or back pain; sharp, intense (in acute prostatitis).
	Low back pain.

SAFETY

May report:	Fever.

SEXUALITY

May report:	Concerns about effects of condition/therapy on sexual abilities.
	Fear of incontinence/dribbling during intimacy.
	Decrease in force of ejaculatory contractions.
May exhibit:	Enlarged, tender prostate.

681

TEACHING/LEARNING

May report: Family history of cancer, hypertension, kidney disease.

Use of antihypertensive or antidepressant medications, urinary antibiotics or antibacterial agents, OTC cold/allergy medications containing sympathomimetics.

Discharge plan considerations: **DRG projected mean length of stay: 2.2 days.**

May need assistance with management of therapy, e.g., catheter.

DIAGNOSTIC STUDIES

Urinalysis: Color yellow, dark brown, dark or bright red (bloody); appearance may be cloudy; pH 7 or greater (suggests infection); bacteria, WBCs, RBCs may be present microscopically.

Urine culture: May reveal *Staphylococcus aureus, Proteus, Klebsiella, Pseudomonas,* or *Escherichia coli.*

Urine cytology: To rule out bladder cancer.

BUN/Cr: Elevated if renal function is compromised.

Serum acid phosphatase/prostatic specific antigen: Increased because of cellular growth and hormonal influences in cancer of the prostate (may indicate metastasis to the bone).

WBC: May be greater than 11,000, indicating infection if patient is not immunosuppressed.

Urinary flow rate determination: Assesses degree of bladder obstruction.

IVP with postvoiding film: Shows delayed emptying of bladder, varying degrees of urinary tract obstruction, and presence of prostatic enlargement, bladder diverticuli, and abnormal thickening of bladder muscle.

Voiding cystourethrography: May be used instead of IVP to visualize bladder and urethra because it uses local dyes.

Cystometrogram: Measures pressure and volume in the bladder to identify bladder dysfunction unrelated to BPH.

Cystourethroscopy: To view degree of prostatic enlargement and bladder-wall changes (contraindicated in presence of acute UTI due to risk of Gram-negative sepsis).

Cystometry: Evaluates detrusor muscle function and tone.

Transrectal ultrasound: Measures size of prostate, amount of residual urine; locates lesions unrelated to BPH.

NURSING PRIORITIES

1. Relieve acute urinary retention.
2. Promote comfort.
3. Prevent complications.
4. Assist patient to deal with psychosocial concerns.
5. Provide information about disease process/prognosis and treatment needs.

DISCHARGE GOALS

1. Voiding pattern normalized.
2. Pain/discomfort relieved.
3. Complications prevented/minimized.
4. Dealing with situation realistically.
5. Disease process/prognosis and therapeutic regimen understood.

NURSING DIAGNOSIS:	URINARY RETENTION [ACUTE/CHRONIC]
May be related to:	Mechanical obstruction; enlarged prostate.

	Decompensation of detrusor musculature.
	Inability of bladder to contract adequately.
Possibly evidenced by:	Frequency, hesitancy, inability to empty bladder completely; incontinence/dribbling.
	Bladder distention, residual urine.
DESIRED OUTCOMES/ EVALUATION CRITERIA— PATIENT WILL:	Void in sufficient amounts with no palpable bladder distention.
	Demonstrate postvoid residuals of less than 50 ml; with absence of dribbling/overflow.

ACTIONS/INTERVENTIONS	RATIONALE
Independent	
Encourage patient to void every 2–4 hours and when urge is noted.	May minimize urinary retention/overdistention of the bladder.
Ask patient about stress incontinence.	High urethral pressure inhibits bladder emptying or can inhibit voiding until abdominal pressure increases enough for urine to be involuntarily lost.
Observe urinary stream, noting size and force.	Useful in evaluating degree of obstruction and choice of intervention.
Monitor and document time and amount of each voiding. Note diminished urinary output and changes in specific gravity.	Urinary retention increases pressure within the upper urinary tract, which may compromise renal function. Any deficit in blood flow to the kidney impairs its ability to filter and concentrate substances.
Percuss/palpate suprapubic area.	A distended bladder can be felt in the suprapubic area.
Force fluids up to 3000 ml daily, within cardiac tolerance, if indicated.	Increased circulating fluid maintains renal perfusion and flushes kidneys and bladder of bacterial growth. *Note:* Initially, fluids may be restricted to prevent additional bladder distention until adequate urinary flow is reestablished.
Monitor vital signs closely. Observe for hypertension, peripheral/dependent edema, changes in mentation. Weigh daily. Maintain accurate I&O.	Loss of kidney function results in decreased fluid elimination and accumulation of toxic wastes; may progress to complete renal shutdown.
Provide/encourage meticulous catheter and perineal care.	Reduces risk of ascending infection.
Provide sitz bath as indicated.	Promotes muscle relaxation, decreases edema, and may enhance voiding effort.
Collaborative	
Administer medications as indicated:	
Antispasmodics, e.g., oxybutynin chloride (Ditropan);	Relieves bladder spasms related to irritation by the catheter.

683

ACTIONS/INTERVENTIONS	RATIONALE
Independent	
Rectal suppositories (B&O);	Suppositories are absorbed easily through mucosa into bladder tissue to produce muscle relaxation/relieve spasms.
Antibiotics and antibacterials;	Given to combat infection. May be used prophylactically.
Phenoxybenzamine (Dibenzyline);	May be given to make urinating easier by relaxing prostatic smooth muscle and decreasing resistance to flow of urine. Used with caution as it does not shrink the gland and has unpleasant side effects such as dizziness and fatigue.
Alpha-adrenergic antagonists, e.g., prazosin (Minipress), terazosin (Hytrin).	Studies indicate that these drugs may be as effective as Dibenzyline with fewer side effects.
Catheterize for residual urine and leave indwelling catheter as indicated.	Relieves/prevents urinary retention and rules out presence of ureteral stricture. *Note:* Bladder decompression should be done in increments of 200 ml to prevent hematuria (rupture of blood vessels in the mucosa of the overdistended bladder) and syncope (excessive autonomic stimulation). Coudé catheter may be required as the curved tip eases passage of the tube through the prostatic urethra.
Irrigate catheter as indicated.	Maintains patency/urinary flow.
Monitor laboratory studies, e.g.:	
BUN, Cr, electrolytes;	Prostatic enlargement (obstruction) eventually causes dilatation of upper urinary tract (ureters and kidneys), potentially impairing kidney function and leading to uremia.
Urinalysis and culture.	Urinary stasis potentiates bacterial growth, increasing risk of UTI.
Prepare for/assist with urinary drainage, e.g.:	
Cystostomy;	May be indicated to drain bladder during acute episode with azotemia or when surgery is contraindicated because of patient's health status.
Experimental procedures, e.g.:	
Transurethral hyperthermia;	Heating the central portion of the prostate by the insertion of a heating element through the urethra tends to shrink the prostate. Treatments are carried out 1–2 times/wk for several weeks to achieve desired results.
Cryosurgery;	Freezing the prostatic capsule causes sloughing of prostatic tissue relieving obstruction. This procedure is not as effective as a TURP and is reserved for individuals who are deemed a poor anesthetic risk.
Balloon urethroplasty/transurethral dilatation of the prostate.	Inflation of a balloon-tipped catheter within the obstructed area displaces prostatic tissue, thus improving urinary flow.

NURSING DIAGNOSIS:	PAIN [ACUTE]
May be related to:	Mucosal irritation: bladder distention, renal colic; urinary infection; radiation therapy.
Possibly evidenced by:	Reports of pain (bladder/rectal spasm).
	Narrowed focus; altered muscle tone, grimacing; distraction behaviors, restlessness.
	Autonomic responses.
DESIRED OUTCOMES/ EVALUATION CRITERIA— PATIENT WILL:	Report pain relieved/controlled.
	Appear relaxed.
	Be able to sleep/rest appropriately.

ACTIONS/INTERVENTIONS

Independent

Assess pain, noting location, intensity (scale of 0–10), duration.

Tape drainage tube to thigh and catheter to the abdomen (if traction not required).

Maintain bed rest when indicated.

Provide comfort measures, e.g., back rub; helping patient assume position of comfort; encouraging use of relaxation/deep-breathing exercises; diversional activities.

Encourage use of sitz baths, warm soaks to perineum.

Collaborative

Insert catheter and attach to straight drainage.

Do prostatic massage.

Administer medications as indicated:

Narcotics, e.g., meperidine (Demerol);

Antibacterials, e.g., methenamine hippurate (Hiprex);

Antispasmodics and bladder sedatives, e.g., flavoxate (Urispas); oxybutynin (Ditropan).

RATIONALE

Provides information to aid in determining choice/ effectiveness of interventions.

Prevents pull on the bladder and erosion of the penile–scrotal junction.

Bed rest may be needed initially during acute retention phase. However, early ambulation can help restore normal voiding patterns and relieve colicky pain.

Promotes relaxation, refocuses attention, and may enhance coping abilities.

Promotes muscle relaxation.

Draining bladder reduces bladder tension and irritability.

Aids in evacuation of ducts of gland to relieve congestion/inflammation. Contraindicated if infection is present.

Given to relieve severe pain, provide physical and mental relaxation.

Reduces bacteria present in urinary tract as well as those introduced by drainage system.

Relieves bladder irritability.

NURSING DIAGNOSIS:	FLUID VOLUME DEFICIT, HIGH RISK FOR
Risk factors may include:	Postobstructive diuresis from rapid drainage of a chronically overdistended bladder.
	Endocrine, electrolyte imbalances (renal dysfunction).
Possibly evidenced by:	[Not applicable; presence of signs and symptoms establishes an actual diagnosis.]
DESIRED OUTCOMES/ EVALUATION CRITERIA— PATIENT WILL:	Maintain adequate hydration as evidenced by stable vital signs, palpable peripheral pulses, good capillary refill, and moist mucous membranes.

ACTIONS/INTERVENTIONS	RATIONALE
Independent	
Monitor output carefully, hourly if indicated. Note outputs of 100–200 ml/h.	Rapid diuresis could cause the patient's total fluid volume to become depleted, because insufficient amounts of sodium are resorbed in renal tubules.
Encourage increased oral intake based on individual needs.	Patient may have restricted oral intake in an attempt to control urinary symptoms, reducing homeostatic reserves and increasing risk of dehydration/ hypovolemia.
Monitor BP, pulse frequently. Evaluate capillary refill and oral mucous membranes.	Enables early detection/intervention of systemic hypovolemia.
Promote bed rest with head elevated.	Decreases cardiac workload, facilitating circulatory homeostasis.
Collaborative	
Monitor electrolytes, especially sodium.	As fluid is pulled from extracellular spaces, sodium may follow the shift, causing hyponatremia.
Administer IV fluids (hypertonic saline) as needed.	Replaces fluid and sodium losses to prevent/correct hypovolemia.

NURSING DIAGNOSIS:	FEAR/ANXIETY [SPECIFY LEVEL]
May be related to:	Change in health status: possibility of surgical procedure/malignancy.
	Embarrassment/loss of dignity associated with genital exposure before, during, and after treatment; concern about sexual ability.
Possibly evidenced by:	Increased tension, apprehension, worry.
	Expressed concerns regarding perceived changes.
	Fear of unspecific consequences.

DESIRED OUTCOMES/ EVALUATION CRITERIA— PATIENT WILL:	Appear relaxed.
	Verbalize accurate knowledge of the situation.
	Demonstrate appropriate range of feelings and lessened fear.
	Report anxiety is reduced to a manageable level.

ACTIONS/INTERVENTIONS	RATIONALE
Independent	
Be available to the patient. Establish trusting relationship with patient/SO.	Demonstrates concern and willingness to help. Helpful in discussing sensitive subjects.
Provide information about specific procedures and tests and what to expect afterward, e.g., catheter, bloody urine, bladder irritation. Be aware of how much information the patient wants.	Helps patient understand purpose of what is being done, and reduces concerns associated with the unknown, including fear of cancer. However, overload of information is not helpful and may increase anxiety.
Maintain matter-of-fact attitude in doing procedures/dealing with patient. Protect patient's privacy.	Communicates acceptance and eases patient's embarrassment.
Encourage patient/SO to verbalize concerns/feelings.	Defines the problem, providing opportunity to answer questions, clarify misconceptions, and problem solve solutions.
Reinforce previous information patient has been given.	Allows the patient to deal with reality and strengthens trust in caregivers and information presented.

NURSING DIAGNOSIS:	KNOWLEDGE DEFICIT [LEARNING NEED], REGARDING CONDITION, PROGNOSIS, AND TREATMENT NEEDS
May be related to:	Lack of exposure/recall, information misinterpretation.
	Unfamiliarity with information resources.
	Concern about sensitive area.
Possibly evidenced by:	Questions, request for information.
	Verbalization of the problem/nonverbal indicators.
	Inaccurate follow-through of instructions, development of preventable complications.
DESIRED OUTCOMES/ EVALUATION CRITERIA— PATIENT WILL:	Verbalize understanding of disease process/prognosis.
	Identify relationship of signs/symptoms to the disease process.
	Initiate necessary lifestyle/behavior changes.
	Participate in treatment regimen.

ACTIONS/INTERVENTIONS	RATIONALE
Independent	
Review disease process, patient expectations.	Provides knowledge base on which patient can make informed therapy choices.
Encourage verbalization of fears/feelings and concerns.	Helping patient work through feelings can be vital to rehabilitation.
Give information that the condition is not sexually transmitted.	May be an unspoken fear.
Recommend avoiding spicy foods, coffee, alcohol, long automobile rides, rapid intake of fluids (particularly alcohol).	May cause prostatic irritation with resulting congestion. Sudden increase in urinary flow can cause bladder distention and loss of bladder tone, resulting in episodes of acute urinary retention.
Address sexual concerns, e.g., that during acute episodes of prostatitis, intercourse is avoided but may be helpful in treatment of chronic condition.	Sexual activity can increase pain during acute episodes but may serve as massaging agent in presence of chronic disease.
Provide information about basic sexual anatomy. Encourage questions and promote a dialog about concerns.	Having information about anatomy involved helps patient understand the implications of proposed treatments, as they might affect sexual performance.
Review signs/symptoms requiring medical evaluation, e.g., cloudy, odorous urine; diminished urinary output, inability to void; presence of fever/chills.	Prompt interventions may prevent more serious complications.
Discuss necessity of notifying other health care providers of diagnosis.	Reduces risk of inappropriate therapy; e.g., use of decongestants, anticholinergics, and antidepressants increases urinary retention and may precipitate an acute episode.
Reinforce importance of medical follow-up for at least 6 months–1 year, including rectal examination, urinalysis.	Recurrence of hypertrophy and/or infection (caused by same or different organisms) is not uncommon and will require changes in therapeutic regimen to prevent serious complications.

Prostatectomy

Surgical resection of the portion of the prostate gland encroaching on the urethra to improve urinary flow and relieve acute urinary retention.

Transurethral Resection of the Prostate (TURP)
Obstructive prostatic tissue of the medial lobe surrounding the urethra is removed by means of a cysto-scope/resectoscope introduced through the urethra.

Suprapubic/Open Prostatectomy
Indicated for masses exceeding 60 g/2 oz. Obstructing prostatic tissue is removed through a low midline incision made through the bladder. This approach is preferred if bladder stones are present.

Retropubic Prostatectomy
Hypertrophied prostatic tissue mass (located high in the pelvic region) is removed through a low abdominal incision without opening the bladder.

Perineal Prostatectomy
Large prostatic masses low in the pelvic area are removed through an incision between the scrotum and the rectum. This radical procedure is done for cancer and may result in impotence.

RELATED CONCERNS

Cancer, p 1014
Psychosocial Aspects of Acute Care, p 899
Surgical Intervention, p 918

PATIENT ASSESSMENT DATA BASE

Refer to CP Benign Prostate Hypertrophy, p 681 for assessment information.

Discharge Plan Considerations   **DRG projected mean length of stay: 4.2 days.**

NURSING PRIORITIES

1. Maintain homeostasis/hemodynamic stability.
2. Promote comfort.
3. Prevent complications.
4. Provide information about surgical procedure/prognosis, treatment, and rehabilitation needs.

DISCHARGE GOALS

1. Urinary flow restored/enhanced.
2. Pain relieved/controlled.
3. Complications prevented/minimized.
4. Procedure/prognosis, therapeutic regimen, and rehabilitation needs understood.

NURSING DIAGNOSIS:	URINARY ELIMINATION: ALTERED
May be related to:	Mechanical obstruction: blood clots, edema, trauma, surgical procedure.
	Pressure and irritation of catheter/balloon.
	Loss of bladder tone due to preoperative overdistention or continued decompression.

Possibly evidenced by:	Frequency, urgency, hesitancy, dysuria, incontinence, retention.
	Bladder fullness; suprapubic discomfort.
DESIRED OUTCOMES/ EVALUATION CRITERIA— PATIENT WILL:	Void normal amounts without retention.
	Demonstrate behaviors to regain bladder/urinary control.

ACTIONS/INTERVENTIONS	RATIONALE

Independent

Assess urine output and catheter/drainage system, especially during bladder irrigation.	Retention can occur because of edema of the surgical area, blood clots, and bladder spasms.
Assist patient to assume normal position to void, e.g., stand, walk to bathroom at frequent intervals after catheter is removed.	Encourages passage of urine and promotes sense of normality.
Note time, amount of voiding, and size of stream after catheter is removed. Note reports of bladder fullness; inability to void, urgency.	The catheter is usually removed 2–5 days after surgery, but voiding may continue to be a problem for some time because of urethral edema and loss of bladder tone.
Encourage patient to void when urge is noted but not more than every 2–4 hours per protocol.	Voiding with urge prevents urinary retention. Limiting voids to every 4 hours (if tolerated), increases bladder tone, and aids in bladder retraining.
Measure residual volumes if suprapubic catheter present.	Monitors effectiveness of bladder emptying. Residuals greater than 50 ml suggest need for continuation of catheter until bladder tone improves.
Encourage fluid intake to 3000 ml as tolerated. Limit fluids in evening, after catheter removal.	Maintains adequate hydration and renal perfusion for urinary flow. "Scheduling" fluid intake reduces need to void/interrupt sleep during the night.
Instruct patient in perineal exercises, e.g., tightening buttocks, stopping and starting urine stream.	Helps to regain bladder/sphincter/urinary control, minimizing incontinence.
Advise patient that "dribbling" is to be expected after catheter is removed and should resolve as recuperation progresses.	Information helps patient to deal with the problem. Normal functioning may return in 2–3 weeks but can take up to 8 months following perineal approach.

Collaborative

Maintain continuous bladder irrigation (CBI), as indicated in early postoperative period.	Flushes bladder of blood clots and debris to maintain patency of the catheter/urinary flow.

NURSING DIAGNOSIS:	FLUID VOLUME DEFICIT, HIGH RISK FOR
Risk factors may include:	Vascular nature of surgical area; difficulty controlling bleeding.
	Restricted intake preoperatively.

Possibly evidenced by:	[Not applicable; presence of signs and symptoms establishes an actual diagnosis.]
DESIRED OUTCOMES/ EVALUATION CRITERIA— PATIENT WILL:	Maintain adequate hydration as evidenced by stable vital signs, palpable peripheral pulses, good capillary refill, moist mucous membranes, and appropriate UO. Display no active bleeding.

ACTIONS/INTERVENTIONS	RATIONALE
Independent	
Anchor catheter, avoid excessive manipulation.	Movement/pulling of catheter may cause bleeding or clot formation and plugging of the catheter, with bladder distention.
Monitor I&O.	Indicator of fluid balance and replacement needs. With bladder irrigations, monitoring is essential for estimating blood loss and accurately assessing urine output.
Observe catheter drainage, noting excessive/continued bleeding.	Bleeding is not unusual during first 24 hours for all but the perineal approach. Continued/heavy bleeding or recurrence of active bleeding requires medical evaluation/intervention.
Evaluate color, consistency of urine, e.g.:	
Bright red with bright red clots;	Usually indicates arterial bleeding and requires aggressive therapy.
Increased viscosity, dark burgundy with dark clots;	Suggests venous source (the most common type of bleeding), which usually subsides on its own.
Bleeding with absence of clots.	May indicate blood dyscrasias or systemic clotting problems.
Inspect dressings/wound drains. Weigh dressings if indicated. Note hematoma formation.	Bleeding may be evident or sequestered within tissues of the perineum.
Monitor vital signs, noting increased pulse and respiration, decreased BP, diaphoresis, pallor, delayed capillary refill, and dry mucous membranes.	Dehydration/hypovolemia requires prompt intervention to prevent impending shock. *Note:* Hypertension, bradycardia, n/v suggests "TURP syndrome," requiring immediate medical intervention.
Investigate restlessness, confusion, changes in behavior.	May reflect decreased cerebral perfusion (hypovolemia) or indicate cerebral edema from excessive solution absorbed into the venous sinusoids during TUR procedure ("TURP syndrome").
Encourage fluid intake to 3000 ml/d unless contraindicated.	Flushes kidneys/bladder of bacteria and debris but may result in water intoxication/fluid overload if not monitored closely.
Avoid rectal temperatures and use of rectal tubes/ enemas.	May result in referred irritation to prostatic bed and increased pressure on prostatic capsule with risk of bleeding.

ACTIONS/INTERVENTIONS	RATIONALE
Collaborative	
Monitor laboratory studies as indicated, e.g.:	
Hb/Hct, RBCs;	Useful in evaluating blood losses/replacement needs.
Coagulation studies, platelet count.	May indicate developing complications, e.g., depletion of clotting factors, DIC.
Administer IV therapy/blood products as indicated.	May need additional fluids, if oral intake inadequate, or blood products, if losses are excessive.
Maintain traction on indwelling catheter; tape catheter to inner thigh.	Traction on the 30-ml balloon positioned in the prostatic urethral fossa will create pressure on the arterial supply of the prostatic capsule to help prevent/control bleeding.
Release traction within 4–5 hours. Document period of application and release of traction, if used.	Prolonged traction may cause permanent trauma/problems with urinary control.
Administer stool softeners, laxatives as indicated.	Prevention of constipation/straining for stool reduces risk of rectal–perineal bleeding.

NURSING DIAGNOSIS:	INFECTION, HIGH RISK FOR
Risk factors may include:	Invasive procedures: instrumentation during surgery, catheter, frequent bladder irrigation.
	Traumatized tissue, surgical incision (e.g., perineal).
Possibly evidenced by:	[Not applicable; presence of signs and symptoms establishes an actual diagnosis.]
DESIRED OUTCOMES/ EVALUATION CRITERIA— PATIENT WILL:	Achieve timely healing.
	Experience no signs of infection.

ACTIONS/INTERVENTIONS	RATIONALE
Independent	
Maintain sterile catheter system; provide regular catheter/meatal care with soap and water, applying antibiotic ointment around catheter site.	Prevents introduction of bacteria and resultant infection/sepsis.
Ambulate with drainage bag dependent.	Avoids backward reflux of urine, which may introduce bacteria into the bladder.
Monitor vital signs, noting low-grade fever, chills, rapid pulse and respiration, restlessness, irritability, disorientation.	Patient who has had cystoscopy and/or TUR of the prostate are at increased risk for surgical/septic shock related to manipulation/instrumentation.
Observe drainage from wounds, around suprapubic catheter.	Presence of drains, suprapubic incision increases risk of infection, as indicated by erythema, purulent drainage.

692

ACTIONS/INTERVENTIONS

Independent

Change dressings frequently (supra/retropubic and perineal incisions), cleaning and drying skin thoroughly each time.

Use ostomy-type skin barriers.

Collaborative

Administer antibiotics as indicated.

RATIONALE

Wet dressings cause skin irritation and provide media for bacterial growth, increasing risk of wound infection.

Provides protection for surrounding skin, preventing excoriation and reducing risk of infection.

May be given prophylactically due to increased risk of infection with prostatectomy.

NURSING DIAGNOSIS:	PAIN, [ACUTE]
May be related to:	Irritation of the bladder mucosa; reflex muscle spasm associated with surgical procedure and/or pressure from bladder balloon (traction).
Possibly evidenced by:	Reports of painful bladder spasms.
	Facial grimacing, guarding, restlessness.
	Autonomic responses.
DESIRED OUTCOMES/ EVALUATION CRITERIA— PATIENT WILL:	Report pain is relieved/controlled.
	Demonstrate use of relaxation skills and diversional activities as indicated for individual situation.
	Appear relaxed, sleep/rest appropriately.

ACTIONS/INTERVENTIONS

Independent

Assess pain, noting location, intensity (0–10 scale).

Maintain patency of catheter and drainage system. Keep tubings free of kinks and clots.

Promote intake of up to 3000 ml/d as tolerated.

Give patient accurate information about catheter, drainage, and bladder spasms.

Provide comfort measures (Therapeutic Touch, position changes, back rub) and diversional activities. Encourage use of relaxation techniques,

RATIONALE

Sharp, intermittent pain with urge to void/passage of urine around catheter suggests bladder spasms, which tend to be more severe with suprapubic or TUR approaches (usually decrease by the end of 48 hours).

Maintaining a properly functioning catheter and drainage system decreases risk of bladder distention/spasm.

Decreases irritation by maintaining a constant flow of fluid over the bladder mucosa.

Allays anxiety and promotes cooperation with necessary procedures.

Reduces muscle tension, refocuses attention, and may enhance coping abilities.

693

ACTIONS/INTERVENTIONS

Independent

including deep-breathing exercises, visualization, guided imagery.

Provide sitz baths or heat lamp if indicated.

Collaborative

Administer antispasmodics, e.g.:

Oxybutynin chloride (Ditropan); B&O suppositories;

Propantheline bromide (Pro-Banthine).

RATIONALE

Promotes tissue perfusion and resolution of edema, and enhances healing (perineal approach).

Relaxes smooth muscle, to provide relief of spasms and associated pain.

Relieves bladder spasms by anticholinergic action. Usually discontinued 24–48 hours before anticipated removal of catheter to promote normal bladder contraction.

NURSING DIAGNOSIS:	SEXUAL DYSFUNCTION, HIGH RISK FOR
Risk factors may include:	Situational crisis (incontinence, leakage of urine after catheter removal, involvement of genital area). Threat to self-concept/change in health status.
Possibly evidenced by:	[Not applicable; presence of signs and symptoms establishes an actual diagnosis.]
DESIRED OUTCOMES/ EVALUATION CRITERIA— PATIENT WILL:	Appear relaxed and report anxiety is reduced to a manageable level. Verbalize understanding of individual situation. Demonstrate problem-solving skills.

ACTIONS/INTERVENTIONS

Independent

Provide openings for patient/ SO to talk about concerns of incontinence and sexual functioning.

Give accurate information about expectation of return of sexual function.

Discuss basic anatomy. Be honest in answers to patient's questions.

RATIONALE

May have anxieties about the effects of surgery and may be hesitant about asking necessary questions. Anxiety may have affected ability to access information given previously.

Physiologic impotence occurs when the perineal nerves are cut during radical procedures; in other approaches, sexual activity can usually be resumed in 6–8 weeks. *Note:* Penile prosthesis may be recommended to facilitate erection and correct impotence following radical perineal procedure.

The nerve plexus that controls erection runs posteriorly to the prostate through the capsule. In procedures that do not involve the prostatic capsule, impotence and sterility usually are not conse-

ACTIONS/INTERVENTIONS

Independent

Discuss retrograde ejaculation if transurethral/suprapubic approach is used.

Instruct in perineal and interruption/continuation of urinary stream exercises.

Collaborative

Refer to sexual counselor as indicated.

RATIONALE

quences. Surgical procedure may not provide a permanent cure, and hypertrophy may recur.

Seminal fluid goes into the bladder and is excreted with the urine. This does not interfere with sexual functioning but will decrease fertility and cause urine to be cloudy.

Promotes regaining muscular control of urinary continence and sexual function.

Persistent/unresolved problems may require professional intervention.

NURSING DIAGNOSIS:	KNOWLEDGE DEFICIT [LEARNING NEED], REGARDING CONDITION, PROGNOSIS, AND TREATMENT NEEDS
May be related to:	Lack of exposure/recall; information misinterpretation. Unfamiliarity with information resources.
Possibly evidenced by:	Questions, request for information, statement of misconception. Verbalization of the problem. Inaccurate follow-through of instruction/development of preventable complications.
DESIRED OUTCOMES/EVALUATION CRITERIA—PATIENT WILL:	Verbalize understanding of surgical procedure and treatment. Correctly perform necessary procedures and explain reasons for actions. Initiate necessary lifestyle changes. Participate in treatment regimen.

ACTIONS/INTERVENTIONS

Independent

Review implications of procedure and future expectations.

Stress necessity of good nutrition; encourage inclusion of fruits, increased fiber in diet.

Discuss initial activity restrictions, e.g., avoidance of heavy lifting, strenuous exercise, prolonged sitting/long automobile trips, climbing more than 2 flights of stairs at a single time.

RATIONALE

Provides knowledge base on which patient can make informed choices.

Promotes healing and prevents constipation, reducing risk of postoperative bleeding.

Increased abdominal pressure/straining places stress on the bladder and prostate, potentiating risk of bleeding.

695

ACTIONS/INTERVENTIONS	RATIONALE
Independent	
Encourage continuation of perineal exercises.	Facilitates urinary control and alleviation of incontinence.
Instruct in urinary catheter care if present. Identify source for supplies/support.	Promotes independence and competent self-care.
Instruct patient to avoid tub baths after discharge.	Decreases the possibility of infection, introduction of bacteria.
Review signs/symptoms requiring medical evaluation, e.g., erythema, purulent drainage from wound sites; changes in character/amount of urine, presence of urgency/frequency; heavy bleeding, fever/chills.	Prompt intervention may prevent serious complications. *Note:* Urine may appear cloudy for several weeks until postoperative healing occurs and may appear cloudy after intercourse because of retrograde ejaculation.

Urolithiasis (Renal Calculi) _____

Kidney stones (calculi) are formed of mineral deposits, most commonly Ca^{2+} oxalate and Ca^{2+} phosphate; however, uric acid and other crystals are also calculus formers. Although renal calculi can form anywhere in the urinary tract, they are most commonly found in the renal pelvis and calyces. Renal calculi can remain asymptomatic until passed into a ureter and/or urine flow is obstructed, when the potential for renal damage is acute.

RELATED CONCERNS:

Acid/Base Imbalances, p 1082
Fluid and Electrolyte Imbalances, p 1054
Psychosocial Aspects of Acute Care, p 899
Renal Failure: Acute, p 618

PATIENT ASSESSMENT DATA BASE

Dependent on size, location, and etiology of calculi.

ACTIVITY/REST

May report: Sedentary occupation, occupation in which patient is exposed to high environmental temperatures.

Activity restrictions/immobility due to a preexisting condition (e.g., debilitating disease, spinal cord injury).

CIRCULATION

May exhibit: Elevated BP/pulse (pain, anxiety, kidney failure).

Warm, flushed skin; pallor.

ELIMINATION

May report: History of recent/chronic UTI; previous obstruction (calculi).

Decreased urinary output, bladder fullness.

Burning, urgency with urination.

Diarrhea.

May exhibit: Oliguria, hematuria, pyuria.

Alterations in voiding pattern.

FOOD/FLUID

May report: Nausea/vomiting, abdominal tenderness.

Diet high in purines, calcium oxalate, and/or phosphates.

Insufficient fluid intake; does not drink fluids well.

May exhibit: Abdominal distention; decreased/absent bowel sounds.

Vomiting.

PAIN/COMFORT

May report: Acute episode of excruciating, colicky pain. Location is dependent on stone location, e.g., in the flank in the region of the costovertebral angle; may radiate to back, abdomen, and down to the groin/genitalia. Constant dull pain suggests calculi located in the renal pelvis or calyces.

697

Pain may be described as acute, severe not relieved by positioning or any other measures.

May exhibit: Guarding; distraction behaviors.

Tenderness in renal areas on palpation.

SAFETY

May report: Use of alcohol.

Fever; chills.

TEACHING/LEARNING

May report: Family history of calculi, kidney disease, hypertension, gout, chronic UTI.

History of small-bowel disease, previous abdominal surgery, hyperparathyroidism.

Use of antibiotics, antihypertensives, sodium bicarbonate, allopurinol, phosphates, thiazides, excessive intake of calcium or vitamin D.

Discharge Plan Considerations: **DRG projected mean length of stay: 3.2 days.**

DIAGNOSTIC STUDIES

Urinalysis: Color may be yellow, dark brown, bloody; commonly shows RBCs, WBCs, crystals (cystine, uric acid, calcium oxalate), casts, minerals, bacteria, pus; pH may be acid (promotes cystine and uric acid stones) or alkaline (promotes magnesium, ammonium phosphate, or calcium phosphate stones).

Urine (24-hour): Cr, uric acid, calcium, phosphorus, oxalate, or cystine may be elevated.

Urine culture: May reveal UTI *(Staphylococcus aureus, Proteus, Klebsiella, Pseudomonas).*

Biochemical survey: Elevated levels of magnesium, calcium, uric acid, phosphates, protein, electrolytes.

Serum and urine BUN/Cr: Abnormal (high in serum/low in urine) secondary to high obstructive stone in kidney causing ischemia/necrosis.

Serum chloride and bicarbonate levels: Elevation of chloride and decreased levels of bicarbonate suggest developing renal tubular acidosis.

CBC: WBC may be increased indicating infection/septicemia.

RBC: Usually normal.

Hb/Hct: Abnormal if patient is severely dehydrated or polycythemia is present (encourages precipitation of solids), or anemic (hemorrhage, kidney dysfunction/failure).

Parathyroid hormone: May be increased if kidney failure present. (PTH stimulates reabsorption of calcium from bones increasing circulating serum and urine calcium.)

KUB x-ray: Shows presence of calculi and/or anatomic changes in the area of the kidneys or along the course of the ureter.

IVP: Provides rapid confirmation of urolithiasis as a cause of abdominal or flank pain. Shows abnormalities in anatomic structures (distended ureter) and outline of calculi.

Cystoureteroscopy: Direct visualization of bladder and ureter may reveal stone and/or obstructive effects.

CT scan: Identifies/delineates calculi and other masses; kidney, ureteral, and bladder distention.

Ultrasound of kidney: To determine obstructive changes, location of stone.

NURSING PRIORITIES

1. Alleviate pain.
2. Maintain adequate renal functioning.
3. Prevent complications.
4. Provide information about disease process/prognosis and treatment needs.

DISCHARGE GOALS

1. Pain relieved/controlled.
2. Fluid/electrolyte balance maintained.
3. Complications prevented/minimized.
4. Disease process/prognosis and therapeutic regimen understood.

NURSING DIAGNOSIS:	PAIN, [ACUTE]
May be related to:	Increased frequency/force of ureteral contractions.
	Tissue trauma, edema formation; cellular ischemia.
Possibly evidenced by:	Reports of colicky pain.
	Guarding/distraction behaviors, restlessness, moaning, self-focusing, facial mask of pain, muscle tension.
	Autonomic responses.
DESIRED OUTCOMES/ EVALUATION CRITERIA— PATIENT WILL:	Report pain is relieved with spasms controlled.
	Appear relaxed, able to sleep/rest appropriately.

ACTIONS/INTERVENTIONS	RATIONALE
Independent	
Document location, duration, intensity (0–10 scale), and radiation. Note nonverbal signs, e.g., elevated BP and pulse, restlessness, moaning, thrashing about.	Helps evaluate site of obstruction and progress of calculi movement. Flank pain often radiates to back, groin, genitalia due to proximity of nerve plexus and blood vessels supplying other areas. Sudden, severe pain may precipitate apprehension, restlessness, severe anxiety.
Explain cause of pain and importance of notifying staff of changes in pain occurrence/characteristics.	Provides opportunity for timely administration of analgesia (helpful in enhancing the patient's coping ability and may reduce anxiety) and alerts staff to possibility of passing of stone/developing complications. Sudden cessation of pain usually indicates stone passage.
Provide comfort measures, e.g., back rub, restful environment.	Promotes relaxation, reduces muscle tension, and enhances coping.
Assist with/encourage use of focused breathing, guided imagery, diversional activities.	Redirects attention and aids in muscle relaxation.
Encourage/assist with frequent ambulation as indicated and increased fluid intake of at least 3–4 L/d within cardiac tolerance.	Vigorous hydration promotes passing of stone, prevents urinary stasis, and aids in prevention of further stone formation.
Note reports of increased/persistent abdominal pain.	Complete obstruction of ureter can cause perforation and extravasation of urine into perirenal space. This represents an acute surgical emergency.

699

ACTIONS/INTERVENTIONS	RATIONALE

Collaborative

Administer medications as indicated:

Narcotics, e.g., meperidine (Demerol), morphine;	Usually given during acute episode to decrease ureteral colic and promote muscle/mental relaxation.
Antispasmodics, e.g., flavoxate (Urispas); oxybutynin (Ditropan);	Decreasing reflex spasm may decrease colic and pain.
Corticosteroids.	May be used to reduce tissue edema to facilitate movement of stone.
Apply warm compresses to back.	Relieves muscle tension and may reduce reflex spasms.
Maintain patency of catheters when used.	Prevents urinary stasis/retention, reduces risk of increased renal pressure and infection.

NURSING DIAGNOSIS:	**URINARY ELIMINATION: ALTERED**
May be related to:	Stimulation of the bladder by calculi, renal or ureteral irritation.
	Mechanical obstruction, inflammation.
Possibly evidenced by:	Urgency and frequency; oliguria (retention).
	Hematuria.
DESIRED OUTCOMES/ EVALUATION CRITERIA— PATIENT WILL:	Void in normal amounts and usual pattern.
	Experience no signs of obstruction.

ACTIONS/INTERVENTIONS	RATIONALE

Independent

Monitor I&O and characteristics of urine.	Provides information about kidney function and presence of complications, e.g., infection and hemorrhage. Bleeding may indicate increased obstruction or irritation of ureter. Note: Hemorrhage due to ureteral ulceration is rare.
Determine patient's normal voiding pattern and note variations.	Calculi may cause nerve excitability, which causes sensations of urgent need to void. Usually frequency and urgency increase as calculus nears ureterovesical junction.
Encourage increased fluid intake.	Increased hydration flushes bacteria, blood, and debris and may facilitate stone passage.
Strain all urine. Document any stones expelled and send to laboratory for analysis.	Retrieval of calculi allows for identification of type of stone and influences choice of therapy.
Investigate reports of bladder fullness; palpate for suprapubic distention. Note decreased urine output, presence of periorbital/dependent edema.	Urinary retention may develop, causing tissue distention (bladder/kidney) and potentiates risk of infection, renal failure.

ACTIONS/INTERVENTIONS	RATIONALE

Independent

Observe for changes in mental status, behavior, or level of consciousness.

Accumulation of uremic wastes and electrolyte imbalances can be toxic to the CNS.

Collaborative

Monitor laboratory studies, e.g., electrolytes, BUN, Cr.

Elevated BUN, Cr, and certain electrolytes indicate kidney dysfunction.

Obtain urine for culture and sensitivities.

Determines presence of UTI, which may be causing/complicating symptoms.

Administer medications as indicated, e.g.:

Acetazolamide (Diamox), allopurinol (Zyloprim);

Increases urine pH (alkalinity) to reduce formation of acid stones.

Hydrochlorothiazide (Esidrix, HydroDIURIL), chlorthalidone (Hygroton);

May be used to prevent urinary stasis and decrease calcium stone formation if not due to underlying disease process such as primary hyperthyroidism or vitamin D abnormalities.

Ammonium chloride; potassium or sodium phosphate (Sal-Hepatica);

Reduces phosphate stone formation.

Antigout agent, e.g., allopurinol (Zyloprim);

Lowers uric acid production/potential of stone formation.

Antibiotics.

Presence of UTI/alkaline urine potentiates stone formation.

Sodium bicarbonate;

Replace losses incurred during bicarbonate wasting and/or alkalinization of urine may reduce/prevent formation of some calculi.

Ascorbic acid;

Acidifies urine to prevent recurrence of alkaline stone formation.

Maintain patency of indwelling catheters (ureteral, urethral, or nephrostomy) when used.

May be required to facilitate urine flow/prevent retention and corresponding complications. Note: Tubes may be occluded by stone fragments.

Irrigate with acid or alkaline solutions as indicated.

Changing urine pH may help dissolve stones and prevent further stone formation.

Prepare patient for/assist with endoscopic procedures, e.g.:

Basket procedure;

Calculi in the distal and mid ureter may be removed by endoscopic cystoscope with capture of the stone in a basketing catheter.

Ureteral stents;

Catheters are positioned above the stone to promote urethral dilation/stone passage. Continuous or intermittent irrigation can be carried out to flush ureters and adjust pH of urine.

Percutaneous or open pyelolithotomy, nephrolithotomy, ureterolithotomy.

Surgery may be necessary to remove stone that is too large to pass through ureters.

Percutaneous ultrasonic lithotripsy.

Invasive shock wave treatment for stones in renal pelvis/calyx or upper ureters.

701

ACTIONS/INTERVENTIONS

Collaborative

Extracorporeal shock-wave lithotripsy (ESWL).

RATIONALE

Noninvasive procedure in which kidney stones are pulverized by shock waves delivered from outside the body.

NURSING DIAGNOSIS:	FLUID VOLUME DEFICIT, HIGH RISK FOR
Risk factors may include:	Nausea/vomiting (generalized abdominal and pelvic nerve irritation from renal or ureteral colic).
	Postobstructive diuresis.
Possibly evidenced by:	[Not applicable; presence of signs or symptoms establishes an actual diagnosis.]
DESIRED OUTCOMES/ EVALUATION CRITERIA— PATIENT WILL:	Maintain adequate fluid balance as evidenced by vital signs and weight within patient's normal range, palpable peripheral pulses, moist mucous membranes, good skin turgor.

ACTIONS/INTERVENTIONS

Independent

Monitor I&O.

Document incidence of vomiting, diarrhea. Note characteristics and frequency of vomiting and diarrhea, as well as accompanying or precipitating events.

Increase fluid intake to 3–4 L/d within cardiac tolerance.

Monitor vital signs. Evaluate pulses, capillary refill, skin turgor, and mucous membranes.

Weigh daily.

Collaborative

Monitor Hb/Hct, electrolytes.

RATIONALE

Comparing actual and anticipated output may aid in evaluating presence/degree of renal stasis/impairment. *Note:* Impaired kidney functioning and decreased urinary output can result in higher circulating volumes with signs/symptoms of CHF.

Nausea/vomiting and diarrhea are commonly associated with renal colic because celiac ganglion serves both kidneys and stomach. Documentation may help rule out other abdominal occurrences as a cause for pain or pinpoint calculi.

Maintains fluid balance for homeostasis as well as "washing" action that may flush the stone(s) out. Dehydration and electrolyte imbalance may occur secondary to excessive fluid loss (vomiting and diarrhea).

Indicators of hydration/circulating volume and need for intervention. *Note:* Decreased GFR stimulates production of renin, which acts to raise BP in an effort to increase renal blood flow.

Rapid weight gain may be related to water retention.

Assesses hydration and effectiveness of/need of interventions.

ACTIONS/INTERVENTIONS

Collaborative

Administer IV fluids.

Administer appropriate diet, clear liquids, bland foods as tolerated.

Administer medications as indicated: antiemetics, e.g., prochlorperazine (Compazine).

RATIONALE

Maintains circulating volume (if oral intake is insufficient) promoting renal function.

Easily digested foods decrease GI activity/irritation and helps maintain fluid and nutritional balance.

Reduces nausea/vomiting.

NURSING DIAGNOSIS:	KNOWLEDGE DEFICIT [LEARNING NEED] REGARDING CONDITION, PROGNOSIS, AND TREATMENT NEEDS
May be related to:	Lack of exposure/recall; information misinterpretation.
	Unfamiliarity with information resources.
Possibly evidenced by:	Questions; request for information; statement of misconception.
	Inaccurate follow-through of instructions, development of preventable complications.
DESIRED OUTCOMES/ EVALUATION CRITERIA— PATIENT WILL:	Verbalize understanding of disease process.
	Correlate symptoms with causative factors.
	Initiate necessary lifestyle changes and participate in treatment regimen.

ACTIONS/INTERVENTIONS

Independent

Review disease process and future expectations.

Stress importance of increased fluid intake, e.g., 3–4 L/d or as much as 6–8 L/d. Encourage patient to notice dry mouth, excessive diuresis/diaphoresis and to increase fluid intake whether or not feeling thirsty.

Review dietary regimen, as individually appropriate:

  Low-purine diet, e.g., limited lean meat, turkey, legumes, whole grains, alcohol;

  Low-calcium diet, e.g., limited milk, cheese, green leafy vegetables, yogurt;

  Low-oxalate diet, e.g., restrict chocolate, caffeine-containing beverages, beets, spinach.

RATIONALE

Provides knowledge base on which patient can make informed choices.

Flushes renal system decreasing opportunity for urinary stasis and stone formation. Increased fluid losses/dehydration require additional intake beyond usual daily needs.

Diet depends on the type of stone. Understanding reason for restrictions provides opportunity for patient to make informed choices, increase cooperation with regimen and may prevent recurrence.

Decreases oral intake of uric acid precursors.

Reduces risk of calcium stone formation.

Reduces calcium oxalate stone formation.

ACTIONS/INTERVENTIONS	RATIONALE

Independent

Shorr regimen: low-calcium/phosphorus diet with aluminum carbonate gel 30–40 ml, 30 minutes pc/hs.	Prevents phosphatic calculi by forming an insoluble precipitate in the GI tract, reducing the load to the kidney nephron. Also effective against other forms of calcium calculi. *Note:* May cause constipation.
Discuss medication regimen, avoidance of OTC drugs and reading of all product/food ingredient labels.	Drugs will be given to acidify or alkalize urine, dependent on underlying cause of stone formation. Ingestion of products containing individually contraindicated ingredients (e.g., calcium, phosphorus) potentiates recurrence of stones.
Encourage regular activity/exercise program.	Inactivity contributes to stone formation through calcium shifts and urinary stasis.
Active-listen concerns about therapeutic regimen/lifestyle changes.	Helps patient work through feelings and gain a sense of control over what is happening.
Identify signs/symptoms requiring medical evaluation, e.g., recurrent pain, hematuria, oliguria.	With increased probability of recurrence of stones, prompt interventions may prevent serious complications.
Demonstrate proper care of incisions/catheters if present.	Promotes competent self-care and independence.

Bibliography

General References

Bellak, JP and Bamford, PA: Nursing Assessment: A Multidimensional Approach. Jones & Bartlett, Boston, 1987.
Berkow, R (ed): The Merck Manual, ed 15. Merck Sharp & Dohme Research Laboratories, Rahway, NJ, 1987.
Cella, JH and Watson, J: Nurse's Manual of Laboratory Tests. FA Davis, Philadelphia, 1989.
Condon, RE and Nyhus, LM (eds): Manual of Surgical Therapeutics, ed 7. Little, Brown & Co, Boston, 1988.
Deglin, JH and Vallerand, AH: Davis's Drug Guide for Nurses, ed 3. FA Davis, Philadelphia, 1992.
Diseases and Disorders Handbook, ed 3. Springhouse Corp, Springhouse, PA, 1989.
Doenges, ME and Moorhouse, MF: Nurse's Pocket Guide: Nursing Diagnoses with Interventions, ed 3. FA Davis, Philadelphia, 1991.
Dunagan, WC and Ridner, ML (eds): Manual of Medical Therapeutics, ed 26. Little, Brown & Co, Boston, 1989.
Fischbach, F: A Manual of Laboratory and Diagnostic Tests, ed 4. JB Lippincott, Philadelphia, 1992.
Guyton, AC: Textbook of Medical Physiology, ed 8. WB Saunders, Philadelphia, 1991.
Kuhn, MM: Pharmacotherapeutics: A Nursing Process Approach, ed 2. FA Davis, Philadelphia,1991.
Professional Guide to Diseases, ed 3. Springhouse Corp, Springhouse, PA, 1989.
Suddarth, DS (ed): The Lippincott Manual of Nursing Practice, ed 5. JB Lippincott, Philadelphia, 1991.
Thomas, CL (ed): Taber's Cyclopedic Medical Dictionary, ed 17. FA Davis, Philadelphia, 1993.
Thompson, JM, et al: Mosby's Manual of Clinical Nursing, ed 2. CV Mosby, St Louis, 1989.

Books

Lancaster, LE (ed): Causes of Renal Failure: Core Curriculum for Nephrology Nursing, ed 2. ANNA, Putnam, NJ, 1990.

Articles

Baer, CL: Acute renal failure: Recognizing and reversing its deadly course. Nursing90 20(6):34, 1990.
Brennan, C: Lithotripter treatment of kidney stones in outpatient surgery. J Post Anesth Nurs 4(3):170, 1989.
Cotton, SJ and Holechek, MJ: Management of anemia using recombinant human erythropoietin in patients on chronic dialysis. ANNA J 16(7):463, 1989.
Chen, HY, Birkett, NJ, and Rakowski-Reinhardt, AD: A tool for assessing inadequate dialysis. ANNA J 16(2):75, 1989.
Faller, NA and Lawrence, KG: How to stabilize a percutaneous tube. Nursing92 22(7):52, 1992.

Gallagher, MT and Kahn, C: Lasers: Scalpels of light. RN 53(5):46, 1990.

Greig, BJ: A new option for cystectomy patients. RN 53(9):34, 1990.

Kadas, N: Reducing fluid overload without hemodialysis. RN 49(5):27, 1986.

Madda, MA: Helping ostomy patients manage medications. Nursing91 21(3):47, 1991.

Mackety, CJ: Lasers in urology. Nurs Clin N Am 25(3):697, 1990.

Molzahn, AE: Primary nursing and patient compliance in a hemodialysis unit. ANNA J 16(4):267, 1989.

Montgomery, BA: Consult stat—A better nephrostomy and biliary drainage setup. RN 52(3):96, 1989.

Moore, CG: Comparison of Blisterfilm and gauze for peritoneal catheter exit site care. ANNA J 16(7):475, 1989.

Motes, CE: Discontinuation of dialysis. ANNA J 16(6):413, 1989.

Piccard, VT, et al: Transfusion therapy: Associated risks and alternative approaches. ANNA J 17(6):457, 1990.

Robinson, J, et al: A care plan for self-administration of Epoetin Alfa. ANNA J 18(6):573, 1991.

Smith, BS and Winslow, EH: Cognitive changes in chronic renal patients during hemodialysis. ANNA J 17(4):283, 1990.

Snyder, TE: An exercise program for dialysis patient. AJN 89(3):362, 1989.

Van Niel, J: What's wrong with this peristomal skin. AJN 21(12):44, 1991.

Willis, D: Taming the overgrown prostate. AJN 22(2):34, 1992.

Wozniak-Petrofsky, J: BPH—Treating older men's most common problem. RN 54(7):32, 1991.

Zorzanello, MM: Preventing acute renal failure in patients with chronic renal insufficiency: Nursing implications. ANNA J 16(6):433, 1989.

CHAPTER **11**
ENDOCRINOLOGY

Addison's Disease (Adrenal Insufficiency/Crisis) _____

The primary form of this disease is caused by atrophy or destruction of the adrenal tissues (e.g., autoimmune response, TB, hemorrhagic infarction, malignancy) or surgical removal.

The secondary form results from pituitary dysfunction/suppression, causing decreased secretion/levels of ACTH; but usually normal secretion of aldosterone remains.

Adrenal insufficiency can occur when a patient abruptly stops taking steroid medications, or when trauma, surgery, or other physiologic stress exhausts body stores of glucocorticoids in a person with adrenal hypofunction. This quickly leads to adrenal crisis.

RELATED CONCERNS

Fluid and Electrolyte Imbalances, p 1054
Psychosocial Aspects of Acute Care, p 899

PATIENT ASSESSMENT DATA BASE

ACTIVITY/REST

May report:	Exhaustion, muscle aches/weakness (progressively worse throughout the day).
	Inability to be active/work.
May exhibit:	Increased heart/pulse rate with minimal activity.
	Decreased strength, ROM.
	Depression, difficulty concentrating, decreased/lack of initiative.
	Lethargy.

CIRCULATION

May exhibit:	Hypotension, including postural.
	Tachycardia, dysrhythmias, diminished heart sounds.
	Weak peripheral pulses.
	Capillary refill may be delayed.
	Extremities cool; cyanosis, pallor.
	Mucous membranes bluish-black or slate gray (increased pigmentation).

EGO INTEGRITY

May report: History of recent/multiple stress factors, including physical illness/surgery, change in lifestyle.
Inability to cope with stress.

May exhibit: Anxiety, irritability, depression, emotional instability.

ELIMINATION

May report: Diarrhea alternating with constipation.
Abdominal cramps.
Changes in frequency, character of urine.

May exhibit: Diuresis, followed by oliguria.

FOOD/FLUID

May report: Marked anorexia (cardinal symptom); nausea/vomiting.
Salt craving.
Marked weight loss.

May exhibit: Poor skin turgor, dry mucous membranes.

NEUROSENSORY

May report: Dizziness, syncope, trembling.
Headaches along with diaphoresis.
Muscle weakness.
Decreased tolerance to cold or stress.
Tingling/numbness/weakness.

May exhibit: Disorientation to time, place, and person (low sodium level), lethargy, mental fatigue, irritability, apprehension/anxiety, coma (crisis).
Paresthesias, paralysis; asthenia (crisis).
Sense of taste/smell exaggerated; acuity of hearing increased.

PAIN/COMFORT

May report: Muscle aches, abdominal cramping, headache.
Severe back, abdominal, extremity pain (crisis).

RESPIRATION

May report: Dyspnea.

May exhibit: Increased respiratory rate, tachypnea.
Breath sounds: crackles, rhonchi (infection).

SAFETY

May report: Intolerance of heat, hot weather.

May exhibit: Hyperpigmentation of skin (brown, tan, or bronze), diffuse or patchy.
Temperature elevation; fever followed by hypothermia (crisis).
Muscle wasting.
Gait disturbances.

SEXUALITY

May report: History of premature menopause; amenorrhea.

Loss of secondary sex characteristics, e.g., decreased body hair (especially in women).

Loss of libido.

TEACHING/LEARNING

May report: Family history of diabetes, TB, cancer.

History of thyroiditis, DM, TB, pernicious anemia.

Discharge Plan Considerations: **DRG projected mean length of stay: 4.3 days.**

May need assistance with medication regimen, self-care activities, home-maker/maintenance tasks.

DIAGNOSTIC STUDIES

Hormone levels:

Plasma cortisol: Decreased with no response to IM (primary) or IV (secondary) ACTH administration.

ACTH: Markedly increased (primary) or decreased (secondary).

ADH: Increased.

Aldosterone: Decreased.

Electrolytes: Serum levels may be normal or sodium somewhat reduced and potassium slightly elevated. However, profound sodium and potassium abnormalities can occur in response to absence of aldosterone and cortisol deficiency (may precipitate/result from crisis).

Glucose: Hypoglycemia.

BUN/Cr: May be elevated (decreased renal perfusion).

ABGs: Metabolic acidosis.

CBC: Normocytic, normochromic anemia (may be masked by decreased fluid volume) and Hct elevated (hemoconcentration). Lymphocyte count may be low, eosinophils elevated.

Urine (24-hour): 17-ketosteroids, 17-hydroxycorticoids, and 17-ketogenic steroids decreased. Free cortisol level decreased. Note: Failure to achieve a rise in urine steroid levels after test administration of ACTH indicates primary Addison's disease (permanent adrenal gland atrophy), while increased levels suggest a secondary cause of hormone suppression. Urine sodium increased.

X-ray: Small heart, adrenal calcifications, or TB (pulmonary, renal) may be noted.

NURSING PRIORITIES

1. Maintain fluid and electrolyte balance.
2. Improve nutritional status.
3. Prevent complications/crisis.
4. Support adjustment to condition.
5. Provide information about disease process/prognosis and lifelong therapy needs.

DISCHARGE GOALS

1. Homeostasis achieved.
2. Complications prevented/minimized.
3. ADLs managed by self/with assistance.
4. Dealing realistically with current situation.
5. Disease process/prognosis and therapeutic regimen understood.

NURSING DIAGNOSIS:	FLUID VOLUME DEFICIT, [REGULATORY FAILURE]
May be related to:	Excessive sodium and water losses via kidney, sweat glands, GI tract (aldosterone deficit).
Possibly evidenced by:	Nausea/vomiting; weakness, thirst; weight loss. Diarrhea; excessive urination, dilute urine. Postural hypotension; tachycardia; weak, thready pulses.
DESIRED OUTCOMES/ EVALUATION CRITERIA— PATIENT WILL:	Demonstrate improved fluid balance, as evidenced by individually adequate urinary output, stable vital signs, palpable peripheral pulses, good skin turgor and capillary refill, moist mucous membranes.

ACTIONS/INTERVENTIONS	RATIONALE
Independent	
Obtain history from patient/SO related to the duration and intensity of present symptoms, e.g., vomiting, excessive urination.	Assists in estimation of total volume depletion.
Monitor vital signs, noting postural BP changes, strength of peripheral pulses.	Postural hypotension is due in part to hypovolemia that results from aldosterone deficiency and from the reduced cardiac output that results from cortisol deficiency. Pulse may be weak, easily obliterated.
Measure I&O. Weigh patient daily.	Provides ongoing estimate of volume replacement needs and effectiveness of therapy. Initial weight gain usually results from sodium and water retention related to steroid replacement therapy.
Assess patient for thirst; weak, rapid, thready pulse; delayed capillary refill; poor skin turgor; and dry mucous membranes. Note skin color and temperature.	Indicates extent of hypovolemia and influences replacement needs.
Investigate changes in mentation/sensorium.	Severe dehydration impairs cardiac output and tissue perfusion, especially in the brain.
Auscultate bowel sounds. Note reports of nausea, presence of vomiting and diarrhea.	Impaired GI function can increase fluid/electrolyte losses and influence choice of routes for fluid and nutrient replacement.
Provide mouth care frequently.	Helps to reduce discomfort of dehydration and prevent mucous membrane breakdown.
Maintain comfortable environment. Cover patient with light blanket/sheet.	Avoids overheating, which could promote further fluid loss.
Promote bed rest, assist with position changes and self-care activities.	Minimizes orthostatic hypotension, reducing risk of loss of consciousness and injury.
Encourage oral fluids up to 3000 ml/d as soon as patient can tolerate them.	Relief of GI symptoms and return of bowel function permits oral replacement of fluids/electrolytes.

709

ACTIONS/INTERVENTIONS	RATIONALE

Independent

Reposition frequently. Massage bony prominences.	Severe dehydration can greatly compromise circulation, and skin breakdown can occur rapidly.
Observe for fatigue, crackles, edema, increased heart rate.	Rapid replacement of fluids may lead to CHF in presence of cardiac strain.

Collaborative

Administer fluids, e.g.:

0.9% saline;	Patient may require up to 4–6 L of fluid to replace losses. IV saline should be given rapidly in rates of up to 500–1000 ml/h for a few hours to replace the sodium deficit.
Glucose solutions.	Added to help relieve hypoglycemia.

Administer medications as indicated:

Cortisone (Cortone) or hydrocortisone (Cortef);	Drugs of choice to replace cortisol deficits and promote sodium resorption, which may reduce fluid losses and maintain cardiac output. *Note:* Patient may need salt restriction and potassium supplement if hypertension occurs, if long-term cortisone therapy is needed and/or patient is taking a potassium-wasting diuretic.
Mineralocorticoids, e.g., fludrocortisone (Florinef); deoxycorticosterone (Cortate, DOCA-A).	Begun after completion of high-dose hydrocortisone therapy, the dosage of these potent salt-retaining steroids are adjusted according to their effect on BP, serum electrolyte levels, and alleviation of symptoms. *Note:* Not required in secondary adrenal insufficiency, because mineralocorticoid secretion is intact.
Insert/maintain indwelling urinary catheter and NG tube as indicated.	Facilitates an accurate measurement of output, provides gastric decompression, limiting vomiting.

Monitor laboratory studies, e.g.:

Hct;	Elevated levels reflecting hemoconcentration should return to normal as rehydration occurs.
BUN/Cr;	Elevated values may reflect cellular breakdown from dehydration or signal the onset of renal failure.
Serum osmolality;	Elevation reflects to dehydration.
Sodium;	Hyponatremia reflects urinary loss due to impaired tubule reabsorption.
Potassium.	Decreased aldosterone levels allow sodium and water to be depleted while potassium is retained, resulting in hyperkalemia.

NURSING DIAGNOSIS:	NUTRITION, ALTERED: LESS THAN BODY REQUIREMENTS
May be related to:	Glucocorticoid deficiency; abnormal fat, protein, and carbohydrate metabolism. Nausea/vomiting, anorexia.
Possibly evidenced by:	Weight loss, muscle wasting, abdominal cramps, and diarrhea. Severe hypoglycemia.
DESIRED OUTCOMES/ EVALUATION CRITERIA— PATIENT WILL:	Report relief of nausea/vomiting. Demonstrate stable weight or weight gain toward desired goal with absence of presenting signs and normalization of laboratory values.

ACTIONS/INTERVENTIONS	RATIONALE
Independent	
Auscultate bowel sounds and assess for abdominal pain, nausea/vomiting.	Cortisol deficit can cause severe GI symptoms, affecting ingestion and absorption of nutrients.
Note presence of cool/clammy skin, changes in level of consciousness, rapid pulse, irritability, headache, shakiness.	Symptoms of hypoglycemia that signal the need for glucose and may indicate a need for more glucocorticoids.
Monitor dietary intake and weigh daily.	Profound anorexia, weakness, and loss of cortisol-regulating metabolism of nutrients can result in weight loss and serious malnutrition. *Note:* Rapid weight gain may reflect fluid retention/effects of glucocorticoid replacement.
Record incidence, amount/other characteristics of vomiting.	This helps to determine degree of digestion/absorption of nutrients.
Provide/assist with mouth care.	A clean mouth can stimulate appetite.
Provide an environment conducive to eating, i.e., unrushed atmosphere, absence of noxious odors, socialization.	May increase appetite, improve intake.
Obtain information about food preferences.	May stimulate appetite and facilitate intake when preferences are incorporated into meal plan.
Include SO in meal planning as indicated.	Understanding and involvement provides support and may enhance cooperation with diet.
Collaborative	
Maintain NPO status as indicated.	Promotes GI rest; reduces discomfort and fluid/electrolyte loss associated with vomiting.
Perform fingerstick glucose testing as indicated.	Serves as an ongoing assessment of serum glucose level/therapy needs. If decreased, dietary as

ACTIONS/INTERVENTIONS	RATIONALE
Collaborative	
	well as glucocorticoid adjustments may need to be made.
Administer IV glucose and medications as indicated:	Corrects hypoglycemia; provides energy source for cellular function.
Glucocorticoids;	Stimulates gluconeogenesis; decreases utilization of glucose and promotes glucose storage as glycogen. Regular administration of drug is necessary for appropriate carbohydrate, protein, and fat metabolism.
Androgens, e.g., testosterone.	May be useful in debilitated/malnourished patients to improve appetite, foster a positive nitrogen balance, improve muscle tone/strength, and enhance sense of well-being.
Consult with dietitian/nutritional support team.	Useful in determining individual nutritional/caloric needs and most appropriate route.
Provide liquids as tolerated; progress to small, frequent feedings of foods high in calories/protein when oral intake is resumed.	When n/v and pain subside, beverages and small portions of solid foods can replace IV fluids. Increased caloric intake may be needed to foster weight gain and prevent hypoglycemia.
Increase sodium in diet, e.g., meats, fish, poultry, milk, eggs.	May help to prevent/correct hyponatremia.
Monitor Hb/Hct.	Presence of anemia can be due to nutritional deficits or may be attributed to a dilutional factor, which may occur from fluid retention associated with glucocorticoid administration.

NURSING DIAGNOSIS:	FATIGUE
May be related to:	Decreased metabolic energy production.
	Altered body chemistry: fluid, electrolyte, and glucose imbalance.
Possibly evidenced by:	Unremitting/overwhelming lack of energy.
	Inability to maintain usual routines, decreased performance.
	Impaired ability to concentrate, lethargy, disinterest in surroundings.
DESIRED OUTCOMES/ EVALUATION CRITERIA— PATIENT WILL:	Report feeling rested, an increased energy level, and a decreased sense of fatigue.
	Verbalize factors that contribute to fatigue.
	Display improved ability to participate in desired activities.

ACTIONS/INTERVENTIONS

Independent

Discuss/review patient's fatigue level and identify activities that worsen fatigue.

Monitor vital signs before and after activity. Observe for tachycardia, hypotension, pallor.

Discuss the need for activity and plan the schedule with the patient. Identify activities that lead to fatigue.

Encourage patient to alternate periods of rest with activity.

Discuss ways of conserving energy (e.g., sitting, rather than standing during activities), assist with/provide self-care as necessary.

Provide adequate time for patient to participate in/complete self-care tasks. Increase patient's involvement as tolerated.

RATIONALE

Patient usually has decreased energy, muscle fatigue, which becomes progressively worse during the day due to disease process and sodium/potassium imbalance.

Circulatory collapse can occur as a result of activity stress if cardiac output is diminished.

Even though patient may initially feel too weak to engage in activity, gradual resumption of activity while receiving hormone replacement therapy improves muscle tone and strength, lessening fatigue. In addition, it provides hope that ability to perform desired activities will return.

Minimizes fatigue and prevents strain on the heart.

Patient will be able to accomplish more with a decreased expenditure of energy.

Increases confidence level and self-esteem as well as activity tolerance level.

NURSING DIAGNOSIS:	CARDIAC OUTPUT, DECREASED, HIGH RISK FOR
Risk factors may include:	Decreased venous return/circulating volume. Alterations in rate, rhythm, conduction (electrolyte imbalance). Inotropic changes in size/strength of cardiac muscle; abnormal metabolism with insufficient energy for cellular function (e.g., hypoglycemia).
Possibly evidenced by:	[Not applicable; presence of signs and symptoms establishes an actual diagnosis.]
DESIRED OUTCOMES/ EVALUATION CRITERIA— PATIENT WILL:	Demonstrate adequate cardiac output, as evidenced by vital signs within normal range, palpable peripheral pulses, brisk capillary refill, and usual mentation.

ACTIONS/INTERVENTIONS

Independent

Monitor vital signs; heart rate/rhythm, documenting dysrhythmias.

RATIONALE

Heart rate will elevate initially to compensate for hypovolemia and decreased cardiac output. Development of cardiac muscle failure/Addisonian crisis may cause sudden and profound hypotension. Irregular heart rate could result in decreased cardiac output or lead to MI. PVCs and depressed

ACTIONS/INTERVENTIONS	RATIONALE
Independent	
	T waves may be present if patient is hypokalemic, or peaked T waves will occur with hyperkalemia.
Measure CVP if available.	CVP provides a more direct measurement of fluid volume and developing complications, e.g., cardiac failure.
Monitor temperature, noting sudden changes.	Sudden hyperpyrexia can occur, followed by hypothermia, as a result of hormonal, fluid, and electrolyte imbalance, affecting heart rate and cardiac output.
Assess skin color, temperature, capillary refill, peripheral pulses.	Pallor, cool/clammy skin, delayed capillary refill, weak/thready pulses may indicate impending shock.
Investigate changes in mentation and reports of severe abdominal, back, or leg pain.	Mental changes (irritability, anxiety, apprehension) may be profound, reflecting decreased cardiac output/cerebral and peripheral perfusion and/or severe hypoglycemia.
Measure urinary output.	Although polyuria is usual, a decreasing urinary output suggests reduced kidney perfusion, reflecting decreased cardiac output.
Place in quiet/cool room, avoiding loud noises and excessive activity. Avoid stressful topics and actions. Maintain bed rest; assist with or perform all care activities.	Patient's normal response to stressors is lacking, and stimuli that usually would not be of concern can negatively affect the patient.
Monitor for hypertension, dependent edema, crackles, weight gain, severe headache, irritability/confusion.	Excessive administration of corticosteroids and/or overzealous sodium and fluid replacement may potentiate fluid excess and cardiac failure.
Collaborative	
Administer IV fluids, blood, saline solutions, and volume expanders as necessary. Avoid use of hypotonic or potassium-containing fluids.	Restoring circulating volume usually improves cardiac output. Because hyperkalemia is often present, exogenous potassium may cause severe dysrhythmias, cardiac arrest.
Administer medications as indicated:	
Hydrocortisone sodium succinate;	Rapid infusion of approximately 25–50 mg over 30–60 minutes, then 75–150 mg in next 4–8 hours may prevent cardiovascular collapse.
Vasopressors, e.g., dopamine (Intropin);	Increases peripheral vascular resistance and venous return to improve cardiac output and BP.
Antipyretics, e.g., acetaminophen.	Fever greater than 40.6°C (105°F) occasionally occurs, contributing to stress and continuing sodium/water losses.
Provide supplemental O_2.	Maximizes oxygenation; may help to reduce cardiac workload.
Monitor serum potassium.	Patient is prone to hyperkalemia because as sodium levels decrease (secondary to an aldosterone deficit), potassium is retained by the kidneys.

NURSING DIAGNOSIS:	THOUGHT PROCESSES, ALTERED, HIGH RISK FOR
Risk factors may include:	Decreased sodium levels, hypoglycemia, dehydration, acid/base imbalance.
Possibly evidenced by:	[Not applicable; presence of signs and symptoms establishes an actual diagnosis.]
DESIRED OUTCOMES/ EVALUATION CRITERIA— PATIENT WILL:	Maintain usual level of mentation. Experience no injury.

ACTIONS/INTERVENTIONS	RATIONALE
Independent	
Assign one nurse from each shift on a consistent basis if possible.	Provides best opportunity for early recognition of CNS changes and promotes a trusting relationship.
Monitor vital and neurologic signs.	Provides baseline for comparison/recognition of abnormal findings. *Note:* High temperature may affect mentation.
Address patient by name. Reorient to place, person, and time as needed. Give short explanations.	Helps to maintain orientation and decrease confusion.
Maintain consistent routine as possible. Schedule nursing time to provide for frequent rest periods.	Promotes orientation; prevents excessive fatigue.
Encourage patient to perform self-care to extent possible, with sufficient time to complete tasks.	Helps to keep the patient in touch with reality and maintain orientation to the environment.
Protect the patient from injury, e.g., place bed in low position with side rails raised; assist with ambulation, changes in position; use restraints judiciously; provide padded bed rails (seizure precautions).	Disorientation increases risk of injury, especially at night. Seizure precautions may be necessary to prevent physical injury, aspiration, and so forth.
Collaborative	
Monitor laboratory studies, e.g., blood glucose, serum osmolality, Hb/Hct.	As fluid, electrolyte, and acid/base imbalances are corrected, thought processes should improve. Continued changes in mentation require further evaluation.

NURSING DIAGNOSIS:	SELF-ESTEEM, SITUATIONAL LOW, HIGH RISK FOR
Risk factors may include:	Presence of physical condition requiring lifelong therapy. Changes in skin pigmentation, weight, secondary sex characteristics, and role functioning.
Possibly evidenced by:	[Not applicable; presence of signs and symptoms establishes an actual diagnosis.]

ACTIONS/INTERVENTIONS	RATIONALE
Independent	
Arrange short periods of uninterrupted time and encourage patient to express feelings about effects of condition, e.g., change in appearance or roles, effect of illness on job. Demonstrate a caring, nonjudgmental manner.	Fosters rapport and promotes openness on the part of the patient. Helps in evaluating how much of a problem the various changes are to the patient.
Reduce excess stimuli in environment; provide private room if indicated. Encourage use of stress-management skills, e.g., relaxation techniques, visualization, guided imagery.	Minimizes feelings of stress, frustration; enhances coping abilities and promotes sense of control.
Encourage patient to enlist the aid of SO in dealing with stress.	Patient will not feel as alone if he or she confides in others and asks for assistance in problem-solving. This also fosters understanding and a feeling of usefulness on the part of SO.
Encourage patient to make choices related to and participate in self-care.	May help to increase confidence level, improve self-esteem, decrease preoccupation with the changes, and enhance sense of control.
Point out improvements that are occurring with treatment, e.g., decreasing skin pigmentation, weight gain, increasing hair growth (if male hormones have been given), resumption of the normal menstrual cycle.	These comments may lift patient's spirits and promote self-esteem.
Suggest visit with person whose disease is controlled and whose symptoms have subsided.	May be encouraging to the patient to see the results of treatment.
Collaborative	
Refer to social services, counseling, support groups as needed.	A comprehensive approach may be needed for patient to maintain/regain coping behaviors.

NURSING DIAGNOSIS:	**KNOWLEDGE DEFICIT [LEARNING NEED], REGARDING CONDITION, PROGNOSIS, AND TREATMENT NEEDS**
May be related to:	Lack of exposure/recall; information misinterpretation. Cognitive limitation.
Possibly evidenced by:	Questions, request for information, verbalization of the problem. Inaccurate follow-through of instruction; development of preventable complications.

DESIRED OUTCOMES/ EVALUATION CRITERIA— PATIENT WILL:	Verbalize understanding of disease process and treatment.
	Identify relationship of signs/symptoms to disease process and correlate symptoms with causative factors.
	Identify stress situations and specific actions to deal with them.
	Initiate necessary lifestyle changes and participate in treatment regimen.

ACTIONS/INTERVENTIONS	RATIONALE

Independent

ACTIONS/INTERVENTIONS	RATIONALE
Review disease process and future expectations.	Provides knowledge base on which patient can make informed choices.
Encourage patient to remain as active as possible, to maintain a regular schedule for eating, sleeping, and exercise.	Helps to promote feelings of well-being and good health and to understand that irregular physical activity may increase hormonal needs.
Explain reason for excessive fluid loss. Recommend that patient monitor I&O and weight as applicable and to increase glucose, fluid, and salt intake during periods of stress, GI upset, excessive sweating (strenuous exercise, hot environment).	Knowledge may help prevent the problem in the future, and participation helps promote compliance with the therapy and provides opportunity for early recognition of changes.
Discuss dietary regimen, e.g., regular, nutritious diet with high carbohydrates and protein. Recommend inclusion of high carbohydrate snacks between meals.	Prevents weight loss and reduces risk of hypoglycemia.
Review hormone replacement therapy and necessity of adherence to drug schedule:	Helps patient to understand reasons for treatment (daily medication enables patient to live normal, active life), which can enhance cooperation.
Take medications at mealtime/with snacks or with antacids.	Reduces GI upset and risk of peptic ulcer formation.
Take two thirds of cortisol dose in the morning, one third in the late afternoon, or fludrocortisone in the morning.	Mimics the body's natural secretion of corticoids.
Avoid omitting a dose of the drug; take IM form of drug when ill (deep gluteal administration).	Failure to comply with replacement regimen places the patient at risk for crisis. *Note:* SC injection potentiates risk of sterile abscess and tissue atrophy.
Stress need to wear an identification bracelet and to carry emergency drugs, e.g., IM or IV dexamethasone sodium (Decajet, Decadron Phosphate).	Assists with prompt/appropriate intervention in case of emergency.
Define and problem solve ways to limit/control stressors, e.g., infection, dental work, trauma/accidents, personal or family crises, increased activity, prolonged exposure to hot temperatures.	The dosage of glucocortocoids may need to be adjusted (doubled or tripled) during periods of stress, and closer monitoring of general condition by health care provider may be needed.
Discuss feelings related to taking drugs for the rest of the patient's life.	Discussing these factors may help patient to incorporate necessary changes into lifestyle.

717

ACTIONS/INTERVENTIONS	RATIONALE
Independent	
Identify signs and symptoms requiring medical evaluation, e.g., nausea/vomiting, anorexia, weight loss, diarrhea, weakness, excess urination, irregular heartbeat; or weight gain and puffy face, neck, legs, or feet.	Prompt recognition of imbalance between hormone replacement and body needs (underdosing/overdosing) may prevent development of life-threatening situation.
Stress importance of avoiding exposure to infection (crowds, persons with infectious processes; maintaining good handwashing/personal practices) and prompt reporting of signs of infection.	Suppression of the inflammatory response increases risk of infection and possibility of progression to a life-threatening situation.
Discuss necessity of regular medical follow-up.	Facilitates control of chronic condition and prevention of complications.

Hyperthyroidism (Thyrotoxicosis, Graves' Disease) _____

Hyperthyroidism is a metabolic imbalance that results from overproduction of thyroid hormone. The most common form is Graves' disease, but other forms of hyperthyroidism include toxic adenoma, TSH-secreting pituitary tumor, subacute or silent thyroiditis, and some forms of thyroid cancer.

    Most people with classic hyperthyroidism rarely need hospitalization. Critically ill patients with hyperthyroidism are those with extreme manifestations of thyrotoxicosis plus a significant concurrent illness.

    Thyroid storm is a rarely encountered manifestation of hyperthyroidism, which can be precipitated by such events as thyroid ablation (surgical or radioiodine), medication overdosage, and trauma. This condition constitutes a medical emergency.

RELATED CONCERNS

Psychosocial Aspects of Acute Care, p 899
Thyroidectomy, p 731

PATIENT ASSESSMENT DATA BASE

Data are dependent on the severity/duration of hormone imbalance and involvement of other organs.

ACTIVITY/REST

May report:	Nervousness, increased irritability, insomnia.
	Muscle weakness, incoordination.
	Extreme fatigue.
May exhibit:	Muscle atrophy.

CIRCULATION

May report:	Palpitations.
	Chest pain (angina).
May exhibit:	Dysrhythmias (atrial fibrillation); gallop rhythm, murmurs.
	Elevated BP with widened pulse pressure.
	Tachycardia at rest.
	Circulatory collapse, shock (thyrotoxic crisis).

ELIMINATION

May report:	Urinating in large amounts.
	Stool changes; diarrhea.

EGO INTEGRITY

May report:	Recent stressful experience, e.g., emotional/physical.
May exhibit:	Emotional lability (mild euphoria to delirium); depression.

FOOD/FLUID

May report:	Recent/sudden weight loss.
	Increased appetite; large meals, frequent meals; thirst.
	Nausea/vomiting.
May exhibit:	Enlarged thyroid; goiter.
	Nonpitting fullness, especially in pretibial area.

NEUROSENSORY

May exhibit: Rapid and hoarse speech.

Mental status and behavior alterations, e.g., confusion, disorientation, nervousness, irritability, delirium, frank psychosis, stupor, coma.

Fine tremor in hands; purposeless, quick, jerky movements of body parts. Hyperactive DTRs.

PAIN/COMFORT

May report: Orbital pain, photophobia (eye involvement).

RESPIRATION

May exhibit: Increased respiratory rate, tachypnea.

Dyspnea.

Pulmonary edema (thyrotoxic crisis).

SAFETY

May report: Heat intolerance, excessive sweating.

Allergy to iodine (may be used in testing).

May exhibit: Elevated temperature (above 100°F), diaphoresis.

Skin smooth, warm, and flushed; hair fine, silky, straight.

Exophthalmia; lid retraction; conjunctival irritation, tearing.

Pruritic, erythematous lesions (often in pretibial area) that become brawny.

SEXUALITY

May report: Decreased libido.

Hypomenorrhea, amenorrhea.

Impotence.

TEACHING/LEARNING

May report: Family history of thyroid problems.

History of hypothyroidism, thyroid hormone replacement therapy or antithyroid therapy, premature withdrawal of antithyroid drugs, recent partial thyroidectomy.

History of insulin-induced hypoglycemia, cardiac disorders or surgery, recent illness (pneumonia), trauma; x-ray contrast studies.

Discharge Plan Considerations: **DRG projected mean length of stay: 4.3 days.**

May require assistance with treatment regimen, self-care activities, homemaker/maintenance tasks.

DIAGNOSTIC STUDIES

RAI uptake test: High in Graves' disease and toxic nodular goiter; low in thyroiditis.

Serum T_4 and T_3: Increased.

Serum free T_4 and T_3: Increased.

TSH: Suppressed and does not respond to thyroid releasing hormone (TRH).

Thyroglobulin: Increased.

TRH stimulation: Hyperthyroidism is indicated if TSH fails to rise after administration of TRH.

Thyroid ^{131}I uptake: Increased.

Protein-bound iodine: Increased.

Blood sugar: Elevated (related to adrenal involvement).

Plasma cortisol: Low levels (less adrenal reserve).

Alkaline phosphatase and serum calcium: Increased.

Liver function tests: Abnormal.

Electrolytes: Hyponatremia may reflect adrenal response or dilutional effect in fluid replacement therapy. Hypokalemia occurs owing to GI losses and diuresis.

Serum catecholamines: Decreased.

Urine creatinine: Increased.

ECG: Atrial fibrillations; shorter systole time; cardiomegaly, heart enlarged with fibrosis and necrosis (late signs or in elderly with masked hyperthyroidism).

NURSING PRIORITIES

1. Reduce metabolic demands and support cardiovascular function.
2. Provide psychologic support.
3. Prevent complications.
4. Provide information about disease process/prognosis and therapy needs.

DISCHARGE GOALS

1. Homeostasis achieved.
2. Patient dealing with current situation.
3. Complications prevented/minimized.
4. Disease process/prognosis and therapeutic regimen understood.

NURSING DIAGNOSIS:	CARDIAC OUTPUT, DECREASED, HIGH RISK FOR
Risk factors may include:	Uncontrolled hyperthyroidism, hypermetabolic state. Increasing cardiac workload. Changes in venous return and systemic vascular resistance. Alterations in rate, rhythm, conduction.
Possibly evidenced by:	[Not applicable; presence of signs and symptoms establishes an actual diagnosis.]
DESIRED OUTCOMES/ EVALUATION CRITERIA— PATIENT WILL:	Maintain adequate cardiac output for tissue needs as evidenced by stable vital signs, palpable peripheral pulses, good capillary refill, usual mentation, and absence of dysrhythmias.

ACTIONS/INTERVENTIONS	RATIONALE
Independent	
Monitor BP lying/sitting and standing, if able. Note widened pulse pressure.	General/orthostatic hypotension may occur as a result of excessive peripheral vasodilation and decreased circulating volume. Widened pulse pres-

ACTIONS/INTERVENTIONS	RATIONALE
Independent	
	sure reflects compensatory increase in stroke volume and decreased systemic vascular resistance.
Monitor CVP if available.	Provides more direct measure of circulating volume and cardiac function.
Investigate reports of chest pain/angina.	May reflect increased myocardial oxygen demands/ischemia.
Assess pulse/heart rate while patient is sleeping.	Provides a more accurate assessment of tachycardia.
Auscultate heart sounds, noting extra heart sounds, development of gallops and systolic murmurs.	Prominent S_1 and murmurs are associated with forceful cardiac output of hypermetabolic state; development of S_3 may warn of impending cardiac failure.
Monitor ECG, noting rate/rhythm. Document dysrhythmias.	Tachycardia (greater than normally expected with fever/increased circulatory demand) may reflect direct myocardial stimulation by thyroid hormone. Dysrhythmias often occur and may compromise cardiac function/output.
Auscultate breath sounds, noting adventitious sounds (e.g., crackles).	Early sign of pulmonary congestion, reflecting developing cardiac failure.
Monitor temperature; provide cool environment; limit bed linens/clothes; administer tepid sponge baths.	Fever (may exceed 104°F) may occur as a result of excessive hormone levels and can aggravate diuresis/dehydration and cause increased peripheral vasodilation, venous pooling, and hypotension.
Observe signs/symptoms of severe thirst, dry mucous membranes, weak/thready pulse, poor capillary refill, decreased urinary output, and hypotension.	Rapid dehydration can occur, which reduces circulating volume and compromises cardiac output.
Record I&O. Note urine specific gravity.	Significant fluid losses (through vomiting, diarrhea, diuresis, diaphoresis) can lead to profound dehydration, concentrated urine, and weight loss.
Weigh daily. Encourage chair/bed rest; limit nonessential activity.	Activity increases metabolic/circulatory demands, which may potentiate cardiac failure.
Note history of asthma/bronchoconstrictive disease, pregnancy, sinus bradycardia/heart blocks, advanced heart failure.	Presence of these conditions affect choice of therapy; e.g., use of β-adrenergic blocking agents is contraindicated.
Observe for adverse side effects of adrenergic antagonists, e.g., severe decrease in pulse, BP; signs of vascular congestion/CHF; cardiac arrest.	Indicates need for reduction/discontinuation of therapy.
Collaborative	
Administer IV fluids as indicated.	Rapid fluid replacement may be necessary to improve circulating volume but must be balanced against signs of cardiac failure/need for inotropic support.
Administer medications as indicated:	
β-blockers, e.g., propranolol (Inderal); atenolol (Tenormin); nadolol (Corgard);	Given to control thyrotoxic effects of tachycardia, tremors, and nervousness and is first drug of

ACTIONS/INTERVENTIONS	RATIONALE
Collaborative	
	choice for acute storm. Decreases heart rate/cardiac work by blocking β-adrenergic receptor sites and blocking conversion of T_4 to T_3. *Note:* If severe bradycardia develops, atropine may be required.
Thyroid hormone antagonists, e.g., propylthiouracil (PTU); methimazole (Tapazole);	Blocks thyroid hormone synthesis and inhibits peripheral conversion of T_4 to T_3. May be definitive treatment or used to prepare patient for surgery; but effect is slow and so may not relieve thyroid storm. *Note:* Once PTU therapy is begun, abrupt withdrawal may precipitate thyroid crisis.
Sodium iodine (Lugol's solution) or supersaturated potassium iodide (SSKI) po.	Temporarily acts to prevent release of thyroid hormone into circulation by increasing the amount of thyroid hormone stored within the gland. May interfere with RAI treatment and may exacerbate the disease in some people. May be used as surgical preparation to decrease size and vascularity of the gland or to treat thyroid storm. *Note:* Should be started 1–3 hours after initiation of antithyroid drug therapy to minimize hormone formation from the iodine.
RAI (^{131}INal or ^{125}INal);	Destroys functioning gland tissue. Peak results take 6–12 weeks (several treatments may be necessary).
Corticosteroids, e.g., dexamethazone (Decadron);	Provides glucocorticol support. Decreases hyperthermia; relieves relative adrenal insufficiency; inhibits calcium absorption; and reduces peripheral conversion of T_3 from T_4.
Digoxin (Lanoxin);	Digitalization may be required in CHF patients before β-adrenergic blocking therapy can be considered/safely initiated.
Furosemide (Lasix);	Diuresis may be necessary if CHF occurs. *Note:* It also may be effective in reducing calcium level if neuromuscular function is impaired.
Acetaminophen (Tylenol);	Drug of choice to reduce temperature and associated metabolic demands. Aspirin is contraindicated because it actually increases level of circulating thyroid hormones by blocking binding of T_3 and T_4 with thyroid-binding proteins.
Sedative, barbiturates;	Promotes rest, thereby reducing metabolic demands/cardiac workload.
Muscle relaxants.	Reduces shivering associated with hyperthermia, which can further increase metabolic demands.
Monitor laboratory studies, as indicated, e.g.:	
Serum potassium (replace as indicated);	Hypokalemia resulting from intestinal losses, altered intake, or diuretic therapy may cause dysrhythmias and compromise cardiac function/output.

723

ACTIONS/INTERVENTIONS	RATIONALE
Collaborative	
Serum calcium;	Elevation may alter cardiac contractility.
Sputum culture.	Pulmonary infection is most frequent precipitating factor of crisis.
Review serial ECGs;	May demonstrate effects of electrolyte imbalance or ischemic changes reflecting inadequate myocardial oxygen supply in presence of increased metabolic demands.
Chest x-rays.	Cardiac enlargement may occur in response to increased circulatory demands. Pulmonary congestion may be noted with cardiac decompensation.
Provide supplemental O_2 as indicated.	May be necessary to support increased metabolic demands/O_2 consumption.
Provide hypothermia blanket as indicated.	Occasionally used to lower uncontrolled hyperthermia (104°F and greater) to reduce metabolic demands/O_2 consumption, and cardiac workload.
Administer/assist with transfusions/plasmapheresis, hemoperfusion, dialysis.	May be done to achieve rapid depletion of extrathyroidal hormone pool in desperately ill/comatose patient.
Prepare for surgery.	Subtotal thyroidectomy (removal of five sixths of the gland) may be treatment of choice for hyperthyroidism once euthyroid state is achieved.

NURSING DIAGNOSIS:	FATIGUE
May be related to:	Hypermetabolic state with increased energy requirements.
	Irritability of CNS; altered body chemistry.
Possibly evidenced by:	Verbalization of overwhelming lack of energy to maintain usual routine, decreased performance.
	Emotional lability/irritability; nervousness, tension.
	Jittery behavior.
	Impaired ability to concentrate.
DESIRED OUTCOMES/ EVALUATION CRITERIA— PATIENT WILL:	Verbalize increase in level of energy.
	Display improved ability to participate in desired activities.

ACTIONS/INTERVENTIONS	RATIONALE
Independent	
Monitor vital signs, noting pulse rate at rest as well as when active.	Pulse is typically elevated and even at rest, tachycardia (up to 160) may be noted.

ACTIONS/INTERVENTIONS

Independent

Note development of tachypnea, dyspnea, pallor, and cyanosis.

Provide for quiet environment; cool room, decreased sensory stimuli, soothing colors, quiet music.

Encourage patient to restrict activity and rest in bed as much as possible.

Provide comfort measures, e.g., judicious touch/massage, cool showers.

Provide for diversional activities that are calming, e.g., reading, radio, television.

Avoid topics that irritate or upset the patient. Discuss ways to respond to these feelings.

Discuss with SO reasons for fatigue and emotional lability.

Collaborative

Administer medications as indicated:

Sedatives, e.g., phenobarbital (Luminal); tranquilizers, e.g., chlordiazepoxide (Librium).

RATIONALE

O_2 demand and consumption is increased in hypermetabolic state, potentiating risk of hypoxia with activity.

Reduces stimuli that may aggravate agitation, hyperactivity, and insomnia.

Helps counteract effects of increased metabolism.

May decrease nervous energy, promoting relaxation.

Allows for use of nervous energy in a constructive manner and may reduce anxiety.

Increased irritability of the CNS may cause patient to be easily excited, agitated, and prone to emotional outbursts.

Understanding that the behavior is physically based may enhance coping with current situation and encourage SO to respond positively and provide support for the patient.

Combats nervousness, hyperactivity, and insomnia.

NURSING DIAGNOSIS:	NUTRITION, ALTERED: LESS THAN BODY REQUIREMENTS, HIGH RISK FOR
Risk factors may include:	Increased metabolism (increased appetite/intake with loss of weight).
	Nausea/vomiting, diarrhea.
	Relative insulin insufficiency; hyperglycemia.
Possibly evidenced by:	[Not applicable; presence of signs and symptoms establishes an actual diagnosis.]
DESIRED OUTCOMES/ EVALUATION CRITERIA— PATIENT WILL:	Demonstrate stable weight with normal laboratory values and be free of signs of malnutrition.

ACTIONS/INTERVENTIONS

Independent

Auscultate bowel sounds.

RATIONALE

Hyperactive bowel sounds reflect increased gastric motility, which can reduce/alter absorption.

ACTIONS/INTERVENTIONS

Independent

Note reports of anorexia, generalized weakness/aches, abdominal pain; presence of nausea/vomiting.

Monitor daily food intake. Weigh daily and report losses.

Encourage patient to eat and increase number of meals and snacks, using high-calorie foods that are easily digested.

Avoid foods that increase peristalsis (e.g., tea, coffee, fibrous and highly seasoned foods) and fluids that cause diarrhea (e.g., apple/prune).

Collaborative

Consult with dietitian to provide diet high in calories, protein, carbohydrates, and vitamins.

Administer medications as indicated:

Glucose, vitamin B complex.

Insulin (small doses).

RATIONALE

Increased adrenergic activity can cause impaired insulin secretion/resistance, resulting in hyperglycemia, polydipsia, polyuria; changes in respiratory rate/depth.

Continued weight loss in face of adequate caloric intake may indicate failure of antithyroid therapy.

Aids in keeping caloric intake high enough to keep up with rapid expenditure of calories caused by hypermetabolic state.

Increased motility of GI tract may result in diarrhea and impair absorption of needed nutrients.

May need assistance to assure adequate intake of nutrients, identify appropriate supplements.

Given to meet energy requirements and prevent or correct hypoglycemia.

Aids in controlling serum glucose if elevated.

NURSING DIAGNOSIS:	TISSUE INTEGRITY, IMPAIRED, HIGH RISK FOR
Risk factors may include:	Alterations of protective mechanisms of eye: Impaired closure of eyelid/exophthalmos.
Possibly evidenced by:	[Not applicable; presence of signs and symptoms establishes an actual diagnosis.]
DESIRED OUTCOMES/ EVALUATION CRITERIA— PATIENT WILL:	Maintain moist eye membranes, free of ulcerations. Identify measures to provide protection for eyes and prevent complications.

ACTIONS/INTERVENTIONS

Independent

Observe for periorbital edema, lid lag, wide-eyed stare, excessive tearing; Note reports of photophobia, feeling of foreign object in eye; eye pain.

Evaluate visual acuity; note reports of blurred or double vision.

RATIONALE

Common manifestations of excessive adrenergic stimulation related to thyrotoxicosis, requiring supportive interventions until therapeutic resolution of crisis state relieves symptomatology.

Infiltrative ophthalmopathy (Graves' disease) is the result of increased retro-orbital tissue, creating exophthalmos and lymphocytic infiltration of extraocular muscles, which causes weakness.

ACTIONS/INTERVENTIONS	RATIONALE
Independent	
	Corresponding visual impairment may worsen or improve independent of therapy and clinical course of disease.
Encourage use of dark glasses when awake and taping the eyelids shut during sleep as needed.	Protects exposed cornea if patient is unable to close eyelids completely due to edema/fibrosis of fat pads.
Elevate the head of the bed and restrict salt intake if indicated.	Decreases tissue edema when appropriate, e.g., CHF, which can aggravate existing exophthalmos.
Instruct the patient in extraocular muscle exercises if appropriate.	Improves circulation and maintains mobility of the eyelids.
Provide opportunity for patient to discuss feelings about altered appearance and measures to enhance self-image.	Protruding eyes may be viewed as unattractive. Appearance can be enhanced with proper use of makeup, overall grooming, and use of shaded glasses.
Collaborative	
Administer medications as indicated:	
Methylcellulose drops;	Lubricates the eyes.
ACTH, prednisone;	Given to decrease rapidly progressive and marked inflammation.
Antithyroid drugs;	May decrease signs/symptoms or prevent worsening of the condition.
Diuretics.	Can decrease edema in mild involvement.
Prepare for surgery as indicated.	Eyelids may need to be sutured shut temporarily to protect the corneas until edema resolves (rare); or increasing space within sinus cavity and adjusting musculature may return eye to a more normal position.

NURSING DIAGNOSIS:	**ANXIETY [SPECIFY LEVEL]**
May be related to:	Physiologic factors: Hypermetabolic state (CNS stimulation), pseudocatecholamine effect of thyroid hormones.
Possibly evidenced by:	Increased feelings of apprehension, shakiness, loss of control, panic.
	Changes in cognition, distortion of environmental stimuli.
	Extraneous movements, restlessness, tremors.
DESIRED OUTCOMES/ EVALUATION CRITERIA— PATIENT WILL:	Appear relaxed.
	Report anxiety reduced to a manageable level.
	Identify healthy ways to deal with feelings.

ACTIONS/INTERVENTIONS	RATIONALE
Independent	
Observe behavior indicative of level of anxiety.	Mild anxiety may be displayed by irritability and insomnia. Severe anxiety progressing to panic state may produce feelings of impending doom, terror, inability to speak or move, shouting/swearing.
Monitor physical responses, noting palpitations, repetitive movements, hyperventilation, insomnia.	Increased number of β-adrenergic receptor sites, coupled with effects of excess thyroid hormones, produces clinical manifestations of catecholamine excess even when normal levels of nor-epinephrine/epinephrine exist.
Stay with patient, maintaining calm manner. Acknowledge fear and allow patient's behavior to belong to the patient.	Affirms to patient/SO that although patient feels out of control, environment is safe. Avoiding personal responses to inappropriate remarks or actions prevents conflicts/overreaction to stressful situation.
Describe/explain procedures, surrounding environment or sounds that may be heard by the patient.	Provides accurate information, which reduces distortions/misinterpretations, that can contribute to anxiety/fear reactions.
Speak in brief statements, using simple words.	Attention span may be shortened, concentration reduced, limiting ability to assimilate information.
Reduce external stimuli: Place in quiet room; provide soft, soothing music; reduce bright lights; reduce number of persons contacting patient.	Creates a therapeutic environment; shows recognition that unit activity/personnel may increase patient's anxiety.
Discuss with patient/SO reasons for emotional lability/psychotic reaction. (Refer to ND: Thought Processes, Altered high risk for, this page.)	Understanding that behavior is physically based, can allow for different responses/approaches, acceptance of situation.
Reinforce expectation that emotional control should return as drug therapy progresses.	Provides information and reassures patient that the situation is temporary and will improve with treatment.
Collaborative	
Administer antianxiety medications (tranquilizers, sedatives) and monitor effects.	May be used in conjunction with medical regimen to reduce effects of hyperthyroid secretion.
Refer to support systems as needed, e.g., counseling, social services, pastoral care.	Ongoing therapy support may be desired/required by patient/SO if crisis precipitates lifestyle alterations.

NURSING DIAGNOSIS:	THOUGHT PROCESSES, ALTERED, HIGH RISK FOR
Risk factors may include:	Physiologic changes: Increased CNS stimulation/accelerated mental activity.
	Altered sleep patterns.
Possibly evidenced by:	[Not applicable; presence of signs and symptoms establishes an actual diagnosis.]

DESIRED OUTCOMES/ EVALUATION CRITERIA— PATIENT WILL:	Maintain usual reality orientation. Recognize changes in thinking/behavior and causative factors.

ACTIONS/INTERVENTIONS	RATIONALE

Independent

Assess thinking processes, e.g., memory, attention span, orientation to person/place/time.	Determines extent of interference with sensory processing.
Note changes in behavior.	May be hypervigilant, restless, extremely sensitive, or crying or may develop frank psychosis.
Assess level of anxiety. (Refer to ND: Anxiety, p 727.	Anxiety may alter thought processes.
Provide quiet environment; decreased stimuli, cool room, dim lights. Limit procedures/personnel.	Reduction of external stimuli may decrease hyperactivity/reflexia, CNS irritability, auditory/visual hallucinations.
Reorient to person/place/time.	Helps to establish and maintain awareness of reality/environment.
Present reality concisely and briefly without challenging illogical thinking.	Limits defensive reaction.
Provide clock, calendar, room with outside window; alter level of lighting to simulate day/night	Promotes continual orientation cues to assist patient in maintaining sense of normality.
Provide safety measures, e.g., padded side rails, soft restraints, close supervision.	Prevents injury to patient who may be hallucinating/disoriented.
Encourage visits by family/SO. Provide support as needed.	Aids in maintaining socialization and orientation. *Note:* Patient's agitation/psychotic behavior may precipitate family quarrels/conflicts.

Collaborative

Administer medications as indicated, e.g., sedatives/tranquilizers/antipsychotic drugs.	Promotes relaxation, reduces CNS hyperactivity/agitation to inhance thought processes.

NURSING DIAGNOSIS:	KNOWLEDGE DEFICIT [LEARNING NEED], REGARDING CONDITION, PROGNOSIS, AND TREATMENT NEEDS
May be related to:	Lack of exposure/recall. Information misinterpretation. Unfamiliarity with information resources.
Possibly evidenced by:	Questions; request for information; statement of misconception. Inaccurate follow-through of instructions/development of preventable complications.

ACTIONS/INTERVENTIONS	RATIONALE
Independent	
Review disease process and future expectations.	Provides knowledge base on which patient can make informed choices.
Provide information appropriate to individual situation.	Severity of condition, cause, age, and concurrent complications determines course of treatment.
Identify stressors, and discuss precipitators of thyroid crises, e.g., personal/social and job concerns, infection, pregnancy.	Psychogenic factors are often of prime importance in the occurrence/exacerbation of this disease.
Provide information about signs/symptoms of hypothyroidism and the need for continuing follow-up care.	The patient who has been treated for hyperthyroidism needs to be aware of possible development of hypothyroidism, which can occur immediately after treatment or as long as 5 years later.
Discuss drug therapy, including need for adhering to regimen, and expected therapeutic and side effects.	Antithyroid medication (either as primary therapy or in preparation for thyroidectomy), requires adherence to a medical regimen over an extended period to inhibit hormone production. Agranulocytosis is the most serious side effect that can occur, and alternative drugs may be given when problems arise.
Identify signs/symptoms requiring medical evaluation, e.g., fever, sore throat, and skin eruptions.	Early identification of toxic reactions (thiourea therapy) and intervention are important in preventing development of agranulocytosis.
Explain need to check with physician/pharmacist before taking other prescribed or OTC drugs.	Antithyroid medications can affect or be affected by numerous other medications, requiring monitoring of medication levels, side effects, and interactions.
Emphasize importance of planned rest periods.	Prevents undue fatigue; reduces metabolic demands. As euthyroid state is achieved, stamina and activity level will increase.
Review need for nutritious diet and periodic review of nutrient needs; avoid caffeine, red/yellow food dyes, artificial preservatives.	Provides adequate nutrients to support hypermetabolic state. As hormonal imbalance is corrected, diet will need to be readjusted to prevent excessive weight gain. Irritants and stimulants should be limited to avoid cumulative systemic effects.
Stress necessity of continued medical follow-up.	Necessary for monitoring effectiveness of therapy and prevention of potentially fatal complications.

Thyroidectomy _____

Thyroidectomy, while rare, may be performed for patients with thyroid cancer, hyperthyroidism and drug reactions to antithyroid agents, pregnant women who can't be managed with drugs, patients who do not want radiation therapy, and those with large goiters who do not respond to antithyroid drugs. The two types of thyroidectomy include:

Total thyroidectomy: The gland is removed completely. Usually done in the case of malignancy. Thyroid replacement therapy is necessary for life.

Subtotal thyroidectomy: Up to five sixths of the gland is removed when antithyroid drugs do not correct hyperthyroidism or RAI therapy is contraindicated.

RELATED CONCERNS

Cancer, p 1014
Hyperthyroidism, p 719
Psychosocial Aspects of Acute Care, p 899
Surgical Intervention, p 918

PATIENT ASSESSMENT DATA BASE

Refer to CP: Hyperthyroidism, p 719 for assessment information.

Discharge Plan Considerations: **DRG projected mean length of stay: 3.0 days.**

NURSING PRIORITIES

1. Reverse hyperthyroid state preoperatively.
2. Prevent complications.
3. Relieve pain.
4. Provide information about surgical procedure, prognosis, and treatment needs.

DISCHARGE GOALS

1. Complications prevented/minimized.
2. Pain alleviated.
3. Surgical procedure/prognosis and therapeutic regimen understood.

NURSING DIAGNOSIS:	AIRWAY CLEARANCE, INEFFECTIVE, HIGH RISK FOR
Risk factors may include:	Tracheal obstruction; swelling, bleeding, laryngeal spasms.
Possibly evidenced by:	[Not applicable; presence of signs and symptoms establishes an actual diagnosis.]
DESIRED OUTCOMES/ EVALUATION CRITERIA— PATIENT WILL:	Maintain patent airway, with aspiration prevented.

731

ACTIONS/INTERVENTIONS	RATIONALE
Independent	
Monitor respiratory rate, depth and work of breathing.	Respirations may remain somewhat rapid, but development of respiratory distress is indicative of tracheal compression from edema or hemorrhage.
Auscultate breath sounds, noting presence of rhonchi.	Rhonchi may indicate airway obstruction/accumulation of copious thick secretions.
Assess for dyspnea, stridor, "crowing," and cyanosis. Note quality of voice.	Indicators of tracheal obstruction/laryngeal spasm, requiring prompt evaluation and intervention.
Caution patient to avoid bending neck; support head with pillows.	Reduces likelihood of tension on surgical wound.
Assist with repositioning, deep-breathing exercises and/or coughing as indicated.	Maintains clear airway and ventilation. Although coughing is not encouraged and may be painful, it may be needed to clear secretions.
Suction mouth and trachea as indicated, noting color and characteristics of sputum.	Edema/pain may impair patient's ability to clear own airway.
Check dressing frequently, especially posterior portion.	If bleeding occurs, anterior dressing may appear dry as blood pools dependently.
Investigate reports of difficulty swallowing, drooling of oral secretions.	May indicate edema/sequestered bleeding in tissues surrounding operative site.
Keep tracheostomy tray at bedside.	Compromised airway may create a life-threatening situation requiring emergency procedure.
Collaborative	
Provide steam inhalation; humidify room air.	Reduces discomfort of sore throat and tissue edema and promotes expectoration of secretions.
Assist with/prepare for procedures, e.g.;	
Tracheostomy;	May be necessary to maintain airway if obstructed by edema of glottis or hemorrhage.
Return to surgery.	May require ligation of bleeding vessels.

NURSING DIAGNOSIS:	COMMUNICATION, IMPAIRED: VERBAL
May be related to:	Vocal cord injury/laryngeal nerve damage.
	Tissue edema; pain.
	Discomfort.
Possibly evidenced by:	Impaired articulation, does not/cannot speak; use of nonverbal cues such as gestures.
DESIRED OUTCOMES/ EVALUATION CRITERIA— PATIENT WILL:	Establish method of communication in which needs can be understood.

ACTIONS/INTERVENTIONS

Independent

Assess speech periodically; encourage voice rest.

Keep communication simple; ask yes/no questions.

Provide alternate methods of communication as appropriate, e.g., slate board, letter/picture board. Place IV line to minimize interference with written communication.

Anticipate needs as possible. Visit patient frequently.

Post notice of patient's voice limitations at central station and answer call bell promptly.

Maintain quiet environment.

RATIONALE

Hoarseness and sore throat may occur secondary to tissue edema or surgical damage to recurrent laryngeal nerve and may last several days. Permanent nerve damage can occur (rare) that causes paralysis of vocal cords and/or compression of the trachea.

Reduces demand for response; promotes voice rest.

Facilitates expression of needs.

Reduces anxiety and patient's need to communicate.

Prevents patient straining voice to make needs known/summon assistance.

Enhances ability to hear whispered communication and reduces necessity for patient to raise/strain voice to be heard.

NURSING DIAGNOSIS:	INJURY, HIGH RISK FOR [TETANY]
Risk factors may include:	Chemical imbalance: Excessive CNS stimulation.
Possibly evidenced by:	[Not applicable; presence of signs and symptoms establishes an actual diagnosis.]
DESIRED OUTCOMES/ EVALUATION CRITERIA— PATIENT WILL:	Demonstrate absence of injury with complications minimized/controlled.

ACTIONS/INTERVENTIONS

Independent

Monitor vital signs noting elevating temperature, tachycardia (140–200/min), dysrhythmias, respiratory distress, cyanosis (developing pulmonary edema/CHF).

Evaluate reflexes periodically. Observe for neuromuscular irritability, e.g., twitching, numbness, paresthesias, positive Chvostek's and Trousseau's signs, seizure activity.

Keep side rails raised/padded, bed in low position and airway at bedside. Avoid use of restraints.

RATIONALE

Manipulation of gland during subtotal thyroidectomy may result in increased hormone release, causing thyroid storm.

Hypocalcemia with tetany (usually transient) may occur 1–7 days postoperatively and indicates hypoparathyroidism, which can occur as a result of inadvertent trauma to/partial-to-total removal of parathyroid gland(s) during surgery.

Reduces potential for injury if seizures occur.

ACTIONS/INTERVENTIONS	RATIONALE

Collaborative

Monitor serum calcium levels.	Patients with levels less than 7.5 mg/100 ml generally require replacement therapy.
Administer medications as indicated:	
Calcium (gluconate, lactate);	Corrects deficiency, which is usually temporary but may be permanent. *Note:* Use with caution in digitalized patient as calcium increases cardiac sensitivity to digitalis, potentiating risk of toxicity.
Phosphate-binding agents;	Helpful in lowering elevated phosphorus levels associated with hypocalcemia.
Sedatives;	Promotes rest, reducing exogenous stimulation.
Anticonvulsants.	Controls seizures until corrective therapy is successful.

NURSING DIAGNOSIS:	**PAIN, [ACUTE]**
May be related to:	Surgical interruption/manipulation of tissues/muscles.
	Postoperative edema.
Possibly evidenced by:	Reports of pain.
	Narrowed focus; guarding behavior; restlessness.
	Autonomic responses.
DESIRED OUTCOMES/ EVALUATION CRITERIA— PATIENT WILL:	Report pain is relieved/controlled.
	Demonstrate use of relaxation skills and diversional activities appropriate to situation.

ACTIONS/INTERVENTIONS	RATIONALE

Independent

Assess verbal/nonverbal reports of pain, noting location, intensity (0–10 scale), and duration.	Useful in evaluating pain, choice of interventions, effectiveness of therapy.
Place in semi-Fowler's position and support head/neck with sandbags or small pillows.	Prevents hyperextension of the neck and protects integrity of the suture line.
Maintain head/neck in neutral position and support during position changes. Instruct patient to use hands to support neck during movement and to avoid hyperextension of neck.	Prevents stress on the suture line and reduces muscle tension.
Keep call bell and frequently needed items within easy reach.	Limits stretching, muscle strain in operative area.
Give cool liquids po or soft foods, such as ice cream or popsicles.	Soothing to sore throat but soft foods may be tolerated better if patient experiences difficulty swallowing.

ACTIONS/INTERVENTIONS

Independent

Encourage patient to use relaxation techniques, e.g., guided imagery, soft music, progressive relaxation.

Collaborative

Administer analgesics and/or analgesic throat sprays/lozenges as necessary.

Provide ice collar if indicated.

RATIONALE

Helps to refocus attention and assists patient to manage pain/discomfort more effectively.

Reduces pain and discomfort; enhances rest.

Reduces tissue edema and decreases perception of pain.

NURSING DIAGNOSIS:	KNOWLEDGE DEFICIT [LEARNING NEED], REGARDING CONDITION, PROGNOSIS, AND TREATMENT NEEDS
May be related to:	Lack of exposure/recall, misinterpretation.
	Unfamiliarity with information resources.
Possibly evidenced by:	Questions; request for information; statement of misconception.
	Inaccurate follow-through of instructions/development of preventable complications.
DESIRED OUTCOMES/ EVALUATION CRITERIA— PATIENT WILL:	Verbalize understanding of surgical procedure and treatment.
	Participate in treatment regimen.
	Initiate necessary lifestyle changes.

ACTIONS/INTERVENTIONS

Independent

Review surgical procedure and future expectations.

Discuss need for well-balanced, nutritious diet and when appropriate, inclusion of iodized salt.

Recommend avoidance of goitrogenic foods, e.g., excessive ingestion of seafood, soybeans, turnips.

Identify foods high in calcium (e.g., dairy products) and vitamin D (e.g., fortified dairy products, egg yolks, liver).

Encourage progressive general exercise program.

RATIONALE

Provides knowledge base on which patient can make informed decisions.

Promotes healing and helps patient to regain/maintain appropriate weight. Use of iodized salt is often sufficient to meet iodine needs unless salt is restricted for other health care problems, e.g., CHF.

Contraindicated after partial thyroidectomy because these foods inhibit thyroid activity.

Maximizes supply and absorption of calcium if parathyroid function is impaired.

In patients with subtotal thyroidectomy, exercise can stimulate the thyroid gland and production of hormones, facilitating recovery of general well-being.

ACTIONS/INTERVENTIONS	RATIONALE
Independent	
Review postoperative exercises to be instituted after incision heals, e.g., flexion, extension, rotation, and lateral movement of head and neck.	Regular ROM exercises strengthen neck muscles, enhance circulation and healing process.
Review importance of rest and relaxation, avoiding stressful situations and emotional outbursts.	Effects of hyperthyroidism usually subside completely, but it takes some time for the body to recover.
Instruct in incisional care, e.g., cleansing, dressing application.	Enables patient to provide competent self-care.
Give information about the use of loose-fitting scarves to cover scar. Avoid the use of jewelry.	Covers the incision without aggravating healing or precipitating infections of suture line.
Apply cold cream after sutures have been removed.	Softens tissues and may help to minimize scarring.
Discuss possibility of change in voice.	Alteration in vocal cord function may cause changes in pitch and quality of voice, which may be temporary or permanent.
Review drug therapy and the necessity of continuing even when feeling well.	If thyroid replacement is needed because of surgical removal of gland, patient needs to understand rationale for replacement therapy and consequences of failure to routinely take medication.
Identify signs/symptoms requiring medical evaluation, e.g., fever, chills, continued/purulent wound drainage, erythema, gaps in wound edges; sudden weight loss, intolerance to heat, n/v, diarrhea, insomnia, weight gain, fatigue, intolerance to cold, constipation, drowsiness.	Early recognition of developing complications such as infection, hyperthyroidism, or hypothyroidism may prevent progression to life-threatening situation. *Note:* As many as 43% of patients with subtotal thyroidectomy will have hypothyroidism in time.
Stress necessity of continued medical follow-up.	Provides opportunity for evaluating effectiveness of therapy and prevention of complications.

Diabetes Mellitus/Diabetic Ketoacidosis _____

DKA is a life-threatening emergency caused by a relative or absolute deficiency of insulin. DKA occurs in patients with IDDM (also called type I diabetes). Conditions or situations known to accelerate lack of insulin include: (1) undiagnosed type I diabetes; (2) imbalance between food and insulin; (3) adolescence and puberty; (4) exercise in uncontrolled diabetes; and (5) stress associated with illness, infection, trauma, or emotional distress.

RELATED CONCERNS

Fluid and Electrolyte Imbalances, p 1054
Psychosocial Aspects of Acute Care, p 899

PATIENT ASSESSMENT DATA BASE

Data are dependent on the severity and duration of metabolic imbalance and effects on organ function.

ACTIVITY/REST

May report: Weakness, exhaustion, difficulty walking/moving.
Muscle cramps, decreased muscle tone. Sleep/rest disturbances.

May exhibit: Tachycardia and tachypnea at rest or with activity.
Lethargy/disorientation, coma.
Decreased muscle strength.

CIRCULATION

May report: History of hypertension; acute MI.
Claudication, numbness, tingling of extremities.
Leg ulcers, slow healing.

May exhibit: Tachycardia.
Postural BP changes; hypertension.
Decreased/absent pulses.
Dysrhythmias.
Crackles; JVD (CHF).
Hot, dry, flushed skin; sunken eyeballs.

EGO INTEGRITY

May report: Stress; dependence on others.
Financial concerns related to condition.

May exhibit: Anxiety, irritability.

ELIMINATION

May report: Change in usual voiding pattern (polyuria), nocturia.
Pain/burning, difficulty voiding (infection), recent/recurrent UTI.
Abdominal tenderness.
Diarrhea.

May exhibit: Pale, yellow, dilute urine; polyuria (may progress to oliguria/anuria if severe hypovolemia occurs).

Cloudy, odorous urine (infection).

Firm abdomen, bloating.

Bowel sounds diminished; hyperactive (diarrhea).

FOOD/FLUID

May report:	Loss of appetite.
	Nausea/vomiting.
	Not following diet; increased intake of glucose/carbohydrates.
	Weight loss over a period of days/weeks.
	Thirst.
	Use of diuretics (thiazides).
May exhibit:	Dry/cracked skin, poor skin turgor.
	Abdominal rigidity/distention, vomiting.
	Enlarged thyroid (increased metabolic needs with increased blood sugar).
	Halitosis/sweet, fruity odor (acetone breath).

NEUROSENSORY

May report:	Fainting spells/dizziness.
	Headaches.
	Tingling, numbness, weakness in muscles, paresthesias.
	Visual disturbances.
May exhibit:	Disorientation; drowsiness, lethargy, stupor/coma (later stages).
	Memory impairment (recent, remote); confusion.
	DTRs decreased (coma).
	Seizure activity (late stages of DKA).

PAIN/COMFORT

May report:	Abdominal bloating/pain (mild/severe).
May exhibit:	Facial grimacing with palpation; guarding.

RESPIRATION

May report:	Air hunger.
	Cough, with/without purulent sputum (infection).
May exhibit:	Increased respiratory rate, tachypnea; deep, rapid (Kussmaul's) respirations (metabolic acidosis).
	Rhonchi, wheezes.
	Yellow or green sputum (infection).

SAFETY

May report:	Dry, itching skin; skin ulcerations.
May exhibit:	Fever, diaphoresis.
	Skin breakdown, lesions/ulcerations.
	Decreased general strength/ROM.
	Paresthesia/paralysis of muscles including respiratory musculature (if potassium levels are markedly decreased).

SEXUALITY

May report: Vaginal discharge (prone to infection).

Problems with impotence; female orgasmic difficulty.

TEACHING/LEARNING

May report: Familial risk factors; DM, heart disease, strokes, hypertension.

Slow/delayed healing.

Use of drugs, e.g., steroids, thiazide diuretics; Dilantin and phenobarbital (can increase glucose levels).

May/may not be taking diabetic medications as ordered.

Discharge Plan Considerations: **DRG projected mean length of stay: 5.9 days.**

May need assistance with dietary regimen, medication administration/supplies, self-care, glucose monitoring.

DIAGNOSTIC STUDIES

Serum glucose: Increased 200–1000 mg/dL, or more.

Plasma acetone (ketones): Strongly positive.

Free fatty acids: Lipids and cholesterol level elevated.

Serum osmolality: Elevated but usually less than 330 mOsm/L.

Electrolytes:

  Sodium: May be normal, elevated, or decreased.

  Potassium: Normal or falsely elevated (cellular shifts), then decreased.

  Phosphorus: Frequently decreased.

Glycosylated hemoglobin: Levels 2 to 4 times normal reflect poor control of DM during past 4 months (life span of RBCs) and is therefore useful in differentiating inadequate control versus incident-related DKA (e.g., current URI).

ABGs: Usually reflects low pH and decreased HCO_3 (metabolic acidosis) with compensatory respiratory alkalosis.

CBC: Hct may be elevated (dehydration); leukocytosis suggests hemoconcentration, response to stress, or infection.

BUN: May be normal or elevated (dehydration/decreased renal perfusion).

Serum amylase: May be elevated indicating acute pancreatitis as cause of DKA.

Serum insulin: May be decreased/absent (type I) or normal to high (type II), indicating insulin insufficiency/improper utilization (endogenous/exogenous). Insulin resistance may develop secondary to formation of antibodies.

Thyroid function tests: Increased thyroid activity can increase blood glucose and insulin needs.

Urine: Positive for sugar and acetone; specific gravity and osmolality may be elevated.

Cultures and sensitivities: Possible UTI, respiratory, or wound infections.

NURSING PRIORITIES

1. Restore fluid/electrolyte, and acid/base balance.
2. Correct/reverse metabolic abnormalities.
3. Identify/assist with management of underlying cause/disease.
4. Prevent complications.
5. Provide information about disease process/prognosis, self-care, and treatment needs.

DISCHARGE GOALS

1. Homeostasis achieved.
2. Causative/precipitating factors corrected/controlled.
3. Complications prevented/minimized.
4. Disease process/prognosis, self-care needs, and therapeutic regimen understood.

NURSING DIAGNOSIS:	FLUID VOLUME DEFICIT, [REGULATORY FAILURE]
May be related to:	Osmotic diuresis (from hyperglycemia).
	Excessive gastric losses: Diarrhea, vomiting.
	Restricted intake: Nausea, confusion.
Possibly evidenced by:	Increased urinary output, dilute urine.
	Weakness; thirst; sudden weight loss.
	Dry skin/mucous membranes, poor skin turgor.
	Hypotension, tachycardia, delayed capillary refill.
DESIRED OUTCOMES/ EVALUATION CRITERIA— PATIENT WILL:	*Demonstrate adequate hydration as evidenced by stable vital signs, palpable peripheral pulses, good skin turgor and capillary refill, individually appropriate urinary output, and electrolyte levels within normal range.*

ACTIONS/INTERVENTIONS	RATIONALE
Independent	
Obtain history from patient/SO related to duration/ intensity of symptoms such as vomiting, excessive urination.	Assists in estimation of total volume depletion. Symptoms may have been present for varying amounts of time (hours–days). Presence of infectious process results in fever and hypermetabolic state, increasing insensible fluid losses.
Monitor vital signs; note orthostatic BP changes;	Hypovolemia may be manifested by hypotension and tachycardia. Estimates of severity of hypovolemia may be made when patient's systolic BP drops more than 10 mm Hg from a recumbent to a sitting/standing position. *Note:* Cardiac neuropathy may block reflexes that normally increase heart rate.
Respiratory pattern, e.g., Kussmaul's respirations; acetone breath;	Lungs remove carbonic acid through respirations, producing a compensatory respiratory alkalosis for ketoacidosis. Acetone breath is due to breakdown of acetoacetic acid and should diminish as ketosis is corrected.
Respiratory rate and quality; use of accessory muscles, periods of apnea, and appearance of cyanosis;	Correction of hyperglycemia and acidosis will cause the respiratory rate and pattern to approach normal. However, increased work of breathing; shallow, rapid respirations; and presence of cyanosis may indicate respiratory fatigue and/or

ACTIONS/INTERVENTIONS

Independent

Temperature, skin color/moisture.

Assess peripheral pulses, capillary refill, skin turgor, and mucous membranes.

Monitor I&O; note urine specific gravity.

Weigh daily.

Maintain fluid intake of at least 2500 ml/d within cardiac tolerance when oral intake is resumed.

Promote comfortable environment. Cover patient with light sheets.

Investigate changes in mentation/sensorium.

Note reports of nausea, abdominal pain; presence of vomiting and gastric distention.

Observe for increased fatigue, crackles, edema, increased weight, bounding pulse, vascular distention.

Collaborative

Administer fluids as indicated:

Normal or half-normal saline with/without dextrose;

Albumin, plasma, dextran.

Insert/maintain urinary catheter.

Monitor laboratory studies, e.g.:

Hct;

RATIONALE

that patient is losing ability to compensate for acidosis.

Although fever, chills, and diaphoresis are common with infectious process, fever with flushed, dry skin may reflect dehydration.

Indicators of level of hydration, adequacy of circulating volume.

Provides ongoing estimate of volume replacement needs, kidney function, and effectiveness of therapy.

Provides the best assessment of current fluid status and adequacy of fluid replacement.

Maintains hydration/circulating volume.

Avoids overheating of patient, which could promote further fluid loss.

Changes in mentation can be due to abnormally high or low glucose, electrolyte abnormalities, acidosis, decreased cerebral perfusion, or developing hypoxia. Regardless of the cause, impaired consciousness can predispose the patient to aspiration.

Fluid and electrolyte deficits alter gastric motility, frequently resulting in vomiting and potentiating the fluid/electrolyte losses.

Rapid fluid replacement may potentiate overload and CHF.

Type and amount of fluid are dependent on degree of deficit and individual patient response.

Plasma expanders may occasionally be needed if the deficit is life-threatening/BP does not normalize with rehydration efforts.

Provides for accurate/ongoing measurement of urinary output, especially if autonomic neuropathies result in neurogenic bladder (urinary retention/overflow incontinence). May be removed when patient is stable to reduce risk of infection.

Assesses level of hydration and is often elevated because of hemoconcentration that occurs after osmotic diuresis.

741

ACTIONS/INTERVENTIONS	RATIONALE
Collaborative	
BUN/Cr;	Elevated values may reflect cellular breakdown from dehydration or signal the onset of renal failure.
Serum osmolality;	Elevated due to hyperglycemia and dehydration.
Sodium;	May be decreased reflecting shift of fluids from the intracellular compartment (osmotic diuresis). High sodium values reflect severe fluid loss/dehydration, or sodium reabsorption in response to aldosterone secretion.
Potassium.	Initially, intravascular hyperkalemia occurs in response to acidosis, but as this potassium is lost in the urine, the absolute potassium level in the body is depleted. As insulin is replaced and acidosis is corrected, serum potassium deficit becomes apparent.
Administer potassium and other electrolytes via IV and/or by oral route as indicated.	Potassium should be added to the IV (as soon as urinary flow is adequate) to prevent hypokalemia. *Note:* Potassium phosphate may be given if IV fluids contain sodium chloride in order to prevent chloride overload.
Administer bicarbonate if pH is less than 7.0.	Given with caution to help correct acidosis in the presence of hypotension or shock.
Insert NG tube and attach to suction as indicated.	Decompresses stomach and may relieve vomiting.

NURSING DIAGNOSIS:	**NUTRITION, ALTERED: LESS THAN BODY REQUIREMENTS**
May be related to:	Insulin deficiency (decreased uptake and utilization of glucose by the tissues resulting in increased protein/fat metabolism).
	Decreased oral intake; anorexia, nausea, gastric fullness, abdominal pain; altered consciousness.
	Hypermetabolic state: Release of stress hormones (e.g., epinephrine, cortisol, and growth hormone), infectious process.
Possibly evidenced by:	Reported inadequate food intake, lack of interest in food.
	Recent weight loss; weakness, fatigue, poor muscle tone.
	Diarrhea.
	Increased ketones (end products of fat metabolism).
DESIRED OUTCOMES/ EVALUATION CRITERIA— PATIENT WILL:	Ingest appropriate amounts of calories/nutrients.
	Display usual energy level.
	Demonstrate stabilized weight or gain toward usual/desired range with normal laboratory values.

ACTIONS/INTERVENTIONS	RATIONALE

Independent

Weigh daily or as indicated.

Assesses adequacy of nutritional intake (absorption and utilization).

Ascertain patient's dietary program and usual pattern; compare with recent intake.

Identifies deficits and deviations from therapeutic needs.

Auscultate bowel sounds. Note reports of abdominal pain/bloating, nausea, vomiting of undigested food. Maintain NPO status as indicated.

Hyperglycemia and fluid and electrolyte disturbances can decrease gastric motility/function (distention or ileus) affecting choice of interventions. *Note:* Long-term difficulties with decreased gastric emptying and poor intestinal motility suggest autonomic neuropathies affecting the GI tract and requiring symptomatic treatment.

Provide liquids containing nutrients and electrolytes as soon as patient can tolerate oral fluids; progress to more solid food as tolerated.

Oral route is preferred when patient is alert and bowel function is restored.

Identify food preferences, including ethnic/cultural needs.

If patient's food preferences can be incorporated into the meal plan, cooperation may be facilitated after discharge.

Include SO in meal planning as indicated.

Promotes sense of involvement; provides information for SO to understand nutritional needs of the patient. *Note:* Various methods available for dietary planning include exchange list, point system, glycemic index, or preselected menus.

Observe for signs of hypoglycemia, e.g., changes in level of consciousness, cool/clammy skin, rapid pulse, hunger, irritability, anxiety, headache, lightheadedness, shakiness.

Once carbohydrate metabolism begins (blood glucose level reduced), and as insulin is being given, hypoglycemia can occur. If patient is comatose, hypoglycemia may occur without notable change in level of consciousness. This potentially life-threatening emergency should be assessed and treated quickly per protocol. *Note:* Type I diabetics of long-standing may not display usual signs of hypoglycemia because normal response to low blood sugar may be diminished.

Collaborative

Perform fingerstick glucose testing.

Bedside analysis of serum glucose is more accurate (displays current levels) than monitoring urine sugar, which is not sensitive enough to detect fluctuations in serum levels and can be affected by patient's individual renal threshold or the presence of urinary retention/renal failure. *Note:* Some studies have found that a urine glucose of 20% may be correlated to a blood glucose of 140–360 mg/dl.

Monitor laboratory studies, e.g., serum glucose, acetone, pH, HCO_3.

Blood sugar will decrease slowly with controlled fluid replacement and insulin therapy. With the administration of optimal insulin dosages, glucose can then enter the cells and be used for energy. When this happens, acetone levels decrease and acidosis is corrected.

Administer regular insulin by intermittent or continuous IV method, e.g., IV bolus followed by a con-

Regular insulin has a rapid onset and thus will quickly help move glucose into cells. The IV route

743

ACTIONS/INTERVENTIONS	RATIONALE

Collaborative

tinuous drip via pump of approximately 5–10 U/h until glucose reaches 250 mg/dL.	is the initial route of choice, because absorption from subcutaneous tissues may be erratic. Many believe the continuous method is the optimal way to facilitate transition to carbohydrate metabolism and reduce incidence of hypoglycemia.
Administer glucose solutions, e.g., dextrose and half normal saline.	Glucose solutions are added after insulin and fluids have brought the blood glucose to approximately 250/dL. As carbohydrate metabolism approaches normal, care must be taken to avoid hypoglycemia.
Consult with dietitian.	Useful in calculating and adjusting diet to meet patient's needs; answers questions and can assist patient/SO in developing meal plans.
Provide diet of approximately 60% carbohydrates, 20% proteins, 20% fats in designated number of meals/snacks.	Complex carbohydrates (e.g., corn, peas, carrots, broccoli, dried beans, oats, apples) decrease glucose levels/insulin needs, reduce serum cholesterol levels, and promote satiation. Food intake will be scheduled according to specific insulin characteristics (e.g., peak effect) and individual patient response. *Note:* HS snack of complex carbohydrates is especially important (if insulin is given in divided doses) to prevent hypoglycemia during sleep and potential Somogyi response.
Administer metoclopramide (Reglan); tetracycline.	May be useful in treating symptoms related to autonomic neuropathies affecting GI tract, thus enhancing oral intake and absorption of nutrients.

NURSING DIAGNOSIS:	**INFECTION, HIGH RISK FOR [SEPSIS]**
Risk factors may include:	High glucose levels, decreased leukocyte function, alterations in circulation.
	Preexisting respiratory infection, or UTI.
Possibly evidenced by:	[Not applicable; presence of signs and symptoms establishes an actual diagnosis.]
DESIRED OUTCOMES/ EVALUATION CRITERIA— PATIENT WILL:	Identify interventions to prevent/reduce risk of infection.
	Demonstrate techniques, lifestyle changes to prevent development of infection.

ACTIONS/INTERVENTIONS	RATIONALE

Independent

Observe for signs of infection and inflammation, e.g., fever, flushed appearance, wound drainage, purulent sputum, cloudy urine.	Patient may be admitted with infection, which could have precipitated the ketoacidotic state, or may develop a nosocomial infection.

ACTIONS/INTERVENTIONS	RATIONALE
Independent	
Promote good hand washing by staff and patient.	Reduces risk of cross-contamination.
Maintain aseptic technique for IV insertion procedure, administration of medications, and providing maintenance care. Rotate IV sites as indicated.	High glucose in the blood creates an excellent medium for bacterial growth.
Provide catheter/perineal care. Teach the female patient to clean from front to back after elimination.	Minimizes risk of UTI. Comatose patient may be at particular risk if urinary retention occurred prior to hospitalization. *Note:* Elderly female diabetic patients are especially prone to urinary tract/vaginal infections such as yeast.
Provide conscientious skin care; massage bony areas. Keep the skin dry, linens dry and wrinkle-free.	Peripheral circulation may be impaired, which places the patient at increased risk for skin irritation/breakdown and infection.
Auscultate breath sounds.	Rhonchi indicates accumulation of secretions possibly related to pneumonia/bronchitis (may have precipitated the DKA). Pulmonary congestion/edema (crackles) may result from rapid fluid replacement/CHF.
Place in semi-Fowler's position.	Facilitates lung expansion; reduces risk of aspiration.
Reposition and encourage coughing/deep breathing if patient is alert and cooperative. Otherwise, suction airway, using sterile technique, as needed.	Aids in ventilating all lung areas and mobilization of secretions. Prevents stasis of secretions with increased risk of infection.
Provide tissues and trash bag in a convenient location for sputum and other secretions.	Minimizes spread of infection.
Assist with oral hygiene.	Reduces risk of oral/gum disease.
Encourage adequate dietary and fluid intake (approximately 3000 ml/d if not contraindicated).	Decreases susceptibility to infection. Increased urinary flow prevents stasis, and aids in maintaining urine pH/acidity, reducing bacteria growth and flushing organisms out of system.
Collaborative	
Obtain specimens for culture and sensitivities as indicated.	Identifies organism(s) so most appropriate drug therapy can be instituted.
Administer antibiotics as appropriate.	Early treatment may help prevent sepsis.

NURSING DIAGNOSIS:	SENSORY-PERCEPTUAL ALTERATION: (SPECIFY), HIGH RISK FOR
Risk factors may include:	Endogenous chemical alteration: Glucose/insulin and/or electrolyte imbalance.
Possibly evidenced by:	[Not applicable; presence of signs and symptoms establishes an actual diagnosis.]

ACTIONS/INTERVENTIONS	RATIONALE

Independent

Monitor vital signs and mental status.	Baseline from which to compare abnormal findings; e.g., high temperature may affect mentation.
Address patient by name, reorient as needed, to place, person, and time. Give short explanations, speaking slowly and enunciating clearly.	Decreases confusion and helps to maintain contact with reality.
Schedule nursing time to provide for uninterrupted rest periods.	Promotes restful sleep, reduces fatigue, and may improve cognition.
Keep patient's routine as consistent as possible. Encourage participation in ADLs as able.	Helps keep the patient in touch with reality and maintain orientation to the environment.
Protect patient from injury (use of restraints) when level of consciousness is impaired. Pad bed rails and provide soft airway if patient is prone to seizures.	Disoriented patient is prone to injury, especially at night, and precautions need to be taken as indicated. Seizure precautions need to be taken to prevent physical injury, aspiration, and so forth.
Evaluate visual acuity as indicated.	Retinal edema/detachment, hemorrhage, presence of cataracts or temporary paralysis of extraocular muscles may impair vision requiring corrective therapy and/or supportive care.
Investigate reports of hyperesthesia, pain, or sensory loss in the feet/legs. Look for ulcers, reddened areas, pressure points, loss of pedal pulses.	Peripheral neuropathies may result in severe discomfort, lack of/distortion of tactile sensation potentiating risk of dermal injury and impaired balance. *Note:* Mononeuropathy affects a single nerve (most often femoral or cranial), causing sudden pain and loss of motor/sensory function along affected nerve path.
Provide bed cradle. Keep hands/feet warm, avoiding exposure to cool drafts/hot water or use of heating pad.	Reduces discomfort and potential for dermal injury. *Note:* Sudden development of cold hands/feet may reflect hypoglycemia, suggesting need to evaluate serum glucose level.
Assist with ambulation/position changes.	Promotes patient safety, especially when sense of balance is affected.

Collaborative

Carry out prescribed regimen for correcting DKA as indicated.	Alteration in thought processes/potential for seizure activity is usually alleviated once hyperosmolar state is corrected.
Monitor laboratory values, e.g., blood glucose, serum osmolality, Hb/Hct, BUN/Cr.	Imbalances can impair mentation. *Note:* If fluid is replaced too quickly, excess water may enter brain cells and cause alteration in the level of consciousness (water intoxication).
Assist with local nerve block, maintenance of TENS unit.	May provide relief of discomfort associated with neuropathies.

NURSING DIAGNOSIS:	FATIGUE
May be related to:	Decreased metabolic energy production.
	Altered body chemistry: Insufficient insulin.
	Increased energy demands: Hypermetabolic state/infection.
Possibly evidenced by:	Overwhelming lack of energy, inability to maintain usual routines, decreased performance, accident-prone.
	Impaired ability to concentrate, listlessness, disinterest in surroundings.
DESIRED OUTCOMES/ EVALUATION CRITERIA— PATIENT WILL:	Verbalize increase in level of energy.
	Display improved ability to participate in desired activities.

ACTIONS/INTERVENTIONS	RATIONALE
Independent	
Discuss with patient the need for activity. Plan schedule with patient and identify activities that lead to fatigue.	Education may provide motivation to increase activity level even though patient may feel too weak initially.
Alternate activity with periods of rest/uninterrupted sleep.	Prevents excessive fatigue.
Monitor pulse, respiratory rate, and BP before/after activity.	Indicates physiologic levels of tolerance.
Discuss ways of conserving energy while bathing, transferring, and so on.	Patient will be able to accomplish more with a decreased expenditure of energy.
Increase patient participation in ADLs as tolerated.	Increases confidence level/self-esteem as well as tolerance level.

NURSING DIAGNOSIS:	POWERLESSNESS
May be related to:	Long-term/progressive illness that is not curable.
	Dependence on others.
Possibly evidenced by:	Reluctance to express true feelings; expressions of having no control/influence over situation.
	Apathy, withdrawal, anger.
	Does not monitor progress, nonparticipation in care/decision making.
	Depression over physical deterioration/complications despite patient cooperation with regimen.

DESIRED OUTCOMES/ EVALUATION CRITERIA— PATIENT WILL:	Acknowledge feelings of helplessness. Identify healthy ways to deal with feelings. Assist in planning own care and independently take responsibility for self-care activities.

ACTIONS/INTERVENTIONS	RATIONALE
Independent	
Encourage patient/SO to express feelings about hospitalization and disease in general.	Identifies concerns and facilitates problem solving.
Acknowledge normality of feelings.	Recognition that reactions are normal can help the patient to problem solve and seek help as needed. Diabetic control is a full-time job that serves as a constant reminder of both presence of disease as well as threat to patient's health/life.
Assess how patient has handled problems in the past. Identify locus of control.	Knowledge of individual's style helps to determine needs for treatment goals. Patient whose locus of control is internal usually looks at ways to gain control over own treatment program. Patient who operates with an external locus of control wants to be cared for by others and may project blame for circumstances onto external factors.
Provide opportunity for SO to express concerns and discuss ways in which they can be helpful to the patient.	Enhances sense of being involved and gives SO a chance to problem-solve solutions to help patient prevent recurrence.
Ascertain expectations/goals of patient/SO.	Unrealistic expectations/pressure from others or self may result in feelings of frustration/loss of control and may impair coping abilities. *Note:* Even with rigid adherence to medical regimen, complications/setbacks may occur.
Determine whether a change in relationship with SO has occurred.	Constant energy and thought required for diabetic control often shifts the focus of a relationship. Development of psychologic concerns/visceral neuropathies affecting self-concept (especially sexual role function) may add further stress.
Encourage patient to make decisions related to care, e.g., ambulation, time for activities, and so forth.	Communicates to patient that some control can be exercised over care.
Support participation in self-care and give positive feedback for efforts.	Promotes feeling of control over situation.

NURSING DIAGNOSIS:	**KNOWLEDGE DEFICIT [LEARNING NEED], REGARDING DISEASE, PROGNOSIS, AND TREATMENT NEEDS**
May be related to:	Lack of exposure/recall, information misinterpretation. Unfamiliarity with information resources.

Possibly evidenced by:	Questions/request for information, verbalization of the problem.
	Inaccurate follow-through of instructions, development of preventable complications.
DESIRED OUTCOMES/ EVALUATION CRITERIA— PATIENT WILL:	Verbalize understanding of disease process.
	Identify relationship of signs/symptoms to the disease process and correlate symptoms with causative factors.
	Correctly perform necessary procedures and explain reasons for the actions.
	Initiate necessary lifestyle changes and participate in treatment regimen.

ACTIONS/INTERVENTIONS	RATIONALE
Independent	
Create an environment of trust by listening to concerns, being available.	Rapport and respect need to be established before patient will be willing to take part in the learning process.
Work with patient in setting mutual goals for learning.	Participation in the planning promotes enthusiasm and cooperation with the principles learned.
Select a variety of teaching strategies, e.g., demonstrate needed skills and have patient do return demonstration, incorporate new skills into the hospital routine.	Use of different means of accessing information promotes learner retention.
Discuss essential elements, e.g.:	
What is a normal glucose blood level and how it compares with the patient's level, the type of DM the patient has, the relationship between insulin deficiency and a high glucose level.	Provides knowledge base on which patient can make informed lifestyle choices.
Reasons for the ketoacidotic episode.	Knowledge of the precipitating factors may help to avoid recurrences.
Acute and chronic complications of the disease, including visual disturbances, neurosensory and cardiovascular changes, renal impairment/hypertension.	Awareness helps patient to be more consistent with care and may prevent/delay onset of complications.
Demonstrate fingerstick testing and have patient return demonstration. Instruct patient to check urine ketones if glucose is greater than 250 mg/dL.	Self-monitoring of blood glucose 4 or more times a day allows flexibility in self-care, promotes tighter control of serum levels (e.g., 60–150 mg/dL) and may prevent/delay development of long-term complications.
Discuss dietary plan, use of high-fiber foods, and ways to deal with meals outside the home.	Awareness of importance of dietary control will aid patient in planning meals/sticking to regimen. Fiber can slow glucose absorption, decreasing fluctuations in serum levels, but may cause GI discomfort, increase flatus, and affect vitamin/mineral absorption.

749

ACTIONS/INTERVENTIONS	RATIONALE

Independent

Review medication regimen, including onset, peak, and duration of prescribed insulin, as applicable, with patient/SO.

Understanding all aspects of drug usage promotes proper use. Dose algorithms are created, taking into account drug dosages established during inpatient evaluation, usual amount and schedule of physical activity, and meal plan. Including SO provides additional support/resource for patient.

Review self-administration of insulin and care of equipment. Have patient demonstrate procedure (e.g., drawing up and injection or use of continuous pump).

Identifies understanding and correctness of procedure or potential problems (e.g., vision, memory, and so on) so that alternate solutions can be found for insulin administration.

Stress importance and necessity of maintaining diary of glucose testing, medication dose/time, dietary intake, activity, feelings/sensations, life events.

Aids in creating overall picture of patient situation to achieve better disease control and promotes self-care/independence.

Discuss factors that play a part in diabetic control, e.g., exercise (aerobic versus isometric), stress, surgery, and illness. Review "Sick Day" rules.

This information promotes diabetic control and can greatly reduce the occurrence of ketoacidosis. *Note:* Aerobic exercise (e.g., walking, swimming) promotes effective use of insulin, lowering glucose levels, and strengthens the cardiovascular system. A "sick day" management plan helps maintain equilibrium during illness, minor surgery, severe emotional stress, or any condition that might send glucose spiraling upward.

Review effects of smoking on insulin use. Encourage cessation of smoking.

Nicotine constricts the small blood vessels, and insulin absorption is delayed for as long as these vessels remain constricted. *Note:* Insulin absorption may be reduced by as much as 30% below normal in the first 30 minutes after smoking.

Establish regular exercise/activity schedule and identify corresponding insulin concerns.

Exercise times should not coincide with the peak action of insulin. A snack should be ingested before or during exercise as needed, and rotation of injection sites should avoid the muscle group that will be used in the activity (e.g., abdominal site is preferred over thigh/arm before jogging or swimming) to prevent accelerated uptake of insulin.

Identify the symptoms of hypoglycemia (e.g., weakness, dizziness, lethargy, hunger, irritability, diaphoresis, pallor, tachycardia, tremors, headache, changes in mentation) and explain causes.

May promote early detection and treatment, preventing/limiting occurrence. *Note:* Early morning hyperglycemia may reflect the dawn phenomenon (indicating need for additional insulin) or a rebound response to hypoglycemia during sleep (Somogyi effect), requiring a decrease in insulin dosage/change in diet (e.g., HS snack). Testing serum levels at 3 AM aids in identifying the specific problem.

Instruct in importance of routine examination of the feet and proper foot care. Demonstrate ways to examine feet; inspect shoes for fit; and care for toenails, calluses, and corns. Encourage use of natural fiber stockings.

Prevents/delays complications associated with peripheral neuropathies and/or circulatory impairment, especially cellulitis, gangrene, and amputation.

ACTIONS/INTERVENTIONS	RATIONALE
Independent	
Stress importance of regular eye examinations, especially for patients who have had type I diabetes for 5 years or more.	Changes in vision may be gradual and are more pronounced in persons with poorly controlled DM. Problems include changes in visual acuity and may progress to retinopathy and blindness.
Arrange for vision aids when needed, e.g., magnifying sleeve for insulin syringe, large print instructions, one-touch glucose meters.	Adaptive aids have been developed in recent years to help the visually impaired manage their own DM more effectively.
Discuss sexual functioning and answer questions patient/SO may have.	Not infrequently, impotence occurs (may be first symptom of onset of DM). *Note:* Counseling and/or use of penile prosthesis may be of benefit.
Stress importance of use of identification bracelet.	Can promote quick entry into the health system and appropriate care with fewer resultant complications in the event of an emergency.
Recommend avoidance of OTC drugs without prior approval of health care provider.	These products may contain sugars/interact with prescribed medications.
Discuss importance of follow-up care.	Helps to maintain tighter control of disease process and may prevent exacerbations of DM, retarding development of systemic complications.
Review signs/symptoms requiring medical evaluation, e.g., fever; cold/flu symptoms; cloudy/odorous urine, painful urination; delayed healing of cuts/sores; sensory changes (pain/tingling) of lower extremities; changes in blood sugar level, presence of ketones in urine.	Prompt intervention may prevent development of more serious/life-threatening complications.
Demonstrate stress management techniques, e.g., deep-breathing exercises, guided imagery, visualization.	Promotes relaxation and control of stress response, which may help to limit incidence of glucose/insulin imbalances.
Identify community resources, e.g., American Diabetic Association, VNA, weight-loss/stop-smoking clinic, contact person/diabetic instructor.	Continued support is usually necessary to sustain lifestyle changes and promote well-being.

Bibliography

General References

Bellak, JP and Bamford, PA: Nursing Assessment: A Multidimensional Approach. Jones & Bartlett, Boston, 1987.

Berkow, R (ed): The Merck Manual, ed 15. Merck Sharp & Dohme Research Laboratories, Rahway, NJ, 1987.

Cella, JH and Watson, J: Nurse's Manual of Laboratory Tests. FA Davis, Philadelphia, 1989.

Condon, RE and Nyhus, LM (eds): Manual of Surgical Therapeutics, ed 7. Little, Brown & Co, Boston, 1988.

Deglin, JH and Vallerand, AH: Davis's Drug Guide for Nurses, ed 3. FA Davis, Philadelphia, 1992.

Diseases and Disorders Handbook, ed 3. Springhouse Corp, Springhouse, PA, 1989.

Doenges, ME and Moorhouse, MF: Nurse's Pocket Guide: Nursing Diagnoses with Interventions, ed 3. FA Davis, Philadelphia, 1991.

Dunagan, WC and Ridner, ML (eds): Manual of Medical Therapeutics, ed 26. Little, Brown & Co, Boston, 1989.

Fischbach, F: A Manual of Laboratory and Diagnostic Tests, ed 4. JB Lippincott, Philadelphia, 1992.

Guyton, AC: Textbook of Medical Physiology, ed 8. WB Saunders, Philadelphia, 1991.

Kuhn, MM: Pharmacotherapeutics: A Nursing Process Approach, ed 2. FA Davis, Philadelphia, 1991.

Professional Guide to Diseases, ed 3. Springhouse Corp, Springhouse, PA, 1989.

Suddarth, DS (ed): The Lippincott Manual of Nursing Practice, ed 5. JB Lippincott, Philadelphia, 1991.

Thomas, CL (ed): Taber's Cyclopedic Medical Dictionary, ed 17. FA Davis, Philadelphia, 1993.
Thompson, JM, et al: Mosby's Manual of Clinical Nursing, ed 2. CV Mosby, St Louis, 1989.

Books

Drug Information for the Health Care Professional, ed 11, Vol IB. USPDI, 1991.

Articles

Becker, S: The risks and rewards of pancreatic transplant. RN 52(7):54, 1989.
Casey, CA: Diabetes: Complications that can cripple. RN 55(8):36, 1992.
Christensen, MH, et al. How to care for the diabetic foot. AJN 91(3):50, 1991.
Epstein, CD: Fluid volume deficit for the adrenal crisis patient. Dimens Crit Care 10(4):210, 1991.
Handerhan, B: Recognizing adrenal crisis. Nursing92 22(4):33, 1992.
Hardcastle, W: Management of Addison's disease. Nursing 3(41):7, 1989.
Herget, MJ and Williams, AS: New aids for low-vision diabetics. AJN 89(10):1319, 1989.
Isley, WL: Thyroid disorders. Crit Care Nurse Q 13(3):39, 1990.
Martinelli, AM and Fontana, JL: Thyroid storm: Potential perioperative crisis. AORN J 52(2):305, 1990.
Lockhart, JS and Griffin, CW: ACTION STAT! Posthyroidectomy respiratory distress. Nursing87 12(7):33, 1987.
Mackowiak, L and McCarthy, R: Managing diabetes on "sick days." AJN 89(7):950, 1989.
Peterson, A and Drass, J: Managing acute complications of diabetes. Nursing91 21(2):34, 1991.
Robertson, C: Coping with chronic complications. RN 52(9):34, 1989.
Sabo, CE and Michael, SR: Diabetic ketoacidosis: Pathophysiology, nursing diagnosis and nursing interventions. Focus on Critical Care 16(1):21, 1989.
Sabo, CE and Michael, SR: Managing DKA and preventing a recurrence. Nursing89 19(2):50, 1989.
Tomky, D: Tapping the full power of insulin pumps. RN

CHAPTER 12

REPRODUCTIVE

Hysterectomy

Hysterectomy is the surgical removal of the uterus, most commonly performed for malignancies and certain nonmalignant conditions (e.g., endometriosis/tumors), to control life-threatening bleeding/hemorrhage, and in the event of intractable pelvic infection or irreparable rupture of the uterus.

Abdominal hysterectomy types include the following:

Subtotal (partial): Body of the uterus is removed; cervical stump remains.

Total: Removal of the uterus and cervix.

Total with bilateral salpingo-oophorectomy: Removal of uterus, cervix, fallopian tubes, and ovaries is the treatment of choice for invasive cancer, fibroid tumors that are rapidly growing or produce severe abnormal bleeding, and endometriosis invading other pelvic organs.

Vaginal hysterectomy may be done in certain conditions, such as uterine prolapse, cystocele/rectocele, carcinoma in situ, and high-risk obesity. It is contraindicated if the diagnosis is obscure.

RELATED CONCERNS

Cancer, p 1014

Psychosocial Aspects of Acute Care, p 899

Surgical Intervention, p 918 (for general considerations and interventions)

Thrombophlebitis: Deep Vein Thrombosis, p 135

PATIENT ASSESSMENT DATA BASE

Data are dependent on the underlying disease process/need for surgical intervention (e.g., cancer, prolapse, dysfunctional uterine bleeding, severe endometriosis or pelvic infections unresponsive to medical management) and associated complications (e.g., anemia).

TEACHING/LEARNING

Discharge Plan Considerations: **DRG projected mean length of stay: 5.4 days.**

May need temporary help with transportation; homemaker/maintenance tasks.

DIAGNOSTIC STUDIES

Pap smear: Cellular dysplasia reflects possibility of/presence of cancer.

Ultrasound or CT scan: Aids in identifying size/location of mass.

Laparoscopy: Done to visualize tumors, bleeding, endometrial changes. Laparotomy may be done for staging cancer or to assess effects of chemotherapy.

D&C with biopsy (endometrial/cervical): Permits histopathologic study of cells to determine presence/location of cancer.

Schiller's test (staining of cervix with iodine): Useful in identifying abnormal cells.

CBC: Decreased Hb may reflect chronic anemia, while decreased Hct suggests active blood loss. WBC elevation may indicate inflammation/infectious process.

NURSING PRIORITIES

1. Support adaptation to change.
2. Prevent complications.
3. Provide information about procedure/prognosis and treatment needs.

DISCHARGE GOALS

1. Dealing realistically with situation.
2. Complications prevented/minimized.
3. Procedure/prognosis and therapeutic regimen understood.

NURSING DIAGNOSIS:	**SELF-ESTEEM, DISTURBANCE IN: (SPECIFY)**
May be related to:	Concerns about inability to have children, changes in femininity, effect on sexual relationship.
	Religious conflicts.
Possibly evidenced by:	Expressions of specific concerns/vague comments about result of surgery; fear of rejection or of reaction of SO.
	Withdrawal, depression.
DESIRED OUTCOMES/ EVALUATION CRITERIA— PATIENT WILL:	Verbalize concerns and indicate healthy ways of dealing with them.
	Verbalize acceptance of self in situation and adaptation to change in body/self-image.

ACTIONS/INTERVENTIONS	RATIONALE
Independent	
Provide time to listen to concerns and fears of patient and SO. Discuss patient's perceptions of self related to anticipated changes and her specific lifestyle.	Conveys interest and concern; provides opportunity to correct misconceptions, e.g., women may fear loss of femininity and sexuality, weight gain, and menopausal body changes.
Assess emotional stress the patient is experiencing. Identify meaning of loss for patient/SO. Encourage patient to vent feelings appropriately.	Nurses need to be aware of what this operation means to the patient to avoid inadvertent casualness or oversolicitude. Depending on the reason for the surgery (e.g., cancer or long-term heavy bleeding) the woman can be frightened or relieved. She may fear inability to fulfill her reproductive role and may experience grief over loss.

ACTIONS/INTERVENTIONS

Independent

Provide accurate information, reinforcing information previously given.

Ascertain individual strengths and identify previous positive coping behaviors.

Provide open environment for patient to discuss concerns about sexuality.

Note withdrawn behavior, negative self-talk, use of denial, or overconcern with actual/perceived changes.

Collaborative

Refer to professional counseling as necessary.

RATIONALE

Provides opportunity for patient to question and assimilate information.

Helpful to build on strengths already available for patient to use in coping with current situation.

Promotes sharing of beliefs/values about sensitive subject and identifies misconceptions/myths that may interfere with adjustment to situation. (Refer to ND: Sexual Dysfunction, high risk for p 758.)

Identifies stage of grief/need for interventions.

May need additional help to resolve feelings about loss.

NURSING DIAGNOSIS:	URINARY ELIMINATION, ALTERED/URINARY RETENTION [ACUTE]
May be related to:	Mechanical trauma, surgical manipulation, presence of local tissue edema, hematoma. Sensory/motor impairment: Nerve paralysis.
Possibly evidenced by:	Sensation of bladder fullness, urgency. Small frequent voiding or absence of urinary output. Overflow incontinence. Bladder distention.
DESIRED OUTCOMES/ EVALUATION CRITERIA— PATIENT WILL:	Empty bladder regularly and completely.

ACTIONS/INTERVENTIONS

Independent

Note voiding pattern and monitor urinary output.

Palpate bladder. Investigate reports of discomfort, fullness, inability to void.

Provide routine voiding measures, e.g., privacy, normal position, running water in sink, pouring warm water over perineum.

RATIONALE

May indicate urine retention if voiding frequently in small/insufficient amounts (<100 ml).

Perception of bladder fullness, distension of bladder above symphysis pubis indicates urinary retention.

Promotes relaxation of perineal muscles and may facilitate voiding efforts.

ACTIONS/INTERVENTIONS	RATIONALE

Independent

Provide good perianal cleansing care and catheter care (when present).	Promotes cleanliness reducing risk of ascending UTI.
Assess urine characteristics, noting color, clarity, odor.	Urinary retention, vaginal drainage, and possible presence of intermittent/indwelling catheter increase risk of infection, especially if patient has perineal sutures.

Collaborative

Catheterize when indicated/per protocol if patient is unable to void or is uncomfortable.	Edema or interference with nerve supply may cause bladder atony/urinary retention requiring decompression of the bladder. *Note:* Indwelling urethral or suprapubic catheter may be inserted intraoperatively if complications are anticipated.
Decompress bladder slowly.	When large amount of urine has accumulated, rapid bladder decompression releases pressure on pelvic vessels promoting venous pooling.
Maintain patency of indwelling catheter; keep drainage tubing free of kinks.	Promotes free drainage of urine, reducing risk of urinary stasis/retention and infection.
Check residual urine volume after voiding as indicated.	May not be emptying bladder completely; retention of urine increases possibility for infection and is uncomfortable/painful.

NURSING DIAGNOSIS:	**CONSTIPATION/DIARRHEA, HIGH RISK FOR**
Risk factors may include:	Physical factors: abdominal surgery, with manipulation of bowel, weakening of abdominal musculature.
	Pain/discomfort in abdomen or perineal area.
	Changes in dietary intake.
Possibly evidenced by:	[Not applicable; presence of signs and symptoms establishes an actual diagnosis.]
DESIRED OUTCOMES/ EVALUATION CRITERIA— PATIENT WILL:	Display active bowel sounds/peristaltic activity.
	Maintain usual pattern of elimination.

ACTIONS/INTERVENTIONS	RATIONALE

Independent

Auscultate bowel sounds. Note abdominal distention, presence of nausea/vomiting.	Indicators of presence/resolution of ileus, affecting choice of interventions.
Assist patient with sitting on edge of bed and walking.	Early ambulation helps stimulate intestinal function and return of peristalsis.
Encourage adequate fluid intake, including fruit juices, when oral intake is resumed.	Promotes softer stool; may aid in stimulating peristalsis.

ACTIONS/INTERVENTIONS

Independent

Provide sitz baths.

Collaborative

Restrict oral intake as indicated.

Maintain NG tube, if present.

Provide clear/full liquids and advance to solid foods as tolerated.

Use rectal tube; apply heat to the abdomen, if appropriate.

Administer medications, e.g., stool softeners, mineral oil, laxatives as indicated.

RATIONALE

Promotes muscle relaxation, minimizes discomfort.

Prevents nausea/vomiting until peristalsis returns (1–2 days).

May be inserted in surgery to decompress stomach.

When peristalsis begins, food and fluid intake promote resumption of normal bowel elimination.

Promotes the passage of flatus.

Promotes formation/passage of softer stool.

NURSING DIAGNOSIS:	TISSUE PERFUSION, ALTERED: (SPECIFY), HIGH RISK FOR
Risk factors may include:	Hypovolemia. Reduction/interruption of blood flow: Pelvic congestion, postoperative tissue inflammation, venous stasis. Intraoperative trauma or pressure on pelvic/calf vessels/lithotomy position during vaginal hysterectomy.
Possibly evidenced by:	[Not applicable; presence of signs and symptoms establishes an actual diagnosis.]
DESIRED OUTCOMES/ EVALUATION CRITERIA— PATIENT WILL:	Demonstrate adequate perfusion, as evidenced by stable vital signs, palpable pulses, good capillary refill, usual mentation, individually adequate urinary output and free of edema, signs of thrombus formation.

ACTIONS/INTERVENTIONS

Independent

Monitor vital signs; palpate peripheral pulses, and note capillary refill; assess urinary output/characteristics. Evaluate changes in mentation.

Inspect dressings and perineal pads, noting color, amount, and odor of drainage. Weigh pads and compare with dry weight, if patient is bleeding heavily.

Turn patient and encourage frequent coughing and deep-breathing exercises.

Avoid high-Fowler's position and pressure under the knees or crossing of legs.

RATIONALE

Indicators of adequacy of systemic perfusion, fluid/blood needs, and developing complications.

Proximity of large blood vessels to operative site and/or potential for alteration of clotting mechanism (e.g., cancer) increase risk of postoperative hemorrhage.

Prevents stasis of secretions and respiratory complications.

Creates vascular stasis by increasing pelvic congestion and pooling of blood in the extremities, potentiating risk of thrombus formation.

ACTIONS/INTERVENTIONS

Independent

Assist with/instruct in foot and leg exercises and ambulate as soon as able.

Check for Homans' sign. Note erythema, swelling of extremity, or complaints of sudden chest pain with dyspnea.

Collaborative

Administer IV fluids, blood products as indicated.

Apply antiembolus stockings.

Assist with/encourage use of incentive spirometer.

RATIONALE

Movement enhances circulation and prevents stasis complications.

May be indicative of development of thrombophlebitis/pulmonary embolus.

Replacement of blood losses maintains circulating volume and tissue perfusion.

Aids in venous return; reduces stasis and risk of thrombosis.

Promotes lung expansion/minimizes atelectasis.

NURSING DIAGNOSIS:	SEXUAL DYSFUNCTION, HIGH RISK FOR
Risk factors may include:	Altered body structure/function, e.g., shortening of vaginal canal; changes in hormone levels, decreased libido.
	Possible change in sexual response pattern, e.g., absence of rhythmic uterine contractions during orgasm; vaginal discomfort/pain (dyspareunia).
Possibly evidenced by:	[Not applicable; presence of signs and symptoms establishes an actual diagnosis.]
DESIRED OUTCOMES/ EVALUATION CRITERIA— PATIENT WILL:	Verbalize understanding of changes in sexual anatomy/function.
	Discuss concerns about body image, sex role, desirability as a sexual partner with SO.
	Identify satisfying/acceptable sexual practices and some alternative ways of dealing with sexual expression.

ACTIONS/INTERVENTIONS

Independent

Listen to comments of patient/SO.

Assess patient/SO information regarding sexual anatomy/function and effects of surgical procedure.

RATIONALE

Sexual concerns are often disguised as humor and/or offhand remarks.

May have misinformation/misconceptions that can affect adjustment. Negative expectations are associated with poor overall outcome. Changes in hormone levels can affect libido and/or decrease suppleness of the vagina. Although a shortened vagina can eventually stretch, initially intercourse may be uncomfortable/painful.

ACTIONS/INTERVENTIONS

Independent

Identify cultural/value factors and conflicts present.

Assist patient to be aware/deal with stage of grieving.

Encourage patient to share thoughts/concerns with partner.

Problem-solve solutions to potential problems, e.g., postponing sexual intercourse when fatigued, substituting alternate means of expression, positions that avoid pressure on abdominal incision, use of vaginal lubricant.

Discuss expected physical sensations/discomforts, changes in response as appropriate to the individual.

Collaborative

Refer to counselor/sex therapist as needed.

RATIONALE

May affect return to satisfying sexual relationship.

Acknowledging normal process of grieving for actual/perceived changes may enhance coping and facilitate resolution.

Open communication can identify areas of agreement/problems and promote discussion and resolution.

Assists patient to return to desired/satisfying sexual activity.

Vaginal pain may be marked following vaginal procedure or sensory loss may occur due to surgical trauma. Although sensory loss is usually temporary, it may take weeks/months to resolve. In addition, changes in vaginal size, altered hormone levels, and loss of sensation of rhythmic contractions of the uterus during orgasm can impair sexual satisfaction. *Note:* Many women experience few negative effects because fear of pregnancy is gone and relieved symptoms often improve enjoyment of intercourse.

May need additional assistance to promote a satisfactory outcome.

NURSING DIAGNOSIS:	KNOWLEDGE DEFICIT [LEARNING NEED], REGARDING CONDITION, PROGNOSIS, AND TREATMENT NEEDS
May be related to:	Lack of exposure/recall.
	Information misinterpretation.
	Unfamiliarity with information resources.
Possibly evidenced by:	Questions/request for information; statement of misconception.
	Inaccurate follow-through of instructions, development of preventable complications.
DESIRED OUTCOMES/ EVALUATION CRITERIA— PATIENT WILL:	Verbalize understanding of condition.
	Identify relationship of signs/symptoms related to surgical procedure and actions to deal with them.

ACTIONS/INTERVENTIONS	RATIONALE
Independent	
Review effects of surgical procedure and future expectations; e.g., patient needs to know she will no longer menstruate or bear children, whether surgical menopause will occur, and the possible need for hormonal replacement.	Provides knowledge base on which patient can make informed choices.
Discuss complexity of problems anticipated during recovery, e.g., emotional lability and expectation of feelings of depression/sadness; excessive fatigue, sleep disturbances, urinary problems.	Physical, emotional, and social factors can have a cumulative effect, which may delay recovery, especially if hysterectomy was performed because of cancer. Providing an opportunity for problem solving may facilitate the process. Patient/SO may benefit from the knowledge that a period of emotional lability is normal and expected during recovery.
Discuss resumption of activity. Encourage light activities initially, with frequent rest periods and increased activities/exercise as tolerated. Stress importance of individual response in recuperation.	Patient can expect to feel tired when she goes home and needs to plan a gradual resumption of activities, with return to work an individual matter. Prevents excessive fatigue; conserves energy for healing/tissue regeneration. *Note:* Some studies suggest that recovery from hysterectomy (especially when oophorectomy is done) may take 4 times as long as recovery from other major surgeries (12 months versus 3 months).
Identify individual restrictions, e.g., avoiding heavy lifting and strenuous activities (such as vacuuming, straining at stool); prolonged sitting/driving. Avoid tub baths/douching until physician allows.	Strenuous activity intensifies fatigue and may delay healing. Activities that increase intra-abdominal pressure can strain surgical repairs, and prolonged sitting potentiates risk of thrombus formation. Showers are permitted, but tub baths/douching may cause vaginal irritation or incisional infections as well as be a safety hazard.
Review recommendations fo resumption of sexual intercourse. (Refer to ND: Sexual Dysfunction, high risk for, p 758.)	When sexual activity is cleared by the physician, it is best to resume activity easily and gently, using alternate coital positions or expressing sexual feelings in other ways.
Identify dietary needs, e.g., high protein, additional iron.	Facilitates healing/tissue regeneration and helps correct anemia if present.
Review replacement hormone therapy. Discuss possibility of "hot flashes" even though ovaries may remain.	Total hysterectomy with bilateral salpingo-oophorectomy (surgically induced menopause) requires replacement hormones. In addition, hormone replacement may be needed after subtotal procedures because a portion of the blood supply to the ovaries is clamped during the procedure, possibly impairing long-term function.
Encourage taking prescribed drug(s) routinely (e.g., with meals).	Taking hormones with meals establishes routine for taking drug and reduces potential for initial nausea.
Discuss potential side effects, e.g., weight gain, increased skin pigmentation or acne, breast tenderness, headaches, photosensitivity.	Development of some side effects is expected but may require problem solving such as change in dosage or use of sunscreen.

ACTIONS/INTERVENTIONS	RATIONALE

Independent

Recommend cessation of smoking when receiving estrogen therapy.	Some studies suggest an increased risk of thrombophlebitis, MI, CVA, and pulmonary emboli associated with smoking and concurrent estrogen therapy.
Review incisional care when appropriate.	Facilitates competent self-care, promoting independence.
Stress importance of follow-up care.	Provides opportunity to ask questions and clear up misunderstandings as well as detect any beginning complications.
Identify signs/symptoms requiring medical evaluation, e.g., fever/chills, change in character of vaginal/wound drainage; bright bleeding.	Early recognition and treatment of developing complications such as infection/hemorrhage may prevent life-threatening situations. *Note:* Hemorrhage may occur as late as 2 weeks postoperatively.

Mastectomy

The choice of treatment for breast cancer depends on tumor type, size, and location, as well as clinical characteristics (staging). Therapy may include surgical intervention with/without radiation, chemotherapy, and hormone therapy. The use of bone marrow transplantation is under investigation.

Types of surgery are generally grouped into three categories: radical mastectomy, total mastectomy, and more limited procedures (e.g., segmental, lumpectomy). Total (simple) mastectomy removes all breast tissue, but all or most axillary lymph nodes and chest muscles are left intact. Modified radical mastectomy removes the entire breast, some or most lymph nodes, and sometimes the pectoralis minor chest muscles. Major chest muscles are left intact. Radical (Halsted's) mastectomy is a procedure that is rarely performed as it requires removal of the entire breast, skin, major and minor pectoral muscles, axillary lymph nodes, and sometimes internal mammary or supraclavicular lymph nodes. Limited procedures (i.e., lumpectomy) may be done on an outpatient basis as only the tumor and some surrounding tissue are removed. Lumpectomy is reserved for well-defined nonmetastatic tumors of less than 5 cm in size that do not involve the nipple. The procedure may be diagnostic (determines cell type) and/or curative when combined with radiation therapy.

RELATED CONCERNS

Cancer, p 1014 (for additional nursing interventions regarding cancer treatment)
Psychosocial Aspects of Acute Care, p 899
Surgical Intervention, p 918

PATIENT ASSESSMENT DATA BASE

ACTIVITY/REST

May report:	Work, activity involving frequent/repetitive arm movements.
	Sleep style (e.g., sleeping on stomach).

CIRCULATION

May exhibit:	Unilateral engorgement in affected arm (invaded lymph system).

FOOD/FLUID

May report:	Loss of appetite, recent weight loss.

EGO INTEGRITY

May report:	Constant stressors in work/home life.
	Stress/fear involving diagnosis, prognosis, future expectations.

PAIN/COMFORT

May report:	Pain in advanced/metastatic disease. (Localized pain rarely occurs in early malignancy.)
	Some experience discomfort or "funny feeling" in breast tissue.
	Heavy, painful breasts premenstrually usually indicate fibrocystic disease.

SAFETY

May exhibit:	Nodular axillary masses.
	Edema, erythema of involved skin.

SEXUALITY

May report: Presence of a breast lump; changes in breast symmetry or size.

Changes in breast skin color or temperature; unusual nipple discharge; itching, burning, or retracted nipple.

History of early menarche (younger than age 12); late menopause (after age 50); late first pregnancy (after age 35).

Concerns about sexuality/intimacy.

May exhibit: Change in breast contour/mass, asymmetry.

Dimpling, puckering of skin; changes in skin color/texture, swelling, redness or heat in breast.

Retraction of nipple; discharge from nipple (serous, serosanguinous, sanguinous, watery discharge increase likelihood of cancer, especially when accompanied by lump).

TEACHING/LEARNING

May report: Family history of breast cancer (mother, sister, maternal aunt, or grandmother).

Previous unilateral breast cancer, endometrial or ovarian cancer.

Discharge Plan Considerations: **DRG projected mean length of stay: 4.0 days.**

May need assistance with treatments/rehabilitation, decisions, self-care activities, homemaker/maintenance tasks.

DIAGNOSTIC STUDIES

Mammography: Visualizes internal structure of the breast; is capable of detecting nonpalpable cancers or tumors that are in early stages of development.

Galactography (ductography): Contrast mammograms obtained by injecting dye into a draining duct).

Ultrasound: May be helpful in distinguishing between solid masses and cysts and in women whose breast tissue is dense; complements findings of mammography.

Xeroradiography: Reveals increased circulation around tumor site.

Thermography: Identifies rapidly growing tumors as "hot spots" because of increased blood supply and corresponding higher skin temperature.

Diaphanography (transillumination): Identifies tumor or mass by differentiating the way that tissues transmit and scatter light. Procedure remains experimental and is considered less accurate than mammography.

CT scan and MRI: Scanning techniques that can detect breast disease, especially larger masses; or tumors in small, dense breasts that are difficult to examine by mammography. These techniques are not suitable for routine screening and are not a substitute for mammography.

Breast biopsy (needle or excisional): Provides definitive diagnosis of mass and is useful for histologic classification, staging, and selection of appropriate therapies.

Hormone receptor assays: Reveal whether cells of excised tumor or biopsy specimens contain hormone receptors (estrogen and progesterone). In malignant cells, the estrogen-plus receptor complex stimulates cell growth and division. About two thirds of all women with breast cancer are estrogen-receptor positive and tend to respond favorably to hormone therapy following primary therapy to extend the disease-free period and survival.

Chest x-ray, liver function studies, CBC, and bone scan: Done to assess for presence of metastasis.

NURSING PRIORITIES

1. Assist patient/SO in dealing with stress of situation/prognosis.
2. Prevent complications.

3. Establish individualized rehabilitation program.
4. Provide information about disease process, procedure, prognosis, and treatment needs.

DISCHARGE GOALS

1. Dealing realistically with situation.
2. Complications prevented/minimized.
3. Exercise regimen initiated.
4. Disease process, surgical procedure, prognosis, and therapeutic regimen understood.

PREOPERATIVE

NURSING DIAGNOSIS:	FEAR/ANXIETY [SPECIFY LEVEL]
May be related to:	Threat of death, e.g., extent of disease.
	Threat to self-concept: Change of body image; scarring, loss of body part, sexual attractiveness.
	Change in health status.
Possibly evidenced by:	Increased tension; apprehension; feelings of helplessness/inadequacy.
	Decreased self-assurance.
	Self-focus; restlessness; sympathetic stimulation.
	Expressed concerns regarding actual/anticipated changes in life.
DESIRED OUTCOMES/ EVALUATION CRITERIA— PATIENT WILL:	Acknowledge and discuss concerns.
	Demonstrate appropriate range of feelings.
	Report fear and anxiety are reduced to a manageable level.

ACTIONS/INTERVENTIONS	RATIONALE
Independent	
Ascertain what information patient has about diagnosis, expected surgical intervention, and future therapies. Note presence of denial or extreme anxiety.	Provides knowledge base for the nurse to enable reinforcement of needed information and helps to identify patient with high anxiety, low capacity for information processing, and need for special attention. *Note:* Denial may be useful as a coping method for a time, but extreme anxiety needs to be dealt with immediately.
Explain purpose and preparation for diagnostic tests.	Clear understanding of procedures and what is happening increases feelings of control and lessens anxiety.
Provide an atmosphere of concern, openness, and availability as well as privacy for the patient/SO. Suggest that SO be present as much as possible/desired.	Time and privacy are needed to provide support, discuss feelings of anticipated loss and other concerns. Therapeutic communication skills, open questions, listening, and so forth, facilitate this process.

ACTIONS/INTERVENTIONS	RATIONALE

Independent

Encourage questions and provide time for expression of fears. Tell patient that stress related to breast cancer can persist for many months and to seek help/support.

Provides opportunity to identify and clarify misconceptions and offer emotional support.

Assess degree of support available to the patient. Give information about community resources, such as Reach to Recovery, YWCA Encore program. Encourage/provide for visit with a woman who has recovered from a mastectomy.

Can be a helpful resource when patient is ready. A peer who has experienced the same process serves as a role model and can provide validity to the comments, hope for recovery/normal future.

Discuss/explain role of rehabilitation after surgery.

Rehabilitation is an essential component of therapy intended to meet physical, social, emotional, and vocational needs so that the patient can achieve the best possible level of physical and emotional functioning.

POSTOPERATIVE

NURSING DIAGNOSIS:	**SKIN/TISSUE INTEGRITY, IMPAIRED**
May be related to:	Surgical removal of skin/tissue; altered circulation, presence of edema, drainage; changes in skin elasticity, sensation; tissue destruction (radiation).
Possibly evidenced by:	Disruption of skin surface, destruction of skin layers/subcutaneous tissues.
DESIRED OUTCOMES/ EVALUATION CRITERIA— PATIENT WILL:	Achieve timely wound healing, free of purulent drainage or erythema.
	Demonstrate behaviors/techniques to promote healing/ prevent complications.

ACTIONS/INTERVENTIONS	RATIONALE

Independent

Assess dressings/wound for characteristics of drainage. Monitor amount of edema, redness, and pain in the incision and arm. Monitor temperature.

Use of dressings depends on the extent of surgery and the type of wound closure. (Pressure dressings are usually applied initially and are reinforced, not changed.) Drainage occurs because of the trauma of the procedure and manipulation of the numerous blood vessels and lymphatics in the area. Early recognition of developing infection can enable quickly instituted treatment.

Place in semi-Fowler's position on back or unaffected side with arm elevated and supported by pillows.

Assists with drainage of fluid through use of gravity.

Do not take BP, inject medications, or insert IVs in affected arm.

Increases potential of constriction, infection, and lymphedema on affected side.

ACTIONS/INTERVENTIONS	RATIONALE
Independent	
Inspect donor/graft site (if done) for color, blister formation; note drainage from donor site.	Color will be affected by availability of circulatory supply. Blister formation provides a site for bacterial growth/infection.
Empty wound drains, periodically noting amount and characteristics of drainage.	Drainage of accumulated fluids (e.g., lymph, blood) enhances healing and reduces the susceptibility to infection. Suction devices (e.g., Hemovac, Jackson Pratt) are often inserted during surgery to maintain negative pressure in wound. Tubes are usually removed around the third day or when drainage ceases.
Encourage wearing of loose-fitting/nonconstrictive clothing. Tell patient not to wear wristwatch or other jewelry on affected arm.	Reduces pressure on compromised tissues, which may improve circulation/healing.
Collaborative	
Administer antibiotics as indicated.	May be given prophylactically or to treat specific infection and enhance healing.

NURSING DIAGNOSIS:	PAIN, [ACUTE]
May be related to:	Surgical procedure; tissue trauma, interruption of nerves, dissection of muscles.
Possibly evidenced by:	Reports of stiffness, numbness in chest area, shoulder/arm pain; alteration of muscle tone.
	Self-focusing; distraction/guarding behavior.
DESIRED OUTCOMES/ EVALUATION CRITERIA— PATIENT WILL:	Express reduction in pain/discomfort.
	Appear relaxed, able to sleep/rest appropriately.

ACTIONS/INTERVENTIONS	RATIONALE
Independent	
Assess reports of pain, noting location, duration, and intensity (0–10 scale). Note verbal and nonverbal clues.	Aids in identifying degree of discomfort and need for/effectiveness of analgesia. The amount of tissue, muscle, and lymphatic system removed can affect the amount of pain experienced. Destruction of nerves in axillary region causes numbness in upper arm and scapular region, which may be more intolerable than surgical pain. *Note:* Pain in chest wall can occur from muscle tension, be affected by extremes in heat and cold, and continue for several months.
Discuss normality of phantom breast sensations.	Provides reassurance that sensations are not imaginary and that relief can be obtained.
Assist patient to find position of comfort.	Elevation of arm, size of dressings, and presence of drains affects patient's ability to relax and rest/sleep effectively.

ACTIONS/INTERVENTIONS

Independent

Provide basic comfort measures (e.g., repositioning on back or unaffected side, backrub) and diversional activities. Encourage early ambulation and use of relaxation techniques, guided imagery, Therapeutic Touch.

Splint/support chest during coughing/deep-breathing exercises.

Give appropriate pain medication on a regular schedule before pain is severe and before activities are scheduled.

Collaborative

Administer narcotics/analgesics as indicated.

RATIONALE

Promotes relaxation, helps to refocus attention, and may enhance coping abilities.

Facilitates participation in activity without undue discomfort.

Maintains comfort level and permits patient to exercise arm and to ambulate without pain hindering efforts.

Provides relief of discomfort/pain and facilitates rest, participation in postoperative therapy.

NURSING DIAGNOSIS:	SELF-ESTEEM, DISTURBANCE IN: [SPECIFY]
May be related to:	Biophysical: Disfiguring surgical procedure.
	Psychosocial: Concern about sexual attractiveness.
Possibly evidenced by:	Actual change in structure/body contour.
	Verbalization of fear of rejection or of reaction by others, change in social involvement.
	Negative feelings about body, preoccupation with change or loss, not looking at body, nonparticipation in therapy.
DESIRED OUTCOMES/ EVALUATION CRITERIA— PATIENT WILL:	Demonstrate movement toward acceptance of self in situation.
	Recognize and incorporate change into self-concept without negating self-esteem.
	Set realistic goals and actively participate in therapy program.

ACTIONS/INTERVENTIONS

Independent

Encourage questions about current situation and future expectations. Provide emotional support when surgical dressings are removed.

Identify role concerns as woman, wife, mother, career woman, and so forth.

Encourage patient to express feelings, e.g., anger, hostility, and grief.

RATIONALE

Loss of the breast causes many reactions, including feeling disfigured, fear of viewing scar, and fear of partner's reaction to change in body.

May reveal how patient's self-view has been altered.

Loss of body part, disfigurement, and perceived loss of sexual desirability engender grieving process that needs to be dealt with so that patient can

767

ACTIONS/INTERVENTIONS	RATIONALE
Independent	
	make plans for the future. *Note:* Grief may resurface when subsequent procedures are done (e.g., fitting for prosthesis, reconstructive procedure).
Discuss signs/symptoms of depression with patient/SO.	Common reaction to this type of procedure and needs to be recognized and acknowledged.
Provide positive reinforcement for gains/improvement and participation in self-care/treatment program.	Encourages continuation of healthy behaviors.
Review possibilities for reconstructive surgery and/or prosthetic augmentation.	If feasible, reconstruction provides less disfiguring/"near normal" cosmetic result. Variations in skin flap may be done for facilitation of future reconstructive process. *Note:* Although reconstruction is usually not done for 3–6 months, prolonged delay may result in increased tension in relationships and impair patient's incorporation of changes into self-concept.
Ascertain feelings/concerns of partner regarding sexual aspects, and provide information and support.	Negative responses directed at the patient may actually reflect partner's concern about hurting patient, fear of cancer/death, difficulty in dealing with personality/behavior changes in patient, or inability to look at operative area.
Discuss and refer to support groups including "Men in Our Lives" for SO.	Provides a place to exchange concerns and feelings with others who have had a similar experience and identifies ways SO can facilitate patient's recovery.
Collaborative	
Provide temporary soft prosthesis, if indicated.	Prosthesis of nylon and Dacron fluff may be worn in bra until incision heals if reconstructive surgery is not performed at the time of mastectomy. This may promote social acceptance and allow patient to feel more comfortable about body image at the time of discharge.

NURSING DIAGNOSIS:	PHYSICAL MOBILITY, IMPAIRED
May be related to:	Neuromuscular impairment; pain/discomfort; edema formation.
Possibly evidenced by:	Reluctance to attempt movement.
	Limited ROM; decreased muscle mass/strength.
DESIRED OUTCOMES/ EVALUATION CRITERIA— PATIENT WILL:	Display willingness to participate in therapy.
	Demonstrate techniques that enable resumption of activities.
	Increase strength of affected body parts.

ACTIONS/INTERVENTIONS	RATIONALE

Independent

Elevate affected arm as indicated. Begin passive ROM (e.g., flexion/extension of elbow, pronation/supination of wrist, clenching/extending fingers) as soon as possible.

Promotes venous return, lessening possibility of lymphedema. Early postoperative exercises are usually started in the first 24 hours to prevent joint stiffness that can further limit movement/mobility.

Have patient move fingers, noting sensations and color of hand on affected side.

Lack of movement may reflect problems with the intercostal brachial nerve, and discoloration can indicate impaired circulation.

Encourage patient to use affected arm for personal hygiene, e.g., feeding, combing hair, washing face.

Increases circulation, helps minimize edema, and maintains strength and function of the arm and hand. These activities use the arm without abduction, which can stress the suture line in the early postoperative period.

Help with self-care activities as necessary.

Conserves patient's energy; prevents undue fatigue.

Assist with ambulation and encourage correct posture.

Patient will feel unbalanced and may need assistance until accustomed to change. Keeping back straight prevents shoulder from moving forward, avoiding permanent limitation in movement and posture.

Advance exercise as indicated, e.g., active extension of arm and rotation of shoulder while lying in bed, pendulum swings, rope turning, elevating arms to touch fingertips behind head.

Prevents joint stiffness, increases circulation, and maintains muscle tone of the shoulders and arm.

Progress to hand climbing (walking fingers up wall), clasping hands behind head, and full abduction exercises as soon as patient can manage.

Since this group of exercises can cause excessive tension on the incision, they are usually delayed until healing process is well-established.

Evaluate presence/degree of exercise-related pain and changes in joint mobility. Measure upper arm and forearm if edema develops.

Monitors progression/resolution of complications. May need to postpone increasing exercises and wait until further healing occurs.

Discuss types of exercises to be done at home to regain strength and enhance circulation in the affected arm.

Exercise program needs to be continued to regain optimal function of the affected side.

Coordinate exercise program into self-care and homemaker activities, e.g., dressing self, washing, swimming, dusting, mopping.

Patient is usually more willing to participate or finds it easier to maintain an exercise program that fits into lifestyle and accomplishes tasks as well.

Assist patient to identify signs and symptoms of shoulder tension, e.g., inability to maintain posture, burning sensation in postscapular region. Instruct patient to avoid sitting or holding arm in dependent position for extended periods.

Altered weight and support puts tension on surrounding structures.

Collaborative

Administer medications as indicated, e.g.:

Analgesics;

Pain needs to be controlled prior to exercise or patient may not participate optimally and incentive to exercise may be lost.

Diuretics.

May be useful in treating and preventing fluid accumulation/lymphedema.

ACTIONS/INTERVENTIONS

Collaborative

Maintain integrity of elastic bandages or custom-fitted pressure-gradient elastic sleeve.

Refer to physical/occupational therapist.

RATIONALE

Promotes venous return and decreases risk/effects of edema formation.

Provides individual exercise program. Assesses limitations/restrictions regarding employment requirements.

NURSING DIAGNOSIS:	KNOWLEDGE DEFICIT [LEARNING NEED] REGARDING CONDITION, PROGNOSIS, AND TREATMENT NEEDS
May be related to:	Lack of exposure/recall.
	Information misinterpretation.
Possibly evidenced by:	Questions/request for information; statement of misconception.
	Inaccurate follow-through of instructions/development of preventable complications.
DESIRED OUTCOMES/ EVALUATION CRITERIA— PATIENT WILL:	Verbalize understanding of disease process and treatment.
	Perform necessary procedures correctly and explain reasons for actions.
	Initiate necessary lifestyle changes and participate in treatment regimen.

ACTIONS/INTERVENTIONS

Independent

Review disease process, surgical procedure, and future expectations.

Discuss necessity for well-balanced, nutritious meals and adequate fluid intake.

Suggest alternating schedule of frequent rest and activity periods especially in situations when sitting is prolonged.

Instruct patient to protect hands and arms when gardening; use thimble when sewing; use potholders when handling hot items; use plastic gloves when doing dishes; and so forth. Do not carry purse or wear jewelry/wristwatch on affected side.

Warn against having blood withdrawn or receiving IV fluids/medications or BP measurements on the affected side.

RATIONALE

Provides knowledge base on which patient can make informed choices including participation in radiation/chemotherapy programs.

Provides optimal nutrition and maintains circulating volume to enhance tissue regeneration/healing process.

Prevents/limits fatigue, promotes healing, and enhances feelings of general well-being. Sitting with arms and head extended intensifies stress on affected structures, creating muscle tension/stiffness, and may interfere with healing.

Compromised lymphatic system causes tissues to be more susceptible to infection and/or injury, which may lead to lymphedema.

May restrict the circulation and increase risk of infection when the lymphatic system is compromised.

ACTIONS/INTERVENTIONS	RATIONALE
Independent	
Recommend wearing of a Medic-Alert device.	Prevents unnecessary trauma (e.g., BPs, injections) to affected arm.
Demonstrate use of intermittent compression as appropriate.	Pneumatic device aid is occasionally used in managing lymphedema by promoting circulation and venous return.
Suggest gentle massage of healed incision with emollients.	Stimulates circulation; promotes elasticity of skin; and reduces discomfort associated with phantom breast sensations.
Recommend use of sexual positions that avoid pressure on chest wall. Encourage alternate forms of sexual expression (cuddling, touching) during initial healing process/while operative area is still tender.	Promotes feelings of femininity and sense of ability to resume sexual activities.
Encourage regular self-examination of remaining breast. Determine recommended schedule for mammography.	Identifies changes in breast tissue indicative of recurrent/new tumor development.
Stress importance of regular medical follow-up.	Other treatment may be required as adjunctive therapy, such as radiation. Recurrence of malignant breast tumors also can be identified and managed by oncologist.
Identify signs/symptoms requiring medical evaluation, e.g., breast or arm red, warm, and swollen; edema, purulent wound drainage, fever/chills.	Lymphangitis can occur as a result of infection, causing lymphedema.

Bibliography

General References

Bellak, JP and Bamford, PA: Nursing Assessment: A Multidimensional Approach. Jones & Bartlett, Boston, 1987.
Berkow, R (ed): The Merck Manual, ed 15. Merck Sharp & Dohme Research Laboratories, Rahway, NJ, 1987.
Cella, JH and Watson, J: Nurse's Manual of Laboratory Tests. FA Davis, Philadelphia, 1989.
Condon, RE and Nyhus, LM (eds): Manual of Surgical Therapeutics, ed 7. Little, Brown & Co, Boston, 1988.
Deglin, JH, Vallerand, AH, and Russin, MM: Davis's Drug Guide for Nurses, ed 2. FA Davis, Philadelphia, 1991.
Diseases and Disorders Handbook, ed 3. Springhouse Corp, Springhouse, PA, 1989.
Doenges, ME and Moorhouse, MF: Nurse's Pocket Guide: Nursing Diagnoses with Interventions, ed 3. FA Davis, Philadelphia, 1991.
Dunagan, WC and Ridner, ML (eds): Manual of Medical Therapeutics, ed 26. Little, Brown & Co, Boston, 1989.
Fischbach, F: A Manual of Laboratory and Diagnostic Tests, ed 4. JB Lippincott, Philadelphia, 1992.
Guyton, AC: Textbook of Medical Physiology, ed 8. WB Saunders, Philadelphia, 1991.
Kuhn, MM: Pharmacotherapeutics: A Nursing Process Approach, ed 2. FA Davis, Philadelphia,1991.
Professional Guide to Diseases, ed 3. Springhouse Corp, Springhouse, PA, 1989.
Suddarth, DS (ed): The Lippincott Manual of Nursing Practice, ed 5. JB Lippincott, Philadelphia, 1991.
Thomas, CL (ed): Taber's Cyclopedic Medical Dictionary, ed 17. FA Davis, Philadelphia, 1993.
Thompson, JM, et al: Mosby's Manual of Clinical Nursing, ed 2. CV Mosby, St Louis, 1989.

Articles

Gribbin, ME. Could you detect these oncological crises? RN 53(7): 37, 1990.
Leis, HP: When is nipple discharge a sign of cancer? Medical Aspects of Human Sexuality 25(7): 32, 1991.
Rust, DL and Kloppenborg, EM: Don't underestimate the lumpectomy patient's needs. RN 53(3): 58, 1990.
Smith, RP: The Pap smear. Med Aspects of Human Sexuality 24(7): 11, 1990.
Walters, P: Chemo: A nurse's guide to action, administration and side effects. RN 53(2): 52, 1990.

CHAPTER 13

ORTHOPEDIC AND CONNECTIVE TISSUE DISORDERS

Fractures

A fracture is a discontinuity or break in a bone. There are more than 150 fracture classifications. Five major ones are as follows:

1. *Incomplete:* Fracture involves only a portion of the cross-section of the bone. One side breaks; the other usually just bends (greenstick).
2. *Complete:* Fracture line involves entire cross-section of the bone, and bone fragments are usually displaced.
3. *Closed (simple):* The fracture does not extend through the skin.
4. *Open (compound):* Bone fragments extend through the muscle and skin, which is potentially infected.
5. *Pathologic:* Fracture occurs in diseased bone (such as cancer, osteoporosis), with no or only minimal trauma.

RELATED CONCERNS

PATIENT ASSESSMENT DATA BASE

Symptoms of fracture depend on the site, severity, type, and amount of damage to other structures.

ACTIVITY/REST

May exhibit: Restricted/loss of function of affected part (may be immediate, owing to the fracture, or develop secondarily, from tissue swelling, pain).

CIRCULATION

May exhibit: Hypertension (occasionally seen as a response to pain/anxiety) or hypotension (blood loss).

Tachycardia (stress response, hypovolemia).

Pulse reduced/absent distal to injury; delayed capillary refill, pallor of affected part.

Tissue swelling or hematoma mass at site of injury.

NEUROSENSORY

May report: Loss of motion/sensation, muscle spasms.

Numbness/tingling (paresthesias).

May exhibit: Local deformities; abnormal angulation, shortening, rotation, crepitation (grating sound), muscle spasms, visible weakness/loss of function.

Agitation (may be related to pain/anxiety or other trauma).

PAIN/COMFORT

May report: Sudden severe pain at the time of injury (may be localized to the area of tissue/skeletal damage; can diminish upon immobilization); absence of pain suggests nerve damage.

Muscle spasms/cramping (after immobilization).

SAFETY

May exhibit: Skin lacerations, tissue avulsion, bleeding, color changes.

Localized swelling (may increase gradually or suddenly).

TEACHING/LEARNING

May report: Circumstances of injury.

Discharge Plan Considerations: **DRG projected mean length of stay: Femur 7.8 days; hip/pelvis, 6.7 days; all other, 4.4 days if hospitalization required.**

May require assistance with transportation, self-care activities, and homemaker/maintenance tasks.

DIAGNOSTIC STUDIES

X-ray examinations: Determine location/extent of fractures/trauma.

Bone scans, tomograms, CT/MRI scans: Visualize fractures; may also be used to identify soft-tissue damage.

Arteriograms: May be done if vascular damage is suspected.

CBC: Hct may be increased (hemoconcentration) or decreased (signifying hemorrhage at the fracture site or distant organs in multiple trauma). Increased WBC count is a normal stress response after trauma.

Cr: Muscle trauma increases load of Cr for renal clearance.

Coagulation profile: Alterations may occur owing to blood loss, multiple transfusions, or liver injury.

NURSING PRIORITIES

1. Prevent further bone/tissue injury.
2. Alleviate pain.
3. Prevent complications.
4. Provide information about condition/prognosis and treatment needs.

DISCHARGE GOALS

1. Fracture stabilized.
2. Pain controlled.
3. Complications prevented/minimized.
4. Condition, prognosis, and therapeutic regimen understood.

NURSING DIAGNOSIS:	TRAUMA, HIGH RISK FOR [ADDITIONAL]
Risk factors may include:	Loss of skeletal integrity (fractures).
Possibly evidenced by:	[Not applicable; presence of signs and symptoms establishes an actual diagnosis.]
DESIRED OUTCOMES/ EVALUATION CRITERIA— PATIENT WILL:	Maintain stabilization and alignment of fracture(s). Demonstrate body mechanics that promote stability at fracture site. Display callus formation/beginning union at fracture site as appropriate.

ACTIONS/INTERVENTIONS	RATIONALE
Independent	
Maintain bed/limb rest as indicated. Provide support of joints above and below fracture site when moving/turning.	Promotes stability; reduces possibility of disturbing alignment/healing.
Place a bedboard under the mattress or place patient on orthopedic bed.	Soft or sagging mattress may deform a wet (green) cast, crack a dry cast, or interfere with pull of traction.
Casts/Splints	
Support fracture site with pillows/folded blankets. Maintain neutral position of affected part with sandbags, splints, trochanter roll, footboard.	Prevents unnecessary movement and disruption of alignment. Proper placement of pillows also can prevent pressure deformities in the drying cast.
Use sufficient personnel for turning. Avoid using abduction bar for turning patient with spica cast.	Hip/body or multiple casts can be extremely heavy and cumbersome. Failure to properly support limbs in casts may cause the cast to break.
Evaluate splinted extremity for resolution of edema.	Coaptation splint (e.g., Jones-Sugar tong) may be used to provide immobilization of fracture while excessive tissue swelling is present. As edema subsides, readjustment of splint or application of plaster cast may be required for continued alignment of fracture.

ACTIONS/INTERVENTIONS	RATIONALE
Independent	
Traction	
Maintain position/integrity of traction (e.g., Buck's, Dunlop, Pearson, Russell).	Traction permits pull on the long axis of the fractured bone and overcomes muscle tension/shortening to facilitate alignment/union. Skeletal traction (pins, wires, tongs) permits use of greater weight for traction pull than can be applied to skin tissues.
Ascertain that all clamps are functional. Lubricate pulleys and check ropes for fraying. Secure and wrap knots with adhesive tape.	Assures that traction setup is functioning properly to avoid interruption of fracture approximation.
Keep ropes unobstructed with weights hanging free; avoid lifting/releasing weights.	Optimal amount of traction weight is maintained. *Note:* Assuring free movement of weights during repositioning of patient avoids sudden excess pull on fracture with associated pain and muscle spasm.
Assist with placement of lifts under bed wheels if indicated.	Helps maintain proper patient position and function of traction by providing counterbalance.
Position the patient so that appropriate pull is maintained on the long axis of the bone.	Promotes bone alignment and reduced complications (e.g., delayed healing/nonunion).
Review restrictions imposed by therapy, e.g., not bending at waist/sitting up with Buck's traction or not turning below the waist with Russell traction.	Maintains integrity of pull of traction.
Assess integrity of external fixation device.	Hoffman traction provides stabilization and rigid support for fractured bone without use of ropes, pulleys, or weights, thus allowing for greater patient mobility/comfort and facilitating wound care. Loose or excessively tightened clamps/nuts can alter the compression of the frame, causing misalignment.
Collaborative	
Review follow-up/serial x-rays.	Provides visual evidence of beginning callus formation/healing process to determine level of activity and need for changes in/additional therapy.
Initiate/maintain electrical stimulation if used.	May be indicated to promote bone growth in presence of delayed healing/nonunion.

NURSING DIAGNOSIS:	PAIN, [ACUTE]
May be related to:	Muscle spasms.
	Movement of bone fragments, edema, and injury to the soft tissue.
	Traction/immobility device.
	Stress, anxiety.

ACTIONS/INTERVENTIONS	RATIONALE
Independent	
Maintain immobilization of affected part by means of bed rest, cast, splint, traction. (Refer to ND: Trauma, high risk for, [Additional], p 774.)	Relieves pain and prevents bone displacement/extension of tissue injury.
Elevate and support injured extremity.	Promotes venous return, decreases edema, and may reduce pain.
Avoid use of plastic sheets/pillows under limbs in cast.	Can increase discomfort by enhancing heat production in the drying cast.
Elevate bed covers; keep linens off toes.	Maintains body warmth without discomfort of pressure of bedclothes on affected parts.
Evaluate reports of pain/discomfort, noting location and characteristics, including intensity (0–10 scale). Note nonverbal pain cues (changes in vital signs and emotions/behavior).	Influences choice of/monitors effectiveness of interventions. Level of anxiety may affect perception of/reaction to pain.
Encourage patient to discuss problems related to injury.	Helps to alleviate anxiety. Patient may feel need to relive the accident experience.
Explain procedures before beginning them.	Allows patient to prepare mentally for activity as well as to participate in controlling level of discomfort.
Medicate before care activities.	Promotes muscle relaxation and enhances participation.
Perform and supervise active/passive ROM exercises.	Maintains strength/mobility of unaffected muscles and facilitates resolution of inflammation in injured tissues.
Provide alternate comfort measures, e.g., massage, backrub, position changes.	Improves general circulation; reduces areas of local pressure and muscle fatigue.
Encourage use of stress management techniques, e.g., progressive relaxation, deep-breathing exercises, visualization/guided imagery, Therapeutic Touch.	Refocuses attention, promotes sense of control, and may enhance coping abilities in the management of pain, which is likely to persist for an extended period.

ACTIONS/INTERVENTIONS

Independent

Identify diversional activities appropriate for patient age, physical abilities, and personal preferences.

Investigate any reports of unusual/sudden pain or deep, progressive/poorly localized pain unrelieved by analgesics.

Collaborative

Apply cold/ice pack first 24–48 hours and as necessary.

Administer medications as indicated: narcotic and non-narcotic analgesics; injectable NSAID, e.g., ketorolac (Toradol); and/or muscle relaxants, e.g., cyclobenzaprine (Flexeril), hydroxyzine (Vistaril). Administer narcotics around the clock for 3–5 days.

Administer/monitor PCA if indicated.

RATIONALE

Prevents boredom, reduces tension, and can increase muscle strength; may enhance self-esteem and coping abilities.

May signal a developing complication; e.g., infection, tissue ischemia, compartmental syndrome. (Refer to ND: Tissue Perfusion, altered: peripheral high risk for, on this page.)

Reduces edema/hematoma formation, decreases pain sensation.

Given to reduce pain and/or muscle spasms. Studies of Toradol have proven it to be effective in alleviating bone pain, with longer action and fewer side effects when compared with narcotic agents. *Note:* Vistaril is often used to potentiate effects of narcotics to improve/prolong pain relief.

Routinely administered or PCA maintains adequate blood level of analgesia, preventing fluctuations in pain relief with associated muscle tension/spasms.

NURSING DIAGNOSIS:	**PERIPHERAL NEUROVASCULAR DYSFUNCTION, HIGH RISK FOR**
Risk factors may include:	Reduction/interruption of blood flow: direct vascular injury, tissue trauma, excessive edema, thrombus formation. Hypovolemia.
Possibly evidenced by:	[Not applicable; presence of signs and symptoms establishes an actual diagnosis.]
DESIRED OUTCOMES/ EVALUATION CRITERIA— PATIENT WILL:	Maintain tissue perfusion as evidenced by palpable pulses, skin warm/dry, normal sensation, usual sensorium, stable vital signs, and adequate urinary output for individual situation.

ACTIONS/INTERVENTIONS

Independent

Remove jewelry from affected limb.

Evaluate presence/quality of peripheral pulse distal to injury via palpation/Doppler. Compare with normal limb.

RATIONALE

May restrict circulation when edema occurs.

Decreased/absent pulse may reflect vascular injury and necessitates immediate medical evaluation of circulatory status. Be aware that occasionally a pulse may be palpated even though circulation is blocked by a soft clot through which pulsations may be felt. In addition, perfusion

ACTIONS/INTERVENTIONS

Independent

Assess capillary return, skin color, and warmth distal to the fracture.

Perform neurovascular assessments, noting changes in motor/sensory function. Ask patient to localize pain/discomfort.

Test sensation of peroneal nerve by pinch/pinprick in the dorsal web between the first and second toe and assess ability to dorsiflex toes if indicated.

Assess tissues around cast edges for rough places/pressure points. Investigate reports of "burning sensation" under cast.

Monitor position/location of supporting ring of splints/sling.

Maintain elevation of injured extremity(ies) unless contraindicated by confirmed presence of compartment syndrome.

Assess entire length of injured extremity for swelling/edema formation. Measure injured extremity and compare with uninjured extremity. Note appearance/spread of hematoma.

Note reports of pain extreme for type of injury or increasing pain on passive movement of extremity, development of paresthesia, muscle tension/tenderness with erythema, and change in pulse quality distal to injury. Do not elevate extremity. Report symptoms to physician at once.

Investigate sudden signs of limb ischemia, e.g., decreased skin temperature, pallor, and increased pain.

Encourage patient to routinely exercise digits/joints distal to injury. Ambulate as soon as possible.

Investigate tenderness, swelling, pain on dorsiflexion of foot (positive Homans' sign).

RATIONALE

through larger arteries may continue after increased compartment pressure has collapsed the arteriole/venule circulation in the muscle.

Return of color should be rapid (3–5 seconds). White, cool skin indicates arterial impairment. Cyanosis suggests venous impairment. *Note:* Peripheral pulses, capillary refill, skin color, and sensation may be normal even in presence of compartmental syndrome, because superficial circulation is usually not compromised.

Impaired feeling, numbness, tingling, increased/ diffuse pain occurs when circulation to nerves is inadequate or nerves are damaged.

Length and position of peroneal nerve increases risk of its injury in the presence of leg fracture, edema/compartmental syndrome, or malposition of traction apparatus.

These factors may be the cause of or be indicative of tissue pressure/ischemia, leading to breakdown/necrosis.

Traction apparatus can cause pressure on vessels/nerves, particularly in the axilla and groin, resulting in ischemia and possible permanent nerve damage.

Promotes venous drainage/decreases edema. *Note:* In presence of increased compartment pressure, elevation of the extremity actually impedes arterial flow, decreasing perfusion.

Increasing circumference of injured extremity may suggest general tissue swelling/edema but may reflect hemorrhage. *Note:* A 1-in increase in an adult thigh can equal approximately 1 unit of sequestered blood.

Continued bleeding/edema formation within a muscle enclosed by tight fascia can result in impaired blood flow and ischemic myositis or compartmental syndrome, necessitating emergency interventions to relieve pressure/restore circulation. *Note:* This condition constitutes a medical emergency and requires immediate interventions.

Fracture dislocations of joints (especially the knee) may cause damage to adjacent arteries, with resulting loss of distal blood flow.

Enhances circulation and reduces pooling of blood, especially in the lower extremities.

There is an increased potential for thrombophlebitis and pulmonary emboli in patients immobile for 5 days or more.

ACTIONS/INTERVENTIONS	RATIONALE
Independent	
Monitor vital signs. Note signs of general pallor/cyanosis, cool skin, changes in mentation.	Inadequate circulating volume will compromise systemic tissue perfusion.
Test stools/gastric aspirant for occult blood. Note continued bleeding at trauma/injection site(s) and oozing from mucous membranes.	Increased incidence of gastric bleeding accompanies fractures/trauma and may be related to stress or occasionally reflects a clotting disorder requiring further evaluation.
Collaborative	
Apply ice bags around fracture site as indicated.	Reduces edema/hematoma formation, which could impair circulation.
Split/bivalve cast as needed.	May be done on an emergency basis to relieve restriction of circulation resulting from edema formation in injured extremity.
Assist with/monitor intracompartmental pressures.	Elevation of pressure (usually to 30 mm Hg or more) indicates need for prompt evaluation and intervention.
Prepare for surgical intervention (e.g., fibulectomy/fasciotomy) as indicated.	Failure to relieve pressure/correct compartmental syndrome within 4 to 6 hours of onset can result in severe contractures/loss of function and disfigurement of extremity distal to injury or even necessitate amputation.
Monitor Hb/Hct, coagulation studies, e.g., protime levels.	Assists in calculation of blood loss and needs/effectiveness of replacement therapy.
Administer IV fluids/blood products as needed.	Maintains circulating volume, enhancing tissue perfusion.
Administer sodium warfarin (Coumadin) if indicated.	May be given prophylactically to reduce threat of deep venous thrombus.
Apply antiembolic hose/sequential pressure hose as indicated.	Decreases venous pooling and may enhance venous return, thereby reducing risk of thrombus formation.

NURSING DIAGNOSIS:	GAS EXCHANGE, IMPAIRED, HIGH RISK FOR
Risk factors may include:	Altered blood flow; blood/fat emboli.
	Alveolar/capillary membrane changes: Interstitial, pulmonary edema, congestion.
Possibly evidenced by:	[Not applicable; presence of signs and symptoms establishes an actual diagnosis.]
DESIRED OUTCOMES/ EVALUATION CRITERIA— PATIENT WILL:	Maintain adequate respiratory function, as evidenced by absence of dyspnea/cyanosis; respiratory rate and ABGs within patient's normal range.

ACTIONS/INTERVENTIONS	RATIONALE
Independent	
Monitor respiratory rate and effort. Note stridor, use of accessory muscles, retractions, development of central cyanosis.	Tachypnea, dyspnea, and changes in mentation are early signs of respiratory insufficiency and may be the only indicator of developing pulmonary emboli in the early stage. Remaining signs/symptoms reflect advanced respiratory distress/impending failure.
Auscultate breath sounds noting development of unequal, hyperresonant sounds; also note presence of crackles/rhonchi/wheezes and inspiratory crowing/croupy sounds.	Changes in/presence of adventitious breath sounds reflects developing respiratory complications, e.g., atelectasis, pneumonia, emboli, ARDS. Inspiratory crowing reflects upper airway edema and is suggestive of fat emboli.
Handle injured tissues/bones gently, especially during first several days.	This may prevent the development of fat emboli (usually seen in first 12–72 hours), which are closely associated with fractures, especially of the long bone and pelvis.
Instruct and assist with deep-breathing and coughing exercises. Reposition frequently.	Promotes alveolar ventilation and perfusion. Repositioning promotes drainage of secretions and decreases congestion in dependent lung areas.
Note increasing restlessness, confusion, lethargy, stupor.	Impaired gas exchange/presence of pulmonary emboli can cause deterioration in the patient's level of consciousness as hypoxemia/acidosis develops.
Observe sputum for signs of blood.	Hemoptysis may occur with pulmonary emboli.
Inspect skin for petechiae above nipple line; in axilla, spreading to abdomen/trunk; buccal mucosa, hard palate; conjunctival sacs and retina.	This is the most characteristic sign of fat emboli, which may appear within 2–3 days after injury.
Collaborative	
Assist with incentive spirometry.	Maximizes ventilation/oxygenation and minimizes atelectasis.
Administer supplemental O_2 if indicated.	Increases available O_2 for optimal tissue oxygenation.
Monitor laboratory studies, e.g.:	
Serial ABGs.	Decreased PaO_2 and increased $PaCO_2$ indicate impaired gas exchange/developing failure.
Hb, calcium, ESR, serum lipase, fat screen, platelets.	Anemia, hypocalcemia, elevated ESR and lipase levels, fat globules in blood/urine/sputum, and decreased platelet count (thrombocytopenia) are often associated with fat emboli.
Administer medications as indicated:	
Low-dose heparin;	Blocks the clotting cycle and prevents clot propagation in presence of thrombophlebitis.
Corticosteroids.	Steroids have been used with some success to prevent/treat fat embolus.

NURSING DIAGNOSIS:	PHYSICAL MOBILITY, IMPAIRED
May be related to:	Neuromuscular skeletal impairment; pain/discomfort; restrictive therapies (limb immobilization).
	Psychologic immobility.
Possibly evidenced by:	Inability to purposefully move within the physical environment, imposed restrictions.
	Reluctance to attempt movement; limited ROM.
	Decreased muscle strength/control.
DESIRED OUTCOMES/ EVALUATION CRITERIA— PATIENT WILL:	Regain/maintain mobility at the highest possible level.
	Maintain position of function.
	Increase strength/function of affected and compensatory body parts.
	Demonstrate techniques that enable resumption of activities.

ACTIONS/INTERVENTIONS	RATIONALE
Independent	
Assess degree of immobility produced by injury/treatment and note patient's perception of immobility.	Patient may be restricted by self-view/self-perception out of proportion with actual physical limitations, requiring information/interventions to promote progress toward wellness.
Encourage participation in diversional/recreational activities. Maintain stimulating environment, e.g., radio, TV, newspapers, personal possessions/pictures, clock, calendar, visits from family/friends.	Provides opportunity for release of energy, refocuses attention, enhances patient's sense of self-control/selfworth, and aids in reducing social isolation.
Instruct patient in/assist with active/passive ROM exercises of affected and unaffected extremities.	Increases blood flow to muscles and bone to improve muscle tone, maintain joint mobility; prevent contractures/atrophy, and calcium resorption from disuse.
Encourage use of isometric exercises starting with the unaffected limb.	Isometrics contract muscles without bending joints or moving limbs and helps to maintain muscle strength and mass. *Note:* These exercises are contraindicated while acute bleeding/edema is present.
Provide footboard, wrist splints, trochanter/hand rolls as appropriate.	Useful in maintaining functional position of extremities, hands/feet and preventing complications (e.g., contractures/foot-drop).
Place in supine position periodically if possible, when traction is used to stabilize lower limb fractures.	Reduces risk of flexion contracture of hip.

ACTIONS/INTERVENTIONS	RATIONALE
Independent	
Instruct in/encourage use of trapeze and "post position" for lower limb fractures.	Facilitates movement during hygiene/skin care, and linen changes; reduces discomfort of remaining flat in bed. "Postposition" involves placing the uninjured foot flat on the bed with the knee bent while grasping the trapeze and lifting the body off the bed.
Assist with/encourage self-care/hygiene (e.g., bathing, shaving).	Improves muscle strength and circulation, enhances patient control in situation, and promotes self-directed wellness.
Provide/assist with mobility by means of wheelchair, walker, crutches, canes as soon as possible. Instruct in safe use of mobility aids.	Early mobility reduces complications of bed rest (e.g., phlebitis), and promotes healing and normalization of organ function. Learning the correct way to use aids is important to maintain optimal mobility and patient safety.
Monitor BP with resumption of activity. Note complaints of dizziness.	Postural hypotension is a common problem following prolonged bed rest and may require specific interventions (e.g., tilt table with gradual elevation to upright position).
Reposition periodically and encourage coughing/deep-breathing exercises.	Prevents/reduces incidence of skin/respiratory complications (e.g., decubitus, atelectasis, pneumonia).
Auscultate bowel sounds. Monitor elimination habits and provide for regular bowel routine. Place on bedside commode, if feasible, or use fracture pan. Provide privacy.	Bed rest, use of analgesics, and changes in dietary habits can slow peristalsis and produce constipation. Nursing measures that facilitate elimination may prevent/limit complications. Fracture pan limits flexion of hips and lessens pressure on lumbar region/lower extremity cast.
Encourage increased fluid intake to 2000–3000 ml/d, including acid/ash juices.	Keeps the body well-hydrated, decreasing risk of urinary infection, stone formation, and constipation.
Provide diet high in proteins, carbohydrates, vitamins, and minerals. Keep protein content reduced until after first BM.	In the presence of musculoskeletal injuries, nutrients required for healing are rapidly depleted, often resulting in a weight loss of as much as 20–30 lb during skeletal traction. This can have a profound effect on muscle mass, tone, and strength. *Note:* Protein foods increase contents in small bowel, resulting in gas formation and constipation. Therefore, GI function should be fully restored before protein foods are increased.
Increase the amount of roughage in the diet. Limit gas-forming foods.	Adding bulk to stool helps prevent constipation. Gas-forming foods may cause abdominal distention, especially in presence of decreased intestinal motility.
Collaborative	
Consult with physical/occupational therapist and/or rehabilitation specialist.	Useful in creating individualized activity/exercise program. Patient may require long-term assistance with movement, strengthening, and weight-bearing activities, as well as use of adjuncts, e.g., walk-

ACTIONS/INTERVENTIONS	RATIONALE
Collaborative	
	ers, crutches, canes; elevated toilet seats; pickup sticks/reachers, special eating utensils.
Initiate bowel program (stool softeners, enemas, laxatives) as indicated.	Done to promote regular bowel evacuation.
Refer to psychiatric nurse clinical specialist/therapist as indicated.	Patient/SO may require more intensive treatment to deal with reality of current condition/prognosis, prolonged immobility, perceived loss of control.

NURSING DIAGNOSIS:	**SKIN/TISSUE INTEGRITY, IMPAIRED: ACTUAL/HIGH RISK FOR**
May be related to:	Puncture injury; compound fracture; surgical repair; insertion of traction pins, wires, screws.
	Altered sensation, circulation; accumulation of excretions/secretions.
	Physical immobilization.
Possibly evidenced by:	Reports of itching, pain, numbness, pressure of affected/surrounding area.
	Disruption of skin surface; invasion of body structures; destruction of skin layers/tissues.
DESIRED OUTCOMES/ EVALUATION CRITERIA— PATIENT WILL:	Verbalize relief of discomfort.
	Demonstrate behaviors/techniques to prevent skin breakdown/facilitate healing as indicated.
	Achieve timely wound/lesion healing if present.

ACTIONS/INTERVENTIONS	RATIONALE
Independent	
Examine the skin for open wounds, foreign bodies, rashes, bleeding, discoloration, duskiness, blanching.	Provides information regarding skin circulation and problems that may be caused by application and/or restriction of cast/splint or traction apparatus; or edema formation that may require further medical intervention.
Massage skin and bony prominences. Keep the bed dry and free of wrinkles. Place water pads/ other padding under elbow/heels as indicated.	Reduces pressure on susceptible areas and risk of abrasions/skin breakdown.
Reposition frequently. Encourage use of trapeze if possible.	Lessens constant pressure on same areas and minimizes risk of skin breakdown. Use of trapeze may reduce risk of abrasions to elbows/heels.
Assess position of splint ring of traction device.	Improper positioning may cause skin injury/breakdown.

ACTIONS/INTERVENTIONS	RATIONALE

Independent

Cast application and skin care:

Cleanse skin with soap and water. Rub gently with alcohol and/or dust with small amount of a borate or stearate of zinc powder;

Provides a dry, clean area for cast application. *Note:* Too much powder may cake when it comes in contact with water/perspiration.

Cut a length of stockinette to cover the area and extend several inches beyond the cast;

Useful for padding bony prominences, finishing cast edges, and protecting the skin.

Use palm of hand to apply, hold or move cast, and support on pillows after application;

Prevents indentations/flattening over bony prominences and weight-bearing areas (e.g., back of heels), which would cause abrasions/tissue trauma. An improperly shaped or dried cast is irritating to the underlying skin and may lead to circulatory impairment.

Trim excess plaster from edges of cast as soon as casting is completed;

Uneven plaster is irritating to the skin and may result in abrasions.

Promote cast drying by removing bed linen, exposing to circulating air;

Prevents skin breakdown caused by prolonged moisture trapped under cast.

Observe for potential pressure areas, especially at the edges of and under the splint/cast;

Pressure can cause ulcerations, necrosis, and/or nerve palsies. These problems may be painless when nerve damage is present.

Pad (petal) the edges of the cast with waterproof tape;

Provides an effective barrier to cast flaking and moisture. Helps prevent breakdown of cast material at edges and reduces skin irritation/excoriation.

Cleanse excess plaster from skin while still wet, if possible;

Dry plaster may flake into completed cast and cause skin damage.

Protect cast and skin in perineal area. Provide frequent pericare;

Prevents tissue breakdown and infection by fecal contamination.

Instruct patient/SO to avoid inserting objects inside casts;

"Scratching an itch" may cause tissue injury.

Massage the skin around the cast edges with alcohol;

Has a drying effect, which toughens the skin. Creams and lotions are not recommended because excessive oils can seal cast perimeter, not allowing the cast to "breathe." Powders are not recommended because of potential for excessive accumulation inside the cast.

Turn frequently to include the uninvolved side and prone position with patient's feet over the end of the mattress.

Minimizes pressure on feet and around cast edges.

Skin traction application and skin care:

Cleanse the skin with warm soapy water;

Reduces level of contaminants on skin.

Apply tincture of benzoin;

"Toughens" the skin for application of skin traction.

Apply commercial skin traction tapes (or make some with strips of moleskin/adhesive tape)

Traction tapes encircling a limb may compromise circulation.

ACTIONS/INTERVENTIONS	RATIONALE

Independent

lengthwise on opposite sides of the affected limb;

Extend the tapes beyond the length of the limb;

Traction is inserted in line with the free ends of the tape.

Mark the line where the tapes extend beyond the extremity;

Allows for quick assessment of slippage.

Place protective padding under the leg and over bony prominences;

Minimizes pressure on these areas.

Wrap the limb circumference, including tapes and padding, with elastic bandages, being careful to wrap snugly but not too tightly;

Provides for appropriate traction pull without compromising circulation.

Palpate taped tissues daily and document any tenderness or pain;

If area under tapes is tender, suspect skin irritation, and prepare to remove the bandage system.

Remove skin traction every 24 hours, per protocol; inspect and give skin care.

Maintains skin integrity.

Skeletal traction application and skin care:

Bend wire ends or cover ends of wires/pins with rubber or cork protectors or needle caps;

Prevents injury to other body parts.

Pad slings/frame with sheepskin, foam.

Prevents excessive pressure on skin and promotes moisture evaporation that reduces risk of excoriation.

Collaborative

Use foam mattress, sheepskins, flotation pads, or air mattress as indicated.

Because of immobilization of body parts, bony prominences other than those affected by the casting may suffer from decreased circulation.

Monovalve, bivalve, or cut a window in the cast, per protocol.

Allows the release of pressure and provides access for wound/skin care.

NURSING DIAGNOSIS:	INFECTION, HIGH RISK FOR
Risk factors may include:	Inadequate primary defenses: Broken skin, traumatized tissues; environmental exposure.
	Invasive procedures, skeletal traction.
Possibly evidenced by:	[Not applicable; presence of signs and symptoms establishes an actual diagnosis.]
DESIRED OUTCOMES/ EVALUATION CRITERIA— PATIENT WILL:	Achieve timely wound healing, free of purulent drainage or erythema, and be afebrile.

ACTIONS/INTERVENTIONS	RATIONALE

Independent

Inspect the skin for preexisting irritation or breaks in continuity.	Pins or wires should not be inserted through skin infections, rashes, or abrasions (may lead to bone infection).
Assess pin sites/skin areas noting reports of increased pain/burning sensation or presence of edema, erythema, foul odor/drainage.	May indicate onset of local infection/tissue necrosis, which can lead to osteomyelitis.
Provide sterile pin/wound care according to protocol, and exercise meticulous hand washing.	May prevent cross-contamination and possibility of infection.
Instruct patient not to touch the insertion sites.	Minimizes opportunity for contamination.
Line perineal cast edges with plastic wrap.	Damp, soiled casts can promote growth of bacteria.
Observe wounds for formation of bullae, crepitation, bronze discoloration of skin, frothy/fruity-smelling drainage.	Signs suggestive of gas gangrene infection.
Assess muscle tone, DTRs, and ability to speak.	Muscle rigidity, tonic spasms of jaw muscles, and dysphagia reflect development of tetanus.
Monitor vital signs. Note presence of chills, fever, malaise, changes in mentation.	Hypotension, confusion may be seen with gas gangrene; tachycardia and chills/fever reflect developing sepsis.
Investigate abrupt onset of pain/limitation of movement with localized edema/erythema in injured extremity.	May indicate development of osteomyelitis.
Institute prescribed isolation procedures.	Presence of purulent drainage will require wound/linen precautions to prevent cross-contamination.

Collaborative

Monitor laboratory studies, e.g.:	
CBC;	Anemia may be noted with osteomyelitis; leukocytosis is usually present with infective processes.
ESR;	Elevated in osteomyelitis.
Cultures and sensitivity of wound/serum/bone;	Identifies infective organism.
Radioisotope scans.	Hot spots signify increased areas of vascularity, indicative of osteomyelitis.
Administer medications as indicated, e.g.;	
IV/topical antibiotics;	Wide-spectrum antibiotics may be used prophylactically or may be geared toward a specific microorganism.
Tetanus toxoid.	Given prophylactically because the possibility of tetanus exists with any open wound. *Note:* Risk increases when injury/wound(s) occur in "field conditions" (outdoor/rural areas).
Provide wound/bone irrigations and apply warm/moist soaks as indicated.	Local debridement/cleansing of wounds reduces microorganisms and incidence of systemic infection. Continuous antimicrobial drip into bone may

ACTIONS/INTERVENTIONS

Collaborative

Assist with procedures, e.g., incision/drainage, placement of drains, hyperbaric O_2 therapy.

Prepare for surgery, as indicated.

RATIONALE

be necessary to treat osteomyelitis, especially if blood supply to bone is compromised.

Numerous procedures may be carried out in treatment of local infections, osteomyelitis, gas gangrene.

Sequestrectomy (removal of necrotic bone) is necessary to facilitate healing and prevent extension of infectious process.

NURSING DIAGNOSIS:	**KNOWLEDGE DEFICIT [LEARNING NEED], REGARDING CONDITION, PROGNOSIS, AND TREATMENT NEEDS**
May be related to:	Lack of exposure/recall.
	Information misinterpretation/unfamiliarity with information resources.
Possibly evidenced by:	Questions/request for information, statement of misconception.
	Inaccurate follow-through of instructions/development of preventable complications.
DESIRED OUTCOMES/ EVALUATION CRITERIA— PATIENT WILL:	Verbalize understanding of condition, prognosis, and treatment.
	Correctly perform necessary procedures and explain reasons for actions.

ACTIONS/INTERVENTIONS

Independent

Review pathology, prognosis, and future expectations.

Reinforce methods of mobility and ambulation as instructed by physical therapist when indicated.

Suggest use of a backpack.

RATIONALE

Provides knowledge base on which patient can make informed choices. *Note:* Internal fixation devices can ultimately compromise the bone's strength and intramedullary nails/rods or plates may be removed at a future date.

Most fractures require casts, splints, or braces during the healing process. Further damage and delay in healing could occur secondary to improper use of ambulatory devices.

Provides place to carry necessary articles and leave hands free to manipulate crutches or may prevent undue muscle fatigue when one arm is casted.

787

ACTIONS/INTERVENTIONS	RATIONALE

Independent

List activities the patient can perform independently and those that require assistance.

Organizes activities around need and who is available to provide help.

Identify available community services, e.g., rehabilitation teams, home nursing/homemaker services.

Provides assistance to facilitate self-care and support independence. Promotes optimal self-care and recovery.

Encourage patient to continue active exercises for the joints above and below the fracture.

Prevents joint stiffness, contractures, and muscle wasting, promoting earlier return to ADLs.

Discuss importance of clinical follow-up appointments.

Fracture healing may take as long as a year for completion, and patient cooperation with the medical regimen is helpful for proper union of bone to take place.

Review proper pin/wound care.

Reduces risk of bone/tissue trauma and infection, which can progress to osteomyelitis.

Identify signs and symptoms requiring medical evaluation, e.g., severe pain, fever/chills, foul odors; changes in sensation, swelling, burning, numbness, tingling, skin discoloration, paralysis, white/cool toes or fingertips; warm spots, soft areas, cracks in cast.

Prompt intervention may reduce severity of complications such as infection/impaired circulation. *Note:* Some darkening of the skin may occur normally when walking on the casted extremity or using casted arm; however, this should resolve with rest and elevation.

Discuss care of "green" or wet cast.

Promotes proper curing to prevent cast deformities and associated misalignment/skin irritation. *Note:* Placing a "cooling" cast directly on rubber or plastic pillows traps heat and increases drying time.

Suggest the use of a blow-dryer to dry small areas of dampened casts.

Cautious use can hasten drying.

Demonstrate use of plastic bags to cover plaster cast during wet weather or while bathing. Clean soiled cast with a slightly dampened cloth and some scouring powder.

Protects from moisture, which softens the plaster and weakens the cast. *Note:* Fiberglass casts are being used more frequently because they are not affected by moisture. In addition, their light weight may enhance patient participation in desired activities.

Recommend use of adaptive clothing.

Facilitates dressing/grooming activities.

Suggest ways to cover toes, if appropriate, e.g., stockinette or soft socks.

Helps to maintain warmth/protect from injury.

Discuss post–cast removal instructions:

    Instruct the patient to continue exercises as permitted;

Reduces stiffness and improves strength and function of affected extremity.

    Inform the patient that the skin under the cast is commonly mottled and covered with scales or crusts of dead skin;

It will be several weeks before normal appearance returns.

    Wash the skin gently with soap, povidone-iodine (Betadine), or pHisoHex, and water. Lubricate with a protective emollient;

New skin is extremely tender because it has been protected beneath a cast.

ACTIONS/INTERVENTIONS	RATIONALE

Independent

Inform the patient that muscles may appear flabby and atrophied (less muscle mass). Recommend supporting the joint above and below the affected part and the use of mobility aids, e.g., elastic bandages, splints, braces, crutches, walkers, or canes;

Muscle strength will be reduced and new or different aches and pains may occur for awhile secondary to loss of support.

Elevate the extremity as needed.

Swelling and edema tend to occur after cast removal.

Reconstructive Facial Surgery (Intermaxillary Fixation, Facial Fractures)

As with any bony fracture, stabilization and fixation of the fracture is required to promote healing and preserve function.

RELATED CONCERNS

Craniocerebral Trauma, p 271
Psychosocial Aspects of Acute Care, p 899
Surgical Intervention, p 918 (for general considerations and additional nursing care)

PATIENT ASSESSMENT DATA BASE

EGO INTEGRITY

May report:	Fear of outcome/appearance.
May exhibit:	Increased tension; sympathetic stimulation.

FOOD/FLUID

May exhibit:	Misalignment, asymmetry of jaw; malocclusion of teeth.
	Facial edema.
	Mastication, swallowing problems.

NEUROSENSORY

May report:	Paresthesia of chin, lower lip.
	Changes in vision, e.g., double vision (diplopia) if fracture extends into orbit.
May exhibit:	Unequal eye movement, loss of peripheral vision.

PAIN/COMFORT

May report:	Facial discomfort/pain.
May exhibit:	Guarding affected area.
	Altered facial muscle tone, generalized muscle tension.

RESPIRATION

May exhibit:	Tachypnea; shallow, rapid, or labored respirations.
	Interference with airway patency (misalignment of mandible, swelling of oral tissues).
	Presence of foreign materials, e.g., broken dentures/teeth, vomitus, external debris.
	Crepitus in face/neck.

SAFETY

May report:	Trauma deformities: Recent injury to bony framework, cartilaginous structures, and soft tissues (bruising, lacerations, edema).

TEACHING/LEARNING

May report:	Family/personal history of diabetes or keloid formation.

Discharge Plan Considerations: **DRG projected mean length of stay: 4.1 days.**

May require assistance with food preparation/dietary intake.

DIAGNOSTIC STUDIES

Facial x-rays: Reveal extent of fracture(s).

NURSING PRIORITIES

1. Assure patent airway.
2. Prevent complications.
3. Assist patient to develop realistic expectations/adjust to altered appearance.
4. Provide information about procedure(s)/prognosis and treatment needs.

DISCHARGE GOALS

1. Airway patent.
2. Complications/infection minimized/prevented.
3. Anxiety reduced and patient dealing realistically with situation.
4. Surgical procedure/prognosis and therapeutic regimen understood.

NURSING DIAGNOSIS:	AIRWAY CLEARANCE, INEFFECTIVE, HIGH RISK FOR
Risk factors may include:	Trauma to soft tissues/airway (surgery and/or injuries).
Possibly evidenced by:	[Not applicable; presence of signs and symptoms establishes an actual diagnosis.]
DESIRED OUTCOMES/ EVALUATION CRITERIA— PATIENT WILL:	Maintain/regain patency of airway with normal respiratory pattern, breath sounds clear and noiseless, and aspiration prevented.
	Demonstrate behaviors to improve/maintain patent airway/dispose of secretions.

ACTIONS/INTERVENTIONS	RATIONALE
Independent	
Elevate head of bed 30 degrees.	Promotes drainage of secretions and reduces edema formation; enhances venous/lymphatic drainage and risk of aspiration.
Observe respiratory rate/rhythm. Note use of accessory muscles, nasal flaring, crowing respirations/stridor, hoarseness.	May indicate impending respiratory failure. Trauma to soft tissue and bone usually produces marked edema of facial tissue, which may develop to its maximum 24 hours after the trauma/surgery.
Examine mouth for swelling, discoloration, accumulation of oral secretions or blood. Encourage patient to "push" secretions through clamped jaw. Suction as necessary/teach patient self-suctioning techniques.	Careful examination is required because bleeding may be "hidden." Removal of material keeps the airway clear and reduces risk of aspiration.

791

ACTIONS/INTERVENTIONS	RATIONALE
Independent	
Note patient's report of increasing dysphagia, high-pitched cough, wheezing, facial tissue edema.	May indicate soft-tissue swelling in the posterior pharynx.
Monitor vital signs and changes in mentation.	Tachycardia/increasing restlessness may indicate developing hypoxia/respiratory compromise.
Auscultate breath sounds.	Presence of wheezes/rhonchi suggests retained secretions, indicating need for more aggressive intervention.
Assess color of nail beds, fingers/toes.	Helpful in determining adequacy of oxygenation. *Note:* Face may appear dusky because of venous congestion, rather than hypoxia.
Apply ice bags to operative area as indicated.	Reduces edema/tissue congestion.
Reposition periodically and encourage deep breathing.	Promotes ventilation of all lung segments and mobilization of secretions, reducing risk of atelectasis and pneumonia.
Inform patient s/he will be carefully observed and needs will be met promptly.	May feel fearful about choking or suffocating because of wires.
Encourage fluid intake of at least 2–3 L/d as possible. Avoid carbonated beverages.	Liquefies oral/respiratory secretions to enhance expectoration. Carbonated beverages "foam" in the oropharynx area and may be difficult for patient to handle, thereby compromising airway.
Tend closely when patient is vomiting or taking fluids/food.	Provides reassurance and allows for prompt intervention if problems arise.
Keep wirecutters/scissors at bedside. Post drawing at bedside depicting which wires are to be cut in emergency situation.	When the jaw is wired, there are usually 2–6 major wires/bands that may need cutting to release the jaw and open the airway.
Collaborative	
Provide humidified air or O$_2$ by face tent.	Reduces congestion, moisturizes mucous membranes, and liquefies secretions. Supplemental O$_2$ may improve oxygenation/correct hypoxia.
Maintain NPO and patency of NG tube if used.	Reduces risk of vomiting/regurgitation and aspiration.
Administer antiemetics, e.g., hydroxyzine (Vistaril) as indicated.	Used to prevent vomiting, which may obstruct the airway/cause aspiration.
Assist with procedures as needed:	
Insertion/maintenance of drains/Hemovacs;	Hematoma/drainage in area may need to be evacuated if swelling is compromising airway.
Tracheostomy.	May be needed when airway is threatened by swelling/major facial reconstruction.

NURSING DIAGNOSIS:	TISSUE INTEGRITY, IMPAIRED
May be related to:	Tissue trauma/damage, preexisting injury/intraoperative manipulation.

	Mechanical factors (fixation devices).
	Altered circulation.
	Nutritional deficit.
Possibly evidenced by:	Edema.
	Hematoma, ecchymotic areas.
	Erythema, inflammation.
	Delayed healing.
DESIRED OUTCOMES/ EVALUATION CRITERIA— PATIENT WILL:	Demonstrate behaviors to promote healing.
	Display timely healing of incisional areas without complications.

ACTIONS/INTERVENTIONS	RATIONALE
Independent	
Remind patient (in immediate postoperative period) about fixation devices and that mouth cannot be opened.	Individual coming out of anesthesia may feel panic when s/he cannot open mouth, and struggling to do so can be damaging.
Monitor facial edema. Assess skin/tissue color and temperature around/under dressings. Observe for oral and facial bleeding, drainage. Apply ice packs and maintain pressure dressings to face (when used).	Vascular nature of tissues increases risk of hemorrhage. Ice packs/pressure dressings may be used (12–24 hours) to limit edema formation, but dressings may need to be loosened to prevent compromising circulation to tissues.
Cleanse mouth frequently with lukewarm saline or dilute peroxide solutions, especially after each feeding.	Promotes healing and reduces risk of infection by keeping suture line clean and intact.
Use low-pressure spray (e.g., WaterPik) or soft-bristled, child-sized toothbrush to cleanse area. Brush teeth and gums, around arch bars, other fixation devices.	Removes debris, food particles, reducing risk of inflammation/tissue deterioration, especially of gums.
Avoid use of sponge/cotton-tipped applicators for mouth care and use of lemon-glycerine or commercial mouthwash preparations.	Fibers may lodge under wires/between teeth and irritate fragile tissues. Products containing alcohol are drying to mucous membranes.
Apply bees/dental wax to ends of wires. Instruct patient to remove wax before eating or mouth care.	Protects buccal tissue from injury.
Provide local wound/pin site care if indicated.	Reduces risk of infection/osteomyelitis when wire or pin fixation is used to stabilize facial fractures.
Inspect mouth/sutures. Observe for development of erythema, inflammation, and drainage/ulcerations around gum/suture line. Avoid disturbing sutures.	Early identification and treatment of localized infection can prevent more serious complications, e.g., bacteremia, osteomyelitis, brain infection.
Note continuance or increase in pain, development of throbbing pain; presence of opaque/odoriferous drainage.	May indicate infection. Any jaw fracture involving a tooth-bearing portion is considered a compound fracture, even when there is no break in the soft tissue, because the tooth allows communication be-

ACTIONS/INTERVENTIONS

Independent

Perform neurologic checks as indicated, noting changes in mentation, reports of increased headache, onset of fever. Note rhinorrhea/otorrhea.

Collaborative

Monitor Hct/Hb, clotting studies.

Apply topical ointments to suture lines if indicated, maintaining sterile technique as appropriate.

Administer IV/oral antimicrobials as indicated.

RATIONALE

tween the mouth and the fracture that can lead to infection. This may lead to the development of gangrene (even gas gangrene) or abscess formation that may involve the oropharynx and endanger airway patency.

May indicate meningeal irritation/brain infection as a complication of facial fractures or localized infection. When head injuries have occurred concurrently with facial injuries, cerebrospinal fluid leak indicates communication between brain and outside, predisposing to meningitis.

Abnormalities may indicate bleeding and/or hematoma formation.

May be used to reduce topical bacteria, which interfere with fine-line suture healing.

Reduces risk of/prevents local and systemic infection.

NURSING DIAGNOSIS:	COMMUNICATION, IMPAIRED: VERBAL
May be related to:	Wiring of jaws. Edema of mouth and surrounding structures. Pain of tissue/muscle movement.
Possibly evidenced by:	Inability/reluctance to talk.
DESIRED OUTCOMES/ EVALUATION CRITERIA— PATIENT WILL:	Establish method of communication in which needs can be expressed.

ACTIONS/INTERVENTIONS

Independent

Determine extent of inability to communicate.

Provide alternate means of communication, e.g., pencil and pad, magic slate, picture board. Place call light/bell where patient can reach it; answer promptly.

Validate meaning of attempted communication. Maintain eye contact. Use "Yes" and "No," blink, and so forth.

RATIONALE

Type of injuries/individual situation will dictate needs for assistance.

Enables patient to communicate needs/concerns, and reduces anxiety associated with being alone/unable to summon help.

Conveys interest in individual and desire to communicate, encouraging continued attempts. Limits frustration and fatigue that can occur with lengthy "conversation."

ACTIONS/INTERVENTIONS

Independent

Anticipate needs. Stop in frequently to check on patient.

Place notice at nurses' station and at bedside concerning communication needs and how they are met. Answer summons promptly.

RATIONALE

Reduces anxiety and feelings of powerlessness.

Patient may not be able to enunciate clearly or obtain emergency/needed assistance.

NURSING DIAGNOSIS:	NUTRITION, ALTERED: LESS THAN BODY REQUIREMENTS, HIGH RISK FOR
Risk factors may include:	Biologic factors (structural changes).
	Facial/tissue edema.
	Inability to chew/swallow.
	Anorexia.
Possibly evidenced by:	[Not applicable; presence of signs and symptoms establishes an actual diagnosis.]
DESIRED OUTCOMES/ EVALUATION CRITERIA— PATIENT WILL:	Maintain usual weight as individually appropriate with timely healing and be free of signs of malnutrition.

ACTIONS/INTERVENTIONS

Independent

Weigh as indicated.

Provide ice chips, water, or other beverages as soon as nausea subsides.

Recommend patient lean forward when ingesting food/fluid. Serve each food in an individual container. Instruct patient in use of straw/feeding syringe as indicated. Provide small/frequent "meals" of acceptable consistency, such as pureed or semiliquid.

Avoid temperature extremes of foods/fluids.

Consult with dietitian to provide diet high in calories, vitamins, proteins, and dietary supplements as indicated.

Provide commercial supplements as indicated, e.g., Ensure.

RATIONALE

Monitors weight loss and effectiveness of dietary program.

Maintains adequate fluid intake to prevent dehydration.

Facilitates swallowing and reduces risk of aspiration. Being able to identify various flavors adds to the pleasure of eating when patient is unable to masticate.

Reduces risk of injuring tender mucosal areas.

Adequate nutrition is important to promote healing and combat excessive weight loss (can reach 10–20 lb in a short period). Patient/SO may need assistance in food choices/menu planning to meet individual dietary needs in view of difficulty with ingestion of nutrients.

Decreased energy/easy fatigability may lead to difficulty ingesting adequate nutrients, and use of these specially formulated products can enhance nutritional intake.

NURSING DIAGNOSIS:	PAIN, [ACUTE]
May be related to:	Presence of tissue and bone trauma, wires, edema.
	Nasal congestion/inability to breathe through nose.
	Immobility in jaw (fixation).
Possibly evidenced by:	Reports of pain.
	Narrowed focus, grimacing, facial tension.
	Sympathetic stimulation.
DESIRED OUTCOMES/ EVALUATION CRITERIA— PATIENT WILL:	Report pain is relieved/controlled.
	Follow prescribed pharmacologic regimen.
	Demonstrate use of relaxation techniques.

ACTIONS/INTERVENTIONS	RATIONALE
Independent	
Assess type/location of pain. Note intensity on a 0–10 scale. Note response to medication.	Useful in differentiating postoperative discomfort from developing complications and in evaluating effectiveness of interventions.
Provide information about anticipated discomforts and relieving interventions.	Knowing what to expect can prevent surprises and resultant anxiety.
Provide frequent oral hygiene; lubricate lips.	Reduces discomfort associated with dry mouth/pooled secretions.
Examine mouth for loose or protruding wires. Apply dental wax to wire ends.	Wires may irritate or damage surrounding tissues.
Maintain immobilization of facial fractures by appropriate means, e.g., nasal packing, wires, pins, and so on.	Maintains proper positioning and prevents undue stress on supporting musculature.
Perform passive/active ROM to extremities/joints. Encourage position changes even when up in chair.	Reduces discomfort and stiffness, stimulates circulation that may be sluggish due to bed rest and areas of tissue edema.
Provide comfort measures, e.g., backrub, diversional activities.	Promotes relaxation and refocuses attention.
Allow time for expression of feelings, within level of ability to communicate.	Expression of concerns/fears reduces anxiety/pain cycle.
Encourage use of stress management techniques, e.g., deep breathing, visualization, diversional activities.	Promotes relaxation, refocuses attention, and may enhance coping ability, relieving pain.
Collaborative	
Administer medications as indicated:	
Analgesics;	May be needed to provide relief for pain/discomfort.

ACTIONS/INTERVENTIONS	RATIONALE
Collaborative	
Nasal decongestants;	Helps relieve upper airway congestion/feeling of suffocation. *Note:* Must be used with caution or may be contraindicated because can reduce local blood supply needed for healing.
Steroids, e.g., dexamethasone (Decadron).	Reduces inflammatory response and tissue edema.
Apply cold/warm compresses.	Cold is used initially to prevent/minimize edema formation. Heat enhances circulation, promoting resolution of edema.
Provide supplemental humidification.	Relieves discomfort of dry mucous membranes.

NURSING DIAGNOSIS:	ANXIETY [SPECIFY LEVEL]/FEAR
May be related to:	Situational crisis.
	Perceived threat to self-concept/body image.
	Perceived threat of death (choking/suffocation).
Possibly evidenced by:	Increased tension, apprehension.
	Expressed concern regarding changes.
	Fearfulness.
	Sympathetic stimulation/restlessness.
DESIRED OUTCOMES/ EVALUATION CRITERIA— PATIENT WILL:	Appear relaxed and report anxiety reduced to manageable level.
	Acknowledge and discuss fears.
	Demonstrate appropriate range of feelings.

ACTIONS/INTERVENTIONS	RATIONALE
Independent	
Discuss safety measures, e.g., suctioning secretions, use of wire cutters, suture cleansing. Place necessary articles within reach.	Provides reassurance and reduces anxiety associated with unknown and/or fear of being alone (unsupervised).
Encourage expression of fears/concerns.	Defines problem and influences choice of interventions.
Acknowledge reality/normality of feelings, including anger.	Provides emotional support that can help patient through the initial adjustment as well as throughout recovery.
Give realistic explanation about altered facial appearance, possible nerve involvement, facial droop, uneven smile, presence of circumoral numbness/tingling, altered taste sensation.	Providing honest information about what to expect will help patient/SO to accept and deal with situation more effectively.

ACTIONS/INTERVENTIONS

Independent

Provide patient with mirror on request.

Encourage use of stress management, e.g., deep-breathing, guided imagery, visualization.

RATIONALE

As edema resolves and healing occurs, alterations in facial nerve function may disappear.

Assists in refocusing attention, promotes relaxation, and may enhance coping ability.

NURSING DIAGNOSIS:	KNOWLEDGE DEFICIT [LEARNING NEED], REGARDING CONDITION, PROGNOSIS, AND TREATMENT NEEDS.
May be related to:	Lack of exposure/recall.
	Information misinterpretation.
	Unfamiliarity with information resources.
Possibly evidenced by:	Questions, request for information, statement of misconception.
	Inaccurate follow-through of instruction.
	Development of preventable complications.
DESIRED OUTCOMES/ EVALUATION CRITERIA— PATIENT WILL:	Verbalize understanding of condition/disease process, prognosis, and treatment.
	Correctly perform necessary procedures and explain reasons for the actions.

ACTIONS/INTERVENTIONS

Independent

Review surgical procedure/prognosis and potential complications.

Instruct patient/SO to carry wire cutters at all times and to know which wire(s) to cut.

Review prescribed medications, e.g., vitamin supplements, stool softeners/mild laxatives, use of and cautions about decongestants as indicated.

Stress importance of medical follow-up.

Discuss signs/symptoms to report to health care provider, e.g., increased pain, edema, fever, halitosis/foul odor from mouth.

RATIONALE

Provides knowledge base on which informed choices about future care and outcome can be made.

Permits immediate intervention to maintain airway in case of emergency.

Reinforces information patient needs to promote optimal recuperation and prevent untoward occurrences (including constipation from lack of dietary fiber). Decongestants may occasionally be used to decrease nasal congestion but are contraindicated in some facial fractures.

Necessary for evaluation of healing/jaw stabilization as well as presence of complications, e.g., oral fistula formation, jaw malalignment.

Prompt evaluation and intervention of developing infection reduces risk of more serious complications, e.g., sepsis, osteomyelitis, brain infection.

ACTIONS/INTERVENTIONS	RATIONALE
Independent	
Recommend progressing diet as tolerated.	Muscle stiffness and dental malocclusion may delay capability for eating normal foods for a time (usually 5–6 weeks).
Review dietary needs. Identify high-calorie, low-fiber foods. Provide recipes for blenderized balanced meals. Suggest addition of spices after oral mucosa heals.	Promotes intake of adequate nutrients to meet metabolic needs, especially during time when weight loss is common. Low-fiber foods reduce risk of materials lodging under fixation devices/between teeth and becoming a medium for growth of pathogenic microorganisms. Addition of spices/new recipes may improve appetite and make food more palatable.
Stress importance of good oral hygiene. Demonstrate use of water spray (e.g., WaterPik), dental wax.	Fixation devices usually remain in place 6–8 weeks and are associated with risk of local irritation, inflammation, and local/systemic infection.
Recommend avoidance of alcohol and alcohol-containing products, e.g., mouthwash, liquid decongestants.	Alcohol is drying and may cause irritation to oral mucosa. In addition, alcoholic beverages dull oral sensation and reflexes necessary to protect the airway.
Discuss activity limitations, e.g., swimming, boating, fishing, and so forth, until wires are removed.	Jaw fixation increases risk of aspiration/drowning, as well as potential for infection by bacteria in untreated water or tissue irritation from chlorine.
Suggest restricting/stopping smoking.	Can irritate mucosa and cause vasoconstriction, which may further impair circulation to involved tissues.

Amputation

In general, amputations are caused by accidents, disease, and congenital disorders. For the purpose of this plan of care, amputation refers to the surgical/traumatic removal of a limb. Lower-extremity amputations are performed much more frequently than upper-extremity amputations. Five levels are currently used in lower-extremity amputation: foot and ankle, below knee (BKA), knee disarticulation and above, knee-hip disarticulation; and hemipelvectomy and translumbar amputation. There are two types of amputations: (1) open (provisional), which requires strict aseptic techniques and later revisions and (2) closed, or "flap."

RELATED CONCERNS

Psychosocial Aspects of Acute Care, p 899
Surgical Intervention, p 918

PATIENT ASSESSMENT DATA BASE

Data are dependent on underlying reason for surgical procedure, e.g., severe trauma, peripheral vascular/arterial occlusive disease, diabetic neuropathy, osteomyelitis, cancer.

ACTIVITY/REST

May report: Actual/anticipated limitations imposed by condition/amputation.

EGO INTEGRITY

May report: Concern about anticipated changes in lifestyle, financial situation, reaction of others.

Feelings of helplessness, powerlessness.

May exhibit: Anxiety, apprehension, irritability, anger, fearfulness, withdrawal, false cheerfulness.

SEXUALITY

May report: Concerns about intimate relationships.

SOCIAL INTERACTION

May report: Problems related to illness/condition.

Concern about role function, reaction of others.

TEACHING/LEARNING

Discharge Plan Considerations: **DRG projected mean length of stay: 9.7 days.**

May require assistance with wound care/supplies, adaptation to prosthesis/ambulatory devices, transportation, homemaker/maintenance tasks, possibly self-care activities and vocational retraining.

DIAGNOSTIC STUDIES

Studies are dependent on underlying condition necessitating amputation and are used to determine the appropriate level for amputation.

X-rays: Identify skeletal abnormalities.

CT scan: Identifies neoplastic lesions, osteomyelitis, hematoma formation.

Angiography and blood flow studies: Evaluate alteration in circulation/tissue perfusion and help predict potential for tissue healing after amputation.

Doppler ultrasound, laser doppler flowmetry: Performed to assess and measure blood flow.

Transcutaneous O$_2$ pressure: Maps out areas of greater and lesser perfusion in the involved extremity.

Thermography: Measures temperature differences in the ischemic limb at two sites, from cutaneous tissue to center of bone. The lower the difference between the two readings, the greater the chance for healing.

Plethysmography: Segmental systolic BP measurements to the lower extremity evaluates arterial blood flow.

ESR: Elevation indicates inflammatory response.

Wound cultures: Identify presence of infection and causative organism.

Biopsy: Confirms diagnosis of benign/malignant mass.

WBC/differential: Elevation and "shift to left" suggests infectious process.

NURSING PRIORITIES

1. Support psychologic and physiologic adjustment.
2. Alleviate pain.
3. Prevent complications.
4. Promote mobility/functional abilities.
5. Provide information about surgical procedure/prognosis and treatment needs.

DISCHARGE GOALS

1. Dealing with current situation realistically.
2. Pain relieved/controlled.
3. Complications prevented/minimized.
4. Mobility/function regained or compensated for.
5. Surgical procedure, prognosis, and therapeutic regimen understood.

NURSING DIAGNOSIS:	SELF-ESTEEM/BODY IMAGE DISTURBANCE, ROLE PERFORMANCE, ALTERED
May be related to:	Biophysical factor: loss of body part.
Possibly evidenced by:	Anticipated changes in lifestyle; fear of rejection/reaction by others.
	Negative feelings about body.
	Focus on past strength, function, or appearance.
	Feelings of helplessness, powerlessness.
	Preoccupation with missing body part, not looking at/or touching body part.
	Perceived change in usual patterns of responsibility/physical capacity to resume role.
DESIRED OUTCOMES/ EVALUATION CRITERIA— PATIENT WILL:	Begin to show adaptation and verbalize acceptance of self in situation (amputee).
	Recognize and incorporate changes into self-concept in accurate manner without negating self-esteem.
	Develop realistic plans for adapting to new role/role modifications.

ACTIONS/INTERVENTIONS	RATIONALE
Independent	
Assess/consider the patient's preparation for and view of amputation.	The patient who views amputation as lifesaving or reconstructive will accept the new self more quickly. The patient with traumatic amputation or who considers amputation to be the result of failure in treatment is at greater risk for self-concept disturbances.
Encourage expression of fears, negative feelings, and grief over loss of body part.	Venting emotions helps patient begin to deal with the fact and reality of life without a limb.
Reinforce preoperative information including type/location of amputation, type of prosthetic fitting if appropriate (immediate, delayed), expected postoperative course, including pain control and rehabilitation.	Provides opportunity for patient to question and assimilate information, and begin to deal with changes in body image and function, which can facilitate postoperative recovery.
Assess degree of support available to the patient.	Sufficient support by SO and friends can facilitate rehabilitation process.
Discuss patient's perceptions of self related to change and how patient sees self in usual lifestyle/role functioning.	Aids in defining concerns in relation to previous lifestyle and facilitates problem solving. For example, may fear loss of independence, ability to work, and so forth.
Ascertain individual strengths and identify previous positive coping behaviors.	Helpful to build on strengths that are already available for patient to use in coping with current situation.
Encourage participation in ADLs. Provide opportunities to view/care for stump using the moment to point out positive signs of healing.	Promotes independence and enhances feelings of self-worth. Although integrating of stump into body image can take months or even years, looking at the stump and hearing positive comments (made in a normal, matter-of-fact manner) can help patient with this acceptance.
Encourage/provide for visit by another amputee, especially one who is successfully rehabilitating.	A peer who has been through a similar experience serves as a role model and can provide validity to comments as well as hope for recovery and a normal future.
Provide open environment for patient to discuss concerns about sexuality.	Promotes sharing of beliefs/values about sensitive subject and identifies misconceptions/myths that may interfere with adjustment to situation.
Note withdrawn behavior, negative self-talk, use of denial or overconcern with actual/perceived changes.	Identifies stage of grief/need for interventions.
Collaborative	
Discuss availability of various resources, e.g., psychiatric/sexual counseling, occupational therapist.	May need assistance for these concerns to facilitate optimal adaptation and rehabilitation.

NURSING DIAGNOSIS:	PAIN, [ACUTE]
May be related to:	Physical injury/tissue and nerve trauma.

	Psychologic impact of loss of body part.
Possibly evidenced by:	Reports of pain.
	Narrowed self-focus.
	Autonomic responses, guarding/protective behavior.
DESIRED OUTCOMES/ EVALUATION CRITERIA— PATIENT WILL:	Report pain is relieved/controlled.
	Appear relaxed and able to rest/sleep appropriately.
	Verbalize understanding of phantom pain and methods to provide relief.

ACTIONS/INTERVENTIONS

Independent

Document location and intensity of pain (0–10 scale). Investigate changes in pain characteristics, e.g., numbness, tingling.

Elevate affected part by raising foot of bed slightly or use of pillow/sling for upper-limb amputation.

Acknowledge reality of phantom-limb sensations, that this is usually self-limiting and that various modalities will be tried for pain relief.

Provide comfort measures (e.g., frequent turning, backrub) and diversional activities. Encourage use of stress management techniques (e.g., deep-breathing exercises, visualization, guided imagery) and Therapeutic Touch.

Provide gentle massage to stump as tolerated once dressings are discontinued.

Investigate reports of progressive/poorly localized pain unrelieved by analgesics.

Collaborative

Administer medications, as indicated, e.g.: analgesics, muscle relaxants. Instruct in PCA.

RATIONALE

Aids in evaluating need for and effectiveness of interventions. Changes may indicate developing complications, e.g., necrosis/infection.

Lessens edema formation by enhancing venous return; reduces muscle fatigue and skin/tissue pressure. *Note:* After initial 24 hours and in absence of edema, stump may be extended and kept flat.

Knowing about these sensations allows the patient to understand this is a normal phenomenon that may develop immediately or several weeks postoperatively. Although the sensations usually resolve on their own, some individuals continue to experience the discomfort for several months/years. *Note:* Phantom pain is not well relieved by traditional pain medications. TENS has proven to offer the most effective short-term relief, in addition to managing stump and prosthesis problems.

Refocuses attention, promotes relaxation, may enhance coping abilities and may decrease occurrence of phantom-limb pain.

Enhances circulation; reduces muscle tension.

May indicate developing compartmental syndrome, especially following traumatic injury. (Refer to CP: Fractures; ND: Tissue Perfusion, altered: Peripheral, high risk for, p 777.)

Reduces pain/muscle spasms. *Note:* PCA provides for timely drug administration preventing

803

ACTIONS/INTERVENTIONS	RATIONALE

Collaborative

	fluctuations in pain with associated muscle tension/spasms.
Maintain TENS device if used.	Provides continuous low-level nerve stimulation, blocking transmission of pain sensation.
Provide topical heat as indicated.	May be used to promote muscle relaxation, enhance circulation, and facilitate resolution of edema.

NURSING DIAGNOSIS:	TISSUE PERFUSION, ALTERED: PERIPHERAL, HIGH RISK FOR
Risk factors may include:	Reduced arterial/venous blood flow; tissue edema, hematoma formation.
	Hypovolemia.
Possibly evidenced by:	[Not applicable; presence of signs and symptoms establishes an actual diagnosis.]
DESIRED OUTCOMES/ EVALUATION CRITERIA— PATIENT WILL:	Maintain adequate tissue perfusion as evidenced by palpable peripheral pulses, warm/dry skin, and timely wound healing.

ACTIONS/INTERVENTIONS	RATIONALE

Independent

Monitor vital signs. Palpate peripheral pulses, noting strength and equality.	General indicators of circulatory status and adequacy of perfusion.
Perform periodic neurovascular assessments, e.g., sensation, movement, pulse, skin color and temperature.	Postoperative tissue edema, hematoma formation, or restrictive dressings may impair circulation to stump, resulting in tissue necrosis.
Inspect dressings/drainage device, noting amount and characteristics of drainage.	Continued blood loss may indicate need for additional fluid replacement and evaluation for coagulation defect or surgical intervention to ligate bleeder.
Apply direct pressure to bleeding site, if hemorrhage occurs. Contact physician immediately.	Direct pressure to bleeding site may be followed by application of a bulk dressing secured with an elastic wrap once bleeding is controlled.
Evaluate nonoperated lower limb for inflammation, positive Homans' sign.	Increased incidence of thrombus formation in patients with preexisting peripheral vascular disease/diabetic changes.

Collaborative

Administer IV fluids/blood products as indicated.	Maintains circulating volume to maximize tissue perfusion.

ACTIONS/INTERVENTIONS	RATIONALE

Collaborative

Apply antiembolic/sequential hose to nonoperated leg.

May enhance venous return reducing venous pooling and risk of thrombophlebitis.

Administer low-dose anticoagulant as indicated.

May be useful in preventing thrombus formation without increasing risk of postoperative bleed/hematoma formation.

Monitor laboratory studies, e.g.:

Hb/Hct;

Indicators of hypovolemia/dehydration that can impair tissue perfusion.

PT/APTT.

Evaluates need for/effectiveness of anticoagulant therapy and identifies developing complication, e.g., posttraumatic DIC.

NURSING DIAGNOSIS:	INFECTION, HIGH RISK FOR
Risk factors may include:	Inadequate primary defenses (broken skin, traumatized tissue). Invasive procedures; environmental exposure. Chronic disease, altered nutritional status.
Possibly evidenced by:	[Not applicable; presence of signs and symptoms establishes an actual diagnosis.]
DESIRED OUTCOMES/ EVALUATION CRITERIA— PATIENT WILL:	Achieve timely wound healing; be free of purulent drainage or erythema; and be afebrile.

ACTIONS/INTERVENTIONS	RATIONALE

Independent

Maintain aseptic technique when changing dressings/caring for wound.

Minimizes opportunity for introduction of bacteria.

Inspect dressings and wound; note characteristics of drainage.

Early detection of developing infection provides opportunity for timely intervention and prevention of more serious complications (e.g., osteomyelitis).

Maintain patency and routinely empty drainage device.

Hemovac, Jackson-Pratt drains facilitate removal of drainage, promoting wound healing and reducing risk of infection.

Cover dressing with plastic when using the bedpan or if incontinent.

Prevents contamination in lower-limb amputation.

Expose stump to air; wash with mild soap and water after dressings are discontinued.

Maintains cleanliness, minimizes skin contaminants, and promotes healing of tender/fragile skin.

Monitor vital signs.

Temperature elevation/tachycardia may reflect developing sepsis.

ACTIONS/INTERVENTIONS

Collaborative

Obtain wound/drainage cultures as appropriate.

Administer antibiotics as indicated.

RATIONALE

Identifies presence of infection/specific organisms.

Wide-spectrum antibiotics may be used prophylactically, or antibiotic therapy may be geared toward specific organisms.

NURSING DIAGNOSIS:	PHYSICAL MOBILITY, IMPAIRED
May be related to:	Loss of a limb (particularly a lower extremity); pain/discomfort; perceptual impairment (altered sense of balance).
Possibly evidenced by:	Reluctance to attempt movement.
	Impaired coordination; decreased muscle strength, control, and mass.
DESIRED OUTCOMES/ EVALUATION CRITERIA— PATIENT WILL:	Verbalize understanding of individual situation, treatment regimen, and safety measures.
	Display willingness to participate in activities.
	Maintain position of function as evidenced by absence of contractures.
	Demonstrate techniques/behaviors that enable resumption of activities.

ACTIONS/INTERVENTIONS

Independent

Provide regular stump care, e.g., inspect area, cleanse and dry thoroughly, and rewrap stump with elastic bandage or air splint, or apply a stump shrinker (heavy stockinette sock), for "delayed" prosthesis. Measure circumference periodically.

Rewrap stump immediately with an elastic bandage, elevate if "immediate/early" cast is accidentally dislodged. Prepare for reapplication of cast.

Assist with specified ROM exercises for the affected as well as unaffected limbs beginning early in postoperative stage.

Encourage active/isometric exercises for upper torso and arms.

RATIONALE

Provides opportunity to evaluate healing and note complications (unless covered by immediate prosthesis). Wrapping stump controls edema and helps form stump into conical shape to facilitate fitting of prosthesis. *Note:* Air splint may be preferred, because it permits visual inspection of the wound. Measurement is done to estimate shrinkage to assure proper fit of sock and prosthesis.

Edema will occur rapidly, and rehabilitation can be delayed.

Prevents contracture deformities, which can develop rapidly and could delay prosthesis usage.

Increases muscle strength to facilitate transfers/ambulation.

ACTIONS/INTERVENTIONS	RATIONALE

Independent

Provide trochanter rolls as indicated.

Prevents external rotation of lower-limb stump.

Instruct patient to lie in prone position as tolerated at least twice a day with pillow under abdomen and lower-extremity stump.

Strengthens extensor muscles and prevents flexion contracture of the hip.

Caution against keeping pillows under lower-extremity stump or allowing BKA limb to hang dependently over side of bed or chair.

Use of pillows can cause permanent flexion contracture of hip and a dependent position of stump impairs venous return and may increase edema formation.

Demonstrate/assist with transfer techniques and use of mobility aids, e.g., trapeze, crutches, or walker.

Facilitates self-care and patient's independence. Proper transfer techniques prevent shearing abrasions/dermal injury related to "scooting."

Assist with ambulation.

Reduces potential for injury. Ambulation after lower-limb amputation is dependent on timing of prosthesis placement. For example: (1) *Immediate postoperative fitting:* A rigid plaster of Paris dressing is applied to the stump and a pylon and artificial foot is attached. Weight bearing begins within 24–48 hours. (2) *Early postoperative fitting:* Weight bearing does not occur until 10–30 days postoperatively. (3) *Delayed fitting:* More common in areas that do not have facilities available for immediate/early application of prosthesis or when the condition of the stump and/or the patient precludes these choices. *Note:* Amputation of an upper extremity may initially affect the patient's sense of balance necessitating monitoring/assistance with ambulation.

Help patient continue preoperative muscle exercises as able/when allowed out of bed; e.g., patient should (while holding on to chair for balance) perform abdominal-tightening exercises and knee bends; hop on foot; stand on toes.

Contributes to gaining improved sense of balance and strengthens compensatory body parts.

Instruct patient in stump-conditioning exercises, e.g., pushing the stump against a pillow initially, then progressing to harder surface.

Hardens the stump by toughening the skin and altering feedback of resected nerves to facilitate use of prosthesis.

Collaborative

Refer to rehabilitation team, e.g., physical and occupational therapy.

Provides for creation of exercise/activity program to meet individual needs and strengths, and identifies mobility functional aids to promote independence. Early use of a temporary prosthesis promotes activity and enhances general well-being/positive outlook. *Note:* Vocational counseling/retraining also may be indicated.

Provide foam/flotation mattress.

Reduces pressure on skin/tissues that can impair circulation, potentiating risk of tissue ischemia/breakdown.

NURSING DIAGNOSIS:	KNOWLEDGE DEFICIT [LEARNING NEED] REGARDING CONDITION, PROGNOSIS, AND TREATMENT NEEDS
May be related to:	Lack of exposure/recall.
	Information misinterpretation.
Possibly evidenced by:	Questions/request for information, verbalization of the problem.
	Inaccurate follow-through of instructions/development of preventable complications.
DESIRED OUTCOMES/ EVALUATION CRITERIA— PATIENT WILL:	Verbalize understanding of condition/disease process and treatment.
	Correctly perform necessary procedures and explain reasons for the actions.
	Initiate necessary lifestyle changes and participate in treatment regimen.

ACTIONS/INTERVENTIONS	RATIONALE
Independent	
Review disease process/surgical procedure and future expectations.	Provides knowledge base on which patient can make informed choices.
Instruct in dressing/wound care, inspection of stump using mirror to visualize all areas, skin massage, and appropriate wrapping of the stump.	Promotes competent self-care; facilitates healing and fitting of prosthesis and reduces potential for complications.
Discuss general stump care, e.g.:	
Massaging the stump after dressings are discontinued and suture line is healed;	Massage softens scar and prevents adherence to the bone, decreases tenderness, and stimulates circulation.
Avoiding use of lotions/powders;	Although a small amount of lotion may be indicated if skin is dry, emollients/creams soften skin and may cause maceration when a prosthesis is worn. Powder may cake, potentiating skin irritation.
Wearing only properly fitted, clean, wrinkle-free limb sock;	Stump may continue to shrink for up to 2 years, and an improperly fitting sock or one that is mended or dirty can cause skin irritation/breakdown.
Using clean cotton T-shirt under harness for upper-limb prosthesis.	Absorbs perspiration; prevents skin irritation from harness.
Demonstrate care of prosthetic device. Stress importance of routine maintenance/periodic refitting.	Ensures proper fit, reduces risk of complications, and prolongs life of prosthesis.
Encourage continuation of postoperative exercise program.	Enhances circulation/healing and function of affected part, facilitating adaptation to prosthetic device.

ACTIONS/INTERVENTIONS	RATIONALE
Independent	
Identify techniques to manage phantom pain, e.g., good stump care, properly fitted prosthesis, gentle massage/pressure to stump. Stress control, relaxation training, and various medications that may be used.	Reduces muscle tension and enhances control of situation and coping abilities.
Stress importance of well-balanced diet and adequate fluid intake.	Provides needed nutrients for tissue regeneration/healing, aids in maintaining circulating volume and normal organ function, and aids in maintenance of proper weight (weight changes affect fit of prosthesis).
Recommend cessation of smoking.	Smoking potentiates peripheral vasoconstriction, impairing circulation as well as tissue oxygenation.
Identify signs/symptoms requiring medical evaluation, e.g., edema, erythema, increased/odorous drainage from incision; changes in sensation, movement, skin color; persistent phantom pain.	Prompt intervention may prevent serious complication and/or loss of function. *Note:* Chronic phantom-limb pain may indicate neuroma, requiring surgical resection.
Identify community support and rehabilitation, e.g., certified prosthetist-orthotist, amputee groups, home nursing service, homemaker services as needed.	Facilitates transfer to home, supports independence, and enhances coping.

Total Joint Replacement _____

Joint replacement is indicated for irreversibly damaged joints and unremitting pain (e.g., degenerative and rheumatoid arthritis [RA]); selected fractures (e.g., femoral neck), joint instability, and congenital hip disease. The surgery can be performed on any joint except the spine. Hip and knee replacement is the most common surgery. The prosthesis may be metallic or polyethylene (or a combination) and implanted with an acrylic cement, or it may be a porous, coated implant that encourages bony ingrowth.

RELATED CONCERNS

Cancer, p 1014
Psychosocial Aspects of Acute Care, p 899
Rheumatoid Arthritis, p 875
Surgical Intervention, p 918

PATIENT ASSESSMENT DATA BASE

ACTIVITY/REST

May report: Difficulty with ambulation; stiffness in joints (worse in the morning or after period of inactivity).

History of occupation/participation in sports activities that wears on particular joint.

Inability to participate in occupational/recreational activities at desired level.

Interruption of sleep, delayed falling asleep/awakened by pain. Does not feel well-rested.

CIRCULATION

May exhibit: Presence of edema; diminished pulses in affected joint, limb/digits.

HYGIENE

May report: Difficulty performing ADLs.

Use of special equipment/devices.

Need for assistance.

NEUROSENSORY

May exhibit: Impaired ROM of affected joints.

PAIN/COMFORT

May report: Pain (dull, aching, persistent) in affected joint(s), worsened by movement.

SAFETY

May report: Traumatic injury/fractures affecting the joint.

Bone tumor, congenital deformities.

History of inflammatory, debilitating arthritis (RA or osteoarthritis); aseptic necrosis of the joint head.

TEACHING/LEARNING

May report: Current medication use, e.g., anti-inflammatory, analgesics/narcotics, steroids.

Discharge Plan Considerations:

DRG projected mean length of stay: 10.6 days.

May need assistance with transportation, self-care activities, homemaker/maintenance tasks, possible placement in extended care facility for continued rehabilitation/assistance.

DIAGNOSTIC STUDIES

X-rays and scans of bones/joints: Determine extent of degeneration and rule out malignancy.

NURSING PRIORITIES

1. Prevent complications.
2. Promote optimal mobility.
3. Alleviate pain.
4. Provide information about diagnosis, prognosis, and treatment needs.

DISCHARGE GOALS

1. Complications prevented/minimized.
2. Mobility increased.
3. Pain relieved/controlled.
4. Diagnosis, prognosis, and therapeutic regimen understood.

NURSING DIAGNOSIS: **INFECTION, HIGH RISK FOR**

Risk factors may include:

Inadequate primary defenses (broken skin, exposure of joint).

Inadequate secondary defenses/immunosuppression (long-term corticosteroid use, cancer).

Invasive procedures; surgical manipulation; implantation of foreign body.

Decreased mobility.

Possibly evidenced by: [Not applicable; presence of signs and symptoms establishes an actual diagnosis.]

DESIRED OUTCOMES/ EVALUATION CRITERIA— PATIENT WILL: Achieve timely wound healing, be free of purulent drainage or erythema, and be afebrile.

ACTIONS/INTERVENTIONS	RATIONALE
Independent	
Promote good hand washing by staff and patient.	Reduces risk of cross-contamination.
Use strict aseptic or clean techniques as indicated to reinforce/change dressings and when handling drains. Instruct patient not to touch/scratch incision.	Prevents contamination and risk of wound infection, which could require removal of prosthesis.

ACTIONS/INTERVENTIONS	RATIONALE
Independent	
Maintain patency of drainage devices (e.g., Hemovac/Jackson-Pratt). Note characteristics of wound drainage.	Reduces risk of infection by preventing accumulation of blood and secretions in the joint space (medium for bacterial growth). Purulent, non-serous, odorous drainage is indicative of infection, and continuous drainage from incision may reflect developing skin tract, which can potentiate infectious process.
Assess skin/incision color, temperature and integrity; note presence of erythema/inflammation, loss of wound approximation.	Provides information about status of healing process and alerts staff to early signs of infection.
Investigate reports of increased wound pain, changes in characteristics of pain.	Deep, dull, aching pain in operative area may indicate infection in joint. *Note:* Infection is devastating because joint cannot be saved once infection and prosthetic loss occurs.
Monitor temperature. Note presence of chills.	Although temperature elevations are common in early postoperative phase, elevations occurring 5 or more days postoperatively and/or presence of chills usually indicate developing infection requiring intervention to prevent more serious complications, e.g., sepsis, osteomyelitis, tissue necrosis, and prosthetic failure.
Encourage fluid intake, high-protein diet with roughage.	Maintains fluid and nutritional balance to support tissue perfusion and provide nutrients necessary for cellular regeneration and tissue healing.
Collaborative	
Maintain reverse isolation, if appropriate.	May be done initially to reduce contact with sources of possible infection, especially in elderly, immunosuppressed, or diabetic patient.
Administer antibiotics as indicated.	May be used prophylactically to prevent infection.
Culture drainage routinely/as needed.	Verifies presence of infection; identifies causative organism. Anaerobic or aerobic bacteria may be present, which affect choice of antibiotic and therapy.

NURSING DIAGNOSIS:	PHYSICAL MOBILITY, IMPAIRED
May be related to:	Pain and discomfort, musculoskeletal impairment.
	Surgery/restrictive therapies.
Possibly evidenced by:	Reluctance to attempt movement, difficulty purposefully moving within the physical environment.
	Reports of pain/discomfort on movement.
	Limited ROM; decreased muscle strength/control.

ORTHOPEDIC AND CONNECTIVE TISSUE DISORDERS: Total Joint Replacement

<table>
<tr><td>

DESIRED OUTCOMES/ EVALUATION CRITERIA— PATIENT WILL:

</td><td>

Maintain position of function, as evidenced by absence of contracture.

Display increased strength and function of affected joint and limb.

Verbalize understanding of individual treatment regimen and participate in rehabilitation program.

</td></tr>
</table>

ACTIONS/INTERVENTIONS	RATIONALE
Independent	
Maintain initial bed rest with affected joint in prescribed position and body in alignment.	Provides time for stabilization of prosthesis and recovery from effects of anesthesia, reducing risk of injury. Length of bed rest depends on joint replaced (e.g., usually 24–72 hours for hip).
Limit use of semi/high-Fowler's position, if indicated.	Prolonged hip flexion may strain/dislocate new prosthesis.
Elevate extremity by raising foot of bed slightly, not knee gatch. Limit movement as indicated, e.g., keep operative leg slightly abducted after total hip or knee replacement to prevent crossing of legs/inward rotation of joint.	Enhances venous return to prevent excessive edema formation; may prevent dislocation of prosthesis. Use of knee gatch or pillow under knee can compromise circulation.
Medicate prior to procedures/activities.	Muscle relaxants, narcotics/analgesics decrease pain, reduce muscle tension/spasm, and facilitate participation in therapy.
Turn on unoperated side using adequate number of personnel and maintaining operated extremity in neutral alignment. Support position with pillows/wedges.	Prevents dislocation of hip prosthesis and prolonged skin/tissue pressure reducing risk of tissue ischemia/breakdown.
Demonstrate/assist with transfer techniques and use of mobility aids, e.g., trapeze, walker.	Facilitates self-care and patient's independence. Proper transfer techniques prevent shearing abrasions of skin, and falls.
Inspect skin; observe for reddened areas. Keep linens dry and wrinkle-free. Massage skin/bony prominences routinely.	Prevents skin irritation/breakdown.
Perform/assist with ROM to unaffected joints.	Patient with degenerative joint disease can quickly lose joint function during periods of restricted activity.
Promote participation in routine exercise program, e.g.:	
Total hip: Quadriceps and gluteal muscle setting, hip-hiking, isometrics, leg lifts, dorsiflexion, plantar flexion of the foot. *Total knee:* Quadriceps setting, gluteal contraction, flexion/extension exercises, isometrics.	Strengthens muscle groups, increasing muscle tone and mass; stimulates circulation; prevents decubitus. Active use of the joint may be painful but will not injure the joint. In fact, continuous passive exercise is usually mechanically performed on the knee joint within the first 48–72 hours.
Other joints: Exercises are individually designed, e.g., toes and knee movements (for ankle-joint	Meets individual needs of the joint that is replaced.

ACTIONS/INTERVENTIONS	RATIONALE

Independent

replacement); arm and unaffected fingers (for finger-joint replacement).

Observe appropriate limitations based on specific joint; e.g., avoid marked flexion/rotation of hip and flexion or hyperextension of leg; adhere to weight-bearing restrictions; wear knee immobilizer as indicated.

Joint stress is to be avoided at all times during stabilization period to prevent dislocation of new prosthesis.

Investigate sudden increased pain and shortening of limb and well as changes in skin color, temperature, and sensation.

Indicative of slippage of prosthesis, requiring medical evaluation/intervention.

Encourage participation in ADLs.

Enhances self-esteem; promotes sense of control and independence.

Provide positive reinforcement for efforts.

Promotes a positive attitude and encourages involvement in therapy.

Collaborative

Consult with physical/occupational therapists and rehabilitation specialist.

Useful in creating individualized activity/exercise program. Patient may require ongoing assistance with movement, strengthening, and weight-bearing activities as well as use of adjuncts, e.g., walkers, crutches, canes, elevated toilet seat, pickup sticks, and so on.

Provide foam/flotation mattress.

Reduces skin/tissue pressure; limits feelings of fatigue and general discomfort.

NURSING DIAGNOSIS:	TISSUE PERFUSION, ALTERED: PERIPHERAL HIGH RISK FOR
Risk factors may include:	Reduced arterial/venous blood flow: Trauma to blood vessels; tissue edema, improper location/dislocation of prosthesis.
	Hypovolemia.
Possibly evidenced by:	[Not applicable; presence of signs and symptoms establishes an actual diagnosis.]
DESIRED OUTCOMES/ EVALUATION CRITERIA— PATIENT WILL:	Demonstrate adequate tissue perfusion as evidenced by palpable pulses, skin warm/dry, stable vital signs.

ACTIONS/INTERVENTIONS	RATIONALE

Independent

Palpate pulses. Evaluate capillary refill as well as skin color and temperature. Compare with nonoperated limb.

Diminished/absent pulses, delayed capillary refill time, pallor, blanching, cyanosis, and coldness of skin reflect diminished circulation/perfusion. Com-

ACTIONS/INTERVENTIONS

Independent

Assess motion and sensation of operated extremity.

Test sensation of peroneal nerve by pinch/pinprick in the dorsal web between first and second toe and assess ability to dorsiflex toes after hip/knee replacement.

Monitor vital signs.

Monitor amount and characteristics of drainage on dressings/from suction device. Note swelling in operative area.

Ensure that stabilizing devices (e.g., trochanter rolls, sling on splint device, traction apparatus) are in correct position and are not exerting undue pressure on skin and underlying tissue. Avoid use of pillow or knee gatch under knees.

Evaluate for calf tenderness, positive Homans' sign, and inflammation.

Observe for signs of continued bleeding, oozing from puncture sites/mucous membranes, or ecchymosis following minimal trauma.

Observe for restlessness, confusion, sudden chest pain, dyspnea, tachycardia, fever, development of petechiae.

Collaborative

Administer IV fluids, blood/plasma expanders as needed.

Monitor laboratory studies, e.g.:

Hct;

Coagulation studies.

RATIONALE

parison with unoperated limb provides clues as to whether problem is localized or generalized.

Increasing pain, numbness/tingling, inability to perform expected movements (e.g., flex foot) suggest nerve injury, compromised circulation, or dislocation of prosthesis, requiring immediate intervention.

Position and length of peroneal nerve increases risk of direct injury or compression by tissue edema/hematoma.

Tachycardia and decreasing BP may reflect response to hypovolemia/blood loss or suggest anaphylaxis related to absorption of methylmethacrylate into systemic circulation. *Note:* This occurs less often because of the advent of prosthetics with a porous layer that fosters ingrowth of bone instead of total reliance on adhesives to internally fix the device.

May indicate excessive bleeding/hematoma formation, which can potentiate neurovascular compromise.

Reduces risk of pressure on underlying nerves or compromised circulation to extremities.

Early identification of thrombus development and intervention may prevent embolus formation.

Depression of clotting mechanisms/sensitivity to anticoagulants may result in bleeding episodes that can affect RBC level/circulating volume.

Fat emboli can occur (usually in first 72 hours postoperatively) because of traumatic manipulation of bone marrow during implantation of hip prosthesis.

Restores circulating volume to maintain perfusion.

Usually done 24–48 hours postoperatively for evaluation of blood loss, which can be quite large because of high vascularity of surgical site.

Evaluates presence/degree of alteration in clotting mechanisms and effects of anticoagulant/antiplatelet agents when used.

ACTIONS/INTERVENTIONS

Collaborative

Administer medications as indicated, e.g.: sodium warfarin (Coumadin), heparin, aspirin, low-molecular-weight dextran.

Apply cold/heat as indicated.

Apply elastic leg wraps or antiembolic stockings.

Prepare for surgical procedure as indicated.

RATIONALE

Anticoagulants/antiplatelet agents may be used to reduce risk of thrombophlebitis and fat emboli.

Ice packs are used initially to limit edema/hematoma formation. Heat may then be used to enhance circulation, facilitating resolution of tissue edema.

Promotes venous return and prevents venous stasis, reducing risk of thrombus formation.

Evacuation of hematoma or relocation of prosthesis may be required to correct compromised circulation.

NURSING DIAGNOSIS:	PAIN [ACUTE]
May be related to:	Injuring agents: Biologic, physical/psychologic (e.g., muscle spasms, surgical procedure, preexisting chronic joint diseases, elderly age, anxiety).
Possibly evidenced by:	Reports of pain; distraction/guarding behaviors.
	Narrowed focus/self-focusing.
	Alteration in muscle tone; autonomic responses.
DESIRED OUTCOMES/ EVALUATION CRITERIA— PATIENT WILL:	Report pain relieved/controlled.
	Demonstrate use of relaxation skills and diversional activities as indicated by individual situation.
	Appear relaxed, able to rest/sleep appropriately.

ACTIONS/INTERVENTIONS

Independent

Assess reports of pain, noting intensity (scale of 0–10), duration, and location.

Maintain proper position of operated extremity.

Provide comfort measures (e.g., use of lumbar roll, frequent repositioning, backrub) and diversional activities. Encourage stress management techniques (e.g., progressive relaxation, guided imagery, visualization) and use of Therapeutic Touch.

Medicate prior to activities/procedures.

Investigate reports of sudden, severe joint pain with muscle spasms and changes in joint mobility; sudden, severe chest pain with dyspnea and restlessness.

RATIONALE

Provides information on which to base and monitor effectiveness of interventions.

Reduces muscle spasm and undue tension on new prosthesis and surrounding tissues.

Reduces muscle tension, refocuses attention, promotes sense of control, and may enhance coping abilities in the management of discomfort/pain, which can persist for an extended period.

Reduces muscle tension; facilitates participation.

Early recognition of developing problems, such as dislocation of prosthesis or pulmonary emboli (blood/fat), provides opportunity for prompt intervention and prevention of more serious complications.

ACTIONS/INTERVENTIONS

Collaborative

Administer narcotics, analgesics, and muscle relaxants as needed.

Apply ice packs as indicated.

Maintain TENS unit if used.

Maintain extremity mobilization: e.g., ambulation, physical therapy, exerciser devices, continuous passive-motion devices.

RATIONALE

Relieves surgical pain and reduces muscle tension/spasm, which contributes to overall discomfort.

Promotes vasoconstriction to reduce bleeding/tissue edema in surgical area and lessens perception of discomfort.

Provides constant low-level electrical stimulation to nerves blocking transmission of sensations of pain.

Increases circulation to affected muscles. Minimizes joint stiffness; relieves muscle spasms related to disuse.

NURSING DIAGNOSIS:	KNOWLEDGE DEFICIT [LEARNING NEED], REGARDING CONDITION, PROGNOSIS, AND TREATMENT NEEDS
May be related to:	Lack of exposure/recall.
	Information misinterpretation.
Possibly evidenced by:	Questions/request for information, statement of misconception.
	Inaccurate follow-through of instructions/development of preventable complications.
DESIRED OUTCOMES/ EVALUATION CRITERIA— PATIENT WILL:	Verbalize understanding of surgical procedure and prognosis.
	Correctly perform necessary procedures and explain reasons for the actions.

ACTIONS/INTERVENTIONS

Independent

Review disease process, surgical procedure, and future expectations.

Encourage alternating rest periods with activity.

Stress importance of continuing prescribed exercise/rehabilitation program within patient's tolerance: crutch/cane walking, weight-bearing exercises, stationary bicycling, or swimming.

Review long-term activity limitations, dependent on joint replaced, e.g., sitting for long periods or in

RATIONALE

Provides knowledge base on which patient can make informed choices.

Conserves energy for healing and prevents undue fatigue, which can increase risk of injury/fall.

Increases muscle strength and joint mobility. Some patients may be involved in formal rehabilitation programs or be followed by physical therapists in extended-care facilities. Muscle aching indicates too much weight bearing or activity, signaling a need to cut back.

Prevents undue stress on implant.

ACTIONS/INTERVENTIONS	RATIONALE

Independent

low chair/toilet seat, jogging, jumping, excessive bending, lifting, twisting or crossing legs.

Discuss need for safe environment in home (e.g., removing scatter rugs and unnecessary furniture) and use of assistive devices (e.g., handrails in tub/toilet, raised toilet seat, cane for long walks).

Reduces risk of falls and excessive stress on joints.

Review incisional/wound care.

Promotes independence in self-care, reducing risk of complications.

Stress importance of continuing to wear antiembolic stockings.

Prevents venous pooling; enhances venous return to reduce risk of thrombophlebitis.

Identify signs/symptoms requiring medical evaluation, e.g., fever/chills, incisional inflammation, unusual wound drainage, pain in calf or upper thigh, or development of "strep" throat/dental infections.

Bacterial infections require prompt treatment to prevent progression to osteomyelitis in the operative area and prosthesis failure, which could occur at any time, even years later.

Review drug regimen, e.g., anticoagulants or antibiotics for invasive procedures (e.g., tooth extraction).

Prophylactic therapy may be necessary for a prolonged period after discharge to limit risk of thromboemboli/infection. Procedures known to cause bacteremia can result in osteomyelitis and prosthesis failure.

Identify bleeding precautions, (e.g., use of soft toothbrush, electric razor, avoidance of trauma/forceful blowing of nose), and necessity of routine laboratory follow-up.

Reduces risk of therapy-induced bleeding/hemorrhage.

Encourage intake of balanced diet including roughage and adequate fluids.

Enhances healing and feeling of general well-being. Promotes bowel and bladder function during period of altered activity.

Bibliography

General References

Bellak, JP and Bamford, PA: Nursing Assessment: A Multidimensional Approach. Jones & Bartlett, Boston, 1987.

Berkow, R (ed): The Merck Manual, ed 15. Merck Sharp & Dohme Research Laboratories, Rahway, NJ, 1987.

Cella, JH and Watson, J: Nurse's Manual of Laboratory Tests. FA Davis, Philadelphia, 1989.

Condon, RE, and Nyhus, LM (eds): Manual of Surgical Therapeutics, ed 7. Little, Brown & Co, Boston, 1988.

Deglin, JH and Vallerand, AH: Davis's Drug Guide for Nurses, ed 3. FA Davis, Philadelphia, 1992.

Diseases and Disorders Handbook, ed 3. Springhouse Corp, Springhouse, PA, 1989.

Doenges, ME and Moorhouse, MF: Nurse's Pocket Guide: Nursing Diagnoses with Interventions, ed 3. FA Davis, Philadelphia, 1991.

Dunagan, WC and Ridner, ML (eds): Manual of Medical Therapeutics, ed 26. Little, Brown & Co, Boston, 1989.

Fischbach, F: A Manual of Laboratory and Diagnostic Tests, ed 4. JB Lippincott, Philadelphia, 1992.

Guyton, AC: Textbook of Medical Physiology, ed 8. WB Saunders, Philadelphia, 1991.

Kuhn, MM: Pharmacotherapeutics: A Nursing Process Approach, ed 2. FA Davis, Philadelphia,1991.

Professional Guide to Diseases, ed 3. Springhouse Corp, Springhouse, PA, 1989.

Suddarth, DS (ed): The Lippincott Manual of Nursing Practice, ed 5. JB Lippincott, Philadelphia, 1991.

Thomas, CL (ed): Taber's Cyclopedic Medical Dictionary, ed 17. FA Davis, Philadelphia, 1993.

Thompson, JM, et al: Mosby's Manual of Clinical Nursing, ed 2. CV Mosby, St Louis, 1989.

Articles

Barkett, PA: ACTION STAT! Obstructed airway with wired jaws. Nursing91 21(12):33, 1991.

Broadhurst, C: Adjusting to amputation. Nursing Times 85(43):55, 1989.

Coffey, M: Total knee replacement. Nursing Times 87(36):37, 1991.

Dunajcik, LM: The hip: When the joint must be replaced. RN 52(4):62, 1989.

Kravitz, M: Immune consequences of trauma. Paper presentation at Colorado Nurses' Association Chitaquaqua, Vail, CO, July 1992.

Lenaghan, NA: After the trauma—Managing its effects down to the last letter. Nursing92 22(3):45, 1992.

McHenry, C: Handy work. Nursing Times 87(45):18, 1991.

Meehan, M: Nursing Dx: Potential for aspiration. RN 55(1):30, 1992.

Meyer, C: Nurses vote for the most valuable new drugs. AJN 91(9):33, 1991.

Shearmon, M: Getting Sydney on his feet. Nursing Times 87(15):36, 1991.

Walker, I: Instructions to patients following rhinoplasty. Plastic and Reconstructive Surgeon, Colorado Springs, CO.

Williamson, VC: Amputation of the lower extremity: An overview. Orthopaedic Nursing 11(2):55, 1992.

CHAPTER 14
INTEGUMENTARY DISORDERS

Burns: Thermal/Chemical/Electrical (Acute and Convalescent Phase)

Thermal burns: Injuring agent can be flame, hot liquid, or contact with hot object. Flame burns are associated with smoke/inhalation injury.

Chemical burns: Occur from type/content of injuring agent, as well as concentration and temperature of agent.

Electrical burns: Occur from type/voltage of current that generates heat in proportion to resistance offered and travels the pathway of least resistance (i.e., nerves offer the least resistance and bones the greatest resistance). Underlying injury will be more severe than visible injury.

Superficial partial-thickness burns (first degree): Involve only the epidermis. Wounds appear bright pink to red with minimal edema and no blisters. The skin is often warm/dry.

Moderate partial-thickness burns (second degree): Involve the epidermis and dermis. Wounds appear red to pink with moderate edema and moist, weeping blisters.

Deep partial-thickness burns (second degree): Involve the deep dermis. Wounds appear pink to pale ivory with moderate edema and blisters. These wounds are dryer than the moderate partial thickness burns.

Full-thickness burns (third degree): Involve all layers of skin, subcutaneous fat, and may involve the muscle, nerves, and blood supply. Wound appearance varies from white, cherry red, to brown or black, with blistering uncommon. These wounds have a dry, leathery texture.

Full-thickness burns (fourth degree): Involve all skin layers plus muscle, organ tissue, and bone. Charring occurs.

RELATED CONCERNS

Adult Respiratory Distress Syndrome, p 217
Fluid and Electrolyte Imbalances, p 1054
Psychosocial Aspects of Acute Care, p 899
Sepsis/Septicemia, p 887
Total Nutritional Support, p 1039
Upper Gastrointestinal/Esophageal Bleeding, p 454

PATIENT ASSESSMENT DATA BASE

Data are dependent on type, severity, and body surface area involved.

ACTIVITY/REST

May exhibit: Decreased strength, endurance.

Limited ROM of involved areas.

Impaired muscle mass, altered tone.

CIRCULATION

May exhibit (with burn injury involving more than 20% TBSA):   Hypotension (shock).

Peripheral pulses diminished distal to extremity injury; generalized peripheral vasoconstriction with loss of pulses, mottling of skin and coolness (electrical shock).

Tachycardia (shock/anxiety/pain).

Dysrhythmias (electrical shock).

Tissue edema formation (all burns).

EGO INTEGRITY

May report: Concerns about family, job, finances, disfigurement.

May exhibit: Anxiety, crying, dependency, denial, withdrawal, hostility.

ELIMINATION

May exhibit: Urinary output decreased/absent during emergent phase. Color may be reddish black if myoglobin present, indicating deep-muscle damage.

Diuresis (after capillary leak sealed and fluids mobilized back into circulation).

Bowel sounds decreased/absent, especially in cutaneous burns of greater than 20% as stress reduces gastric motility/peristalsis.

FOOD/FLUID

May exhibit: Generalized tissue edema.

Anorexia, nausea/vomiting.

NEUROSENSORY

May report: Mixed areas of numbness, tingling.

May exhibit: Changes in orientation, affect, behavior.

Decreased DTRs in injured extremities.

Seizure activity (electrical shock).

Corneal lacerations, retinal damage, decreased visual acuity (electrical shock).

Rupture of tympanic membrane (electrical shock).

Paralysis (electrical injury to nerve pathways).

PAIN/COMFORT

May report: Pain varies, e.g., first-degree burns are extremely sensitive to touch, pressure, air movement, and temperature changes; second-degree moderate-thickness burns are very painful, while pain response in second-degree deep-thickness burns is dependent on intactness of nerve endings; third-degree burns are painless.

RESPIRATION

May report: Confinement in a closed space, prolonged exposure (possibility of inhalation injury).

May exhibit: Hoarseness, wheezy cough, carbonaceous particles in sputum, drooling/inability to swallow oral secretions, and cyanosis, indicative of inhalation injury.

Thoracic excursion may be limited in presence of circumferential chest burns.

Upper airway stridor/wheezes (obstruction due to laryngospasm, laryngeal edema).

Breath sounds: Crackles (pulmonary edema), stridor (laryngeal edema), profuse airway secretions (rhonchi).

SAFETY

May exhibit: Skin: General: Exact depth of tissue destruction may not be evident for 3–5 days due to the process of microvascular thromboses in some wounds. Unburned skin areas may be cool/clammy, pale, with slow capillary refill in the presence of decreased cardiac output due to fluid loss/shock state.

Flame injury: There may be areas of mixed depth of injury due to varied intensity of heat produced by burning clothing. Singed nasal hairs; dry, red mucosa of nose and mouth; blisters on posterior pharynx; circumoral and/or circumnasal edema.

Chemical injury: Appearance of wound varies according to causative agent. Skin may be yellowish brown with soft leatherlike texture; blisters, ulcers, necrosis, or thick eschar. Injuries are generally deeper than they appear cutaneously, and tissue destruction can continue for up to 72 hours after injury.

Electrical injury: The external cutaneous injury is usually much less than the underlying necrosis. Appearance of wounds varies and may include entry/exit (explosive) wounds of current, arc burns from current moving in close proximity to body, and thermal burns due to ignition of clothing.

Presence of fractures/dislocations (concurrent falls, motor vehicle accident; tetanic muscle contractions due to electrical shock).

TEACHING/LEARNING

Discharge plan considerations: **DRG projected mean length of stay: Dependent on severity and involvement of other organ systems.**

May require assistance with treatments, wound care/supplies, self-care activities, homemaker/maintenance tasks, transportation, finances, vocational counseling; changes in physical layout of home or living facility other than home during prolonged rehabilitation.

DIAGNOSTIC STUDIES

CBC: Initial increased Hct suggests hemoconcentration due to fluid shift/loss. Later decreased Hct and RBCs may occur due to heat damage to vascular endothelium.

WBCs: Leukocytosis can occur due to loss of cells at wound site and inflammatory response to injury.

ABGs: Baseline especially important with suspicion of inhalation injury. Reduced PaO_2/increased $PaCO_2$ may be seen with carbon monoxide retention. Acidosis may occur due to reduced renal function and loss of compensatory respiratory mechanisms.

COHbg (carboxyhemoglobin): Elevation of greater than 15% indicates carbon monoxide poisoning/inhalation injury.

Serum electrolytes: Potassium may be initially elevated due to injured tissues/RBC destruction and decreased renal function; hypokalemia can occur when diuresis starts; magnesium may be decreased. Sodium initially may be decreased with body water losses; hypernatremia can occur later as renal conservation occurs.

Random urine sodium: Greater than 20 mEq/L indicates excessive fluid resuscitation; less than 10 mEq/L suggests inadequate fluid resuscitation.

Alkaline phosphatase: Elevated due to interstitial fluid shifts/impairment of sodium pump.

Serum glucose: Elevation reflects stress response.

Serum albumin: Albumin/globulin ratio may be reversed due to loss of protein in edema fluid.

BUN/Cr: Elevation reflects decreased renal perfusion/function; however, Cr can elevate because of tissue injury.

Urine: Presence of albumin, Hb, and myoglobin indicates deep-tissue damage and protein loss (especially seen with serious electrical burns). Reddish black color of urine is due to presence of myoglobin. Wound cultures: May be obtained for baseline data and repeated periodically.

Chest x-ray: May appear normal in early postburn period even with inhalation injury; however, a true inhalation injury will present as a progressive whiteout on x-ray (ARDS).

Fiberoptic bronchoscopy: Useful in diagnosing extent of inhalation injury; findings can include edema, hemorrhage, and/or ulceration of upper respiratory tract.

Flow volume loop: Provides noninvasive assessment of effects/extent of inhalation injury.

Lung scan: May be done to determine extent of inhalation injury.

ECG: Signs of myocardial ischemia/dysrhythmias may occur with electrical burns.

Photographs of burns: Provides documentation for later burn wound healing.

NURSING PRIORITIES

1. Maintain patent airway/respiratory function.
2. Restore hemodynamic stability/circulating volume.
3. Alleviate pain.
4. Prevent complications.
5. Provide emotional support for patient/SO.
6. Provide information about condition, prognosis, and treatment.

DISCHARGE GOALS

1. Homeostasis achieved.
2. Pain controlled/reduced.
3. Complications prevented/minimized.
4. Dealing with current situation realistically.
5. Condition/prognosis and therapeutic regimen understood.

NURSING DIAGNOSIS:	AIRWAY CLEARANCE, INEFFECTIVE, HIGH RISK FOR
Risk factors may include:	Tracheobronchial obstruction: Mucosal edema and loss of ciliary action (smoke inhalation); circumferential full-thickness burns of the neck, thorax and chest with compression of the airway or limited chest excursion.
	Trauma: Direct upper-airway injury by flame, steam, hot air, and chemicals/gases.

823

	Fluid shifts, pulmonary edema, decreased lung compliance.
Possibly evidenced by:	[Not applicable; presence of signs and symptoms establishes an actual diagnosis.]
DESIRED OUTCOMES/ EVALUATION CRITERIA— PATIENT WILL:	Demonstrate clear breath sounds, respiratory rate within normal range, free of dyspnea/cyanosis.

ACTIONS/INTERVENTIONS	RATIONALE

Independent

Obtain history of injury. Note presence of preexisting respiratory conditions, history of smoking.	Causative agent, duration of exposure, occurrence in closed or open space indicates probability of inhalation injury. Type of material burned (wood, plastic, wool, and so forth) suggests type of toxic gas exposure. Preexisting conditions increase the risk of respiratory complications.
Assess gag/swallow reflexes; note drooling, inability to swallow, hoarseness, wheezy cough.	Suggestive of inhalation injury.
Monitor respiratory rate, rhythm, depth; note presence of pallor/cyanosis and carbonaceous or pink-tinged sputum.	Tachypnea, use of accessory muscles, presence of cyanosis, and changes in sputum suggest developing respiratory distress/pulmonary edema, and need for medical intervention.
Auscultate lungs, noting stridor, wheezing/crackles, diminished breath sounds, brassy cough.	Airway obstruction/respiratory distress can occur very quickly or may be delayed, e.g., up to 48 hours after burn.
Note presence of pallor or cherry red color of uninjured skin.	Suggests presence of hypoxemia or carbon monoxide.
Elevate head of bed. Avoid use of pillow under head, as indicated.	Promotes optimal lung expansion/respiratory function. When head/neck burns are present, a pillow can inhibit respiration, cause necrosis of burned ear cartilage, and promote neck contractures.
Encourage coughing/deep-breathing exercises and frequent position changes.	Promotes lung expansion, mobilization and drainage of secretions.
Suction (if necessary) with extreme care, maintaining sterile technique.	Helps to maintain clear airway, but should be done cautiously because of mucosal edema and inflammation. Sterile technique reduces risk of infection.
Promote voice rest but assess ability to speak and/or swallow oral secretions periodically.	Increasing hoarseness/decreased ability to swallow suggests increasing tracheal edema and may indicate need for prompt intubation.
Investigate changes in behavior/mentation, e.g., restlessness, agitation, confusion.	Although often related to pain, changes in consciousness may reflect developing/worsening hypoxia.
Monitor 24-hour fluid balance, noting variations/ changes.	Fluid shifts or excess fluid replacement increases risk of pulmonary edema. *Note:* Inhalation injury increases fluid demands as much as 35% or more because of obligatory edema.

ACTIONS/INTERVENTIONS	RATIONALE
Collaborative	
Administer humidified O$_2$ via appropriate mode, e.g., face mask.	O$_2$ corrects hypoxemia/acidosis. Humidity decreases drying of respiratory tract and reduces viscosity of sputum.
Monitor/graph serial ABGs.	Baseline is essential for further assessment of respiratory status and as a guide to treatment. PaO$_2$ less than 50, PaCO$_2$ greater than 50, and decreasing pH reflect smoke inhalation and developing pneumonia/ARDS.
Review serial x-rays.	Changes reflecting atelectasis/pulmonary edema may not occur for 2–3 days after burn.
Provide/assist with chest physiotherapy/incentive spirometry.	Chest physiotherapy drains dependent areas of the lung, while incentive spirometry may be done to improve lung expansion, thereby promoting respiratory function and reducing atelectasis.
Prepare for/assist with intubation or tracheostomy as indicated.	Intubation/mechanical support is required when airway edema or circumferential burn injury interferes with respiratory function/oxygenation.

NURSING DIAGNOSIS:	FLUID VOLUME DEFICIT, HIGH RISK FOR
Risk factors may include:	Loss of fluid through abnormal routes, e.g., wounds.
	Increased need: Hypermetabolic state, insufficient intake.
	Hemorrhagic losses.
Possibly evidenced by:	[Not applicable; presence of signs and symptoms establishes an actual diagnosis.]
DESIRED OUTCOMES/ EVALUATION CRITERIA— PATIENT WILL:	Demonstrate improved fluid balance as evidenced by individually adequate urinary output with normal specific gravity, stable vital signs, moist mucous membranes.

ACTIONS/INTERVENTIONS	RATIONALE
Independent	
Monitor vital signs, CVP. Note capillary refill and strength of peripheral pulses.	Serves as a guide to fluid replacement needs and assesses cardiovascular response. *Note:* Invasive monitoring is indicated for patients with major burns, smoke inhalation, or preexisting cardiac disease although there is an associated increased risk of infection, necessitating careful monitoring and care of insertion site.
Monitor urinary output and specific gravity. Observe urine color and hematest as indicated.	Generally, fluid replacement should be titrated to ensure average urinary output of 30–50 ml/h (in the adult). Urine can appear red to black, with massive muscle destruction due to presence of

ACTIONS/INTERVENTIONS	RATIONALE

Independent

	blood and release of myoglobin. If gross myoglobinuria is present, minimum urinary output should be 75–100 ml/h to prevent tubular damage/necrosis.
Estimate wound drainage and insensible losses.	Increased capillary permeability, protein shifts, inflammatory process, and evaporative losses greatly affect circulating volume and urinary output, especially during initial 24–72 hours after burn.
Maintain cumulative record of amount and type of fluid intake.	Massive/rapid replacement with different types of fluids and fluctuations in rate of administration requires close tabulation to prevent constituent imbalances or fluid overload.
Weigh daily.	Fluid replacement formulas partly depend on admission weight and subsequent changes. A 15%–20% weight gain in the first 72 hours during fluid replacement can be anticipated with return to preburn weight approximately 10 days after burn.
Measure circumference of burned extremities daily as indicated.	May be helpful in estimating extent of edema/fluid shifts affecting circulating volume and urinary output.
Investigate changes in mentation.	Deterioration in the level of consciousness may indicate inadequate circulating volume/reduced cerebral perfusion.
Observe for gastric distention, hematemesis, tarry stools. Hematest NG drainage and stools periodically.	Stress (Curling's) ulcer occurs in up to half of all severely burned patients (can occur as early as first week).

Collaborative

Insert/maintain indwelling urinary catheter.	Allows for close observation of renal function and prevents stasis or reflux of urine. Retention of urine with its byproducts of tissue-cell destruction can lead to renal dysfunction and infection.
Insert/maintain large bore IV catheter(s).	Accommodates rapid infusion of fluids.
Administer calculated IV replacement of fluids, electrolytes, plasma, albumin.	Fluid resuscitation replaces lost fluids/electrolytes and helps to prevent complications, e.g., shock, ATN. Replacement formulas vary (e.g., Brooke, Evans, Parkland) but are based on extent of injury, amount of urinary output and weight. *Note:* Once initial fluid resuscitation has been accomplished, a steady rate of fluid administration is preferred to "boluses," which may increase interstitial fluid shifts and cardiopulmonary congestion.
Monitor laboratory studies (e.g., Hb/Hct, electrolytes, random urine sodium).	Identifies blood loss/RBC destruction, and fluid and electrolyte replacement needs. Urine sodium less than 10 mEq/L suggests inadequate fluid resuscitation. *Note:* During first 24 hours postburn, hemoconcentration is common due to fluid shifts into the interstitial space.

ACTIONS/INTERVENTIONS

Collaborative

Administer medications as indicated:

Diuretics, e.g., mannitol (Osmitrol);

Potassium;

Antacids, e.g., calcium carbonate (Titrilac), ma-galdrate (Riopan); Histamine inhibitors, e.g., cimetidine (Tagamet)/ranitidine (Zantac).

Add electrolytes to water used for wound debride-ment.

RATIONALE

May be indicated to enhance urinary output and clear tubules of debris/prevent necrosis.

Although hyperkalemia often occurs during first 24–48 hours (tissue destruction), subsequent re-placement may be necessary because of large uri-nary losses.

Antacids may reduce gastric acidity, while hista-mine inhibitors decrease production of hydrochlo-ric acid to reduce risk of gastric irritation/bleeding.

Washing solution that approximates tissue fluids may minimize osmotic fluid shifts.

NURSING DIAGNOSIS:	INFECTION, HIGH RISK FOR
Risk factors may include:	Inadequate primary defenses: Destruction of skin barrier, traumatized tissues.
	Inadequate secondary defenses: Decreased Hb, sup-pressed inflammatory response.
	Environmental exposure, invasive procedures.
Possibly evidenced by:	[Not applicable; presence of signs and symptoms estab-lishes an actual diagnosis.]
DESIRED OUTCOMES/ EVALUATION CRITERIA— PATIENT WILL:	Achieve timely wound healing free of purulent exudate and be afebrile.

ACTIONS/INTERVENTIONS

Independent

Implement appropriate isolation techniques as in-dicated.

Stress necessity of good hand-washing technique for all individuals coming in contact with patient.

Use gowns, gloves, masks, and strict aseptic tech-nique during direct wound care and provide sterile or freshly laundered bed linens/gowns.

Monitor/limit visitors, if necessary. Explain isolation procedure to visitors if used.

RATIONALE

Dependent on type/extent of wounds and the choice of wound treatment (e.g., open versus closed); isolation may range from simple wound/ skin to complete/reverse to reduce risk of cross-contamination/exposure to multiple bacterial flora.

Prevents cross-contamination; reduces risk of ac-quired infection.

Prevents exposure to infectious organisms.

Prevents cross-contamination from visitors. Con-cern for risk of infection should be balanced against patients need for family support and so-cialization.

ACTIONS/INTERVENTIONS	RATIONALE

Independent

Shave/clip all hair from around burned areas to include a 1-in border (excluding eyebrows). Shave facial hair (men) and shampoo head daily.

Hair is a good medium for bacterial growth; however, eyebrows act as a protective barrier for the eyes. Regular shampooing decreases bacterial fallout into burned areas.

Examine unburned areas (such as groin, neck creases, mucus membranes, and vaginal discharge) routinely.

Opportunistic infections (e.g., yeast) frequently occur due to depression of the immune system, and/or proliferation of normal body flora during systemic antibiotic therapy.

Provide special care for eyes, e.g., use eye covers and tear formulas as appropriate.

Eyes may be swollen shut and/or become infected by drainage from surrounding burns. If lids are burned, eye covers may be needed to prevent corneal damage.

Prevent skin-to-skin surface contact (e.g., wrap each burned finger/toe separately; do not allow burned ear to touch scalp).

Prevents adherence to surface it may be touching and encourages proper healing. *Note:* Ear cartilage has limited circulation and is prone to pressure necrosis.

Remove dressings and cleanse burned areas in a hydrotherapy/whirlpool tub or in a shower stall with handheld shower head. Maintain temperature of water at 100°F (37.8°C). Wash areas with a mild cleansing agent or surgical soap.

Water softens and aids in removal of dressings and eschar (slough layer of dead skin or tissue). Sources vary as to whether bath or shower is best. Bath has advantage of water providing support for exercising extremities but may promote cross-contamination of wounds. Showering enhances wound inspection and prevents contamination from floating debris.

Debride necrotic/loose tissue (including ruptured blisters) with scissors and forceps. Do not disturb intact blisters if they are smaller than 2–3 cm, do not interfere with joint function, and do not appear infected.

Promotes healing. Prevents autocontamination. Small, intact blisters help to protect skin and increase rate of reepithelization unless the burn injury is the result of chemicals (in which case fluid contained in blisters may continue to cause tissue destruction).

Examine wounds daily, note/document changes in appearance, odor, or quantity of drainage.

Identifies presence of healing (granulation tissue) and provides for early detection of burn-wound infection. Infection in a partial thickness burn may cause conversion of burn to full-thickness injury.

Monitor vital signs for fever, increased respiratory rate/depth in association with changes in sensorium, presence of diarrhea, decreased platelet count, and hyperglycemia with glycosuria.

Indicators of sepsis (often occurs with full-thickness burn) requiring prompt evaluation and intervention. *Note:* Changes in sensorium, bowel habits, and respiratory rate usually precede fever and alteration of laboratory studies.

Collaborative

Place IV/invasive lines in nonburned area.

Decreased risk of infection at insertion site with possibility of progression to septicemia.

Obtain routine cultures and sensitivities of wounds/drainage.

Allows early recognition and specific treatment of wound infection.

Assist with excisional biopsies when infection is suspected.

Bacteria can colonize the wound surface without invading the underlying tissue; therefore, biopsies may be obtained for diagnosing infection.

ACTIONS/INTERVENTIONS	RATIONALE
Collaborative	
Photograph wound initially and at periodic intervals.	Provides baseline and documentation of healing process.
Administer topical agents as indicated, e.g.:	The following agents help to prevent/control wound infections and prevent drying of wound, which can cause further tissue destruction.
Silver sulfadiazine (Silvadene);	Wide-spectrum antimicrobial that is relatively painless but has less eschar penetration than Sulfamylon and may cause rash or depression of WBCs.
Mafenide acetate (Sulfamylon);	Antibiotic of choice with confirmed invasive burn wound infection. Useful against gram-negative/gram-positive organisms. Causes burning/pain on application and for 30 minutes thereafter. Can cause rash, metabolic acidosis, and decreased $PaCO_2$.
Silver nitrate;	Effective against *Staphylococcus aureus, Escherichia coli,* and *Pseudomonas aeruginosa,* but has poor eschar penetration, is painful, and may cause electrolyte imbalance. Dressings must be constantly saturated. Product stains skin/surfaces black.
Providone-iodine (Betadine).	Broad-spectrum antimicrobial but is painful on application, may cause metabolic acidosis/increased iodine absorption, and damage fragile tissues.
Administer medications as appropriate, e.g.;	
Subeschar clysis/systemic antibiotics;	Local and systemic antibiotics are given to control pathogens identified by culture/sensitivity. Subeschar clysis has been found effective against pathogens to prevent sepsis in granulated tissues at the line of demarcation between viable/nonviable tissue.
Tetanus toxoid or clostridial antitoxin as appropriate.	Tissue destruction/altered defense mechanisms increases risk of developing tetanus or gas gangrene, especially in deep burns such as those caused by electricity.

NURSING DIAGNOSIS:	PAIN, [ACUTE]
May be related to:	Destruction of skin/tissues; edema formation.
	Manipulation of injured tissues, e.g., wound debridement.
Possibly evidenced by:	Reports of pain.
	Narrowed focus, facial mask of pain.
	Alteration in muscle tone; autonomic responses.
	Distraction guarding behaviors; anxiety/fear.

ACTIONS/INTERVENTIONS

Independent

Cover wounds as soon as possible unless open-air exposure burn care method required.

Elevate burned extremities periodically.

Provide bed cradle as indicated.

Wrap digits/extremities in position of function (avoiding flexed position of affected joints) using splints and footboards as necessary.

Change position frequently and assist with active and passive ROM as indicated.

Maintain comfortable environmental temperature, provide heat lamps, heat retaining body coverings.

Assess reports of pain, noting location/character and intensity (0–10 scale).

Perform dressing changes and debridement after patient is medicated and/or in hydrotherapy.

Encourage expression of feelings about pain.

Involve patient in determining schedule for activities, treatments, drug administration.

Explain procedures/provide frequent information as appropriate, especially during wound debridement.

Provide basic comfort measures, e.g., massage of uninjured areas, frequent position changes.

RATIONALE

Temperature changes and air movement can cause great pain to exposed nerve endings.

Elevation may be required initially to reduce edema formation; thereafter changes in position and elevation reduce discomfort as well as risk of joint contractures.

Elevation of linens off of wounds may help to reduce pain.

Position of function reduces deformities/contractures and promotes comfort. Although flexed position of injured joints may feel more comfortable, it can lead to flexion contractures.

Movement and exercise reduces joint stiffness and muscle fatigue but type of exercise is dependent on location and extent of injury.

Temperature regulation may be lost with major burns. External heat sources may be necessary to prevent chilling.

Pain is nearly always present to some degree because of varying severity of tissue involvement/destruction but is usually most severe during dressing changes and debridement. Changes in location/character/intensity of pain may indicate developing complications (e.g., limb ischemia) or herald improvement/return of nerve function/sensation.

Reduces severe physical and emotional distress associated with dressing changes and debridement.

Verbalization allows outlet for emotions and may enhance coping mechanisms.

Enhances patient's sense of control and strengthens coping mechanisms.

Empathic support can help to alleviate pain/promote relaxation. Knowing what to expect provides opportunity for patient to prepare self and enhances sense of control.

Promotes relaxation; reduces muscle tension and general fatigue.

ACTIONS/INTERVENTIONS

Independent

Encourage use of stress management techniques, e.g., progressive relaxation, deep breathing, guided imagery, and visualization.

Provide diversional activities appropriate for age/condition.

Promote uninterrupted sleep periods.

Collaborative

Administer analgesics (narcotic and non-narcotic) as indicated.

Provide/instruct in use of PCA.

RATIONALE

Refocuses attention, promotes relaxation, and enhances sense of control, which may reduce pharmacologic dependency.

Helps to lessen concentration on pain experience and refocus attention.

Sleep deprivation can increase perception of pain/reduce coping abilities.

IV method is often used initially to maximize drug effect. Concerns of patient addiction or doubts regarding degree of pain experienced are not valid during emergent/acute phase of care, but narcotics should be decreased as soon as feasible and alternate methods for pain relief initiated.

PCA provides for timely drug administration, preventing fluctuations in intensity of pain, often at lower total dosage than would be given by conventional methods.

NURSING DIAGNOSIS:	TISSUE PERFUSION, ALTERED/PERIPHERAL NEUROVASCULAR DYSFUNCTION, HIGH RISK FOR
Risk factors may include:	Reduction/interruption of arterial/venous blood flow, e.g., circumferential burns of extremities with resultant edema.
	Hypovolemia.
Possibly evidenced by:	[Not applicable; presence of signs and symptoms establishes an actual diagnosis.]
DESIRED OUTCOMES/ EVALUATION CRITERIA— PATIENT WILL:	Maintain palpable peripheral pulses of equal quality/strength; good capillary refill and skin color normal in uninjured areas.

ACTIONS/INTERVENTIONS

Independent

Assess color, sensation, movement, peripheral pulses (via Doppler), and capillary refill on extremities with circumferential burns. Compare with findings of unaffected limb.

Elevate affected extremities, as appropriate. Remove jewelry/arm band. Avoid taping around a burned extremity/digit.

RATIONALE

Edema formation can readily compress blood vessels, thereby impeding circulation and increasing venous stasis/edema. Comparisons with unaffected limbs aid in differentiating localized versus systemic problems (e.g., hypovolemia/decreased cardiac output).

Promotes systemic circulation/venous return and may reduce edema or other deleterious effects of constriction of edematous tissues. Prolonged ele-

831

ACTIONS/INTERVENTIONS	RATIONALE
Independent	
	vation can impair arterial perfusion if BP falls or tissue pressures rise excessively.
Obtain BP in unburned extremity. Remove BP cuff after each reading.	If BP readings must be obtained on an injured extremity, leaving the cuff in place may increase edema formation/reduce perfusion, and convert partial-thickness burn to a more serious injury.
Investigate reports of deep/throbbing ache, numbness.	Indicators of decreased perfusion and/or increased pressure within enclosed space, such as may occur with a circumferential burn of an extremity (compartment syndrome).
Encourage active ROM exercises of unaffected body parts.	Promotes local and systemic circulation.
Investigate irregular pulses.	Cardiac dysrhythmias can occur as a result of electrolyte shifts, electrical injury, or release of myocardial depressant factor, compromising cardiac output/tissue perfusion.
Collaborative	
Maintain fluid replacement per protocol. (Refer to ND: Fluid Volume Deficit, high risk for, p 825.)	Maximizes circulating volume and tissue perfusion.
Monitor electrolytes, especially sodium, potassium, and calcium. Administer replacement therapy as indicated.	Losses/shifts of these electrolytes affect cellular membrane potential/excitability, thereby altering myocardial conductivity, potentiating risk of dysrhythmias, and reducing cardiac output/tissue perfusion.
Avoid use of IM/SC injections.	Altered tissue perfusion and edema formation impair drug absorption. Injections into potential donor sites may render them unusable due to hematoma formation.
Measure intracompartmental pressures as indicated. (Refer to CP: Fractures; ND: Tissue Perfusion, altered, p 777.)	Ischemic myositis may develop due to decreased perfusion.
Assist with/prepare for escharotomy/fasciotomy, as indicated.	Enhances circulation by relieving constriction caused by rigid nonviable tissue (eschar) or edema formation.

NURSING DIAGNOSIS:	**NUTRITION, ALTERED: LESS THAN BODY REQUIREMENTS**
May be related to:	Hypermetabolic state (can be as much as 50%–60% greater than normal proportional to the severity of injury).
	Protein catabolism.
Possibly evidenced by:	Decrease in total body weight, loss of muscle mass/subcutaneous fat, and development of negative nitrogen balance.

DESIRED OUTCOMES/ EVALUATION CRITERIA— PATIENT WILL:	Demonstrate nutritional intake adequate to meet metabolic needs as evidenced by stable weight/muscle-mass measurements, positive nitrogen balance, and tissue regeneration.

ACTIONS/INTERVENTIONS	RATIONALE

Independent

ACTIONS/INTERVENTIONS	RATIONALE
Auscultate bowel sounds, noting hypoactive/absent sounds.	Ileus is often associated with postburn period but usually subsides within 36–48 hours at which time oral feedings can be initiated.
Maintain strict caloric count. Weigh daily. Reassess percent of open body surface area/wounds weekly.	Appropriate guides to proper caloric intake. As burn wound heals, percentage of burned areas is reevaluated to calculate prescribed dietary formulas, and appropriate adjustments are made.
Monitor muscle mass/subcutaneous fat as indicated.	May be useful in estimating body reserves/losses and effectiveness of therapy.
Provide small, frequent meals and snacks.	Helps to prevent gastric distention/discomfort and may enhance intake.
Encourage patient to view diet as a treatment and to make food/beverage choices high in calories/protein.	Calories and proteins are needed to maintain weight, meet metabolic needs, and promote wound healing.
Ascertain food likes/dislikes. Encourage SO to bring food from home, as appropriate.	Provides patient/SO sense of control; enhances participation in care and may improve intake.
Encourage patient to sit up for meals, and visit with others.	Sitting helps to prevent aspiration and aids in proper digestion of food. Socialization promotes relaxation and may enhance intake.
Provide oral hygiene before meals.	Clean mouth/clear palate enhances taste and helps promote a good appetite.
Perform fingerstick glucose, clinitest/acetest as indicated.	Monitors for development of hyperglycemia related to hormonal changes/demands or use of hyperalimentation to meet caloric needs.

Collaborative

ACTIONS/INTERVENTIONS	RATIONALE
Refer to dietitian/nutritional support team.	Useful in establishing individual nutritional needs (based on weight and body surface area of injury) and identifying appropriate routes.
Provide diet high in calories/protein with vitamin supplements.	Calories (3000–5000/d), proteins, and vitamins are needed to meet increased metabolic needs, maintain weight, and encourage tissue regeneration. *Note:* Oral route is most preferable once GI function returns.
Insert/maintain small feeding tube for enteric feedings/supplements if needed.	Provides continuous/supplemental feedings when patient is unable to consume total daily calorie requirements orally. *Note:* Continuous tube feeding during the night increases calorie intake without decreasing appetite and oral intake during the day.

ACTIONS/INTERVENTIONS	RATIONALE
Collaborative	
Administer parenteral hyperalimentation as indicated.	Hyperalimentation will maintain nutritional intake/meet metabolic needs in presence of severe complications or sustained esophageal/gastric injuries that do not permit enteral feedings.
Monitor laboratory studies e.g., serum albumin, Cr, transferrin; urine urea nitrogen.	Indicators of nutritional needs and adequacy of diet/therapy.
Administer insulin as indicated.	Elevated serum glucose levels may develop due to stress response to injury, high caloric intake, pancreatic fatigue.

NURSING DIAGNOSIS:	PHYSICAL MOBILITY, IMPAIRED
May be related to:	Neuromuscular impairment, pain/discomfort, decreased strength and endurance.
	Restrictive therapies, limb immobilization; contractures.
Possibly evidenced by:	Reluctance to move/inability to purposefully move.
	Limited ROM, decreased muscle strength control and/or mass.
DESIRED OUTCOMES/ EVALUATION CRITERIA— PATIENT WILL:	Verbalize and demonstrate willingness to participate in activities.
	Maintain position of function as evidenced by absence of contractures.
	Maintain or increase strength and function of affected and/or compensatory body part.
	Demonstrate techniques/behaviors that enable resumption of activities.

ACTIONS/INTERVENTIONS	RATIONALE
Independent	
Maintain proper body alignment with supports or splints especially for burns over joints.	Promotes functional positioning of extremities and prevents contractures, which are more likely over joints.
Note circulation, motion, and sensation of digits frequently.	Edema may compromise circulation to extremities potentiating tissue necrosis/development of contractures.
Initiate the rehabilitative phase on admission.	It is easier to enlist participation when the patient is aware of the possibilities that exist for recovery.

ACTIONS/INTERVENTIONS	RATIONALE

Independent

Perform ROM exercises consistently, initially passive, then active.

Prevents progressively tightening scar tissue and contractures; enhances maintenance of muscle/joint functioning and reduces loss of calcium from the bone.

Medicate for pain before activity/exercises.

Reduces muscle/tissue stiffness and tension enabling patient to be more active and facilitating participation.

Schedule treatments and care activities to provide periods of uninterrupted rest.

Increases patient's strength and tolerance for activity.

Instruct and assist with mobility aids, e.g., cane, walker, crutches as appropriate.

Promotes safe ambulation.

Encourage family/SO support and assistance with ROM exercises.

Enables family/SO to be active in patient care and provides more constant/consistent therapy.

Incorporate ADLs with physical therapy, hydrotherapy, and nursing care.

Combining activities produces improved results by enhancing effects of each.

Encourage patient participation in all activities as individually able.

Promotes independence, enhances self-esteem, and facilitates recovery process.

Collaborative

Provide foam, water/air mattress or kinetic therapy bed as indicated.

Prevents prolonged pressure on tissues, reducing potential for tissue ischemia/necrosis and decubitus formation.

Excise and cover burn wounds quickly.

Early excision is known to reduce scarring as well as risk of infection, thereby facilitating healing.

Maintain pressure garment when used.

Hypertrophic scarring can develop around grafted areas or at the site of deep, partial-thickness wounds. Pressure dressings minimize scar tissue by keeping it flat, soft, and pliable.

Consult with rehabilitation, physical, and occupational therapists.

Provides integrated activity/exercise program and specific assistive devices based on individual needs and facilitates intensive long-term management of potential deficits.

NURSING DIAGNOSIS:	SKIN INTEGRITY, IMPAIRED: ACTUAL [GRAFTS]
May be related to:	Trauma: Disruption of skin surface with destruction of skin layers (partial/full-thickness burn).
Possibly evidenced by:	Absence of viable tissue.
DESIRED OUTCOMES/ EVALUATION CRITERIA— PATIENT WILL:	Demonstrate tissue regeneration. Achieve timely healing of burned areas.

ACTIONS/INTERVENTIONS	RATIONALE

Independent

Preoperative

Assess/document size, color, depth of wound, noting necrotic tissue and condition of surrounding skin.

Provide baseline information about need for skin grafting and possible clues about circulation in area to support graft.

Provide appropriate burn care and infection control measures. (Refer to ND: Infection, high risk for, p 827.)

Prepares tissues for grafting and reduces risk of infection/graft failure.

Postoperative

Maintain wound covering as indicated, e.g.:

Biosynthetic dressing (Biobrane);

Nylon fabric/silicon membrane containing collagenous porcine peptides that adheres to wound surface until removed or sloughed off by spontaneous skin reepithelialization. Useful for eschar-free partial-thickness burns awaiting autografts because it can remain in place 2–3 weeks or longer, and is permeable to topical antimicrobial agents.

Synthetic dressings, e.g., DuoDerm;

Hydroactive dressing that adheres to the skin to cover small partial-thickness burns and interacts with wound exudate to form a soft gel that facilitates debridement.

Op-Site.

Thin, transparent, elastic, waterproof, occlusive dressing (permeable to moisture and air) that is used to cover clean partial-thickness wounds and clean donor sites.

Elevate grafted area if possible/appropriate. Maintain desired position and immobility of area when indicated.

Reduces swelling/limits risk of graft separation. Movement of tissue under graft can dislodge it, interfering with optimal healing.

Maintain dressings over newly grafted area and/or donor site as indicated, e.g., mesh, petroleum, nonadhesive.

Areas may be covered by translucent, nonreactive surface material (between graft and outer dressing) to eliminate shearing of new epithelium/protect healing tissue.

Keep skin free from pressure.

Promotes circulation and prevents ischemia/necrosis and graft failure.

Evaluate color of grafted and donor sites; note presence/absence of healing.

Evaluates effectiveness of circulation and identifies developing complications.

Wash sites with mild soap, rinse, and lubricate with cream (e.g., Nivea) several times daily, after dressings are removed and healing is accomplished.

Newly grafted skin and healed donor sites require special care to maintain flexibility.

Aspirate blebs under sheet grafts with sterile needle or roll with sterile swab.

Fluid-filled blebs prevent graft adherence to underlying tissue increasing risk of graft failure.

ACTIONS/INTERVENTIONS	RATIONALE

Collaborative

Prepare for/assist with surgical procedure/biologic dressings, e.g.:

Homograft (allograft);

Skin grafts obtained from living persons or cadavers are used as a temporary covering for extensive burns until person's own skin is ready for grafting (test graft), to cover excised wounds immediately after escharotomy, or to protect granulation tissue.

Heterograft (xenograft, porcine);

Skin grafts obtained may be from animal skin with use the same as for homograft or to cover meshed autografts.

Autograft.

Skin graft obtained from uninjured part of patient's own skin; may be full-thickness or partial-thickness.

NURSING DIAGNOSIS:	FEAR/ANXIETY

May be related to: Situational crises: Hospitalization/isolation procedures, interpersonal transmission and contagion, memory of the trauma experience, threat of death and/or disfigurement.

Possibly evidenced by: Expressed concern regarding changes in life, fear of unspecific consequences.

Apprehension; increased tension.

Feelings of helplessness, uncertainty, decreased self-assurance.

Sympathetic stimulation, extraneous movements, restlessness, insomnia.

DESIRED OUTCOMES/ EVALUATION CRITERIA— PATIENT WILL: Verbalize awareness of feelings and healthy ways to deal with them.

Report anxiety/fear reduced to manageable level.

Demonstrate problem-solving skills, effective use of resources.

ACTIONS/INTERVENTIONS	RATIONALE

Independent

Provide frequent explanations and information about care procedures.

Knowing what to expect usually reduces fear and anxiety, clarifies misconceptions, and promotes cooperation.

837

ACTIONS/INTERVENTIONS	RATIONALE
Independent	
Demonstrate willingness to listen and talk to patient when free of painful procedures.	Helps patient/SO to know that support is available and that caregiver is interested in the person, not just care of the burn.
Involve patient/SO in decision-making process whenever possible.	Promotes sense of control and cooperation, decreasing feelings of helplessness/hopelessness.
Assess mental status, including mood/affect, comprehension of events, and content of thoughts, e.g., illusions or manifestations of terror/panic.	Initially, the patient may use denial and repression to reduce and filter information that might be overwhelming. Some patients display calm manner and alert mental status, representing a dissociation from reality, which is also a protective mechanism.
Investigate changes in mentation and presence of hypervigilance/hypovigilance, hallucinations, sleep disturbances (e.g., nightmares), agitation/apathy, disorientation, labile affect, all of which may vary from moment to moment.	Indicators of extreme anxiety/delirium state in which the patient is literally fighting for life. Although cause can be psychologically based, pathologic life-threatening causes (e.g., shock, sepsis, hypoxia) must be ruled out.
Provide constant and consistent orientation.	Helps the patient stay in touch with surroundings and reality.
Encourage the patient to talk about the burn circumstances when ready.	Patient may need to tell the story of what happened over and over to make some sense out of what is a terrifying situation.
Explain to patient what happened. Provide opportunity for questions and give open/honest answers.	Compassionate statements reflecting the reality of the situation can help the patient/SO acknowledge that reality and begin to deal with what has happened.
Identify previous methods of coping/handling of stressful situations.	Past successful behavior can be used to assist in dealing with the present situation.
Assist the family to express their feelings of grief and guilt.	The family may initially be most concerned about the patient dying and/or feel guilty, believing that in some way they could have prevented the incident.
Be nonjudgmental in dealing with the patient and family.	Family relationships are disrupted; financial, lifestyle/role changes make this a difficult time for those involved with the patient, and they may react in many different ways.
Encourage family/SO to visit and discuss family happenings. Remind patient of past and future events.	Maintains contact with a familiar reality, creating a sense of attachment and continuity of life.
Collaborative	
Involve entire burn team in care from admission to discharge, including social worker and psychiatric resources.	Provides a wider support system and promotes continuity of care and coordination of activities.
Administer mild sedation/tranquilizers as indicated, e.g., haloperidol (Haldol) or lorazepam (Ativan).	Antianxiety medications may be necessary for a brief period until patient is more physically stable and internal locus of control is regained.

NURSING DIAGNOSIS:	BODY IMAGE DISTURBANCE, ROLE PERFORMANCE ALTERED
May be related to:	Situational crisis: Traumatic event, dependent patient role; disfigurement, pain.
Possibly evidenced by:	Negative feelings about body/self, fear of rejection/reaction by others.
	Focus on past appearance, abilities; preoccupation with change/loss.
	Change in physical capacity to resume role; change in social involvement.
DESIRED OUTCOMES/ EVALUATION CRITERIA— PATIENT WILL:	Verbalize acceptance of self in situation.
	Talk with family/SO about situation, changes that have occurred.
	Develop realistic goals/plans for the future.
	Incorporate changes into self-concept without negating self-esteem.

ACTIONS/INTERVENTIONS	RATIONALE
Independent	
Assess meaning of loss/change to patient/SO.	Traumatic episode results in sudden, unanticipated changes, creating feelings of grief over actual/perceived losses. This necessitates support to work through to optimal resolution.
Acknowledge and accept expression of feelings of frustration, dependency, anger, grief, and hostility. Note withdrawn behavior and use of denial.	Acceptance of these feelings as a normal response to what has occurred facilitates resolution. It is not helpful or possible to push patient before ready to deal with situation. Denial may be prolonged and be an adaptive mechanism, because patient is not ready to cope with personal problems.
Set limits on maladaptive behavior (e.g., manipulative/aggressive). Maintain nonjudgmental attitude while giving care, and help patient to identify positive behaviors that will aid in recovery.	Patient and SO tend to deal with this crisis in the same way in which they have dealt with problems in the past. Staff may find it difficult and frustrating to handle behavior that is disrupting/not helpful to recuperation but should realize that the behavior is usually directed toward situation and not the caregiver.
Be realistic and positive during treatments, in health teaching, and in setting goals within limitations.	Enhances trust and rapport between patient and nurse.
Provide hope within parameters of individual situation; do not give false reassurance.	Promotes positive attitude and provides opportunity to set goals and plan for future based on reality.

839

ACTIONS/INTERVENTIONS

Independent

Give positive reinforcement of progress and encourage endeavors toward attainment of rehabilitation goals.

Show slides or pictures of burn care/other patient outcomes, being selective in what is shown as appropriate to the individual situation. Encourage discussion of feelings about what they have seen.

Encourage family interaction with each other and with rehabilitation team.

Provide support group for SO. Give them information about how they can be helpful to the patient.

Collaborative

Refer to physical/occupational therapy, vocational counselor, and psychiatric counseling, e.g., clinical specialist psychiatric nurse, social services, psychologist as needed.

RATIONALE

Words of encouragement can support development of positive coping behaviors.

Allows patient/SO to be realistic in expectations. Also assists in demonstration of importance of/necessity for certain devices and procedures.

Maintains/opens lines of communication and provides ongoing support for patient and family.

Promotes ventilation of feelings and allows for more helpful responses to the patient.

Helpful in identifying ways/devices to regain/maintain independence. Patient may need further assistance to resolve emotional problems if they persist (e.g., posttrauma response).

NURSING DIAGNOSIS:	**KNOWLEDGE DEFICIT [LEARNING NEED], REGARDING CONDITION, PROGNOSIS, AND TREATMENT NEEDS**
May be related to:	Lack of exposure/recall.
	Information misinterpretation.
	Unfamiliarity with resources.
Possibly evidenced by:	Questions/request for information, statement of misconception.
	Inaccurate follow-through of instructions/development of preventable complications.
DESIRED OUTCOMES/ EVALUATION CRITERIA— PATIENT WILL:	Verbalize understanding of condition, prognosis, and treatment.
	Correctly perform necessary procedures and explain reasons for actions.
	Initiate necessary lifestyle changes and participate in treatment regimen.

ACTIONS/INTERVENTIONS

Independent

Review condition, prognosis, and future expectations.

RATIONALE

Provides knowledge base on which patient can make informed choices.

ACTIONS/INTERVENTIONS	RATIONALE

Independent

Discuss patient's expectations of returning home, to work, and to normal activities.	Patient frequently has a difficult adjustment to discharge. Problems often occur (e.g., sleep disturbances, nightmares, reliving the accident, difficulty with resumption of intimacy/sexual activity, emotional lability) that interfere with successful adjustment to resuming normal life.
Review proper burn, skin graft and wound care techniques. Identify appropriate sources for outpatient care and supplies.	Promotes competent self-care after discharge and enhances independence.
Discuss skin care, e.g., use of moisturizers and sunscreens.	Itching, blistering, and sensitivity of healing wounds/graft sites can be expected for an extended time.
Explain scarring process and necessity for/proper use of pressure garments when used.	Promotes optimal regrowth of skin, minimizing development of hypertrophic scarring and contractures and facilitating healing process. *Note:* Consistent use of the pressure garment over a long period can reduce the need for reconstructive surgery to release contractures and remove scars.
Encourage continuation of prescribed exercise program and scheduled rest periods.	Maintains mobility, reduces complications, and prevents fatigue, facilitating recovery process.
Identify specific limitations of activity as individually appropriate.	Imposed restrictions are dependent on severity/location of injury and stage of healing.
Stress importance of sustained intake of high protein/calorie diet.	Optimal nutrition enhances tissue regeneration and general feeling of well-being.
Review medications, including purpose, dosage, route, and expected/reportable side effects.	Reiteration allows opportunity for patient to ask questions and be sure understanding is accurate.
Advise patient/SO of potential for exhaustion, boredom, emotional lability, adjustment problems. Provide information about possibility of discussion/interaction with appropriate professional counselors.	Provides perspective to some of the problems patient/SO may encounter and helps them to be aware that help/assistance is available when necessary.
Identify signs/symptoms requiring medical evaluation, e.g., inflammation, increased or changes in wound drainage, fever/chills; changes in pain characteristics or loss of mobility/function.	Early detection of developing complications (e.g., infection, delayed healing) may prevent progression to more serious/life-threatening situations.
Stress necessity/importance of follow-up care/rehabilitation.	Long-term support with continual reevaluation and changes in therapy are required to achieve optimal recovery.
Provide phone number for contact person.	Provides easy access to treatment team to reinforce teaching, clarify misconceptions, and reduce potential for complications.
Identify community resources, e.g., crisis centers, recovery groups, mental health, Red Cross, VNA, Ambli-Cab, homemaker service.	Facilitates transition to home, provides assistance with meeting individual needs, and supports independence.

Bibliography

General References

Bellak, JP and Bamford, PA: Nursing Assessment: A Multidimensional Approach. Jones & Bartlett, Boston, 1987.

Berkow, R (ed): The Merck Manual, ed 15. Merck Sharp & Dohme Research Laboratories, Rahway, NJ, 1987.

Cella, JH and Watson, J: Nurse's Manual of Laboratory Tests. FA Davis, Philadelphia, 1989.

Condon, RE, and Nyhus, LM (eds): Manual of Surgical Therapeutics, ed 7. Little, Brown & Co, Boston, 1988.

Deglin, JH and Vallerand, AH: Davis's Drug Guide for Nurses, ed 3. FA Davis, Philadelphia, 1992.

Diseases and Disorders Handbook, ed 3. Springhouse Corp, Springhouse, PA, 1989.

Doenges, ME and Moorhouse, MF: Nurse's Pocket Guide: Nursing Diagnoses with Interventions, ed 3. FA Davis, Philadelphia, 1991.

Dunagan, WC and Ridner, ML (eds): Manual of Medical Therapeutics, ed 26. Little, Brown & Co, Boston, 1989.

Fischbach, F: A Manual of Laboratory and Diagnostic Tests, ed 4. JB Lippincott, Philadelphia, 1992.

Guyton, AC: Textbook of Medical Physiology, ed 8. WB Saunders, Philadelphia, 1991.

Kuhn, MM: Pharmacotherapeutics: A Nursing Process Approach, ed 2. FA Davis, Philadelphia, 1991.

Professional Guide to Diseases, ed 3. Springhouse Corp, Springhouse, PA, 1989.

Suddarth, DS (ed): The Lippincott Manual of Nursing Practice, ed 5. JB Lippincott, Philadelphia, 1991.

Thomas, CL (ed): Taber's Cyclopedic Medical Dictionary, ed 17. FA Davis, Philadelphia, 1993.

Thompson, JM, et al: Mosby's Manual of Clinical Nursing, ed 2. CV Mosby, St Louis, 1989.

Books

Artz, CP, Moncrief, JA, and Pruett, BA (eds): Burns: A Team Approach. WB Saunders, Philadelphia, 1979.

Carvajal, HF and Parks, DH: Burns in Children: Pediatric Burn Management. Year Book Medical Publishers, Chicago, 1988.

Fisher, SV and Phala, AH (eds): Comprehensive Rehabilitation of Burns. Williams and Wilkins, Baltimore, 1984.

Grossman, JA: Hand Clinics, Vol 6, No 2: Burns of the Upper Extremity. WB Saunders, Philadelphia, 1990.

Rea, RE (ed): Trauma Nursing Core Course Provider Manual, ed 2. Award Printing Corp, Chicago, 1986.

Trofino, RB (ed): Nursing Care of the Burn Injured Patient. FA Davis, Philadelphia, 1991.

Articles

Jepson, DL: How to manage a patient with lightning injury. AJN 92(6):38, 1992.

Martin, LM: Nursing implications of today's burn care technique. RN 52(5):26, 1989.

Smith, GA and Savinski-Bozinko, G: Giving emergency care for burns. Nursing89 19(9):55, 1989.

CHAPTER 15
IMMUNOLOGIC DISORDERS

The HIV-Positive Patient

The individual who is seropositive for HIV, with or without symptoms, is considered to be HIV-positive. This person may live for many years before meeting the Centers for Disease Control (CDC) criteria for a diagnosis of AIDS. While imminent death is not a realistic concern, the patient needs to make major behavioral and lifestyle changes to prolong life expectancy and may have significant problems that require information and assistance. The person who is well-supported medically may survive opportunistic infection episodes for a number of years.

RELATED FACTORS

AIDS, p 850
Pneumonia, microbial, p 162
Psychosocial Aspects of Acute Care, p 889
Sepsis/Septicemia, p 887

PATIENT ASSESSMENT DATA BASE

Refer to CP: AIDS, p 850.
Note: Patient generally not hospitalized except when debilitating illness/infection present.

NURSING DIAGNOSIS:	ADJUSTMENT, IMPAIRED
May be related to:	Life-threatening, stigmatized condition/disease.
	Assault to self-esteem, altered locus of control.
	Incomplete grieving.
	Inadequate support systems.
	Medication side effects (fatigue and depression).
Possibly evidenced by:	Verbalization of nonacceptance/denial of diagnosis.
	Nonexistent or unsuccessful ability to be involved in problem solving or goal setting.

DESIRED OUTCOMES/ EVALUATION CRITERIA— PATIENT WILL:	Extended period of shock, disbelief, or anger regarding health-status change.
	Lack of future-oriented thinking.
	Verbalize understanding of disease process.
	Demonstrate increased trust and participation in development of plan of action.
	Initiate lifestyle changes that will permit adaptation to present life situations.

ACTIONS/INTERVENTIONS	RATIONALE
Independent	
Evaluate patient's ability to understand events and realistically appraise situation.	Provides base to develop plan of action.
Encourage expression of feelings, denial, shock, and fears. Listen without judgment, accepting patient's expressions. Avoid dwelling on future possibilities.	It is important to convey belief in commonality of patient's fears/feelings. Speculating about the future focuses on the negative aspects of what might happen.
Challenge morbid thoughts and reframe into positive statements, i.e., "You know why the virus is going to kill me, I deserve to die for what I've done." Response: "The virus may or may not kill you. It's not smart enough to decide when you may die."	Interrupts morbid thoughts and challenges patient's self-depreciating ideas.
Determine available resources or programs.	Addictive behaviors, ability of IV drug user to obtain clean "works," sexual myths, and perceptions of the use of condoms may need to be addressed.
Assess social system as well as presence of support, perception of losses, and stressors.	Partners, friends, and families will have individual responses dependent on acceptance of the person's lifestyle, knowledge of HIV transmission, and belief in myths.
Encourage patient to participate in support groups.	Long-term support is critical to dealing with and effectively coping with reality.
Discuss meaning of high-risk behavior and barriers to change.	Sexual behavior may be used to express caring as well as to feel connected and less lonely.
Inform patient about interactions between medications, HIV, and emotions.	Fatigue and depression can be side effects of medications as well as of the infection itself. Knowledge that it is usually of short duration can support informed choices/cooperation and promote hope.
Encourage continued use and renewed use of familiar effective coping strategies.	Patient is supported and given strokes for past effective behavior. Positive reinforcement enhances self-esteem.
Explore and practice the potential use of new and different coping strategies.	Using new strategies can be uncomfortable and practice fosters self-confidence.
Help the patient to use humor to combat stigmatization of the disease.	Humor defuses the sense of secretiveness people may place on HIV.
Reinforce structure in daily life. Include exercise as part of routine.	Routines assist the person to focus. Exercise improves sense of wellness.

ACTIONS/INTERVENTIONS

Independent

Assist patient to set limits on acting-out behaviors.

Assist patient to channel anger to healthy activities.

Inform patient about new medical advances/treatments.

Collaborative

Refer to nurse practitioner/clinical specialist, psychologist, social worker knowledgeable of HIV.

RATIONALE

Needs for love, comfort, and companionship that have been met through sexual expression need to be met through other means that carry a reduced risk of HIV transmission.

The increased energy of anger can be used to accomplish other tasks and enhance feelings of self-esteem.

Promotes hope and helps patient to make informed decisions.

May need additional help to adjust to difficult situation.

NURSING DIAGNOSIS:	NUTRITION, ALTERED, LESS THAN BODY REQUIREMENTS, HIGH RISK FOR
Risk factors may include:	Reported inadequate food intake less than recommended daily allowance. Lack of interest in food. Lack of information, misinformation, misconceptions. Reported altered taste sensation (side effects of medications). Loss of weight with adequate food intake; poor muscle tone. Sore, inflamed buccal cavity.
Possibly evidenced by:	[Not applicable; presence of signs and symptoms establishes an actual diagnosis].
DESIRED OUTCOMES/ EVALUATION CRITERIA— PATIENT WILL:	Maintain adequate muscle mass. Maintain weight within 2–3 lb of usual premorbid weight. Demonstrate laboratory values within normal limits. Report improved energy level.

ACTIONS/INTERVENTIONS

Independent

Determine usual weight before patient was diagnosed with HIV.

RATIONALE

Early wasting is not readily determined by normal-weight-to-height charts. Therefore, determining current weight in relation to prediagnosis weight is more useful.

845

ACTIONS/INTERVENTIONS	RATIONALE
Independent	
Establish current anthropometric measurements.	Helps to monitor wasting and determine nutritional needs as illness progresses.
Determine patient's current dietary pattern/intake and knowledge of nutrition. Use an indepth dietary assessment tool.	Identification of these factors helps to plan for individual needs. Patients with HIV infection have documented trace mineral zinc, magnesium, selenium deficits. Alcohol and drug abuse interfere with adequate intake.
Discuss/note nutritional side effects of medications.	Commonly used medications cause anorexia and n/v; some interfere with bone marrow production of RBCs.
Provide information about nutritionally dense high-calorie, high-protein, high-vitamin, and high-mineral foods. Help patient plan ways to maintain/improve intake.	Having this information helps patient to understand importance of well-balanced diet. Some patients may try macrobiotic or other diets believing the diarrhea is caused by lactose intolerance. Eliminating dairy products can have detrimental effects when these components are not replaced.
Stress importance of maintaining balanced/adequate nutritional intake.	Patient may get discouraged with changed status and find it difficult to eat. Knowing how important nutritional intake is to remaining healthy can motivate patient to maintain proper diet.
Assist patient to formulate dietary plan.	Provides guidance and feedback while promoting sense of control, enhancing self-esteem, and possibly improving intake.
Recommend environment conducive to eating, e.g., avoiding cooking odors if bothersome; keeping room well ventilated, removing noxious stimuli. Suggest use of spices, marinating red meat before cooking and/or substituting other protein sources for red meat.	Improves nutritional intake. Medications and disease can change sense of smell and taste. Patient may develop an aversion to red meat.
Collaborative	
Consult with dietitian.	Provides assistance in planning nutritionally sound diet to meet individual needs.
Monitor laboratory values, e.g., Hct, Hb, albumin, potassium, sodium.	In spite of adequate nutritional intake, fluctuations occur and supplemental feedings or vitamins may be needed to prevent further deterioration.

NURSING DIAGNOSIS:	**KNOWLEDGE DEFICIT [LEARNING NEED], REGARDING DISEASE, PROGNOSIS, AND TREATMENT NEEDS**
May be related to:	Lack of exposure/recall.
	Information misinterpretation.
	Unfamiliarity with information resources.
	Cognitive limitation.

Possibly evidenced by:	Statement of misconception/request for information.
	Inaccurate follow-through of instructions/development of preventable complications.
	Inappropriate/exaggerated behaviors (e.g., hostile, agitated, hysterical, apathetic).
DESIRED OUTCOMES/ EVALUATION CRITERIA— PATIENT WILL:	Verbalize understanding of condition/disease process and treatment.
	Identify relationship of signs/symptoms to the disease process and correlate symptoms with causative factors.
	Initiate necessary lifestyle changes.
	Participate in treatment regimen.

ACTIONS/INTERVENTIONS

Independent

Determine current understanding and perception of diagnosis. Discuss difference between HIV-positivity and AIDS.

Assess emotional ability to assimilate information and understand instructions. Respect patient's need to use "denial" coping techniques initially.

Assess potential for inappropriate/high-risk behavior: continued IV drug abuse, unsafe sexual practices.

Provide information about normal immune system/response and how HIV affects it, transmission of the virus, behaviors/factors believed to increase probability of progression. Encourage questions.

Provide realistic, optimistic information during each contact with patient.

Plan short sessions for additional information.

Review signs/symptoms that may be a consequence of HIV infection, e.g., mild persistent fever, anorexia, weight loss, fatigue, night sweats, diarrhea, dry cough, rashes, headaches, and sleep disturbances.

RATIONALE

Provides opportunity to clarify misconceptions/ myths and make informed choices. Allows for development of individualized plan of care.

Initial shock and anxiety can block intake of information. Self-esteem, lifestyle, guilt, and denial of possibility of exposure/own responsibility in acquiring disease become issues. *Note:* Some initial denial may serve as a protective mechanism promoting more effective self-care.

High denial/anger, drug addiction may result in behaviors that are high risk for spread of the virus. A person's sexuality and identity are threatened by the discovery of the diagnosis.

Patient needs to be aware of own personal risk as well as risk to others in order to make immediate and long-range decisions and establish a basis for goal setting. Also, establishes rapport and provides opportunity to identify concerns and assimilate information.

Necessary to provide realistic hope to reduce risk of suicide. Many patients have been exposed to media information about AIDS or have friends/ lovers who have died of the disease. These persons may feel suicidal on being diagnosed.

Patient will need time and repeated contacts to absorb information.

Patient may experience an acute illness 2–6 weeks after becoming infected; however, it is common for infection to be subclinical, with the individual simply feeling unwell.

ACTIONS/INTERVENTIONS	RATIONALE
Independent	
Discuss signs/symptoms that require medical evaluation, e.g., persistent increasing cough or swollen lymph glands, profound fatigue that is unrelieved by rest, weight loss of 10 lb in less than 2 months, severe/persistent diarrhea, fever, blurred vision, skin discoloration or rash that persists or spreads, open sores anywhere.	Early recognition of progression of disease/development of complications provides for timely intervention and may prevent more serious situations.
Stress necessity of practicing safer sex at all times; also stress need to avoid use of illicit IV drugs, or if unwilling to abstain, to avoid sharing needles and to clean "works" with bleach solution, rinsing carefully with water.	Limits spread of virus. Reduces exposure to other infective agents/additional stress to the immune system.
Discuss active changes in sexual behaviors that the patient can make that may satisfy sexual needs and are designed to prevent transmission.	Promotes a sense of responsibility and control and may reduce sexual tensions.
Provide information about necessary lifestyle changes and health maintenance factors:	Evidence suggests that specific dietary and lifestyle factors may affect the progression of HIV infection along the continuum to AIDS.
Avoid crowds and people with infections;	Early detection and treatment of infection is crucial to delay of further impairment of the immune system and development of opportunistic diseases.
Exercise to limit of ability, alternate rest periods with activity, and get adequate sleep;	Avoids undue fatigue; maintains strength and sense of well-being.
Eat regularly, even if appetite is reduced. Try small, frequent meals and snacks;	Physical and psychologic stressors increase metabolic needs; in addition, side effects of medication, presence of n/v, and anorexia often limit oral intake. The result is nutritional deficits that can further impair the immune system.
Practice good oral hygiene and use a soft toothbrush; examine mouth regularly for sores, white film, or changes in color; have regular dental checkups every 6 months;	Poor oral hygiene/dental care can negatively impact oral intake and increase the risk of opportunistic infections.
Examine skin for rashes, bruises, breaks in skin integrity;	May indicate developing complications/increase risk of infection.
Stress importance of follow-up care. Review procedures and tests that will be necessary for periodic assessment of status.	Even though patient may be asymptomatic, periodic evaluation may prevent development of complications/progression of the disease. Knowledge about what to expect promotes sense of control over situation.
Discuss management strategies for persistent signs and symptoms.	Patient involvement in care increases cooperation and satisfaction with care.
Review drug therapies, side effects, and adverse reactions as appropriate, e.g., zidovudine (AZT, Retrovir); dideoxyinosine (ddI, Videx); zalcitabine (ddC, HIVID).	These experimental drugs appear to halt the HIV replication process. Side effects such as symptoms of peripheral neuropathy or pancreatitis necessitate prompt evaluation and possible discontinuation/change in therapy.

ACTIONS/INTERVENTIONS	RATIONALE
Independent	
Provide written information.	Patient may feel overwhelmed, and written materials allow for later review and reinforcement when patient has had an opportunity to calm down.
Encourage contact with SO, family, and friends. Include in discussions/conferences as appropriate.	Many fear telling their SO, family, and friends for fear of rejection; others withdraw as a result of tumultuous feelings. Contact promotes sense of support, concern, involvement, and understanding. Supporting loved ones as they learn of the diagnosis will be beneficial for the long-term support of the patient.
Identify additional resources, e.g., support groups, peer counselors, and mental health professionals.	Patient will experience a variety of emotional and psychologic responses to the diagnosis and may need additional assistance to promote optimal adjustment.

The CDC recommends that the diagnosis of AIDS be reserved for a person who has an opportunistic infection, while having an underlying immunodeficiency (a T-cell count of 200 or less) and being antibody-positive for HIV. Other frequently associated conditions include progressive dementia, wasting syndrome, or Kaposi's sarcoma (KS) (in patients younger than age 60), certain other cancers (e.g., invasive cervical cancer), or dissemination of generally localized diseases (e.g., TB).

Persons with AIDS have generally been found to fall into six categories: homosexual men, bisexual men, IV drug users, recipients of infected blood or blood products, heterosexual partners of a person with HIV infection, and children born to an infected mother. The rate of infection is currently most rapidly expanding in women and minorities.

RELATED FACTORS

Fluid and Electrolyte Imbalances, p 1054
Long-term Care, p 938
Psychosocial Aspects of Acute Care, p 899
Sepsis/Septicemia, p 887
Total Nutritional Support, p 1039
Upper Gastrointestinal/Esophageal Bleeding, p 454
Ventilatory Assistance (Mechanical), p 226

PATIENT ASSESSMENT DATA BASE

Data are dependent on the organs/body tissues involved and the specific opportunistic infection or cancer.

ACTIVITY/REST

May report:	Easily tired, reduced tolerance for usual activities, progressing to profound fatigue/malaise.
	Altered sleep patterns.
May exhibit:	Muscle weakness, wasting of muscle mass.
	Physiologic response to activity, e.g., changes in BP, heart rate, respiration.

CIRCULATION

May report:	Slow healing (if anemic); bleeding longer with injury (less common).
May exhibit:	Tachycardia, postural BP changes.
	Decreased peripheral pulse volume.
	Pallor or cyanosis; delayed capillary refill.

EGO INTEGRITY

May report:	Stress factors related to losses, e.g., family support, relationships, finances, lifestyle concerns, and spiritual distress.
	Concern about appearance: alopecia, disfiguring lesions, weight loss.
	Denial of diagnosis, feelings of powerlessness, hopelessness, helplessness, worthlessness, guilt, loss of control, depression.
May exhibit:	Denial, anxiety, depression, fear, withdrawal.
	Angry behaviors, dejected body posture, crying, poor eye contact.
	Failure to keep appointments or multiple appointments for similar symptoms.

ELIMINATION

May report: Intermittent, persistent, frequent diarrhea with or without abdominal cramping.
Flank pain, burning on urination.

May exhibit: Loose-formed to watery stools with or without mucus or blood.
Frequent, copious diarrhea.
Abdominal tenderness.
Rectal, perianal lesions or abscesses.
Changes in urinary output, color, character.

FOOD/FLUID

May report: Anorexia, changes in taste of foods/food intolerance, nausea/vomiting.
Rapid/progressive weight loss.
Dysphagia, retrosternal pain with swallowing.

May exhibit: Hyperactive bowel sounds.
Weight loss; thin frame; decreased subcutaneous fat/muscle mass.
Poor skin turgor.
Lesions of the oral cavity, white patches, discoloration.
Poor dental/gum health, loss of teeth.
Edema (generalized, dependent).

HYGIENE

May report: Unable to complete ADLs.

May exhibit: Disheveled appearance.
Deficits in many or all personal care, self-care activities.

NEUROSENSORY

May report: Fainting spells/dizziness; headache.
Changes in mental status, loss of mental acuity/ability to solve problems, forgetfulness, poor concentration.
Impaired sensation or sense of position and vibration.
Muscle weakness, tremors, changes in visual acuity.
Numbness, tingling in extremities (feet seem to display earliest changes).

May exhibit: Mental status changes ranging from confusion to dementia, forgetfulness, poor concentration, decreased alertness, apathy, psychomotor retardation/slowed responses.
Paranoid ideation, free-floating anxiety, unrealistic expectations.
Abnormal reflexes, decreased muscle strength, ataxic gait.
Fine/gross motor tremors, focal motor deficits; hemiparesis, seizures.
Retinal hemorrhages and exudates (CMV retinitis).

PAIN/COMFORT

May report: Generalized/localized pain, aching, burning in feet.
Headache (CNS involvement).
Pleuritic chest pain.

851

May exhibit:

Swelling of joints, painful nodules, tenderness.

Decreased ROM, gait changes/limp.

Muscle guarding.

RESPIRATION

May report:

Frequent, persistent URIs.

Progressive shortness of breath.

Cough (ranging from mild to severe); nonproductive/productive of sputum (earliest sign of PCP may be a spasmodic cough on deep breathing).

Congestion or tightness in chest.

May exhibit:

Tachypnea, respiratory distress.

Changes in breath sounds/adventitious breath sounds.

Sputum: yellow (in sputum-producing pneumonia).

SAFETY

May report:

History of falls, burns, episodes of fainting, slow-healing wounds.

History of frequent or multiple blood transfusions (e.g., hemophiliac, major vascular surgery, traumatic incident).

History of immune deficiency diseases, e.g., advanced cancer.

History of/current infection with STDs.

Recurrent fevers; low grade, intermittent temperature elevations/spikes; night sweats.

May exhibit:

Changes in skin integrity: Cuts, ulcerations, rashes, e.g., eczema, exanthems, psoriasis; discolorations; changes in size/color of moles; unexplained, easy bruising.

Rectal, perianal lesions or abscesses.

Nodules, enlarged lymph nodes in two or more areas of the body (e.g., neck, armpits, groin).

Decline in general strength, muscle tone, changes in gait.

SEXUALITY

May report:

History of high-risk behavior, e.g., having sex with a partner who is HIV positive, multiple sexual partners, unprotected sexual activity, and anal sex.

Loss of libido, being too sick for sex.

Inconsistent use of condoms.

Use of birth control pills (enhanced susceptibility to virus in women who are exposed due to increased vaginal dryness/friability).

May exhibit:

Pregnant or at risk for pregnancy.

Genitalia: Skin manifestations (e.g., herpes, warts); discharge.

SOCIAL INTERACTION

May report:

Problems imposed by diagnosis, e.g., loss of family/SO, friends, support. Fear of telling others; fear of rejection/loss of income.

Isolation, loneliness, close friends or sexual partners who have died from AIDS.

Questioning of ability to remain independent, unable to plan.

May exhibit:

Changes in family/SO interaction pattern.

Disorganized activities, altered goal setting.

TEACHING/LEARNING

May report: Failure to comply with treatment, continued high-risk behavior (e.g., sexual or IV drug use)

IV drug use/abuse, current smoking, alcohol abuse.

Evidence of failure to improve from last hospitalization.

Discharge Plan Considerations: **DRG projected mean length of stay: 10.2 days.**

May require assistance with finances, medications/treatments, skin/wound care, equipment/supplies; transportation, food shopping and preparation; self-care, technical nursing procedures, homemaker/maintenance tasks, child care; changes in living facilities.

DIAGNOSTIC STUDIES

CBC: Anemia and idiopathic thrombocytopenia.

WBC: Leukopenia may be present; differential shift to the left suggests infectious process (PCP); shift to the right may be noted. With certain infections, low T-cell count, or T-cell tumor, no shift may occur.

Anergy panel: Cutaneous anergy (lack of reactivity to common antigens to which the patient has been exposed) is a common indicator of depressed cell-mediated immunity.

TB (PPD): To determine exposure and/or in active disease (must be given with anergy panel to determine false-negative result due to deficient immune response). Of AIDS patients, 100% will have active Mycobacterium TB in their lifetime if exposure has occurred.

Serologic:

Serum antibody test: HIV screen by ELISA. A positive test result may be indicative of exposure to HIV but is not diagnostic. (Sensitivity varies with the incidence of false-positive results as high as 25%.)

Western blot test: Confirms diagnosis of HIV.

T-lymphocyte cells: Total count reduced.

T4-helper cells (immune system indicator that mediates several immune system processes and signals B cells to produce antibodies to foreign germs): Numbers less than 200 indicate severe immune deficiency response.

T8 (cytopathic suppressor cells): Reversed ratio (2:1 or greater) of suppressor cells to helper cells (T8 to T4) indicates immune suppression.

P24 (envelope protein of HIV): Increased quantitative values of this protein can be indicative of progression of infection. (May not be detectable during very early stages of HIV infection.)

Ig levels: Usually elevated, especially IgG and IgA, with normal to near normal IgM (indicator of the ability of the body to show whether infectious processing is intact, but is used infrequently because other factors can alter it, e.g., environmental pollutants).

Polymerase chain reaction: Detects viral DNA in presence of small quantities of infected peripheral mononuclear cells.

STD testing: Hepatitis B envelope and core antibodies, syphilis, CMV may be positive.

Cultures: Histologic, cytologic studies of urine, blood, stool, spinal fluid, lesions, sputum, and secretions may be done to identify the opportunistic infection. Some of the most commonly identified are the following:

Protozoa and helminthic infections: PCP cryptosporidiosis, toxoplasmosis.

Fungal infections: Candida albicans (candidiasis), *Cryptococcus neoformans* (cryptococcosis); *Histoplasma capsulatum* (histoplasmosis).

Bacterial infections: Mycobacterium avium-intercellulare, miliary mycobacterial TB, Shigella (shigellosis), Salmonella (salmonellosis).

Viral infections: CMV, herpes simplex, herpes zoster.

Neurologic studies, e.g., EEG, MRI, CT scans of the brain: EMG/nerve conduction studies: Indicated for changes in mentation, fever of undetermined origin and/or changes in sensory/motor function.

Chest x-ray: May initially be normal or may reveal progressive interstitial infiltrates from advanced PCP (most common opportunistic disease) or other pulmonary complications.

853

Pulmonary function tests: Useful in early detection of interstitial pneumonias.

Gallium scan: Diffuse pulmonary uptake occurs in PCP and other forms of pneumonia.

Biopsies: May be done for differential diagnosis of KS or other neoplastic lesions.

Bronchoscopy/tracheobronchial washings: May be done with biopsy when PCP or lung malignancies are suspected (diagnostic confirming test for PCP).

Barium swallow, endoscopy, colonoscopy: May be done to identify opportunistic infection (e.g., Candida, CMV) or to stage KS in the GI system.

NURSING PRIORITIES

1. Prevent/minimize infections.
2. Maintain homeostasis.
3. Promote comfort.
4. Support psychosocial adjustment.
5. Provide information about disease process/prognosis and treatment needs.

DISCHARGE GOALS

1. Infection prevented/resolved.
2. Complications prevented/minimized.
3. Pain/discomfort alleviated.
4. Patient is dealing with current situation realistically.
5. Diagnosis, prognosis, and therapeutic regimen understood.

NURSING DIAGNOSIS:	INFECTION, HIGH RISK FOR (PROGRESSION TO SEPSIS/ONSET OF NEW OPPORTUNISTIC INFECTION)
Risk factors may include:	Inadequate primary defenses: broken skin, traumatized tissue, stasis of body fluids.
	Depression of the immune system; use of antimicrobial agents.
	Environmental exposure, invasive techniques.
	Chronic disease; malnutrition.
Possibly evidenced by:	[Not applicable; presence of signs and symptoms establishes an actual diagnosis.]
DESIRED OUTCOMES/ EVALUATION CRITERIA— PATIENT WILL:	Identify/participate in behaviors to reduce risk of infection.
	Achieve timely healing of wounds/lesions.
	Be afebrile and free of purulent drainage/secretions and other signs of infectious conditions.

ACTIONS/INTERVENTIONS	RATIONALE
Independent	
Wash hands before and after all care contacts. Instruct patient/SO to wash hands as indicated.	Reduces risk of cross-contamination.
Provide a clean, well-ventilated environment. Screen visitors/staff for signs of infection and maintain isolation precautions as indicated.	Reduces number of pathogens presented to the immune system and reduces possibility of patient contracting a nosocomial infection.

ACTIONS/INTERVENTIONS	RATIONALE
Independent	
Discuss extent and rationale for isolation precautions and maintenance of personal hygiene.	Promotes cooperation with regimen and may lessen feelings of isolation.
Monitor vital signs, including temperature.	Provides information for baseline data; frequent temperature elevations/onset of new fever indicates that the body is responding to a new infectious process or that medications are not effectively controlling noncurable infections.
Assess respiratory rate/depth; note dry spasmodic cough on deep inspiration, changes in characteristics of sputum, and presence of wheezes/rhonchi. Initiate respiratory isolation when etiology of productive cough is unknown.	Respiratory congestion/distress may indicate developing PCP, the most common opportunistic disease. However, TB is on the rise and other fungal, viral, and bacterial infections may occur that compromise the respiratory system.
Investigate reports of headache, stiff neck, altered vision. Note changes in mentation and behavior. Monitor for nuchal rigidity/seizure activity.	Neurologic abnormalities are common and may be related to the HIV or secondary infections. Symptoms may vary from subtle changes in mood/sensorium (personality changes or depression)to hallucinations, memory loss, severe dementias, seizures, and loss of vision. CNS infections (encephalitis is the most common) may be caused by protozoa and helminthic organisms or fungus.
Examine skin/oral mucous membranes for white patches/lesions. (Refer to ND: Skin Integrity, Impaired: actual and/or high risk for, p 863 and ND: Oral Mucous Membranes, altered, p 864.)	Oral candidiasis, KS, herpes, CMV, and Cryptococcus are common opportunistic diseases affecting the cutaneous membranes.
Clean nails daily. File, rather than cut, and avoid trimming cuticles.	Reduces risk of transmission of pathogens through breaks in skin. *Note:* Fungal infections along the nail plate are common.
Monitor reports of heartburn, dysphagia, retrosternal pain on swallowing, increased abdominal cramping, profuse diarrhea.	Esophagitis may occur secondary to oral candidiasis or herpes. Cryptosporidiosis is a parasitic infection responsible for watery diarrhea (often greater than 15 L/d).
Inspect wounds/site of invasive devices, noting signs of local inflammation/infection.	Early identification/treatment of secondary infection may prevent sepsis.
Wear gloves and gowns during direct contact with secretions/excretions or anytime there is a break in skin of care giver's hands. Wear mask and protective eyewear to protect nose, mouth, and eyes from secretions during procedures (e.g., suctioning) or when splattering of blood may occur.	Use of masks, gowns, and gloves is required by OSHA (1992) for direct contact with body fluids, e.g., sputum, blood/blood products, semen, vaginal secretions.
Dispose of needles/sharps in rigid, puncture-resistant containers.	Prevents accidental inoculation of care givers. Use of needle cutters and recapping is not to be practiced. *Note:* Accidental inoculations/punctures should be reported immediately and follow-up evaluations done per protocol.
Label blood bags, body fluid containers, soiled dressings/linens, and package appropriately for disposal per isolation protocol.	Prevents cross-contamination and alerts appropriate personnel/departments to exercise specific hazardous materials procedures.

855

ACTIONS/INTERVENTIONS	RATIONALE

Independent

Clean up spills of body fluids/blood with bleach solution (1:10).

Controls microorganisms on hard surfaces.

Collaborative

Monitor laboratory studies, e.g.:

CBC/differential;

Shifts in the differential and changes in WBC count indicates infectious process. Low WBC count or other changes in blood count may be related to treatments/medications.

Culture/sensitivity studies of lesions, blood, urine, and sputum.

May be done to identify cause of fever, diagnose infecting organisms, or determine appropriate course of treatment.

Administer antibiotic antifungal/antimicrobial agents, e.g., trimethroprim (Bactrim, Septra), nystatin (Mycostatin), ketoconazole, pentamidine; or AZT/Retrovir and ganciclovir (Cytovene), or foscarnet (Fascavir), dideoxyinosine (ddI, VIDEX), dideoxycytidine (ddC, HIVID).

Combats infectious process. Some drugs are targeted for specific organisms/affected system. Other drugs are targeted to improve immune function. Although no cure is currently available, agents such as AZT are aimed at blocking the enzyme that enables the virus to enter the genetic material of the T4 cell, thereby retarding the progression of the disease. Ganciclovir is used when CMV is present to prevent blindness/life-threatening dissemination. *Note:* If leukopenia occurs with combined use of AZT and ganciclovir, AZT may be discontinued. Fascavir is available to prevent CMV progression but should be used with caution as it may cause renal toxicity.

NURSING DIAGNOSIS:	FLUID VOLUME DEFICIT, HIGH RISK FOR
Risk factors may include:	Excessive losses: Copious diarrhea, profuse sweating, vomiting.
	Hypermetabolic state, fever.
	Restricted intake: Nausea, anorexia; lethargy.
Possibly evidenced by:	[Not applicable; presence of signs and symptoms establishes an actual diagnosis.]
DESIRED OUTCOMES/ EVALUATION CRITERIA— PATIENT WILL:	Maintain hydration as evidenced by moist mucous membranes, good skin turgor, stable vital signs, individually adequate urinary output.

ACTIONS/INTERVENTIONS	RATIONALE

Independent

Monitor vital signs, including CVP if available. Note hypotension, including postural changes.

Indicators of circulating fluid volume.

ACTIONS/INTERVENTIONS	RATIONALE

Independent

Note temperature elevation and duration of febrile episode. Administer tepid sponge baths as indicated. Keep clothing and linens dry. Maintain comfortable environmental temperature.

Increased metabolic demands and excessive diaphoresis associated with fever result in increased insensible fluid losses.

Assess skin turgor, mucous membranes, and thirst.

Indirect indicators of fluid status.

Measure urinary output and specific gravity. Measure/estimate amount of diarrheal loss. Note insensible losses.

Increased specific gravity/decreasing urinary output reflects altered renal perfusion/circulating volume. *Note:* Monitoring fluid balance is difficult because of excessive GI/insensible losses.

Weigh as indicated.

Although weight loss may reflect muscle wasting, sudden fluctuations reflect state of hydration. Fluid losses associated with diarrhea can quickly create a crisis and become life threatening.

Monitor oral intake and encourage fluids of at least 2500 ml/d.

Maintains fluid balance, reduces thirst, and moisturizes mucous membranes.

Make fluids easily accessible to patient; use fluids that are tolerable to the patient and that replace needed electrolytes, e.g., Gatorade, broth.

Enhances intake. Certain fluids may be too painful to consume (e.g., acidic juices) because of mouth lesions.

Eliminate foods potentiating diarrhea, e.g., spicy/high-fat foods, nuts, cabbage, milk products. Adjust rate/concentration of tube feedings if indicated.

May help reduce diarrhea.

Collaborative

Administer fluids/electrolytes via feeding tube/IV.

May be necessary to support/augment circulating volume, especially if oral intake is inadequate, nausea/vomiting persists.

Monitor laboratory studies as indicated, e.g.:

Hb/Hct.

Useful in estimating fluid needs.

Serum/urine electrolytes.

Alerts to possible electrolyte disturbances and determines replacement needs.

BUN/Cr.

Evaluates renal perfusion/function.

Administer medications as indicated:

Antiemetics, e.g., prochlorperazine maleate (Compazine); trimethobenzamide (Tigan); metoclopramide (Reglan);

Reduces incidence of vomiting to reduce further loss of fluids/electrolytes.

Antidiarrheals, e.g., diphenoxylate (Lomotil), loperamide imodium, paregoric, or antispasmodics, e.g., mepenzolate bromide (Cantil);

Decreases the amount and fluidity of stool; may reduce intestinal spasm and peristalsis. *Note:* Antibiotics may also be used to treat diarrhea if caused by infection.

Antipyretics, e.g., acetaminophen (Tylenol).

Helps to reduce fever and hypermetabolic response, decreasing insensible losses.

Maintain hypothermia blanket if used.

May be necessary when other measures fail to reduce excessive fever.

ACTIONS/INTERVENTIONS	RATIONALE
Independent	
Auscultate breath sounds, noting areas of decreased/absent ventilation and presence of adventitious sounds, e.g., crackles, wheezes, rhonchi.	Suggests developing pulmonary complications/infection, e.g., atelectasis/pneumonia. *Note:* PCP is often advanced before changes in breath sounds occur.
Note rate/depth of respiration, cyanosis, use of accessory muscles/increased work of breathing and presence of dyspnea, anxiety.	Tachypnea, cyanosis, restlessness, and increased work of breathing reflect respiratory distress and need for increased surveillance/medical intervention.
Elevate head of bed. Have patient turn, cough, deep breathe, as indicated.	Promotes optimal pulmonary function, and reduces incidence of aspiration or infection due to atelectasis.
Suction airway as indicated, using sterile technique and observing safety precautions, e.g., mask, protective eyewear.	Assists in clearing the ventilatory passages, thereby facilitating gas exchange and preventing respiratory complications.
Assess changes in level of consciousness.	Hypoxemia can result in changes ranging from anxiety and confusion to unresponsiveness.
Investigate reports of chest pain.	Pleuritic chest pain may reflect nonspecific pneumonitis or pleural effusions associated with malignancies.
Allow adequate rest periods between care activities. Maintain a quiet environment.	Reduces O_2 consumption.
Collaborative	
Monitor/graph serial ABGs/pulse oximetry.	Indicators of respiratory status, treatment needs/effectiveness.

ACTIONS/INTERVENTIONS	RATIONALE
Collaborative	
Review serial chest x-rays.	Presence of diffuse infiltrates may suggest pneumonia or PCP, while areas of congestion/consolidation may reflect other pulmonary complications, e.g., atelectasis or KS lesions.
Instruct in use of incentive spirometer. Provide chest physiotherapy, e.g., percussion, vibration, and postural drainage.	Encourages proper breathing technique and improves lung expansion. Loosens secretions, dislodges mucous plugs to promote airway clearance. *Note:* In the event of multiple skin lesions, chest physiotherapy may be discontinued.
Provide humidified supplemental O_2 via appropriate means, e.g., cannula, mask, intubation/mechanical ventilation.	Maintains effective ventilation/oxygenation to prevent/correct respiratory crisis.
Administer medications as indicated:	
Antimicrobials, e.g.: trimethoprim (Bactrim, Septra); pentamidine isethionate (Pentam);	Choice of therapy is dependent on individual situation/infecting organism(s). *Note:* Bactrim is the drug of choice as a prophylaxis (as the T4 count approaches 200) to prevent PCP pneumonia.
Bronchodilators, expectorants, cough depressants.	May be needed to improve/maintain airway patency or help clear secretions.
Prepare/assist with procedures as indicated, e.g., bronchoscopy.	May be required to clear mucous plugs, obtain specimens for diagnosis (biopsies/lavage).

NURSING DIAGNOSIS:	**INJURY, HIGH RISK FOR, ALTERED CLOTTING FACTORS**
Risk factors may include:	Decreased vitamin K absorption, alteration in hepatic function, presence of autoimmune antiplatelet antibodies, malignancies (KS); and/or circulating endotoxins (sepsis).
Possibly evidenced by:	[Not applicable; presence of signs and symptoms establishes an actual diagnosis.]
DESIRED OUTCOMES/ EVALUATION CRITERIA— PATIENT WILL:	Display homeostasis as evidenced by absence of mucosal bleeding and be free of ecchymosis.

ACTIONS/INTERVENTIONS	RATIONALE
Independent	
Hematest body fluids for occult blood, e.g., urine, stool, vomitus.	Prompt detection of bleeding/initiation of therapy may prevent critical hemorrhage.
Observe for/report epistaxis, hemoptysis, hematuria, nonmenstrual vaginal bleeding, or oozing from lesions/body orifices/IV insertion sites.	Spontaneous bleeding may indicate development of DIC or immune thrombocytopenia.

859

ACTIONS/INTERVENTIONS	RATIONALE
Independent	
Monitor for changes in vital signs and skin color, e.g., BP, pulse, respirations, skin pallor/discoloration.	Presence of bleeding/hemorrhage may lead to circulatory failure/shock.
Monitor for change in level of consciousness and visual disturbances.	Change may reflect cerebral bleeding.
Avoid IM injections, rectal temperatures/suppositories, rectal tubes.	Protects patient from procedure-related causes of bleeding; e.g., insertion of thermometers, rectal tubes can damage or tear rectal mucosa.
Maintain a safe environment; e.g., keep all necessary objects and call bell within patient's reach and keep bed in low position.	Reduces accidental injury, which could result in bleeding.
Maintain bed/chair rest when platelets are below 10,000 or as individually appropriate. Assess medication regimen.	Reduces possibility of injury, although activity needs to be maintained. May need to discontinue or reduce drug, e.g., AZT. *Note:* Patient can have a surprisingly low platelet count without bleeding.
Collaborative	
Review laboratory studies, e.g., PT, PTT, clotting time, platelets, Hb/Hct.	Detects alterations in clotting capability; identifies therapy needs.
Administer blood products as indicated.	Transfusions may be required in the event of persistent/massive spontaneous bleeding.
Avoid use of aspirin products.	Reduces platelet aggregation, impairing/prolonging the coagulation process.

NURSING DIAGNOSIS:	**NUTRITION, ALTERED: LESS THAN BODY REQUIREMENTS**
May be related to:	Inability or altered ability to ingest, digest and/or metabolize nutrients: nausea/vomiting, hyperactive gag reflex, intestinal disturbances.
	Increased metabolic rate/nutritional needs (fever/infection).
Possibly evidenced by:	Weight loss, decreased subcutaneous fat/muscle mass.
	Lack of interest in food, aversion to eating, altered taste sensation.
	Abdominal cramping, hyperactive bowel sounds, diarrhea.
	Sore, inflamed buccal cavity.
DESIRED OUTCOMES/ EVALUATION CRITERIA— PATIENT WILL:	Maintain weight or display weight gain toward desired goal.
	Demonstrate positive nitrogen balance, be free of signs of malnutrition, and display improved energy level.

ACTIONS/INTERVENTIONS	RATIONALE
Independent	
Assess ability to chew, taste, and swallow.	Lesions of the mouth, throat, and esophagus may cause dysphagia, limiting patient's ability to ingest food and reducing desire to eat.
Auscultate bowel sounds.	Hypermotility of intestinal tract is common and is associated with vomiting and diarrhea, which may affect choice of diet/route. *Note:* Lactose intolerance and malabsorption contributes to diarrhea and may necessitate change in diet/supplemental formula (e.g., Resource).
Weigh as indicated. Evaluate weight in terms of premorbid weight. Use serial weights and anthropometric measurements.	Indicator of nutritional needs/adequacy of intake. *Note:* Because of immune suppression, some blood tests normally used for testing nutritional status are not useful.
Remove existing noxious environmental stimuli or conditions that aggravate gag reflex.	Reduces stimulus of the vomiting center in the medulla.
Provide frequent mouth care, observing secretion precautions. Avoid alcohol-containing mouthwashes.	Reduces discomfort associated with nausea/vomiting oral lesions, mucosal dryness, and halitosis. Clean mouth may enhance appetite.
Plan diet with patient/SO; suggest "foods from home" if appropriate. Provide small, frequent meals/snacks of nutritionally dense foods and nonacidic foods and beverages, with choice of foods palatable to patient. Encourage high-calorie/nutrition foods, some of which may be considered appetite stimulants. Note time of day when appetite is best, and try to serve larger meal at that time.	Including patient in planning gives sense of control of environment and may enhance intake. Fulfilling cravings for noninstitutional food may also improve intake.
Assess medications for nutritional side effects.	Prophylactic and therapeutic medications can have nutritional side effects, e.g., AZT (altered taste, nausea/vomiting. Bactrim (anorexia, glucose intolerance, glossitis), pentamidine (altered taste and smell, nausea/vomiting, glucose intolerance).
Limit food(s) that induce nausea/vomiting or are poorly tolerated by the patient because of mouth sores/dysphagia. Avoid serving very hot liquids/foods. Serve foods easy to swallow, e.g., eggs, ice cream, cooked vegetables.	Pain in the mouth or fear of irritating oral lesions may cause the patient to be reluctant to eat. These measures may be helpful in increasing food intake.
Schedule medications between meals (if tolerated) and limit fluid intake with meals, unless fluid has nutritional value.	Gastric fullness diminishes appetite and food intake.
Encourage as much physical activity as possible.	May improve appetite and general feelings of well-being.
Provide rest period before meals. Avoid stressful procedures close to mealtime.	Minimizes fatigue; increases energy available for work of eating.
Encourage patient to sit up for meals.	Facilitates swallowing and reduces risk of aspiration.
Record caloric intake.	Identifies need for supplements or alternate feeding methods.

ACTIONS/INTERVENTIONS	RATIONALE
Collaborative	
Review laboratory studies, e.g., BUN, glucose, liver function studies, electrolytes, protein, and albumin.	Indicates nutritional status and organ function, and identifies replacement needs. *Note:* Nutritional tests can be altered because of disease processes as well as response to some medications/therapies.
Maintain NPO status when appropriate.	May be needed to reduce vomiting.
Insert/maintain NG tube as indicated.	May be needed to reduce n/v, or to administer tube feedings. *Note:* Esophageal irritation from existing infection (Candida/herpes or KS) may provide site for secondary infections/trauma; therefore, tube should be used with caution.
Consult with dietitian/nutritional support team.	Provides for diet based on individual needs/appropriate route.
Administer TPN (hyperalimentation/intralipids) as indicated.	Occasionally parenteral nutrients may be required if oral/enteral feedings are not tolerated.
Administer medications as indicated:	
Antiemetics, e.g., metoclopramide (Reglan);	Reduces incidence of vomiting; promotes gastric function.
Vitamin supplements.	Vitamin deficiencies result from decreased food intake and/or disorders of digestion and absorption in the GI system.

NURSING DIAGNOSIS:	**PAIN, [ACUTE]/CHRONIC**
May be related to:	Tissue inflammation/destruction: Infections, internal/external cutaneous lesions, rectal excoriation, malignancies, necrosis.
	Peripheral neuropathies, myalgias, and arthralgias.
	Abdominal cramping.
Possibly evidenced by:	Reports of pain.
	Self-focusing; narrowed focus, guarding behaviors.
	Alteration in muscle tone; muscle cramping, ataxia, muscle weakness, paresthesias, paralysis.
	Autonomic responses; restlessness.
DESIRED OUTCOMES/ EVALUATION CRITERIA— PATIENT WILL:	Report pain relieved/controlled.
	Demonstrate relaxed posture/facial expression.
	Be able to sleep/rest appropriately.

ACTIONS/INTERVENTIONS	RATIONALE

Independent

Assess pain reports, noting location, intensity (0–10 scale), frequency, and time of onset. Note nonverbal cues, e.g., restlessness, tachycardia, grimacing.

Indicates need for/effectiveness of interventions and may signal development/resolution of complications. *Note:* Chronic pain does not produce autonomic changes.

Encourage verbalization of feelings.

Can reduce anxiety and fear and thereby reduce perception of intensity of pain.

Provide diversional activities, e.g., reading, visiting, television.

Refocuses attention; may enhance coping abilities.

Perform palliative measures e.g., repositioning, massage, ROM of affected joints.

Promotes relaxation/decreases muscle tension.

Apply warm/moist packs to pentamidine injection/IV sites for 20 minutes after administration.

These injections are known to cause pain and sterile abscesses.

Instruct patient in/encourage use of visualization/guided imagery, progressive relaxation, deep-breathing techniques.

Promotes relaxation and feeling of well-being. May decrease the need for narcotic analgesics (CNS depressants) where there is already a neuro/motor degenerative process involved. May not be successful in presence of dementia, even though minor.

Provide oral care. (Refer to ND: Oral Mucous Membranes, altered, p 864.)

Oral ulcerations/lesions may cause severe discomfort.

Collaborative

Administer analgesics/antipyretics, narcotic analgesics. Use PCA or provide around-the-clock analgesia with rescue doses prn.

Provides relief of pain/discomfort; reduces fever. Patient-controlled or around-the-clock medicating keeps the blood level of analgesia stable, preventing cyclic undermedication or overmedication.

NURSING DIAGNOSIS:	**SKIN INTEGRITY, IMPAIRED: ACTUAL AND/OR HIGH RISK FOR**
May be related to:	
Actual:	Immunologic deficit: AIDS-related dermatitis; viral, bacterial and fungal infections (e.g., herpes, Pseudomonas, Candida); opportunistic disease processes (e.g., KS).
Risk factors may include:	Decreased level of activity, altered sensation, skeletal prominence, changes in skin turgor.
	Malnutrition, altered metabolic state.
Possibly evidenced by:	Skin lesions; ulcerations; decubitus ulcer formation (actual).
DESIRED OUTCOMES/ EVALUATION CRITERIA— PATIENT WILL:	Demonstrate behaviors/techniques to prevent skin breakdown/promote healing.
	Display improvement in wound/lesion healing.

ACTIONS/INTERVENTIONS	RATIONALE
Independent	
Assess skin daily. Note color, turgor, circulation, and sensation. Describe lesions and observe changes.	Establishes baseline with which changes in status can be compared and appropriate interventions instituted.
Maintain/instruct in good skin hygiene, e.g., wash thoroughly, pat dry carefully, and massage with lotion or appropriate cream.	Maintaining clean, dry skin provides a barrier to infection. Patting skin dry instead of rubbing reduces risk of dermal trauma to dry/fragile skin. Massaging increases circulation to the skin and promotes comfort. *Note:* Isolation precautions are required, especially when extensive mucocutaneous lesions are present.
Reposition frequently. Use turn sheet as needed. Encourage periodic weight shifts. Protect bony prominences with pillows, heel/elbow pads, sheepskin.	Reduces stress on pressure points, improves blood flow to tissues, and promotes healing.
Maintain clean, dry, wrinkle-free linen.	Skin friction caused by wet or wrinkled sheets leads to irritation and potentiates infection.
Encourage ambulation/out of bed as tolerated.	Decreases pressure on skin from prolonged bed rest.
Cleanse perianal area by removing stool with water and mineral oil. Avoid use of toilet paper if vesicles present. Apply protective creams, e.g., zinc oxide, A&D ointment.	Prevents maceration caused by diarrhea and keeps perianal lesions dry. *Note:* Use of toilet paper may abrade lesions.
File nails regularly.	Long/rough nails increase risk of dermal damage.
Cover open pressure ulcers with sterile dressings or protective barrier, e.g., DuoDerm, as indicated.	May reduce bacterial contamination, promote healing.
Collaborative	
Provide foam/flotation mattress or bed.	Decreases tissue ischemia, reducing pressure on skin, tissue, and lesions.
Obtain cultures of open skin lesions.	Identifies pathogens and appropriate treatment choices.
Apply/administer topical/systemic drugs as indicated.	Used in treatment of skin lesions. *Note:* When multidose ointments are used, care must be taken to avoid cross-contamination.
Cover ulcerated KS lesions with wet-to-wet dressings or antibiotic ointment and nonstick dressing (e.g., Telfa) as indicated.	Protects ulcerated areas from contamination and promotes healing.

NURSING DIAGNOSIS:	**ORAL MUCOUS MEMBRANES, ALTERED**
May be related to:	Immunologic deficit and presence of lesion-causing pathogens, e.g., Candida, herpes, KS.
	Dehydration, malnutrition.

	Ineffective oral hygiene.
	Side effects of drugs, chemotherapy.
Possibly evidenced by:	Open, ulcerated lesions, vesicles.
	Oral pain/discomfort.
	Stomatitis; leukoplakia, gingivitis, carious teeth.
DESIRED OUTCOMES/ EVALUATION CRITERIA— PATIENT WILL:	Display intact mucous membranes, which are pink, moist, and free of inflammation/ulcerations.
	Demonstrate techniques to restore/maintain integrity of oral mucosa.

ACTIONS/INTERVENTIONS	RATIONALE
Independent	
Assess mucous membranes/document all oral lesions. Note reports of pain, swelling, difficulty with chewing/swallowing.	Edema, open lesions, and crusting on oral mucous membranes and throat may cause pain and difficulty with chewing/swallowing.
Provide oral care daily and after food intake, using soft toothbrush, nonabrasive toothpaste, nonalcohol mouthwash, floss, and lip moisturizer.	Alleviates discomfort, promotes feeling of well-being, and prevents acid formation associated with retained food particles.
Rinse oral mucosal lesions with saline/dilute hydrogen peroxide or baking soda solutions.	Reduces spread of lesions and encrustations from candidiasis and promotes comfort.
Suggest use of sugarless gum/candy or commercial salivary substitute.	Stimulates flow of saliva to neutralize acids and protect mucous membranes.
Plan diet to avoid salty, spicy, abrasive, and acidic foods or beverages. Check for temperature tolerance of foods. Offer cool/cold smooth foods.	Abrasive foods may open healing lesions. Open lesions are painful and aggravated by salt, spice, acidic foods/beverages. Extreme cold or heat can cause pain to sensitive mucous membranes.
Encourage oral intake of at least 2500 ml/d.	Maintains hydration; prevents drying of oral cavity.
Encourage patient to refrain from smoking.	Smoke is drying and irritating to mucous membranes.
Collaborative	
Obtain culture specimens of lesions.	Reveals causative agents and identifies appropriate therapies.
Administer medications, as indicated, e.g., nystatin (Mycostatin), ketoconazole (Nizoral).	Specific drug choice is dependent on particular infecting organism(s), e.g., Candida.
Refer for dental consultation, if appropriate.	May require additional therapy to prevent dental losses.

NURSING DIAGNOSIS:	**FATIGUE**
May be related to:	Decreased metabolic energy production, increased energy requirements (hypermetabolic state).

	Overwhelming psychologic/emotional demands.
	Altered body chemistry: Side effects of medication, chemotherapy.
Possibly evidenced by:	Unremitting/overwhelming lack of energy, inability to maintain usual routines, decreased performance, impaired ability to concentrate, lethargy/listlessness.
	Disinterest in surroundings.
DESIRED OUTCOMES/ EVALUATION CRITERIA— PATIENT WILL:	Report improved sense of energy.
	Perform ADLs.
	Participate in desired activities at level of ability.

ACTIONS/INTERVENTIONS	RATIONALE
Independent	
Assess sleep patterns and note changes in thought processes/behaviors.	Multiple factors can aggravate fatigue, including sleep deprivation, CNS disease, emotional distress, and side effects of drugs/chemotherapies.
Plan care to allow for rest periods. Schedule activities for periods when patient has most energy. Involve patient/SO in schedule planning.	Frequent rest periods are needed to restore/conserve energy. Planning will allow patient to be active during times when energy level is higher, which may restore a feeling of well-being and a sense of control.
Establish realistic activity goals with patient.	Provides for a sense of control and feelings of accomplishment. Prevents discouragement from fatigue of overactivity.
Assist with self-care needs; keep bed in low position and travelways clear of furniture; assist with ambulation.	Weakness may make ADLs almost impossible for the patient to complete. Protects patient from injury during activities.
Encourage patient to do whatever possible, e.g., self-care, sit in chair, walk, go out to lunch. Increase activity level as indicated.	May conserve strength, increase stamina, and enable patient to become more active without undue fatigue and discouragement.
Monitor physiologic response to activity, e.g., changes in BP, respiratory rate, or heart rate.	Tolerance varies greatly depending on the stage of the disease process, nutrition state, fluid balance, and number/type of opportunistic diseases that the patient has been subject to.
Encourage nutritional intake. (Refer to ND: Nutrition, Altered: Less than body requirements, p 860.)	Adequate intake/utilization of nutrients is necessary to meet energy needs for activity.
Collaborative	
Provide supplemental O_2 as indicated.	Presence of anemia/hypoxemia reduces O_2 available for cellular uptake and contributes to fatigue.
Refer to physical/occupational therapy.	Programmed daily exercises and activities help patient to maintain/increase strength and muscle tone, enhance sense of well-being.

NURSING DIAGNOSIS:	THOUGHT PROCESSES, ALTERED
May be related to:	Hypoxemia, CNS infection by HIV, brain malignancies, and/or disseminated systemic opportunistic infection, CVA/hemorrhage; vasculitis.
	Alteration of drug metabolism/excretion, accumulation of toxic elements; renal failure, severe electrolyte imbalance, hepatic insufficiency.
Possibly evidenced by:	Altered attention span; distractibility.
	Memory deficit.
	Disorientation; cognitive dissonance; delusional thinking.
	Sleep disturbances.
	Impaired ability to make decisions/problem solve; inability to follow complex commands/mental tasks, loss of impulse control.
DESIRED OUTCOMES/ EVALUATION CRITERIA— PATIENT WILL:	Maintain usual reality orientation and optimal cognitive functioning.

ACTIONS/INTERVENTIONS	RATIONALE
Independent	
Assess mental and neurologic status using appropriate tools. Note changes in orientation, response to stimuli, ability to problem-solve, anxiety, altered sleep patterns, hallucinations, paranoid ideation.	Establishes functional level at time of admission and alerts the nurse to changes in status that may be associated with exacerbation of CNS infection/opportunistic disease, environmental stressors, psychologic stress, or side effects of drug therapy.
Consider effects of emotional distress, e.g., anxiety, grief, anger.	May contribute to reduced alertness, confusion, withdrawal, hypoactivity and require further evaluation and intervention.
Monitor medication regimen and usage.	Actions and interactions of various medications, prolonged drug half-life/altered excretion, results in cumulative effects, potentiating risk of toxic reactions. Some drugs may have adverse side effects; e.g., haloperidol (Haldol) can seriously impair motor function in patients with AIDS dementia complex.
Monitor for signs of CNS infection, e.g., headache, nuchal rigidity, vomiting, fever.	CNS symptoms associated with disseminated meningitis/encephalitis may range from subtle personality changes to confusion, irritability, drowsiness, stupor, seizures, and dementia.
Maintain a pleasant environment with appropriate auditory, visual, and cognitive stimuli.	Providing normal environmental stimuli can help in maintaining some sense of reality orientation.

867

ACTIONS/INTERVENTIONS	RATIONALE

Independent

Provide cues for reorientation, e.g., radio, television, calendars, clocks, room with an outside view. Use patient's name; identify yourself. Maintain consistent personnel and structured schedules as appropriate.

Frequent reorientation to place and time may be necessary, especially during fever/acute CNS involvement. Sense of continuity may reduce associated anxiety.

Discuss use of datebooks, lists, other devices to keep track of activities.

These techniques help patient to manage problems of forgetfulness.

Encourage family/SO to socialize and provide reorientation with current news, family events.

Familiar contacts are often helpful in maintaining reality orientation, especially if patient is hallucinating.

Encourage patient to do as much as possible, e.g., dress and groom daily, see friends, and so forth.

Can help to maintain mental abilities for longer period.

Provide support for SO. Encourage discussion of concerns/fears.

Bizarre behavior/deterioration of abilities may be very frightening for SO and makes management of care/dealing with situation difficult. SO may feel a loss of control as stress, anxiety, burnout, and anticipatory grieving impairs usual coping abilities.

Reduce provocative/noxious stimuli. Maintain bed rest in quiet, darkened room if indicated.

If the patient is prone to agitation, violent behavior, or seizures, reducing external stimuli may be helpful.

Decrease noise, especially at night.

Promotes sleep; reduces cognitive symptoms and sleep deprivation.

Set limits on maladaptive/abusive behavior; avoid open-ended choices.

Provides sense of security/stability in an otherwise confusing situation.

Maintain safe environment: e.g., excess furniture out of the way, call bell within patient's reach, bed in low position/rails up; restriction of smoking (unless monitored by care giver/SO), seizure precautions, soft restraints if indicated.

Decreases the possibility of patient injury.

Provide information about care on an ongoing basis. Answer questions simply and honestly. Repeat explanations as needed.

Can reduce anxiety and fear of unknown; can enhance patient's understanding and involvement/cooperation in treatment when possible.

Discuss causes/future expectations and treatment if dementia is diagnosed. Use concrete terms.

Obtaining information that AZT has been shown to improve cognition can provide hope and control for losses.

Collaborative

Assist with diagnostic studies, e.g., MRI, CT scan spinal tap; and monitor laboratory studies as indicated, e.g., BUN/Cr, electrolytes, ABGs.

Choice of tests/studies are dependent on clinical manifestations and index of suspicion, as changes in mental status may reflect a wide variety of causative factors, e.g., CMV meningitis/encephalitis, drug toxicity, electrolyte imbalances, and altered organ function.

Administer medications as indicated:

   Amphotericin B (Fungizone);

Antifungal useful in treatment of cryptococcosis meningitis.

ACTIONS/INTERVENTIONS	RATIONALE
Collaborative	
AZT(Retrovir);	Shown to improve neurologic and mental functioning.
Antipsychotics, e.g., haloperidol/(Haldol), and/or antianxiety agents, e.g., lorazepam (Ativan).	Cautious use may help with problems of sleeplessness, emotional lability, hallucinations, suspiciousness, and agitation.
Provide controlled environment/behavioral management.	Team approach may be required to protect patient when mental impairment (e.g., delusions) threaten patient safety.
Refer to counseling as indicated.	May help patient gain control in presence of thought disturbances or psychotic symptomatology.

NURSING DIAGNOSIS:	**ANXIETY [SPECIFY LEVEL]/FEAR**
May be related to:	Threat to self-concept, threat of death, change in health/ socioeconomic status, role functioning.
	Interpersonal transmission and contagion.
	Separation from support system.
	Fear of transmission of the disease to family/loved ones.
Possibly evidenced by:	Increased tension, apprehension, feelings of helplessness/ hopelessness.
	Expressed concern regarding changes in life.
	Fear of unspecific consequences.
	Somatic complaints, insomnia; sympathetic stimulation, restlessness.
DESIRED OUTCOMES/ EVALUATION CRITERIA— PATIENT WILL:	Verbalize awareness of feelings and healthy ways to deal with them.
	Display appropriate range of feelings and lessened fear/ anxiety.
	Demonstrate problem-solving skills.
	Use resources effectively.

ACTIONS/INTERVENTIONS	RATIONALE
Independent	
Assure patient of confidentiality within limits of situation.	Provides reassurance and opportunity for patient to problem-solve solutions to anticipated situations.

ACTIONS/INTERVENTIONS	RATIONALE

Independent

Maintain frequent contact with patient. Talk with and touch the patient. Limit use of isolation clothing and masks.

Provides assurance that the patient is not alone or rejected; conveys respect for and acceptance of the person, fostering trust.

Provide accurate, consistent information regarding prognosis. Avoid arguing about patient's perceptions of the situation.

Can reduce anxiety and enable patient to make decisions/choices based on realities.

Be alert to signs of denial/depression (e.g., withdrawal; angry, inappropriate remarks). Determine presence of suicidal ideation and assess potential on a scale of 1–10.

Patient may use defense mechanism of denial and continue to hope that diagnosis is inaccurate. Feelings of guilt and spiritual distress may cause the patient to become withdrawn and believe that suicide is a viable alternative.

Provide open environment in which patient feels safe to discuss feelings or to refrain from talking.

Helps patient to feel accepted in present condition without feeling judged and promotes sense of dignity and control.

Permit expressions of anger, fear, despair without confrontation. Give information that feelings are normal and are to be appropriately expressed.

Acceptance of feelings allows patient to begin to deal with situation.

Recognize and support the stage patient/family are at in the grieving process. (Refer to CP: Cancer, ND: Grieving, Anticipatory, p 1018.)

Choice of interventions is dictated by stage of grief, coping behaviors, e.g., anger/withdrawal, denial.

Explain procedures, providing opportunity for questions and honest answers. Stay with patient during anxiety-producing procedures and consultations.

Accurate information allows the patient to deal more effectively with the reality of the situation, thereby reducing anxiety and fear of the unknown.

Identify and encourage patient interaction with support systems. Encourage verbalization/interaction with family/SO.

Reduces feeling of isolation. If family support systems are not available, outside sources may be needed immediately, e.g., local AIDS task force.

Provide reliable and consistent information and support for SO.

Allows for better interpersonal interaction and reduction of anxiety and fear.

Include SO as indicated when major decisions are to be made.

Ensures a support system for the patient, and allows the SO the chance to participate in patient's life. *Note:* If patient, family, and SO are in conflict, separate care consultations and visiting times may be needed.

Collaborative

Refer to psychiatric counseling (e.g., clinical nurse specialist, psychiatrist, social worker).

May require further assistance in dealing with diagnosis/prognosis, especially when suicidal thoughts are present.

NURSING DIAGNOSIS:	SOCIAL ISOLATION
May be related to:	Altered state of wellness, changes in physical appearance, alterations in mental status.
	Perceptions of unacceptable social or sexual behavior/values.

	Inadequate personal resources/support systems.
	Physical isolation.
Possibly evidenced by:	Expressed feeling of aloneness imposed by others, feelings of rejection.
	Absence of supportive SO: Partners, family, acquaintances/friends.
DESIRED OUTCOMES/ EVALUATION CRITERIA— PATIENT WILL:	Express increased sense of self-worth.
	Participate in activities/programs at level of ability/desire.

ACTIONS/INTERVENTIONS	RATIONALE
Independent	
Ascertain patient's perception of situation.	Isolation may be partly self-imposed as patient fears rejection/reaction of others.
Spend time talking with patient during and between care activities. Be supportive, allowing for verbalization. Treat with dignity and regard for patient's feelings.	Patient may experience physical isolation due to current medical status and some degree of social isolation secondary to diagnosis of AIDS.
Limit/avoid use of mask, gown, and gloves when possible, e.g., when talking to patient.	Reduces patient's sense of physical isolation and provides positive social contact, which may enhance self-esteem.
Identify support systems available to patient, including presence of/relationship with immediate and extended family.	When patient has assistance from SO, feelings of loneliness and rejection will be diminished. *Note:* Patient may not receive usual/needed support for coping with life-threatening illness and associated grief because of fear and lack of understanding (AIDS hysteria).
Explain isolation precautions/procedures to patient/SO.	Gloves, gowns, mask are not routinely required with a diagnosis of AIDS except when contact with secretions/excretions is expected. Misuse of these barriers enhances feelings of emotional as well as physical isolation. When precautions are necessary, explanations help patient understand reasons for procedures and provide feeling of inclusion in what is happening.
Encourage open visitation (as able), telephone contacts, and social activities within tolerated level.	Participation with others can foster a feeling of belonging.
Encourage active role of contact with SO.	Helps to reestablish a feeling of participation in a social relationship. May lessen likelihood of suicide attempts.
Develop a plan of action with patient: Look at available resources; support healthy risk-taking behaviors. Help patient problem-solve solutions to short-term/imposed isolation.	Having a plan promotes a sense of control over own life and gives patient something to look forward to/actions to accomplish.

871

ACTIONS/INTERVENTIONS

Independent

Be alert to verbal/nonverbal cues, e.g., withdrawal, statements of despair, sense of aloneness. Ask the patient if thoughts of suicide are being entertained.

Collaborative

Refer to resources, e.g., social services, counselors, and AIDS organizations/projects (local/national).

Provide for placement in sheltered community when necessary.

RATIONALE

Indicators of despair and suicidal ideation are often present; when these cues are acknowledged by the caregiver, the patient is usually willing to talk about thoughts of suicide, and sense of isolation and hopelessness.

Establishes support systems; may reduce feelings of isolation.

May need more specific care when unable to be maintained at home or when SO cannot manage care.

NURSING DIAGNOSIS:	POWERLESSNESS
May be related to:	Confirmed diagnosis of a terminal disease, incomplete grieving process.
	Social ramifications of AIDS; alteration in body image/desired lifestyle; advancing CNS involvement.
Possibly evidenced by:	Feelings of loss of control over own life.
	Depression over physical deterioration that occurs despite patient compliance with regimen.
	Anger, apathy, withdrawal, passivity.
	Dependence on others for care/decision-making, resulting in resentment, anger, guilt.
DESIRED OUTCOMES/ EVALUATION CRITERIA— PATIENT WILL:	Acknowledge feelings and healthy ways to deal with them.
	Verbalize some sense of control over present situation.
	Make choices related to care and be involved in self-care.

ACTIONS/INTERVENTIONS

Independent

Identify factors that contribute to the patient's feelings of powerlessness, e.g., diagnosis of a terminal illness, lack of support systems, lack of knowledge about present situation.

RATIONALE

Patients with AIDS are usually aware of the current literature and prognosis. Fear of AIDS (by the general population as well as the patient's family/SO) is the most profound cause of the patient's isolation. For some homosexual patients, this may be the first time that the family has been made aware that the patient lives an alternative lifestyle.

ACTIONS/INTERVENTIONS

Independent

Assess degree of feelings of helplessness, e.g., verbal/nonverbal expressions indicating lack of control ("It won't make any difference"), flat affect, lack of communication.

Encourage active role in planning activities, establishing realistic/attainable daily goals. Encourage patient control and responsibility as much as possible. Identify things that the patient can and cannot control.

Encourage living will and durable power of attorney documents, with specific and precise instructions regarding acceptable and nonacceptable procedures to prolong life.

RATIONALE

Determines the status of the individual patient and allows for appropriate intervention when the patient is immobilized by depressed feelings.

May enhance feelings of control and self-worth and sense of personal responsibility.

Many factors associated with the treatments used in this debilitating and often fatal disease process place the patient at the mercy of medical personnel and other unknown people who may be making decisions for and about the patient without regard for the patient's loss of independence.

NURSING DIAGNOSIS:

KNOWLEDGE DEFICIT [LEARNING NEED], REGARDING DISEASE, PROGNOSIS, AND TREATMENT NEEDS

May be related to:

Lack of exposure/recall; information misinterpretation.

Cognitive limitation.

Unfamiliarity with information resources.

Possibly evidenced by:

Questions/request for information; statement of misconception.

Inaccurate follow-through of instructions/development of preventable complications.

DESIRED OUTCOMES/ EVALUATION CRITERIA— PATIENT WILL:

Verbalize understanding of condition/disease process and treatment.

Identify relationship of signs/symptoms to the disease process and correlate symptoms with causative factors.

Correctly perform necessary procedures and explain reasons for actions.

Initiate necessary lifestyle changes and participate in treatment regimen.

ACTIONS/INTERVENTIONS

Independent

Review disease process and future expectations.

Determine level of dependence and physical condition. Note extent of care and support available from family/SO and need for other caregivers.

RATIONALE

Provides knowledge base on which patient can make informed choices.

Helps to plan amount of care and symptom management required and need for additional resources.

ACTIONS/INTERVENTIONS	RATIONALE

Independent

Review modes of transmission of disease.

Corrects myths and misconceptions; promotes safety for patient/others.

Instruct patient and care givers concerning infection control, e.g.: good hand-washing techniques for everyone (patient, family, care givers); use of gloves when handling bedpans, dressings/soiled linens; wearing mask if patient has productive cough; placing soiled/wet linens in plastic bag and separating from family laundry; washing with detergent and hot water; cleaning surfaces with bleach/water solution of 1:10; disinfecting toilet bowl/bedpan with full-strength bleach; preparing patient's food in clean area; washing dishes/utensils in hot soapy water (can be washed with the family dishes).

Reduces transmission of diseases; promotes wellness in presence of reduced ability of immune system to control level of flora.

Stress necessity of daily skin care, including inspecting skin folds, pressure points, and perineum, and of providing adequate cleansing and protective measures, e.g., ointments, padding.

Healthy skin provides barrier to infection. Measures to prevent skin disruption and associated complications are critical.

Ascertain that patient/SO can perform necessary oral and dental care. Review procedures as indicated. Encourage regular dental care.

The oral mucosa can quickly exhibit severe, progressive complications. Studies indicate that 65% of AIDs patients have some oral symptoms. Therefore prevention and early intervention is critical.

Review dietary needs (high-protein and high-calorie) and ways to improve intake when anorexia, diarrhea, weakness, depression interfere with intake.

Promotes adequate nutrition necessary for healing and support of immune system; enhances feeling of well-being.

Discuss medication regimen, interactions, and side effects.

Enhances cooperation with/increases probability of success with therapeutic regimen.

Provide information about symptom management that complements medical regimen, e.g., with intermittent diarrhea, take Lomotil before going to social event.

Provides patient with increased sense of control, reduces risk of embarrassment, and promotes comfort.

Stress importance of adequate rest.

Prevents/reduces fatigue; enhances abilities.

Encourage activity/exercise at level that patient can tolerate.

Stimulates release of endorphins in the brain, enhancing sense of well-being.

Stress necessity of continued health care and follow-up.

Provides opportunity for altering regimen to meet individual/changing needs.

Recommend cessation of smoking.

Smoking increases risk of respiratory infections and can impair immune system (decrease O_2-combining power with RBCs).

Identify signs/symptoms requiring medical evaluation, e.g., persistent fever/night sweats, swollen glands, continued weight loss, diarrhea, skin blotches/lesions, headache, chest pain, dyspnea.

Early recognition of developing complications and timely interventions may prevent progression to life-threatening situation.

Identify community resources, e.g., hospice/residential care centers, VNA, homecare services, Meals-on-Wheels, peer group support.

Facilitates transfer from acute care setting; supports recovery and independence.

Rheumatoid Arthritis

RA is a chronic, systemic inflammatory disease of unknown cause, characterized by destruction and proliferation of the synovial membrane, resulting in joint destruction, ankylosis, and deformity. Immunologic mechanisms appear to play an important role in the initiation and perpetuation of the disease in which spontaneous remissions and unpredictable exacerbations occur.

RELATED CONCERNS

Psychosocial Aspects of Acute Care, p 899
Total Joint Replacement, p 810

PATIENT ASSESSMENT DATA BASE

Data are dependent on severity and involvement of other organs (e.g., eyes, heart, lungs, kidneys), stage (i.e., acute exacerbation or remission), and coexistence of other forms of arthritis.

ACTIVITY/REST

May report:	Joint pain with motion, or tenderness, worsened by stress placed on joint; morning stiffness, usually occurs bilaterally and symmetrically.
	Functional limitations affecting lifestyle, leisure time, occupation.
	Fatigue.
May exhibit:	Malaise.
	Limited ROM; atrophy of muscle, skin; joint and muscle contractures/deformities.

CARDIOVASCULAR

May report:	Raynaud's phenomenon of fingers/toes (i.e., intermittent pallor, cyanosis, then redness of digits before color returns to normal).

EGO INTEGRITY

May report:	Acute/chronic stress factors; e.g., financial, employment, disability, relationship factors.
	Hopelessness and powerlessness (incapacitating situation).
	Threat to self-concept, body image, personal identity (e.g., dependence on others).

FOOD/FLUID

May report:	Inability to obtain/consume adequate food/fluids; nausea.
	Anorexia.
	Difficulty chewing (TMJ involvement).
May exhibit:	Weight loss.
	Dryness of mucous membranes.

HYGIENE

May report:	Varying difficulty performing self-care activities. Dependence on others.

NEUROSENSORY

May report:	Numbness/tingling of hands and feet, loss of sensation in fingers.
May exhibit:	Symmetric joint swelling.

875

PAIN/COMFORT

May report: Acute episodes of pain (may/may not be accompanied by soft-tissue swelling in joints).

Chronic aching pain and stiffness (mornings are most difficult).

SAFETY

May report: Shiny, taut skin; subcutaneous nodules.

Skin/periarticular local warmth, erythema.

Skin lesions, leg ulcers.

Difficulty managing homemaker/maintenance tasks.

Persistent low-grade fever.

Dryness of eyes and mucous membranes.

SOCIAL INTERACTION

May report: Impaired interactions with family/others; change in roles; isolation.

TEACHING/LEARNING

May report: Familial history of RA (in juvenile onset).

Use of health foods, vitamins, untested arthritis "cures".

History of pericarditis, valvular lesions; pulmonary fibrosis, pleuritis.

Discharge Plan   **DRG projected mean length of stay: 4.8 days.**
Considerations: May require assistance with transportation, self-care activities, and homemaker/ maintenance tasks; changes in physical layout of home.

DIAGNOSTIC STUDIES

Rheumatoid factor: Positive in 80%–95% of cases.

Latex fixation: Positive in 75% of typical cases.

Agglutination reactions: Positive in more than 50% of typical cases.

ESR: Usually greatly increased (80–100 mm/h). May return to normal as symptoms improve.

C-reactive protein: Positive during exacerbations.

WBC: Elevated when inflammatory processes are present.

CBC: Usually reveals moderate anemia.

Ig (IgM and IgG): Elevation strongly suggests autoimmune process as cause for RA.

X-rays of involved joints: Reveals soft-tissue swelling, erosion of joints, and osteoporosis of adjacent bone (early changes) progressing to bone-cyst formation, narrowing of joint space, and subluxation. Concurrent osteoarthritic changes.

Radionuclide scans: Identify inflamed synovium.

Direct arthroscopy: Visualization of area reveals bone irregularities/degeneration of joint.

Synovia/fluid aspirate: May reveal volume greater than normal; opaque, cloudy, yellow appearance (inflammatory response, bleeding, degenerative waste products); elevated WBCs and leukocytes; decreased viscosity and complement (C_3 and C_4).

Synovial membrane biopsy: Reveals inflammatory changes and development of pannus.

NURSING PRIORITIES

1. Alleviate pain.
2. Increase mobility.

3. Promote positive self-concept.
4. Support independence.
5. Provide information about disease process/prognosis and treatment needs.

DISCHARGE GOALS

1. Pain relieved/controlled.
2. Patient is dealing realistically with current situation.
3. Patient is managing ADLs by self/with assistance as appropriate.
4. Disease process/prognosis and therapeutic regimen understood.

NURSING DIAGNOSIS:	**PAIN [ACUTE]/CHRONIC**
May be related to:	Injuring agents: Distention of tissues by accumulation of fluid/inflammatory process, destruction of joint.
Possibly evidenced by:	Reports of pain/discomfort, fatigue. Self/narrowed focus. Distraction behaviors/autonomic responses. Guarding/protective behavior.
DESIRED OUTCOMES/ EVALUATION CRITERIA— PATIENT WILL:	Report pain is relieved/controlled. Appear relaxed, able to sleep/rest and participate in activities appropriately. Follow prescribed pharmacologic regimen. Incorporate relaxation skills and diversional activities into pain control program.

ACTIONS/INTERVENTIONS	RATIONALE
Independent	
Investigate reports of pain, noting location and intensity (scale of 0–10). Note precipitating factors and nonverbal pain cues.	Helpful in determining pain management needs and effectiveness of program.
Provide firm mattress/bedboards, small pillow. Elevate bed linens as needed.	Soft/sagging mattress, large pillows prevent maintenance of proper body alignment, placing stress on affected joints. Elevation of bed linens reduces pressure on inflamed/painful joints.
Have patient assume position of comfort while in bed or sitting in chair. Promote bed rest as indicated.	In severe disease/acute exacerbation, total bed rest may be necessary (until objective and subjective improvements are noted) to limit pain/injury to joint.
Place/monitor use of pillows, sandbags, trochanter rolls, splints, braces.	Rests painful joints and maintains neutral position. *Note:* Use of splints can decrease pain and may reduce damage to joint. However, prolonged inactivity can result in loss of joint mobility/function.

877

ACTIONS/INTERVENTIONS	RATIONALE

Independent

Encourage frequent changes of position. Assist patient to move in bed, supporting affected joints above and below, avoiding jerky movements.

Prevents general fatigue and joint stiffness. Stabilizes joint, decreasing joint movement/pain.

Recommend patient take warm bath or shower on arising and/or at bedtime. Apply warm moist compresses to affected joints several times a day. Monitor water temperature of compress, baths, and so on.

Heat promotes muscle relaxation and mobility, decreases pain, and relieves morning stiffness. Sensitivity to heat may be diminished and dermal injury may occur.

Provide gentle massage.

Promotes relaxation/reduces muscle tension.

Encourage use of stress management techniques, e.g., progressive relaxation, Therapeutic Touch, biofeedback, visualization, guided imagery, self-hypnosis, and controlled breathing.

Promotes relaxation, provides sense of control, and may enhance coping abilities.

Involve in diversional activities appropriate for individual situation.

Refocuses attention, provides stimulation, and enhances self-esteem and feelings of general well-being.

Medicate prior to planned activities/exercises as indicated.

Promotes relaxation, reduces muscle tension/spasms, facilitating participation in therapy.

Collaborative

Administer medications as indicated, e.g.:

  Acetylsalicylates (aspirin);

ASA exerts an anti-inflammatory and mild analgesic effect decreasing stiffness and increasing mobility. ASA must be taken regularly to sustain a therapeutic blood level. Research indicates that ASA has the lowest "toxicity index" of commonly prescribed NSAIDs.

  Other NSAIDs, e.g., ibuprofen (Motrin); naproxen (Naprosyn); sulindac (Clinoril); piroxicam (Feldene); fenoprofen (Nalfon);

May be used when patient does not respond to aspirin or to enhance effects of aspirin. *Note:* These drugs are listed in ascending order of relative severity of side effects ("toxicity index").

  D-penicillamine (Cuprimine);

May control systemic effects of RA if other therapies have not been successful. High rate of side effects (e.g., thrombocytopenia, leukopenia, aplastic anemia) necessitates close monitoring. *Note:* Drug should be given between meals because drug absorption is impaired by food as well as antacids and iron products.

  Antacids;

Given with NSAID agents to minimize gastric irritation/discomfort.

  Codeine products.

Although narcotics are generally contraindicated because of chronic nature of condition, short-term use may be required during periods of acute exacerbation to control severe pain.

Assist with physical therapy, e.g., paraffin glove, whirlpool baths.

Provides sustained heat to affected joints. *Note:* Heat may be contraindicated in the presence of hot, swollen joints.

ACTIONS/INTERVENTIONS

Collaborative

Apply ice or cold packs when indicated.

Maintain TENS unit if used.

Prepare for surgical interventions, e.g., synovectomy.

RATIONALE

Cold may relieve pain and swelling during acute episodes.

Constant low-level electrical stimulus blocks transmission of pain sensations.

Removal of inflamed synovium can alleviate pain and limit progression of degenerative changes.

NURSING DIAGNOSIS:	PHYSICAL MOBILITY, IMPAIRED
May be related to:	Skeletal deformity.
	Pain, discomfort.
	Intolerance to activity; decreased muscle strength.
Possibly evidenced by:	Reluctance to attempt movement/inability to purposefully move within the physical environment.
	Limited ROM, impaired coordination, decreased muscle strength/control and mass [late stages].
DESIRED OUTCOMES/ EVALUATION CRITERIA— PATIENT WILL:	Maintain position of function with absence/limitation of contractures.
	Maintain or increase strength and function of affected and/or compensatory body part.
	Demonstrate techniques/behaviors that enable resumption/continuation of activities.

ACTIONS/INTERVENTIONS

Independent

Evaluate/continuously monitor degree of joint inflammation/pain.

Maintain bed/chair rest when indicated. Schedule activities providing frequent rest periods and uninterrupted nighttime sleep.

Assist with active/passive ROM as well as resistive exercises and isometrics when able.

Reposition frequently with adequate personnel. Demonstrate/assist with transfer techniques and use of mobility aids, e.g., trapeze.

Position with pillows, sandbags, trochanter rolls, splints, braces.

RATIONALE

Level of activity/exercise is dependent on progression/resolution of inflammatory process.

Systemic rest is mandatory during acute exacerbations and important throughout all phases of disease to prevent fatigue, maintain strength.

Maintains/improves joint function, muscle strength, and general stamina. *Note:* Inadequate exercise leads to joint stiffening, whereas excessive activity can damage joints.

Relieves pressure on tissues and promotes circulation. Facilitates self-care and patient's independence. Proper transfer techniques prevent shearing abrasions of skin.

Promotes joint stability (reducing risk of injury) and maintains proper joint position and body alignment, minimizing contractures.

ACTIONS/INTERVENTIONS	RATIONALE

Independent

Use small/thin pillow under neck.	Prevents flexion of neck.
Encourage patient to maintain upright and erect posture when sitting, standing, walking.	Maximizes joint function, maintains mobility.
Provide safe environment, e.g., raised chairs/toilet seat, use of handrails in tub/shower and toilet, proper use of mobility aids/wheelchair safety.	Avoids accidental injuries/falls.

Collaborative

Consult with physical/occupational therapists and vocational specialist.	Useful in formulating exercise/activity program based on individual needs and in identifying mobility devices/adjuncts.
Provide foam/alternating pressure mattress.	Decreases pressure on fragile tissues to reduce risks of immobility/development of decubitus.
Administer medications as indicated:	
Antirheumatic agents, e.g., gold, sodium thiomaleate (Myochrysine) or auranofin (Ridaura);	Chrysotherapy (gold salts) may produce dramatic/sustained remission but may result in rebound inflammation if discontinued or serious side effects occur, e.g., nitritoid crisis with dizziness, blurred vision, flushing, progressing to anaphylactic shock.
Steroids.	May be necessary to suppress acute systemic inflammation.
Prepare for surgical interventions, e.g.:	
Arthroplasty;	Correction of periarticular weakness and subluxation promotes joint stability.
Tunnel release procedures, tendon repair, ganglionectomy;	Corrects associated connective tissue defects; enhances function and mobility.
Joint implant.	Replacement may be needed to restore optimal functioning and mobility.

NURSING DIAGNOSIS:	BODY IMAGE DISTURBANCE/ROLE PERFORMANCE ALTERED
May be related to:	Changes in ability to perform usual tasks.
	Increased energy expenditure; impaired mobility.
Possibly evidenced by:	Change in structure/function of affected parts.
	Negative self-talk, focus on past strength/function, appearance.
	Change in lifestyle/physical ability to resume roles, loss of employment, dependence on SO for assistance.
	Change in social involvement; sense of isolation.
	Feelings of helplessness, hopelessness.

DESIRED OUTCOMES/ EVALUATION CRITERIA— PATIENT WILL:	Verbalize increased confidence in ability to deal with illness, changes in lifestyle, and possible limitations. Formulate realistic goals/plans for future.

ACTIONS/INTERVENTIONS	RATIONALE
Independent	
Encourage verbalization about concerns of disease process, future expectations.	Provides opportunity to identify fears/misconceptions and deal with them directly.
Discuss meaning of loss/change to patient/SO. Ascertain how patient views self in usual lifestyle functioning, including sexual aspects.	Identifying how illness affects perception of self and interactions with others will determine need for further intervention/counseling.
Discuss patient's perception of how SO perceives limitations.	Verbal/nonverbal cues from SO may have a major impact on how patient views self.
Acknowledge and accept feelings of grief, hostility, dependency.	Constant pain is wearing, and feelings of anger and hostility are common. Acceptance provides feedback that feelings are normal.
Note withdrawn behavior, use of denial, or over-concern with body/changes.	May suggest emotional exhaustion or maladaptive coping methods, requiring more in-depth intervention/psychologic support.
Set limits on maladaptive behavior. Assist patient to identify positive behaviors that will aid in coping.	Helps patient to maintain self-control, which enhances self-esteem.
Involve patient in planning care and scheduling activities.	Enhances feelings of competency/self-worth, encourages independence, and encourages participation in therapy.
Assist with grooming needs as necessary.	Maintaining appearance enhances self-image.
Give positive reinforcement for accomplishments.	Allows patient to feel good about self. Reinforces positive behavior. Enhances self-confidence.
Collaborative	
Refer to psychiatric counseling, e.g., clinical specialist psychiatric nurse, psychiatrist/psychologist, social worker.	Patient/SO may require ongoing support to deal with long-term/debilitating process.
Administer medications as indicated, e.g.: antianxiety and mood-elevating drugs.	May be needed in presence of severe depression until patient develops more effective coping skills.

NURSING DIAGNOSIS:	**SELF-CARE DEFICIT: (SPECIFY)**
May be related to:	Musculoskeletal impairment; decreased strength, endurance, pain on movement. Depression.
Possibly evidenced by:	Inability to manage ADLs (feeding, bathing, dressing, and toileting).

ACTIONS/INTERVENTIONS	RATIONALE
Independent	
Discuss usual level of functioning (0–4) prior to onset/exacerbation of illness and potential changes now anticipated.	May be able to continue usual activities with necessary adaptations to current limitations.
Maintain mobility, pain control, and exercise program.	Supports physical/emotional independence.
Assess barriers to participation in self-care. Identify/plan for environmental modifications.	Prepares for increased independence, which enhances self-esteem.
Allow patient sufficient time to complete tasks to fullest extent of ability. Capitalize on individual strengths.	May need more time to complete tasks by self but provides an opportunity for greater sense of self-confidence and self-worth.
Collaborative	
Consult with occupational therapists.	Useful for determining assistive devices to meet individual needs, e.g., button hook, long-handled shoe horn, reacher, handheld shower head.
Arrange home-health evaluation prior to discharge with follow-up afterward.	Identifies problems that may be encountered because of current level of disability. Provides for more successful team efforts with others who are involved in care, e.g., occupational therapy team.
Arrange for consult with other agencies, e.g., Meals-on-Wheels, home care service, nutritionist.	May need additional kinds of assistance to continue in home setting.

ACTIONS/INTERVENTIONS

Independent

Assess level of physical functioning.

Evaluate environment to assess ability to care for self.

Determine financial resources to meet needs of individual situation. Identify support systems available to patient, e.g., extended family, friends/neighbors.

Develop plan for maintaining a clean, healthful environment, e.g., sharing of household repair/tasks between family members or by contract services.

Identify sources for necessary equipment, e.g., lifts, elevated toilet seat, wheelchair.

Collaborative

Coordinate home evaluation by occupational therapist.

Identify/meet with community resources, e.g., VNA, homemaker service, social services, senior citizens groups.

RATIONALE

Identifies degree of assistance/support required.

Determines feasibility of remaining in/changing home layout to meet individual needs.

Availability of personal resources/community supports will affect ability to problem-solve solutions.

Assures that needs will be met on an ongoing basis.

Provides opportunity to acquire equipment before discharge.

Useful for identifying adaptive equipment, ways to modify tasks to maintain independence.

Can facilitate transfer to/support continuation in home setting.

NURSING DIAGNOSIS:	KNOWLEDGE DEFICIT [LEARNING NEED], REGARDING DISEASE, PROGNOSIS, TREATMENT NEEDS
May be related to:	Lack of exposure/recall.
	Information misinterpretation.
Possibly evidenced by:	Questions/request for information, statement of misconception.
	Inaccurate follow-through of instruction/development of preventable complications.
DESIRED OUTCOMES/ EVALUATION CRITERIA— PATIENT WILL:	Verbalize understanding of condition/prognosis, treatment.
	Develop a plan for self-care, including lifestyle modifications consistent with mobility and/or activity restrictions.

ACTIONS/INTERVENTIONS

Independent

Review disease process, prognosis, and future expectations.

Discuss patient's role in management of disease process through diet, medication, and balanced program of exercise and rest.

RATIONALE

Provides knowledge base on which patient can make informed choices.

Goal of disease control is to suppress inflammation in joints/other tissues to maintain joint function and prevent deformities.

ACTIONS/INTERVENTIONS	RATIONALE
Independent	
Assist in planning a realistic and integrated schedule of activity, rest, personal care, drug administration, physical therapy, and stress management.	Provides structure and defuses anxiety when managing a complex chronic disease process.
Stress importance of continued pharmacotherapeutic management.	Benefits of drug therapy are dependent on correct dosage; e.g., aspirin must be taken regularly to sustain therapeutic blood levels of 18–25 mg.
Recommend use of enteric coated/buffered aspirin or nonacetylated salicylates, e.g., choline salicylate (Arthropan) or choline magnesium trisalicylate (Trilisate).	Coated/buffered preparations ingested with food, minimize gastric irritation, reducing risk of bleeding/hemorrhage. *Note:* Nonacetylated products have a longer half-life, requiring less frequent administration in addition to producing less gastric irritation.
Suggest ingestion of medications with meals, milk products, or antacids and at bedtime.	Limits gastric irritation. Reduction of pain at HS enhances sleep and increased blood level decreases early-morning stiffness.
Identify adverse drug effects, e.g., tinnitus, gastric intolerance, GI bleeding, purpuric rash.	Prolonged, maximal doses of aspirin may result in overdose. Tinnitus usually indicates high therapeutic blood levels. If tinnitus occurs, the dosage is usually decreased by 1 tablet every 2–3 days until it stops.
Stress importance of reading product labels and refraining from OTC drug usage without prior medical approval.	Many products contain hidden salicylates (e.g., cold remedies, antidiarrheals) that increase risk of drug overdose/harmful side effects.
Review importance of balanced diet with foods high in vitamins, protein, and iron.	Promotes general well-being and tissue repair/regeneration.
Encourage obese patient to lose weight and supply with weight reduction information as appropriate.	Weight loss will reduce stress on joints, especially hips, knees, ankles, feet.
Provide information about assistive devices, e.g., wheeled dolly/wagon for moving items, pickup sticks, light-weight dishes and pans, raised toilet seats, safety handlebars.	Reduces force exerted on joints and enables individual to participate more comfortably in needed/desired activities.
Discuss energy-saving techniques, e.g., sitting instead of standing to prepare meals and shower.	Prevents fatigue; facilitates self-care and independence.
Encourage maintenance of correct body position and posture both at rest and during activity, e.g., keeping joints extended, not flexed, wearing splints for prescribed periods, avoiding remaining in a single position for extended periods, positioning hands near center of body during use, and sliding rather than lifting objects when possible.	Good body mechanics must become a part of the patient's lifestyle to lessen joint stress and pain.
Review necessity of frequent inspection of skin and meticulous skin care under splints, casts, supporting devices. Demonstrate proper padding.	Reduces risk of skin irritation/breakdown.
Discuss necessity of medical follow-up/laboratory studies, e.g., ESR, salicylate levels, PT.	Drug therapy requires frequent assessment/refinement to assure optimal effect and to prevent overdose/dangerous side effects, e.g., aspirin prolongs

ACTIONS/INTERVENTIONS	RATIONALE
Independent	
	PT, increasing risk of bleeding. Chrysotherapy depresses platelets, potentiating risk of thrombocytopenia.
Provide for sexual counseling as necessary.	Information about different positions and techniques and/or other options for sexual fulfillment may enhance personal relationships and feelings of self-worth/self-esteem.
Identify community resources, e.g., Arthritis Foundation.	Assistance/support from others promotes maximal recovery.

Bibliography

General References

Bellak, JP and Bamford, PA: Nursing Assessment: A Multidimensional Approach. Jones & Bartlett, Boston, 1987.

Berkow, R (ed): The Merck Manual, ed 15. Merck Sharp & Dohme Research Laboratories, Rahway, NJ, 1987.

Cella, JH and Watson, J: Nurse's Manual of Laboratory Tests. FA Davis, Philadelphia, 1989.

Condon, RE and Nyhus, LM (eds): Manual of Surgical Therapeutics, ed 7. Little, Brown & Co, Boston, 1988.

Deglin, JH and Vallerand, AH: Davis's Drug Guide for Nurses, ed 3. FA Davis, Philadelphia, 1992.

Diseases and Disorders Handbook, ed 3. Springhouse Corp, Springhouse, PA, 1989.

Doenges, ME and Moorhouse, MF: Nurse's Pocket Guide: Nursing Diagnoses with Interventions, ed 3. FA Davis, Philadelphia, 1991.

Dunagan, WC and Ridner, ML (eds): Manual of Medical Therapeutics, ed 26. Little, Brown & Co, Boston, 1989.

Fischbach, F: A Manual of Laboratory and Diagnostic Tests, ed 4. JB Lippincott, Philadelphia, 1992.

Guyton, AC: Textbook of Medical Physiology, ed 8. WB Saunders, Philadelphia, 1991.

Kuhn, MM: Pharmacotherapeutics: A Nursing Process Approach, ed 2. FA Davis, Philadelphia, 1991.

Professional Guide to Diseases, ed 3. Springhouse Corp, Springhouse, PA, 1989.

Suddarth, DS (ed): The Lippincott Manual of Nursing Practice, ed 5. JB Lippincott, Philadelphia, 1991.

Thomas, CL (ed): Taber's Cyclopedic Medical Dictionary, ed 17. FA Davis, Philadelphia, 1993.

Thompson, JM, et al: Mosby's Manual of Clinical Nursing, ed 2. CV Mosby, St Louis, 1989.

Books

Brassell, MP: Pharmacologic Management of Rheumatic Diseases. pp 43–51.

Cohen, PT, Sande, MA, and Bolberding, PA: The AIDS Knowledge Base. Medical Publishing Group, Massachusetts Medical Society, 1990.

Dilley, JW, Pies, C, and Helquist, M: Face to Face: A Guide to AIDS Counseling. AIDS Health Project. University of California, San Francisco, 1989.

Fitzpatrick, TB and Freedburg, IM: Dermatology in General Medicine, ed 3. 1987, pp 1841–1851.

Flaskerud, J and Ungvarski, P: HIV/AIDS: A Guide to Nursing Care, ed 2. WB Saunders, Philadelphia, 1992.

Kelley: Textbook of Rheumatology, ed 3. 1989, pp 1232–1235.

Phipps, W, et al (eds): Medical Surgical Nursing Concepts and Clinical Practice, ed 4. CV Mosby, St Louis, 1991.

Register, C: Living with Chronic Illness: Days of Patience and Passion. Bantam Books, 1992.

Schroeder, SA, et al (eds): Current Medical Diagnosis and Treatment. Appleton & Lange, Norwalk, 1990. Thorn, K: Applying Medical Case Management: AIDS. Thorn Publishing, 1990.

Articles

Brunton, JA (ed): NSAID toxicity: Which ones are worse? Internal Medicine Alert 14(2):9, 1992.

Cerrato, PL: Nutrition and HIV: What to tell your patients. RN 54(4):73, 1991.

Ince, S: Rheumatoid arthritis: Dispelling the "old age" myth. Weight Watcher's: Womens Health and Fitness News. May 4, 1989.

Keithley, JK, et al: Nutritional alterations in persons with HIV infection. IMAGE 24(3):183–188, 1992.

McGuire, L: The power of non-narcotic pain relievers. RN 53(4):28, 1990.

McHenry, C: Handy work. Nursing Times 87(45):18, 1991.

O'Brien, LM and Bartlett, KA: TB plus HIV spells trouble. AJN 92(5):28, 1992.

Santangelo, J and Schnack, J: Primary care intervention and case management for adults with early HIV infection. Nurse Pract June: 9, 1991.

Scherer, P: How AIDS attacks the brain. AJN 90(1):44, 1990.

Scherer, P: How HIV attacks the peripheral nervous system. AJN 90(5):67, 1990.

Soloway, B and Hect, FM: Changing approaches to prophylaxis for pneumocystis carinii pneumonia. AIDS Clinical Care 4(8):61, 1992.

Wicklund, S and Devroye, M (eds): Nurse's drug alert—Methotrexate therapy and arthritic joint degeneration. AJN 12(3):333, 1988.

CHAPTER 16

SYSTEMIC INFECTIONS

Sepsis/Septicemia

Sepsis is a syndrome characterized by clinical signs and symptoms of severe infection, which may progress to septicemia and septic shock. Septicemia implies the presence of a systemic infection of the blood caused by rapidly multiplying microorganisms or their toxins, which can result in profound physiologic changes. The pathogens can be bacteria, fungi, viruses, or rickettsiae. The most common causes of septicemia are gram-negative organisms. If the defense system of the body is not effective in controlling the invading microorganisms, septic shock may result, characterized by altered hemodynamics, impaired cellular function, and multiple system failure.

RELATED CONCERNS

Adult Respiratory Distress Syndrome p 217
AIDS, p 850
Inflammatory Cardiac Conditions, p 126
Intracranial Infections, p 307
Peritonitis, p 514
Pneumonia, Microbial, p 162
Psychosocial Aspects of Acute Care, p 899
Pulmonary Tuberculosis, p 241
Renal Failure: Acute, p 618
Total Nutritional Support, p 1039

PATIENT ASSESSMENT DATA BASE

Data are dependent on the type, location, duration of the infective process and organ involvement.

ACTIVITY/REST

May report: Malaise.

CIRCULATION

May exhibit: BP normal/slightly low normal range (as long as cardiac output remains elevated).

Peripheral pulses bounding, rapid (hyperdynamic phase); weak/thready/easily obliterated, extreme tachycardia (shock).

Heart sounds: dysrhythmias and development of S_3 suggest myocardial dysfunction, effects of acidosis/electrolyte imbalance.

Skin warm, dry, flushed (vasodilation), pale, cold, clammy, mottled (vasoconstriction).

ELIMINATION

May report:	Diarrhea.

FOOD/FLUID

May report:	Anorexia; nausea/vomiting.
May exhibit:	Weight loss, decreased subcutaneous fat/muscle mass (malnutrition).
	Urinary output decreased, concentrated; progressing to oliguria, anuria.

NEUROSENSORY

May report:	Headache; dizziness, fainting.
May exhibit:	Restlessness, apprehension, confusion, disorientation, delirium/coma.

PAIN/COMFORT

May report:	Abdominal tenderness, localized pain/discomfort.
	Generalized urticaria/pruritus.

RESPIRATION

May exhibit:	Tachypnea with decreased respiratory depth, dyspnea.
	Basilar crackles, rhonchi, wheezes (developing pulmonary complications/onset of cardiac decompensation).

SAFETY

May report:	Immunosuppression: Cancer therapies, corticosteroid use.
	Recent/current infection, viral illness.
May exhibit:	Temperature: Usually elevated (101°F or greater) but may be normal in elderly or compromised patient; occasionally subnormal (under 98.6°F).
	Shaking chills.
	Poor/delayed wound healing, purulent drainage, localized erythema.
	Macular erythematous rash.

SEXUALITY

May report:	Perineal pruritus.
	Recent childbirth/abortion.
May exhibit:	Maceration of vulva, purulent vaginal drainage.

TEACHING/LEARNING

May report:	Chronic/debilitating health problems, e.g., liver, renal, cardiac disease; cancer, DM, alcoholism.
	History of splenectomy.
	Recent surgery/invasive procedures, traumatic wounds.
	Antibiotic use (recent or long-term).

Discharge Plan Considerations: DRG projected mean length of stay: 7.5 days.

May require assistance with wound care/supplies, treatments, self-care, and homemaker tasks.

DIAGNOSTIC STUDIES

Cultures (wound, sputum, urine, blood): May identify organism(s) causing the sepsis. Sensitivity determines most effective drug choices. Catheter/intravascular line tips may need to be removed and cultured if the portal of entry is unknown.

WBC: Hct may be elevated in hypovolemic states due to hemoconcentration. Leukopenia (decreased WBCs) occurs early, followed by a rebound leukocytosis (15,000–30,000) with increased bands (shift to the left) indicating rapid production of immature WBCs.

Serum electrolytes: Various imbalances may occur due to acidosis, fluid shifts, and altered renal function.

Clotting studies:

Platelets: Decreased levels (thrombocytopenia) can occur due to platelet aggregation.

PT/PTT may be prolonged indicating coagulopathy associated with liver ischemia/circulating toxins/shock state.

Serum lactate: Elevated in metabolic acidosis, liver dysfunction, shock.

Serum glucose: Hyperglycemia occurs reflecting gluconeogenesis and glycogenolysis in the liver in response to cellular starvation/alteration in metabolism.

BUN/Cr: Increased levels are associated with dehydration, renal impairment/failure, and liver dysfunction/failure.

ABGs: Respiratory alkalosis and hypoxemia may occur early. In later stages, hypoxemia, respiratory acidosis, and metabolic acidosis occur due to failure of compensatory mechanisms.

Urinalysis: Presence of WBCs/bacteria suggests infection. Protein and RBCs are often present.

X-rays: Abdominal and lower chest films indicating free air in the abdomen may suggest infection due to perforated abdominal/pelvic organ.

ECG: May show ST-segment and T-wave changes and dysrhythmia resembling myocardial infarction.

NURSING PRIORITIES

1. Eliminate infection.
2. Support tissue perfusion/circulatory volume.
3. Prevent complications.
4. Provide information about disease process, prognosis, and treatment needs.

DISCHARGE GOALS

1. Infection eliminated/controlled.
2. Homeostasis maintained.
3. Complications prevented/minimized.
4. Disease process, prognosis, and therapeutic regimen understood.

NURSING DIAGNOSIS:	INFECTION, HIGH RISK FOR [PROGRESSION OF SEPSIS TO SEPTIC SHOCK, DEVELOPMENT OF OPPORTUNISTIC INFECTIONS]
May be related to:	Compromised immune system.
	Failure to recognize/treat infection, and/or exercise proper preventive measures.

889

ACTIONS/INTERVENTIONS	RATIONALE
Independent	
Provide isolation/monitor visitors as indicated.	Wound/linen isolation and hand washing may be all that is required for draining wounds, while reverse isolation/restriction of visitors may be needed to protect the immunosuppressed patient. Reduces risk of opportunistic infections.
Wash hands before/after each care activity even if sterile gloves are used.	Reduces risk of cross-contamination.
Encourage frequent change of position, deep breathing/coughing.	Good pulmonary toilet may prevent pneumonia.
Encourage patient to cover mouth and nose with tissue during coughs/sneezes.	Prevents spread of infection via airborne droplets.
Limit use of invasive devices/procedures when possible.	Reduces number of sites for entry of opportunistic organisms.
Inspect wounds/site of invasive devices daily, paying particular attention to hyperalimentation lines.	Note signs of local inflammation/infection, changes in character of wound drainage or sputum, urine. May provide clue to portal of entry, type of infecting organism(s), as well as early identification of secondary infections. *Note:* High nutrient content of TPN provides excellent media for bacterial growth.
Use sterile technique when changing dressings/ suctioning/providing site care, e.g., invasive line, urinary catheter.	Prevents introduction of bacteria, reducing risk of nosocomial infection.
Wear gloves/gowns when caring for open wounds/ anticipating direct contact with secretions or excretions.	Prevents spread of infection/cross-contamination.
Dispose of soiled dressings/materials in double bag.	Reduces contamination/soilage of area; limits spread of airborne organisms.
Monitor temperature trends.	Fever (101°F–105°F/38.5°C–40°C) is caused by the effect of endotoxins on the hypothalamus and pyrogen-released endorphins. Hypothermia (less than 96°F/36°C) is a grave sign reflecting advancing shock state/decreased tissue perfusion.
Observe for shaking chills and profuse diaphoresis.	Chills often precede temperature spikes in presence of generalized infection.

ACTIONS/INTERVENTIONS

Independent

Monitor for signs of deterioration of condition/failure to improve during therapy.

Inspect oral cavity for white plaques (thrush). Investigate reports of vaginal/perineal itching or burning.

Collaborative

Obtain specimens of urine, blood, sputum, wound, invasive lines/tubes as indicated for Gram stain, culture, and sensitivity.

Administer anti-infective medications as indicated: Broad-spectrum antibiotics, e.g., methicillin (Staphcillin); Gram-negative, e.g., ticarcillin disodium (Ticar); Gram-positive, e.g., nafcillin (Nafcil), vancomycin (Vancocin); aminoglycosides, e.g., tobramycin (Nebcin), gentamicin (Garamycin); cephalosporins, e.g., cefotaxime (Claforan);

Immune globulins as appropriate.

Assist with/prepare for incision and drainage of wound, irrigation, application of warm/moist soaks as indicated.

RATIONALE

May reflect inappropriate/inadequate antibiotic therapy or overgrowth of resistant/opportunistic organisms.

Depression of immune system and use of antibiotics increases risk of secondary infections, particularly yeast.

Identification of portal of entry and organism causing the septicemia is crucial to effective treatment.

Specific antibiotics are determined by culture results, but therapy is usually initiated prior to obtaining results, using broad-spectrum antibiotics and/or based on most likely infecting organisms. Concomitant use of antimicrobials is often beneficial, but dosage must be balanced against renal function/clearance.

May boost/provide temporary immunity to general infection or specific illness, e.g., varicella zoster, rabies.

Facilitates removal of purulent material/necrotic tissue and promotes healing.

NURSING DIAGNOSIS: HYPERTHERMIA

May be related to: Increased metabolic rate, illness.

Dehydration.

Direct effect of circulating endotoxins on the hypothalamus, altering temperature regulation.

Possibly evidenced by: Increase in body temperature greater than normal range.

Flushed skin, warm to touch.

Increased respiratory rate, tachycardia.

DESIRED OUTCOMES/ EVALUATION CRITERIA— PATIENT WILL: Demonstrate temperature within normal range, be free of chills.

Experience no associated complications.

ACTIONS/INTERVENTIONS

Independent

Monitor patient temperature (degree and pattern); note shaking chills/profuse diaphoresis.

RATIONALE

Temperature of 102°F–106°F (38.9°C–41.1°C) suggests acute infectious disease process. Fever pattern may aid in diagnosis; e.g., sustained or

ACTIONS/INTERVENTIONS	RATIONALE

Independent

continuous fever curves lasting more than 24 hours suggest pneumococcal pneumonia, scarlet or typhoid fever; remittent fever (varying only a few degrees in either direction) reflects pulmonary infections; intermittent curves or fever that returns to normal once in 24-hour period suggest septic episode, septic endocarditis, or TB. Chills often precede temperature spikes. *Note:* Use of antipyretics alters fever patterns and may be restricted until diagnosis is made or if fever remains greater than 102°F (38.9°C).

Monitor environmental temperature; limit/add bed linens as indicated.	Room temperature/number of blankets should be altered to maintain near normal temperature.
Provide tepid sponge baths; avoid use of alcohol.	May help reduce fever. *Note:* Use of ice water/alcohol may cause chills, actually elevating temperature. In addition, alcohol is very drying to skin.

Collaborative

Administer antipyretics, e.g., ASA (aspirin), acetaminophen (Tylenol).	Used to reduce fever by its central action on the hypothalamus, although fever may be beneficial in limiting growth of organisms and enhancing autodestruction of infected cells.
Provide cooling blanket.	Used to reduce fever usually greater than 104°F–105°F (39.5°C–40°C), when brain damage/seizures can occur.

NURSING DIAGNOSIS:	**TISSUE PERFUSION, ALTERED, HIGH RISK FOR**
Risk factors may include:	Relative/actual hypovolemia.
	Reduction of arterial/venous blood flow: Selective vasoconstriction, vascular occlusion (intimal damage/microemboli).
Possibly evidenced by:	[Not applicable; presence of signs and symptoms establishes an actual diagnosis.]
DESIRED OUTCOMES/ EVALUATION CRITERIA— PATIENT WILL:	Display adequate perfusion as evidenced by stable vital signs, palpable peripheral pulses, skin warm and dry, usual level of consciousness, individually appropriate urinary output and active bowel sounds.

ACTIONS/INTERVENTIONS	RATIONALE

Independent

Maintain bed rest; assist with care activities.	Decreases myocardial workload and O_2 consumption, maximizing effectiveness of tissue perfusion.

ACTIONS/INTERVENTIONS	RATIONALE

Independent

Monitor trends in BP, noting progressive hypotension and changes in pulse pressure.	Hypotension develops as microorganisms invade the bloodstream, stimulating release or activation of chemical and hormonal substances, which initially results in peripheral vasodilation, decreased systemic vascular resistance, and relative hypovolemia. As shock progresses, cardiac output becomes severely depressed because of major alterations in contractility and preload/afterload, producing profound hypotension.
Monitor heart rate, rhythm. Note dysrhythmias.	Tachycardia occurs, due to sympathetic nervous system stimulation secondary to stress response and to compensate for the relative hypovolemia and hypotension. Cardiac dysrhythmias can occur as a result of hypoxia, acid–base/electrolyte imbalance, and/or low-flow perfusion state.
Note quality/strength of peripheral pulses.	Initially the pulse is strong/bounding because of increased cardiac output. Pulse may become weak/thready because of sustained hypotension, decreased cardiac output, and peripheral vasoconstriction if the shock state progresses.
Assess respiratory rate, depth and quality. Note onset of severe dyspnea.	Increased respirations occur in response to direct effects of endotoxins on the respiratory center in the brain, as well as developing hypoxia, stress, and fever. Respiration can become shallow as respiratory insufficiency develops, creating risk of acute respiratory failure. (Refer to ND: Gas Exchange, Impaired, p 895.)
Investigate changes in sensorium, e.g., mental cloudiness, agitation, restlessness, personality changes, delirium, stupor, coma.	Changes reflect alterations in cerebral perfusion, hypoxemia, and/or acidosis.
Assess skin for changes in color, temperature, moisture.	Compensatory mechanism of vasodilatation results in warm, dry, pink skin, which is characteristic of hyperperfusion in hyperdynamic phase of early septic shock. If shock state progresses, compensatory vasoconstriction occurs, shunting blood to vital organs, reducing peripheral blood flow, and creating cool, clammy, pale/dusky skin.
Record hourly urinary output and specific gravity.	Decreasing urinary output with increased specific gravity indicates diminished renal perfusion related to fluid shifts and selective vasoconstriction. There may be transient polyuria during hyperdynamic phase (while cardiac output is elevated) but may progress to oliguria.
Auscultate bowel sounds.	Reduced blood flow to the mesentery (splanchnic vasoconstriction) decreases peristalsis and may lead to paralytic ileus.
Monitor gastric pH as indicated. Hematest gastric secretions/stools for occult blood.	Stress of illness and use of steroids increase risk of gastric mucosal erosion/bleeding.

ACTIONS/INTERVENTIONS	RATIONALE
Independent	
Evaluate lower extremities for local tissue swelling, erythema, positive Homans' sign.	Venous stasis and infectious process may result in the development of thrombosis.
Monitor for signs of bleeding, e.g., oozing from puncture sites/suture lines, petechiae, ecchymoses, hematuria, epistaxis, hemoptysis, hematemesis.	Coagulopathy/DIC may occur related to accelerated clotting in the microcirculation (activation of chemical mediators, vascular insufficiency, and cell destruction), creating a life-threatening hemorrhagic situation/multiple emboli.
Note drug effects, and monitor for signs of toxicity.	Massive doses of antibiotics are often ordered. These have potentially toxic effects when hepatic/renal perfusion is compromised.
Collaborative	
Administer parenteral fluids. (Refer to ND: Fluid Volume Deficit, high risk for, this page.)	To maintain tissue perfusion, large amounts of fluid may be required to support circulating volume.
Administer drugs as indicated:	
Corticosteroids;	Although controversial, steroids may be given for the potential advantages of decreased capillary permeability, increased renal perfusion, and inhibition of microemboli formation.
$NaHCO_3$;	Impaired tissue perfusion and production of lactate results in metabolic acidosis, requiring base replacement therapy.
Antacids: e.g., aluminum hydroxide (Amphojel).	Decreases potential for gastric bleeding related to stress response/altered perfusion.
Monitor laboratory studies, e.g., ABGs, lactate levels.	Development of respiratory/metabolic acidosis reflects loss of compensatory mechanisms, e.g., decreased renal perfusion/hydrogen excretion; and accumulation of lactic acid due to circulatory shunting/stagnation.
Administer supplemental O_2.	Maximizes O_2 available for cellular uptake.
Maintain body temperature, using adjunctive aids as necessary. (Refer to ND: Hyperthermia, p 891.)	Temperature elevations increase metabolic/O_2 demands beyond cellular resources, hastening tissue ischemia/cellular destruction.
Transfer to critical care setting as indicated.	Progressive deterioration will require more aggressive therapy (e.g., hemodynamic monitoring and vasoactive drugs).

NURSING DIAGNOSIS:	FLUID VOLUME DEFICIT, HIGH RISK FOR
Risk factors may include:	Marked increase in vascular compartment/massive vasodilatation.
	Capillary permeability/fluid leaks into the interstitial space (third-spacing).
Possibly evidenced by:	[Not applicable; presence of signs and symptoms establishes an actual diagnosis.]

DESIRED OUTCOMES/ EVALUATION CRITERIA— PATIENT WILL:	Maintain adequate circulatory volume as evidenced by vital signs within patient's normal range, palpable peripheral pulses of good quality, and individually appropriate urinary output.

ACTIONS/INTERVENTIONS

Independent

Measure/record urinary output and specific gravity. Note cumulative I&O imbalances (including all/insensible losses), and correlate with daily weight. Encourage oral fluids to tolerance.

Monitor BP and heart rate. Measure CVP.

Palpate peripheral pulses.

Assess for dry mucous membranes, poor skin turgor, and thirst.

Observe for dependent/peripheral edema in sacrum, scrotum, back, legs.

Collaborative

Administer IV fluids, e.g., crystalloids (D5W, NS) and colloids (albumin, fresh frozen plasma) as indicated.

Monitor laboratory values, e.g.:

Hct/RBC count;

BUN/Cr.

RATIONALE

Decreasing urinary output with a high specific gravity suggests hypovolemia. Continued positive fluid balance with corresponding weight gain may indicate third spacing and tissue edema, suggesting need to alter fluid therapy/replacement components.

Reduction in the circulating fluid volume reduces BP/CVP, initiating compensatory mechanisms of tachycardia to improve cardiac output and increase systemic BP.

Weak, easily obliterated pulses suggest hypovolemia.

Hypovolemia/third spacing of fluid gives rise to signs of dehydration.

Fluid losses from the vascular compartment into the interstitial space create tissue edema.

Large volumes of fluid may be required to overcome relative hypovolemia (peripheral vasodilation); replace losses from increased capillary permeability (e.g., sequestration of fluid in the peritoneal cavity) and increased insensible sources (e.g., fever/diaphoresis).

Evaluates changes in hydration/blood viscosity.

Moderate elevations of BUN reflect dehydration, high values of BUN/Cr may indicate renal dysfunction/failure.

NURSING DIAGNOSIS:	GAS EXCHANGE, IMPAIRED, HIGH RISK FOR
Risk factors may include:	Altered O_2 supply: Effects of endotoxins on the respiratory center in the medulla (resulting in hyperventilation/respiratory alkalosis); hypoventilation.
	Altered blood flow (changes in vascular resistance), alveolar–capillary membrane changes (increased capillary permeability leading to pulmonary congestion).
	Interference with O_2 delivery/utilization in the tissues (endotoxin-induced damage to the cells/capillaries).

895

ACTIONS/INTERVENTIONS

Independent

Maintain patent airway. Place patient in position of comfort with head of bed elevated.

Monitor respiratory rate and depth. Note use of accessory muscles/work of breathing.

Auscultate breath sounds. Note crackles, wheezes, areas of decreased/absent ventilation.

Note presence of circumoral cyanosis.

Investigate alterations in sensorium: agitation, confusion, personality changes, delirium, stupor, coma.

Note cough and purulent sputum production.

Reposition frequently. Encourage cough and deep-breathing exercises. Suction with lavage, as indicated.

Collaborative

Monitor ABGs/pulse oximetry.

Administer supplemental O_2 via appropriate route, e.g., nasal cannula, mask, high-flow rebreathing mask.

RATIONALE

Enhances lung expansion, respiratory effort.

Rapid/shallow respirations occur because of hypoxemia, stress, and circulating endotoxins. Hypoventilation and dyspnea reflect ineffective compensatory mechanisms and are an indication that ventilatory support is needed.

Respiratory distress and the presence of adventitious sounds are indicators of pulmonary congestion/interstitial edema, atelectasis. *Note:* Respiratory complications, including pneumonia and ARDS are a prime cause of death.

Reflects inadequate systemic oxygenation/hypoxemia.

Cerebral function is very sensitive to decreases in oxygenation (e.g., hypoxemia/reduced perfusion).

Pneumonia is a common nosocomial infection, which can occur by aspiration of oropharyngeal organisms or spread from other sites.

Good pulmonary toilet is necessary for reducing ventilation/perfusion imbalance, mobilizing and facilitating removal of secretions, to maximize gas exchange.

Hypoxemia is related to decreased ventilation/pulmonary changes (e.g., interstitial edema, atelectasis, and pulmonary shunting) and increased demands (e.g., fever). Respiratory acidosis (pH below 7.35 and $PaCO_2$ greater than 40 mm Hg) occurs because of hypoventilation and ventilation–perfusion imbalance. As septic condition worsens, metabolic acidosis (pH below 7.35 and HCO_3 less than 22–24 mEq/L) arises due to buildup of lactic acid from anaerobic metabolism.

Necessary for correction of hypoxemia with failing respiratory effort/progressing acidosis. *Note:* Intubation/mechanical ventilation may be required if respiratory failure develops.

ACTIONS/INTERVENTIONS	RATIONALE
Collaborative	
Review chest x-rays.	Changes reflect progression/resolution of pulmonary complications, e.g., infiltrates/edema.

NURSING DIAGNOSIS:	**KNOWLEDGE DEFICIT [LEARNING NEED], REGARDING ILLNESS, PROGNOSIS, AND TREATMENT NEEDS**
May be related to:	Lack of exposure/recall; information misinterpretation.
	Cognitive limitation.
Possibly evidenced by:	Questions/request for information, statement of misconception.
	Inaccurate follow-through of instructions/development of preventable complications.
DESIRED OUTCOMES/ EVALUATION CRITERIA— PATIENT WILL:	Verbalize understanding of disease process and prognosis.
	Correctly perform necessary procedures and explain reasons for the actions.
	Initiate necessary lifestyle changes.
	Participate in treatment regimen.

ACTIONS/INTERVENTIONS	RATIONALE
Independent	
Review disease process and future expectations.	Provides knowledge base on which patient can make informed choices.
Review individual risk factors and mode of transmission/portal of entry of infections.	Glucocorticoid therapy, kidney/liver dysfunction, neoplastic disease, rheumatic heart disease, valve dysfunction, and DM may predispose to septicemia. Being aware of how infection is transmitted provides opportunity to plan for/institute protective measures.
Provide information about drug therapy, interactions, side effects, and importance of adherence to regimen.	Promotes understanding of and enhances cooperation in treatment/prophylaxis and reduces risk of recurrence and complications.
Discuss need for good nutritional intake/balanced diet.	Necessary for optimal healing and general well-being.
Encourage adequate rest periods with scheduled activities.	Prevents fatigue, conserves energy, and promotes healing.
Review necessity of personal hygiene and environmental cleanliness.	Helps to control environmental exposure by diminishing the number of pathogens present.
Discuss proper use or avoidance of tampons as indicated.	Superabsorbent tampons/infrequent changing potentiates risk of *Staphylococcus aureus* infection (toxic shock syndrome).

897

ACTIONS/INTERVENTIONS	RATIONALE

Independent

Identify signs/symptoms requiring medical evaluation, e.g., persistent temperature elevation(s), tachycardia, syncope, rashes of unknown origin, unexplained fatigue, anorexia, increased thirst, and changes in bladder function.

Early recognition of developing/recurring infection allows for timely intervention and reduces risk for progression to life-threatening situation.

Stress importance of prophylactic immunization/antibiotic therapy as needed.

Used for prevention of infection.

Bibliography

General References

Bellak, JP and Bamford, PA: Nursing Assessment: A Multidimensional Approach. Jones & Bartlett, Boston, 1987.
Berkow, R (ed): The Merck Manual, ed 15. Merck Sharp & Dohme Research Laboratories, Rahway, NJ, 1987.
Cella, JH and Watson, J: Nurse's Manual of Laboratory Tests. FA Davis, Philadelphia, 1989.
Condon, RE, and Nyhus, LM (eds): Manual of Surgical Therapeutics, ed 7. Little, Brown & Co, Boston, 1988.
Deglin, JH and Vallerand, AH: Davis's Drug Guide for Nurses, ed 3. FA Davis, Philadelphia, 1992.
Diseases and Disorders Handbook, ed 3. Springhouse Corp, Springhouse, PA, 1989.
Doenges, ME and Moorhouse, MF: Nurse's Pocket Guide: Nursing Diagnoses with Interventions, ed 3. FA Davis, Philadelphia, 1991.
Dunagan, WC and Ridner, ML (eds): Manual of Medical Therapeutics, ed 26. Little, Brown & Co, Boston, 1989.
Fischbach, F: A Manual of Laboratory and Diagnostic Tests, ed 4. JB Lippincott, Philadelphia, 1992.
Guyton, AC: Textbook of Medical Physiology, ed 8. WB Saunders, Philadelphia, 1991.
Kuhn, MM: Pharmacotherapeutics: A Nursing Process Approach, ed 2. FA Davis, Philadelphia,1991.
Professional Guide to Diseases, ed 3. Springhouse Corp, Springhouse, PA, 1989.
Suddarth, DS (ed): The Lippincott Manual of Nursing Practice, ed 5. JB Lippincott, Philadelphia, 1991.
Thomas, CL (ed): Taber's Cyclopedic Medical Dictionary, ed 17. FA Davis, Philadelphia, 1993.
Thompson, JM, et al: Mosby's Manual of Clinical Nursing, ed 2. CV Mosby, St Louis, 1989.

Articles

Czurylo, KT, Pfeiffer, AM, and Steffen, M: Dealing with a hidden hazard: MRSA. Nursing91 21(12):68, 1991.
Jackson, MM and Lynch, P: Infection control: In search of a rational approach. AJN 90(10):65, 1990.
McMorrow, ME and Conney-Daniello, M: When to suspect septic shock. RN 54(10): 32, 1991.

CHAPTER 17

GENERAL

Psychosocial Aspects of Acute Care _____

The emotional response of the patient in the acute care setting is of extreme importance. The mind–body–spirit connection is well established; for example, when a physiologic response occurs, there is a corresponding psychologic response. Also, there are physiologic conditions that have a psychologic component, for example, the emotional instability of Cushing's syndrome, steroid therapy, or the irritability of hypoglycemia. Rapid growth of the field of psychoneuroimmunology is regularly providing new information about these issues.

Although the stress of illness is well recognized, the effect on the individual is unpredictable. Values of caregivers and patients/SOs, sensitivity to different cultures, language barriers (including difficulties that people have in talking about their bodies) impact the care a patient expects and receives. It is not necessarily the event, but rather the patient's perception of the event, that creates problems, and unmet psychologic needs drain energy resources needed for healing.

With the expanding technology in health care, ethical issues are more hotly debated.

RELATED CONCERNS

This is an aspect of all care and plans of care.

ASSESSMENT FACTORS TO BE CONSIDERED

INDIVIDUAL

Age and sex.
Religious affiliation: Church attendance, importance of religion in patient's life, belief in life after death.
Level of knowledge/education. Way the individual accesses information, e.g., auditory, visual, kinesthetic.
Patient's dominant language? Is s/he literate?
Patterns of communication with SOs, with health care givers? Style of speech?
Perception of body and its functions. When well? In illness? This illness?
How does patient define and perceive illness?
How is patient experiencing illness versus what illness actually is?
Emotional response to current treatment and hospitalization?
Past experience with illness, hospitalization, and health care systems?
Describe emotional reaction in feeling (sensory) terms: e.g., States "I feel scared."
Behavior when anxious, afraid, impatient, or angry.

SIGNIFICANT OTHERS

Marital status. Who are SOs? Nuclear family? Extended family? Recurring or patterned relationships?
Family developmental cycle: Just married? Children? (young, adolescent, leaving/returning home) Retired?
Patient's role in family tasks and functions.
How are SOs affected by the illness and prognosis?
What are the interaction processes within the family?
Lifestyle differences that need to be considered. Dietary? Spiritual? Sexual preference? Other community
   (e.g., religious order, communes, retirement center)?

SOCIOECONOMIC

Employment; finances.
Environmental factors: Home, work, and recreation.
Out of usual environment (on vacation, visiting).
Social class; value system.
Social acceptability of disease/condition (e.g., STDs, HIV, obesity, substance abuse).

CULTURAL

Ethnic background.
Health-seeking behaviors; illness referral system.
Values related to health and treatment.
Cultural factors related to illness in general and to pain response.
Beliefs regarding caring and curing.

DISEASE (ILLNESS)

Kind/cause of illness. How has it been treated? Will it be treated? Should it be treated? Anticipated re-
   sponse to treatment? What is the threat to others?
Is this an acute or a chronic illness? Is it inherited?
If terminal illness, what do the patient and SO know and anticipate?
Is the condition "appropriate" to the afflicted individual, e.g., multiple sclerosis, DM, cancer.
Illness related to personality factors, such as type A (may be myth or valid)?

NURSE-RELATED

Basic knowledge of human responses and how the current situation is related to response of the individual.
Basic knowledge of biologic, psychologic, social, and cultural issues.
Knowledge and use of therapeutic communication skills.
Knowledge of own value and belief systems.
Willingness to look at own behavior in relation to interaction with others and make changes as necessary.
Respect of patient's privacy; confidentiality.

NURSING PRIORITIES

1. Reduce anxiety/fear.
2. Support grieving process.
3. Facilitate integration of self-concept and body-image changes.
4. Encourage effective coping skills of patient/SO.
5. Promote safe environment/patient well-being.

NURSING DIAGNOSIS:	ANXIETY [SPECIFY LEVEL]/FEAR
May be related to:	Unconscious conflict about essential values.
	Situational and/or maturational crises; interpersonal transmission and contagion.
	Threat to self-concept; threat of death; change in health status; unmet needs.
	Separation from support system; knowledge deficit.
	Sensory impairment; environmental stimuli.
Possibly evidenced by:	Reports of increased tension; feelings of helplessness.
	Inadequacy; apprehension, uncertainty, being scared; overexcitedness.
	Expressed concern regarding changes in life events; dread of an identifiable problem recognized by the patient; fear of unspecific consequences.
	Focus on self; fight/flight behavior.
	Facial tension; sympathetic stimulation; extraneous movements.
DESIRED OUTCOMES/ EVALUATION CRITERIA— PATIENT WILL:	Acknowledge and discuss fears.
	Appear relaxed and report anxiety is reduced to a manageable level.
	Verbalize awareness of feelings of anxiety and healthy ways to deal with them.
	Demonstrate problem solving and use resources effectively.

ACTIONS/INTERVENTIONS	RATIONALE
Independent	
Note palpitations, elevated pulse/respiratory rate.	Changes in vital signs may suggest the degree of anxiety being experienced by the patient or reflect the impact of physiologic factors, e.g., endocrine imbalances.
Acknowledge fear/anxieties. Validate observations with patient, e.g., "You seem to be afraid?"	Feelings are real, and it is helpful to bring them out in the open so they can be discussed and dealt with.
Assess degree/reality of threat to patient and level of anxiety (e.g., mild, moderate, severe) by observing behavior such as clenched hands, wide eyes, startle response, furrowed brow, clinging to family/staff, or physical/verbal lashing out.	Individual responses can vary according to culturally learned patterns. Distorted perceptions of the situation may magnify feelings.

901

ACTIONS/INTERVENTIONS	RATIONALE

Independent

Note narrowed focus of attention (e.g., patient concentrates on one thing at a time).

Narrowed focus usually reflects extreme fear/panic.

Observe speech content and patterns: rapidity/slowed, pressured, words used, repetition, laughter.

Provides clues about such factors as the level of anxiety, ability to comprehend, brain damage, or possible language differences.

Assess severity of pain when present. Delay gathering of information if pain is severe.

Severe pain and anxiety leave little energy for thinking and other activities.

Identify patient's/SO's perception(s) of the situation.

Regardless of the reality of the situation, perception affects how each individual deals with the illness/stress.

Acknowledge reality of the situation as the patient sees it, without challenging the belief.

Patient may need to deny reality until ready to deal with it. It is not helpful to force the patient to face facts.

Evaluate coping/defense mechanisms being used to deal with the perceived or real threat.

May be dealing well with the situation at the moment; e.g., denial and regression may be helpful coping mechanisms for a time. However, use of such mechanisms divert energy the patient needs for healing, and problems need to be dealt with at some point in time.

Review coping mechanisms used in the past, e.g., problem-solving skills, recognizing/asking for help.

Provides opportunity to build on resources the patient/SO may have used successfully.

Maintain frequent contact with the patient/SO. Be available for listening and talking as needed.

Establishes rapport, promotes expression of feelings, and helps patient and SO look at realities of the illness/treatment without confronting issues they are not ready to deal with.

Acknowledge feelings as expressed (e.g., Active-listen, reflection). If actions are unacceptable, take necessary steps to control/deal with behavior. (Refer to ND: Violence, high risk for, p 913.)

Often acknowledging feelings will enable patient to deal more appropriately with situation. May need chemical/physical control for brief periods.

Identify ways in which patient can get help when needed.

Provides assurance that staff is available for assistance/support.

Stay with or arrange to have someone stay with patient as indicated.

Continuous support may help patient regain internal locus of control and reduce anxiety/fear to a manageable level.

Provide accurate information as appropriate and when requested by the patient/SO. Answer questions freely and honestly and in language that is understandable by all. Repeat information as necessary; correct misconceptions.

Complex and/or anxiety-provoking information can be given in manageable amounts over an extended period. As opportunities arise and facts are given, individuals will accept what they are ready for. *Note:* Words/phrases may have different meanings for each individual; therefore, clarification is necessary to ensure understanding.

Avoid empty reassurances, e.g., statements of "everything will be all right." Instead, provide specific information: e.g., "Your heart rate is regular, your pain is being easily controlled, and that is what we want."

It is not possible for the nurse to know how the specific situation will be resolved, and false reassurances may be interpreted as lack of understanding or honesty, further isolating the patient. Sharing observations used in assessing condition/prognosis provides opportunity for patient/SO to feel reassured.

ACTIONS/INTERVENTIONS	RATIONALE

Independent

Note expressions of concern/anger about treatment or staff.

Anxiety about self and outcome may be masked by comments/angry outbursts directed at therapy/caregivers.

Ask the patient/SO to identify what they can/cannot do about what is happening.

Assists in identifying areas in which control is available as well as those in which control is not possible.

Provide as much order and predictability as possible in scheduling care/activities, visitors.

Helps patient anticipate and prepare for difficult treatments/movements as well as look forward to pleasant occurrences.

Instruct in ways to use positive self-talk, e.g., "I know I can manage this pain for now."

Internal dialog is often negative. When this is shared out loud, the patient becomes aware and can be directed in the use of positive self-talk, which can help reduce anxiety.

Encourage/instruct in mental imagery/relaxation methods; e.g., imaging a pleasant place, use of music/tapes, slow breathing, and meditation.

Promotes release of endorphins and aids in developing internal locus of control, reducing anxiety. May enhance coping skills, allowing body to go about its work of healing.

Use touch, Therapeutic Touch, massage, and other adjunctive therapies as indicated.

Aids in meeting basic human need, decreasing sense of isolation, and assisting the patient to feel less anxious. *Note:* Therapeutic Touch is a method of using the hands to direct human energies to help or to heal.

Collaborative

Administer medications as needed: e.g., diazepam (Valium); × 3 clorazepate dipotassium (Tranxene); chlordiazepoxide (Librium); alprazolam (Xanax).

Antianxiety agents may be useful for brief periods to assist the patient/SO to reduce anxiety to manageable levels, providing opportunity for initiation of patient's own coping skills.

NURSING DIAGNOSIS:	GRIEVING [SPECIFY]
May be related to:	Actual or perceived loss; chronic and/or fatal illness.
	Thwarted grieving response to a loss; lack of resolution of previous grieving response/absence of anticipatory grieving.
Possibly evidenced by:	Verbal expression of distress/unresolved issues.
	Denial of loss.
	Altered eating habits, sleep/dream patterns, activity levels, libido.
	Crying; labile affect; feelings of sorrow, guilt, anger.
	Difficulty in expressing loss; alterations in concentration and/or pursuit of tasks.

ACTIONS/INTERVENTIONS

Independent

Provide open environment in which the patient feels free to realistically discuss feelings and concerns.

Identify stage of grieving/dysfunction:

Denial: Be aware of avoidance behaviors; anger, withdrawal, and so forth. Allow patient to talk about what s/he chooses, and do not try to force patient to "face the facts";

Anger: Note behaviors of withdrawal, lack of co-operation, and direct expression of anger. Be alert to body language and check meaning with the patient. Encourage/allow verbalization of anger with acknowledgment of feelings and setting of limits regarding destructive behavior;

Bargaining: Be aware of statements such as "...if I do this, that will fix my problem". Allow verbalization without confrontation about realities;

Depression: Give patient permission to be where s/he is. Provide comfort and availability as well as caring for physical needs;

Acceptance: Respect the patient's needs and wishes for quiet, privacy, and/or talking.

Active-listen patient's concerns and be available for help as necessary.

Identify and problem-solve solutions to existing physical responses, e.g., eating, sleeping, activity levels, and sexual desire.

RATIONALE

Therapeutic communication skills such as Active-listening, silence, being available, and acceptance can allow the patient the opportunity to talk freely and deal with the perceived/actual loss.

Awareness allows for appropriate choice of interventions as individuals handle grief in many different ways.

Denying the reality of diagnosis and/or prognosis is an important phase in which the patient protects self from the pain and reality of the threat of loss. Each person does this in an individual manner based on previous experiences with loss and cultural/religious factors.

Denial gives way to feelings of anger, rage, guilt, and resentment. Patient may find it difficult to express anger directly and may feel guilty about feeling angry. Although staff may have difficulty dealing with angry behaviors, acceptance of it allows patient to work through the anger and move on to more effective coping behaviors.

Bargaining with care providers or God often occurs and may be helpful in beginning resolution and acceptance. Patient may be working through feelings of guilt about things done or undone.

When patient can no longer deny the reality of the loss, feelings of helplessness and hopelessness replace feelings of anger. The patient needs information that this is a normal progression of feelings.

Having worked through the denial, anger and depression, patient often prefers to be alone and does not want to talk much at this point. Patient may still cling to hope, which can be sustaining through whatever is happening at this point.

The process of grieving does not proceed in an orderly fashion, but fluctuates with various aspects of all stages present at one time or another. If process is dysfunctional or prolonged, more aggressive interventions may be required to facilitate the process.

May need additional assistance to deal with the physical aspects of grieving.

ACTIONS/INTERVENTIONS	RATIONALE
Independent	
Assess needs of SO and assist as indicated.	Identification of problems indicating dysfunctional grieving allows for individual interventions.
Collaborative	
Refer to other resources, e.g., counseling, psychotherapy as indicated.	May need additional help to resolve grief, make plans, and look toward the future.

NURSING DIAGNOSIS:	SELF-ESTEEM, SITUATIONAL LOW
May be related to:	Biophysical, psychosocial, cognitive perceptual, cultural, and/or spiritual crisis, e.g., changes in body image, role performance, personal identity.
	Perceived/anticipated failure at life event(s).
Possibly evidenced by:	Negating self-appraisal in response to life events.
	Verbalization of negative feelings about the self (helplessness, uselessness); focus on past abilities, strengths, function or appearance; preoccupation with change/loss.
	Evaluates self as unable to handle situations/events.
	Fear of rejection/reaction by others.
	Difficulty making decisions.
DESIRED OUTCOMES/ EVALUATION CRITERIA— PATIENT WILL:	Verbalize realistic view and acceptance of self in situation.
	Identify existing strengths and view self as capable person.
	Recognize and incorporate change into self-concept in accurate manner without negating self-esteem.
	Demonstrate adaptation to changes/events that have occurred as evidenced by setting of realistic goals and active participation in work/play/personal relationships.

ACTIONS/INTERVENTIONS	RATIONALE
Independent	
Ask what the patient would like to be called.	Shows courtesy/respect and acknowledges person.
Identify SO from whom the patient derives comfort and who should be notified in case of emergency.	Allows provisions to be made for specific person(s) to visit or remain close and provide needed support for patient. *Note:* May or may not be legal next of kin.
Active-listen patient concerns and fears.	Conveys sense of caring and can more effectively identify the needs and problems as well as patient's coping strategies and how effective they are. Provides opportunity to duplicate and begin a problem-solving process.

ACTIONS/INTERVENTIONS	RATIONALE
Independent	
Encourage verbalization of feelings, accepting what is said.	Helps patient/SO begin to adapt to change and reduces anxiety about altered function/lifestyle.
Discuss stages of grief and the importance of grief work. (Refer to ND: Grieving [specify], p 903.)	Grieving is a necessary step for integration of change/loss into self-concept.
Provide nonthreatening environment.	Promotes feelings of safety, encouraging verbalization.
Observe nonverbal communication, e.g., body posture and movements, eye contact, gestures, use of touch.	Nonverbal language is a large portion of communication and therefore is extremely important. How the person uses touch provides information about how it is accepted and how comfortable the individual is with being touched.
Reflect back to the patient what has been said, for clarification and verification.	Information must be validated by the patient as assumptions may be inaccurate.
Observe and describe behavior in objective terms.	All behavior has meaning, some of which is obvious and some of which needs to be identified. This is a process of educated guesswork and needs to be validated by the patient.
Identify age and developmental level.	Age is an indicator of the stage of life patient is experiencing, e.g., adolescence, middle age. However, developmental level may be more important than chronologic age in anticipating and identifying some of patient's needs. Some degree of regression occurs during illness, dependent on many factors such as the normal coping skills of the individual and the severity of the illness.
Discuss patient's view of body image and how illness/condition might affect it.	The patient's perception of a change in body image may occur suddenly or over time (e.g., actual loss of a body part through injury/surgery or a perceived loss, a heart attack) or be a continuous subtle process (e.g., chronic illness, eating disorders, or aging). Awareness can alert the nurse to the need for appropriate interventions tailored to the individual need.
Encourage discussion of physical changes in a simple, direct, and factual manner. Give realistic feedback and discuss future options, e.g., rehabilitation services.	Provides opportunity to begin incorporating actual changes in an accepting and hopeful atmosphere.
Acknowledge efforts at problem-solving, resolution of current situation, and future planning.	Provides encouragement and reinforces continuation of desired behaviors.
Recognize patient's pace for adaptation to demands of current situation.	Failure to acknowledge patient's need to take time and/or pressuring patient to "get on with it" conveys a lack of acceptance of the person as an individual and may result in feelings of lowered self-esteem.
Introduce tasks at patient's level of functioning, progressing to more complex activities as tolerated.	Provides for success experiences, reaffirming capabilities and enhancing self-esteem.

ACTIONS/INTERVENTIONS	RATIONALE

Independent

Ascertain how the patient sees own role within the family system, e.g., breadwinner, homemaker, husband/wife.

Illness may create a temporary or permanent problem in role expectations. Sexual role and how the patient views self in relation to the current illness also play important parts in recovery.

Assist patient/SO with clarifying expected roles and those that may need to be relinquished or altered.

Provides opportunity to identify misconceptions and begin to look at options; promotes reality orientation.

Assess impact of illness/surgery on sexuality.

Sexuality encompasses the whole person in the total environment. Many times problems of illness are superimposed on already existing problems of sexuality and can impact patient's sense of self-worth. Some problems are more obvious than others, such as illness involving the reproductive parts of the body. Others are less obvious, such as sexual values, role in family, e.g., mother, wage earner, single parent, and so on.

Be alert to comments and innuendos, which may mean the patient has a concern in this area.

People are often reluctant and/or embarrassed to ask direct questions about sexual/sexuality concerns.

Be aware of nurse's feelings about dealing with the subject of sexuality.

Nurses/caregivers are often as reluctant and embarrassed in dealing with sexuality issues as most patients.

Provide information and referral to hospital and community resources.

Enables patient/SO to be in contact with interested groups with access to assistive and supportive devices, services and counseling.

Collaborative

Refer to psychiatric support/therapy group, social services, as indicated.

May be needed to assist patient/SO to achieve optimal recovery.

Refer to appropriate resources for sex therapy as need indicates.

May be someone with comfort level and knowledge who is available or may be necessary to refer to professional resources for additional help and support.

NURSING DIAGNOSIS:	COPING, INEFFECTIVE INDIVIDUAL/DECISIONAL CONFLICT
May be related to:	Situational crises/personal vulnerability; multiple life changes/maturational crises.
	Inadequate coping methods.
	Inadequate support systems.
	No vacations/inadequate relaxation.
	Impairment of nervous system; memory loss; impaired adaptive behaviors and problem-solving skills.
	Severe pain/overwhelming threat to self.

907

	Unclear personal values/beliefs; perceived threat to value system; lack of experience/interference with decision making; lack of information.
Possibly evidenced by:	Verbalization of inability to cope/asking for help.
	Muscular tension, frequent headaches/neckaches.
	Chronic worry, fatigue, insomnia, anxiety/depression.
	Poor self-esteem.
	Inappropriate use of defense mechanisms; inability to meet role expectations, basic needs, problem-solve.
	Alteration in social participation; change in usual communication patterns.
	High illness/accident rate; overeating; excessive smoking/drinking.
	Destructive behavior toward self or others.
	Uncertainty about choices; vacillation between alternative actions; delayed decision making.
DESIRED OUTCOMES/ EVALUATION CRITERIA— PATIENT WILL:	Identify ineffective coping behaviors and consequences.
	Verbalize awareness of own coping/problem-solving abilities.
	Meet psychologic needs as evidenced by appropriate expression of feelings, identification of options, and use of resources.
	Make decisions and express satisfaction with choices.

ACTIONS/INTERVENTIONS	RATIONALE
Independent	
Review pathophysiology affecting the patient and extent of feelings of hopelessness/helplessness/loss of control over life, level of anxiety.	Indicators of degree of disequilibrium and need for intervention to prevent or resolve the crisis.
Establish therapeutic nurse–patient relationship.	Patient may feel freer in the context of this relationship to verbalize feelings of helplessness/powerlessness, and to discuss changes that may be necessary in the patient's life.
Note expressions of indecision, dependence on others, and inability to manage own ADLs.	May indicate need to lean on others for a time. Early recognition and intervention can help patient regain equilibrium.
Assess presence of positive coping skills, e.g., use of relaxation techniques, willingness to express feelings.	When the individual has coping skills that have been successful in the past, they may be used in the current situation to relieve tension and preserve the individual's sense of control.

ACTIONS/INTERVENTIONS	RATIONALE
Independent	
Encourage patient to talk about what is happening at this time and what has occurred to precipitate feelings of helplessness and anxiety.	Provides clues to assist patient to develop coping skills and regain equilibrium.
Correct misperceptions patient may have. Provide factual information.	Assists in identification and correction of perception of reality and enables problem solving to begin.
Provide quiet, nonstimulating environment. Determine what patient needs, and provide if possible. Give simple, factual information about what patient can expect and repeat as necessary.	Decreases anxiety and provides control for the patient during crisis situation.
Allow patient to be dependent in the beginning with gradual resumption of independence in ADLs, self-care, and other activities. Make opportunities for patient to make decisions about care when possible, accepting choice not to do so.	Promotes feelings of security (patient will know nurse will provide safety). As control is regained, patient has the opportunity to develop adaptive coping/problem-solving skills.
Accept verbal expressions of anger, setting limits on maladaptive behavior.	Verbalizing angry feelings is an important process for resolution of grief and loss. However, preventing destructive actions (such as striking out at others) preserves patient's self-esteem.
Discuss feelings of self-blame/projection of blame on others.	While these mechanisms may be protective at the moment of crisis, they are counter-productive and intensify feelings of helplessness and hopelessness.
Note expressions of inability to find meaning in life/reason for living, feelings of futility or alienation from God.	Crisis situation may evoke questioning of spiritual beliefs affecting ability to cope with current situation and plan for the future.
Problem-solve solutions for current situation. Provide information/support and reinforce reality as patient begins to ask questions; look at what is happening.	Helping patient/SO to brainstorm possible solutions (giving consideration to the pros and cons of each) promotes feelings of self-control/esteem.
Identify new coping behaviors patient is displaying and reinforce positive adaptation.	During crisis, patient develops new ways of dealing with problems, which can assist with resolution of current situation as well as future crises.

NURSING DIAGNOSIS:	**FAMILY COPING, INEFFECTIVE, COMPROMISED/ DISABLING/CAREGIVER ROLE STRAIN**
May be related to:	Inadequate or incorrect information or understanding by a primary person.
	Temporary preoccupation by significant person who is trying to manage emotional conflicts and personal suffering and is unable to perceive or to act effectively with regard to patient's needs; do not have enough resources to provide the care needed.

	Temporary family disorganization and role changes; feel that care giving interferes with other important roles in their lives.
	Patient providing little support in turn for the primary person.
	Prolonged disease/disability progression that exhausts the supportive capacity of significant persons.
	Significant person with chronically unexpressed feelings of guilt, anxiety, hostility, despair.
	Highly ambivalent family relationships; feel stress or nervousness in their relationship with the care receiver.
Possibly evidenced by:	Patient expresses/confirms a concern or complains about SO's response to patient's health problem, despair about family reactions/lack of involvement; past history of poor relationship between caregiver and care receiver.
	Neglectful relationships with other family members.
	SO describes preoccupation about personal reactions; displays intolerance, abandonment, rejection; care giver is not developmentally ready for caregiver role.
	SO attempts assistive/supportive behaviors with less than satisfactory results; withdraws or enters into limited or temporary personal communication with patient; displays protective behavior disproportionate (too little or too much) to patient's abilities or need for autonomy.
DESIRED OUTCOMES/ EVALUATION CRITERIA— FAMILY/CAREGIVER WILL:	Identify resources within themselves to deal with situation.
	Provide opportunity for patient to deal with situation in own way.
	Express more realistic understanding and expectations of the patient; visit regularly and participate positively in care of patient, within limits of abilities.

ACTIONS/INTERVENTIONS	RATIONALE
Independent	
Assess level of anxiety present in family/SO.	Anxiety level needs to be dealt with before problem solving can begin. Individuals may be so preoccupied with own reactions to situation that they are unable to respond to another's needs.
Establish rapport and acknowledge difficulty of the situation for the family.	May assist SO to accept what is happening and be willing to share problems with staff.
Assess preillness/current behaviors that are interfering with the care/recovery of the patient.	Information about family problems (e.g., divorce/ separation, alcoholism, drug abuse, abusive situation) will be helpful in developing an appropriate plan of care.

910

ACTIONS/INTERVENTIONS

Independent

Determine current knowledge of the situation.

Assess current actions of SO and how they are received by patient.

Involve SO in information giving, problem-solving, and care of patient as feasible.

Encourage seeking help appropriately. Give information about persons and agencies available to them.

RATIONALE

Provides information on which to begin planning care and make informed decisions. Lack of information can interfere with caregiver's/care receiver's response to illness situation.

SO may be trying to be helpful but is not perceived as helpful by the patient. May be withdrawn or may be too protective.

Information can reduce feelings of helplessness and uselessness. Involvement in care enhances feelings of control and self-worth.

Permission to seek help as needed allows them to choose to take advantage of what is available.

NURSING DIAGNOSIS:	FAMILY COPING: POTENTIAL FOR GROWTH
May be related to:	Basic needs are sufficiently gratified and adaptive tasks effectively addressed to enable goals of self-actualization to surface.
	Willingness to deal with one's own needs and to begin to problem-solve with the patient.
Possibly evidenced by:	Family member attempting to describe growth impact of crisis on his/her own values, priorities, goals, or relationships.
	Family member moving in direction of health-promoting and enriching lifestyle and generally choosing experiences that optimize wellness.
DESIRED OUTCOMES/ EVALUATION CRITERIA— FAMILY WILL:	Express willingness to look at own role in family's growth.
	Undertake tasks leading to change.
	Verbalize feelings of self-confidence and satisfaction with progress being made.

ACTIONS/INTERVENTIONS

Independent

Provide opportunities for family to talk with patient and/or staff.

Listen to family's expressions of hope, planning, effect on relationships/life.

RATIONALE

Reduces anxiety and allows expression of what has been learned and how they are managing, as well as opportunity to make plans for the future and share support.

Provides clues to avenues to explore for assistance with growth.

ACTIONS/INTERVENTIONS

Independent

Provide opportunities for and instruction in how SOs can care for patient. Discuss ways in which they can support patient in meeting own needs.

Provide a role model with which family may identify.

Assist family to develop effective communication skills of Active-listening, "I-messages," and problem solving.

Collaborative

Refer to support group(s) and other resources as indicated.

RATIONALE

Enhances feelings of control and involvement in situation in which SOs cannot do many things. Also provides opportunity to learn how to be most helpful when patient is discharged.

Having a positive example can help with adoption of new behaviors to promote growth.

Helps individuals to express needs and wants in ways that will develop family cohesiveness. Promotes solutions in which everyone wins.

Provides opportunities for sharing experiences; provides mutual support and practical problem solving; and can aid in decreasing alienation and helplessness.

NURSING DIAGNOSIS:	NONCOMPLIANCE [COMPLIANCE, ALTERED] (SPECIFY)
May be related to:	Patient value system: Health beliefs, spiritual values, cultural influences.
	Patient and provider relationships.
	Fear/anxiety; side effects of therapy.
Possibly evidenced by:	Statements of unwillingness to follow treatment regimen.
	Behavior indicative of failure to adhere to treatment regimen, e.g., not keeping appointments.
	Evidence of development of complications; failure to progress.
DESIRED OUTCOMES/ EVALUATION CRITERIA PATIENT WILL:	Participate in the development of goals and treatment plan.
	Verbalize accurate knowledge of disease and understanding of treatment regimen.
	Make choices at level of readiness based on accurate information.

ACTIONS/INTERVENTIONS

Independent

Determine reason(s) for behavior/problems that are interfering with treatment. Assess level of anxiety, locus of control, sense of powerlessness, and so forth.

RATIONALE

Many factors may be involved in behavior that is disruptive to the treatment regimen (e.g., fear, pain, anxiety, hypoxemia, chemical imbalance).

ACTIONS/INTERVENTIONS	RATIONALE

Independent

Review patient's/SO's knowledge and understanding of the need for treatment/medication as well as consequences of actions/choices.

Provides opportunities to clarify viewpoints/misconceptions. Verifies that patient/SO has accurate/factual information with which to make informed choices.

Determine cultural, spiritual, and health beliefs.

Provides insight into thoughts/factors related to individual situation. Beliefs will impact patient's perception of situation and participation in treatment regimen.

Note length of illness/prognosis.

Patients tend to become passive and dependent in long-term, debilitating illness.

Assess support systems available to the patient.

Access to helpful resources may assist patient in meeting treatment goals/provide purpose for living. Presence of caring/empathic family/SO(s) can help patient in process of recovery.

Review treatment plan with patient/SO. Establish graduated goals or modified regimen as necessary; work out alternate solutions.

Provides opportunities to exchange accurate information and to clarify viewpoints/misconceptions. Promotes patient involvement/independence; provides opportunity for compromise, and may enhance cooperation with regimen.

Contract with the patient for participation in care.

Patient who agrees to own responsibility is more apt to cooperate.

Accept the patient's choice/point of view, even it if appears to be self-destructive, e.g., decision to continue smoking.

Confrontation is not beneficial and may actually be detrimental to future cooperation and goal achievement.

Develop a system for self-monitoring. Share data pertinent to patient's condition, e.g., laboratory results, BP readings.

Provides a sense of control and enables patient to follow own progress and to assist with making choices.

Have same personnel care for patient as much as possible.

Enables relationship to develop in which the patient can begin to trust/participate in care.

Be aware of own (caregiver's) response to patient's treatment choices (e.g., refusal of blood or chemotherapy, Living Will).

Negative feelings regarding these choices may be expressed in judgmental behaviors that block or interfere with patient's wishes, comfort, and/or care.

NURSING DIAGNOSIS:	VIOLENCE, HIGH RISK FOR, DIRECTED AT SELF/OTHERS
Risk factors may include:	Attempt to deal with the threat to self-concept that illness can represent.
	Antisocial character; catatonic/manic excitement; panic states; rage reactions.
	Suicidal ideation/behavior, depression.

	Hormonal imbalance; temporal lobe epilepsy; toxic reactions to medication.
	Negative role modeling; developmental crisis.
[Possible indicators:]	Suspicion of others, paranoid ideation, delusions, hallucinations.
	Expressed intent or desire to harm self/others (directly or indirectly); hostile verbalizations.
	Body language: Rigid posture, clenched fists, facial expressions.
	Increased motor activity, excitement, irritability, agitation.
	Overt and aggressive acts; self-destructive behavior.
	Substance abuse/withdrawal.
DESIRED OUTCOMES/ EVALUATION CRITERIA— PATIENT WILL:	Acknowledge realities of the situation.
	Verbalize understanding of reason(s) for behavior/precipitating factors.
	Express increased self-concept/esteem.
	Demonstrate self-control, as evidenced by relaxed posture, nonviolent behavior.

ACTIONS/INTERVENTIONS	RATIONALE
Independent	
Observe for early signs of distress.	Irritability, pacing, shouting/cursing, lack of cooperation and demanding behavior may all be signs of increasing anxiety.
Help patient identify more adequate solutions. Give as much autonomy as is possible in the situation.	Enhances feelings of power and control in a situation in which many things are not within individual's control.
Provide protection within the environment, e.g., constant observation, removal of objects that might be used to harm self/others.	May need more structure to maintain control until own internal locus of control is regained.
Give permission to express angry feelings in acceptable ways. Make time to listen to verbalization of these feelings.	Encouraging acceptable expression can be helpful in defusing feelings of helplessness and anger, as well as decreasing guilt.
Accept patient's anger without reacting on an emotional basis.	Responding with anger is not helpful in resolving the situation and may result in escalating patient's behavior.
Remain calm and state limits on behavior in a firm manner. Be truthful.	Understanding that helplessness and fear underlie this behavior can be helpful.
Assume that the patient has control and is responsible for own behavior.	Often enables the individual to exercise control. Note: When violent behavior is the result of drugs, patient may not be able to respond appropriately.

ACTIONS/INTERVENTIONS	RATIONALE

Independent

Identify conditions that may interfere with ability to control own behavior.

Tell patient to "stop."

Use an organized team approach when necessary to subdue patient with force. Tell patient clearly and concisely what is happening.

Hold patient; place in restraints or seclusion if necessary. Do so in a calm, positive, nonstimulating/nonpunitive manner.

Apply and adjust restraint devices properly.

Document precise reason for restraints, actions taken. Check restraints frequently per hospital protocol, each time documenting the condition and how long the restraints are used.

Monitor for suicidal intent, e.g., morbid or anxious feelings while with the patient; warning from the patient, "It doesn't matter, I'd be better off dead."; mood swings, putting affairs in order, previous suicide attempt.

Assess suicidal intent (1–10 scale) by asking directly if patient is thinking of killing self, has plan, means, and so on.

Collaborative

Refer to psychiatric resource(s), e.g., clinical specialist psychiatric nurse, psychiatrist, psychologist, social worker.

Administer medications, e.g., tranquilizers, sedatives, narcotics.

Acute or chronic brain syndrome/drug-induced or postsurgical confusion may precipitate violent behavior that is difficult to control.

May be sufficient to help patient control own actions if exhibiting hostile actions. *Note:* Patient is often afraid of own actions and wants staff to set limits.

Knowing and practicing these actions before they are needed helps to prevent untoward problems. Keeping patient informed can help patient to regain internal control.

As a last resort, physical restraint may be necessary while the patient regains control. *Note:* These measures are meant to protect the patient, not punish the behavior.

It is important to maintain body alignment and patient comfort.

Restraints are to be used for very specific reasons, which need to be clearly documented to avoid overuse or misuse.

Indicators of need for further assessment, evaluation, and intervention/psychiatric care.

Provides guidelines for necessity/urgency of interventions. Direct questioning is most helpful when done in a caring, concerned manner.

More in-depth assistance may be needed to deal with patient and defuse situation.

May be indicated to quiet/control behavior. *Note:* May need to be withheld if they are suspected to be the cause of/contribute to the behavior.

NURSING DIAGNOSIS:	POST-TRAUMA RESPONSE
May be related to:	Disasters (e.g., floods, earthquakes, tornadoes, airplane crashes, combat); wars, epidemics, rape, incest, assault, torture, catastrophic illness or accident, being held hostage.

Possibly evidenced by:	Reexperiencing traumatic event (may be identified in cognitive, affective, and/or sensory–motor activities, e.g., flashbacks, intrusive thoughts, repetitive dreams or nightmares, excessive verbalization of the traumatic event, verbalization of survival guilt or guilt about behavior required for survival).
	Altered lifestyle (self-destructiveness); loss of interest in usual activities; loss of feeling of intimacy/sexuality; development of phobia; poor impulse control/irritability and explosiveness.
	Disturbance of mood, e.g., depression, anxiety, embarrassment, fear, self-blame, low self-esteem.
	Cognitive disruption: Confusion, loss of memory/concentration, indecisiveness.
DESIRED OUTCOMES/ EVALUATION CRITERIA— PATIENT WILL:	Verbalize reduced anxiety/fear.
	Demonstrate ability to deal with emotional reactions in an individually appropriate manner.
	Express own feelings/reactions; avoid projection.
	Demonstrate appropriate changes in lifestyle/getting support from SO as needed.
	Participate in plans for follow-up care/counseling.

ACTIONS/INTERVENTIONS	RATIONALE
Independent	
Determine when incident occurred: present or past.	Manifestations of acute and chronic post-trauma responses may require different interventions.
Assess physical trauma if present and individual reaction to occurrence, e.g., physical symptoms such as numbness, headache, tightness in chest, and psychologic responses of anger, shock, acute anxiety, confusion, denial.	Provides information on which to develop plan of care, make informed choices.
Evaluate behavior (e.g., calm/agitated, excited/hysterical; inappropriate laughter, crying), expressions of disbelief and/or self-blame.	Indicators of extent of individual response to traumatic incident and degree of disorganization.
Note ethnic background/cultural perceptions and beliefs about the incident.	May influence patient's response to what has happened, e.g., may believe it is retribution from God.
Assess signs/stage of grieving.	Patient may be suffering from sense of loss of self and/or others.
Tell patient that painful emotional reactions are normal. Phrase this information in neutral terms: "You may or may not experience...."	Understanding that experiencing these uncomfortable feelings is not unusual after traumatic event may reduce patient's anxiety/fear of "going crazy" and enhance coping.

ACTIONS/INTERVENTIONS	RATIONALE

Independent

Discuss things patient can do to feel better, e.g., physical exercise alternated with relaxation; keeping busy with normal activities; talking to others; acknowledging that it is all right to feel upset; writing about the experience in a journal; being kind to yourself.

Enhances sense of control and helps patient achieve resolution of uncomfortable feelings. Often when the patient begins these activities within the first 24 hours of the event, further therapy may not be required.

Identify supportive persons for patient.

Having positive support systems can help patient reach optimal recovery.

Note signs of severe/prolonged depression, note presence of flashbacks, nightmares, chronic pain, somatic complaints.

If patient did not deal with trauma when it occurred, behavioral manifestations may reveal extent of problem in the present.

Collaborative

Refer to counselors/therapists for further therapy, e.g., psychotherapy (in conjunction with medications); implosive therapy, flooding, hypnosis, Rolfing, memory work, or cognitive restructuring as indicated.

When post-trauma response has become chronic, patient may need more in-depth assistance from sensitive, trained individuals who are skilled in dealing with these problems.

Surgical Intervention _____

Surgery may be needed to diagnose or cure a specific disease process, correct a structural deformity, or restore a functional process; may be performed in the acute care center or an ambulatory surgical setting.

RELATED CONCERNS

PATIENT ASSESSMENT DATA BASE

Data are dependent on the duration/severity of underlying problem and involvement of other body systems. Refer to specific plans of care for data and diagnostic studies relevant to the procedure and additional nursing diagnoses.

CIRCULATION

May report: History of cardiac problems, CHF, pulmonary edema, peripheral vascular disease, or vascular stasis (increases risk of thrombus formation).

EGO INTEGRITY

May report: Feelings of anxiety, fear, anger, apathy.

Multiple stress factors, e.g., financial, relationship, lifestyle.

May exhibit: Restlessness, increased tension/irritability.

Sympathetic stimulation.

FOOD/FLUID

May report: Pancreatic insufficiency/DM (predisposing to hypoglycemia/ketoacidosis).

May exhibit: Malnutrition (including obesity).

Dry mucous membranes (limited intake/NPO period preoperatively).

RESPIRATION

May report: Infections, chronic conditions/cough, smoking.

SAFETFY

May report: Allergies or sensitivities to medications, food, tape, and solution(s).

Immune deficiencies (increases risk of systemic infections and delayed healing). Presence of cancer/recent cancer therapy.

Family history of malignant hyperthermia/reaction to anesthesia.

	History of hepatic disease (affects drug detoxification and may alter coagulation).
	History of blood transfusion(s)/transfusion reaction.
May exhibit:	Presence of existing infectious process; fever.

TEACHING/LEARNING

May report:	Use of anticoagulants, steroids, antibiotics, antihypertensives, cardiotonic glycosides, antidysrhythmics, bronchodilators, diuretics, decongestants, analgesics, anti-inflammatories, anticonvulsants, or tranquilizers as well as OTC, street, or recreational drugs.
	Use of alcohol (risk of liver damage affecting coagulation and choice of anesthesia, as well as potential for postoperative withdrawal).
Discharge Plan Considerations:	**DRG projected mean length of stay: 2.6 days for inpatient procedures.**
	May require assistance with transportation, dressing(s)/supplies, self-care, and homemaker/maintenance tasks. Possible placement in rehabilitation/long-term facility.

DIAGNOSTIC STUDIES

General preoperative requirements may include: Urinalysis, CBC, PT, PTT, chest x-ray. Other studies are dependent on type of operative procedure, current medications, systemic processes, age, and weight, e.g., BUN, Cr, glucose, ABGs, electrolytes, thyroid studies. Deviations from normal should be corrected if possible prior to safe administration of anesthetic agents.

Urinalysis: Presence of WBCs or bacteria indicates infection.

Pregnancy test: Positive results affect timing of procedure and choice of pharmacologic agents.

CBC: WBC elevation is indicative of inflammatory process (may be diagnostic, e.g., appendicitis); decreased WBC count suggests viral processes (requiring evaluation because immune system may be dysfunctional). Low Hb suggests anemia/blood loss (impairs tissue oxygenation and reduces the Hb available to bind with inhalation anesthetics); may suggest need for cross-match/blood transfusion. Hct elevation may indicate dehydration; decreased Hct suggests fluid overload.

Electrolytes: Imbalances impair organ function, e.g., decreased potassium affects cardiac muscle contractility, leading to decreased cardiac output.

ABGs: Evaluates current respiratory status.

Coagulation times: May be prolonged, interfering with intraoperative/postoperative hemostasis.

Chest x-ray: Should be free of infiltrates, pneumonia; used for identification of masses and COPD.

ECG: Abnormal findings require attention prior to administering anesthetics.

NURSING PRIORITIES

1. Reduce anxiety and emotional trauma.
2. Provide for physical safety.
3. Prevent complications.
4. Alleviate pain.
5. Facilitate recovery process.
6. Provide information about disease process/surgical procedure, prognosis, and treatment needs.

DISCHARGE GOALS

1. Patient is dealing realistically with current situation.
2. Injury prevented.
3. Complications prevented/minimized.
4. Pain relieved/controlled.
5. Wound healing/organ function progressing toward normal.
6. Disease process/surgical procedure, prognosis, and therapeutic regimen understood.

PREOPERATIVE

NURSING DIAGNOSIS:	**KNOWLEDGE DEFICIT [LEARNING NEED] REGARDING CONDITION, PROGNOSIS, AND TREATMENT NEEDS**
May be related to:	Lack of exposure/recall, information misinterpretation.
	Unfamiliarity with information resources.
Possibly evidenced by:	Statement of the problem/concerns, misconceptions.
	Request for information.
	Inappropriate, exaggerated behaviors (e.g., agitated, apathetic, hostile).
	Inaccurate follow-through of instructions/development of preventable complications.
DESIRED OUTCOMES/ EVALUATION CRITERIA— PATIENT WILL:	Verbalize understanding of disease process/perioperative process and postoperative expectations.
	Correctly perform necessary procedures and explain reasons for the actions.
	Initiate necessary lifestyle changes and participate in treatment regimen.

ACTIONS/INTERVENTIONS	RATIONALE
Independent	
Assess patient's level of understanding.	Facilitates planning of preoperative teaching program.
Review specific pathology and anticipated surgical procedure.	Provides knowledge base on which patient can make informed therapy choices and consent for procedure, and presents opportunity to clarify misconceptions.
Use resource teaching materials, audiovisuals as available.	Specifically designed materials can facilitate the patient's learning.
Implement individualized preoperative teaching program: Preoperative/postoperative procedures and restrictions, e.g., urinary and bowel changes, dietary considerations, activity levels/transfers, respiratory and cardiovascular exercises, pain control.	Enhances patient's understanding/control and enables participation in postoperative care. Explanation of anticipated IV lines and tubes (e.g., NG tubes, drains, and catheters) can relieve stress related to the unknown/unexpected. Increased understanding of the importance of performing activities and cooperating with restrictions reduces the possibility of postoperative complications and promotes a rapid return to normal body function.
Provide opportunity to practice coughing, deep-breathing, and muscular exercises.	Enhances learning and continuation of activity postoperatively.

ACTIONS/INTERVENTIONS

Independent

Inform patient/SO about itinerary, physician/SO communications.

RATIONALE

Logistical information about OR schedule and places (e.g., recovery room, postoperative room assignment) as well as where and when the surgeon will communicate with SO relieves stress and miscommunications, preventing confusion and doubt over patient's well-being.

NURSING DIAGNOSIS:	FEAR/ANXIETY (SPECIFY LEVEL)
May be related to:	Situational crisis; unfamiliarity with environment.
	Threat of death; change in health status.
	Separation from usual support systems.
Possibly evidenced by:	Increased tension, apprehension, decreased self-assurance.
	Expressed concern regarding changes, fear of consequences.
	Facial tension, restlessness, focus on self.
	Sympathetic stimulation.
DESIRED OUTCOMES/ EVALUATION CRITERIA— PATIENT WILL:	Acknowledge feelings and identify healthy ways to deal with them.
	Appear relaxed, able to rest/sleep appropriately.
	Report decreased fear and anxiety reduced to a manageable level.

ACTIONS/INTERVENTIONS

Independent

Provide for visit with OR personnel before surgery when possible. Discuss anticipated things that may frighten/concern patient, e.g., masks, lights, IVs, BP cuff, electrodes, bovie pad, autoclave noises, child crying.

Inform patient/SO of nurse's intraoperative advocate role.

Identify fear levels that may necessitate postponement of surgical procedure.

Validate source of fear. Provide accurate, factual information. Active-listen concerns.

RATIONALE

Can provide reassurance and alleviate patient's anxiety, as well as provide information for formulating intraoperative care. Acknowledges that foreign environment may be frightening, alleviates associated fears.

Develops trust/rapport, decreasing fear of loss of control in a foreign environment.

Overwhelming or persistent fears result in excessive stress reaction, potentiating risk of adverse reaction to procedure/anesthetic agents.

Identification of specific fear helps patient to deal realistically with it, e.g., misidentification/wrong operation, dismemberment, disfigurement, loss of dignity/control, or being awake/aware with local anesthesia. Patient may have misinterpreted pre-

921

ACTIONS/INTERVENTIONS	RATIONALE
Independent	operative information or have misinformation regarding surgery/disease process. Previous experiences, family/acquaintances fears may be unresolved.
Note expressions of distress/feelings of helplessness, preoccupation with anticipated change/loss, choked feelings.	Patient may already be grieving the loss represented by the anticipated surgical procedure/diagnosis/prognosis of illness.
Tell patient anticipating local/spinal anesthesia that drowsiness/sleep occurs, that more sedation may be requested and will be given if needed, and that surgical drapes will block view of the operative field.	Reduces anxiety/fear that patient may "see" the procedure.
Introduce staff at time of transfer to operating suite.	Establishes rapport and psychologic comfort.
Compare surgery schedule, chart, patient identification band, and signed operative consent.	Provides for positive identification, reducing fear that wrong procedure may be done.
Prevent unnecessary body exposure during transfer and in OR suite.	Patients are concerned about loss of dignity and inability to exercise control.
Give simple, concise directions/explanations to sedated patient. Review environmental concerns as needed.	Impairment of thought processes makes it difficult for patient to understand lengthy instructions.
Control external stimuli.	Extraneous noises and commotion may accelerate anxiety.
Collaborative	
Refer to pastor/spiritual care, psychiatric nurse clinical specialist, psychiatric counseling if indicated.	Professional counseling may be required for patient to resolve fear.
Discuss postponement/cancellation of surgery with physician, anesthesiologist, patient, and family as appropriate.	May be necessary if overwhelming fears are not reduced/resolved.
Administer medications as indicated, e.g.: sedatives, hypnotics;	Used to promote sleep the evening before surgery; may enhance coping abilities.
IV tranquilizers.	May be needed in the holding area to reduce nervousness and provide comfort. *Note:* Respiratory depression/bradycardia may occur necessitating prompt intervention.

INTRAOPERATIVE

NURSING DIAGNOSIS:	INJURY, HIGH RISK FOR
Risk factors may include:	Interactive conditions between individual and environment.
	External environment, e.g., physical design, structure of environment, exposure to equipment, instrumentation, positioning, use of pharmaceutical agents.

	Internal environment, e.g., tissue hypoxia, abnormal blood profile/altered clotting factors, broken skin.
Possibly evidenced by:	[Not applicable; presence of signs and symptoms establishes an actual diagnosis.]
DESIRED OUTCOMES/ EVALUATION CRITERIA— CAREGIVER WILL:	Identify individual risk factors. Modify environment as indicated to enhance safety and use resources appropriately.

ACTIONS/INTERVENTIONS	RATIONALE

Independent

Remove partial plates or bridges preoperatively per protocol. Inform anesthesiologist of loose teeth.	Foreign bodies may be aspirated during endotracheal intubation/extubation.
Remove artificial devices preoperatively or after induction, dependent on sensory/perceptual alterations and mobility impairment.	Contact lenses may cause corneal abrasions while under anesthesia; eyeglasses and hearing aids are obstructive and may break; however, patients may feel more in control of environment if hearing and visual aids are left on as long as possible. Artificial limbs may be damaged and skin integrity impaired if left on.
Remove jewelry preoperatively.	Metals conduct electrical current and provide an electrocautery hazard. In addition, loss or damage to patient's personal property can easily occur in the foreign environment.
Verify patient identity and scheduled operative procedure by comparing patient chart, arm band, and surgical schedule. Verbally ascertain correct name, procedure, and physician.	Assures correct patient and procedure.
Give simple and concise directions to the sedated patient.	Impairment of thought process makes it difficult for patient to understand lengthy directions.
Stabilize both patient cart and OR table when transferring patient to and from OR table, using adequate numbers of personnel for transfer and support of extremities.	Unstabilized cart/table can separate, causing patient to fall. Both side rails must be in the down position for caregiver(s) to assist patient transfer and prevent loss of balance.
Anticipate movement of extraneous lines and tubes during the transfer and secure or guide them into position.	Prevents undue tension and dislocation of IV lines, NG tubes, catheters, and chest tubes; maintains gravity drainage when appropriate.
Secure patient on OR table with safety belt over thighs as appropriate, explaining necessity for restraint.	OR tables and arm boards are narrow, and patient or extremity may fall off, causing injury, especially during fasciculation. Sedated or emerging patient may become resistive or combative, furthering potential for injury.
Prepare equipment and padding for required position, according to operative procedure and patient's specific needs.	Depending on individual patient's size, weight, and preexisting conditions, extra padding materials may be required to protect bony prominences, prevent circulatory compromise/nerve pressure, or allow for optimum chest expansion for ventilation.

923

ACTIONS/INTERVENTIONS	RATIONALE

Independent

Position extremities so they may be periodically checked for safety, circulation, nerve pressure, and alignment. Periodically check peripheral pulses.

Prevents accidental trauma, e.g., hands, fingers, and toes could inadvertently be scraped, pinched, or amputated by moving table attachments; positional pressure of brachial plexus, peroneal, and ulnar nerves can cause serious problems with extremities; prolonged plantar flexion may result in foot-drop.

Prevent pooling of prep solutions under and around patient.

Antiseptic solutions may chemically burn skin as well as conduct electricity.

Assist with induction as needed; e.g., stand by to apply cricoid pressure during intubation or stabilize position during lumbar puncture for spinal block.

Facilitates safe administration of anesthesia.

Ascertain electrical safety of equipment used in surgical procedure, e.g., intact cords, grounds, medical engineering verification labels.

Malfunction of equipment can occur during the operative procedure, causing not only delays and unnecessary anesthesia but also injury or death, e.g., short circuits, faulty grounds, laser malfunction, or laser misalignment. Periodic electrical safety checks are imperative for all OR equipment.

Place dispersive electrode (electrocautery pad) over greatest available muscle mass, ensuring its contact.

Provides a ground for maximum conductivity to prevent electrical burns.

Verify credentials of laser operators for specific wave length laser required for particular procedure.

Due to the potential hazards of laser, physician and equipment operators must be certified in the use and safety requirements of specific wave length laser and procedure, i.e., open, endoscopic, abdominal, laryngeal, intrauterine.

Confirm presence of fire extinguishers and wet fire smothering materials when lasers are used intraoperatively.

Laser beam may inadvertently contact and ignite combustibles outside of surgical field, i.e., drapes, sponges.

Apply patient eye protection before laser activation.

Eye protection for specific laser wave length must be used to prevent injury.

Protect surrounding skin and anatomy appropriately, i.e., wet towels, sponges, dams, cottonoids.

Prevents inadvertent skin integrity disruption, hair ignition, and adjacent anatomy injury in area of laser beam use.

Monitor I&O during procedure.

Potential for fluid volume deficit exists, affecting safety of anesthesia, organ function, and patient well-being.

Confirm and document correct sponge, instrument, needle, and blade counts.

Foreign bodies remaining in body cavities at closure not only cause inflammation, infection, perforation, and abscess formation, but also may result in disastrous complications, leading to death.

Handle, label, and document specimens appropriately, ensuring proper medium and transport for tests required.

Proper identification of specimens to patient is imperative. Frozen sections, preserved or fresh examination, and cultures all have different requirements. OR nurse advocate must be knowledgeable of specific hospital laboratory requirements for validity of examination.

ACTIONS/INTERVENTIONS

Collaborative

Recommend position changes to anesthesiologist and/or surgeon as appropriate.

Limit/avoid use of epinephrine to Fluothane-anesthetized patient.

RATIONALE

Close attention to proper positioning can prevent muscle strain, nerve damage, circulatory compromise, and undue pressure on skin/bony prominences. Although the anesthesiologist is usually responsible for positioning, the nurse may be able to see/have more time to note patient needs.

Fluothane sensitizes the myocardium to catecholamines and may produce dysrhythmias.

NURSING DIAGNOSIS:	**INFECTION, HIGH RISK FOR**
Risk factors may include:	Broken skin, traumatized tissues, stasis of body fluids.
	Presence of pathogens/contaminants, environmental exposure, invasive procedures.
Possibly evidenced by:	[Not applicable; presence of signs and symptoms establishes an actual diagnosis.]
DESIRED OUTCOMES/ EVALUATION CRITERIA— CAREGIVER WILL:	Identify individual risk factors and interventions to reduce potential for infection.
	Maintain safe aseptic environment.

ACTIONS/INTERVENTIONS

Independent

Adhere to facility infection control, sterilization, and aseptic policies/procedures.

Verify sterility of all manufacturers' items.

Review laboratory studies for possibility of systemic infections.

Verify that preoperative skin, vaginal, and bowel cleansing procedures have been done as needed.

Prepare operative site according to specific procedures.

RATIONALE

Established mechanisms designed to prevent infection.

Prepackaged items may appear to be sterile, however, each item must be scrutinized for manufacturer's statement of sterility, breaks in packaging, environmental effect on package, and delivery techniques. Package sterilization/expiration dates, lot/serial numbers must be documented on implant items for further follow-up if necessary.

Increased WBC may indicate ongoing infection, which the operative procedure will alleviate (e.g., appendicitis, abscess, inflammation from trauma); or presence of systemic/organ infection, which may contraindicate surgical procedure and/or anesthesia (e.g., pneumonia, kidney).

Cleansing reduces bacterial counts on the skin, vaginal mucosa, and alimentary tract.

Minimizes bacterial counts at operative site.

ACTIONS/INTERVENTIONS	RATIONALE
Independent	
Examine skin for breaks or ongoing infection.	Disruptions of skin integrity at or near the operative site are sources of contamination to the wound. Careful shaving/clipping is imperative to prevent abrasions and nicks in the skin.
Maintain dependent gravity drainage of indwelling catheters, tubes, and/or positive pressure of parenteral or irrigation lines.	Prevents stasis and reflux of body fluids.
Identify breaks in aseptic technique and resolve immediately on occurrence.	Contamination by environmental/personnel contact renders the sterile field unsterile thereby increasing the risk of infection.
Contain contaminated fluids/materials in specific site in operating room suite, and dispose of according to hospital protocol.	Containment of blood and body fluids, tissue and materials in contact with an infected wound/patient will prevent spread of infection to environment/other patients/personnel.
Provide sterile dressing.	Prevents environmental contamination of fresh wound.
Collaborative	
Do copious wound irrigation, e.g., saline, water, antibiotic, or antiseptic.	May be used intraoperatively to reduce bacterial counts at the site and cleanse the wound of debris, e.g., bone, ischemic tissue, bowel contaminants, toxins.
Obtain specimens for cultures/Gram stain.	Immediate identification of type of infective organism by Gram stain allows prompt treatment while more specific identification by cultures can be obtained in hours/days.
Administer antibiotics as indicated.	May be given prophylactically for suspected infection or contamination.

NURSING DIAGNOSIS:	**BODY TEMPERATURE, ALTERED, HIGH RISK FOR**
Risk factors may include:	Exposure to cool environment.
	Use of medications, anesthetic agents.
	Extremes of age, weight.
	Dehydration.
Possibly evidenced by:	[Not applicable; presence of signs and symptoms establishes an actual diagnosis.]
DESIRED OUTCOMES/ EVALUATION CRITERIA— PATIENT WILL:	Maintain body temperature within normal range.

ACTIONS/INTERVENTIONS	RATIONALE

Independent

Note preoperative temperature.

Used as baseline for monitoring intraoperative temperature. Preoperative temperature elevations are indicative of disease process, e.g., appendicitis, abscess, or systemic disease requiring treatment preoperatively and possibly postoperatively.

Assess environmental temperature and modify as needed, e.g., providing warming and cooling blankets, increasing room temperature.

May assist in maintaining/stabilizing patient's temperature.

Cover skin areas outside of operative field.

Heat losses will occur as skin (e.g., legs, arms, head) is exposed to cool environment.

Provide cooling measures for patient with preoperative temperature elevations.

Cool irrigations and exposure of skin surfaces to air may be required to decrease temperature.

Note rapid temperature elevation/persistent high fever and treat promptly per protocol.

Malignant hyperthermia must be recognized and treated promptly to avoid serious complications.

Apply warm blankets at emergence from anesthesia.

Inhalation anesthetics depress the hypothalamus, resulting in poor body temperature regulation.

Collaborative

Monitor temperature throughout intraoperative phase.

Continuous warm/cool humidified inhalation anesthetics are used to maintain humidity and temperature balance within the tracheobronchial tree. Temperature elevation intraoperatively may indicate adverse response to anesthesia. *Note:* Use of atropine or scopolamine may further increase temperature.

Place warming/cooling blanket under patient. Provide iced saline as indicated.

Maintains steady body temperature in cool environment of OR suite and/or fever. *Note:* Lavage of body cavity with iced saline may help reduce hyperthermic responses.

Obtain dantrolene (Dantrium) for IV administration.

Immediate action to control temperature is necessary to prevent death from malignant hyperthermia.

POSTOPERATIVE

NURSING DIAGNOSIS:	BREATHING PATTERN, INEFFECTIVE
May be related to:	Neuromuscular, perceptual/cognitive impairment.
	Decreased lung expansion, energy.
	Tracheobr onchial obstruction.
Possibly evidenced by:	Changes in respiratory rate and depth.
	Reduced vital capacity, apnea, cyanosis, noisy respirations.

ACTIONS/INTERVENTIONS	RATIONALE
Independent	
Maintain patent airway by head tilt, jaw hyperextension, oral pharyngeal airway.	Prevents airway obstruction.
Auscultate breath sounds. Listen for gurgling, wheezing, crowing, and/or silence after extubation.	Lack of breath sounds is indicative of obstruction by mucus or tongue and may be corrected by positioning and/or suctioning. Diminished breath sounds suggest atelectasis. Wheezing indicates bronchospasm, whereas crowing or silence reflects partial-to-total laryngospasm.
Observe respiratory rate, depth, use of accessory muscles, chest expansion, retraction or flaring of nostrils, skin color, and airflow.	Ascertains effectiveness of respirations immediately so corrective measures can be initiated.
Monitor vital signs continuously.	Increased respirations, tachycardia, and/or bradycardia suggest hypoxia.
Position patient appropriately dependent on respiratory effort and type of surgery.	Head elevation and left lateral Sims' position prevent aspiration of vomitus; proper positioning enhances ventilation to lower lobes and relieves pressure on diaphragm.
Observe for return of muscle function, especially respiratory.	After administration of intraoperative muscle relaxants, return of muscle function occurs first to the diaphragm, intercostals, and larynx; followed by large muscle groups, neck, shoulders, and abdominal muscles; then by midsize muscles, tongue, pharynx, extensors, and flexors; and finally by eyes, mouth, face, and fingers.
Initiate stir-up regimen as soon as patient is reactive and continue into the postoperative period.	Active deep ventilation inflates alveoli, breaks up secretions, increases O_2 transfer, and removes anesthetic gases; coughing enhances removal of secretions from the pulmonary system.
Observe for excessive somnolence.	Narcotic-induced respiratory depression or presence of muscle relaxants in the system may be cyclical in recurrence, creating sine-wave pattern of depression and reemergence. In addition, pentothal is absorbed in the fatty tissues, and as circulation improves, it may be redistributed throughout the bloodstream.
Suction as necessary.	Airway obstruction can occur because of blood or mucus in throat or trachea.
Collaborative	
Administer supplemental O_2 as indicated.	Maximizes O_2 for uptake to bind with Hb in place of anesthetic gases to enhance removal of inhalation agents.

928

ACTIONS/INTERVENTIONS

Collaborative

Administer IV medications, e.g., naloxone (Narcan) or doxapram (Dopram).

Provide/maintain ventilator assistance.

Assist with use of respiratory aids, e.g., incentive spirometer, blow bottles.

RATIONALE

Narcan reverses narcotic-induced CNS depression, and Dopram stimulates respiratory muscles. Both drugs are cyclical in nature, and respiratory depression may return.

Dependent on cause of respiratory depression or type of surgery (e.g., pulmonary, extensive abdominal, cardiac), endotracheal tube may be left in place and mechanical ventilation maintained for a time.

Maximal respiratory efforts reduce potential for atelectasis and infection.

NURSING DIAGNOSIS:	SENSORY-PERCEPTUAL ALTERATION: (SPECIFY)/THOUGHT PROCESSES, ALTERED
May be related to:	Chemical alteration: Use of pharmaceutical agents, hypoxia.
	Therapeutically restricted environments; excessive sensory stimuli.
	Physiologic stress.
Possibly evidenced by:	Disorientation to person, place, time; change in usual response to stimuli, impaired ability to concentrate, reason, make decisions.
	Motor incoordination.
DESIRED OUTCOMES/ EVALUATION CRITERIA— PATIENT WILL:	Regain usual level of consciousness/mentation.
	Recognize limitations and seek assistance as necessary.

ACTIONS/INTERVENTIONS

Independent

Reorient patient continuously when coming out from under anesthesia; confirm that surgery is completed.

Speak in normal, clear voice without shouting, being aware of what you are saying. Minimize discussion of negatives (e.g., patient/personnel problems) within patient's hearing. Explain procedures even if patient does not seem aware.

Evaluate sensation/movement of extremities and trunk as appropriate.

RATIONALE

As patient regains consciousness, support and assurance will help to alleviate anxiety.

Cannot tell when patient is aware, but sense of hearing returns first; so it is important not to say things that may be misinterpreted. Providing information helps patient to preserve dignity and to prepare for activity.

Return of function following local or spinal nerve blocks is dependent on type/amount of agent used and duration of procedure.

929

ACTIONS/INTERVENTIONS	RATIONALE

Independent

Use bedrail padding, restraints as necessary.	Provides for patient safety during emergence stage. Prevents injury to head and extremities if patient becomes combative while disoriented.
Secure parenteral lines, endotracheal tube, catheters, if present, and check for patency.	Disoriented patient may pull on lines and drainage systems, disconnecting or kinking them.
Maintain quiet, calm environment.	External stimuli, e.g., noise, lights, touch may cause psychic aberrations when dissociative anesthetics (e.g., ketamine) have been administered.
Observe for hallucinations, delusions, depression, or an excited state.	May develop following trauma and indicate delirium. In patient who has used alcohol to excess, may suggest impending delirium tremens.
Reassess return of sensory abilities and thought processes thoroughly prior to discharge, as indicated.	Ambulatory surgical patient must be able to care for self with the help of SO (if available) to prevent personal injury after discharge.

Collaborative

Maintain extended stay in postoperative recovery area prior to discharge.	Disorientation may persist, and SO may not be able to protect the patient at home.

NURSING DIAGNOSIS:	FLUID VOLUME DEFICIT, HIGH RISK FOR
Risk factors may include:	Restriction of oral intake (disease process/medical procedure/presence of nausea).
	Loss of fluid through abnormal routes, e.g., indwelling tubes, drains; normal routes, e.g., vomiting.
	Loss of vascular integrity, changes in clotting ability.
	Extremes of age and weight.
Possibly evidenced by:	[Not applicable; presence of signs and symptoms establishes an actual diagnosis.]
DESIRED OUTCOMES/ EVALUATION CRITERIA— PATIENT WILL:	Demonstrate adequate fluid balance, as evidenced by stable vital signs, palpable pulses of good quality, normal skin turgor, moist mucous membranes, and individually appropriate urinary output.

ACTIONS/INTERVENTIONS	RATIONALE

Independent

Measure and record I&O (including GI losses). Review intraoperative record.	Accurate documentation helps identify fluid losses/replacement needs and influences choice of interventions.

ACTIONS/INTERVENTIONS	RATIONALE
Independent	
Assess urinary output specifically for type of operative procedure done.	May be decreased or absent after procedures on the genitourinary system and/or adjacent structures (e.g., ureteroplasty, ureterolithotomy, abdominal or vaginal hysterectomy), indicating malfunction or obstruction of the urinary system.
Provide voiding assistance measures as needed, e.g., privacy, sitting position, running water in sink, pouring warm water over perineum.	Promotes relaxation of perineal muscles and may facilitate voiding efforts.
Monitor vital signs.	Hypotension, tachycardia, increased respirations may indicate fluid deficit, e.g., dehydration/hypovolemia.
Note presence of nausea/vomiting, patient history of motion sickness.	Women, obese patients, and those prone to motion sickness have a higher risk of postoperative nausea/vomiting. In addition, the longer the duration of anesthesia, the greater the risk for nausea. *Note:* Nausea occurring during first 12 to 24 hours postoperatively is frequently related to anesthesia (including regional anesthesia). Nausea persisting more than 3 days postoperatively may be related to the choice of narcotic for pain control or other drug therapy.
Inspect dressings, drainage devices at regular intervals. Assess wound for swelling.	Excessive bleeding can lead to hypovolemia/circulatory collapse. Local swelling may indicate hematoma formation/hemorrhage. *Note:* Bleeding into a cavity (e.g., retroperitoneal) may be hidden and only diagnosed via vital sign depression, patient reports of pressure sensation in affected area.
Monitor skin temperature, palpate peripheral pulses.	Cool/clammy skin, weak pulses indicate decreased peripheral circulation and need for additional fluid replacement.
Collaborative	
Administer parenteral fluids, blood products, and/or plasma expanders as indicated. Increase IV rate if needed.	Replaces documented fluid loss. Timely replacement of circulating volume decreases potential for complications of deficit, e.g., electrolyte imbalance, dehydration, cardiovascular collapse. *Note:* Increased volume may be required initially to support circulating volume/prevent hypotension because of decreased vasomotor tone following Fluothane administration.
Insert urinary catheter with or without urimeter as necessary.	Provides mechanism for accurate monitoring of urinary output.
Resume oral intake gradually as indicated.	Oral intake is dependent on return of GI function.
Administer antiemetics as appropriate.	Relieves nausea/vomiting, which may impair intake/add to fluid losses. *Note:* Naloxone (Narcan) may relieve nausea related to use of regional anesthesia agents, e.g., Duramorph, Sublimaze.

931

ACTIONS/INTERVENTIONS	RATIONALE

Collaborative

Monitor laboratory studies, e.g., Hb/Hct. Compare preoperative and postoperative blood studies.	Indicators of hydration/circulating volume. Preoperative anemia and/or low Hct combined with unreplaced fluid losses intraoperatively will further potentiate deficit.

NURSING DIAGNOSIS:	**PAIN [ACUTE]**
May be related to:	Disruption of skin, tissue, and muscle integrity, musculoskeletal/bone trauma.
	Presence of tubes and drains.
Possibly evidenced by:	Reports of pain.
	Alteration in muscle tone; facial mask of pain.
	Distraction/guarding/protective behaviors.
	Self-focusing; narrowed focus.
	Autonomic responses.
DESIRED OUTCOMES/ EVALUATION CRITERIA— PATIENT WILL:	Report pain relieved/controlled.
	Appear relaxed, able to rest/sleep and participate in activities appropriately.

ACTIONS/INTERVENTIONS	RATIONALE

Independent

Note patient's age, weight, coexisting medical/psychologic problems, idiosyncratic sensitivity to analgesics, and intraoperative course (e.g., size/location of incision, drain placement, anesthetic agents) used.	Approach to postoperative pain management is based on multiple variable factors.
Review intraoperative/recovery room record for type of anesthesia and medications previously administered.	Presence of narcotics and droperidol in system will potentiate narcotic analgesia, whereas patients anesthetized with Fluothane and Ethrane have no residual analgesic effects. In addition, intraoperative local/regional blocks have varying duration, e.g., 1–2 hours for regionals or up to 2–6 hours for locals.
Evaluate pain regularly (e.g., every 2 hours × 12) noting characteristics, location, and intensity (0–10 scale).	Provides information about need for/effectiveness of interventions. *Note:* A frontal and/or occipital headache may develop 24–72 hours following spinal anesthesia, necessitating recumbent position, increased fluid intake, and notification of the anesthesiologist.
Note presence of anxiety/fear, and relate with nature and preparation for procedure.	Concern about the unknown (e.g., outcome of a biopsy) and/or inadequate preparation (e.g., emer-

ACTIONS/INTERVENTIONS	RATIONALE
Independent	
	gency appendectomy) can heighten patient's perception of pain.
Assess vital signs, noting tachycardia, hypertension, and increased respiration, even if patient denies pain.	May indicate acute pain and discomfort. *Note:* Some patients may have a slightly lowered BP, which returns to normal range after pain relief is achieved.
Assess causes of possible discomfort other than operative procedure.	Discomfort can be caused/aggravated by presence of nonpatent indwelling catheters, NG tube, parenteral lines, (bladder pain, gastric fluid and gas accumulation, and infiltration of IV fluids/medications.)
Provide information about transitory nature of discomfort, as appropriate.	Understanding the cause of the discomfort (e.g., sore muscles from administration of succinylcholine may persist up to 48 hours postoperatively, sinus headache associated with nitrous oxide and sore throat due to intubation are transitory) provides emotional reassurance. *Note:* Paresthesia of body parts suggests nerve injury. Symptoms may last hours or months and require additional evaluation.
Reposition as indicated, e.g., semi-Fowler's; lateral Sims'.	May relieve pain and enhance circulation. Semi-Fowler's position will relieve abdominal muscle tension and arthritic back muscle tension, whereas lateral Sims' will relieve dorsal pressures.
Encourage use of relaxation techniques, e.g., deep-breathing exercises, guided imagery, visualization.	Relieves muscle and emotional tension; enhances sense of control and may improve coping abilities.
Provide regular oral care, occasional ice chips/sips of fluids as tolerated.	Reduces discomfort associated with dry mucous membranes due to anesthetic agents, oral restrictions.
Observe effects of analgesia.	Respirations may decrease on administration of narcotic, and synergistic effects with anesthetic agents may occur.
Collaborative	
Administer medications as indicated:	
Analgesics IV (after reviewing anesthesia record for contraindications and/or presence of agents that may potentiate analgesia); provide around-the-clock analgesia with intermittent rescue doses;	Analgesics given IV reach the pain centers immediately, providing more effective relief with small doses of medication. IM administration takes longer, and its effectiveness is dependent on absorption rates and circulation. *Note:* Narcotic dosage should be reduced by one fourth to one third after use of Innovar or Inapsine to prevent profound tranquilization during first 10 hours postoperatively. Current research supports need to administer analgesics around the clock instead of prn in order to *prevent* rather than merely treat pain.

933

ACTIONS/INTERVENTIONS	RATIONALE

Independent

Patient-controlled analgesia;	Use of PCA necessitates detailed instruction in its use and must be monitored closely but is considered very effective in managing acute postoperative pain with smaller amounts of narcotic.
Local anesthetics, e.g., epidural block.	Analgesics may be injected into the operative site, or nerves to the site may be kept blocked in the immediate postoperative phase to prevent pain.

NURSING DIAGNOSIS:	*SKIN/TISSUE INTEGRITY, IMPAIRED*
May be related to:	*Mechanical interruption of skin/tissues.*
	Altered circulation, effects of medication; accumulation of drainage; altered metabolic state.
Possibly evidenced by:	*Disruption of skin surface/layers and tissues.*
DESIRED OUTCOMES/ EVALUATION CRITERIA— PATIENT WILL:	*Achieve timely wound healing.*
	Demonstrate behaviors/techniques to promote healing and to prevent complications.

ACTIONS/INTERVENTIONS	RATIONALE

Independent

Reinforce initial dressing/change as indicated. Use strict aseptic techniques.	Protects wound from mechanical injury and contamination. Prevents accumulation of fluids that may cause excoriation.
Gently remove tape (in direction of hair growth) and dressings when changing.	Reduces risk of skin trauma and disruption of wound.
Apply skin sealants/barriers before tape if needed. Use paper/silk (hypoallergenic) tape or Montgomery straps/elastic netting for dressings requiring frequent changing.	Reduces potential for skin trauma/abrasions and provides additional protection for delicate skin/tissues.
Check tension of dressings. Apply tape at center of incision to outer margin of dressing. Avoid wrapping tape around extremity.	Can impair/occlude circulation to wound as well as distal portion of extremity.
Inspect wound regularly, noting characteristics and integrity.	Early recognition of delayed healing/developing complications may prevent a more serious situation.
Assess amount and characteristics of drainage.	Decreasing drainage suggests evolution of healing process, while continued drainage or presence of bloody/odoriferous exudate suggests complications (e.g., fistula formation, hemorrhage, infection).
Maintain patency of drainage tubes; apply collection bag over drains/incisions in presence of copious or caustic drainage.	Facilitates approximation of wound edges; reduces risk of infection and chemical injury to skin/tissues.

ACTIONS/INTERVENTIONS	RATIONALE

Independent

Elevate operative area as appropriate.

Promotes venous return and limits edema formation. *Note:* Elevation in presence of venous insufficiency may be detrimental.

Splint abdominal and chest incisions/area with pillow or pad during coughing/movement.

Equalizes pressure on the wound, minimizing risk of dehiscence/rupture.

Caution patient not to touch wound.

Prevents contamination of wound.

Leave wound open to air as soon as possible, or cover with small gauze/Telfa pad as needed.

Aids in drying wound and facilitates healing processes. Light covering may be necessary to prevent irritation if sutures/wound edges rub against linens.

Cleanse skin surface with diluted hydrogen peroxide, or running water and mild soap after incision is sealed.

Reduces skin contaminants; aids in removal of exudate.

Collaborative

Apply ice if appropriate.

Reduces edema formation that may cause undue pressure on incision during initial postoperative period.

Use abdominal binder if indicated.

Provides additional support for high-risk incisions (e.g., obese patient).

Irrigate wound; assist with debridement as needed.

Removes infectious exudate/necrotic tissue to promote healing.

NURSING DIAGNOSIS:	TISSUE PERFUSION, ALTERED, HIGH RISK FOR
Risk factors may include:	Interruption of flow: Arterial, venous. Hypovolemia.
Possibly evidenced by:	[Not applicable; presence of signs and symptoms establishes an actual diagnosis.]
DESIRED OUTCOMES/ EVALUATION CRITERIA— PATIENT WILL:	Demonstrate adequate perfusion evidenced by stable vital signs, peripheral pulses present and strong; skin warm/dry; usual mentation and individually appropriate urinary output.

ACTIONS/INTERVENTIONS	RATIONALE

Independent

Change position slowly in bed and at transfer (especially Fluothane-anesthetized patient).

Vasoconstrictor mechanisms are depressed and quick movement may lead to hypotension.

Assist with ROM exercises, including active ankle/leg exercises.

Stimulates peripheral circulation, aids in preventing venous stasis to reduce risk of thrombus formation.

935

ACTIONS/INTERVENTIONS	RATIONALE
Independent	
Encourage/assist with early ambulation.	Enhances circulation and return of normal organ function.
Avoid use of knee gatch/pillow under knees. Caution patient against crossing legs or sitting with legs dependent for prolonged period.	Prevents stasis of venous circulation and reduces risk of thrombophlebitis.
Assess lower extremities for erythema, positive Homans' sign.	Circulation may be restricted by some positions used during surgery, while anesthetics and decreased activity alter vasomotor tone, potentiating vascular pooling and increasing risks of thrombus formation.
Monitor vital signs; palpate peripheral pulses; note skin temperature/color and capillary refill. Evaluate urinary output/time of voiding.	Indicators of adequacy of circulating volume and tissue perfusion/organ function.
Collaborative	
Administer IV fluids/blood products as needed.	Maintains circulating volume; supports perfusion.
Apply antiembolic hose as indicated.	Promotes venous return and prevents venous stasis of legs to reduce risk of thrombosis.

NURSING DIAGNOSIS:	KNOWLEDGE DEFICIT [LEARNING NEED] REGARDING CONDITION/SITUATION, PROGNOSIS, TREATMENT NEEDS
May be related to:	Lack of exposure/lack of recall, information misinterpretation.
	Unfamiliarity with information resources.
	Cognitive limitation.
Possibly evidenced by:	Questions/request for information.
	Statement of misconception.
	Inaccurate follow-through of instructions/development of preventable complications.
DESIRED OUTCOMES/ EVALUATION CRITERIA— PATIENT WILL:	Verbalize understanding of condition, effects of procedure and treatment.
	Correctly perform necessary procedures and explain reasons for actions.
	Initiate necessary lifestyle changes and participate in treatment regimen.

ACTIONS/INTERVENTIONS	RATIONALE
Independent	
Review specific surgery performed/procedure done and future expectations.	Provides knowledge base on which patient can make informed choices.
Review and have patient/SO demonstrate dressing/wound care when indicated. Identify source for supplies.	Promotes competent self-care and enhances independence.
Review avoidance of environmental risk factors, e.g., exposure to crowds/persons with infections.	Reduces potential for acquired infections.
Discuss drug therapy, including use of prescribed and OTC analgesics.	Enhances cooperation with regimen; reduces risk of adverse reactions/untoward effects.
Identify specific activity limitations.	Prevents undue strain on operative site.
Recommend planned/progressive exercise.	Promotes return of normal function and enhances feelings of general well-being.
Schedule adequate rest periods.	Prevents fatigue and conserves energy for healing.
Review importance of nutritious diet and adequate fluid intake.	Provides elements necessary for tissue regeneration/healing and support of tissue perfusion and organ function.
Encourage cessation of smoking.	Increases risk of pulmonary infections. Causes vasoconstriction and reduces oxygen-binding capacity of blood, affecting cellular perfusion and potentially impairing healing.
Identify signs/symptoms requiring medical evaluation, e.g., nausea/vomiting; difficulty voiding; fever, continued/odoriferous wound drainage; incisional swelling, erythema or separation of edges; unresolved or changes in characteristics of pain.	Early recognition and treatment of developing complications (e.g., ileus, urinary retention, infection, delayed healing) may prevent progression to more serious or life-threatening situation.
Stress necessity of follow-up visits.	Monitors progress of healing and evaluates effectiveness of regimen.
Include SO in teaching program. Provide written instructions/teaching materials.	Provides additional resource for reference after discharge.
Identify available resources, e.g., homecare services, visiting nurse, Meals-On-Wheels, outpatient therapy, contact phone number for questions.	Enhances support for patient during recovery period and provides additional evaluation of ongoing needs/new concerns.

Long-Term Care

Patients in the acute care setting may be discharged to an extended care facility. Patients requiring relatively short-term rehabilitation as well as those needing long-term care/permanent nursing care are included in this group. Coordination and knowledge are essential in providing continuity and quality care for these patients. The needs of the patient (e.g., physical, occupational, and rehabilitation therapy) are frequently the deciding factors in the choice of placement.

RELATED CONCERNS

AIDS, p 850
Alzheimer's Disease, p 372
Cerebrovascular Accident/Stroke, p 290
Craniocerebral Trauma, p 271
Fractures, p 772
Multiple Sclerosis, p 391
Psychosocial Aspects of Acute Care, p 889
Spinal Cord Injury, p 337

PATIENT ASSESSMENT DATA BASE

Data are dependent on underlying physical/psychosocial conditions necessitating continuation of structured care.

TEACHING/LEARNING

Discharge Plan Considerations: **Projected mean length of stay: Dependent on underlying disease/condition and individual care needs. Therefore, this may be temporary or permanent placement.**

May require assistance with treatments, self-care activities, homemaker/maintenance tasks or alternate living arrangements (e.g., group home).

DIAGNOSTIC STUDIES

ECG: Provides baseline data; detects abnormalities.

Chest x-ray: Reveals size of heart, lung abnormalities/disease conditions, changes of the large blood vessels and bony structure of the chest.

Visual acuity testing: Identifies cataracts/other vision problems.

Tonometer test: Measures intraocular pressure.

CBC: Reveals problems such as infection, anemia, other abnormalities.

Chemistry profile: Evaluates general organ function/imbalances.

Pulse oximetry: Determines oxygenation, respiratory function.

Communicable disease screen: TB, HIV, RPR, hepatitis.

Drug screen: As indicated by usage to identify therapeutic or toxic levels.

Urinalysis: Provides information about kidney function; determines presence of UTI or DM.

NURSING PRIORITIES

1. Promote physiologic and psychologic well-being.
2. Provide for security and safety.
3. Prevent complications of disease and/or aging process.
4. Promote effective coping skills and independence.
5. Encourage continuation of "healthy" habits, participation in plan of care to meet individual needs and wishes.

DISCHARGE GOALS

1. Patient is dealing realistically with current situation.
2. Homeostasis maintained.
3. Injury prevented.
4. Complications prevented/minimized.
5. Patient is meeting ADLs by self/with assistance as necessary.

NURSING DIAGNOSIS:	ANXIETY [SPECIFY LEVEL]/FEAR
May be related to:	Change in health status, role functioning, interaction patterns, socioeconomic status, environment.
	Unmet needs; recent life changes, loss of friends/SO.
Possibly evidenced by:	Apprehension, restlessness, repetitive questioning; pacing, purposeless activity; insomnia.
	Various behaviors (appears overexcited, withdrawn, worried, fearful); presence of facial tension, trembling, hand tremors.
	Expressed concern regarding changes in life events.
	Focus on self; lack of interest in activity.
DESIRED OUTCOMES/ EVALUATION CRITERIA— PATIENT WILL:	Appear relaxed.
	Report anxiety is reduced to a manageable level.
	Demonstrate problem-solving skills and use resources effectively.

ACTIONS/INTERVENTIONS

Independent

Provide patient/SO with copy of "Patients' Bill of Rights" and review it with them. Discuss facility's rules, e.g., visiting, off-grounds visits.

Determine patient/SO attitude toward admission to facility and expectations for the future.

Help family/SO to be honest with patient regarding admission.

Assess level of anxiety and discuss reasons when possible.

RATIONALE

Provides information that can foster confidence that individual rights do continue in this setting and the patient is still "his or her own person" and has some control over what happens.

If this is expected to be a temporary placement, patient/SO concerns will be different than if placement is permanent. When patient is giving up own home and way of life, feelings of helplessness, loss, and grief are to be expected.

Family may have difficulty dealing with decision/reality of permanent placement and may avoid discussing situation with patient.

Identifying specific problems will enable individual to deal more realistically with them.

939

ACTIONS/INTERVENTIONS

Independent

Make time to listen to patient about concerns, and encourage free expression of feelings, e.g., anger, hostility, fear, and loneliness.

Acknowledge reality of situation and feelings of patient. Accept expressions of anger while limiting aggressive, acting-out behavior.

Develop nurse/patient relationship.

Orient to physical aspects of facility, schedules, and activities. Introduce to roommate(s) and staff. Give explanation of roles.

Provide above information in written or taped form as well.

Give careful thought to room placement. Provide help and encouragement in placing own belongings around room. Do not transfer from one room to another without patient approval/documentable need.

Collaborative

Refer to social service or other appropriate agency for assistance. Have social worker discuss ramifications of Medicare/Medicaid if patient is eligible for these resources.

RATIONALE

Being available in this way allows patient to feel accepted, begin to acknowledge and deal with feelings related to circumstances of admission.

Permission to express feelings allows for beginning resolution. Acceptance promotes sense of self-worth. *Note:* Psychosocial and/or physiologic disturbances can occur as a result of transfer from one environment to another (i.e., relocation stress syndrome).

Trusting relationships among patient/SO/staff promotes optimal care and support.

Getting acquainted is an important part of admission. Knowledge of where things are and who patient can expect assistance from can be helpful in reducing anxiety.

Overload of information is difficult to remember. Patient can refer to written or taped material as needed to refresh memory/learn new information.

Location, roommate compatibility, and place for personal belongings are important considerations for helping the patient feel "at home." Changes are often met with resistance and can result in emotional upset and decline in physical condition.

Often patient is not aware of the resources available, and providing current information about individual coverage/limitations and other possible sources of support will assist with adjustment to new situation.

NURSING DIAGNOSIS:	GRIEVING, ANTICIPATORY
May be related to:	Perceived, actual or potential loss of physiopsychosocial well-being, personal possessions, or SO; cultural beliefs about aging.
Possibly evidenced by:	Denial of feelings, depression, sorrow, guilt.
	Alterations in activity level, sleep patterns, eating habits, libido.
DESIRED OUTCOMES/ EVALUATION CRITERIA— PATIENT WILL:	Identify and express feelings appropriately; progress through the grieving process.
	Enjoy the present and plan for the future, one day at a time.

ACTIONS/INTERVENTIONS	RATIONALE
Independent	
Assess emotional state.	Anxiety and depression are common reactions to changes/losses associated with long-term illness or debilitating condition. In addition, changes in neurotransmitter levels (e.g., increased MAO and serotonin levels with decreased norepinephrine) may potentiate depression in elderly patients.
Make time to listen to the patient. Encourage free expression of hopeless feelings and desire to die.	It is more helpful to allow these feelings to be expressed and dealt with than to deny them.
Assess suicidal potential.	May be related to physical disease, social isolation, and grief. *Note:* Studies indicate women are 3 times as likely to attempt suicide, however, men are 3 times as likely to succeed.
Involve SO in discussions and activities to the level of their willingness.	When SOs are involved, there is more potential for successful problem solving. *Note:* SO may not be available or may not choose to be involved.
Provide liberal touching/hugs as individually accepted.	Conveys sense of concern/closeness to reduce feelings of isolation and enhance sense of self-worth. *Note:* Touch may be viewed as a threat by some patients and escalate feelings of anger.
Collaborative	
Refer to other resources as indicated, e.g., clinical specialist, nurse, social worker.	May need further assistance to resolve some problems.
Assist with/plan for specifics as necessary (e.g., advanced directives (to determine code status/ Living Will wishes), making of will, funeral arrangements).	Having these issues resolved can help patient/SO deal with the grieving process and may provide peace of mind.

NURSING DIAGNOSIS:	**THOUGHT PROCESSES, ALTERED**
May be related to:	Physiologic changes of aging, loss of cells/brain atrophy, decreased blood supply, altered sensory input.
	Pain; effects of medications.
	Psychologic conflicts: disrupted life pattern.
Possibly evidenced by:	Slower reaction times, gradual memory loss, altered attention span; disorientation; inability to follow.
	Altered sleep patterns.
	Personality changes.
DESIRED OUTCOMES/ EVALUATION CRITERIA— PATIENT WILL:	Maintain usual reality orientation.
	Recognize changes in thinking and behavior.
	Identify interventions to deal effectively with situation/ deficits.

ACTIONS/INTERVENTIONS	RATIONALE
Independent	
Allow adequate time for patient to respond to questions/comments and to make decisions.	Reaction time may be slowed with aging (changes in metabolism/cerebral blood flow) or with brain injuries and some neuromuscular conditions.
Discuss happenings of the past. Place familiar objects in room. Encourage the display of photographs/photo albums, frequent visits from SO/ friends.	Events of the past may be more readily recalled by the patient, because long-term memory usually remains intact. Reminiscence/life review and companionship are beneficial to the elderly patient.
Note patient's problem of short-term memory loss, and provide with aids (e.g., calendars, clocks, room signs, pictures) to assist in continual reorientation.	Short-term memory loss presents a challenge for nursing care, especially if the patient cannot remember such things as how to use the call bell or how to get to the bathroom. This problem is not in patient's control but may be less frustrating if simple reminders are used. It may be helpful for older person to know that short-term memory loss is common and is not necessarily a sign of "senility."
Evaluate individual stress level and deal with it appropriately.	Stress level may be greatly increased because of recent losses, e.g., poor health, death of spouse/ companion, loss of home. In addition, some conflicts that occur with age come from previously unresolved problems that may need to be dealt with now.
Assess physical status/psychiatric symptoms. Institute interventions appropriate to findings.	Not all mental changes are the result of aging, and it is important to rule out physical causes before accepting these as unchangeable. May be metabolic, toxic, drug-induced (e.g., antiparkinson agents, tricyclic antidepressants), or the result of infectious, cardiac, or respiratory disorders.
Reorient to person/place/time as appropriate.	Helps patient maintain focus.
Have patient repeat verbal/written instructions.	Verifies hearing/ability to read and comprehend.
Note cyclic changes in mentation/behavior, e.g., evening confusion, picking at bedclothes, banging on side rails, pacing, shouting, wandering aimlessly.	"Sundown syndrome" may occur in response to visual/hearing deficits enhanced by declining light, fatigue, inflexible institution schedules, peak/ trough drug levels, dehydration, and electrolytes imbalances.
Involve in regular exercise and activity programs.	Studies suggest withdrawn and inactive patients are at greater risk of evening confusion.
Schedule at least one rest period per day.	Prevents fatigue; enhances general well-being.
Provide brighter lighting in room/area by midafternoon (e.g., 3 PM) or earlier on cloudy/winter days.	Maximizes visual perception; may limit evening confusion.
Turn off lights at bedtime. Provide night lights where appropriate.	Reinforces "sleep time" while meeting safety needs.
Support patient's involvement in own care. Provide opportunity for choices on a daily basis.	Choice is a necessary component in everyday life. Cognitively impaired patients may respond with aggressive behavior as they lose control in their lives.

NURSING DIAGNOSIS:	FAMILY COPING, INEFFECTIVE, COMPROMISED
May be related to:	Placement of family member in LTC facility.
	Temporary family disorganization and role changes.
	Situational crises SO may be facing.
	Patient providing little support for SO.
	Prolonged disease or disability progression that exhausts the supportive capacity of SOs.
Possibly evidenced by:	SO describes significant preoccupation with personal reactions, e.g., fear, anticipatory grief, guilt, anxiety.
	SO attempts assistive/supportive behaviors with unsatisfactory results.
	SO withdraws from patient.
	SO displays protective behavior disproportionate (too little or too much) to patient's abilities/need for autonomy.
DESIRED OUTCOMES/ EVALUATION CRITERIA— FAMILY WILL:	Identify/verbalize resources within themselves to deal with the situation.
	Interact appropriately with the patient and staff, providing support and assistance as indicated.
	Verbalize knowledge and understanding of situation.

ACTIONS/INTERVENTIONS

Independent

Introduce staff and provide SO with information about facility and care. Be available for questions. Provide tour of facility.

Encourage SO participation in care at level of desire and capability and within limits of safety. Include in social events/celebrations.

Accept choices of SO regarding level of involvement in care.

Evaluate SO's/caregiver's level of stress/coping abilities especially prior to planning for discharge.

RATIONALE

Helpful to establish beginning relationships. Offers opportunities for enhancing feelings of involvement.

Helps family to feel at ease and allows them to feel supportive and a part of the patient's life.

Families may choose to ignore patient or may project feelings of guilt regarding placing patient in LTC by criticizing staff. *Note:* Feelings of dissatisfaction with the staff may be transferred back to the patient.

Caring for/about patients with chronic/debilitating conditions places a heavy strain on SO. Although support groups may be very helpful, learning stress management techniques may be more effective in strengthening individual coping as the focus is on the SO rather than the SO/patient relationship.

943

ACTIONS/INTERVENTIONS

Independent

Be aware of staff's own feelings of anger and frustration about patient's/SO's choices and goals that differ from staff, and deal with appropriately.

Collaborative

Inform SO of services available to them (meal tickets, family cooking time, group care conference, VNA, caseworker, social services).

RATIONALE

Group care conferences or individual counseling may be helpful in problem solving.

Promotes feeling of involvement; eases transition in adjustment to patient's admission.

NURSING DIAGNOSIS:	INJURY, HIGH RISK FOR [DRUG TOXICITY]
Risk factors may include:	Reduced metabolism; impaired circulation; precarious physiologic balance, presence of multiple diseases/organ involvement. Use of multiple prescribed/OTC drugs.
Possibly evidenced by:	[Not applicable; presence of signs and symptoms establishes an actual diagnosis.]
DESIRED OUTCOMES/ EVALUATION CRITERIA— PATIENT WILL:	Maintain prescribed drug regimen free of untoward side effects.

ACTIONS/INTERVENTIONS

Independent

Determine allergies and other drug history.

Use resources (e.g., drug manuals, pharmacist) for information about toxic symptoms and side effects. List drug actions and interactions and idiosyncracies, e.g., medications that are given with or without foods, as well as those that should not be crushed.

Discuss self-administration of/access to OTC products.

Identify swallowing problems or reluctance to take tablets or capsules.

Give pills in a spoonful of soft foods, e.g., applesauce, ice cream; or use liquid form of medication if available.

RATIONALE

Avoids repetition/creation of problems.

Provides information about drugs being taken and identifies possible interactions. Toxicity can be increased in the debilitated and older patient with symptoms not as apparent.

Limits interference with prescribed regimen/desired drug action and organ function. May prevent inadvertent overdosing/toxic reactions. *Note:* Appropriate use of OTC products kept at bedside or via free access at nurses' station fosters independence as well as enhances sense of control and self-esteem.

May not be able to or want to take medication.

Ensures proper dosage if patient is unable to/ does not like to swallow pills.

ACTIONS/INTERVENTIONS	RATIONALE
Independent	
Open capsules or crush tablets only when appropriate.	Should not be done unless absolutely necessary as this may alter absorption of medications, e.g., enteric-coated tablets may be absorbed in stomach when crushed, instead of the intestines.
Make sure medication has been swallowed.	Ensures effective therapeutic use of medication and prevents hoarding.
Observe for changes in condition/behavior.	Behavior may be only indication of drug toxicity, and early identification of problems provides for appropriate intervention. *Note:* Elderly individuals have increased sensitivity to anticholinergic effects of medications. Therefore, use of anticholinergics, antiparkinson agents, benzodiazepines, CNS depressants, and tricyclic antidepressants may cause delirium/confusion.
Use discretion in the administration of sedatives.	A quiet place where the patient can pace or seclusion may be more helpful. If patient is destructive or excessively disruptive, pharmacologic or mechanical control measures may be required. Convenience of the staff is never a reason for sedating patients; however, patient safety and rights of other patients need to be taken into consideration.
Collaborative	
Review drug regimen routinely with physician and pharmacist.	Provides opportunity to alter therapy (e.g., reduce dosage, discontinue medications) as patient's needs and organ functions change.
Obtain serum drug levels as indicated.	Determines therapeutic/toxicity levels.

NURSING DIAGNOSIS:	**COMMUNICATION, IMPAIRED VERBAL**
May be related to:	Degenerative changes (e.g., reduced cerebral circulation, hearing loss); progressive neurologic disease (e.g., Parkinson's disease, Alzheimer's disease).
	Laryngectomy/tracheostomy; stroke.
Possibly evidenced by:	Impaired articulation; difficulty with phonation; inability to modulate speech, find words, name, or identify objects.
	Diminished hearing ability.
	Aphasia, dysarthria.
DESIRED OUTCOMES/ EVALUATION CRITERIA— PATIENT WILL:	Establish method of communication by which needs can be expressed.
	Demonstrate congruent verbal and nonverbal communication.

ACTIONS/INTERVENTIONS	RATIONALE

Independent

Assess reason for lack of communication, including CNS and neuromuscular functioning, gag/swallow reflexes, hearing, teeth/mouth problems.	Identification of the problem is essential to appropriate intervention. Sometimes patients do not want to talk, may think they talk when they do not, may expect others to know what they want, may not be able to comprehend or be understood.
Check for excess cerumen.	Hardened earwax may decrease hearing acuity and causes tinnitus.
Ascertain if patient has/uses hearing aids.	Patient may have, but not use hearing aid (e.g., may not fit well, may need batteries).
Be aware that behavioral problems may indicate hearing loss.	Anger, explosive temper outbursts, frustration, embarrassment, depression, withdrawal, and paranoia may be attempts to deal with communication problems.
Determine whether patient is bilingual or whether English is primary language.	With declining cerebral function/diminished thought processes, increased level of stress, patient may mix languages/revert to original language.
Investigate how SO communicates with the patient.	Provides opportunity to develop/continue effective communication patterns, which have already been established.
Assess patient knowledge base and level of comprehension. Treat the patient as an adult, avoiding pity and impatience.	Knowing how much to expect of the patient can help to avoid frustration and unreasonable demands for performance. However, having an expectation that the patient will understand may help to raise level of performance.
Establish therapeutic nurse–patient relationship through Active-listening, being available for problem solving.	Aids in dealing with communication problems.
Make patient aware of presence when entering the room by turning a light off and on/touching patient or mattress as appropriate.	Getting attention is the first step in communication.
Make eye contact, lower self to patient's level, and speak face to face.	Conveys interest and promotes contact.
Speak slowly and distinctly, using simple sentences, yes-or-no questions. Avoid speaking loudly or shouting. Supplement with written communication when possible/needed. Allow sufficient time for reply; remain relaxed with patient.	Assists in comprehension and overall communication. Patient may respond poorly to high-pitched sounds; shouting also obscures consonants and amplifies vowels.
Use other creative measures to assist in communication, e.g., picture chart/alphabet board, sign language, lip reading when appropriate.	Many options are available, depending on individual situation. *Note:* Sign language also may be used effectively with other than hearing-impaired individuals.

Collaborative

Refer to speech therapists, ear, nose, and throat physician, or for audiometry as needed to deter-	May be helpful to patient and staff in improving communication. Testing may ascertain precise na-

ACTIONS/INTERVENTIONS	RATIONALE

Collaborative

mine extent of hearing loss and whether a hearing aid is appropriate.

ture of the hearing deficit. Some sources believe 90% of the patients in LTC facilities have some degree of hearing loss (presbycusis) as this is a common age change. Hearing aids are most effective with conductive losses and may help with sensorineural losses.

NURSING DIAGNOSIS:	SLEEP PATTERN DISTURBANCE
May be related to:	Internal factors: Illness, psychologic stress, inactivity. External factors: Environmental changes, facility routines.
Possibly evidenced by:	Complaints of difficulty in falling asleep/not feeling well-rested. Interrupted sleep, awakening earlier than desired. Change in behavior/performance increasing irritability, listlessness.
DESIRED OUTCOMES/ EVALUATION CRITERIA— PATIENT WILL:	Report improvement in sleep/rest pattern. Verbalize increased sense of well-being and feeling rested.

ACTIONS/INTERVENTIONS	RATIONALE

Independent

Determine usual sleep habits and changes that are occurring.

Assesses need for and identifies appropriate interventions.

Provide comfortable bedding and some of own possessions, e.g., pillow, afghan.

Increases comfort for sleep as well as physiologic/psychologic support.

Establish new sleep routine incorporating old pattern and new environment.

When new routine contains as many aspects of old habits as possible, stress and related anxiety may be reduced.

Match with roommate who has similar sleep patterns and nocturnal needs.

Decreases likelihood that "night owl" roommate may delay patient falling asleep or create interruptions that cause awakening.

Encourage some light physical activity during the day. Make sure patient stops activity several hours before bedtime.

Daytime activity can help patient expend energy and be ready for nighttime sleep. However, continuation of activity close to bedtime may act as a stimulant, delaying sleep.

Promote bedtime comfort regimens, e.g., warm bath and massage, a glass of warm milk, wine or brandy at bedtime.

Promotes a relaxing soothing effect. *Note:* Milk has soporific qualities, enhancing synthesis of serotonin, a neurotransmitter that helps patient fall asleep faster and sleep longer.

947

ACTIONS/INTERVENTIONS

Independent

Instruct in relaxation measures.

Reduce noise and light.

Encourage position of comfort, assist in turning.

Use side rails as indicated; lower bed when possible.

Avoid interruptions when possible (e.g., awakening for medications or therapies).

Collaborative

Administer sedatives, hypnotics, as indicated.

RATIONALE

Helps to induce sleep.

Provides atmosphere conducive to sleep.

Repositioning alters areas of pressure and promotes rest.

May have fear of falling because of change in size and height of bed. Side rails provide safety and may be used to assist with turning. *Note:* Some people do better with no side rails and tend to fall when climbing over side rails.

Uninterrupted sleep is more restful, and patient may be unable to return to sleep when wakened.

May be given to help patient sleep/rest during transition period from home to new setting. *Note:* Avoid habitual use, because these drugs decrease REM sleep time.

NURSING DIAGNOSIS:	NUTRITION, ALTERED: LESS/MORE THAN BODY REQUIREMENTS
May be related to:	Impaired dentition; dulling of senses of smell and taste.
	Cognitive limitations, depression.
	Inability to feed self effectively.
	Sedentary activity level.
Possibly evidenced by:	Reported/observed dysfunctional eating patterns.
	Weight under/over ideal for height and frame.
	Poor muscle tone, pale conjunctiva/mucous membranes.
DESIRED OUTCOMES/ EVALUATION CRITERIA— PATIENT WILL:	Maintain normal weight or progress toward weight goal with normalization of laboratory values and be free of signs of malnutrition/obesity.
	Demonstrate eating patterns/behaviors to maintain appropriate weight.

ACTIONS/INTERVENTIONS

Independent

Assess causes of weight loss/gain, e.g., dysphagia caused by neurogenic/psychogenic disturbances, tumors, muscular dysfunction, or dysfunctional eating patterns related to depression.

RATIONALE

Aids in creating plan of care/choice of interventions.

ACTIONS/INTERVENTIONS	RATIONALE
Independent	
Check state of patient's dental health periodically, including fit and condition of dentures, if present.	Oral infections/dental problems, shrinking gums and loose-fitting dentures decrease patient's ability to chew.
Weigh on admission and on a regular basis.	Monitors nutritional state and effectiveness of interventions.
Observe condition of skin; note muscle wasting, brittle nails, dry, lifeless hair, and signs of poor healing.	Reflects lack of adequate nutrition.
Evaluate activity pattern.	Extremes of exercise (e.g., sedentary life, continuous pacing) affect caloric needs.
Incorporate favorite foods and maintain as near normal food consistency as possible, e.g., soft or finely ground food with gravy or liquid added. Avoid baby food whenever possible.	Aids in maintaining intake, especially when mouth and dental problems exist. Baby food is often unpalatable and can decrease appetite and lower self-esteem.
Encourage the use of spices (other than sodium) to patient's personal taste.	Reduction in number and acuity of taste buds results in food tasting bland and decreases enjoyment of food and desire to eat.
Provide small, frequent feedings as indicated.	Decreased gastric motility causes patient to feel full and reduces intake.
Serve hot foods hot and cold foods cold.	Food is more palatable and enjoyment may increase appetite.
Promote a pleasant environment for eating, with company if possible.	Eating is in part a social event, and appetite can improve with increased socialization.
Have snack foods (e.g., cheese, crackers, soup, fruit) available on a 24-hour basis.	Helps meet individual needs and enhances intake.
Encourage exercise and activity program within individual ability.	Promotes sense of well-being and may improve appetite.
Collaborative	
Consult with dietitian.	Aids in establishing specific nutritional program to meet individual patient needs.
Provide balanced diet with individually appropriate protein, complex carbohydrates, and calories. Include supplements between meals as indicated.	Adjustments may be needed to deal with the body's decreased ability to process protein, as well as decreased metabolic rate and levels of activity. *Note:* Elderly individuals have delayed insulin release by the pancreas and reduced peripheral sensitivity to insulin decreasing their glucose tolerance.
Refer for dental care routinely and as needed.	Maintenance of oral/dental health and good dentition can enhance intake.

NURSING DIAGNOSIS:	SELF-CARE DEFICIT: (SPECIFY)
May be related to:	Depression, discouragement, loss of mobility, general debilitation; perceptual/cognitive impairment.

Possibly evidenced by:	Inability to manage ADLs; unkempt appearance.
DESIRED OUTCOMES/ EVALUATION CRITERIA— PATIENT WILL:	Perform *self-care* activities within level of own ability.
	Demonstrate techniques/lifestyle changes to meet own needs.
	Use resources effectively.

ACTIONS/INTERVENTIONS

Independent

Determine current capabilities (0–4 scale) and barriers to participation in care.

Involve patient in formulation of plan of care at level of ability.

Encourage self-care. Work with present abilities; do not pressure patient beyond capabilities. Provide adequate time for patient to complete tasks. Have expectation of improvement and assist as needed.

Provide and promote privacy, including during bathing/showering.

Use specialized equipment as needed, e.g., tub transfer seat, grab bars, raised toilet seat.

Give tub bath, using a 2-person or mechanical lift if necessary. Use shower chair and spray attachment, as appropriate. Avoid chilling.

Shampoo/style hair as needed. Provide/assist with manicure.

Encourage use of barber/beauty salon if able.

Acquire clothing with modified fasteners as indicated.

Encourage/assist with routine mouth/teeth care daily.

Collaborative

Consult with physical/occupational therapist and rehabilitation specialist.

RATIONALE

Identifies need for/level of interventions required.

Enhances sense of control and aids in cooperation and development of independence.

Doing for oneself enhances feeling of self-worth. Failure can produce discouragement and depression.

Modesty may lead to reluctance to participate in care or perform activities in the presence of others.

Enhances ability to move/perform activities safely.

Provides safety for those who cannot get into the tub alone. Shower may be more feasible for some patients though it may be less beneficial/desirable to the patient. Elderly/debilitated patients are more prone to chilling.

Aids in maintaining appearance. Shampooing may be required more/less frequently than bathing schedule.

Enhances self-image and self-esteem, preserving dignity of the patient.

Use of Velcro instead of buttons/shoe laces can facilitate process of dressing/undressing.

Reduces risk of gum disease/tooth loss; promotes proper fitting of dentures.

Useful in establishing exercise/activity program and in identifying assistive devices to meet individual needs/facilitate independence.

NURSING DIAGNOSIS:	**SKIN INTEGRITY, IMPAIRED, HIGH RISK FOR**
Risk factors may include:	General debilitation; reduced mobility; changes in skin and muscle mass associated with aging, sensory/motor deficits.

Altered circulation; edema; poor nutrition.

Excretions/secretions (bladder and bowel incontinence).

Problems with self-care.

Possibly evidenced by: [Not applicable; presence of signs and symptoms establishes an actual diagnosis.]

DESIRED OUTCOMES/ EVALUATION CRITERIA— PATIENT WILL:

Maintain intact skin.

Identify individual risk factors.

Demonstrate behaviors/techniques to prevent skin breakdown/facilitate healing.

ACTIONS/INTERVENTIONS	RATIONALE
Independent	
Anticipate and use preventive measures in patients who are at risk for skin breakdown, such as anyone who is thin, obese, aging, or debilitated.	Decubitus ulcers are difficult to heal, and prevention is the best treatment.
Assess nutritional status and initiate corrective measures as indicated. Provide balanced diet, e.g., adequate protein, vitamins, and minerals.	A positive nitrogen balance and improved nutritional state can help prevent skin breakdown and promote ulcer healing. *Note:* May need additional calories and protein if draining ulcer present.
Maintain strict skin hygiene, using mild, nondetergent soap (if any), drying gently and thoroughly, and lubricating with lotion or emollient.	A daily bath is usually not necessary in elderly patients because there is atrophy of sebaceous and sweat glands, and bathing may create dry-skin problems. However, as epidermis thins with age, cleansing and use of lubricants keeps skin soft/pliable and protects susceptible skin from breakdown.
Change position frequently in bed and chair. Recommend 10 minutes of exercise each hour and/or perform passive ROM.	Improves circulation, muscle tone, and joint motion and promotes patient participation.
Use a rotation schedule in turning patient. Use draw/turn sheet. Pay close attention to patient's comfort level.	Allows for longer periods free of pressure; prevents shearing or tearing motions that can damage fragile tissues. *Note:* Use of prone position is dependent on patient tolerance and should be maintained for only a short time.
Massage bony prominences gently with lotion or cream.	Enhances circulation to tissues, increases vascular tone, and reduces tissue edema. *Note:* Contraindicated if area is pink/red as cellular damage may occur. Massage *around* area may stimulate circulation to impaired tissues.
Keep sheets and bedclothes clean, dry, and free from wrinkles, crumbs, and other irritating material.	Avoids friction/abrasions of skin.
Use elbow/heel protectors, foam/water or gel pads, sheepskin for positioning in bed and when up in chair.	Reduces risk of tissue abrasions and decreases pressure that can impair cellular blood flow. Promotes circulation of air along skin surface to dissipate heat/moisture.

951

ACTIONS/INTERVENTIONS	RATIONALE

Independent

Provide for safety during ambulation.

Loss of muscle control and debilitation may result in impaired coordination.

Limit exposure to temperature extremes/use of heating pad or ice pack.

Decreased sensitivity to pain/heat/cold increases risk of tissue trauma.

Examine feet and nails routinely and provide foot and nail care as indicated:

Foot problems are common among patients who are bedfast/debilitated.

Keep nails cut short and smooth;

Jagged, rough nails can cause tissue damage/infection by scratching adjacent skin areas.

Use lotion, softening cream on feet;

Prevents drying/cracking of skin; promotes maintenance of healthy skin.

Check for fissures between toes. Swab with hydrogen peroxide or dust with antiseptic powder and place a wisp of cotton between the toes;

Prevents spread of infection and/or tissue injury.

Rub feet with witch hazel or a mentholated preparation and have patient wear lightweight cotton stockings.

Even though rash may not be present, burning and itching may be a problem. *Note:* Witch hazel may be contraindicated if skin is dry.

Inspect skin surface/folds (especially when diapers are used) and bony prominences routinely. Increase preventive measures when reddened areas are noticed.

Skin breakdown can occur quickly with potential for infection and necrosis, possibly involving muscle and bone. There is increased risk of redness/irritation around legs due to elastic bands in adult diapers/continence pads.

Continue regimen for redness and irritation when break in skin occurs.

Aggressive measures are important because decubitus can develop in a matter of a few hours.

Observe for decubitus ulcer development, and treat immediately according to protocol.

Timely intervention may prevent extensive damage.

Collaborative

Provide waterbed, alternating pressure/eggcrate mattress, padded chair.

Provides protection and improves circulation by decreasing amount of pressure on tissues.

Monitor Hb/Hct and blood sugar levels.

Anemia and elevated blood sugar levels are factors in skin breakdown and can impair healing.

Refer to podiatrist as indicated.

May need professional care for such problems as ingrown toenails, corns, bony changes, skin/tissue ulceration.

Provide whirlpool treatments as appropriate.

Increases circulation and has a debriding action.

Assist with topical applications; skin barrier dressings (Duoderm, Opsite); collagenase therapy; absorbable gelatin sponges (Gelfoam); aerosol sprays.

Although there are differing opinions about the efficacy of these agents, individual or combination use may enhance healing.

Administer iron and vitamin C supplements.

Aids in healing/cellular regeneration.

Prepare for/assist with skin grafting. (Refer to CP: Burns, ND: Skin Integrity, Impaired, p 835.)

May be needed to close large ulcers.

NURSING DIAGNOSIS:	URINARY ELIMINATION: ALTERED, HIGH RISK FOR
Risk factors may include:	Changes in fluid/nutritional pattern.
	Neuromuscular changes.
	Perceptual/cognitive impairment.
Possibly evidenced by:	[Not applicable; presence of signs and symptoms establishes an actual diagnosis.]
DESIRED OUTCOMES/ EVALUATION CRITERIA— PATIENT WILL:	Maintain/regain effective pattern of elimination.
	Initiate necessary lifestyle changes.
	Participate in treatment regimen to correct/control situation, e.g., bladder training program or use of indwelling catheter.

ACTIONS/INTERVENTIONS	RATIONALE
Independent	
Monitor voiding pattern. Identify possible reasons for changes, e.g., disorientation, neuromuscular impairment, psychotropic medications.	This information is essential to plan for care and influences choice of individual interventions.
Palpate bladder. Observe for "overflow" voiding; determine frequency and timing of dribbling/voiding.	Bladder distention indicates urinary retention, which may cause incontinence and infection.
Promote fluid intake of 2000–3000 ml/d within cardiac tolerance; include fruit juices, especially cranberry juice. Schedule fluid intake times appropriately.	Maintains adequate hydration and promotes kidney function. Acid–ash juices act as an internal pH acidifier, retarding bacterial growth. *Note:* Patient may decrease fluid intake in an attempt to control incontinence and become dehydrated. Instead, fluids may be scheduled to decrease frequency of incontinence (e.g., limit fluids after 6 PM to reduce need to void during the night).
Institute bladder program (including scheduled voiding times, Kegel exercise) involving patient and staff in a positive manner.	Regular toileting times may help to control incontinence. Program is more apt to be successful when positive attitudes and cooperation are present.
Assist patient to sit upright on bedpan/commode.	Provides functional position for voiding.
Provide/encourage perineal care daily and p.r.n.	Reduces risk of contamination/ascending infection.
Use adult diapers during day if needed. Keep patient clean and dry. Provide frequent skin care.	When training is unsuccessful, this is the preferred method of management. *Note:* Using incontinence pads during night exposes skin to air, reducing risk of irritation.
Avoid verbal or nonverbal signs of rejection, disgust, or disapproval over failures.	Expressions of disapproval lower self-esteem and are not helpful to a successful program.
Provide regular catheter care and maintain patency if indwelling catheter is present.	Prevents infection and/or minimizes reflux.

ACTIONS/INTERVENTIONS	RATIONALE
Collaborative	
Administer medications as indicated, e.g., oxybutynin chloride (Ditropan);	Promotes sphincter control.
Vitamin C, methenamine hippurate (Hiprex), methenamine mendelate (Mandelamine).	Bladder pH acidifiers retard bacterial growth.
Maintain indwelling catheter/provide intermittent catheterization.	May be used if continence cannot be maintained to prevent skin breakdown and resultant problems.
Irrigate catheter with acetic acid, if indicated.	May be done to maintain acid pH and retard bacterial growth.

NURSING DIAGNOSIS:	CONSTIPATION/DIARRHEA, HIGH RISK FOR
Risk factors may include:	Changes in/inadequate nutritional/fluid intake; poor muscle tone; change in level of activity.
	Medication side effects.
	Perceptual/cognitive impairment, depression.
	Lack of privacy.
Possibly evidenced by:	[Not applicable; presence of signs and symptoms establishes an actual diagnosis.]
DESIRED OUTCOMES/ EVALUATION CRITERIA— PATIENT WILL:	Establish/maintain normal patterns of bowel functioning.
	Demonstrate changes in lifestyle as necessitated by risk or contributing factors.
	Participate in bowel program, as indicated.

ACTIONS/INTERVENTIONS	RATIONALE
Independent	
Ascertain usual bowel pattern and aids used (e.g., previous long-term laxative use). Compare with current routine.	Determines extent of problem and indicates need for/type of interventions appropriate. Many patients may already be laxative-dependent, and it is important to reestablish as near normal functioning as possible.
Assess reasons for problems; rule out medical causes, e.g., bowel obstruction, cancer, hemorrhoids, drugs, impaction.	Identification/treatment of underlying medical condition is necessary to achieve optimal bowel function.
Determine presence of food/drug sensitivities.	May contribute to diarrhea.
Institute individualized program of exercise, rest, diet, and bowel retraining.	Depends on the needs of the patient. Loss of muscular tone reduces peristalsis or may impair control of rectal sphincter.
Provide diet high in bulk in the form of whole-grain cereals, breads, fresh fruits (especially prunes, plums).	Improves stool consistency, promotes evacuation.

ACTIONS/INTERVENTIONS

Independent

Decrease or eliminate foods such as dairy products.

Encourage increased fluid intake.

Use adult diapers, if needed. Keep patient clean and dry. Provide frequent perineal care. Apply skin protective ointment to anal area.

Keep air freshener in room/at bedside or in bathroom.

Give emotional support to patient. Avoid "blaming" (talk/actions) if incontinence occurs.

Collaborative

Administer medications as indicated:

Bulk-providers/stool softeners, e.g., Metamucil;

Camphorated tincture of opium (Paregoric), diphenoxylate with atropine (Lomotil).

RATIONALE

These foods are known to be constipating.

Promotes normal stool consistency.

Prevents skin breakdown.

Limits noxious odors and may help reduce patient embarrassment/concern.

Decreases feelings of frustration and embarrassment.

Promotes regularity by increasing bulk and/or improving stool consistency.

May be needed on a short-term basis when diarrhea persists.

NURSING DIAGNOSIS:	PHYSICAL MOBILITY, IMPAIRED
May be related to:	Decreased strength and endurance, neuromuscular impairment.
	Pain/discomfort.
	Perceptual/cognitive impairment.
Possibly evidenced by:	Impaired coordination, limited ROM; decreased muscle mass, strength, control.
	Reluctance to attempt movement; inability to purposefully move.
DESIRED OUTCOMES/ EVALUATION CRITERIA— PATIENT WILL:	Verbalize willingness to and participate in activities.
	Demonstrate techniques/behaviors that enable continuation or resumption of activities.
	Maintain/increase strength and function of affected body parts.

ACTIONS/INTERVENTIONS

Independent

Determine functional ability (0–4 scale) and reasons for impairment.

RATIONALE

Identifies need for/degree of intervention required.

955

ACTIONS/INTERVENTIONS	RATIONALE
Independent	
Note emotional/behavioral responses to altered ability.	Physical changes and loss of independence often create feelings of anger, frustration, and depression that may be manifested as reluctance to engage in activity.
Plan activities/visits with adequate rest periods as necessary.	Prevents fatigue; conserves energy for continued participation.
Encourage participation in self-care, occupational/recreational activities.	Promotes independence and self-esteem; may enhance willingness to participate.
Assist with transfers and ambulation if indicated; show patient/SO ways to move safely.	Prevents accidental falls/injury.
Obtain supportive shoes and well-fitting, nonskid slippers.	Assists patient to walk with a firm step/maintain sense of balance and prevents slipping.
Remove extraneous furniture from pathways.	Prevents patient from bumping into furniture and reduces risk of falling/injuring self.
Encourage use of hand rails in hallway, stairwells, and bathrooms.	Promotes independence in mobility; reduces risk of falls.
Review safe use of mobility aids/adjunctive devices, e.g., walkers, braces, prosthetics.	Facilitates activity, reduces risk of injury.
Provide chairs with firm, high seats and lifting chairs when indicated.	Facilitates rising from seated position.
Provide for environmental changes to meet visual deficiencies.	Prevents accidents and sensory deprivation. If patient is blind, will need assistance and ongoing orientation to surroundings.
Speak to patient when entering the room, and let patient know when leaving.	Special actions help patient who cannot see to know when someone is there.
Encourage the patient with glasses/contacts to wear them. Be sure glasses are kept clean.	Optimal visual acuity facilitates participation in activities and reduces risk of falls/injury.
Determine reason if glasses are not being worn.	Patient may not be wearing glasses because they need adjustment or change in correction.
Collaborative	
Consult with physical/occupational therapist, rehabilitation specialist.	Useful in creating individual exercise/activity program and identifying adjunctive aids.
Arrange for eye examination as necessary.	Identifies specific vision problem, e.g., myopia, hyperopia, presbyopia, astigmatism, cataract and glaucoma development, tunnel vision, and blindness.

NURSING DIAGNOSIS:	DIVERSIONAL ACTIVITY DEFICIT
May be related to:	Environmental lack of diversional activity; long-term care requirements.
	Physical limitations; psychologic condition, e.g., depression.

Possibly evidenced by:	Statements of boredom, depression, lack of energy.
	Disinterest, lethargy, withdrawn behavior, hostility.
DESIRED OUTCOMES/ EVALUATION CRITERIA— PATIENT WILL:	Recognize own response and initiate appropriate coping actions.
	Engage in satisfying activities within personal limitations.

ACTIONS/INTERVENTIONS	RATIONALE
Independent	
Determine avocation/hobbies patient previously pursued. Incorporate activities, if appropriate, into present program.	Encourages involvement and helps to stimulate patient mentally/physically to improve overall condition and sense of well-being.
Encourage participation in mix of activities/stimuli, e.g., music, news program, educational presentations, crafts as appropriate.	Offering different activities helps patient to try out new ideas and develop new interests. Activities need to be personally meaningful for the patient to derive the most enjoyment from them (e.g., talking or Braille books for the blind, closed-captioned TV broadcasts for the deaf/hearing impaired).
Provide change of scenery when possible; alter personal environment; encourage trips to shop/ participate in local/family events.	Stimulates energy and provides new outlook for patient.
Collaborative	
Refer to occupational therapist, activity director.	Can introduce and design new programs to provide positive stimuli for the patient.

NURSING DIAGNOSIS:	**SEXUALITY PATTERNS, ALTERED, HIGH RISK FOR**
Risk factors may include:	Biopsychosocial alteration of sexuality.
	Interference in psychologic/physical well-being; self-image.
	Lack of privacy/SO.
Possibly evidenced by:	[Not applicable; presence of signs and symptoms establishes an actual diagnosis.]
DESIRED OUTCOMES/ EVALUATION CRITERIA— PATIENT WILL:	Verbalize knowledge and understanding of sexual limitations, difficulties, or changes that have occurred.
	Demonstrate improved communication and relationship skills.

ACTIONS/INTERVENTIONS	RATIONALE

Independent

Note patient/SO cues regarding sexuality.	May be concerned that condition/environmental restrictions may interfere with sexual function or ability, but be afraid to ask directly.
Evaluate cultural and religious/value factors and conflicts that may be present.	Affects patient's perception of existing problems.
Assess developmental and lifestyle issues.	Factors such as menopause and aging, adolescence and young adulthood need to be taken into consideration with regard to sexual concerns about illness and long-term care.
Provide atmosphere in which discussion of sexuality is encouraged/permitted.	When concerns are identified and discussed, problem solving can occur.
Provide privacy for patient/SO.	Demonstrates acceptance of need for intimacy and provides opportunity to continue previous patterns of interaction as much as possible.

Collaborative

Refer to sex counselor/therapist, family therapy when needed.	May require additional assistance for resolution of problems.

NURSING DIAGNOSIS:	**HEALTH MAINTENANCE, ALTERED**
May be related to:	Lack of, or significant alteration in, communication skills.
	Complete or partial lack of gross and/or fine motor skills.
	Perceptual/cognitive impairment, lack of ability to make deliberate/thoughtful judgments.
	Lack of material resources.
Possibly evidenced by:	Demonstrated lack of knowledge regarding basic health practices.
	Reported/observed inability to take responsibility for meeting basic health needs; impairment of personal support system.
	Demonstrated lack of behaviors adaptive to internal or external environmental changes.
DESIRED OUTCOMES/ EVALUATION CRITERIA— PATIENT WILL:	Verbalize understanding of factors contributing to current situation.
	Adopt lifestyle changes supporting individual health care goals.
	Assume responsibility for own health care needs when possible.

ACTIONS/INTERVENTIONS	RATIONALE

Independent

Assess level of adaptive behavior; knowledge and skills about health maintenance, environment, and safety.

Identifies areas of concern/need and aids in choice of interventions.

Provide information about individual health care needs.

Provides knowledge base and encourages participation in decision making.

Note patient's previous use of professional services, and continue as appropriate. Include in choice of new health care providers as able.

Preserves continuity and promotes independence in meeting own health care needs.

Maintain adequate hydration and balanced diet with sufficient protein intake.

Promotes general well-being and aids in disease prevention.

Schedule adequate rest with progressive activity program.

Prevents fatigue and enhances general well-being.

Promote good hand washing and personal hygiene. Use aseptic techniques as necessary.

Prevents contamination/cross-contamination, reducing risk of illness/infection.

Protect from exposure to infections; avoid extremes of temperature. Recommend the wearing of masks/other interventions as indicated.

With age, immune protective responses slow down and physiologic reactions to temperature extremes may be impaired. As organ function decreases and natural antibodies decline, patients are at increased risk for infection. Staff and/or visitors with colds/other infections may expose patient to these illnesses.

Encourage cessation of smoking.

Smokers are prone to bronchitis and ineffective clearing of secretions.

Encourage reporting of signs/symptoms as they occur.

Provides opportunity for early recognition of developing complications and timely intervention to prevent serious illness.

Observe for/monitor changes in vital signs, e.g., temperature elevation.

Early identification of onset of illness allows for timely intervention and may prevent serious complications. *Note:* Elderly persons often display subnormal temperatures, so presence of a low-grade fever may be of serious concern.

Collaborative

Administer medications as indicated:

Immunizations, e.g., *Haemophilus influenzae,* flu, pneumonia;

Reduces risk of acquiring contagious/potentially life-threatening diseases.

Antibiotics.

May be used prophylactically (rare) and to treat infections.

Schedule preventive/routine health care appointments based on individual needs, e.g., with cardiologist, podiatrist, ophthalmologist, dentist.

Promotes optimal recovery/maintenance of health.

Alcoholism [Acute]: Intoxication/Overdose _____

Alcohol is a CNS depressant drug that is used socially in our society for many reasons, e.g., to enhance the flavor of food, encourage relaxation and conviviality, for feelings of celebration, and as a sacred ritual in some religious ceremonies. Therapeutically, it is the major ingredient in many OTC/prescription medications. It can be harmless, enjoyable, and sometimes beneficial when used responsibly and in moderation. Like other mind-altering drugs, however, it has the potential for abuse and is the most widely abused drug in the United States.

Although patients are not generally admitted to the acute care setting with this diagnosis, withdrawal from alcohol may occur secondarily during hospitalization for other illnesses/conditions.

RELATED CONCERNS

Psychosocial Aspects of Acute Care, p 899
Substance Dependence/Abuse Rehabilitation, p 1000

PATIENT ASSESSMENT DATA BASE

Data are dependent on the duration/extent of use of alcohol, concurrent use of other drugs, and degree of organ involvement.

ACTIVITY/REST

May report: Difficulty sleeping. Not feeling well rested.

CIRCULATION

May exhibit: Generalized tissue edema (due to protein deficiencies).

Peripheral pulses weak, irregular, or rapid.

Hypertension common in early withdrawal stage but may become labile/progress to hypotension.

Tachycardia common during acute withdrawal; numerous dysrhythmias may be identified. (Other abnormalities depend on underlying heart disease.)

EGO INTEGRITY

May report: Feelings of guilt/shame; defensiveness about drinking.

Denial, rationalization.

ELIMINATION

May report: Diarrhea.

Constant upper abdominal pain and tenderness radiating to the back (pancreatic inflammation).

FOOD/FLUID

May report: Nausea/vomiting; food intolerance.

May exhibit: Gastric distention; ascites, liver enlargement (seen in cirrhosis with long-term use).

Muscle wasting, dry/dull hair, swollen salivary glands, inflamed buccal cavity, capillary fragility (malnutrition).

Bowel sounds varied, related to gastric complications, such as gastric hemorrhage or distention.

NEUROSENSORY

May report: "Internal shakes."

Headache, dizziness, blurred vision; "blackouts."

May exhibit: Psychopathology, e.g., paranoid schizophrenia, major depression (may indicate dual diagnosis).

Level of consciousness/orientation: Confusion, stupor, hyperactivity, distorted thought processes, slurred/incoherent speech.

Memory loss/confabulation.

Affect/mood/behavior: May be fearful, anxious, easily startled, inappropriate, silly, euphoric, irritable, physically/verbally abusive, depressed, and/or paranoid.

Hallucinations—visual, tactile, olfactory and auditory, e.g., patient may be picking items out of air or responding verbally to unseen person/voices.

Nystagmus (associated with cranial nerve palsy).

Pupil constriction (may indicate CNS depression).

Arcus senilis (ringlike opacity of the cornea): Although normal in aging populations, suggests alcohol-related changes in younger patients.

Fine motor tremors of face, tongue, and hands; seizures (commonly grand mal).

Gait unsteady (ataxia); may be due to thiamine deficiency or cerebellar degeneration (Wernicke's encephalopathy).

RESPIRATION

May report: History of smoking, recurrent/chronic respiratory problems.

May exhibit: Tachypnea (hyperactive state of alcohol withdrawal).

Cheyne-Stokes respirations or respiratory depression.

Breath sounds: Diminished/adventitious sounds (suggests pulmonary complications, e.g., respiratory depression, pneumonia).

SAFETY

May report: History of recurrent trauma such as falls, fractures, lacerations, burns, blackouts, or automobile accidents.

May exhibit: Skin: Flushed face/palms of hands, scars, ecchymotic areas, cigarette burns on fingers, spider nevus (impaired portal circulation); fissures at corners of mouth (vitamin deficiency).

Fractures—healed or new (signs of recent/recurrent trauma).

Temperature elevation (dehydration and sympathetic stimulation); flushing/diaphoresis (suggests presence of infection).

Suicidal ideation/suicide attempts (some research suggests alcoholic suicide attempts are 30% higher than national average for general population).

SOCIAL INTERACTION

May report: Frequent sick days off work/school; fighting with others, arrests (disorderly conduct, motor vehicle violations/DUIs).

That alcohol intake does not have any significant effect on present condition (denial).

Dysfunctional family system of origin; problems in current relationships.

Mood changes.

TEACHING/LEARNING

May report:　　　　History of alcohol and/or other drug use/abuse.

Ignorance and/or denial of addiction to alcohol, or inability to cut down or stop drinking despite repeated efforts.

Large amount of alcohol consumed in last 24–48 hours, previous periods of abstinence/withdrawal.

Previous hospitalizations for alcoholism/alcohol-related diseases, e.g., cirrhosis, esophageal varices.

Family history of alcoholism.

Discharge Plan Considerations:　　　**DRG projected mean length of stay: 4.5 days.**

May require assistance to maintain abstinence and begin to participate in rehabilitation program.

DIAGNOSTIC STUDIES

Blood alcohol/drug levels: Alcohol level may/may not be severely elevated, depending on amount consumed and time between consumption and testing. In addition to alcohol, numerous controlled substances may be identified in a poly-drug screen, e.g., amphetamine, cocaine, morphine, Percodan, Quaalude.

CBC: Decreased Hb/Hct may reflect such problems as iron-deficiency anemia or acute/chronic GI bleeding. WBC count may be increased with infection or decreased if immunosuppressed.

Glucose: Hyperglycemia/hypoglycemia may be present, related to pancreatitis, malnutrition, or depletion of liver glycogen stores.

Electrolytes: Hypokalemia and hypomagnesemia are common.

Liver function tests: CPK, LDH, AST/SGOT, ALT/SGPT and amylase may be elevated, reflecting liver or pancreatic damage.

Nutritional tests: Albumin is low and total protein may be decreased. Vitamin deficiencies are usually present, reflecting malnutrition/malabsorption.

Urinalysis: Infection may be identified; ketones may be present, related to breakdown of fatty acids in malnutrition (pseudodiabetic condition).

Chest x-ray: May reveal right lower lobe pneumonia (malnutrition, depressed immune system, aspiration) or chronic lung disorders associated with tobacco use.

ECG: Dysrhythmias, cardiomyopathies, and/or ischemia may be present owing to direct effect of alcohol on the cardiac muscle and/or conduction system, as well as effects of electrolyte imbalance.

Addiction Severity Index: An assessment tool that produces a "problem severity profile" of the patient, including chemical, medical, psychologic, legal, family/social, and employment/support aspects, indicating areas of treatment needs.

NURSING PRIORITIES

1. Maintain physiologic stability during acute withdrawal phase.
2. Promote patient safety.
3. Provide appropriate referral and follow-up.
4. Encourage/support SO involvement in "Intervention" (confrontation) process.
5. Provide information about condition/prognosis and treatment needs.

DISCHARGE GOALS

1. Homeostasis achieved.
2. Complications prevented/resolved.

3. Sobriety being maintained on a day-to-day basis.
4. Transferred to rehabilitation program/attending group therapy, e.g., Alcoholics Anonymous.
5. Condition, prognosis, and therapeutic regimen understood.

NURSING DIAGNOSIS:	**BREATHING PATTERN, INEFFECTIVE, HIGH RISK FOR**
Risk factors may include:	Direct effect of alcohol toxicity on respiratory center and/or sedative drugs given to decrease alcohol withdrawal symptoms. Tracheobronchial obstruction. Presence of chronic respiratory problems, inflammatory process. Decreased energy/fatigue.
Possibly evidenced by:	[Not applicable; presence of signs and symptoms establishes an actual diagnosis.]
DESIRED OUTCOMES/ EVALUATION CRITERIA— PATIENT WILL:	Maintain effective breathing pattern with respiratory rate within normal range; lungs clear, free of cyanosis and other signs/symptoms of hypoxia.

ACTIONS/INTERVENTIONS

Independent

Monitor respiratory rate/depth and pattern as indicated. Note periods of apnea, Cheyne-Stokes respirations.

Elevate head of bed.

Encourage cough/deep-breathing exercises and frequent position changes.

Auscultate breath sounds. Note presence of adventitious sounds, e.g., rhonchi, wheezes.

Have suction equipment, airway adjuncts available.

RATIONALE

Frequent assessment is important because toxicity levels may change rapidly. Hyperventilation is common during acute withdrawal phase. Kussmaul respirations are sometimes present due to acidotic state associated with vomiting and malnutrition. However, marked respiratory depression can occur due to CNS depressant effects from alcohol. This may be compounded by drugs used to control alcohol withdrawal symptoms.

Decreases possibility of aspiration; lowers diaphragm to enhance lung inflation.

Facilitates lung expansion and mobilization of secretions to reduce risk of atelectasis/pneumonia.

Patient is at risk for atelectasis related to hypoventilation and pneumonia. Right lower lobe pneumonia is common in alcohol-debilitated patients and is often due to chronic aspiration. Chronic lung diseases are also common, e.g., emphysema, bronchitis.

Sedative effects of alcohol/drugs potentiates risk of aspiration, relaxation of oropharyngeal muscles, and respiratory depression, requiring intervention to prevent respiratory arrest.

963

ACTIONS/INTERVENTIONS

Collaborative

Administer supplemental O_2 if necessary.

Review chest x-rays, ABGs/pulse oximetry as indicated.

RATIONALE

Hypoxia may occur with CNS/respiratory depression.

Monitors presence of secondary complications such as atelectasis/pneumonia; evaluates effectiveness of respiratory effort.

NURSING DIAGNOSIS:	CARDIAC OUTPUT, DECREASED, HIGH RISK FOR
Risk factors may include:	Direct effect of alcohol on the heart muscle.
	Altered systemic vascular resistance.
	Electrical alterations in rate; rhythm; conduction.
Possibly evidenced by:	[Not applicable; presence of signs and symptoms establishes an actual diagnosis.]
DESIRED OUTCOMES/ EVALUATION CRITERIA— PATIENT WILL:	Display vital signs within patient's normal range; absence of/reduced frequency of dysrhythmias.
	Demonstrate an increase in activity tolerance.
	Verbalize understanding of the effect of alcohol on the heart.

ACTIONS/INTERVENTIONS

Independent

Monitor vital signs frequently during acute withdrawal.

Monitor cardiac rate/rhythm. Document irregularities/dysrhythmias.

Monitor body temperature.

RATIONALE

Hypertension frequently occurs in acute withdrawal phase. Extreme hyperexcitability, accompanied by catecholamine release and increased peripheral vascular resistance, raises BP (and heart rate), but BP may become labile/progress to hypotension. *Note:* May have underlying cardiovascular disease, which is compounded by alcohol withdrawal.

Long-term alcohol abuse may result in cardiomyopathy/CHF. Tachycardia is common due to sympathetic response to increased circulating catecholamines. Irregularities/dysrhythmias may develop with electrolyte shifts/imbalance. All of these may have an adverse effect on cardiac function/output.

Elevation may occur due to sympathetic stimulation, dehydration, and/or infections, causing vasodilation and compromising venous return/cardiac output.

ACTIONS/INTERVENTIONS	RATIONALE

Independent

Monitor I&O. Note 24-hour fluid balance.

Preexisting dehydration, vomiting, fever, and diaphoresis may result in decreased circulating volume that can compromise cardiovascular function. *Note:* Hydration is difficult to assess in the alcoholic patient because the usual indicators are not reliable, and overhydration is a risk in the presence of compromised cardiac function.

Be prepared for/assist in cardiopulmonary resuscitation.

Causes of death during acute withdrawal stages include cardiac dysrhythmias, respiratory depression/arrest, oversedation, excessive psychomotor activity, severe dehydration or overhydration, and massive infections. Mortality for unrecognized/untreated DTs may be as high as 5%–25%.

Collaborative

Monitor laboratory studies, e.g., serum electrolyte levels.

Electrolyte imbalance, e.g., potassium/magnesium, potentiate risk of cardiac dysrhythmias and CNS excitability.

Administer medications as indicated, e.g.:

Clonidine (Catapres).

Provides for greater mean reductions in heart rate and systolic BP with less nausea/vomiting.

Potassium.

Corrects deficits that can result in life-threatening dysrhythmias.

NURSING DIAGNOSIS:	INJURY, HIGH RISK FOR [SPECIFY]
Risk factors may include:	Cessation of alcohol intake with varied autonomic nervous system responses to the system's suddenly altered state.
	Involuntary clonic/tonic muscle activity (seizures).
	Equilibrium/balancing difficulties, reduced muscle and hand/eye coordination.
Possibly evidenced by:	[Not applicable; presence of signs and symptoms establishes an actual diagnosis.]
DESIRED OUTCOMES/ EVALUATION CRITERIA— PATIENT WILL:	Demonstrate absence of untoward effects of withdrawal. Experience no physical injury.

ACTIONS/INTERVENTIONS	RATIONALE

Independent

Identify stage of alcohol withdrawal symptoms, i.e., stage I is associated with signs/symptoms of hyperactivity (e.g., tremors, sleeplessness, nausea/vomiting, diaphoresis, tachycardia, hypertension).

Prompt recognition and intervention may halt progression of symptoms and enhance recovery/improve prognosis. In addition, recurrence/progression of symptoms indicate need for changes in

ACTIONS/INTERVENTIONS

Independent

Stage II is manifested by increased hyperactivity plus hallucinations and/or seizure activity. Stage III symptoms include DTs and extreme autonomic hyperactivity with profound confusion, anxiety, insomnia, fever.

Monitor/document seizure activity. Maintain patent airway. Provide environmental safety, e.g., padded side rails, bed in low position.

Check deep-tendon reflexes. Assess gait, if possible.

Assist with ambulation and self-care activities as needed.

Provide for environmental safety when indicated. (Refer to ND: Sensory-Perceptual Alteration p 967.)

Collaborative

Administer IV/PO fluids with caution, as indicated.

Administer medications as indicated:

Benzodiazepines, e.g., chlordiazepoxide (Librium), diazepam (Valium), clonazepam (Klonopin);

Oxazepam (Serax);

Phenobarbital;

Magnesium sulfate.

RATIONALE

drug therapy/more intense treatment to prevent death.

Grand mal seizures are most common and may be related to decreased magnesium levels, hypoglycemia, elevated blood alcohol, or history of seizures. *Note:* In absence of history of or other pathology causing seizures, they usually stop spontaneously, requiring only symptomatic treatment.

Reflexes may be depressed, absent, or hyperactive. Peripheral neuropathies are common, especially in malnourished patient. Ataxia (gait disturbance) is associated with Wernicke's syndrome (thiamine deficiency) and cerebellar degeneration.

Prevents falls with resultant injury.

May be required when equilibrium, hand/eye coordination problems exist.

Cautious replacemen.t corrects dehydration and promotes renal clearance of toxins while reducing risk of overhydration.

Commonly used to control neuronal hyperactivity that occurs as alcohol is detoxified. IV/PO administration is preferred route, because IM absorption is unpredictable. Muscle-relaxant qualities are particularly helpful to patient in controlling "the shakes," trembling, and ataxic quality of movements. Patient may initially require large doses to achieve desired effect, and then drugs may be tapered and discontinued, usually within 96 hours. *Note:* These agents must be used cautiously in patient with hepatic disease as they are metabolized by the liver.

Although less dramatic for control of withdrawal symptoms, may be drug of choice in patient with liver disease because of its shorter half-life.

Useful in suppressing withdrawal symptoms as well as an effective anticonvulsant. Use must be monitored so that exacerbation of respiratory depression is prevented.

Reduces tremors and seizure activity by decreasing neuromuscular excitability.

NURSING DIAGNOSIS:	SENSORY-PERCEPTUAL ALTERATION: (SPECIFY)
May be related to:	Chemical alteration: Exogenous (e.g., alcohol consumption/sudden cessation) and endogenous (e.g., electrolyte imbalance, elevated ammonia and BUN).
	Sleep deprivation.
	Psychologic stress (anxiety/fear).
Possibly evidenced by:	Disorientation to time/place or person.
	Changes in usual response to stimuli; exaggerated emotional responses, change in behavior.
	Bizarre thinking.
	Fear/anxiety.
DESIRED OUTCOMES/ EVALUATION CRITERIA— PATIENT WILL:	Regain/maintain usual level of consciousness.
	Report absence of/reduced hallucinations.
	Identify external factors that affect sensory-perceptual abilities.

ACTIONS/INTERVENTIONS	RATIONALE
Independent	
Assess level of consciousness; ability to speak, response to stimuli/commands.	Speech may be garbled, confused, or slurred. Response to commands may reveal inability to concentrate, impaired judgment, or muscle coordination deficits.
Observe behavioral responses, e.g., hyperactivity, disorientation, confusion, sleeplessness, irritability.	Hyperactivity related to CNS disturbances may escalate rapidly. Sleeplessness is common due to loss of sedative effect gained from alcohol usually consumed prior to bedtime. Sleep deprivation may aggravate disorientation/confusion. Progression of symptoms may indicate impending hallucinations (stage II) or DTs (stage III).
Note onset of hallucinations. Document as auditory, visual, and/or tactile.	Auditory hallucinations are reported to be more frightening/threatening to patient. Visual hallucinations occur more at night and often include insects, animals, or faces of friends/enemies. Patients are frequently observed "picking the air." Yelling may occur if patient is calling for help from perceived threat (usually seen in stage III).
Provide quiet environment. Speak in calm, quiet voice. Regulate lighting as indicated. Turn off radio/TV during sleep.	Reduces external stimuli during hyperactive stage. Patient may become more delirious when surroundings cannot be seen, but some respond better to quiet, darkened room.
Provide care by same personnel whenever possible.	Promotes recognition of caregivers and a sense of consistency, which may reduce fear.

967

ACTIONS/INTERVENTIONS	RATIONALE

Independent

Encourage SO to stay with patient whenever possible.

May have a calming effect, and may provide a reorienting influence.

Reorient frequently to person, place, time, and surrounding environment as indicated.

May reduce confusion, prevent/limit misinterpretation of external stimuli.

Avoid bedside discussion about patient or topics unrelated to the patient that do not include the patient.

Patient may hear and misinterpret conversation, which can aggravate hallucinations.

Provide environmental safety, e.g., place bed in low position, leave doors in full open or closed position, observe frequently, place call light/bell within reach, remove articles that can harm patient.

Patient may have distorted sense of reality, be fearful, or be suicidal, requiring protection from self.

Collaborative

Provide seclusion, restraints as necessary.

Patients with excessive psychomotor activity, severe hallucinations, violent behavior, and/or suicidal gestures may respond better to seclusion. Restraints are usually ineffective and add to patient's agitation, but occasionally may be required to prevent self-harm.

Monitor laboratory studies, e.g., electrolytes, liver function studies, ammonia, BUN, glucose, ABGs, magnesium levels.

Changes in organ function may precipitate or potentiate sensory-perceptual deficits. Electrolyte imbalance is common. Liver function is often impaired in the chronic alcoholic. Ammonia intoxication can occur if the liver is unable to convert ammonia to urea. Ketoacidosis is sometimes present without glycosuria; however, hyperglycemia or hypoglycemia may occur, suggesting pancreatitis or impaired gluconeogenesis in the liver. Hypoxemia and hypercarbia are common manifestations in chronic alcoholics who are also heavy smokers.

Administer medications as indicated: e.g.:

Minor tranquilizers as indicated. (Refer to ND: Anxiety [Specify Level]/Fear), p 970);

Reduces hyperactivity, promoting relaxation/sleep. Drugs that have little effect on dreaming may be desired to allow dream recovery (REM rebound) to occur, which has previously been suppressed by alcohol use.

Thiamine, C and B complex, multivitamins, Stresstabs.

Vitamin deficiency (especially thiamine) is associated with ataxia, loss of eye movement and pupillary response, palpitations, postural hypotension, and exertional dyspnea.

NURSING DIAGNOSIS: **NUTRITION, ALTERED: LESS THAN BODY REQUIREMENTS**

May be related to: Poor dietary intake (replaced by alcohol consumption).

Effects of alcohol on organs involved in digestion, e.g., stomach, pancreas, liver; interference with absorption and metabolism of nutrients and amino acids; and increased loss of vitamins in the urine.

Possibly evidenced by: Reports of inadequate food intake, altered taste sensation, abdominal pain, lack of interest in food.

Body weight 20% or more under ideal.

Pale conjunctiva and mucous membranes; sore inflamed buccal cavity/cheilosis.

Poor muscle tone, skin turgor.

Hyperactive bowel sounds, diarrhea.

Third spacing of circulating blood volume (e.g., edema of extremities, ascites).

Presence of neuropathies.

Laboratory evidence of decreased RBC count (and anemias), vitamin deficiencies, reduced serum albumin, or electrolyte imbalance.

DESIRED OUTCOMES/ EVALUATION CRITERIA— PATIENT WILL: Demonstrate stable weight or progressive weight gain toward goal with normalization of laboratory values and absence of signs of malnutrition.

Verbalize understanding of effects of alcohol ingestion and reduced dietary intake on nutritional status.

Demonstrate behaviors, lifestyle changes to regain/maintain appropriate weight.

ACTIONS/INTERVENTIONS	RATIONALE
Independent	
Evaluate presence/quality of bowel sounds. Note abdominal distention, tenderness.	Irritation of gastric mucosa is common and may result in epigastric pain, nausea, and hyperactive bowel sounds. More serious effects on GI system may occur secondary to cirrhosis and hepatitis.
Note presence of nausea/vomiting, diarrhea.	Nausea/vomiting are often among first signs of alcohol withdrawal and may interfere with achieving adequate nutritional intake.
Assess ability to feed self.	Tremors, altered mentation, or hallucinations may interfere with ingestion of nutrients and indicate need for assistance.
Provide frequent, small, easily digested feedings/snacks and advance as tolerated.	May limit distress; may enhance intake and tolerance of nutrients. As appetite and ability to tolerate food increases, diet should be adjusted to provide the necessary calories and nutrition for cellular repair and restoration of energy.

969

ACTIONS/INTERVENTIONS	RATIONALE
Collaborative	
Review laboratory studies, e.g., AST/SGOT, ALT/SGPT LDH, serum albumin, transferrin.	Assesses liver function, adequacy of nutritional intake; influences choice of diet and need for/effectiveness of supplemental therapy.
Refer to dietitian/nutritional support team.	Useful in establishing individual nutritional program.
Provide diet high in protein with at least half of calories obtained from carbohydrates.	Stabilizes blood sugar, thereby reducing risk of hypoglycemia while providing for energy needs and cellular regeneration.
Administer medications as indicated, e.g.:	
Antacids, antiemetics, antidiarrheals;	Reduces gastric irritation and effects of sympathetic stimulation.
Vitamins, thiamine.	Replace losses. *Note:* All patients should receive thiamine, because vitamin deficiencies (either clinical or subclinical) exist in most, if not all, chronic alcoholics.
Institute/maintain NPO status as indicated.	Provides GI rest to reduce harmful effects of gastric/pancreatic stimulation in presence of GI bleeding or excessive vomiting.

NURSING DIAGNOSIS:	ANXIETY [SPECIFY LEVEL]/FEAR
May be related to:	Cessation of alcohol intake/physiologic withdrawal.
	Situational crisis (hospitalization).
	Threat to self-concept, perceived threat of death.
Possibly evidenced by:	Feelings of inadequacy, shame, self-disgust, and remorse.
	Increased helplessness/hopelessness with loss of control of own life.
	Increased tension, apprehension.
	Fear of unspecified consequences.
DESIRED OUTCOMES/ EVALUATION CRITERIA— PATIENT WILL:	Verbalize reduction of fear and anxiety to an acceptable and manageable level.
	Express sense of regaining some control of situation/life.
	Demonstrate problem-solving skills and use resources effectively.

ACTIONS/INTERVENTIONS	RATIONALE
Independent	
Identify cause of anxiety, involving patient in the process. Explain that alcohol withdrawal increases	Person in acute phase of withdrawal may be unable to identify and/or accept what is happening.

ACTIONS/INTERVENTIONS	RATIONALE

Independent

anxiety and uneasiness. Reassess level of anxiety on an ongoing basis.

Anxiety may be physiologically or environmentally caused. Continued alcohol toxicity will be manifested by increased anxiety and agitation as effects of tranquilizers wear off.

Develop a trusting relationship through frequent contact. Project an accepting attitude about alcoholism.

Provides patient with a sense of humanness, helping to decrease paranoia and distrust. Patient will be able to detect biased or condescending attitude of caregivers.

Inform patient about what you plan to do and why. Include patient in planning process and provide choices when possible.

Enhances sense of trust, and may increase cooperation or reduce anxiety. Provides sense of control over self in circumstance where loss of control is a significant factor.

Reorient frequently. (Refer to ND: Sensory-Perceptual Alteration, p 967.)

Patient may experience periods of confusion resulting in increased anxiety.

Collaborative

Administer medications as indicated:

    Benzodiazepines, e.g., chlordiazepoxide (Librium), diazepam (Valium).

Minor tranquilizers are given during acute withdrawal to help patient relax, be less hyperactive, and feel more in control.

Arrange "Intervention" (confrontation) to assist patient to accept that substance use is creating a problem.

Process of Intervention, wherein SOs, supported by staff, provide information about how patient's drinking and behavior has affected each one of them, helps patient acknowledge that drinking is a problem and has resulted in current situational crisis.

Provide consultation for referral to detoxification/crisis center for ongoing treatment program as soon as medically stable (e.g., oriented to reality).

Patient is more likely to contract for treatment while still "hurting" and experiencing fear and anxiety from last drinking episode. Motivation decreases as well-being increases and person again feels able to control the problem. Direct contact with available treatment resources provides realistic picture of help. Decreases time for patient to "think about it"/change mind or restructure and strengthen denial systems.

Hallucinogens (LSD, PCP, Cannabis): Intoxication/Overdose ___

Hallucinogenic substances are capable of distorting an individual's perception of reality, altering sensory perception, and inducing hallucinations. For this reason, they are referred to as "mind expanding." They are highly unpredictable in the effects they may induce each time they are used and adverse reactions, including "flashbacks," can recur at any time, even without current use of the drug. Hallucinogens have been used as part of religious ceremonies and at social gatherings by native Americans for more than 2000 years. Therapeutic uses for LSD have been proposed, however, more research is required. At this time, no real evidence speaks to the safety and efficacy of the drug in humans.

Of the drugs that produce mood and perceptual changes varying from sensory illusion to hallucinations, the most popular and well-known are LSD and other LSD-like hallucinogenic drugs, e.g, MDA, MDMA (Ecstasy), mescaline, synthetic THC, DOM (STP), morning glory seeds, nutmeg; PCP; and cannabis (marijuana, hashish, THC).

RELATED CONCERNS

Depressants, p 993
Psychosocial Aspects of Acute Care, p 899
Stimulants, p 983
Substance Dependence/Abuse Rehabilitation, p 1000

PATIENT ASSESSMENT DATA BASE

Factors that can affect the kind of reaction (positive or negative) experienced by the hallucinogen user include individual circadian rhythms (fatigue), previous drug-taking experience, personality, mood, expectations, and concurrent use of alcohol/other drugs can compound symptoms/reactions. One's educational level can also cause different perceptions.

ACTIVITY/REST

May report: Insomnia.

May exhibit: Disturbances of sleep/wakefulness.

Hyperactivity (LSD, mescaline, PCP).

CIRCULATORY

May report: Palpitations.

May exhibit: Increased vital signs (LSD).

Decreased diastolic BP (cannabis, high-dose PCP); hypertension, hypertensive crisis (low-to-moderate dose PCP).

Tachycardia; possible dysrhythmias (high-dose PCP).

EGO INTEGRITY

May report: Euphoria, anxiety, suspiciousness.

May exhibit: Highly dependent nature, with characteristics of poor impulse control, low frustration tolerance, low self-esteem; depersonalization.

Weak superego possibly resulting in absence of guilt feelings for behavior or self reproach, excessive guilt, fearfulness.

Moods reflecting depression or anxiety.

Preoccupation with the idea that brain is destroyed and/or will not return to a normal state.

FOOD/FLUID

May report: Increased appetite (cannabis).

Nausea/vomiting, increased salivation.

NEUROSENSORY

May report: Blurred vision, altered depth perception.

Dizziness, headache (LSD).

Flashback (spontaneous transitory recurrence of a drug-induced experience [LSD] in a drug-free state).

"Bad trips" (self-limiting and confined to period of intoxication.

LSD: Three kinds: (1) bad body trip, e.g., "my body is purple"; (2) bad environment trip, visual distortions so real the person thinks he or she is going crazy; (3) bad mind trip, e.g., unexpected subconscious material bursts forth into consciousness, as in, "I'm responsible for my mother's death."

PCP: Aggravates any underlying psychopathology.

Cannabis: Rare; however, when they do occur, panic attacks are usually seen.

May exhibit: Eyes: Pupil constriction, vertical and horizontal nystagmus (PCP); pupillary dilation, catatonic staring (LSD, mescaline).

Muscle incoordination/tremors, seizures; increased muscle strength may be noted with PCP due to the anesthetic effect that deadens pain perception; deep-tendon reflexes increased (low-to-moderate dose PCP) or depressed (high-dose PCP); opisthotonos (body-arching spasm).

Level of consciousness: Usually responsive; coma may be noted (especially if intracranial hemorrhage occurs with PCP); slurred speech, mutism.

Mental status: Perceptual changes, e.g., sensation of slowed time, perceptions enhanced (colors richer, music more profound, smells and tastes heightened), synesthesia (merging of senses, colors are "heard" or sounds are "seen"), changes in body image, depersonalization.

Delirium with clouded state of consciousness (sensory misperception, disorientation, and memory impairment, difficulty in sustaining attention, disordered stream of thought, psychomotor activity); delusions, illusions, hallucinations (rare with cannabis intoxication). May occur within 24 hours after use or after recovery; may occur days after PCP has been taken.

Delusions occurring in a normal state of consciousness may persist beyond 24 hours after cessation of hallucinogen use; persecutory delusions can follow cannabis use immediately or may occur during the course of cannabis intoxication.

Mood: Euphoria/dysphoria, anxiety, emotional lability, apathy, grandiosity.

Behavioral findings: May include assaultiveness, bizarre behavior, impulsivity, unpredictability, belligerence, impaired judgment, paranoid ideation, panic attacks.

PAIN/COMFORT

May report: Decreased awareness of pain.

Sudden, intense chest pain or persistent chest discomfort (if drug is smoked).

RESPIRATION

May exhibit: Decreased rate/depth of respiration (PCP, heavy cannabis use).

Rhonchi, gurgling sounds.

SAFETY

May exhibit: Skin: Diaphoretic.

Eyes: Conjunctival redness (cannabis).

SOCIAL INTERACTION

May report: Dysfunctional family system; one parent who is absent or who is an overpowering tyrant and/or one who is weak and ineffectual.

Substance abuse as the primary coping method.

Overwhelming peer pressure leading to involvement with drugs.

Impaired social or occupational functioning (fights, loss of friends, absence from work, loss of job, or legal difficulties).

TEACHING/LEARNING

May report: Family history of substance abuse.

Discharge Plan Considerations: **DRG projected mean length of stay: 4.5 days.**

May need assistance with abstinence and/or transfer to rehabilitation program.

DIAGNOSTIC STUDIES

Drug screen/urinalysis: To identify drug(s) being used.

Addiction Severity Index: To assess substance abuse and determine treatment needs.

NURSING PRIORITIES

1. Protect patient/others from injury.
2. Promote physiologic/psychologic stability.
3. Provide appropriate referral and follow-up.
4. Support patient/family in "Intervention" (confrontation) process for decision to stop using drugs.
5. Provide information about dependency/prognosis and treatment needs.

DISCHARGE GOALS

1. Homeostasis achieved.
2. Complications prevented/resolved.
3. Abstinence from drug(s) maintained.
4. Dependency condition, prognosis, and therapeutic regimen understood.
5. Enrolled in/transferred to drug rehabilitation program.

NURSING DIAGNOSIS:	VIOLENCE, HIGH RISK FOR, DIRECTED AT SELF/OTHERS
Risk factors may include:	Chemical alteration, exogenous (CNS stimulants/mind-altering drug); toxic reaction to drug(s).
	Organic brain syndrome (drug anesthetizes mind and body).
	Psychologic state (narrowed perceptual field).

[Possible indicators]:	Synesthesias, hallucinations, illusions, visual/auditory distortions; panic state; suspiciousness of others, paranoid ideation, delusions.
	Hostile threatening verbalizations; unpredictable behavior.
	Change in behavior pattern; exaggerated emotional response.
	Increased motor activity, pacing, excitement, irritability, agitation.
	Overt and aggressive acts; self-destructive behavior.
	Increasing anxiety, fear, and feelings of loss of control.
	Decreased response to pain.
DESIRED OUTCOMES/ EVALUATION CRITERIA— PATIENT WILL:	Demonstrate self-control, as evidenced by relaxed posture, free of violent behavior.
	Acknowledge reality of situation and understanding of relationship of behavior to drug use.
	Participate in treatment program.

ACTIONS/INTERVENTIONS	RATIONALE
Independent	
Place in darkened, quiet, nonthreatening environment with a nonintrusive observer.	Lowered stimulation can decrease the degree of confusion and fear, thus reducing chance of violent response. Use of an observer promotes safety. *Note:* PCP users often seek/or are brought for help only after the situation has gotten out of hand, and it is therefore important to take safe action immediately.
Speak in a soft, nonthreatening voice. Use "Talk-downs" when LSD has been taken. If technique is tried with other drugs (PCP) and agitation increases, stop immediately.	Nonthreatening communication may have a calming effect. However, "Talk-downs" (the use of orientation, support and reassuring words/touch) may be deleterious in the presence of PCP intoxication, resulting in an increase in the user's agitation level.
Observe for escalating anxiety, fear, irritability, and agitation.	May indicate potential for violent behavior. *Note:* Patient is not in complete control because of drug use.
Accept patient's anger, without reacting on an emotional basis.	Responding emotionally on a personal level is not constructive and may escalate reactions.
Provide protection within the environment via constant observation and removal of objects that may be used to hurt self or others.	Reduces risk of injury to patient and/or staff. Patient may not feel pain and may not be able to follow directions because of the drug.
Observe behavior before administering medication.	A period of drug-free observation should precede any decision to administer medications (e.g., tranquilizers), so that a clear clinical picture can develop. In addition, because it is not known what other drugs may also have been ingested, it is not generally advisable to add another drug.

975

ACTIONS/INTERVENTIONS	RATIONALE
Collaborative	
Administer medications as necessary, e.g.:	
Diazepam (Valium);	Used to reduce muscle spasms and/or restlessness in PCP user.
Haloperidol (Haldol).	Preferred to control psychosis and assaultive behavior.
Avoid use of phenothiazine neuroleptics.	Drugs such as chlorpromazine (Thorazine) should probably be avoided because of the possibility of potentiating PCP anticholinergic effects.
Apply restraints, if needed and document reason(s) for use.	Restraints should be avoided in a frightened, hallucinating patient but may be necessary because of potential injury to self or others, or when other dangerous drugs have been taken. PCP users are unpredictable; so it is best to err on the side of safety (using restraints with sufficient documentation) rather than risking injury.

NURSING DIAGNOSIS:	**TRAUMA/SUFFOCATION/POISONING, HIGH RISK FOR**
Risk factors may include:	Muscle incoordination; reduced hand/eye coordination.
	Decreased response to/perception of pain, reduced temperature/tactile sensation.
	Clouded sensorium and impaired judgment; unfamiliar environment; fear.
	Clonic movements, muscle rigidity (may precede/occur with generalized seizure activity).
	Internal factors, host: Psychologic perception (hallucinations).
	Interactive conditions between individual and environment that impose a risk to the defensive and adaptive resources of the individual, e.g., placing hand in open flame, "flying out of window."
Possibly evidenced by:	[Not applicable; presence of signs and symptoms establishes an actual diagnosis.]
DESIRED OUTCOMES/ EVALUATION CRITERIA— PATIENT WILL:	Verbalize understanding of factors (e.g., drug use) that contribute to possibility of injury and take steps to correct situation.
	Demonstrate behaviors and lifestyle changes necessary to minimize and/or prevent injury.
	Maintain/achieve physiologic stability, as evidenced by patent airway and adequate respiratory/cardiac function.

ACTIONS/INTERVENTIONS	RATIONALE
Independent	
Ascertain what drugs have been taken.	Necessary for appropriate intervention/anticipation of needs. Lethal overdoses of hallucinogenic drugs (except for MDA, "angel dust", PCP) are rare; however, caution must be taken because adulterants such as sedative-hypnotics, anticholinergics, and strychnine are often used for "cutting" the drug. *Note:* Two reasons one might not know what drug was taken are (1) that the patient lies because of legal concerns or feels embarrassed and (2) that the person who sold the drugs to the patient either did not know what it was or lied to the patient. In either case, the nurse should listen to the patient but be aware that the information the patient gives may not be accurate.
Anticipate some form of unpredictability and be prepared for the unexpected, including physiologic as well as psychologic emergencies.	These drugs are dangerous and they do lead to bizarre thinking/harmful behavior.
Maintain patient under close observation. Note precursors that might indicate increasing agitation, e.g., body tension, rising voice tone, quickening movements.	These drugs alter thinking and many are anesthetic; therefore the patient may hurt self because of bizarre thinking, e.g., attempt to jump out window or escape from restraints.
Remove objects that may be used to hurt self or others.	Provides protection within the environment.
Provide a hockey/bicycle helmet as indicated.	If patient is banging head against hard objects, a helmet can decrease the potential for/severity of injury.
Monitor vital signs, respiratory rate/depth and rhythm.	Decreased diastolic BP (cannabis) or hypertensive crisis (PCP) may develop. Bradypnea/respiratory arrest can occur, especially with PCP or heavy cannabis use.
Assess gag/swallow response and character of respirations.	Hypersalivation and vomiting, especially in the presence of ineffective cough and/or loss of muscle tone may result in occlusion of airway, crowing/gurgling/choked respirations and respiratory arrest.
Position patient on side.	Facilitates drainage of vomitus and buildup of saliva, and prevents aspiration in sedated/comatose patient.
Encourage taking fluids frequently, if patient is able to swallow safely.	Adequate hydration keeps secretions loose and easier to expectorate and enhances renal clearance of drugs.
Have emergency equipment (including airway adjunct/suction) and medications available.	Toxic effects of several of these drugs on the heart and respiratory system may result in cardiac/respiratory arrest, requiring prompt intervention to prevent death.
Collaborative	
Administer IV fluids and ammonium chloride or ascorbic acid, as indicated.	Forced diuresis and acidifying urine enhance renal clearance of PCP. (Effects are dose-related: > 5

977

ACTIONS/INTERVENTIONS	RATIONALE
Collaborative	
	mg = low dose; > 10 mg = high dose; > 20 mg can lead to hypertensive crisis, coma/death due to respiratory/cardiac failure).
Administer medications as indicated, e.g., diazepam (Valium).	May be useful to reduce agitation and hyperactivity once drug(s) used are identified.
Apply restraints with caution when used.	May prevent injury to self or others. However, restraints should be avoided, if possible, in a frightened, hallucinating patient as they can increase agitation.

NURSING DIAGNOSIS:	**TISSUE PERFUSION, ALTERED: CEREBRAL, HIGH RISK FOR**
Risk factors may include:	Alterations in blood flow (hypertensive crisis).
Possibly evidenced by:	[Not applicable; presence of signs and symptoms establishes an actual diagnosis.]
DESIRED OUTCOMES/ EVALUATION CRITERIA— PATIENT WILL:	Regain/maintain usual level of consciousness free of adverse neurologic symptoms/complications.

ACTIONS/INTERVENTIONS	RATIONALE
Independent	
Elevate head of the bed; keep head in midline position.	Enhances venous drainage, thereby reducing risk of vascular congestion, increasing intracranial pressure, and possibility of hemorrhage in PCP intoxication.
Observe for pupillary or vital sign changes, decreased level of consciousness and/or motor function.	Provides for early detection and intervention to minimize intracranial pressure/injury.
Encourage rest and quiet. Reduce environmental stimuli.	Promotes relaxation and may assist with lowering of BP.
Monitor BP.	Evaluates need for/effectiveness of interventions.
Collaborative	
Administer antihypertensive medications, e.g., diazoxide (Hyperstat) and hydralazine (Apresoline).	Effective in lowering BP to prevent hypertensive crisis, which can be associated with PCP intoxication.

NURSING DIAGNOSIS:	THOUGHT PROCESSES, ALTERED
May be related to:	Physiologic changes (use of hallucinogenic substance).
	Impaired judgment with loss of memory.
Possibly evidenced by:	Inaccurate interpretation of environment, memory impairment, bizarre thinking, disorientation.
	Inability to make decisions; unpredictable behavior.
	Cognitive dissonance; distractibility.
	Inappropriate/nonreality-based thinking.
	Sleep deprivation.
	Inability to communicate needs/desires effectively (mutism or confusion).
DESIRED OUTCOMES/ EVALUATION CRITERIA— PATIENT WILL:	Exhibit return of memory and ability to function.
	Communicate effectively.
	Report absence of visual/auditory distortions.
	Verbalize understanding that the drug is the cause of/contributes to alteration in perception.

ACTIONS/INTERVENTIONS	RATIONALE
Independent	
Observe closely; do not leave unattended; make sure restraints are secure when used. Remove objects from the environment that patient could use to harm self and others. (Refer to ND: Violence, High Risk For, Directed at Self/Others, p 974.)	PCP alters thinking, is an anesthetic, and patient may hurt self via attempt to jump out window, jump in front of cars, escape from restraints, and so forth. Removal of potentially harmful objects provides for protection and safety.
Anticipate some form of unpredictable behavior and be prepared for the unexpected.	Use of hallucinogens can lead to bizarre thinking/harmful responses.
Tell patient that current thoughts and feelings are a result of the drug if indicated.	This information may be helpful to the patient who can accept it; however, it may cause agitation.
Allow patient to sleep whenever possible.	Sleep cycle is often disturbed and patient will need sleep after being agitated and expending excessive amounts of energy. Sleeping also provides time for drug(s) to clear system.
Observe for psychotic indicators, e.g., paranoia, delusions, hallucinations.	Overdose may precipitate psychotic episode, which may clear within hours to days. When psychosis remains, preexisting condition (e.g., schizophrenia) may have been precipitated.
Note altered speech ability/patterns. Refer to loss of speech as temporary.	Mutism and confusion may occur, and information may reassure patient that problem is drug-induced and that it will improve with time. *Note:* "Talk-down" approach may agitate the patient and should be used with caution.

979

ACTIONS/INTERVENTIONS

Independent

Anticipate patient's needs and allow more time for patient to respond to any necessary questions and/or comments.

Collaborative

Administer medications as indicated, e.g.: diazepam (Valium) or chlordiazepoxide (Librium).

RATIONALE

May reduce need to communicate in presence of confusion/interference with memory. Adequate time allows full expression. *Note:* Be aware that touching and/or physical closeness may increase anxiety and agitation.

Chronic PCP users in whom psychiatric complications develop may require further treatment for the thought disorder or depressive illness. The response may be very slow because of the persistence of PCP in the body tissues, sometimes for a period of several months.

NURSING DIAGNOSIS:	ANXIETY [SPECIFY LEVEL]/FEAR
May be related to:	Situational crisis; threat to/change in health status.
	Perceived threat of death.
	Inexperience or unfamiliarity with the effect of drug(s), (e.g., PCP, LSD).
	Impaired thought processes; sensory impairment.
Possibly evidenced by:	Assumptions of "losing my mind, losing control"; verbalized concern about unknown consequences/outcomes.
	Sympathetic stimulation, e.g., cardiovascular excitation, superficial vasoconstriction, pupil dilation, vomiting/diarrhea, restlessness, trembling.
	Preoccupation with feelings of impending doom; apprehension.
	Attack behavior.
DESIRED OUTCOMES/ EVALUATION CRITERIA— PATIENT WILL:	Verbalize awareness/cause of feelings of anxiety.
	Report anxiety reduced to a manageable level.
	Appear relaxed.
	Identify the fear and verbalize feelings of control of self and situation.

ACTIONS/INTERVENTIONS

Independent

Assess level of anxiety on an ongoing basis.

RATIONALE

Increased anxiety may lead to agitation and violent behavior because patient is not in complete control of actions/responses.

ACTIONS/INTERVENTIONS	RATIONALE
Independent	
Place in darkened, quiet, nonthreatening environment with a nonintrusive observer.	Lowered stimulation decreases the likelihood of confusion and fear.
Orient person to surroundings, time, and who is with the patient. Speak in soft voice, in a nonthreatening manner.	Knowing where one is can increase the feeling of security when experiencing a "bad trip."
Use "Talk-downs" with caution, telling the patient that the ingested drug is the cause of feelings of anxiety, the effects are only temporary, and permanent damage should not occur.	Reassurance can be the single most important therapeutic intervention. "Talk-downs" are effective with persons who have taken LSD or similar substances. If the patient can realize that the perceptions are drug related, then an increase in control can take place. However, in some situations (e.g., PCP) "Talk-downs" can result in an increase in fear and agitation.
Encourage verbal expression of changes in perception that are occurring.	Can be used for assessment and provides guidance on direction for support.
Collaborative	
Administer sedatives if necessary, e.g., diazepam (Valium) or chlordiazepoxide (Librium).	These are drugs of choice to be used in extreme cases to calm patient. *Note:* Medications are often discouraged because "bad trips" are usually self-limiting, and time is the best remedy for treating negative effects.

NURSING DIAGNOSIS:	SELF-CARE DEFICIT: (SPECIFY)
May be related to:	Perceptual/cognitive impairment.
	Therapeutic management (restraints).
Possibly evidenced by:	Inability to meet own physical needs.
DESIRED OUTCOMES/ EVALUATION CRITERIA— PATIENT WILL:	Resume/perform self-care activities within level of own ability. Verbalize commitment to lifestyle changes to meet self-care needs.

ACTIONS/INTERVENTIONS	RATIONALE
Independent	
Provide care as needed/permitted.	Patient may be agitated and care will need to be postponed until control is regained.
Involve patient in formulation of plan of care, as possible.	Enables patient to participate at level of ability and enhances sense of control. *Note:* PCP user is often unable to interact without becoming agitated.
Work with patient's present abilities. Do not pressure to perform beyond capabilities.	Failure can produce discouragement, depression, and agitation.

ACTIONS/INTERVENTIONS	RATIONALE
Independent	
Provide and promote privacy within limits of safety needs.	Important to enhance self-esteem.
Collaborative	
Problem-solve with patient, using input from other team members as indicated.	Multidisciplinary approach with involvement of everyone who is caring for the patient, along with the patient, increases probability of plan being effective/successful.

Stimulants (Amphetamines, Cocaine, Caffeine, Tobacco): Intoxication/Overdose

Stimulants are natural and man-made drugs that speed up the nervous system. They can be swallowed, injected, inhaled, or smoked. These substances are identified by behavioral stimulation and psychomotor agitation that they induce. They differ widely in their molecular structures and in their mechanisms of action. The two most prevalent and widely used stimulants are caffeine and nicotine. Caffeine is readily available as a common ingredient in coffee, tea, colas, and chocolate. Nicotine is a primary substance in tobacco products. These are generally accepted as a part of our culture and are not usually seen in overdose situations. Other more potent stimulants (e.g., cocaine, amphetamines, and nonamphetamine stimulants) are regulated by the Controlled Substances Act. They are available for therapeutic purposes by prescription only, but are also widely available on the illicit market. The potential for overdose and even death is high.

RELATED CONCERNS

Depressants, p 993
Pneumonia, Microbial, p 162
Psychosocial Aspects of Acute Care, p 899
Substance Dependence/Abuse Rehabilitation, p 1000

PATIENT ASSESSMENT DATA BASE

Data are dependent on stage of withdrawal, concurrent use of alcohol/other drugs or contaminants in drug "cut."

ACTIVITY/REST

May report:	Insomnia; hypersomnia, nightmares.
May exhibit:	Anxiety.
	Hyperactivity, increased alertness, or falling asleep during activities.
	Inability to tolerate or to correct chronic fatigue (depression and/or loneliness may be a factor).

CIRCULATION

May exhibit:	Elevated BP, tachycardia, cardiac dysrhythmias.
	Diaphoresis.

EGO INTEGRITY

May exhibit:	Underdeveloped ego; highly dependent nature, with characteristics of poor impulse control, low frustration tolerance, and low self-esteem; weak superego.
	Absence of guilt feelings for behavior.
	May be seen or view self as susceptible to influence by others, having an inability to say "no." Need to feel elated, sociable, happy with self; desire to prove self-worth, improve self-esteem.

FOOD/FLUID

May report:	Nausea/vomiting, anorexia.
May exhibit:	Weight loss; thin, cachectic appearance.

NEUROSENSORY

May report: Emotional/psychologic symptoms, e.g., elation, grandiosity, loquacity, hypervigilance.

Numbness in hands and feet. Twitching, jerking in face, neck, arms, hands.

May exhibit: Pupillary dilation.

Tremors, convulsions, coma.

Delirium with tactile and olfactory hallucinations as well as hallucinations of insects or vermin crawling in/under the skin (formication); labile affect, violent or aggressive behavior, symptoms of a paranoid delusional disorder (amphetamine or similarly acting substances).

Fixed delusional system of a persecutory nature, lasting weeks to a year or more.

Psychosis: Can occur with a one-time high dose of amphetamine (especially with IV administration) or with long-term use at moderate or high doses.

Ideas of reference.

Aggressiveness, hostility, violence, quick response to anger; psychomotor agitation.

Stereotyped compulsive motor behavior, e.g., sorting, taking things apart and putting them back together, moving mouth from side to side in a stereotypic grimacing pattern.

Anxiety; impaired judgment and perception.

Compulsion regarding stimulant use, or denial of powerlessness over the stimulant (use of drug for celebration or crisis; believing drug can be used in regulated quantities, often resulting in binge use).

May think of recovery process as notion of willpower, subject to impulse control.

PAIN/COMFORT

May report: Bone pain.

RESPIRATION

May exhibit: Tachypnea, coughing.

Nasal rhinitis (chronic cocaine use).

Chronic/recurrent bronchiolitis; pneumonia.

Pulmonary hemorrhage.

SAFETY

May report: History of accidents, involvement with legal system.

May exhibit: Elevated temperature.

Fever/chills.

Nasal damage (if drug is snorted).

Evidence of trauma, e.g., bruises, lacerations, burns.

SEXUALITY

May report: Pregnancy.

Diminished/enhanced sexual desire. Disinhibition regarding sexual behavior.

SOCIAL INTERACTION

May report: Dysfunctional family system (family of origin).

Impairment in relation, social, or occupational functioning.

TEACHING/LEARNING

May report: Pattern of habitual use of the particular drug or pathologic abuse, with inability to reduce or to stop use, occurring for at least 1 month duration.

Intoxication throughout the day, sometimes with daily involvement.

Episodes of overdose in which hallucinations and delusions occur (cocaine).

Previous hospitalization or having been in residential treatment program.

Health beliefs about use of drugs, e.g., "diet pills are OK to use to lose weight."

Attendance at recovery groups, e.g., Narcotics/Alcoholics Anonymous, or other drug-specific recovery groups.

Discharge Plan Considerations: **DRG projected mean length of stay: 4.5 days.**

May need assistance to maintain abstinence and begin to participate in rehabilitation program.

DIAGNOSTIC STUDIES

Blood and urine screens: For presence of drug(s).

Tests for hepatitis and HIV may be routine in known IV drug users or when the patient is at high risk.

ASI: Produces a "problem severity profile," which indicates areas of treatment needs.

NURSING PRIORITIES

1. Maintain physiologic stability.
2. Promote safety and security.
3. Prevent complications.
4. Support patient's acceptance of reality of situation.
5. Promote family involvement in "Intervention"/treatment process.
6. Provide information about dependency, prognosis, and treatment needs.

DISCHARGE GOALS

1. Homeostasis maintained.
2. Complications prevented/resolved.
3. Patient is dealing with situation realistically/planning for the future.
4. Abstinence from drug(s) maintained on a day-to-day basis.
5. Transferred to rehabilitation program/attending group.
6. Dependence condition, prognosis, and therapeutic regimen understood.

NURSING DIAGNOSIS:	CARDIAC OUTPUT, DECREASED, HIGH RISK FOR
Risk factors may include:	Drug (e.g., cocaine) effect on myocardium (dependent on drug purity/quantity ingested).
	Preexisting myocardiopathy (with or without previous prolonged drug abuse).
	Alterations in electrical rate/rhythm/conduction.

985

Possibly evidenced by:	[Not applicable; presence of signs and symptoms establishes an actual diagnosis.]
DESIRED OUTCOMES/ EVALUATION CRITERIA— PATIENT WILL:	Report absence of chest pain.
	Demonstrate adequate cardiac output free of signs of shock, dysrhythmias.

ACTIONS/INTERVENTIONS	RATIONALE
Independent	
Monitor BP.	BP fluctuations can be extreme with both hypertension and hypotension affecting cardiac output.
Monitor cardiac rate and rhythm. Document dysrhythmias.	Ventricular dysrhythmias/cardiac arrest may occur at any time, especially with toxic levels of certain drugs, e.g., cocaine, crack, crank, ice, and other amphetamines.
Investigate reports of chest pain, indigestion/heartburn.	Incidence of myocardial infarction is increased in cocaine users.
Have emergency equipment/medications available.	Prompt treatment of dysrhythmias may prevent cardiac arrest.
Collaborative	
Administer supplemental O_2 as needed.	Tachycardia and other cardiac dysrhythmias may be improved/decreased with increased O_2 delivery to tissues.
Administer medications as indicated, e.g.:	
Propranolol (Inderal);	Beta-adrenergic blocker that reduces cardiac O_2 demand by blocking catecholamine-induced increases in heart rate, BP, and force of myocardial contraction.
Antidysrhythmics, e.g., bretylium (Bretylate).	May be used to control/prevent ventricular dysrhythmias.

NURSING DIAGNOSIS:	**VIOLENCE, HIGH RISK FOR, DIRECTED AT SELF/OTHERS**
Risk factors may include:	Toxic reaction to drug, withdrawal from drug.
	Panic state, profound depression/suicidal behavior.
	Organic brain syndrome.
[Possible indicators]:	Overt and aggressive acts.
	Increased motor activity.
	Possession of destructive means.
	Suspicion of others, paranoid ideation, delusions, and hallucinations.
	Expressed intent directly/indirectly.

DESIRED OUTCOMES/ EVALUATION CRITERIA— PATIENT WILL:	Acknowledge fearfulness and realities of situation. Verbalize understanding of behavior and precipitating factors. Demonstrate self control.

ACTIONS/INTERVENTIONS

Independent

Obtain information specific to pattern of drug use over past month, what drugs have been used together, in addition to immunization history, allergies, medications used for other purposes.

Decrease stimuli, provide quiet in own room or place in stimulus-reduction room with supervision.

Allow SO to remain in room during procedures when appropriate.

Remove potentially harmful objects from environment.

Explain consistent rules of unit, e.g., no violence, no threats.

Maintain high staff profile in situations in which potential violence can occur.

Provide opportunities for verbal expression of aggressive feelings.

Assist patient in identifying what provokes anger.

Provide outlets for expression that involve physical activity, e.g., stationary bicycle, racquetball/basketball/volleyball.

Discuss consequences of aggressive behavior.

Be alert to violence potential, e.g., increased pacing, verbalization of delusional persecutory content, hypervigilance regarding specific persons in the milieu, gesturing aggressively, threatening others verbally or physically.

Isolate immediately if patient becomes violent, using adequate staff trained in assaultive management. Maintain calm, nonpunitive attitude.

Negotiate conditions for coming out of isolation/ "quiet time" when the patient is calm, based on agreement of social appropriateness.

RATIONALE

Initial factual history can reveal information essential to treatment needs. Where person obtained drug could assist in investigating possible "cut" with other drugs.

Reduces reactivity; enhances calm feelings.

Can provide a calming effect to see someone that patient knows/cares about and may trust.

Reduces opportunity for patient to harm others or carry out suicidal ideas. Patient may be suicidal when/if rebound CNS depression occurs secondary to stimulant withdrawal.

Secure environment enhances sense of safety, which can decrease perceived threat. Enhances opportunity for patient to learn ways to cope with aggressive feelings before reacting.

May prevent onset of violence.

Encouragement of new avenue of expression helps patient learn new coping skills.

Awareness of reaction is the first step in learning change.

Being physically active in protected environment can lessen aggressive drive.

Learning choices assists patient to gain control of situation and self.

Recognizing potential and assisting patient to gain control can be more effective prior to violent outbreak.

Patient will feel safer if others take control until internal locus of control can be regained. An attitude of acceptance is important while refusing to tolerate the violent behavior. *Note:* Use of seclusion and restraints may exacerbate hyperactivity.

Clear expectations aid patient in feeling secure about own control.

987

ACTIONS/INTERVENTIONS

Independent

Build trust: follow through on commitments/agreements, maintain consistent staff and frequent brief contact with patient.

Collaborative

Administer medications as indicated, e.g.:

    Chlorpromazine (Thorazine); haloperidol (Haldol);

    Diazepam (Valium), chlordiazepoxide (Librium).

RATIONALE

Trust is essential to working with all patients. Brief contacts can prevent overstimulation.

Short-term use of major tranquilizers during acute intoxication/psychosis assists patient in gaining self-control; promotes sedation/rest when agitated, assaultive, overstimulated. *Note:* Thorazine may cause postural hypotension, and Haldol may provoke acute extrapyramidal reaction, requiring additional evaluation/medication.

Occasionally useful for treatment of acute cocaine intoxication. Either drug is useful for preventing DTs when substance use is combined with alcohol.

NURSING DIAGNOSIS:	SENSORY-PERCEPTUAL ALTERATION: (SPECIFY)
May be related to:	Chemical alteration: exogenous (CNS stimulants or depressants, mind-altering drugs).
	Altered sensory reception, transmission and/or integration: Altered status of sense organs.
Possibly evidenced by:	Bizarre thinking, anxiety/panic.
	Preoccupation with/appears to be responding to internal stimuli from hallucinatory experiences, e.g., "listening pose," laughing and talking to self, stopping in midsentence and listening, "picking" at self and clothing, trying to "get away from bugs."
	Changes in sensory acuity, decreased pain perception.
DESIRED OUTCOMES/ EVALUATION CRITERIA— PATIENT WILL:	Distinguish reality from altered perceptions.
	State awareness that hallucinations may result from stimulant use.

ACTIONS/INTERVENTIONS

Independent

Notice patient's preoccupation, responses, gesturing, social skill.

Assist patient in checking perceptions verbally; provide reality information.

RATIONALE

Helps to assess whether or not patient is hallucinating without overstimulating verbally.

Can calm the patient and provide reassurance of safety and that formication (illusion of insects crawling on the body) or other misperceptions are not occurring.

ACTIONS/INTERVENTIONS

Independent

Acknowledge patient's emotional state; reassure regarding safety.

Explore ways of calming and relaxing patient.

Be aware that altered sensation and perception may cause injury, e.g., be alert for patient burning self with cigarette, excessive scratching at skin to rid self of insects or drug (which may feel as though it is in the skin), accidentally harming self through poor judgment or misperceptions. (Refer to ND: Violence, High Risk For: Directed At Self/ Others, p 986.)

Inform patient (if calm enough) of temporary nature of hallucinations that have resulted from stimulant use.

RATIONALE

Empathetic response can diminish intensity of fear.

Relaxation can promote positive outlook, distracting from negativity and enhancing clarity of perceptions.

Amphetamine use causes impaired judgment, increasing risk of injury/self-harm. Overdose of many stimulants causes frightening hallucinations, often of large insects crawling on skin.

Learning cause, effect, and possible temporary nature of misperceptions may reduce fear, anxiety, and negativity. May inject hope and positive attitude.

NURSING DIAGNOSIS:	**FEAR/ANXIETY [SPECIFY LEVEL]**
May be related to:	Paranoid delusions associated with stimulant use.
Possibly evidenced by:	Feelings/beliefs that others are conspiring against or are about to kill patient.
DESIRED OUTCOMES/ EVALUATION CRITERIA— PATIENT WILL:	Recognize frightening feelings before preoccupying self or becoming violent.
	Discuss reality base of persecutory fears with staff.
	Report fear/anxiety reduced to manageable level.
	Demonstrate appropriate range of feelings and appear relaxed.

ACTIONS/INTERVENTIONS

Independent

Establish consistent staff. Build trust by being reliable, honest, genuine, prompt.

Acknowledge awareness of patient's feelings, e.g., fear, terror, overwhelmed, panic, anxiety, confusion.

Be concrete, clear in communication. Assess patient's readiness for humor and/or touch.

RATIONALE

Trust and rapport are necessary for overcoming fear.

Empathy can assist patient to tolerate/deal with own feelings.

Fear negatively influences one's ability to laugh. Fear is serious to the perceiver and must be respected. Touch can be misinterpreted/increase anxiety.

ACTIONS/INTERVENTIONS

Independent

Encourage verbalization of fears/anxieties.

Assist patient in reality checking fears. Use gentle confrontation.

RATIONALE

Venting feelings to trusted staff can lessen intensity of fearfulness. Provides opportunity to clarify misunderstandings and comfort patient.

Patient can reduce fear if s/he understands difference between reality and delusions. Should be used cautiously because reality checking a delusional system puts trust at risk.

NURSING DIAGNOSIS:	NUTRITION, ALTERED: LESS THAN BODY REQUIREMENTS
May be related to:	Anorexia (stimulant use).
	Insufficient/inappropriate use of financial resources.
Possibly evidenced by:	Reported inadequate intake.
	Lack of interest in food; weight loss.
	Poor muscle tone.
	Signs/laboratory evidence of vitamin deficiencies.
DESIRED OUTCOMES/ EVALUATION CRITERIA— PATIENT WILL:	Demonstrate progressive weight gain toward goal.
	Verbalize understanding of causative factors and individual needs.
	Identify appropriate dietary choices, lifestyle changes to regain/maintain desired weight.

ACTIONS/INTERVENTIONS

Independent

Ascertain dietary intake pattern over past several weeks.

Discuss needs/likes/dislikes about food choices.

Anticipate hyperphagia and weigh every other day.

Provide meals in a relaxed, nonstimulating environment.

Encourage frequent nutritional snacks, small nutritious meals.

Collaborative

Obtain/review routine laboratory work, e.g., CBC, serum protein, albumin, UA.

RATIONALE

Stimulants cause decreased appetite and impaired judgment regarding nutritional needs.

Will be more likely to maintain desired intake if individual preferences are considered.

Overeating may be a consequence of stimulant withdrawal and may result in sudden/inappropriate weight gain.

Stimulus reduction aids relaxation and ability to focus on eating.

Small amounts of food frequently can prevent/reduce GI distress.

Assessment of nutritional state is necessary to treat preexisting deficiencies, rule out anemia, dehydration, or ketosis.

ACTIONS/INTERVENTIONS	RATIONALE
Collaborative	
Consult with dietitian.	Useful in establishing individual nutritional needs/dietary program.

NURSING DIAGNOSIS:	INFECTION, HIGH RISK FOR
Risk factors may include:	IV drug use techniques; impurities of injected drugs.
	Localized trauma; nasal septum damage (snorting cocaine).
	Malnutrition; altered immune state.
Possibly evidenced by:	[Not applicable; presence of signs and symptoms establishes an actual diagnosis.]
DESIRED OUTCOMES/ EVALUATION CRITERIA— PATIENT WILL:	Verbalize understanding of individual risk factors.
	Identify interventions to prevent/reduce risk factors.
	Demonstrate lifestyle changes to promote safe environment.
	Achieve timely healing of infectious process if present/develops and is afebrile.

ACTIONS/INTERVENTIONS	RATIONALE
Independent	
Assess skin integrity and character. Assist as needed with body and oral hygiene; provide clean clothes, properly fitting shoes.	Maintaining skin integrity requires cleanliness. If sores are present, they may need care to prevent infection.
Use blood/body fluid precautions as appropriate.	Protects caregiver from possible contamination by infectious disease viruses, e.g., hepatitis, HIV.
Monitor vital signs. Assess level of consciousness.	Abnormal signs, including fever, can indicate presence of infection. Cerebral complications, e.g., meningitis, brain abscess, may occur, affecting mentation. *Note:* Fever is also a symptom of toxic CNS effect.
Investigate recurrent cough; note characteristics of sputum. Auscultate breath sounds.	These patients are at increased risk for development of pulmonary infections.
Observe for nasal stuffiness, pain, bleeding, abnormal mucus production.	Cocaine snorting can cause erosion of the nasal septum, requiring additional therapy/interventions.
Investigate complaints of acute/chronic bone pain, tenderness, guarding with movement, regional muscle spasm.	Symptoms of osteomyelitis usually due to hematogenous spread of bacteria, most often affecting lumbar vertebrae.
Ascertain health status of family members/SO currently in contact with patient.	May expose patient to diseases such as colds, hepatitis, AIDS.

991

ACTIONS/INTERVENTIONS

Collaborative

Review laboratory studies, e.g., UA, CBC, SMA, RPR, ESR, ELISA/Western Blot test.

RATIONALE

May identify complications of IV drug use such as hepatitis, nephritis, tetanus, vasculitis, septicemia, subacute bacterial endocarditis, embolic phenomena, malaria. Toxic allergic reactions may result from other substances in the "cut" and immunologic abnormalities may occur due to repeated antigenic stimulation. *Note:* IV needle drug users are at high risk for contamination with HIV and hepatitis viruses.

NURSING DIAGNOSIS:	SLEEP PATTERN DISTURBANCE
May be related to:	CNS sensory alterations: External factor (stimulant use), internal factors (psychologic stress).
Possibly evidenced by:	Altered sleep cycle; initial signs of insomnia and then hypersomnia.
	Constant alertness; racing thoughts that prevent rest.
	Denial of need to sleep or reports of inability to stay awake.
DESIRED OUTCOMES/ EVALUATION CRITERIA— PATIENT WILL:	Sleep 6 to 8 hours at night.
	Rest minimally, appropriately, during the day.
	Verbalize feeling rested when awakens.

ACTIONS/INTERVENTIONS

Independent

Establish sleep cycle in which patient sleeps at night, is awake during day with brief rest periods as needed.

Decrease external stimuli and enhance relaxation prior to bedtime; encourage use of presleep routines, e.g., hot bath, warm milk, stretching.

Provide opportunities for fresh air, mild exercise, noncaffeinated beverages, quiet environment as patient can tolerate.

RATIONALE

Adequate rest and sleep can improve emotional state. Restoration of regular pattern is a priority in a sleep-deprived stimulant user.

Patient may need calming in order to attempt rest.

Promotes drowsiness/desire for sleep.

Depressants (Benzodiazepines, Barbiturates, Opioids): Intoxication/Overdose _____

CNS depressants are drugs that slow down the central nervous system. They are usually divided into 4 types: barbiturates, tranquilizers, sedative-hypnotics, and narcotics (e.g., morphine, heroin).

CNS depressants prescribed for symptoms of anxiety, depression, and sleep disturbances are among the most widely used and abused drugs. These drugs are very likely to be abused when the underlying conditions remain untreated. Sometimes these drugs are used in conjunction with stimulants, with the user developing a pattern of taking a stimulant to be "up," then needing the depressant drug to "come down."

Several principles apply to all CNS depressants: (1) The effects are interactive and cumulative with one another and with the behavioral state of the user; (2) there is no specific antagonist that will specifically block the action of these drugs; (3) low doses produce an initial excitatory response; (4) they are capable of producing physiologic and psychologic dependency; and (5) cross-tolerance and cross-dependence may exist between various CNS depressants. While the margin of safety of these drugs is great, they have a characteristic syndrome of withdrawal that can be very severe.

RELATED CONCERNS:

Stimulants, p 983
Substance Dependence/Abuse Rehabilitation, p 1000
Pneumonia, Microbial, p 162
Psychosocial Aspects of Acute Care, p 899

PATIENT ASSESSMENT DATA BASE

Data are dependent on stage of withdrawal and concurrent use of alcohol/other drugs.

ACTIVITY/REST

May report:	Interference with sleep pattern.
	General malaise.
May exhibit:	Lethargy, drowsiness, somnolence.

CIRCULATION

May exhibit:	Tachycardia (suggests withdrawal syndrome); atrial fibrillation, ventricular dysrhythmias.
	Hypotension.

EGO INTEGRITY

May report:	Substance use for stress management.
	Feelings of helplessness, hopelessness, powerlessness.
May exhibit:	Underdeveloped ego; highly dependent nature, with characteristics of poor impulse control, low frustration tolerance, and low self-esteem.
	Weak superego, with absence of guilt feelings.
	Psychostructural factors (e.g., personality) are seen as significant with substance use/abuse (maladaptive coping mechanisms).

ELIMINATION

May report:	Diarrhea, occassionally constipation.

FOOD/FLUID

May report: Nausea.

May exhibit: Vomiting.

NEUROSENSORY

May report: Twitching.

May exhibit: Mental status: Confusion, concentration and memory problems; impaired judgment with some affective change; alterations in consciousness, from extreme agitation to coma.

Behavior: Mood swings, lack of motivation, aggression, combativeness (related to general "disinhibiting" effect of the drug, loss of impulse control).

Temporary psychosis with acute onset of auditory hallucinations and paranoid delusions (unexplained neuropsychiatric presentation may be indicative of drug use).

Psychomotor activity increased.

Hypersensitivity, e.g., anxiety, tremors, hypotension, irritability, restlessness, and seizures.

Pupils small/pinpoint constriction (opiates), dilated (barbiturates).

Gait unsteady/staggering, loss of coordination; positive Romberg's sign.

Slurred speech.

PAIN/COMFORT

May report: Headache, abdominal pain/severe cramping.

Muscle aches.

Deep muscle/bone pain (methadone abusers).

RESPIRATION

May report: Continued rhinorrhea, excessive lacrimation, sneezing.

May exhibit: Respiratory depression (noted in overdose).

Increased rate (withdrawal syndrome).

SAFETY

May report: Hot/cold flashes.

May exhibit: Thermoregulation instability with hyperpyrexia, hypothermia.

Skin: Piloerection ("gooseflesh"); puncture wounds on arms, hands, legs, under tongue, indicating IV drug use.

SOCIAL INTERACTION

May report: Dysfunctional family of origin system.

History from family member/SO(s) may reveal dysfunctional patterns of interaction.

TEACHING/LEARNING

May report: Preexisting physical/psychologic conditions.

Family history of substance use/abuse.

History of chronic condition/disease process.

Discharge Plan Considerations: **DRG projected mean length of stay: 4.5 days.**

May need assistance to maintain abstinence and begin to participate in rehabilitation program.

DIAGNOSTIC STUDIES

Drug screen: Identifies drug(s) being used.

STD screening: To determine presence of HIV, hepatitis B, and so on.

ASI: Produces a "problem severity profile," which indicates areas of treatment needs.

NURSING PRIORITIES

1. Promote physiologic stability.
2. Protect patient from injury.
3. Provide appropriate referral and follow-up.
4. Promote family involvement in the withdrawal/rehabilitation process.
5. Provide information about dependency/prognosis and treatment needs.

DISCHARGE GOALS

1. Homeostasis achieved.
2. Complications prevented/resolved.
3. Abstinence from drug(s) initiated/maintained.
4. Transferred to rehabilitation program/attending group therapy, e.g., Narcotics Anonymous.
5. Dependency condition, prognosis, and therapeutic regimen understood.

NURSING DIAGNOSIS:	**TRAUMA/SUFFOCATION/POISONING, HIGH RISK FOR**
Risk factors may include:	CNS depression (effect of overdose).
	CNS agitation (effect of abrupt withdrawal).
	Hypersensitivity to the drug(s).
	Psychologic stress (narrowed perceptual fields seen with anxiety).
Possibly evidenced by:	[Not applicable; presence of signs and symptoms establishes an actual diagnosis.]
DESIRED OUTCOMES/ EVALUATION CRITERIA— PATIENT WILL:	Verbalize understanding of risks of taking drugs.
	Refrain from acting on hallucinations/impaired judgment.
	Complete withdrawal without injury to self/development of complications.

ACTIONS/INTERVENTIONS	RATIONALE
Independent	
Determine degree of impairment by talking to patient/SO, noting when person was last seen well; also note sleep patterns and duration of problems.	Information provides an approximate time frame for impairment, with sleep disruption often the first observable sign of a problem. Prescription infor-

995

ACTIONS/INTERVENTIONS

Independent

Identify drug(s) taken, when taken, and route used if possible.

Assess level of consciousness, e.g., agitated, stuporous, lethargic, confused, or unconscious. Note pinpoint pupils.

Evaluate for evidence of head trauma.

Determine when food was last eaten. Note reports of nausea.

Monitor temperature as indicated. Observe for signs of dehydration.

Monitor BP, pulse, respirations.

Provide quiet, lighted room e.g., an isolation room with simple furniture.

Observe patient at all times; use staff or family member as available.

Reorient to surroundings and circumstances as needed.

Note presence of tremors.

Provide seizure precautions, e.g., padded side rails, bed in low position, airway adjunct/suction at bedside.

Note changes in behavior indicative of psychosis, e.g., distorted reality, altered mood, impaired language and memory.

Assess emotional state, noting psychiatric history and suicide gestures/attempts. Note use/abuse of other substances.

Determine history of hallucinations.

RATIONALE

mation provides clues to identify drug(s) and amount taken.

Helpful to identify interventions for specific drug. Determining drug(s) taken may be difficult outside of blood/urine testing because the patient may not feel free to tell because of embarrassment or for legal reasons, or may not know what has been ingested.

May be indicator of degree of intoxication and level of intervention required. Constricted pupils are a classic sign of opioid (heroin) use.

Important for differential diagnosis to prevent incorrect treatment/interventions.

Presence of food in the stomach may slow absorption of drug(s) into the bloodstream; however, if level of consciousness is depressed, the risk of vomiting and aspiration is increased.

Hypothermia may be seen in intoxication, while hyperpyrexia may occur with withdrawal or indicate infectious process. *Note:* Dehydration often accompanies hyperpyrexia, requiring additional intervention/fluid replacement.

Changes depend on drug taken, e.g., diazepam (Valium) may be evidenced by hypotension, tachycardia.

Reduces stimuli, internal or external, that may lead to injury as the patient responds.

Patient with varying level of consciousness should not be left alone because of the danger of accidental injury.

Maintaining contact provides reassurance, reduces anxiety when consciousness returns.

Involuntary movements of one or more parts of the body may result from abrupt removal of drug.

Precautions can prevent injury if seizures occur during withdrawal.

Drug intoxication can precipitate altered perceptions/psychotic behavior.

Patterns of drug use will indicate likelihood of intentional or accidental overdose. Substance abuse/suicide attempts may be symptom of or response to underlying psychiatric illness or to hallucinations caused by sensitivity to drug.

May be auditory, visual, tactile, and very frightening. May also trigger suicidal/homicidal behavior.

ACTIONS/INTERVENTIONS	RATIONALE
Independent	
Institute suicide precautions, as indicated.	May need environmental restraints to protect patient until own coping abilities improve and internal locus of control is regained.
Collaborative	
Start/maintain IV line.	Provides easy access for emergency treatment.
Administer 50% glucose IV with thiamine added.	Acute thiamine deficiency and hypoglycemia may mimic drug intoxication if patient is comatose.
Assist with gastric lavage if indicated.	May be done when drug has been recently ingested, or when consciousness is depressed making vomiting hazardous, or when induced emesis has failed.
Administer medication per current treatment/protocol:	
Emetics, e.g., apomorphine, syrup of ipecac;	Induced vomiting is an efficient and effective way to empty the stomach when the patient is fully conscious. It is of questionable value unless performed very soon after drug ingestion because of rapid GI absorption.
Activated charcoal;	Binds with many substances in the GI tract, reducing absorption of ingested drug(s).
Phenobarbital;	Prolonged effect provides smoother sedation for agitated patient without "high" of more rapidly acting drugs, and also has an anticonvulsant effect.
Methadone.	Replaces heroin or other narcotic analgesics in detoxification program, reducing/minimizing withdrawal symptoms.
Assist with barbiturate detoxification program.	Reintoxication should be done before drug withdrawal is attempted. This establishes an independent estimate of prior drug use and provides a baseline to begin the detoxification schedule. Reintoxication is done so the drug can be withdrawn on a strict schedule and should begin as soon as there are signs of abstinence syndrome e.g., nystagmus, slurred speech, ataxia on backward and frontward tandem gait.
Prepare for/assist with dialysis if indicated.	Occasionally effective for clearance of toxic/lethal levels of phenobarbital.
Refer to rehabilitation program, involve in "Intervention" (confrontation) and/or therapy as indicated.	Patient will need ongoing assistance to acknowledge and maintain drug-free existence.

NURSING DIAGNOSIS:	**BREATHING PATTERN, INEFFECTIVE/GAS EXCHANGE, IMPAIRED, HIGH RISK FOR**
Risk factors may include:	Neuromuscular impairment.

	Decreased energy/fatigue.
	Inflammatory process.
	Decreased lung expansion.
Possibly evidenced by:	[Not applicable; presence of signs and symptoms establishes an actual diagnosis.]
DESIRED OUTCOMES/ EVALUATION CRITERIA— PATIENT WILL:	Establish normal/effective breathing pattern with absence of cyanosis/symptoms of respiratory distress.

ACTIONS/INTERVENTIONS	RATIONALE
Independent	
Monitor respiratory rate, depth, rhythm, and breath sounds.	Sedative/depressant effects on CNS may result in loss of airway patency and/or respiratory depression. Prompt treatment is necessary to prevent respiratory arrest. *Note:* Acute pulmonary edema is a common complication in heroin overdose/intoxication.
Have suction equipment/airway adjuncts available.	Sedative effects of drugs, increased salivation, and vomiting potentiate risk of aspiration. Relaxation of oropharyngeal muscles and respiratory depression require prompt intervention to prevent respiratory arrest.
Collaborative	
Administer medications as indicated, e.g., naloxone (Narcan).	Narcotic antagonist that can reverse effects of respiratory depression in opioid intoxication. *Note:* May trigger acute withdrawal syndrome.
Provide supplemental oxygen.	May be necessary to improve oxygen intake in presence of respiratory depression.
Review chest x-ray.	Common complications of depressant (opiate) abuse include pneumonia, aspiration pneumonitis, lung abscess, atelectasis, which will require specific treatment.
Monitor ABGs/pulse oximetry, pulmonary function studies when indicated.	Chronic addiction may result in decreased vital capacity and pulmonary diffusion, affecting gas exchange. Presence of septic pulmonary emboli or pulmonary fibrosis (from talc granulomatosis occurring in IV drug abuse) may further compromise respiratory function.

NURSING DIAGNOSIS:	**INFECTION, HIGH RISK FOR**
Risk factors may include:	IV drug use techniques; impurities in injected drugs.

Localized trauma.

Malnutrition; altered immune state.

Possibly evidenced by: [Not applicable; presence of signs and symptoms establishes an actual diagnosis.]

DESIRED OUTCOMES/ EVALUATION CRITERIA— PATIENT WILL: Verbalize understanding of and demonstrate lifestyle changes to reduce risk factor(s).

Achieve timely healing of infectious process if present or develops, and be afebrile.

ACTIONS/INTERVENTIONS	RATIONALE

Independent

Refer to CP: Stimulants, ND: Infection, high risk for, p 991 for interventions specific to this nursing diagnosis.

Substance Dependence/Abuse Rehabilitation _____

This disorder is a continuum of phases incorporating a cluster of cognitive, behavioral, and physiologic symptoms that include loss of control over use of the substance and a continued use of the substance despite adverse consequences. A number of factors have been implicated in the predisposition to abuse substances, e.g., biologic, biochemical, psychologic (including developmental), personality, sociocultural and conditioning, cultural and ethnic influences. However, no single theory adequately explains the etiology of this problem.

Alcohol; amphetamines or similarly acting sympathomimetics; cannabis, cocaine, hallucinogens, barbiturates, opioids; sedatives/hypnotics/anxiolytics are drugs that are subject to abuse.

RELATED CONCERNS

Alcoholism, p 960
Depressants, p 993
Hallucinogens, p 972
Psychosocial Aspects of Acute Care, p 899
Stimulants, p 983

PATIENT ASSESSMENT DATA BASE

Refer to appropriate acute CP as indicated.

TEACHING/LEARNING

Discharge Plan Considerations: **DRG projected mean length of stay: 13.5 days.**
May need assistance with long-range plan for recovery.

DIAGNOSTIC STUDIES

ASI assessment tool: Produces a "problem severity profile" of the patient, including chemical, medical, psychologic, legal, family/social and employment/support aspects, indicating areas of treatment needs.

NURSING PRIORITIES

1. Provide support for decision to stop substance use.
2. Strengthen individual coping skills.
3. Facilitate learning of new ways to reduce anxiety.
4. Promote family involvement in rehabilitation program.
5. Facilitate family growth/development.
6. Provide information about condition, prognosis, and treatment needs.

DISCHARGE GOALS

1. Responsibility for own life and behavior assumed.
2. Plan to maintain substance-free life formulated.
3. Family relationships/codependency issues being addressed.
4. Treatment program successfully begun.
5. Condition, prognosis, and therapeutic regimen understood.

NURSING DIAGNOSIS:	DENIAL/COPING, INDIVIDUAL, INEFFECTIVE
	Personal vulnerability; difficulty handling new situations.
May be related to:	Previous ineffective/inadequate coping skills with substitution of drug(s).
	Anxiety/fear.
Possibly evidenced by:	Denial (one of the strongest and most resistant symptoms of substance abuse); lack of acceptance that drug use is causing the present situation.
	Use of manipulation to avoid responsibility for self.
	Altered social patterns/participation.
	Impaired adaptive behavior and problem-solving skills.
	Decreased ability to handle stress of illness/hospitalization.
	Financial affairs in disarray; employment difficulties e.g., losing time on job/not maintaining steady employment, poor work performance, on-the-job injuries.
DESIRED OUTCOMES/ EVALUATION CRITERIA— PATIENT WILL:	Verbalize awareness of relationship of substance abuse to current situation.
	Identify ineffective coping behaviors/consequences.
	Use effective coping skills/problem solving.
	Initiate necessary lifestyle changes.
	Attend support group (e.g., Cocaine/Narcotics/Alcoholics Anonymous) regularly.

ACTIONS/INTERVENTIONS	RATIONALE
Independent	
Ascertain what name patient would like to be addressed by.	Shows courtesy and respect. Gives sense of orientation and control.
Determine understanding of current situation and previous/other methods of coping with life's problems.	Provides information about degree of denial; identifies coping skills that may be used in present plan of care.
Confront and examine denial in peer group.	Because denial is the major defense mechanism in addictive disease, confrontation by peers can help the patient accept the reality that drug use is a major problem.
Remain nonjudgmental. Be alert to changes in behavior, e.g., restlessness, increased tension.	Confrontation can lead to increased agitation, which may compromise safety of patient/staff.
Provide positive feedback for expressing awareness of denial in self/others.	Positive feedback is necessary to enhance self-esteem and to reinforce insight into behavior.

1001

ACTIONS/INTERVENTIONS	RATIONALE
Independent	
Maintain firm expectation that patient attend recovery support/therapy groups regularly.	Attending is related to admitting need for help, to working with denial, and for maintenance of a long-term drug-free existence.
Structure diversional activity that relates to recovery (e.g., social activity within support group) wherein issues of being chemically free are examined.	Discovery of alternative methods of recreation and for coping with drug hunger can remind patient that addiction is a lifelong process and opportunity for changing patterns is available.
Use peer support to examine ways of coping with drug hunger.	Addictive self-help groups are valuable for learning and promoting abstinence in each member with understanding and support as well as peer pressure.
Provide information about addictive use versus experimental, occasional use; biochemical/genetic disorder theory (genetic predisposition); use activated by environment; pharmacology of stimulant; compulsive desire as a lifelong occurrence.	Progression of use continuum in the addict is from experimental/recreational to addictive use. Comprehending this process is important in combating denial. Education may relieve patient of guilt and blame, may help awareness of recurring addictive characteristics.
Encourage and support patient's taking responsibility for own recovery (e.g., development of alternative behaviors to drug use). Assist patient to learn own responsibility for recovering.	Denial can be replaced with responsible action when patient accepts the reality of own responsibility.
Set limits and confront efforts to get care giver to grant special privileges, making excuses for not following through on behaviors agreed on and attempting to continue drug use.	Patient has learned manipulative behavior throughout life and needs to learn a new way of getting needs met. Following through on consequences of failure to maintain limits can help the patient to change ineffective behaviors.
Assist patient to learn/encourage use of relaxation skills, guided imagery, visualizations.	Helps patient to relax, develop new ways to deal with stress, problem-solve.
Be aware of staff enabling behaviors and feelings.	Lack of understanding of enabling and codependence can result in nontherapeutic approaches to addicts.
Collaborative	
Administer medications as indicated, e.g.:	
disulfiram (Antabuse);	This drug can be helpful in maintaining abstinence from alcohol while other therapy is undertaken. By inhibiting alcohol oxidation, the drug leads to an accumulation of acetaldehyde with a highly unpleasant reaction if alcohol is consumed.
Methadone.	This drug is thought to blunt the craving for/diminish the effects of heroin and is used to assist in withdrawal and long-term maintenance programs. It has fewer side effects and allows the individual to maintain daily activities and ultimately withdraw from drug use.
Encourage involvement with self-help associations, e.g., Alcoholics/Narcotics Anonymous.	Puts patient in direct contact with support systems necessary for managing sobriety/drug-free life.

NURSING DIAGNOSIS:	**POWERLESSNESS**
May be related to:	Substance addiction with/without periods of abstinence.
	Episodic compulsive indulgence; attempts at recovery.
	Lifestyle of helplessness.
Possibly evidenced by:	Ineffective recovery attempts; statements of inability to stop behavior/requests for help.
	Continuous/constant thinking about drug and/or obtaining drug.
	Alteration in personal, occupational, and social life.
DESIRED OUTCOMES/ EVALUATION CRITERIA— PATIENT WILL:	Admit inability to control drug habit, surrender to powerlessness over addiction.
	Verbalize acceptance of need for treatment and awareness that willpower alone cannot control abstinence.
	Engage in peer support.
	Demonstrate active participation in program.
	Regain and maintain healthy state with a drug-free lifestyle.

ACTIONS/INTERVENTIONS	RATIONALE
Independent	
Use crisis intervention techniques:	Patient is more amenable to acceptance of need for treatment at this time.
Assist patient to recognize problem exists;	While patient is hurting, it is easier to admit drug(s) is a problem.
Identify goals for change;	Helpful in planning direction for care, promoting belief that change can occur.
Discuss alternative solutions;	Brainstorming helps creatively identify possibilities and provides sense of control.
Assist in selecting most appropriate alternative;	As possibilities are discussed, the most useful solution becomes clear.
Support decision and implementation of selected alternative(s).	Helps the patient to persevere in process of change.
Discuss need for help in a caring, nonjudgmental way.	A caring confrontive manner is more therapeutic because the patient may respond defensively to a moralistic attitude, blocking recovery.
Discuss ways in which drug has interfered with life occupation, personal/interpersonal relationships.	Awareness of how the drug has controlled life is important in combatting denial/sense of powerlessness.

1003

ACTIONS/INTERVENTIONS	RATIONALE

Independent

Explore support in peer group. Encourage sharing about drug hunger, situations that increase the desire to indulge, ways that substance has influenced life.

May need assistance in expressing self, speaking about powerlessness, admitting need for help in order to face up to problem and begin resolution.

Assist patient to learn ways to enhance health and structure healthy diversion from drug use, e.g., a balanced diet, adequate rest, acupuncture, biofeedback, deep meditative techniques, exercise (e.g., walking, slow/long distance running).

Learning to empower self in constructive areas can strengthen ability to continue recovery. These activities help restore natural biochemical balance, aid detoxification, and manage stress, anxiety, use of free time. These diversions can increase self-confidence, thereby improving self-esteem. *Note: Release of endorphins from lengthy exercise can create a feeling of well-being.*

Assist patient in self-examination of spirituality, faith.

Surrendering to and faith in a power greater than oneself has been found to be effective in substance recovery; may decrease sense of powerlessness.

Assist patient to learn assertive communication.

Effective in assisting in ability to refuse use, to stop relationships with users and dealers, to build healthy relationships, regain control of own life.

Provide treatment information on an ongoing basis.

Helps patient know what to expect. Creates opportunity for patient to be a part of what is happening and make informed choices about participation/outcomes.

Collaborative

Refer to/assist with making appointment to treatment program for continuation after discharge, e.g., partial hospitalization drug treatment programs, Narcotics/Alcoholics Anonymous.

Follow-through on appointments may be easier than making the initial contact, and continuing treatment is essential to positive outcome.

NURSING DIAGNOSIS:	NUTRITION, ALTERED: LESS THAN BODY REQUIREMENTS
May be related to:	Insufficient dietary intake to meet metabolic needs for psychologic, physiologic, or economic reasons.
Possibly evidenced by:	Weight loss; weight less than norm for height/body build; decreased subcutaneous fat/muscle mass.
	Reported altered taste sensation; lack of interest in food.
	Poor muscle tone.
	Sore, inflamed buccal cavity.
	Laboratory evidence of protein/vitamin deficiencies.

DESIRED OUTCOMES/ EVALUATION CRITERIA— PATIENT WILL:	Demonstrate progressive weight gain toward goal with normalization of laboratory values and absence of signs of malnutrition.
	Verbalize understanding of effects of substance abuse, reduced dietary intake on nutritional status.
	Demonstrate behaviors, lifestyle changes to regain and maintain appropriate weight.

ACTIONS/INTERVENTIONS	RATIONALE

Independent

Assess height/weight, age, body build, strength, activity/rest level. Note condition of oral cavity.	Provides information about individual on which to base caloric needs/dietary plan. Type of diet/foods may be affected by condition of mucous membranes and teeth.
Take anthropometric measurements e.g., triceps skinfold.	Calculates subcutaneous fat and muscle mass to aid in determining dietary needs.
Note total daily calorie intake; maintain a diary of intake, times, and patterns of eating.	Information about patient's dietary pattern will identify nutritional needs/deficiencies.
Evaluate energy expenditure (e.g., pacing or sedentary), and establish an individualized exercise program.	Activity level affects nutritional needs. Exercise enhances muscle tone, may stimulate appetite.
Provide opportunity to choose foods/snacks to meet dietary plan.	Enhances participation/sense of control and may promote resolution of nutritional deficiencies.
Weigh weekly and record.	Provides information regarding effectiveness of dietary plan.

Collaborative

Consult with dietitian.	Useful in establishing individual dietary needs/ plan. Provides additional resource for learning.
Review laboratory work as indicated, e.g., glucose, serum albumin, electrolytes.	Identifies anemias, electrolyte imbalances, other abnormalities that may be present, requiring specific therapy.
Refer for dental consultation as necessary.	Teeth are essential to good nutritional intake and dental hygiene/care is often a neglected area in this population.

NURSING DIAGNOSIS:	SELF-ESTEEM, DISTURBANCE/SITUATIONAL LOW
May be related to:	Social stigma attached to substance abuse.
	Social expectation that one control behavior.
	Biochemical body change (e.g., withdrawal from alcohol/other drugs).
	Situational crisis with loss of control over life events.

Possibly evidenced by:	Not taking responsibility for self/self-care; lack of follow-through.
	Self-destructive behavior.
	Change in usual role patterns or responsibility (family, job, legal).
	Confusion about self, purpose or direction in life.
	Denial that substance use is a problem.
DESIRED OUTCOMES/ EVALUATION CRITERIA— PATIENT WILL:	Identify feelings and methods for coping with negative perception of self.
	Verbalize acceptance of self as is and an increased sense of self-esteem.
	Set goals and participate in realistic planning for lifestyle changes necessary to live without drugs.

ACTIONS/INTERVENTIONS	RATIONALE
Independent	
Provide opportunity for and encourage verbalization/discussion of individual situation.	Patient often has difficulty expressing self, even more difficulty accepting the degree of importance substance has assumed in life and its relationship to present situation.
Assess mental status. Note presence of other psychiatric disorders (dual diagnosis).	Many patients use substances (alcohol and other drugs) to seek relief from depression or anxiety. *Note:* Approximately 60% of substance-dependent patients also have mental illness problems, and there is an increasing awareness that treatment for both is imperative.
Spend time with patient. Discuss patient's behavior/use of substance in a nonjudgmental way.	Presence of the nurse conveys acceptance of the individual as a worthwhile person. Discussion provides opportunity for insight into the problems abuse has created for the patient.
Provide reinforcement for positive actions and encourage patient to accept this input.	Failure and lack of self-esteem have been problems for this patient, who needs to learn to accept self as an individual with positive attributes.
Observe family interactions, SO dynamics/support.	Substance abuse is a family disease, and how the members act and react to the patient's behavior affects the course of the disease and how patient sees self. Many unconsciously become "enablers," helping the individual to cover up the consequences of the abuse. (Refer to ND: Family Coping, Ineffective, Compromised/Disabling, p 1007.)
Encourage expression of feelings of guilt, shame, and anger.	The patient often has lost respect for self and believes that the situation is hopeless. Expression of these feelings helps the patient to begin to accept responsibility for self and take steps to make changes.

ACTIONS/INTERVENTIONS	RATIONALE

Independent

Help the patient to acknowledge that substance use is the problem and that problems can be dealt with without the use of drugs. Confront the use of defenses, e.g., denial, projection, rationalization.

When drugs can no longer be blamed for the problems that exist, the patient can begin to deal with the problems and live without substance use. Confrontation helps the patient accept the reality of the problems as they exist.

Ask the patient to list and review past accomplishments and positive happenings.

There are things in everyone's life that have been successful. Often when self-esteem is low, it is difficult to remember these successes or to view them as successes.

Use techniques of role rehearsal.

Assists patient to practice the development of skills to cope with new role as a person who no longer uses or needs drugs to handle life's problems.

Collaborative

Involve in group therapy.

Group sharing helps encourage verbalization as other members of group are in various stages of abstinence from drugs and can address the patient's concerns/denial. The patient can gain new skills, hope, and a sense of family/community from group participation.

Refer to other resources, such as Narcotics/Alcoholics Anonymous.

One of the oldest and most popular forms of group treatment, which uses a basic strategy known as the Twelve Steps. The patient admits powerlessness over drug, and, although not necessary, may seek help from a "higher power." Members help one another, and meetings are available at many different times and places in most communities. The philosophy of "one day at a time" helps attain the goal of abstinence.

Formulate plan to treat other mental illness problems.

Patients who seek relief for other mental health problems through drugs will continue to do so once discharged. Both the substance use and the mental health problems need to be treated together to maximize abstinence potential.

Administer antipsychotic medications as necessary.

Prolonged/profound psychosis following LSD or PCP use can be treated with these drugs as it is probably the result of an underlying functional psychosis that has now emerged. *Note:* Avoid the use of phenothiazines as they may decrease seizure threshold and cause hypotension in the presence of LSD/PCP.

NURSING DIAGNOSIS:	FAMILY COPING, INEFFECTIVE: COMPROMISED/DISABLING/CAREGIVER ROLE STRAIN
May be related to:	Personal vulnerability of individual family members; codependency issues.

1007

Situational crises.

Compromised social systems; family disorganization/role changes.

Prolonged disease progression that exhausts supportive capability of family members.

SO(s) with chronically unexpressed feelings of guilt, anger, hostility, despair.

Possibly evidenced by: Denial (one of the strongest and most resistant symptoms); lack of acceptance that drinking/drug use is causing the present situation, or belief that all problems are due to substance use.

Severely dysfunctional family, e.g., family violence, spouse/child abuse, separation/divorce, children displaying acting-out behaviors.

Financial affairs in disarray; employment difficulties.

Altered social patterns/participation.

SO demonstrating enabling or codependent behaviors, e.g., avoiding and shielding, attempting to control, taking over responsibilities, rationalizing and accepting, cooperating and collaborating, rescuing and subserving.

DESIRED OUTCOMES/ EVALUATION CRITERIA— FAMILY WILL: Verbalize understanding of dynamics of codependence and participate in individual and family programs.

Identify ineffective coping behaviors/consequences.

Demonstrate/plan for necessary lifestyle changes.

Take action to change self-destructive behaviors/alter behavior that contributes to partner's/SO's addiction.

ACTIONS/INTERVENTIONS	RATIONALE
Independent	
Assess family history; explore roles of family members, circumstances involving drug use, strengths, areas for growth.	Determines areas for focus, potential for change.
Explore how the SO has coped with the addict's habit, e.g., denial, repression, rationalization, hurt, loneliness, projection.	The codependent person also suffers from the same feelings as the patient (e.g., anxiety, self-hatred, helplessness, low self-worth, guilt) and needs help in learning new/effective coping skills.
Determine understanding of current situation and previous methods of coping with life's problems.	Provides information on which to base present plan of care.
Assess current level of functioning of family members.	Affects individual's ability to cope with situation.

ACTIONS/INTERVENTIONS	RATIONALE
Independent	
Determine extent of "enabling" behaviors being evidenced by family members; explore with individual and patient.	"Enabling" is doing for the patient what s/he needs to do for self. People want to be helpful and do not want to feel powerless to help their loved one to stop drinking and change the behavior that is so destructive. However, the substance abuser often does rely on others to cover up own inability to cope with daily responsibilities.
Provide information about enabling behavior, addictive disease characteristics for both user and nonuser person who is codependent.	Awareness and knowledge provide opportunity for individuals to begin the process of change.
Provide factual information to patient and family about the effects of addictive behaviors on the family and what to expect after discharge.	Many patients/SOs are not aware of the nature of addiction. If patient is using legally obtained drugs, may believe this does not constitute abuse.
Encourage SOs to be aware of their own feelings, look at the situation with perspective and objectivity. They can ask themselves: "Am I being conned? Am I acting out of fear, shame, guilt, or anger? Do I have a need to control?"	When the codependent family members become aware of their own actions that perpetuate the addict's problems, they need to decide to change themselves. If they change, the patient can then face the consequences of the patient's own actions and may choose to get well.
Provide support for partner(s) who are codependent. Encourage group work.	Families/SOs need support as much as the person who is addicted in order to produce change.
Assist the partner who is codependent to become aware that patient's abstinence and drug use is not the partner's responsibility.	Partners need to learn that user's habit may or may not change despite partner's involvement in treatment.
Help the recovering (former user) person who is codependent to distinguish between destructive aspects of enabling behavior and genuine motivation to aid the user.	Enabling behavior can be partner's attempts at personal survival.
Note how the partner who is codependent relates to the treatment team/staff.	Determines enabling style. A parallel exists between how partner relates to user and to staff, based on partner's feelings about self and situation.
Assess conflicting feelings the person who is codependent may have about treatment, e.g., feelings similar to those of abuser (blend of anger, guilt, fear, exhaustion, embarrassment, loneliness, distrust, grief, and possibly relief).	Useful in establishing the need for therapy for the person who is codependent. This person's own identity may have been lost, s/he may fear self-disclosure to staff, and may have difficulty giving up the dependent relationship.
Involve SO in discharge referral plans.	Drug abuse is a family illness. Because the family has been so involved in dealing with the substance abuse behavior, they need help adjusting to the new behavior of sobriety/abstinence. Incidence of recovery is almost doubled when the family is treated along with the patient.
Be aware of staff's enabling behaviors and feelings about patient, and partners who are codependent.	Lack of understanding of enabling and codependence can result in nontherapeutic approaches to addicts and their families.

1009

ACTIONS/INTERVENTIONS

Collaborative

Encourage involvement with self-help associations, Alcoholics/Narcotics Anonymous, Al-Anon, Al-A-teen, and professional family therapy.

RATIONALE

Puts patient/family in direct contact with support systems necessary for continued sobriety and to assist with problem resolution.

NURSING DIAGNOSIS:	SEXUAL DYSFUNCTION
May be related to:	Altered body function: neurologic damage and debilitating effects of drug use (particularly alcohol and opiates).
Possibly evidenced by:	Progressive interference with sexual functioning.
	In men: A significant degree of testicular atrophy is noted (testes are smaller and softer than normal); gynecomastia (breast enlargement); impotence/decreased sperm counts.
	In women: Loss of body hair, thin soft skin, and spider angioma (elevated estrogen); amenorrhea/increase in miscarriages.
DESIRED OUTCOMES/ EVALUATION CRITERIA— PATIENT WILL:	Verbally acknowledge effects of drug use on sexual functioning/reproduction.
	Identify interventions to correct/overcome individual situation.

ACTIONS/INTERVENTIONS

Independent

Assess patient's current information and have patient describe problem in own words.

Encourage and accept individual expressions of concern.

Provide education opportunity (e.g., pamphlets, consultation from appropriate persons) for patient to learn effects of drug on sexual functioning.

Provide information about individual's condition.

Provide information about effects of drugs on the reproductive system/fetus (e.g., increased risk of

RATIONALE

Determines level of knowledge, what patient perceives own needs are.

Most people find it difficult to talk about this sensitive subject and may not ask directly for information.

Much of denial and hesitancy to seek treatment may be reduced as a result of sufficient and appropriate information.

Sexual functioning may have been affected by drug (alcohol) intake, physiologic and/or psychologic factors (such as stress). Information will assist patient to understand own situation and identify actions to be taken.

Awareness of the negative effects of alcohol/other drugs on reproduction may motivate patient to

ACTIONS/INTERVENTIONS

Independent

premature birth, brain damage and fetal malformation). Assess drinking/drug history of pregnant patient.

Discuss prognosis for sexual dysfunction, e.g., impotence/low sexual desire.

Collaborative

Refer for sexual counseling, if indicated.

Review results of sonogram if pregnant.

RATIONALE

stop using drug(s). When patient is pregnant, identification of potential problems aids in planning for future fetal needs/concerns.

In about 50% of cases, impotence is reversed with abstinence from drug(s); in 25% the return to normal functioning is delayed; and approximately 25% remain impotent.

Patient may need additional assistance to resolve more severe problems/situations. Patient may have difficulty adjusting if drug has improved sexual experience (e.g., heroin decreases dyspareunia in women/premature ejaculation in men). Further, the patient may have engaged enjoyably in bizarre erotic and sexual behavior under influence of the stimulant drug; patient may have found no substitute for the drug, may have driven a partner away, and may have no motivation to adjust to sexual experience without drugs.

Assesses fetal growth and development to identify possibility of fetal alcohol syndrome and future needs.

NURSING DIAGNOSIS:	KNOWLEDGE DEFICIT [LEARNING NEED] REGARDING CONDITION, PROGNOSIS, AND TREATMENT NEEDS
May be related to:	Lack of information; information misinterpretation.
	Cognitive limitations/interference with learning (other mental illness problems/organic brain syndrome); lack of recall.
Possibly evidenced by:	Statements of concern; questions/misconceptions.
	Inaccurate follow-through of instructions/development of preventable complications.
	Continued use in spite of complications/bad trips.
DESIRED OUTCOMES/ EVALUATION CRITERIA— PATIENT WILL:	Verbalize understanding of own condition/disease process, prognosis, and treatment plan.
	Identify/initiate necessary lifestyle changes to remain drug-free.
	Participate in treatment program.

ACTIONS/INTERVENTIONS	RATIONALE
Independent	
Be aware of and deal with anxiety of patient and family members.	Anxiety can interfere with ability to hear and assimilate information.
Provide an active role for the patient/SO in the learning process, e.g., discussions, group participation, role playing.	Learning is enhanced when persons are actively involved.
Provide written and verbal information as indicated. Include list of articles and books related to patient/family needs and encourage reading and discussing what they learn.	Helps patient/SO to make informed choices about future. Bibliotherapy can be a useful addition to other therapy approaches.
Assess patient's knowledge of own situation, e.g., disease, complications, and needed changes in lifestyle.	Assists in planning for long-range changes necessary for maintaining sobriety/drug-free status. Patient may have street knowledge of the drug but be ignorant of medical facts.
Review condition and prognosis/future expectations.	Provides knowledge base on which patient can make informed choices.
Time activities to individual needs.	Facilitates learning as information is more readily assimilated when pacing is considered.
Discuss relationship of drug use to current situation.	Often patient has misperception (denial) of real reason for admission to the medical (psychiatric) setting.
Discuss effects of drug(s) used, e.g., PCP is deposited in body fat and may reactivate (flashbacks) even after long interval of abstinence; alcohol use may result in mental deterioration, liver involvement/damage; cocaine can damage post-capillary vessels, increase platelet aggregation, promoting thromboses and infarction of skin/internal organs, causing localized atrophie blanche or sclerodermatous lesions.	Information will help patient understand possible long-term effects of drug use.
Discuss potential for reemergence of withdrawal symptoms in stimulant abuse as early as 3 months or as late as 9–12 months.	While symptoms of intoxication may have passed, patient may manifest denial, drug hunger, periods of "flare up" wherein there is a delayed recurrence of withdrawal symptoms, e.g., anxiety, depression, irritability, sleep disturbance, compulsiveness with food (especially sugars).
Inform patient of effects of Antabuse with alcohol intake and importance of avoiding use of alcohol-containing products, e.g., cough syrups or foods/candy.	Interaction of alcohol and Antabuse results in nausea and hypotension, which may produce fatal shock. Individuals on Antabuse are sensitive to alcohol on a continuum with some being able to drink on the drug, and others can have a reaction with only slight exposure, e.g., alcohol-containing foods or products such as aftershave. Reactions appear to be dose-related as well.
Review specific aftercare needs; e.g., PCP user should drink cranberry juice and continue use of ascorbic acid; alcohol abuser with liver damage	Promotes individualized care related to specific situation. Cranberry juice and ascorbic acid enhance clearance of PCP from the system. Substances

ACTIONS/INTERVENTIONS	RATIONALE
Independent	
should refrain from drugs/anesthetics/household cleaning products detoxified in the liver.	that have the potential for liver damage are more dangerous in the presence of already damaged liver.
Discuss variety of helpful organizations and programs that are available for assistance/referral.	Long-term support is necessary to maintain optimal recovery. Psychosocial needs may require addressing as well as other issues.

Cancer

Cancer is a general term used to describe a disturbance of cellular growth and refers to a group of diseases and not a single disease entity. There are currently more than 150 different known types of cancer. Because cancer is a cellular disease, it can arise from any body tissue, with manifestations that are the result of failure to control the proliferation and maturation of cells.

There are four main classifications of cancer according to tissue type: (1) lymphomas (cancers originating in infection-fighting organs); (2) leukemias (cancers originating in blood-forming organs); (3) sarcomas (cancers originating in bones, muscle, or connective tissue); and (4) carcinomas (cancers originating in epithelial cells). Within these broad categories, a cancer is classified by histology, stage, and grade.

Through years of observation and documentation, it has been noted that the metastatic behavior of cancers varied according to the primary site of diagnosis. This behavior pattern is known as the "natural history." An example is the metastatic pattern for primary breast cancer: breast-bone-lung-liver-brain. Knowledge of the etiology and natural history of a cancer type is important in planning the patient's care and in evaluation of the patient's progress, prognosis, and physical complaints.

RELATED CONCERNS

Leukemias, p 601
Lung Cancer: Surgical Intervention, p 184
Lymphomas, p 611
Mastectomy, p 762
Psychosocial Aspects of Acute Care, p 899
Radical Neck Surgery, p 202
Sepsis/Septicemia, p 887
Total Nutritional Support, p 1039

PATIENT ASSESSMENT DATA BASE

Refer to appropriate plans of care for additional assessment information.

ACTIVITY/REST

May report:	Weakness and/or fatigue.
	Changes in rest pattern and usual hours of sleep per night; presence of factors affecting sleep, e.g., pain, anxiety, night sweats.
	Limitations of participation in hobbies, exercise.
	Occupation or profession with environmental carcinogen exposure, high stress level.

CIRCULATION

May report:	Palpitations, chest pain on exertion.
May exhibit:	Changes in BP.

EGO INTEGRITY

May report:	Stress factors (financial, job, role changes) and ways of handling stress (e.g., smoking, drinking, delay in seeking treatment, religious/spiritual belief).
	Concern about changes in appearance, e.g., alopecia, disfiguring lesions, surgery.
	Denial of diagnosis, feelings of powerlessness, hopelessness, helplessness, worthlessness, guilt, loss of control, depression.
May exhibit:	Denial, withdrawal, anger.

ELIMINATION

May report: Changes in bowel pattern, e.g., blood in stools, pain with defecation.

Changes in urinary elimination, e.g., pain or burning on urination, hematuria, frequent micturition.

May exhibit: Changes in bowel sounds, abdominal distention.

FOOD/FLUID

May report: Poor dietary habits (e.g., low-fiber, high-fat, additives, preservatives).

Anorexia, nausea/vomiting.

Food intolerances.

Changes in weight; severe weight loss, cachexia, wasting of muscle mass.

May exhibit: Changes in skin moisture/turgor; edema.

NEUROSENSORY

May report: Dizziness; syncope.

PAIN/COMFORT

May report: No pain, or varying degrees, e.g., mild discomfort to severe pain (associated with disease process).

RESPIRATION

May report: Smoking (tobacco, marijuana, living with someone who smokes).

Asbestos exposure.

SAFETY

May report: Exposure to toxic chemicals, carcinogens.

Excessive/prolonged sun exposure.

May exhibit: Fever.

Skin rashes, ulcerations.

SEXUALITY

May report: Sexual concerns, e.g., impact on relationship, change in level of satisfaction. Nulligravida greater than 30 years of age.

Multigravida, multiple sex partners, early sexual activity. Genital herpes.

SOCIAL INTERACTION

May report: Inadequate/weak support system.

Marital history (regarding in-home satisfaction, support, or help).

Concerns about role function/responsibility.

TEACHING/LEARNING

May report: Family history of cancer, e.g., mother or aunt with breast cancer.

Primary site: Of primary disease, date discovered/diagnosed.

1015

Metastatic disease: Additional sites involved; if none, natural history of primary will provide important information for looking for metastasis.

Treatment history: Previous treatment for cancer-place and treatments given.

Discharge Plan Considerations:

DRG projected mean length of stay: Dependent on specific system affected and therapeutic needs. Refer to appropriate resources.

May require assistance with finances, medications/treatments, wound care/supplies, transportation, food shopping and preparation, self-care, homemaker/maintenance tasks, provision for child care; changes in living facilities/hospice.

DIAGNOSTIC STUDIES

Test selection depends on history, clinical manifestations, and index of suspicion for a particular cancer.

Scans (e.g., MRI, CT, gallium) and ultrasound: May be done for diagnostic purposes, identification of metastasis, and evaluation of response to treatment.

Biopsy (aspiration, excision, needle, punch): Done to differentiate diagnosis and delineate treatment and may be taken from bone marrow, skin, organ, and so forth. Examples: Bone marrow is done in myeloproliferative diseases for diagnosis; in solid tumors for staging.

Tumor markers (substances produced and secreted by tumor cells and found in serum, e.g., CEA, prostate specific antigen, alpha-fetoprotein, HCG, prostatic acid phosphatase, calcitonin, pancreatic oncofetal antigen, CA 15-3, CA 19-9, CA 125 and so on): Can help in diagnosing cancer but are more useful as prognostic indices and/or therapeutic monitors. Estrogen and progesterone receptors are assays done on breast tissue to provide information about whether or not hormonal manipulation would be therapeutic in metastatic disease control.

Screening chemistry tests: e.g., electrolytes (sodium, potassium, calcium); renal tests (BUN/Cr); liver tests (bilirubin, AST/SGOT alkaline phosphatase, LDH); bone tests (alkaline phosphatase, calcium).

CBC with differential and platelets: May reveal anemia, changes in RBCs and WBCs; reduced or increased platelets.

Chest x-ray: Screens for primary or metastatic disease of lungs.

NURSING PRIORITIES

1. Support adaptation and independence.
2. Promote comfort.
3. Maintain optimal physiologic functioning.
4. Prevent complications.
5. Provide information about disease process/condition, prognosis, and treatment needs.

DISCHARGE GOALS

1. Patient is dealing with current situation realistically.
2. Pain alleviated/controlled.
3. Homeostasis achieved.
4. Complications prevented/minimized.
5. Disease process/condition, prognosis, and therapeutic choices and regimen understood.

NURSING DIAGNOSIS:	FEAR/ANXIETY (SPECIFY LEVEL)
May be related to:	Situational crisis (cancer).
	Threat to/change in health/socioeconomic status, role functioning, interaction patterns.

	Threat of death.
	Separation from family (hospitalization, treatments) interpersonal transmission/contagion of feelings.
Possibly evidenced by:	Increased tension, shakiness, apprehension, restlessness.
	Expressed concerns regarding changes in life events.
	Feelings of helplessness, hopelessness, inadequacy.
	Sympathetic stimulation, somatic complaints.
DESIRED OUTCOMES/ EVALUATION CRITERIA— PATIENT WILL:	Display appropriate range of feelings and lessened fear.
	Appear relaxed and report anxiety is reduced to a manageable level.
	Demonstrate use of effective coping mechanisms and active participation in treatment regimen.

ACTIONS/INTERVENTIONS	RATIONALE
Independent	
Review patient's/SO's previous experience with cancer. Determine what the doctor has told patient and what conclusion patient has reached.	Assists in identification of fear(s) and misconceptions based on experience with cancer.
Encourage patient to share thoughts and feelings.	Provides opportunity to examine realistic fears as well as misconceptions about diagnosis.
Provide open environment in which patient feels safe to discuss feelings or to refrain from talking.	Helps patient to feel accepted in present condition without feeling judged and promotes sense of dignity and control.
Maintain frequent contact with patient. Talk with and touch patient as appropriate.	Provides assurance that the patient is not alone or rejected; conveys respect for and acceptance of the person, fostering trust.
Be aware of effects of isolation on patient when required for immunosuppression or radiation implant. Limit use of isolation clothing/masks as possible.	Sensory deprivation may result when sufficient stimulation is not available and may intensify feelings of anxiety/fear.
Assist patient/SO in recognizing and clarifying fears to begin developing coping strategies for dealing with these fears.	Coping skills are often impaired after diagnosis and during different phases of treatment. Support and counseling are often necessary to enable individual to recognize and deal with fear and to realize that control/coping strategies are available.
Provide accurate, consistent information regarding prognosis. Avoid arguing about patient's perceptions of situation.	Can reduce anxiety and enable patient to make decisions/choices based on realities.
Permit expressions of anger, fear, despair without confrontation. Give information that feelings are normal and are to be appropriately expressed.	Acceptance of feelings allows patient to begin to deal with situation.
Explain the recommended treatment, its purpose and potential side effects. Help patient prepare for treatments.	The goal of cancer treatment is to destroy malignant cells while minimizing damage to normal ones. Treatment may include surgery (curative,

1017

ACTIONS/INTERVENTIONS

Independent

Explain procedures, providing opportunity for questions and honest answers. Stay with patient during anxiety-producing procedures and consultations.

Provide primary or consistent caregivers whenever possible.

Promote calm, quiet environment.

Identify stage/degree of grief patient and SO are currently experiencing. (Refer to ND: Grieving, Anticipatory, this page.)

Note ineffective coping, e.g., poor social interactions, helplessness, giving up everyday functions and usual sources of gratification.

Be alert to signs of denial/depression, e.g., withdrawal, anger, inappropriate remarks. Determine presence of suicidal ideation and assess potential on a scale of 1–10.

Encourage and foster patient interaction with support systems.

Provide reliable and consistent information and support for SO.

Include SO as indicated when major decisions are to be made.

RATIONALE

preventive, palliative) as well as chemotherapy, radiation (internal, external) or newer/organ specific treatments such as whole-body hyperthermia or biotherapy. Bone marrow transplant may be recommended for some types of cancer.

Accurate information allows patient to deal more effectively with reality of situation, thereby reducing anxiety and fear of the unknown.

May help reduce anxiety by fostering therapeutic relationship and facilitating continuity of care.

Facilitates rest, conserves energy, and may enhance coping abilities.

Choice of interventions are dictated by stage of grief, coping behaviors, e.g., anger/withdrawal, denial.

Identifies individual problems and provides support for patient/SO in using effective coping skills.

Patient may use defense mechanism of denial and express hope that diagnosis is inaccurate. Feelings of guilt, spiritual distress, physical symptoms, or lack of cure may cause the patient to become withdrawn and believe that suicide is a viable alternative.

Reduces feelings of isolation. If family support systems are not available, outside sources may be needed immediately, e.g., local cancer support groups.

Allows for better interpersonal interaction and reduction of anxiety and fear.

Ensures a support system for the patient and allows the SO to be involved appropriately.

NURSING DIAGNOSIS:	GRIEVING, ANTICIPATORY
May be related to:	Anticipated loss of physiologic well-being (e.g., loss of body part; change in body function); change in lifestyle.
	Perceived potential death of patient.
Possibly evidenced by:	Changes in eating habits, alterations in sleep patterns, activity levels, libido, and communication patterns.
	Denial of potential loss, choked feelings, anger.

DESIRED OUTCOMES/ EVALUATION CRITERIA— PATIENT WILL:	Identify and express feelings appropriately. Continue normal life activities, looking toward/planning for the future, one day at a time. Verbalize understanding of the dying process and feelings of being supported in grief work.

ACTIONS/INTERVENTIONS	RATIONALE

Independent

Expect initial shock and disbelief following diagnosis of cancer and/or traumatizing procedures (e.g., disfiguring surgery, colostomy, amputation).	Few patients are fully prepared for reality of the changes that can occur.
Assess patient/SO for stage of grief currently being experienced. Explain process as appropriate.	Knowledge about the grieving process reinforces the normality of feelings/reactions being experienced and can help patient deal more effectively with them.
Provide open, nonjudgmental environment. Use therapeutic communication skills of Active-listening acknowledgement, and so on.	Promotes and encourages realistic dialogue about feelings and concerns.
Encourage verbalization of thoughts/concerns and accept expressions of sadness, anger, rejection. Acknowledge normality of these feelings.	Patient may feel supported in expression of feelings by the understanding that deep and often conflicting emotions are normal and experienced by others in this difficult situation.
Be aware of mood swings, hostility, and other acting-out behavior. Set limits on inappropriate behavior, correct negative thinking.	Indicators of ineffective coping and need for additional interventions. Preventing destructive actions enables patient to maintain control and sense of self-esteem.
Be aware of debilitating depression. Ask patient direct questions about state of mind.	Studies show that many cancer patients are at high risk for suicide. They are especially vulnerable when recently diagnosed and/or discharged from hospital.
Visit frequently and provide physical contact as appropriate/desired. Move patient closer to nurses station if frightened; leave door open if comfortable for patient.	Helps reduce feelings of isolation and abandonment.
Reinforce teaching regarding disease process and treatments and provide information as requested/appropriate about dying. Be honest; do not give false hope while providing emotional support.	Patient/SO benefit from factual information. Individuals may ask direct questions about death, and honest answers promote trust and provide reassurance that correct information will be given.
Review past life experiences, role changes, and coping skills. Talk about things that interest the patient.	Opportunity to identify skills that may help individuals cope with grief of current situation more effectively.
Identify positive aspects of the situation.	Possibility of remission and slow progression of disease and/or new therapies can offer hope for the future.
Discuss ways patient/SO can plan together for the future. Encourage setting of realistic goals.	Having a part in problem solving/planning can provide a sense of control over anticipated events.

1019

ACTIONS/INTERVENTIONS

Independent

Assist patient/SO to identify strengths in self/situation and support systems.

Encourage participation in care and treatment decisions.

Note evidence of conflict, expressions of anger and statements of despair, guilt, hopelessness, "nothing to live for."

Assess way that patient/SO understand and respond to death, e.g., cultural expectations, learned behaviors, experience with death (close family members/friends), beliefs about life after death, faith in higher being (God).

Provide open environment for discussion with patient/SO (when appropriate) about desires/plans pertaining to death; e.g., making will, burial arrangements, tissue donation, death benefits, insurance, time for family gatherings.

Be aware of own feelings about cancer, impending death. Accept whatever methods patient/SO have chosen to help each other through process.

Collaborative

Refer to appropriate counselor as needed (e.g., psychiatric clinical nurse specialist, social worker, psychologist, clergyman).

Refer to community hospice program, if appropriate, or VNA, home health agency service as needed.

RATIONALE

Recognizing these resources provides opportunity to work through feelings of grief.

Allows patient to retain some control over life.

Interpersonal conflicts/angry behavior may be patient's ways of expressing/dealing with feelings of despair/spiritual distress and could be indicative of suicidal ideation.

These factors affect how each individual deals with the possibility of death and influences how they may respond and interact.

If the patient/SO are mutually aware of impending death, they may more easily deal with unfinished business or desired activities.

Caregiver's anxiety and unwillingness to accept reality of possibility of own death may block ability to be helpful to the patient/SO, necessitating enlisting the aid of others to provide needed support.

Can help to alleviate distress or palliate feelings of grief to facilitate coping and foster growth.

Provides support in meeting physical and emotional needs of patient/SO, and can supplement the care family and friends are able to give.

NURSING DIAGNOSIS:	**SELF-ESTEEM, DISTURBANCE**
May be related to:	Biophysical: Disfiguring surgery, chemotherapy or radiotherapy side effects, e.g., loss of hair, nausea/vomiting, weight loss, anorexia, impotence, sterility, overwhelming fatigue, uncontrolled pain.
	Psychosocial: Threat of death; feelings of lack of control and doubt regarding acceptance by others; fear and anxiety.
Possibly evidenced by:	Verbalization of change in lifestyle; fear of rejection/reaction of others; negative feelings about body; feelings of helplessness, hopelessness, powerlessness.
	Preoccupation with change or loss.

Not taking responsibility for self-care, lack of follow-through.

Change in self-perception/other's perception of role.

DESIRED OUTCOMES/ EVALUATION CRITERIA— PATIENT WILL:

Verbalize understanding of body changes, acceptance of self in situation.

Begin to develop coping mechanisms to deal effectively with problems.

Demonstrate adaptation to changes/events that have occurred as evidenced by setting of realistic goals and active participation in work/play/personal relationships as appropriate.

ACTIONS/INTERVENTIONS	RATIONALE
Independent	
Discuss with patient/SO how the diagnosis and treatment are affecting the patient's personal life/home and work activities.	Aids in defining concerns to begin problem-solving process.
Review anticipated side effects associated with a particular treatment, including possible effects on sexual activity and sense of attractiveness/desirability, e.g., alopecia, disfiguring surgery. Tell patient that not all side effects occur.	Anticipatory guidance can help patient/SO begin the process of adaptation to new state and to prepare for some side effects, e.g., buy a wig before radiation, schedule time off from work as indicated. (Refer to ND: Sexuality Patterns, Altered, high risk for, p 1034.)
Encourage discussion of/problem-solve concerns about effects of cancer/treatments on role as homemaker, wage earner, parent, and so forth.	May help reduce problems that interfere with acceptance of treatment or stimulate progression of disease.
Acknowledge difficulties patient may be experiencing. Give information that counseling is often necessary and important in the adaptation process.	Validates reality of patient's feelings and gives permission to take whatever measures are necessary to cope with what is happening.
Evaluate support structures available to and used by patient/SO.	Helps with planning for care while hospitalized as well as after discharge.
Provide emotional support for patient/SO during diagnostic tests and treatment phase.	Although some patients adapt/adjust to cancer effects or side effects of therapy, many need additional support during this period.
Use touch during interactions, if acceptable to patient, and maintain eye contact.	Affirmation of individuality and acceptance are important in reducing patient's feelings of insecurity and self-doubt.
Collaborative	
Refer patient/SO to supportive group programs (e.g., CanSurmount, I Can Cope, Reach to Recovery, Encore).	Group support is usually very beneficial for both patient/SO, providing contact with other patients with cancer at various levels of treatment and/or recovery.

ACTIONS/INTERVENTIONS

RATIONALE

Collaborative

Refer to professional counseling if indicated.

May be necessary to regain and maintain a positive psychosocial structure if patient/SO support systems are deteriorating.

NURSING DIAGNOSIS:	PAIN, [ACUTE]
May be related to:	Disease process (compression/destruction of nerve tissue, infiltration of nerves or their vascular supply, obstruction of a nerve pathway, inflammation).
	Side effects of various cancer therapy agents.
Possibly evidenced by:	Reports of pain.
	Self-focusing/narrowed focus.
	Alteration in muscle tone; facial mask of pain.
	Distraction/guarding behaviors.
	Autonomic responses, restlessness.
DESIRED OUTCOMES/ EVALUATION CRITERIA— PATIENT WILL:	Report maximal pain relief/control with minimal interference with ADLs.
	Follow prescribed pharmacologic regimen.
	Demonstrate use of relaxation skills and diversional activities as indicated for individual situation.

ACTIONS/INTERVENTIONS

RATIONALE

Independent

Determine pain history, e.g., location of pain, frequency, duration, and intensity (0–10 scale), and relief measures used.

Information provides baseline data to evaluate need for/effectiveness of interventions. *Note:* The pain experience is an individualized one composed of both physical and emotional responses.

Evaluate/be aware of particular therapies, i.e., surgery, radiation, chemotherapy, biotherapy. Teach patient/SO what to expect.

A wide range of discomforts are common (e.g., incisional pain, burning skin, low back pain, headaches) depending on the procedure/agent being used.

Provide basic comfort measures (e.g., repositioning, backrub) and diversional activities (e.g., music, television).

Promotes relaxation and helps refocus attention.

Encourage use of stress management skills (e.g., relaxation techniques, visualization, guided imagery), laughter, music, and Therapeutic Touch.

Enables patient to participate actively and enhances sense of control.

Evaluate pain relief/control. Adjust medication regimen as necessary.

Goal is maximum pain control with minimum interference with ADLs.

ACTIONS/INTERVENTIONS	RATIONALE
Collaborative	
Develop pain management plan with the patient and physician.	An organized plan improves chance for pain control. Particularly with chronic pain, patient/SO must be active participants in pain management at home.
Administer analgesics as indicated, e.g.: Brompton's cocktail, morphine, methadone, or specific IV narcotic mixtures. Give doses to provide analgesia around the clock. Convert from short-acting to long-acting analgesics when indicated.	Pain is a frequent complication of cancer, although individual responses differ. As changes in the disease/treatment occur, adjustments in dosage and delivery will be needed. *Note:* Addiction to or dependency on drug is not a concern.
Provide/instruct in use of PCA as appropriate.	Patient-controlled analgesia provides for timely drug administration, preventing fluctuations in intensity of pain, often at lower total dosage than would be given by conventional methods.
Prepare for/assist with procedures, e.g., nerve blocks, cordotomy, commissural myelotomy.	May be used in severe/intractable pain unresponsive to other measures.

NURSING DIAGNOSIS:	**NUTRITION, ALTERED: LESS THAN BODY REQUIREMENTS**
May be related to:	Hypermetabolic state associated with cancer.
	Consequences of chemotherapy, radiation, surgery, e.g., anorexia, gastric irritation, taste distortions, nausea.
	Emotional distress, fatigue, poorly controlled pain.
Possibly evidenced by:	Reported inadequate food intake, altered taste sensation, loss of interest in food, perceived/actual inability to ingest food.
	Body weight 20% or more under ideal for height and frame, decreased subcutaneous fat/muscle mass.
	Sore, inflamed buccal cavity.
	Diarrhea and/or constipation, abdominal cramping.
DESIRED OUTCOMES/ EVALUATION CRITERIA— PATIENT WILL:	Demonstrate stable weight, progressive weight gain toward goal with normalization of laboratory values and free of signs of malnutrition.
	Verbalize understanding of individual interferences to adequate intake.
	Participate in specific interventions to stimulate appetite/ increase dietary intake.

1023

ACTIONS/INTERVENTIONS	RATIONALE
Independent	
Monitor daily food intake; have patient keep food diary as indicated.	Identifies nutritional strengths/deficiencies.
Measure height, weight and tricep skinfold thickness (or other anthropometric measurements as appropriate). Ascertain amount of recent weight loss. Weigh daily or as indicated.	If these measurements fall below minimum standards, patient's chief source of stored energy (fat tissue) is depleted.
Assess for pallor, delayed wound healing, enlarged parotid glands.	Helps in identification of protein-calorie malnutrition, especially when weight and anthropometric measurements are less than normal.
Encourage patient to eat high-calorie nutrient-rich diet, with adequate fluid intake. Encourage use of supplements and frequent/smaller meals spaced throughout the day.	Metabolic tissue needs are increased as well as fluids (to eliminate waste products). Supplements can play an important role in maintaining adequate caloric and protein intake.
Adjust diet prior to and immediately after treatment, e.g., clear, cool liquids, light/bland foods, dry crackers, toast, carbonated drinks. Give liquids 1 hour before or 1 hour after meals.	The effectiveness of diet adjustment is very individualized in relief of posttherapy nausea. Patients must experiment to find best solution/combination.
Control environmental factors (e.g., strong/noxious odors or noise). Avoid overly sweet, fatty, or spicy foods.	Can trigger nausea/vomiting response.
Create pleasant dining atmosphere; encourage patient to share meals with family/friends.	Makes mealtime more enjoyable, which may enhance intake.
Encourage use of relaxation techniques, visualization, guided imagery, moderate exercise before meals.	May prevent onset or reduce severity of nausea, decrease anorexia, and enable patient to increase oral intake.
Identify the patient who experiences anticipatory nausea/vomiting.	Psychogenic nausea/vomiting occurring before chemotherapy begins generally does not respond to antiemetic drugs. Change of treatment environment or patient routine on treatment day may be effective.
Encourage open communication regarding anorexia problem.	Often a source of emotional distress, especially for SO who wants to feed patient frequently. When patient refuses, SO may feel rejected/frustrated.
Administer antiemetic on a regular schedule before/during and after administration of antineoplastic agent as appropriate.	Nasuea/vomiting are frequently the most disabling and psychologically stressful side effects of chemotherapy.
Evaluate effectiveness of antiemetic.	Individuals respond differently to all medications. Firstline antiemetics may not work, requiring alteration in or combination drug therapy.
Hematest stools, gastric secretions.	Certain therapies (e.g., antimetabolites) inhibit renewal of epithelial cells lining the GI tract, which may cause changes ranging from mild erythema to severe ulceration with bleeding.
Collaborative	
Review laboratory studies as indicated, e.g., total lymphocyte count, serum transferrin, and albumin.	Helps identify the degree of biochemical imbalance/malnutrition and influences choice of dietary

ACTIONS/INTERVENTIONS	RATIONALE
Collaborative	interventions. *Note:* Anticancer treatments can also alter nutrition studies so all results must be correlated with the patients' clinical status.
Administer medications as indicated:	
Phenothiazines, e.g., prochlorperazine (Compazine), thiethylperazine (Torecan); antidopaminergics, e.g., metoclopramide (Reglan), ondansetron (Zofran); antihistamines, e.g., diphenhydramine (Benadryl);	Most antiemetics act to interfere with stimulation of true vomiting center and chemoreceptor trigger zone agents also act peripherally to inhibit reverse peristalsis.
Corticosteroids, e.g., dexamethasone (Decadron); cannabinoids, e.g., 9-tetrahydrocannabinol; benzodiazepines, e.g., diazepam (Valium);	Combination therapy (e.g., Torecan with Decadron or Valium) is often more effective than single agents.
Vitamins, especially A, D, E, and B_6:	Prevents deficit related to decreased absorption of fat-soluble vitamins. Deficiency of B_6 can contribute to/exacerbate depression, irritability.
Antacids.	Minimizes gastric irritation and reduces risk of mucosal ulceration.
Refer to dietitian/nutritional support team.	Provides for specific dietary plan to meet individual needs and reduce problems associated with protein/calorie malnutrition and micronutrient deficiencies.
Insert/maintain NG or feeding tube for enteric feedings, or central line for parenteral hyperalimentation if indicated.	In the presence of severe malnutrition (e.g., loss of 25%–30% body weight in 2 months), or patient has been NPO for 5 days and is unlikely to be able to eat for another week, tube feeding or TPN may be necessary to meet nutritional needs. *Note:* TPN is used with caution as it is associated with a more than 4-fold increase in the risk of significant infection.

NURSING DIAGNOSIS:	**FLUID VOLUME DEFICIT, HIGH RISK FOR**
Risk factors may include:	Excessive losses through normal (e.g., vomiting, diarrhea) and/or abnormal routes (e.g., indwelling tubes, wounds).
	Hypermetabolic state.
	Impaired intake of fluids.
Possibly evidenced by:	[Not applicable; presence of signs and symptoms establishes an actual diagnosis.]
DESIRED OUTCOMES/ EVALUATION CRITERIA— PATIENT WILL:	Display adequate fluid balance as evidenced by stable vital signs, moist mucous membranes, good skin turgor, prompt capillary refill, and individually adequate urinary output.

ACTIONS/INTERVENTIONS	RATIONALE
Independent	
Monitor I&O and specific gravity; include all output sources, e.g., emesis, diarrhea, draining wounds. Calculate 24-hour balance.	Continued negative fluid balance, decreasing renal output and concentration of urine suggests developing dehydration and need for increased fluid replacement.
Weigh as indicated.	Sensitive measurement of fluctuations in fluid balance.
Monitor vital signs. Evaluate peripheral pulses, capillary refill.	Reflects adequacy of circulating volume.
Assess skin turgor and moisture of mucous membranes. Note reports of thirst.	Indirect indicators of hydration status/degree of deficit.
Encourage increased fluid intake to 3000 ml/d as individually appropriate/tolerated.	Assists in maintenance of fluid requirements and reduces risk of harmful side effects, e.g., hemorrhagic cystitis in patient receiving Cyclophosphamide (Cytoxan).
Observe for bleeding tendencies, e.g., oozing from mucous membranes, puncture sites; presence of ecchymosis or petechiae.	Early identification of problems (which may occur as a result of cancer and/or therapies) allows for prompt intervention.
Minimize venipunctures (e.g., combine IV starts with blood draws). Encourage patient to consider central venous catheter placement.	Reduces potential for hemorrhage and infection associated with repeated venous puncture.
Avoid trauma and apply pressure to puncture sites.	Reduces potential for bleeding/hematoma formation.
Collaborative	
Provide IV fluids as indicated.	Given for general hydration as well as to dilute antineoplastic drugs and reduce adverse side effects, e.g., nausea/vomiting, or nephrotoxicity.
Administer antiemetic therapy. (Refer to ND: Nutrition, Altered: Less Than Body Requirements, p 1023.	Alleviation of nausea/vomiting decreases gastric losses and allows for increased oral intake.
Monitor laboratory studies, e.g., CBC, electrolytes, serum albumin.	Provides information about level of hydration and corresponding deficits. *Note:* Malnutrition and effects of decreased albumin levels potentiates fluid shifts/edema formation.
Administer transfusions as indicated, e.g.:	
RBCs;	May be needed to restore blood count and prevent manifestations of anemia often present in cancer patients, e.g., tachycardia, tachypnea, dizziness, and weakness.
Platelets.	Thrombocytopenia (which may occur as a side effect of chemotherapy, radiation, or cancer process) increases the risk of bleeding from mucous membranes and other body sites. Spontaneous bleeding generally occurs with platelets less than 20,000.

ACTIONS/INTERVENTIONS

Collaborative

Avoid use of aspirin, gastric irritants, or platelet inhibitors.

RATIONALE

Potentiates risk of bleeding.

NURSING DIAGNOSIS:	FATIGUE
May be related to:	Decreased metabolic energy production, increased energy requirements (hypermetabolic state).
	Overwhelming psychologic/emotional demands.
	Altered body chemistry: Side effects of medications, chemotherapy.
Possibly evidenced by:	Unremitting/overwhelming lack of energy, inability to maintain usual routines, decreased performance, impaired ability to concentrate, lethargy/listlessness.
	Disinterest in surroundings.
DESIRED OUTCOMES/ EVALUATION CRITERIA:— PATIENT WILL:	Report improved sense of energy.
	Perform ADLs and participate in desired activities at level of ability.

ACTIONS/INTERVENTIONS

Independent

Plan care to allow for rest periods. Schedule activities for periods when patient has most energy. Involve patient/SO in schedule planning.

Establish realistic activity goals with patient.

Assist with self-care needs when indicated; keep bed in low position, pathways clear of furniture; assist with ambulation.

Encourage patient to do whatever possible, e.g., self-bath, sitting up in chair, walking. Increase activity level as able.

Monitor physiologic response to activity, e.g., changes in BP or heart/respiratory rate.

Encourage nutritional intake. (Refer to ND: Nutrition, Altered: Less Than Body Requirements, p 1023.)

RATIONALE

Frequent rest periods are needed to restore/conserve energy. Planning will allow patient to be active during times when energy level is higher, which may restore a feeling of well-being and a sense of control.

Provides for a sense of control and feelings of accomplishment.

Weakness may make ADLs difficult to complete or place the patient at risk for injury during activities.

Enhances strength/stamina and enables patient to become more active without undue fatigue.

Tolerance varies greatly depending on the stage of the disease process, nutrition state, fluid balance, and reaction to therapeutic regimen.

Adequate intake/use of nutrients is necessary to meet energy needs for activity.

ACTIONS/INTERVENTIONS	RATIONALE

Collaborative

Provide supplemental O_2 as indicated.

Presence of anemia/hypoxemia reduces O_2 available for cellular uptake and contributes to fatigue.

Refer to physical/occupational therapy.

Programmed daily exercises and activities help patient to maintain/increase strength and muscle tone, enhance sense of well-being. Use of adaptive devices may help conserve energy.

NURSING DIAGNOSIS:	INFECTION, HIGH RISK FOR
Risk factors may include:	Inadequate secondary defenses and immunosuppression, e.g., bone marrow suppression (dose-limiting side effect of both chemotherapy and radiation). Malnutrition, chronic disease process. Invasive procedures.
Possibly evidenced by:	[Not applicable; presence of signs and symptoms establishes an actual diagnosis.]
DESIRED OUTCOMES/ EVALUATION CRITERIA— PATIENT WILL:	Identify and participate in interventions to prevent/reduce risk of infection. Remain afebrile and achieve timely healing as appropriate.

ACTIONS/INTERVENTIONS	RATIONALE

Independent

Promote good hand-washing procedures by staff and visitors. Screen/limit visitors who may have infections. Place in reverse isolation as indicated.

Protects patient from sources of infection, such as visitors and staff who may have URI.

Emphasize personal hygiene.

Limits potential sources of infection and/or secondary overgrowth.

Monitor temperature.

Temperature elevation may occur (if not masked by corticosteroids or anti-inflammatory drugs) because of various factors, e.g., chemotherapy side effects, disease process, or infection. Early identification of infectious process enables appropriate therapy to be started promptly.

Assess all systems (e.g., skin, respiratory, genitourinary) for signs/symptoms of infection on a continual basis.

Early recognition and intervention may prevent progression to more serious situation/sepsis.

Reposition frequently; keep linens dry and wrinkle-free.

Reduces pressure and irritation to tissues and may prevent skin breakdown (potential site for bacterial growth).

Promote adequate rest/exercise periods.

Limits fatigue, yet encourages sufficient movement to prevent stasis complications, e.g., pneumonia, decubitus, and thrombus formation.

ACTIONS/INTERVENTIONS	RATIONALE

Independent

Stress importance of good oral hygiene.

Development of stomatitis increases risk of infection/secondary overgrowth.

Avoid/limit invasive procedures. Adhere to aseptic techniques.

Reduces risk of contamination, limits portal of entry for infectious agents.

Collaborative

Monitor CBC with differential WBC and granulocyte count and platelets as indicated.

Bone marrow activity may be inhibited by effects of chemotherapy, the disease state, or radiation therapy. Monitoring status of myelosuppression is important, for preventing further complications (e.g., infection, anemia or hemorrhage) and scheduling drug delivery. *Note:* The nadir (point of lowest drop in blood count) is usually seen 7–10 days after administration of chemotherapy.

Obtain cultures as indicated.

Identifies causative organism(s) and appropriate therapy.

Administer antibiotics as indicated.

May be used to treat identified infection or given prophylactically in immunocompromised patient.

NURSING DIAGNOSIS:	ORAL MUCOUS MEMBRANE, ALTERED, HIGH RISK FOR
Risk factors may include:	Side effect of some chemotherapeutic agents (e.g., antimetabolites) and radiation.
Possibly evidenced by:	[Not applicable; presence of signs and symptoms establishes an actual diagnosis.]
DESIRED OUTCOMES/ EVALUATION CRITERIA— PATIENT WILL:	Display intact mucous membranes, which are pink, moist, and free of inflammation/ulcerations.
	Verbalize understanding of causative factors.
	Demonstrate techniques to maintain/restore integrity of oral mucosa.

ACTIONS/INTERVENTIONS	RATIONALE

Independent

Assess dental health and oral hygiene on admission and periodically.

Identifies prophylactic treatment that may be needed prior to initiation of chemotherapy or radiation and provides baseline data in current oral hygiene care.

Assess oral cavity daily, noting changes in mucous membrane integrity (e.g., dry, reddened). Ascertain whether patient notices burning in the mouth, changes in voice quality, ability to swallow,

Inflammation of the oral mucosa (stomatitis) generally occurs 7–14 days after treatment begins, but signs may be seen as early as day 3 to 4, especially if there were any preexisting oral problems.

1029

ACTIONS/INTERVENTIONS	RATIONALE
Independent	
sense of taste, development of thick/viscous saliva.	The range of response extends from mild erythema to severe ulceration, which can be very painful, inhibit oral intake, and be potentially life threatening. Early identification enables prompt treatment.
Discuss with patient areas needing improvement and demonstrate methods for good oral care.	Good care is critical during treatment to control stomatitis complications.
Initiate oral hygiene program to include:	
Avoidance of commercial mouthwashes, lemon/glycerine swabs;	Products containing alcohol or phenol may exacerbate mucous membrane dryness/irritation.
Use of mouthwash made from warm saline, dilute solution of hydrogen peroxide or baking soda and water;	May be soothing to the membranes. Rinsing before meals may improve the patient's sense of taste. Rinsing after meals and at bedtime dilutes oral acids and relieves xerostomia.
Brush with soft toothbrush or toothette;	Prevents trauma to delicate/fragile tissues.
Floss gently or use WaterPik cautiously;	Removes food particles that can promote bacterial growth.
Keep lips moist with lip gloss, KY Jelly, Chapstick, and so forth;	Promotes comfort and prevents drying/cracking of tissues.
Encourage use of mints/hard candy or artificial saliva (Ora-Lube, Salivert) as indicated.	Stimulates/provides moisture to maintain integrity of mucous membranes, especially in presence of dehydration/reduced saliva production.
Instruct regarding dietary changes: e.g., avoid hot or spicy foods, acidic juices; suggest use of straw; ingesting soft or blenderized foods, Popsicles, and ice cream as tolerated.	Severe stomatitis may interfere with nutritional and fluid intake leading to negative nitrogen balance or dehydration. Dietary modifications may make foods easier to swallow and feel soothing.
Encourage fluid intake as individually tolerated.	Adequate hydration helps keep mucous membranes moist, preventing drying/cracking.
Discuss limitation of smoking and alcohol intake.	May cause further irritation and dryness of mucous membranes. *Note:* May need to compromise if these activities are important to patient's emotional status.
Monitor for and explain to patient signs of oral superinfection (e.g., thrush).	Early recognition ensures prompt initiation of treatment.
Collaborative	
Refer to dentist before initiating chemotherapy or head/neck radiation.	Prophylactic examination and repair work prior to therapy reduces risk of infection.
Culture suspicious oral lesions.	Identifies organism(s) responsible for oral infections, and suggests appropriate drug therapy.
Administer medications as indicated, e.g.:	
Analgesic rinses, topical lidocaine (Xylocaine) jelly;	Aggressive analgesia program may be required to relieve intense pain.
Antimicrobial mouthwash preparation, e.g., nystatin (Mycostatin).	May be needed to treat/prevent secondary oral infections, such as Candida, Pseudomonas, herpes simplex.

NURSING DIAGNOSIS:	SKIN/TISSUE INTEGRITY, IMPAIRED, HIGH RISK FOR
Risk factors may include:	Effects of radiation and chemotherapy.
	Immunologic deficit.
	Altered nutritional state, anemia.
Possibly evidenced by:	[Not applicable; presence of signs and symptoms establishes an actual diagnosis.]
DESIRED OUTCOMES/ EVALUATION CRITERIA— PATIENT WILL:	Identify interventions appropriate for specific condition.
	Participate in techniques to prevent complications/promote healing as appropriate.

ACTIONS/INTERVENTIONS	RATIONALE

Independent

Assess skin frequently for side effects of cancer therapy; note breakdown/delayed wound healing. Stress importance of reporting open areas to care giver.	A reddening and/or tanning effect (radiation reaction) may develop within the field of radiation. Dry desquamation (dryness and pruritus), moist desquamation (blistering), ulceration, hair loss, loss of dermis, and sweat glands may also be noted. In addition, skin reactions (e.g., allergic rashes, hyperpigmentation, pruritus, and alopecia) may occur with some chemotherapy agents.
Bathe with lukewarm water and mild soap.	Maintains cleanliness without irritating the skin.
Encourage patient to avoid scratching and to pat skin dry instead of rubbing.	Helps prevent skin friction/trauma.
Turn/reposition frequently.	Promotes circulation and prevents undue pressure on skin/tissues.
Advise patient to avoid any skin creams, ointments, and powders unless physician approves.	May actually increase irritation/reaction.
Review skin care protocol for patient receiving radiation therapy:	Designed to minimize trauma to area of radiation therapy.
Avoid rubbing or use of soap, lotions, or deodorants on area; avoid applying heat or attempting to wash off marks/tattoos placed on skin to identify area of irradiation;	Can potentiate or otherwise interfere with radiation delivery.
Recommend wearing soft, loose clothing next to area; have patient avoid wearing bra if it creates pressure;	Skin is very sensitive during treatment and after, and all irritation should be avoided to prevent dermal injury.
Apply cornstarch to area as needed, and Eucerin (or other recommended cream) to area twice daily after radiation is completed;	Helps to control dampness or pruritus. Maintenance care is required until skin tissues have regenerated and are back to normal.
Review use of sunscreen/block.	Protects skin from ultraviolet rays and reduces risk of recall reactions.

1031

ACTIONS/INTERVENTIONS	RATIONALE

Independent

Review skin care protocol for patient receiving chemotherapy, e.g.:

Use appropriate peripheral or central venous catheter, dilute anticancer drug per protocol and ascertain that IV is infusing well;

Reduces risk of tissue irritation/extravasation of agent into tissues.

Instruct patient to notify caregiver promptly of discomfort at IV insertion site;

Development of irritation indicates need for alteration of rate/dilution of chemotherapy and/or change of IV site to prevent more serious reaction.

Assess skin/IV site and vein for erythema, edema, tenderness; weltlike patches, itching/burning; or swelling, burning, soreness, blisters progressing to ulceration/tissue necrosis.

Presence of phlebitis, vein flare (localized allergic reaction) or extravasation requires immediate discontinuation of antineoplastic agent and medical intervention.

Wash skin immediately with soap and water if antineoplastic agents are spilled on unprotected skin (patient or caregiver).

Dilutes drug to reduce risk of skin irritation/chemical burn.

Advise patients receiving 5FU and methotrexate to avoid sun exposure. Withhold methotrexate if sunburn present.

Sun can cause exacerbation of burn spotting (a side effect of 5-Fluorouracil) or can cause a red "flash" area with methotrexate, which can exacerbate drug's effect.

Review expected dermatologic side effects seen with chemotherapy, e.g., rash, hyperpigmentation, and peeling of palms with 5FU.

Anticipatory guidance helps decrease concern if side effects do occur.

Inform patient that if alopecia occurs, hair could grow back after completion of chemotherapy, but may/may not grow back after radiation therapy.

Anticipatory guidance may help adjustment to/preparation for baldness. Men are often as sensitive to hair loss as women. Radiation's effect on hair follicles may be permanent, depending on rad dosage.

Collaborative

Administer appropriate antidote if extravasation should occur, e.g.:

Reduces local tissue damage.

topical DMSO;

May be useful for mitomycin, doxorubicin (Adriamycin)/daunorubicin. *Note:* Injection of Benadryl may relieve symptoms of vein flare.

Hyaluronidase (Wydase);

Injected subcutaneously for vincristine infiltration.

NaHCO$_3$;

Injected IV and/or into surrounding tissues for Bisantrene.

Thiosulfate.

Injected subcutaneously for nitrogen mustard.

Apply topical ointment, e.g., silver sulfadiazine (Silvadene) as appropriate.

May be used to prevent infection/facilitate healing if chemical burn (extravasation) occurs.

Apply ice pack/warm compresses per protocol.

Controversial intervention is dependent on type of agent used. Ice restricts blood flow, keeping drug localized, while heat enhances dispersion of antidote.

NURSING DIAGNOSIS:	CONSTIPATION/DIARRHEA, HIGH RISK FOR
Risk factors may include:	Irritation of the GI mucosa from either chemotherapy or radiation therapy; malabsorption of fat. Hormone-secreting tumor, carcinoma of colon. Poor fluid intake, low-bulk diet, lack of exercise, use of opiates/narcotics.
Possibly evidenced by:	[Not applicable; presence of signs and symptoms establishes an actual diagnosis.]
DESIRED OUTCOMES/ EVALUATION CRITERIA— PATIENT WILL:	Maintain usual bowel consistency/pattern. Verbalize understanding of factors and appropriate interventions/solutions related to individual situation.

ACTIONS/INTERVENTIONS

Independent

Ascertain usual elimination habits.

Assess bowel sounds and monitor/record bowel movements including frequency, consistency (particularly during first 3–5 days of Vinca alkaloid therapy).

Monitor I&O and weight.

Encourage adequate fluid intake (e.g., 2000 ml/24 h), increased fiber in diet; exercise.

Provide small, frequent meals of foods low in residue (if not contraindicated), maintaining needed protein and carbohydrates (e.g., eggs, cooked cereal, bland cooked vegetables).

Adjust diet as appropriate: avoid foods high in fat (e.g., butter, fried foods, nuts); foods with high-fiber content; those known to cause diarrhea or gas (e.g., cabbage, baked beans, chili); food/fluids high in caffeine; or extremely hot/cold food/fluids.

Check for impaction if patient has not had BM in 3 days or abdominal distention, cramping, headache are present.

Collaborative

Monitor laboratory studies as indicated, e.g., electrolytes.

RATIONALE

Data required as baseline for future evaluation.

Defines problem, i.e., diarrhea, constipation. Note: Constipation is one of the earliest manifestations of neurotoxicity.

Dehydration, weight loss, and electrolyte imbalance are complications of diarrhea. Inadequate fluid intake may potentiate constipation.

May reduce potential for constipation by improving stool consistency and stimulating peristalsis; can prevent dehydration (diarrhea).

Reduces gastric irritation. Use of low-fiber foods can decrease irritability and provide bowel rest when diarrhea present.

GI stimulants that may increase gastric motility/frequency of stools.

Further interventions/alternative bowel care may be needed.

Electrolyte imbalances may be the result of/contribute to altered GI function.

1033

ACTIONS/INTERVENTIONS

Collaborative

Administer IV fluids;

Antidiarrheal agents;

Stool softeners, laxatives, enemas as indicated.

RATIONALE

Prevents dehydration, dilutes chemotherapy agents to diminish side effects.

May be indicated in severe diarrhea.

Prophylactic use may prevent further complications in some patients (e.g., those who will receive Vinca alkaloid, have poor bowel pattern prior to treatment, or have decreased motility).

NURSING DIAGNOSIS:	SEXUALITY PATTERNS, ALTERED, HIGH RISK FOR
Risk factors may include	Knowledge/skill deficit about alternative responses to health-related transitions, altered body function/structure, illness, and medical treatment.
Possibly evidenced by:	Overwhelming fatigue.
	Fear and anxiety.
DESIRED OUTCOMES/ EVALUATION CRITERIA— PATIENT WILL:	Lack of privacy/SO.
	[Not applicable; presence of signs and symptoms establishes an actual diagnosis.]
	Verbalize understanding of effects of cancer and therapeutic regimen on sexuality and measures to correct/deal with problems.
	Maintain sexual activity at a desired level as possible.

ACTIONS/INTERVENTIONS

Independent

Discuss with patient/SO the nature of sexuality and reactions when it is altered or threatened. Provide information about normality of these problems and that many people find it helpful to seek assistance with adaptation process.

Advise patient of side effects of prescribed cancer treatment that are known to affect sexuality.

Provide private time for hospitalized patient. Knock on door and receive permission from patient/SO before entering.

RATIONALE

Acknowledges legitimacy of the problem. Sexuality encompasses the way men and women view themselves as individuals and how they relate between and among themselves in every area of life.

Anticipatory guidance can help patient and SO begin the process of adaptation to new state.

Sexuality needs do not end because the patient is hospitalized. Intimacy needs continue and an open and accepting attitude for the expression of those needs is essential.

NURSING DIAGNOSIS:	FAMILY PROCESS, ALTERED, HIGH RISK FOR
Risk factors may include:	Situational/transitional crises: Long-term illness, change in roles/economic status.
	Developmental: Anticipated loss of a family member.
Possibly evidenced by:	[Not applicable; presence of signs and symptoms establishes an actual diagnosis.]
DESIRED OUTCOMES/ EVALUATION CRITERIA— FAMILY WILL:	Express feelings freely.
	Demonstrate individual involvement in problem-solving process directed at appropriate solutions for the situation.
	Encourage and allow member who is ill to handle situation in own way.

ACTIONS/INTERVENTIONS

Independent

Note components of family, presence of extended family and others, e.g., friends/neighbors.

Identify patterns of communication in family and patterns of interaction between family members.

Assess role expectations of family members and encourage discussion about them.

Assess energy direction, e.g., are efforts at resolution/problem solving purposeful or scattered?

Note cultural/religious beliefs.

Listen for expressions of helplessness.

Deal with family members in a warm, caring, respectful way. Provide information (verbal/written), and reinforce as necessary.

Encourage appropriate expressions of anger without reacting negatively to them.

RATIONALE

Helps to know who is available to assist with care/provide respite, provide support, and be available as needed.

Provides information about effectiveness of communication and identifies problems that may interfere with family's ability to assist patient and adjust positively to diagnosis/treatment of cancer.

Each person may see the situation in own individual manner, and clear identification and sharing of these expectations promotes understanding.

Provides clues about interventions that may be appropriate to assist patient and family in directing energies in a more effective manner.

Affects patient/SO reaction and adjustment to diagnosis, treatment, and outcome of cancer.

Helpless feelings may contribute to difficulty adjusting to diagnosis of cancer and cooperating with treatment regimen.

Provides feeling of empathy and promotes individual's sense of worth and competence in ability to handle current situation.

Feelings of anger are to be expected when individuals are dealing with the difficult/potentially fatal illness of cancer. Appropriate expression enables progress toward resolution of the stages of the grieving process.

1035

ACTIONS/INTERVENTIONS

Independent

Acknowledge difficulties of the situation, e.g., diagnosis and treatment of cancer, possibility of death.

Identify and encourage use of previous successful coping behaviors.

Stress importance of continuous open dialogue between family members.

Collaborative

Refer to support groups, clergy, family therapy as indicated.

RATIONALE

Communicates acceptance of the reality the patient/family are facing.

Most people have developed effective coping skills that can be useful in dealing with current situation.

Promotes understanding and assists family members to maintain clear communication and resolve problems effectively.

May need additional assistance to resolve problems of disorganization that may accompany diagnosis of potentially terminal illness (cancer).

NURSING DIAGNOSIS:	KNOWLEDGE DEFICIT [LEARNING NEED], REGARDING ILLNESS, PROGNOSIS, AND TREATMENT NEEDS
May be related to:	Lack of exposure/recall; information misinterpretation, myths.
	Unfamiliarity with information resources.
	Cognitive limitation.
Possibly evidenced by:	Questions/request for information, verbalization of problem.
	Statement of misconception.
	Inaccurate follow-through of instructions/development of preventable complications.
DESIRED OUTCOMES/ EVALUATION CRITERIA— PATIENT WILL:	Verbalize accurate information about diagnosis and treatment regimen at own level of readiness.
	Correctly perform necessary procedures and explain reasons for the actions.
	Initiate necessary lifestyle changes and participate in treatment regimen.
	Identify/use available resources appropriately.

ACTIONS/INTERVENTIONS

Independent

Review with patient/SO understanding of specific diagnosis, treatment alternatives, and future expectations.

RATIONALE

Validates current level of understanding, identifies learning needs, and provides knowledge base on which patient can make informed decisions.

ACTIONS/INTERVENTIONS	RATIONALE

Independent

Determine patient's perception of cancer and cancer treatment(s); ask about patient's own/previous experience or experience with other people who have (or had) cancer.

Aids in identification of ideas, attitudes, fears, misconceptions, and gaps in knowledge about cancer.

Provide clear, accurate information in a factual but sensitive manner. Answer questions specifically, but do not bombard with unessential details.

Helps with adjustment to the diagnosis of cancer, by providing needed information along with time to absorb it. *Note:* Rate and method of giving information may need to be altered in order to decrease patient's anxiety and enhance ability to assimilate information.

Provide anticipatory guidance with patient/SO regarding treatment protocol, length of therapy, expected results, possible side effects. Be honest with patient.

Patient has the "right to know" (be informed) and participate in decision tree. Accurate and concise information helps to dispel fears and anxiety, helps clarify the expected routine, and enables patient to maintain some degree of control.

Ask patient for verbal feedback, and correct misconception about individual's type of cancer and treatment.

Misconceptions about cancer may be more disturbing than facts and can interfere with treatments/reduce healing.

Outline normally expected limitations (if any) on ADLs (e.g., limit sun exposure, alcohol intake; loss of work time because of in-hospital treatments).

If limitations are required, enables patient/SO to begin to put them into perspective and plan/adapt as indicated.

Provide written materials about cancer, treatment, and available support systems.

Anxiety and preoccupation with thoughts about life and death often interfere with patient's ability to assimilate adequate information. Written, take-home materials provide reinforcement and clarification about information as patient needs it.

Review specific medication regimen and use of OTC drugs.

Enhances ability to manage self-care and avoid potential complications, drug reactions/interactions.

Address specific home care needs, e.g., ability to live alone, perform necessary treatments/procedures, and acquire supplies.

Provides information regarding changes that may be needed in current plan of care to meet therapeutic needs.

Do predischarge home evaluation as indicated.

Aids in transition to home setting by providing information about needed changes in physical layout, acquisition of needed supplies.

Refer to community resources as indicated: e.g., social services, home health, Meals-on-Wheels, local American Cancer Society chapter, hospice center/services.

Promotes competent self-care and optimal independence. Maintains patient in desired/home setting.

Review with patient/SO the importance of maintaining optimal nutritional status.

Promotes well-being, facilitates recovery, and is critical in enabling the patient to tolerate treatments.

Encourage diet variations and experimentation in meal planning and food preparation, e.g., cooking with sweet juices, wine; serving foods cold or at room temperature as appropriate (egg salad, ice cream).

Creativity may enhance flavor and intake, especially when protein foods taste bitter.

1037

ACTIONS/INTERVENTIONS	RATIONALE
Independent	
Recommend cookbooks that are designed for cancer patients.	Helpful in providing specific menu/recipe ideas.
Recommend increased fluid intake and fiber in diet as well as routine exercise.	Improves consistency of stool and stimulates peristalsis.
Instruct patient to assess oral mucous membranes routinely, noting erythema, ulceration.	Early recognition of problems promotes early intervention, minimizing complications that may impair oral intake and provide avenue for systemic infection.
Advise patient concerning skin and hair care: e.g., avoid harsh shampoos, hair dyes, permanents, salt water, chlorinated water; avoid exposure to strong wind and extreme heat or cold; avoid sun exposure to target area for 1 year after end of radiation treatments and apply sunblock (SPF 15 or greater).	Prevents additional hair damage and skin irritation; may prevent recall reactions.
Review signs and symptoms, requiring medical evaluation, e.g., infection, delayed healing, drug reactions, increased pain (dependent on individual situation).	Early identification and treatment may limit severity of complications.
Stress importance of continuing medical follow-up.	Provides ongoing monitoring of progression/resolution of disease process and opportunity for timely diagnosis and treatment of complications. *Note:* Some complications can develop long after therapy is completed, e.g., pathologic fractures, radiation cystitis/nephritis.

Total Nutritional Support: Parenteral/Enteral Feeding _____

Specifically designed nutritional therapy can be administered by the parenteral or enteral route when the use of standard diets via the oral route is inadequate or not possible, to prevent/correct protein-calorie malnutrition.

Enteral nutrition is preferred for the patient who has a functional GI tract but is unable to consume an adequate nutritional intake, or oral intake is contraindicated/impossible. Feeding may be done via NG or orogastric tube, esophagostomy, gastrostomy, duodenostomy, or jejunostomy.

Parenteral nutrition may be chosen because of altered metabolic states or when mechanical or functional abnormalities of the GI tract prevent enteral feeding. Amino acids, fat, carbohydrates, trace elements, vitamins, and electrolytes may be infused via a central or peripheral vein.

RELATED CONCERNS:

Burns, p 820
Cancer, p 1014
Fluid and Electrolyte Imbalances, p 1054
Psychosocial Aspects of Acute Care, p 899
Surgical Intervention, p 918

PATIENT ASSESSMENT DATA BASE

Clinical signs listed below are dependent on degree and duration of malnutrition and include observations indicative of vitamin and mineral as well as protein/calorie deficiency.

ACTIVITY/REST

May exhibit: Muscle wasting (temporal, intercostal, gastrocnemius, dorsum of hand); thin extremities, flaccid muscles, decreased activity tolerance.

CIRCULATION

May exhibit: Tachycardia, bradycardia.

Diaphoresis, cyanosis.

ELIMINATION

May report: Diarrhea or constipation; flatulence associated with food intake.

May exhibit: Abdominal distention/increased girth, ascites; tenderness on palpation. Stools may be loose, hard-formed, fatty, or clay-colored.

FOOD/FLUID

May report: Weight loss of 10% or more of body weight within previous 6 months.

Problems with chewing, swallowing, choking, or saliva production.

Changes in the taste of food; anorexia, nausea/vomiting; inadequate oral intake (NPO) status for 7–10 days, long-term use of 5% dextrose intravenously.

May exhibit: Actual weight (measured) as compared with usual or preillness weight is less than 90% of ideal body weight for height, sex, and age or equal to or greater than 120% of ideal body weight (patient risk in obesity is a tendency to overlook protein and calorie requirements). A distorted actual weight may occur due to the presence of edema, ascites, organomegaly, tumor bulk, anasarca, amputation.

Edentulous or with ill-fitting dentures.

Bowel sounds diminished, hyperactive, or absent.

Thyroid, parotid enlargement.

Lips dry, cracked, red, swollen; angular stomatitis.

Tongue may be smooth, pale, slick, coated. Color often magenta, beefy red. Lingual papillae atrophy/swelling.

Gums swollen/bleeding, multiple caries.

Mucous membranes dry, pale, red, swollen.

NEUROSENSORY

May exhibit: Lethargy, apathy, listlessness, irritability, disorientation, coma.

Gag/swallow reflex may be decreased/absent, e.g., CVA, head trauma, nerve injury.

RESPIRATION

May exhibit: Increased respiratory rate; respiratory distress.

Dyspnea, increased sputum production.

Breath sounds: crackles (protein deficiency-related fluid shifts).

SAFETY

May report: Recent course of radiation therapy (radiation enteritis).

May exhibit: Hair may be fragile, coarse, lackluster. Alopecia, decreased pigmentation may be present.

Skin dry, scaly, tented; "flaky paint" dermatosis; edema; draining or unhealed wounds, pressure sores; ecchymoses, perifollicular petechiae, subcutaneous fat loss. Eyes sunken, dull, dry, with pale conjunctiva; Bitot's spots (triangular, shiny, gray spots on the conjunctiva seen in vitamin A deficiency), or scleral icterus.

Nails may be brittle, thin, flattened, ridged, spoon-shaped.

SEXUALITY

May report: Loss of libido.

Amenorrhea.

TEACHING/LEARNING

May report: History of conditions causing protracted protein losses, e.g., malabsorption or shortgut syndrome with increased diarrhea, acute pancreatitis, renal dialysis, fistulas, draining wounds, thermal injuries.

Presence of factors known to alter nutritional requirements/increase energy demands, e.g., single or multiorgan failure; sepsis; fever; trauma; extensive burns; use of steroids, antitumor agents, immunosuppressants.

Use of medications that cause untoward drug/nutrient interactions, e.g., laxatives, anticonvulsants, diuretics, antacids, narcotics, immunosuppressants, high-dose chemotherapy.

Illness of psychiatric origin, e.g., anorexia nervosa/bulimia.

Educational/social factors, e.g., lack of nutrition knowledge, kitchen facilities, reduced/limited financial resources.

Discharge Plan Considerations: **DRG projected mean length of stay: 6.1 days.**

May require assistance with solution preparation, therapy supplies, and maintenance of feeding device for home nutritional care.

DIAGNOSTIC STUDIES

Anthropometrics: Includes measurement of weight-to-height ratio, osseometry, and ratios of lean-to-fat weight:

Triceps skin fold measurement: Estimates subcutaneous fat stores; fat reserves less than 10th percentile suggest advanced depletion; levels less than the 30th percentile suggest mild-to-moderate depletion.

Midarm muscle circumference: Measures somatic muscle mass and is used in combination with triceps skinfold measurement; a decrease of 15–20 percentiles from the expected value suggests a significant reduction.

Visceral proteins:

Serum albumin (the classic marker measured): Values of 2.7–3.4 g/dl indicate mild depletion; 2.1–2.7 g/dl, moderate depletion; and less than 2.1 g/dl, severe depletion. (Decreased levels are due to poor protein intake, nephrotic syndrome, sepsis, burns, CHF, cirrhosis, eclampsia, protein-losing enteropathy. Above normal values [greater than 4.5 g/dl] are seen in dehydration.)

Serum transferrin: More sensitive to changes in visceral protein stores than albumin; levels of 150–200 mg/dl reflect mild depletion; 100–150 mg/dl, moderate depletion; and 100 mg/dl, severe depletion. (Elevated values are seen with iron deficiency, pregnancy, hypoxia, and chronic blood loss. Decreased values are seen with pernicious anemia, chronic infection, liver disease, iron overload, and protein-losing enteropathy.)

Thyroxine-binding prealbumin: Reflects rapid changes in hepatic protein synthesis and thus is a more sensitive indicator of visceral protein depletion. (Decreased levels less than 200 mEg/ml are noted with cirrhosis, inflammation, and surgical trauma.)

Amino acid profile: Alterations reflect an imbalance of plasma proteins with depressed levels of branch chain amino acids (common with hepatic encephalopathy or sepsis).

Tests of immune system:

Total lymphocyte count: Less than 1500 cells/mm indicates leukopenia and results from decreased generation of T cells, which are very sensitive to malnutrition. (Levels are also altered by infection and administration of immunosuppressants.)

Tests of micronutrients:

Potassium: Deficiency occurs with inadequate intake and with loss of potassium-containing fluids (e.g., urine, diarrhea, vomiting, fistula drainage, continuous NG suctioning). Potassium is also lost from cells during muscle wasting and is excreted by the kidneys.

Sodium: Levels are dependent on state of hydration/presence of active loss as may exist in excessive diuresis, GI suctioning, burns.

Phosphorus: May be decreased reflecting inadequate intake or may be elevated in renal failure.

Magnesium: Deficiency is common in alcoholics, chronic vomiting, diarrhea; may be elevated in renal failure.

Calcium: Levels will be decreased with conditions associated with hypoalbuminemia, e.g., renal failure (majority of calcium is bound to albumin). Absorption is decreased by fat malabsorption and low-protein diet.

Zinc: Deficiency is seen in alcoholic cirrhosis; or may be secondary to hypoalbuminemia and GI losses (diarrhea).

Tests reflecting protein (nitrogen) loss:

Nitrogen balance studies: Nitrogen (protein) excretion via urine, stool and insensible losses often exceed nitrogen intake in the acutely ill, reflecting catabolic response to stress and use of endogenous protein stores for energy production (gluconeogenesis). BUN may be severely decreased as a result of chronic malnutrition and depletion of skeletal protein stores.

24-hour creatinine excretion: Because Cr is concentrated in muscle mass, there is a good correlation between lean body mass and 24-hour Cr excretion. Actual values are compared with ideal values (based on height and weight) times 100, known as the Cr height index: 60%–80% indicates moderate depletion; less than 60%, severe depletion.

Tests of function:

Include Schilling test, D-xylose test, 72-hour stool fat, GI series: determine malabsorption.

Chest x-ray: May be normal or show evidence of pleural effusion; small heart silhouette.

ECG: May be normal or demonstrate low voltage, dysrhythmias/patterns reflective of electrolyte imbalances.

NURSING PRIORITIES

1. Promote consistent intake of estimated calorie and protein requirements.
2. Prevent complications.
3. Minimize energy losses/needs.
4. Provide information about condition, prognosis, and treatment needs.

DISCHARGE GOALS

1. Nutritional intake adequate for individual needs.
2. Complications prevented/minimized.
3. Fatigue alleviated.
4. Condition, prognosis, and therapeutic regimen understood.

NURSING DIAGNOSIS:	**NUTRITION, ALTERED: LESS THAN BODY REQUIREMENTS**
May be related to:	Conditions that interfere with nutrient intake or increase nutrient need/metabolic demand, e.g., cancer and associated treatments, anorexia, surgical procedures, dysphagia/difficulty swallowing, depressed mental status/level of consciousness.
Possibly evidenced by:	Body weight 10% or more under ideal. Decreased subcutaneous fat/muscle mass, poor muscle tone. Changes in gastric motility and stool characteristics.
DESIRED OUTCOMES/ EVALUATION CRITERIA— PATIENT WILL:	Demonstrate stable weight or progressive weight gain toward goal with normalization of laboratory values and be free of signs of malnutrition.

ACTIONS/INTERVENTIONS	RATIONALE
Independent	
General	
Assess nutritional status continually, during daily nursing care, noting energy level; condition of skin, nails, hair, oral cavity, desire to eat/anorexia.	Provides the opportunity to observe deviations from normals/patient baseline and influences choice of interventions.
Weigh daily and compare with admission weight.	Establishes baseline, aids in monitoring effectiveness of therapeutic regimen, and alerts nurse to inappropriate trends in weight loss/gain.

ACTIONS/INTERVENTIONS	RATIONALE

Independent

Document oral intake by use of 24-hour recall, food history, calorie counts .as appropriate.

Identifies imbalance between estimated nutritional requirements and actual intake.

Assure accurate collection of specimens (urine, stool, drainage) for nitrogen balance studies.

Inaccurate collection can alter test results, leading to improper interpretation of patient's current status and needs.

Administer nutritional solutions at prescribed rate via infusion control device as needed. Adjust rate to deliver prescribed hourly rate. Do not increase rate to "catch up."

Nutrition support prescriptions are based on estimated caloric and protein requirements. A consistent rate of nutrient administration will assure proper utilization with fewer side effects, such as hyperglycemia or dumping syndrome. *Note:* Continuous and cyclic infusion of enteral formulas are generally better tolerated than bolus feedings and result in improved absorption.

Be familiar with electrolyte content of nutritional solutions.

Metabolic complications of nutritional support often result from a lack of appreciation of changes that can occur as a result of refeeding, e.g., hyperglycemic, hyperosmotic nonketotic coma, electrolyte imbalances.

Schedule activities with adequate rest periods. Promote relaxation techniques.

Conserves energy/reduces calorie needs. (Refer to ND: Fatigue, p 1050.)

Parenteral
Observe appropriate "hang" time of parenteral solutions per protocol.

Effectiveness of IV vitamins diminishes after 24 hours.

Monitor urine sugar/acetone or fingerstick glucose per protocol.

High glucose content of solutions may lead to pancreatic fatigue, requiring use of supplemental insulin to prevent HHNC. *Note:* Fingerstick determination of glucose level is more accurate/may be preferred over urine testing because of variations in renal glucose threshold.

Enteral
Assess GI function and tolerance to enteral feedings: note bowel sounds; reports of nausea/vomiting, abdominal discomfort; presence of diarrhea/constipation; development of weakness lightheadedness, diaphoresis, tachycardia, abdominal cramping.

Because protein turnover of the GI mucosa occurs approximately every 3 days, the GI tract is at great risk for early dysfunction and atrophy from disease and malnutrition. Intolerance of formula/presence of dumping syndrome may require alteration of rate of administration/concentration of formula or change to parenteral administration.

Check gastric residuals if bolus feedings are done, and as otherwise indicated; hold feeding/return aspirate per protocol for type/rate of feeding used if residual is greater than predetermined level.

Delayed gastric emptying can be caused by a specific disease process, e.g., paralytic ileus/surgery, shock; by drug therapy (especially narcotics); or the protein/fat content of the individual formula. *Note:* Replacement of gastric aspirate reduces loss of gastric acid/electrolytes.

Maintain patency of enteral feeding tubes by flushing with warm water, as indicated.

Enteral formulas contain protein that can clog feeding tubes (silicone more likely than polyurethane tubes) necessitating removal/replacement of tube. *Note:* Cranberry juice or colas are not recommended. Pancrelipase (a pancreatic enzyme) may be effective in clearing tubing of persistent clog.

1043

ACTIONS/INTERVENTIONS	RATIONALE

Independent

Transitional

Stress importance of transition to oral feedings as appropriate.

Although patient may have little interest or desire to eat, transition to oral feedings is preferred in view of potential side effects/complications of nutritional support therapy.

Assess gag reflex, ability to chew/swallow, and motor skills when progressing to transitional feedings.

May require additional interventions, e.g., retraining by dysphagia expert (speech therapist) or long-term nutritional support.

Provide self-help utensils as indicated, e.g., plate guard, utensils with builtup handles, lidded cups.

Patients with neuromuscular deficits, e.g., post-CVA, brain injury, may require use of special aids developed for feeding.

Create optimal environment, e.g., remove noxious stimuli, bedpans, soiled linens. Provide cheerful, attractive tray/table, soft music, companionship.

Encourages patient's attempts to eat, reduces anorexia, and introduces some of the social pleasures usually associated with mealtime.

Allow adequate time for chewing, swallowing, savoring food; provide socialization and feeding assistance as indicated.

Patients need encouragement/assistance to overcome underlying problems such as anorexia, fatigue, muscular weakness.

Offer small, frequent feedings; incorporate patient likes/dislikes in meal planning as much as possible, and include "home foods" as appropriate.

May enhance patient's desire for food and amount of intake.

Provide calorie-containing beverages, when oral intake is possible, e.g., juices/Jello water, dietary supplements (Sustacal, Ensure, Polycase) to beverages/water.

Maximizes calorie intake when oral intake is limited/restricted.

Collaborative

Refer to nutritional team/registered dietitian.

Aids in identification of nutrient deficits and need for parenteral/enteral nutritional intervention.

Calculate basal energy expenditure using formula based on sex, height, weight, age, and estimated energy requirements.

Provides an estimation of calorie and protein needs.

Review results of indirect calorimetry test if available.

Measures O_2 consumption at basal or resting metabolic rate, to aid in estimating calorie/protein requirements.

Assist with insertion and confirm proper placement of infusion line (e.g., chest x-ray for central venous catheter or aspiration of gastric contents from feeding tube) prior to administration of solutions.

Reduces risk of feeding-induced complications, including pneumothorax/hemothorax, hydrothorax, air embolus, arterial puncture (central venous line), or aspiration (NG tube).

Administer dextrose-electrolyte or dextrose-amino acid and lipid emulsions (3-in-1) solutions as indicated.

Solutions provide calories, essential amino acids, and micronutrients, usually combined with lipids for complete nutrition known as total nutrient admixtures. Solutions are modified to meet specific needs, e.g., renal and liver failure (lower protein), respiratory failure (higher fat).

Co-infuse lipid emulsions if 3-in-1 solutions not used.

Useful in meeting excessive calorie requirements (e.g., burns) or as a source of essential fatty acids

ACTIONS/INTERVENTIONS
Collaborative

RATIONALE

during long-term hyperalimentation. *Note:* Lipid solutions may be contraindicated in patients with alterations in fat metabolism or in the presence of pancreatitis, liver damage, anemia, coagulation disorders, pulmonary disease.

Administer medications, as indicated, e.g.:

Multivitamin preparations;

Water-soluble vitamins will be added to parenteral solutions. Other vitamins may be given for identified deficiencies.

Insulin;

High glucose content of solutions may require exogenous insulin for metabolism especially in presence of pancreatic insufficiency or disease. *Note:* Insulin is usually now added directly to parenteral solution.

Diphenoxylate with atropine (Lomotil), camphorated tincture of opium (Paregoric), and metoclopramide (Reglan).

GI side effects of enteral feeding may need to be controlled with antidiarrheal agents (Lomotil/Paregoric) or peristaltic stimulants (Reglan) if more conservative measures such as alteration of rate/strength or type of formula are not successful.

Monitor laboratory studies, e.g., serum glucose, electrolytes, transferrin, albumin, total protein, phosphate, BUN/Cr, liver enzymes, CBC, ABGs.

Untoward metabolic effects of TPN include: hypokalemia, hyponatremia and fluid retention, hyperglycemia, hypophosphatemia, increased CO_2 production resulting in respiratory compromise, elevation of liver function tests, renal dysfunction.

NURSING DIAGNOSIS:	INFECTION, HIGH RISK FOR
Risk factors may include:	Invasive procedures: Insertion of venous catheter; surgically placed gastrostomy/jejunostomy feeding tube.
	Malnutrition; chronic disease.
	Environmental exposure: Access devices in place for extended periods, improper preparation/handling/contamination of the feeding solution.
Possibly evidenced by:	[Not applicable; presence of signs and symptoms establishes an actual diagnosis.]
DESIRED OUTCOMES/ EVALUATION CRITERIA— PATIENT WILL:	Experience no fever or chills.
	Demonstrate clean catheter insertion sites, free of drainage and erythema/edema.

ACTIONS/INTERVENTIONS

Independent

Parenteral

Maintain an optimal aseptic environment during bedside insertion of central venous catheters and during changes of TPN bottles and administration tubing.

Secure external portion of catheter/administration tubing to dressing with tape. Note intactness of skin suture.

Maintain a sterile occlusive dressing over catheter insertion site. Perform central/peripheral venous catheter dressing care per protocol.

Inspect insertion site of catheter for erythema, induration, drainage, tenderness.

Refrigerate premixed solutions prior to use; observe a 24-hour hang time for amino acid or total nutrient admixture solutions and a 12-hour hang time for individual IV fat emulsions.

Monitor temperature and glucose.

Enteral

Keep manipulations of enteral feeding system to a minimum and wash hands before opening system.

Alternate nares for tube placement in long-term NG feedings.

Provide daily/prn site care to abdominally placed feeding tubes.

Refrigerate reconstituted enteral formulas before use; observe a hang time of 4–8 hours; discard unused formula after 24 hours.

Collaborative

Aseptically prepare parenteral solutions/enteral formulas for administration.

RATIONALE

Catheter-related sepsis may result from entry of pathogenic microorganisms through skin insertion tract, or from touch contamination during manipulations of TPN system.

Manipulation of catheter in/out of insertion site can result in tissue trauma (coring) and potentiate entry of skin organisms into catheter tract.

Protects catheter insertion sites from potential sources of contamination. *Note:* Central venous catheter sites can easily become contaminated from tracheostomy or endotracheal secretions or from wounds of the head, neck, and chest.

The catheter is a potential irritant to the surrounding skin and subcutaneous skin tract, and extended use may result in insertion site irritation and infection.

TPN solutions and fat emulsions have been shown to support the growth of a variety of pathogenic organisms once contaminated.

A rise in temperature or loss of glucose tolerance (glycosuria, hyperglycemia) are early indications of possible catheter-related sepsis.

Touch contamination by caregiver during enteral formula administration has been shown to cause contamination of formula.

Reduces risk of trauma/infection of paranasal tissue (especially important in facial trauma/burns).

GI secretions leaking through or around gastrostomy/jejunostomy tube tracts can cause skin breakdown severe enough to require removal of the feeding tube.

Enteral formulas easily support bacterial growth and can be contaminated during formula preparation. For example, bacterial growth has been shown to occur within 4 hours after contamination.

TPN solutions should be prepared under a laminar flow hood in the department of pharmacy. Enteral formulas should be mixed in a clean environment in the dietary or pharmacy department, although with the advent of canned/modular formulas, this may not be necessary. *Note:* Additives to TPN solutions, as a rule, should not be made on the unit because of the potential for contamination and drug incompatibilities.

ACTIONS/INTERVENTIONS	RATIONALE

Collaborative

Notify physician if signs of infection present. Follow protocol for obtaining appropriate culture specimens, e.g., blood, solutions. Change bottle/tubing as indicated.

Necessary to identify source of infection and initiate appropriate therapy. May require removal of TPN line and culture of catheter tip.

Administer antibiotics as indicated.

May be given prophylactically or for specifically identified organism.

NURSING DIAGNOSIS;	INJURY, HIGH RISK FOR, [MULTIFACTOR]
Risk factors may include:	External environment: Catheter-related complications (air emboli and septic thrombophlebitis). Internal factors: Aspiration; effects of therapy/drug interactions.
Possibly evidenced by:	[Not applicable; presence of signs and symptoms establishes an actual diagnosis.]
DESIRED OUTCOMES/ EVALUATION CRITERIA— PATIENT WILL:	Be free of complications associated with nutritional support. Modify environment/correct hazards to enhance safety for in-home therapy.

ACTIONS/INTERVENTIONS	RATIONALE

Independent

Parenteral

Maintain a closed central IV system using Luer-Lok connections/taping of all connections.

Inadvertent disconnection of central IV system can result in lethal air emboli.

Administer appropriate TPN solution via peripheral or central venous route.

Solutions containing high concentrations of dextrose (greater than 10%) must be delivered via a central vein, because they will result in chemical phlebitis when delivered through small peripheral veins.

Monitor for potential drug/nutrient interactions.

Various interactions are possible, for example, digoxin (in conjunction with diuretic therapy) can cause hypomagnesemia; hypokalemia may result from chronic use of laxatives, mineralocorticosteroids, diuretics, or amphotericin.

Assess catheter for signs of displacement out of central venous position, i.e., extended length of catheter on skin surface; leaking of IV solution onto dressing; patient complaints of neck pain, tenderness at catheter site, or swelling of extremity on side of catheter insertion.

Central venous catheter tip may slip out of superior vena cava and migrate into smaller innominate and jugular veins, causing a chemical thrombophlebitis. Incidence of subclavian or superior vena cava thrombosis is increased with extended use of central venous catheters.

1047

ACTIONS/INTERVENTIONS	RATIONALE

Independent

Inspect peripheral TPN catheter site routinely and change sites at least every 3 days or per protocol.

Peripheral TPN solutions (although less hyperosmolar) can still irritate small veins and cause phlebitis. Peripheral venous access is often limited in malnourished patients, but site should still be changed if signs of irritation develop.

Investigate reports of severe chest pain/coughing. Turn patient to left side in Trendelenburg position if indicated and notify physician.

Suggests presence of air embolus requiring immediate intervention to displace air into apex of heart away from the pulmonary artery.

Maintain an occlusive dressing on catheter insertion sites for 24 hours after subclavian catheter is removed.

Extended catheter use may result in development of catheter skin tract. Once the catheter is removed, air embolus is still a potential risk until skin tract has sealed.

Enteral

Assess gastrostomy or jejunostomy tube sites for evidence of malposition.

Indwelling and mushroom catheters are still frequently used for feeding tubes inserted via the abdomen. Migration of the catheter balloon can result in duodenal or jejunal obstruction. Improperly sutured gastrostomy tubes may easily fall out.

Collaborative

Review chest x-ray as indicated.

Central parenteral line placement is routinely confirmed by x-ray.

Consult with pharmacist in regard to site/time of delivery of drugs that might have action adversely affected by enteral formula.

Absorption of vitamin D is impaired by administration of mineral oil (inhibits micelle formation of bile salts) and by neomycin (inactivates bile salts). Aluminum-containing antacids bind with the phosphorus in the feeding solution, potentiating hypophosphatemia.

NURSING DIAGNOSIS:	ASPIRATION, HIGH RISK FOR
Risk factors may include:	Presence of the GI tube, bolus tube feedings, medication administration.
Possibly evidenced by:	Increased intragastric pressure, delayed gastric emptying.
	[Not applicable; presence of signs and symptoms establishes an actual diagnosis.]
DESIRED OUTCOMES/ EVALUATION CRITERIA— PATIENT WILL:	Maintain clear airway, be free of signs of aspiration.

ACTIONS/INTERVENTIONS	RATIONALE

Independent

Confirm placement of nasoenteral feeding tubes. Determine feeding tube position in stomach by

Malplacement of nasoenteral feeding tubes may result in aspiration of enteral formula. Patients at

ACTIONS/INTERVENTIONS	RATIONALE

Independent

x-ray, confirmation of pH of 2 or 3 of the gastric fluid withdrawn through tube, or auscultation of injected air prior to intermittent feedings. Observe for ability to speak/cough.

particular risk include those who are intubated or obtunded; following CVA or surgery of the head/neck, upper GI system.

Maintain aspiration precautions during enteral feedings, e.g.:

Keep head of bed elevated at 30–45 degrees during feeding and at least 1 hour after feeding;

Aspiration of enteral formulas is irritating to the lung parenchyma and may result in pneumonia and respiratory compromise.

Inflate tracheostomy cuff during and for 1 hour after intermittent feeding. Interrupt feeding when patient is in prone position;

Add blue food coloring to enteral formula as indicated.

Helps identify aspiration of enteral formula and/or tracheal esophageal fistula, if discovered in sputum/lung secretions. *Note:* Avoid use of methylene blue dye, which may cause false-positive guaiac test when assessing for GI bleeding.

Monitor gastric residuals after bolus feedings (as previously noted in ND: Nutrition, Altered: Less Than Body Requirements, p 1042.)

Presence of large gastric residuals may potentiate an incompetent esophageal sphincter, leading to vomiting and aspiration.

Note characteristics of sputum/tracheal aspirate. Investigate development of dyspnea, cough, tachypnea, cyanosis. Auscultate breath sounds.

Presence of formula in tracheal secretions or signs/symptoms reflecting respiratory distress suggests aspiration.

Note indicators of NG tube intolerance, e.g., absence of gag reflex, high risk of aspiration, frequent removal of NG feeding tubes.

May require consideration of surgically placed feeding tubes (e.g., gastrostomy, jejunostomy) for patient safety and consistency of enteral formula delivery.

Collaborative

Review abdominal x-ray if done.

Confirmation of gastric feeding tube may be obtained by x-ray.

NURSING DIAGNOSIS:	FLUID VOLUME, ALTERED: [FLUCTUATION]
May be related to:	Active loss and/or failure of regulatory mechanisms (specific to underlying disease process/trauma); complications of nutrition therapy, e.g., high glucose solutions, hyperglycemia (hyperosmolar nonketotic coma and severe dehydration). Inability to obtain/ingest fluids.
Possibly evidenced by:	[Not applicable; presence of signs and symptoms establishes an actual diagnosis.]
DESIRED OUTCOMES/ EVALUATION CRITERIA— PATIENT WILL:	Display moist skin/mucous membranes, stable vital signs, individually adequate urinary output; be free of edema and excessive weight loss/inappropriate gain.

ACTIONS/INTERVENTIONS	RATIONALE
Independent	
Assess for clinical signs of dehydration (e.g., thirst, dry skin/mucous membranes, hypotension); or fluid excess (e.g., peripheral edema, tachycardia, adventitious breath sounds).	Early detection and intervention may prevent occurrence/excessive fluctuation in fluid balance. *Note:* Severely malnourished patients have an increased risk of developing refeeding syndrome, e.g., life-threatening fluid overload, intracellular electrolyte shifts, and cardiac strain occurring during initial 3–5 days of therapy.
Incorporate knowledge of caloric density of enteral formulas into assessment of fluid balance.	Enteric solutions are usually concentrated and do not meet free water needs.
Provide additional water/flush tubing as indicated.	With higher calorie formula, additional water is needed to prevent dehydration/HHNC.
Record I&O; calculate fluid balance. Measure urine specific gravity.	Excessive urinary losses may reflect developing HHNC. Specific gravity is an indicator of hydration and renal function.
Weigh daily or as indicated; evaluate changes.	Rapid weight gain (reflecting fluid retention) can predispose/potentiate CHF or pulmonary edema. Gain of greater than 0.5 lb/d indicates fluid retention and not deposition of lean body mass.
Collaborative	
Monitor laboratory studies, e.g.:	
Serum potassium/phosphorus.	Hypokalemia/phosphatemia can occur due to intracellular shifts during initial refeeding and may compromise cardiac function if not corrected.
Hct.	Reflects hydration/circulating volume.
Serum albumin.	Hypoalbuminemia/decreased colloidal osmotic pressure leads to third spacing of fluid (edema).
Dilute formula or change from hypertonic to isotonic formula as indicated.	May decrease gastric intolerance reducing occurrence of diarrhea and associated fluid losses.

NURSING DIAGNOSIS:	FATIGUE
May be related to:	Decreased metabolic energy production; increased energy requirements (hypermetabolic states, healing process).
	Altered body chemistry: Medications, chemotherapy.
Possibly evidenced by:	Overwhelming lack of energy, inability to maintain usual routines/accomplish routine tasks.
	Lethargy, impaired ability to concentrate.
DESIRED OUTCOMES/ EVALUATION CRITERIA— PATIENT WILL:	Report increased sense of well-being/energy level.
	Demonstrate measurable increase in physical activity.

ACTIONS/INTERVENTIONS	RATIONALE

Independent

Monitor physiologic response to activity, e.g., changes in BP, or heart/respiratory rate.

Tolerance varies greatly, depending on the stage of the disease process, nutritional state, and fluid balance.

Establish realistic activity goals with patient.

Provides for a sense of control and feelings of accomplishment.

Plan care to allow for rest periods. Schedule activities for periods when patient has most energy. Involve patient/SO in schedule planning.

Frequent rest periods are needed to restore/conserve energy. Planning will allow patient to be active during times when energy level is higher, which may restore a feeling of well-being and a sense of control.

Encourage patient to do whatever possible, e.g., self-care, sitting up in chair, walking. Increase activity level as indicated.

Increases strength/stamina and enables patient to become more active without undue fatigue.

Provide passive/active ROM exercises to bedridden patients.

The development of healthy lean muscle mass is dependent on the provision of both isotonic and isometric exercises.

Keep bed in low position, pathways clear of furniture; assist with ambulation.

Protects patient from injury during activities.

Assist with self-care needs as necessary.

Weakness may make ADLs almost impossible for the patient to complete.

Collaborative

Provide supplemental O_2 as indicated.

Presence of anemia/hypoxemia reduces O_2 available for cellular uptake and contributes to fatigue.

Refer to physical/occupational therapy.

Programmed daily exercises and activities help patient to maintain/increase strength and muscle tone and enhance sense of well-being.

NURSING DIAGNOSIS:	**KNOWLEDGE DEFICIT [LEARNING NEED] REGARDING CONDITION, PROGNOSIS, AND TREATMENT NEEDS**
May be related to:	Lack of exposure/recall, information misinterpretation.
	Cognitive limitation.
Possibly evidenced by:	Request for information, questions/statement of misconception.
	Inaccurate follow-through of instructions/development of preventable complications.
DESIRED OUTCOMES/ EVALUATION CRITERIA— PATIENT WILL:	Verbalize understanding of condition/disease process and individual nutritional needs.
	Correctly perform necessary procedures and explain reasons for the actions.

ACTIONS/INTERVENTIONS

Independent

Assess patient's/SO knowledge of nutritional state. Review individual situation, signs/symptoms of malnutrition, future expectations, transitional feeding needs.

Discuss reasons for use of parenteral/enteral nutrition support.

Provide adequate time for patient/SO teaching when patient is going home on enteral/parenteral feedings. Document patient/SO understanding and ability/competence to deliver safe home therapy.

Discuss proper handling, storage, preparation of nutritional solutions or blenderized feedings; also discuss aseptic or clean techniques for care of insertion sites and use of dressings.

Review use/care of nutritional support devices.

Review specific precautions dependent on type of feeding, e.g., checking placement of tube, sitting upright for enteral feeding, maintaining patency of tube, anchoring of tubing.

Demonstrate reinsertion of gastric feeding tube if appropriate.

Identify signs/symptoms requiring medical evaluation, e.g., nausea/vomiting, abdominal cramping/bloating, diarrhea, rapid weight changes; erythema, drainage, foul odor at tube insertion site, fever/chills; coughing/choking or difficulty breathing during enteral feeding.

Instruct patient/SO in glucose monitoring if indicated.

Discuss signs/symptoms and treatment of hyperglycemia/hypoglycemia.

Encourage use of diary for recording test results, physical feelings/reactions, activity level, oral intake if any, I&O, weekly weight.

RATIONALE

Provides information on which the patient/SO can base informed choices. Knowledge of the interaction between malnutrition and illness is helpful to understanding need for special therapy.

May experience anxiety regarding inability to eat and may not comprehend the nutritional value of the prescribed TPN/tube feedings.

Generally, 3–4 days is sufficient for patient/SO to become proficient with tube feedings. Parenteral therapy is more complex and may require a week or longer for patient/SO to feel ready for home management and requires follow-up in the home.

Reduces risk of metabolic complications and infection.

Patient understanding and cooperation is key to the safe insertion and maintenance of nutritional support access devices as well as prevention of complications.

Promotes safe self-care and reduces risk of complications.

Tube may be changed routinely or only inserted for feedings. Intermittent feedings enhance patient mobility and aid in transition to regular feeding pattern.

Early evaluation and treatment of problems (e.g., feeding intolerance, infection, aspiration) may prevent progression to more serious complications.

Timely recognition of changes in blood sugar levels reduces risk of hypoglycemic reactions in patient on hyperalimentation.

Hyperglycemia is more common for patient receiving parenteral feedings and those who have pancreas or liver disease or are on large doses of corticosteroids. Rebound hypoglycemia can occur when feedings are intentionally/accidentally discontinued.

Provides resource for review by health care providers for optimal management of individual situation.

ACTIONS/INTERVENTIONS	RATIONALE

Independent

Recommend daily exercise/activity to tolerance, scheduling of adequate rest periods.

Enhances gastric motility for enteral/transition feedings, promotes feelings of general well-being, and prevents undue fatigue.

Ascertain that all supplies are in place in the home prior to discharge; make arrangements as needed with suppliers, e.g., hospital, pharmacy, medical equipment suppliers.

Provides for successful and competent home therapy.

Refer to nutritional support team, home health care agency, and so on. Provide with immediate access phone numbers.

Patient/SO need readily available support persons to assist with nutrition therapy, equipment problems, and emotional adjustments in long-term/home-based therapy.

Fluid and Electrolyte Imbalances

The body is equipped with homeostatic mechanisms to keep the composition and volume of body fluids within narrow limits of normal. Organs involved in this mechanism include the kidneys, lungs, heart, blood vessels, adrenal glands, parathyroid glands, pituitary gland. Note: Because fluid and electrolyte imbalances usually occur in conjunction with other medical conditions, the following files are offered as a reference. The interventions are presented in a general format for inclusion in the primary plan of care.

RELATED CONCERNS

Plans of care specific to underlying cause.
Acid-Base Imbalances, p 1082
Renal Dialysis, p 646

NURSING PRIORITIES

1. Restore homeostasis.
2. Prevent/minimize complications.
3. Provide information about condition/prognosis and treatment needs as appropriate.

DISCHARGE GOALS

1. Homeostasis restored.
2. Free of complications.
3. Condition/prognosis and treatment needs understood.

HYPERVOLEMIA (EXTRACELLULAR FLUID VOLUME EXCESS)

PREDISPOSING/CONTRIBUTING FACTORS

Excess sodium intake/hypertonic fluid replacement.
Excessive, rapid administration of isotonic parenteral fluids.
Increased release of ADH; excessive ACTH production, hyperaldosteronism.
Decreased plasma proteins as may occur with chronic liver disease with ascites, major abdominal surgery, malnutrition/protein depletion.
Chronic kidney disease/ARF.
CHF.

PATIENT ASSESSMENT DATA BASE

ACTIVITY/REST

May report: Fatigue, generalized weakness.

CIRCULATION

May exhibit: Hypertension, elevated CVP.

Pulse full/bounding; tachycardia usually present; bradycardia (late sign of cardiac decompensation).

Extra heart sounds (S_3).

Edema: Dependent, pitting, facial, periorbital, anasarca. Neck and peripheral vein distention.

1054

ELIMINATION

May report: Decreased urinary output, polyuria if renal function normal.

FOOD/FLUID

May report: Anorexia, nausea/vomiting, thirst.

May exhibit: Abdominal girth increased with visible fluid wave on palpation (ascites).
Acute weight gain, often in excess of 5% of total body weight.
Edema: Initially dependent, may progress to general/anasarca.

NEUROSENSORY

May exhibit: Changes in level of consciousness, from confusion to coma. Aphasia. Seizures.

RESPIRATION

May exhibit: Tachypnea with/without dyspnea, orthopnea; productive cough.
Crackles.

SAFETY

May exhibit: Fever.
Skin changes in color, temperature, turgor, e.g., taut and cool where edematous.

TEACHING/LEARNING

Refer to predisposing/contributing factors.

Discharge Plan Considerations: **DRG projected mean length of stay: 4.1 days.**
May require assistance with changes in therapeutic regimen, dietary management.

DIAGNOSTIC STUDIES

CBC: Hb/Hct and RBC usually decreased (hemodilution).
Serum Sodium: May be high, low, or normal.
Urine Sodium: May be low because of sodium retention.
Total protein: Albumin may be decreased.
Serum osmolality: Usually unchanged, although hypo-osmolality may occur.
Serum Potassium and BUN: Normal or decreased, unless renal damage present.
Urine specific gravity: Decreased.
Chest x-ray: May reveal signs of congestion.

ACTIONS/INTERVENTIONS	RATIONALE
Independent	
Monitor vital signs and CVP.	Tachycardia and hypertension are common manifestations. Tachypnea usually present with/without dyspnea. Elevated CVP may be noted before dyspnea and adventitious breath sounds occur.
Auscultate lungs and heart sounds.	Adventitious sounds (crackles) and extra heart sounds (S_3) are indicative of fluid excess. Pulmonary edema may develop rapidly.

1055

ACTIONS/INTERVENTIONS	RATIONALE

Independent

Assess for presence/location of edema formation.

Edema may be generalized or localized in dependent areas. Elderly patients may develop dependent edema with relatively little excess fluid. *Note:* Patients in a supine position can have an increase of 4–8 L of fluid before edema is readily detected.

Note presence of neck and peripheral vein distention, along with pitting edema, dyspnea.

Signs of cardiac decompensation/CHF.

Maintain accurate I&O. Note decreased urinary output, positive fluid balance on 24-hour calculations.

Decreased renal perfusion, cardiac insufficiency, and fluid shifts may cause decreased urinary output and edema formation.

Weigh as indicated. Be alert for acute or sudden weight gain.

1 L of fluid retention equals a weight gain of 2.2 lb.

Give oral fluids with caution. If fluids are restricted, set up a 24-hour schedule for fluid intake.

Fluid restrictions, as well as extracellular shifts, can cause drying of mucous membranes, and patient may desire more fluids than are prudent.

Monitor infusion rate of parenteral fluids closely; administer via control device/pump as necessary.

Sudden fluid bolus/prolonged excessive administration potentiates volume overload/risk of cardiac decompensation.

Encourage coughing/deep-breathing exercises.

Pulmonary fluid shifts potentiate respiratory complications.

Maintain semi-Fowler's position if dyspnea or ascites is present.

Gravity improves lung expansion by lowering diaphragm and shifting fluid to lower abdominal cavity.

Turn, reposition, and provide skin care at regular intervals.

Reduces pressure and friction on edematous tissue, which is more prone to breakdown than normal tissue.

Promote bedrest. Schedule care to provide frequent rest periods.

Limited cardiac reserves result in fatigue/activity intolerances.

Provide safety precautions as indicated, e.g., use of side rails, bed in low position, frequent observation, soft restraints (if required).

Fluid shifts may cause cerebral edema/changes in mentation, especially in the geriatric population.

Collaborative

Assist with identification/treatment of underlying cause.

Refer to listing of predisposing/contributing factors.

Monitor laboratory studies as indicated, e.g., electrolytes, BUN, ABGs.

Extracellular fluid shifts, sodium/water restriction and renal function all affect serum sodium levels. Potassium deficit may occur with diuretic therapy. BUN may be increased as a result of renal dysfunction/failure. ABGs may reflect metabolic acidosis.

Provide high-protein, low-sodium diet. Restrict fluids as indicated.

Increased serum proteins can enhance colloidal osmotic gradients and promote return of fluid to the vascular space. Restriction of sodium/water decreases extracellular fluid retention.

Administer diuretics: e.g., loop diuretic, furosemide (Lasix); thiazide diuretic, e.g., hydrochlorothiazide

To achieve excretion of excess fluid, either a single diuretic (e.g., thiazide) or a combination of agents

ACTIONS/INTERVENTIONS	RATIONALE

Collaborative

(Esidrex); potassium-sparing diuretic, e.g., spironolactone (Aldactone).

may be selected (e.g., thiazide and spironolactone). The combination can be particularly helpful when two drugs have different sites of action and allow more effective control of fluid excess.

Replace potassium losses as indicated.

Potassium deficit (which may occur if patient is receiving potassium-wasting diuretic) can cause lethal cardiac dysrhythmias if untreated.

Prepare for/assist with dialysis/ultrafiltration, if indicated.

May be done to rapidly reduce fluid overload, especially in the presence of severe cardiac/renal failure.

HYPOVOLEMIA (EXTRACELLULAR FLUID VOLUME DEFICIT)

PREDISPOSING/CONTRIBUTING FACTORS

Excessive losses: Vomiting, gastric suctioning, diarrhea, polyuria, diaphoresis, wounds or burns, intraoperative fluid loss, hemorrhage.
Insufficient/decreased fluid intake, e.g., preoperative/postoperative NPO status.
Systemic infections, fever.
Intestinal obstruction or fistulas.
Pancreatitis, peritonitis, cirrhosis/ascites.
Kidney disease, diabetic ketoacidosis, HHNC, diabetes insipidus.

PATIENT ASSESSMENT DATA BASE

ACTIVITY/REST

May report: Fatigue, generalized weakness.

CIRCULATION

May exhibit: Hypotension, including postural changes.
Pulse weak/thready; tachycardia.
Neck veins flattened; CVP decreased.

ELIMINATION

May report: Constipation or occasionally diarrhea, abdominal cramps.

May exhibit: Urine volume decreased, dark/concentrated color; oliguria (severe fluid depletion).

FOOD/FLUID

May report: Thirst, anorexia, nausea/vomiting.

May exhibit: Weight loss often exceeding 2%–8% of total body weight.
Abdominal distention.
Mucous membranes dry, furrows on tongue; decreased tearing and salivation.
Skin dry with poor turgor; or pale, moist, clammy (shock).

NEUROSENSORY

May report: Tingling of the extremities, vertigo, syncope.

May exhibit: Behavior change, apathy, restlessness, confusion.

RESPIRATION

May exhibit: Tachypnea, rapid/shallow breathing.

SAFETY

May exhibit: Temperature usually subnormal, although fever may occur.

TEACHING/LEARNING

Refer to predisposing/contributing factors.

Discharge Plan Considerations: **DRG projected mean length of stay: 4.1 days.**
May require assistance with changes in therapeutic regimen, dietary management.

DIAGNOSTIC STUDIES

Serum Sodium: May be normal, high, or low.

Urine Sodium: Usually decreased (less than 10 mEq/L when losses are from external causes; usually greater than 20 mEq/L if the cause is renal or adrenal).

CBC: Hb/Hct and RBC usually increased (hemoconcentration); decrease suggests hemorrhage.

Serum glucose: Normal or elevated.

Serum protein: Increased.

BUN and Cr: Increased, with BUN out of proportion to Cr.

Urine specific gravity: Increased.

ACTIONS/INTERVENTIONS	RATIONALE
Independent	
Monitor vital signs and CVP. Note presence/degree of postural BP changes. Observe for temperature elevations/fever.	Tachycardia is present as well as varying degrees of hypotension, depending on degree of fluid deficit. CVP measurements are useful in determining degree of fluid deficit and response to replacement therapy. Fever increases metabolism and exacerbates fluid loss.
Palpate peripheral pulses; note capillary refill, skin color/temperature; assess mentation.	Conditions that contribute to extracellular fluid deficit can result in inadequate organ perfusion to all areas and may cause circulatory collapse/shock.
Monitor urinary output. Measure/estimate fluid losses from all sources, e.g., gastric losses, wound drainage, diaphoresis.	Fluid replacement needs are based on correction of current deficits and ongoing losses. *Note:* A diaphoretic episode requiring a full linen change may represent a fluid loss of as much as 1 L. A decreased urinary output may indicate insufficient renal perfusion/hypovolemia, or polyuria can be present, requiring more aggressive fluid replacement.

ACTIONS/INTERVENTIONS	RATIONALE

Independent

Weigh daily and compare with 24-hour fluid balance. Mark/measure edematous areas, e.g., abdomen, limbs.

Changes in weight may not accurately reflect intravascular volume, e.g., third space fluid accumulation cannot be used by the body for tissue perfusion.

Ascertain patient's beverage preferences, and set up a 24-hour schedule for fluid intake. Encourage foods with high fluid content.

Relieves thirst and discomfort of dry mucous membranes and augments parenteral replacement.

Turn frequently, massage skin, and protect bony prominences.

Tissues are susceptible to breakdown because of vasoconstriction and increased cellular fragility.

Provide skin and mouth care. Bathe every other day using mild soap. Apply lotion as indicated.

Skin and mucous membranes are dry, with decreased elasticity, because of vasoconstriction and reduced intracellular water. Daily bathing may increase dryness.

Provide safety precautions as indicated, e.g., use of side rails, bed in low position, frequent observation, soft restraints (if required).

Decreased cerebral perfusion frequently results in changes in mentation/altered thought processes, requiring protective measures to prevent patient injury.

Investigate reports of sudden/sharp chest pain, dyspnea, cyanosis, increased anxiety, restlessness.

Hemoconcentration (sludging) and increased platelet aggregation may result in systemic emboli formation.

Monitor for sudden/marked elevation of BP, restlessness, moist cough, dyspnea, basalar crackles, frothy sputum.

Too rapid a correction of fluid deficit may compromise the cardiopulmonary system, especially if colloids are used in general fluid replacement (increased osmotic pressure potentiates fluid shifts).

Collaborative

Assist with identification/treatment of underlying cause.

Refer to listing of predisposing/contributing factors.

Monitor laboratory studies as indicated, e.g., electrolytes, glucose, pH/PCO_2, coagulation studies.

Depending on the avenue of fluid loss, differing electrolyte/metabolic imbalances may be present/require correction; e.g., use of glucose solutions in patients with underlying glucose intolerance may result in serum glucose elevation and increased urinary water losses.

Administer IV solutions as indicated:

Isotonic solutions, e.g., 0.9% NaCl (normal saline), 5% dextrose/water;

Crystalloids provide prompt circulatory improvement, although the benefit may be transient (increased renal clearance).

0.45% NaCl ($\frac{1}{2}$ strength saline), lactated Ringer's;

As soon as the patient is normotensive, a hypotonic solution (0.45% NaCl) may be used to provide both electrolytes and free water for renal excretion of metabolic wastes. *Note:* Buffered crystalloids (LR) are used with caution as they may potentiate the risk of metabolic acidosis.

Colloids, e.g., dextran, Plasmanate/albumin, hetastarch (Hespan);

Corrects plasma protein concentration deficits, thereby increasing intravascular osmotic pressure

Collaborative

                       and facilitating return of fluid into vascular compartment.

Whole blood/packed RBC transfusion.   Indicated when hypovolemia is related to active blood loss.

Administer sodium bicarbonate, if indicated.   May be given to correct severe acidosis while correcting fluid balance.

SODIUM

Sodium is the major cation of extracellular fluid and is primarily responsible for osmotic pressure in that compartment. Sodium enhances neuromuscular conduction/transmission of impulses and is essential for maintaining acid/base balance. Normal serum range is 135–145 mEq/L; intracellular, 10 mEq/L. Chloride is carried by Na and will display the same imbalances. Normal serum chloride range is 95–105 mEq/L.

HYPONATREMIA (SODIUM DEFICIT)

PREDISPOSING/CONTRIBUTING FACTORS

Primary hyponatremia (loss of sodium): Lack of sufficient dietary sodium, severe malnutrition, infusion of sodium-free solutions. Excessive sodium loss through heavy sweating (e.g., heat exhaustion), wounds/trauma (hemorrhage), burns, gastric suctioning, vomiting, diarrhea, small-bowel obstruction, peritonitis, salt-wasting renal dysfunction, adrenal insufficiency (Addison's disease).

Dilutional hyponatremia (water gains): Excessive water intake, electrolyte-free IV infusion, water intoxication (IV therapy, tap-water enemas), gastric irrigations with electrolyte-free solutions, presence of tumors or CNS disorders predisposing to SIADH, CHF, renal failure/nephrotic syndrome, hepatic cirrhosis, DM (hyperglycemia), fresh water near-drowning; use of certain drugs, e.g., hypoglycemia medications, barbiturates, antipsychotics, aminophylline, or morphine (may stimulate pituitary gland to secrete excessive amounts of ADH).

Note: A pseudohyponatremia may occur in presence of multiple myeloma, hyperlipidemia, or hypoproteinemia but does not reflect an actual abnormality of water metabolism.

PATIENT ASSESSMENT DATA BASE

GENERAL

ACTIVITY/REST

    May report: Malaise.

                       Generalized weakness, faintness, muscle cramps.

EGO INTEGRITY

    May report: Anxiety.

    May exhibit: Restlessness, apprehension.

FOOD/FLUID

    May report: Nausea, anorexia, thirst.

                       Low-sodium diet.

NEUROSENSORY

May report:	Headache, blurred vision, vertigo.
May exhibit:	Loss of coordination, stupor, coma.
	Use of oral hypoglycemic agent, potent diuretics, NSAIDs.

TEACHING/LEARNING

Refer to predisposing/contributing factors.

Discharge Plan Considerations: **DRG projected mean length of stay: 4.1 days.**
May require assistance with changes in therapeutic regimen, dietary management.

SODIUM/WATER DEFICIT

CIRCULATION

May exhibit:	Hypotension, tachycardia.
	Peripheral pulses diminished.

ELIMINATION

May report:	Abdominal cramping, diarrhea.
May exhibit:	Urinary output decreased.

FOOD/FLUID

May report:	Anorexia, nausea/vomiting.
May exhibit:	Poor skin turgor; soft/sunken eyeballs.
	Mucous membranes dry, decreased saliva/perspiration.

NEUROSENSORY

May exhibit:	Muscle twitching.
	Lethargy, restlessness, confusion, stupor.

RESPIRATION

May exhibit:	Tachypnea.

SAFETY

May exhibit:	Skin flushed, dry, hot.
	Fever.

SODIUM DEFICIT/WATER EXCESS

CIRCULATION

May exhibit:	Hypertension.
	Generalized edema.

ELIMINATION

May exhibit:	Urinary output increased.

SEVERE SODIUM DEFICIT

CIRCULATION

May exhibit: Hypotension with vasomotor collapse.

Rapid thready pulse.

Cold/clammy skin, fingerprinting on sternum; cyanosis.

NEUROSENSORY

May exhibit: Hyperreflexia.

Convulsions/coma.

DIAGNOSTIC STUDIES (Dependent on associated fluid level)

Serum sodium: Decreased, less than 135 mEq/L. (However, signs and symptoms may not occur until level is less than 120 mEq/L).

Urine sodium: Less than 15 mEq/L indicates renal conservation of sodium due to sodium loss from a nonrenal source unless sodium wasting nephropathy present. Urine sodium greater than 20 mEq/L indicates SIADH.

Serum potassium: May be decreased as the kidneys attempt to conserve sodium at the expense of potassium.

Serum chloride/bicarbonate: Levels are decreased, depending on which ion is lost with the sodium.

Osmolality: Commonly low, but may be normal (pseudohyponatremia) or high (HHNC).

Urine osmolality: Usually less than 100 mOsmol/L unless SIADH present in which case it will exceed serum osmolality.

Urine specific gravity: May be decreased (less than 1.010) or increased (greater than 1.020) if SIADH is present.

Hct: Is dependent on fluid balance, e.g., fluid excess versus dehydration.

ACTIONS/INTERVENTIONS	RATIONALE
Independent	
Identify the patient at risk for hypernatremia and the specific cause, e.g., sodium loss or fluid excess.	Provides clues for early intervention.
Monitor I&O. Calculate fluid balance. Weigh daily.	Indicators of fluid balance are important, because either fluid excess or deficit may occur with hyponatremia.
Assess level of consciousness/neuromuscular response.	Sodium deficit may result in decreased mentation (to point of coma), as well as generalized muscle weakness/cramps, convulsions.
Maintain quiet environment; provide safety/seizure precautions.	Reduces CNS stimulation and risk of injury from neurologic complications, e.g., seizures.
Note respiratory rate and depth.	Co-occurring hypochloremia may produce slow/shallow respirations as the body compensates for metabolic alkalosis.
Encourage foods and fluids high in sodium, e.g., milk, meat, eggs, carrots, beets, and celery. Use fruit juices and bouillon instead of plain water.	Unless sodium deficit causes serious symptoms requiring immediate IV replacement, the patient may benefit from slower replacement by oral method or removal of previous salt restriction.
Irrigate NG tube (when used) with normal saline instead of water.	Isotonic irrigation will minimize loss of GI electrolytes.

ACTIONS/INTERVENTIONS	RATIONALE

Collaborative

Assist with identification/treatment of underlying cause.

Refer to listing of predisposing/contributing factors.

Monitor serum and urine electrolytes, osmolality.

Evaluates therapy needs/effectiveness.

Administer/restrict fluids dependent on fluid volume status.

In presence of hypovolemia, volume losses are replaced with isotonic saline (e.g., normal saline), or, on occasion, hypertonic solution (3% NaCl) when hyponatremia is life threatening. In the presence of fluid volume excess, or SIADH, fluid restriction is indicated.

Administer medications as indicated, e.g.:

Furosemide (Lasix);

Effective in reducing fluid excess to correct sodium/water balance.

Sodium chloride;

Used to replace deficits/prevent recurrence in the presence of chronic/ongoing losses.

Potassium chloride;

Corrects potassium deficit, especially when diuretic is used.

Demeclocycline (Declomycin);

Useful in treating chronic SIADH, or when severe water restriction may not be tolerated, e.g., COPD. *Note:* May be contraindicated in patients with liver disease as nephrotoxicity may occur.

Captopril (Capoten).

May be used in combination with a loop diuretic (e.g., Lasix) to correct fluid volume excess especially in the presence of CHF.

Prepare for/assist with dialysis as indicated.

May be done to restore Na balance without increasing fluid level when hyponatremia is severe or response to diuretic therapy is inadequate.

HYPERNATREMIA (SODIUM EXCESS)

PREDISPOSING/CONTRIBUTING FACTORS

Excessive water losses: Polyuria (as may occur with diabetes insipidus); use of osmotic diuretics (such as mannitol); presence of fever, profuse sweating, vomiting, diarrhea. Extracellular fluid volume excesses: e.g., renal disease, congestive heart disease, primary aldosteronism, excessive steroids/Cushing's disease. Excessive ingestion or infusion of sodium; salt water near-drowning.

Insufficient water intake: Administration of tube feedings/high-protein diets with minimal fluid intake, ulcer diets primarily using half and half.

PATIENT ASSESSMENT DATA BASE

SODIUM EXCESS/WATER DEFICIT

ACTIVITY/REST

May report: Weakness.

May exhibit: Muscle rigidity/tremors, generalized weakness.

1063

CIRCULATION

May exhibit: Postural hypotension.
Tachycardia.

ELIMINATION

May exhibit: Urinary output decreased.

FOOD/FLUID

May report: Thirst.

May exhibit: Mucous membranes dry, sticky; tongue rough.

NEUROSENSORY

May exhibit: Irritability, lethargy/coma, seizures.
Delusions, hallucinations.

SAFETY

May exhibit: Hot, dry flushed skin.
Fever.

Sodium/Water Excess

CIRCULATION

May exhibit: Elevated BP, hypertension.

ELIMINATION

May exhibit: Polyuria.

FOOD/FLUID

May report: Thirst.

May exhibit: Skin pale, moist, taut with pitting edema.
Weight gain.

NEUROSENSORY

May exhibit: Confusion, lethargy.
Delusions, hallucinations.

RESPIRATION

May exhibit: Dyspnea.

TEACHING/LEARNING

Refer to predisposing/contributing factors.

Discharge Plan Considerations: **DRG projected mean length of stay: 4.1 days.**
May require assistance with changes in therapeutic regimen, dietary management.

DIAGNOSTIC STUDIES

Serum sodium: Increased, greater than 145 mEq/L. Serum levels greater than 160 mEq/L may be accompanied by severe neurologic signs.

Serum chloride: Increased, greater than 106 mEq/L.

Serum potassium: Decreased.

Serum osmolality: Greater than 295 mOsm/L when dehydrated; lower in presence of extracellular fluid excess, and less than 200 mOsm/L with excessive polyurea.

Hct: May be normal or elevated.

Urine sodium: Less than 50 mEq/L.

Urine chloride: Less than 50 mEq/L.

Urine osmolality: Greater than 800 mOsm/L.

Urine specific gravity: Increased, greater than 1.015, if water deficit present; or less than 1.005 when hypernatremia is due to polyuria.

ACTIONS/INTERVENTIONS	RATIONALE
Independent	
Monitor BP.	Either hypertension or hypotension may be present, depending on the fluid status. Presence of postural hypotension may affect activity tolerance.
Identify patient at risk for hypernatremia and likely cause, e.g., water deficit, sodium excess.	Early identification and intervention prevents serious complications associated with this problem.
Note respiratory rate, depth.	Deep labored respirations with air hunger suggest metabolic acidosis (hyperchloremia), which can lead to cardiopulmonary arrest if not corrected.
Monitor I&O, urine specific gravity. Weigh daily. Assess presence/location of edema.	These parameters are variable depending on fluid status and are indicators of therapy needs/effectiveness.
Assess level of consciousness and muscular strength, tone, movement.	Sodium imbalance may cause changes, which vary from confusion and irritability to seizures and coma. In presence of water deficit, rapid rehydration may cause cerebral edema.
Maintain safety/seizure precautions, as indicated, e.g., bed in low position, use of padded side rails.	Sodium excess/cerebral edema increases risk of convulsions.
Assess skin turgor, color, temperature, and mucous membrane moisture.	Water-deficit hyponatremia manifests by signs of dehydration.
Provide meticulous skin care and frequent repositioning.	Maintains skin integrity.
Provide frequent oral care. Avoid use of mouthwash/rinse that contains alcohol.	Promotes comfort and prevents further drying of mucous membranes.
Offer debilitated patient fluids at regular intervals. Give free water to patient receiving enteral feedings.	May prevent hypernatremia in patient who is unable to perceive or respond to thirst.
Recommend avoidance of foods high in sodium, e.g., canned soups/vegetables, processed foods, snack foods, and condiments.	Reduces risk of sodium-associated complications.

ACTIONS/INTERVENTIONS	RATIONALE
Collaborative	
Assist with identification/treatment of underlying cause.	Refer to listing of predisposing/contributing factors.
Monitor serum electrolytes, osmolality, and ABGs as indicated.	Evaluates therapy needs/effectiveness. *Note:* Co-occurring hyperchloremia may cause metabolic acidosis, requiring buffering, e.g., sodium bicarbonate.
Increase PO/IV fluid intake, e.g., 50% dextrose (in H_2O in presence of dehydration); 0.90% NaCl (if extracellular deficit is present).	Replacement of total body water deficit will gradually restore sodium/water balance. *Note:* Rapid reduction of serum sodium level with corresponding decrease in serum osmolality can cause cerebral edema/convulsions.
Restrict sodium intake and administer diuretics as indicated.	Restriction of sodium intake while promoting renal clearance lowers serum sodium levels in the presence of extracellular fluid excess.

POTASSIUM

Potassium is the major cation of the intracellular fluid and is responsible for maintaining intracellular osmotic pressure. Potassium also regulates neuromuscular excitability, aids in maintenance of acid/base balance, synthesis of protein, and metabolism of carbohydrates. Normal serum range is 3.5–5.0 mEq/L (body total of 42 mEq/L).

HYPOKALEMIA (POTASSIUM DEFICIT)

PREDISPOSING/CONTRIBUTING FACTORS

Renal loss: Use of potassium-wasting diuretics, diuretic phase of ATN, healing phase of burns; diabetic acidosis; Cushing's syndrome; nephritis, hypomagnesemia; use of high-dose sodium penicillins, amphotericin B, steroids.
GI loss: Profuse vomiting, excessive diarrhea, laxative abuse, prolonged gastric suction, inflammatory bowel disease, fistulas.
Liver disease.
Inadequate dietary intake: Anorexia nervosa, starvation, high sodium diet.
Shift into cells: Hyperalimentation, alkalosis, or excessive secretion or administration of insulin.

PATIENT ASSESSMENT DATA BASE

ACTIVITY/REST

May report: Generalized weakness, lethargy, fatigue.

CIRCULATION

May exhibit: Hypotension.
Pulses weak/diminished, irregular.
Heart sounds distant.
Characteristic ECG changes.
Dysrhythmias: PVCs, ventricular tachycardia/fibrillation.

ELIMINATION

May exhibit: Nocturia, polyuria if factors contributing to hypokalemia include CHF or DM. Bowel sounds diminished, decreased bowel motility, paralytic ileus. Abdominal distention.

FOOD/FLUID

May report: Anorexia, nausea/vomiting.

NEUROSENSORY

May report: Paresthesias.

May exhibit: Depressed mental state/confusion, apathy, drowsiness, irritability, coma. Hyporeflexia, tetany, paralysis.

PAIN/COMFORT

May report: Muscle pain/cramps.

RESPIRATION

May exhibit: Hypoventilation/decreased respiratory depth due to muscle weakness/paralysis of diaphragm; apnea, cyanosis.

TEACHING/LEARNING

Refer to predisposing/contributing factors.

Discharge Plan Considerations: **DRG projected mean length of stay: 4.1 days.**
May require assistance with changes in therapeutic regimen, dietary management.

DIAGNOSTIC STUDIES

Serum potassium: Decreased, less than 3.5 mEq/L.

Serum chloride: Often decreased, less than 98 mEq/L.

Serum glucose: May be slightly elevated.

Plasma bicarbonate: Increased, greater than 29 mEq/L.

Urine osmolality: Decreased.

ABGs: pH and bicarbonate may be elevated (metabolic alkalosis).

ECG: Low voltage; flat or inverted T wave, appearance of U wave, depressed ST segment, peaked P waves; prolonged Q-T interval, ventricular dysrhythmias.

ACTIONS/INTERVENTIONS	RATIONALE
Independent	
Monitor heart rate/rhythm.	Changes associated with hypokalemia include abnormalities in both conduction and contractility. Tachycardia may develop, and potentially life-threatening atrial and ventricular dysrhythmias, e.g., PVCs, sinus bradycardia, AV blocks, AV dissociation, ventricular tachycardia.
Monitor respiratory rate, depth, effort. Encourage cough/deep-breathing exercises; reposition frequently.	Respiratory muscle weakness may proceed to paralysis and eventual respiratory arrest.

ACTIONS/INTERVENTIONS	RATIONALE

Independent

Assess level of consciousness and neuromuscular function, e.g., strength, sensation, movement.

Apathy, drowsiness, irritability, tetany, paresthesias, and coma may occur.

Auscultate bowel sounds, noting decrease/absence/change.

Paralytic ileus commonly follows gastric losses through vomiting/gastric suction, protracted diarrhea.

Maintain accurate record of urinary, gastric, and wound losses.

Guide for calculating fluid/potassium replacement needs.

Monitor rate of IV potassium administration using microdrop/minidrop infusion devices. Check for side effects. Provide ice pack as indicated.

Assures controlled delivery of medication to prevent bolus effect and reduce associated discomfort, e.g., burning sensation at IV site. When solution cannot be administered via central vein, and slowing rate is not possible/effective, ice pack to infusion site may help relieve discomfort.

Encourage intake of foods and fluids high in potassium, e.g., bananas, oranges, dried fruits, red meat, turkey, salmon, coffee, colas, tea, leafy vegetables, peas, baked potatoes, tomatoes, winter squash. Discuss use of potassium chloride salt substitutes for patient receiving long-term diuretics.

Potassium may be replaced/level maintained through the diet when the patient is allowed oral food and fluids. Dietary replacement of 40–60 mEq/L/d is typically sufficient if there are no abnormal losses occurring.

Review drug regimen for potassium-wasting drugs, e.g., furosemide (Lasix), hydrochlorothiazide (Diamox), IV catecholamines, gentamicin (Garamycin), carbenicillin (Geocillin), amphotericin B (Fungizone).

If alternate agents (e.g., potassium-sparing diuretics such as Aldactone, Dyrenium, Midamor) cannot be administered, or when high-dose sodium drugs are administered (e.g., carbenicillin), close monitoring and replacement of potassium is necessary.

Dilute liquid and effervescent K^+ supplements (K-Tab, K-Lyte/Cl) with 4 oz water/juice and give after meals.

May prevent/reduce GI irritation and saline laxative effect.

Watch for signs of digitalis intoxication when used (e.g., reports of nausea/vomiting, blurred vision, increasing atrial dysrhythmias, and heart block).

Low potassium enhances effect of digitalis, slowing cardiac conduction. *Note:* Combined effects of digitalis, diuretics, and hypokalemia may produce lethal dysrhythmias.

Observe for signs of metabolic alkalosis, e.g., hypoventilation, tachycardia, dysrhythmias, tetany, changes in mentation.

Frequently associated with hypokalemia.

Collaborative

Assist with identification/treatment of underlying cause.

Refer to listing of predisposing/contributing factors.

Monitor laboratory studies, e.g.:

Serum potassium;

Levels should be checked frequently during replacement therapy, especially in the presence of insufficient renal function. Sudden excess/elevation may cause cardiac dysrhythmias.

ABGs;

Correction of alkalosis will raise serum potassium level and reduce replacement needs. Correction of acidosis will drive potassium back into cells, resulting in decreased serum levels and increased replacement needs.

ACTIONS/INTERVENTIONS	RATIONALE
Collaborative	
Serum magnesium;	Hypomagnesemia exacerbates potassium loss and sodium retention, altering cell membrane excitability (affects cardiac as well as neuromuscular function).
Serum chloride.	Use of diuretics, e.g., Lasix, HydroDIURIL may also cause chloride as well as potassium depletion.
Administer oral and/or IV potassium.	May be required to correct severe/life-threatening deficiencies when changes in medications therapy and/or dietary intake are insufficient. *Note:* Parenteral replacement should not exceed 40 mEq/2 h. Dietary supplementation may also be used to produce a gradual equilibration if patient is able to take oral food and fluids.

HYPERKALEMIA [POTASSIUM EXCESS]

PREDISPOSING/CONTRIBUTING FACTORS

Potassium retention: Decreased renal excretion (e.g., renal disease/acute failure, hypoaldosteronism), hypovolemia, use of potassium-conserving diuretics, especially when associated with potassium supplements.

Excessive potassium intake: Salt substitutes, drugs containing potassium (e.g., penicillin), too rapid IV administration of potassium, massive transfusion of banked blood.

Shift or release of potassium out of cells: Severe catabolism, burns, crush injuries, MI, severe hemolysis, rhabdomyolysis, chemotherapy with cytotoxic drugs, metabolic acidosis, anoxia, insulin deficiency.

PATIENT ASSESSMENT DATA BASE

Data are dependent on degree of elevation as well as length of time condition has existed.

ACTIVITY/REST

May report:	Vague muscular weakness.

CIRCULATION

May exhibit:	Irregular pulse, bradycardia, heart block, asystole.

ELIMINATION

May report:	Abdominal cramps, diarrhea.
May exhibit:	Urine volume decreased. Hyperactive bowel sounds.

FOOD/FLUID

May report:	Nausea/vomiting.

NEUROSENSORY

May report:	Paresthesias (often of face, tongue, hands, feet).

1069

May exhibit:	Decreased deep-tendon reflexes; progressive, ascending flaccid paralysis; twitching, seizures. Apathy, confusion.

TEACHING/LEARNING

Refer to predisposing/contributing factors.

Discharge Plan Considerations:	**DRG projected mean length of stay: 4.1 days.** May require assistance with changes in therapeutic regimen, dietary management.

DIAGNOSTIC STUDIES

Serum potassium: Increased, greater than 5.5 mEq/L.

Renal function studies: May be altered indicating failure.

Leukocyte or thrombocyte count: Elevation may cause a pseudohyperkalemia affecting choice of interventions.

ECG changes: T waves tall and peaked/tented, prolonged P-R interval, loss of P waves, widening of QRS complex, shortened Q-T interval, and ST-segment depression; atrial/ventricular dysrhythmias, e.g., bradycardia, atrial arrest, complete heart block, ventricular fibrillation, cardiac arrest.

ACTIONS/INTERVENTIONS	RATIONALE
Independent	
Identify the patient at risk; or the cause of the hyperkalemia, e.g., excessive intake of potassium or decreased excretion.	Influences choice of interventions. Early identification and treatment can prevent complication.
Take measures/teach patient about use of potassium-containing salts, taking potassium supplements safely, and so forth.	The patient is often able to prevent hyperkalemia through management of supplements, diets, and other medications.
Monitor respiratory rate and depth. Elevate head of bed. Encourage cough/deep-breathing exercises.	Patients may hypoventilate and retain CO_2, leading to respiratory acidosis. Muscular weakness can affect respiratory muscles and lead to respiratory complications of infection/respiratory failure.
Monitor heart rate/rhythm. Be aware that cardiac arrest can occur.	Excess potassium depresses myocardial conduction. Bradycardia can progress to cardiac fibrillation/arrest.
Monitor urinary output.	In kidney failure, potassium is retained because of improper excretion. Potassium should not be given if oliguria or anuria is present.
Assess level of consciousness, neuromuscular function, e.g., movement, strength, sensation.	Patient is usually awake and alert, while muscular paresthesia, weakness, and flaccid paralysis may occur.
Assist with active/passive ROM exercises.	Improves muscular tone and reduces muscle cramps and pain.
Encourage frequent rest periods; assist with care activities, as indicated.	General muscle weakness decreases activity tolerance.
Review drug regimen for medications containing/affecting potassium excretion, e.g., penicillin G, Aldactone, Midamor, Dyazide, Maxzide.	Requires regular monitoring of potassium levels, and may require alternate drug choices or changes in dosage/frequency.

ACTIONS/INTERVENTIONS	RATIONALE

Independent

Identify/discontinue dietary sources of potassium, e.g., tomatoes, broccoli, orange juice, bananas, bran, chocolate, coffee, tea, eggs, dairy products, dried fruits.

Facilitates reduction of potassium level and may prevent recurrence of hyperkalemia.

Stress importance of patient notifying future care givers when chronic condition potentiates development of hyperkalemia, e.g., oliguric renal failure.

May help prevent recurrence.

Collaborative

Assist with identification/treatment of underlying cause.

Refer to listing of predisposing/contributing factors.

Monitor laboratory results, e.g., serum potassium, ABGs, BUN/Cr, glucose as indicated.

Evaluates therapy needs/effectiveness. Note: Hypoventilation may result in respiratory acidosis, thereby increasing serum potassium levels.

Administer medications as indicated:

Diuretics, e.g., furosemide (Lasix);

Promotes renal clearance and excretion of potassium.

IV glucose with insulin, sodium bicarbonate;

Short-term emergency measure to move potassium into the cell, thus reducing toxic serum level. *Note:* Use with caution in presence of CHF or hypernatremia.

Calcium gluconate;

Temporary stop-gap measure that antagonizes toxic potassium depressant effects on heart and stimulates cardiac contractility. *Note:* Calcium is contraindicated in patients on digitalis because it increases the cardiotonic effects of the drug and may cause dysrhythmias.

Sodium chloride;

Enhances renal excretion of potassium.

Sodium polystyrene sulfonate (Kayexelate), orally per NG tube or rectally.

Resin that exchanges potassium for sodium or calcium in the GI tract. Sorbitol enhances evacuation. *Note:* Use cautiously in patients with CHF, edema, and in the elderly because it contains sodium. In addition, Kayexelate may cause hyperchloremia.

Restrict potassium-containing fluids and salt substitutes. Increase carbohydrates/fats and foods low in potassium, e.g., canned fruits, refined cereals, apple/cranberry juice.

Reduces exogenous sources of potassium and prevents catabolic tissue breakdown with release of cellular potassium.

Infuse potassium-based medication/solutions slowly.

Prevents administration of concentrated bolus, allows time for kidneys to clear excess free potassium.

Provide fresh blood or washed RBCs (when possible) if transfusions required.

Fresh blood has less potassium than banked blood, because breakdown of older RBCs releases potassium.

Prepare for/assist with dialysis (peritoneal or hemodialysis).

May be required when more conservative methods fail or are contraindicated, e.g., severe CHF.

CALCIUM

Calcium is involved in bone formation/reabsorption, neural transmission/muscle contraction, regulation of enzyme systems and is a coenzyme in blood coagulation. Normal serum levels are 4.5–5.3 mEq/L (ionized), or 8.5–10.5 mg/dL (total). The ionized calcium is physiologically active and clinically important, especially in critically ill patients. The total serum calcium is directly related to the serum albumin, follows it, and must be considered if only total serum readings are available. Some factors that alter the percentage of ionized calcium are changes in pH (affects how much calcium is bound to protein), or increased serum levels of fatty acids, lactate, and bicarbonate.

HYPOCALCEMIA (CALCIUM DEFICIT)

PREDISPOSING/CONTRIBUTING FACTORS

Primary or surgical hypoparathyroidism; transient hypocalcemia following thyroidectomy; hyperphosphatemia, hypomagnesemia.

Massive SC tissue infections, acute pancreatitis, burns, peritonitis, malignancies.

Excessive GI losses: Draining fistula, diarrhea, fat malabsorption syndromes, chronic laxative use (particularly phosphate-containing laxatives/enemas).

Extreme stress situations with mobilization and excretion of calcium.

Diuretic and terminal phase of renal failure.

Inadequate dietary intake, lack of milk/vitamin D, excessive protein diet.

Alcoholism: Primary effect of ethanol, plus intestinal malabsorption, hypomagnesemia, hypoalbuminemia, and pancreatitis.

Use of anticonvulsants, antibiotics, corticosteroids; loop diuretics, drugs that lower serum magnesium.

Infusion of citrated blood, calcium-free infusions; rapid infusion of Plasmanate.

Malignant neoplasms with bone metastases.

Alkalosis.

PATIENT ASSESSMENT DATA BASE

(Dependent on duration, severity, and rate of development)

CIRCULATION

May exhibit: Hypotension.

Pulses weak/decreased, irregular (weak cardiac contraction/premature dysrhythmias).

ELIMINATION

May report: Diarrhea, abdominal pain.

May exhibit: Abdominal distention (paralytic ileus).

FOOD/FLUID

May report: Nausea/vomiting.

NEUROSENSORY

May report: Circumoral paresthesia, numbness and tingling of fingers and toes; muscle cramps.

May exhibit: Anxiety, confusion, irritability, depression, hallucinations, psychoses.

Muscle spasms (carpopedal and laryngeal), increased deep-tendon reflexes; tetany, tonic/clonic seizures, positive Trousseau's and Chvostek's signs.

RESPIRATION

May exhibit: Labored shallow breathing.

SAFETY

May exhibit: Bleeding with no or minimal trauma.

TEACHING/LEARNING

Refer to predisposing/contributing factors.

Discharge Plan Considerations: **DRG projected mean length of stay: 4.1 days.**
May require assistance with changes in therapeutic regimen, dietary management.

DIAGNOSTIC STUDIES

Ca^{2+}: Decreased, less than 4.5 mEq/L (ionized), or 8.5 mg/dl (total).

Urine Sulkowitch test: Shows no precipitate.

ECG: Prolonged Q-T interval (characteristic but not necessarily diagnostic). In severe deficiency, T waves may flatten or invert giving appearance of hypokalemia or myocardial ischemia; ventricular tachycardia may develop.

ACTIONS/INTERVENTIONS	RATIONALE
Independent	
Monitor heart rate/rhythm.	Calcium deficit along with associated hypomagnesemia weakens cardiac muscle/contractility.
Assess respiratory rate, rhythm, effort. Have tracheostomy equipment available.	Laryngeal stridor may develop and result in respiratory emergency/arrest.
Observe for neuromuscular irritability, e.g., tetany, seizures. Assess for presence of Chvostek's/Trousseau's signs.	Calcium deficit causes repetitive and uncontrolled nerve transmission leading to muscle spasms and hyperirritability.
Provide quiet environment and seizure precautions.	Reduces CNS stimulation and protects patient from potential injury.
Promote relaxation/stress reduction techniques, e.g., deep-breathing exercises, guided imagery, visualization.	Tetany can be potentiated by hyperventilation and stress. *Note:* Direct pressure on the nerves (e.g., tightening BP cuff) may also cause tetany.
Check for bleeding from any source (mucous membranes, puncture sites, wounds/incisions, and so on). Note presence of ecchymosis, petechiae.	Alterations in coagulation can occur as a result of calcium deficiency.
Review patient's drug regimen, e.g., use of insulin, mithramycin, parathyroid injection, digitalis.	Some drugs can lower magnesium levels. Digitalis is enhanced by calcium, and, in patient receiving calcium, digitalis intoxication may develop.
Discuss use of laxatives/antacids.	Those containing phosphate may negatively affect calcium metabolism.
Review dietary intake of vitamins and fat.	Insufficient ingestion of vitamin D and fat impairs absorption of calcium.
Identify sources to increase calcium and vitamin D in diet, e.g., dairy products, beans, cauliflower, eggs, oranges, pineapples, sardines, shellfish. Restrict intake of phosphorus, e.g., barley, bran, whole wheat, rye, liver, nuts, chocolate.	Vitamin D aids in absorption of calcium from intestinal tract. Phosphorus competes with calcium for intestinal absorption.

1073

ACTIONS/INTERVENTIONS	RATIONALE

Independent

Encourage use of calcium-containing antacids if needed (e.g., Titralac, Dicarbosil, Tums).	Possible sources for oral replacement to help maintain calcium levels.
Stress importance of meeting calcium needs.	Adverse effects of long-term deficiency include tooth decay, eczema, cataracts, and osteoporosis.

Collaborative

Assist with identification/treatment of underlying cause.	Refer to listing of predisposing/contributing factors.
Monitor laboratory studies, e.g.:	
Serum calcium and magnesium; serum albumin, ABGs;	Evaluates therapy needs/effectiveness. *Note:* Low serum albumin levels or serum pH affects calcium levels, e.g., a low albumin level causes a deceptively low calcium level; alkalosis causes surplus bicarbonate to bind with free calcium, impairing function; acidosis frees calcium, potentiating hypercalcemia.
PT, platelets.	Calcium is an essential part of the clotting mechanism and deficit may lead to excessive bleeding.
Administer the following:	
Calcium gluconate/chloride/gluceptate IV;	Provides rapid treatment in acute calcium deficit (especially in presence of tetany/convulsions).
Oral preparations, e.g., calcium lactate/carbonate;	Oral preparations are useful in correcting subacute deficiencies.
Magnesium sulfate IV/PO if indicated;	Hypomagnesemia is a precipitating factor in calcium deficit.
Vitamin D supplement (e.g., calcitriol).	May be used in combination with calcium therapy to enhance calcium absorption once concomitant phosphate deficiency is corrected.

HYPERCALCEMIA (CALCIUM EXCESS)

PREDISPOSING/CONTRIBUTING FACTORS

Hyperparathyroidism, hyperthyroidism, multiple myeloma/other malignancies, renal disease, skeletal muscle paralysis, parathyroid tumor, sarcoidosis, adrenal insufficiency, TB.

Excessive/prolonged use of vitamins A and D and calcium-containing antacids; prolonged use of thiazide diuretics, lithium.

Multiple fractures, bone tumors, osteoporosis, osteomalacia, prolonged immobilization causing release of calcium stores.

Milk-alkali syndrome as a side effect of prolonged milk/antacid ulcer therapy.

Hypophosphatasia, hyperproteinemia.

Anticancer drugs, e.g., tamoxifen, androgens/estrogens.

PATIENT ASSESSMENT DATA BASE

ACTIVITY/REST

May report: General malaise, fatigue/weakness.

May exhibit:	Incoordination, ataxia.

CIRCULATION

May exhibit:	Hypertension.
	Irregular pulse, dysrhythmias, bradycardia.

ELIMINATION

May report:	Constipation or diarrhea.
May exhibit:	Polyuria, nocturia.
	Kidney stones/calculi.

FOOD/FLUID

May report:	Anorexia, nausea/vomiting.
	Thirst.
	Abdominal pain.
May exhibit:	Poor skin turgor, dry mucous membranes.

NEUROSENSORY

May report:	Headache.
May exhibit:	Hypotonicity/muscular relaxation, flaccid paralysis, depressed/absent deep-tendon reflexes.
	Drowsiness, lethargy, apathy, paranoia, personality changes, memory loss, depression, psychosis, stupor/coma (with high calcium levels).
	Slurred speech.

PAIN/COMFORT

May report:	Epigastric, deep flank, or bone/joint pain.

TEACHING/LEARNING

	Refer to predisposing/contributing factors.
Discharge Plan Considerations:	**DRG projected mean length of stay: 4.1 days.**
	May require assistance with changes in therapeutic regimen, dietary management.

DIAGNOSTIC STUDIES

Serum calcium: Increased, greater than 5.8 mEq/L (ionized) or 10.5 mg/dl (total).

BUN: Increased (calculi can damage kidney).

Serum phosphorus: Decreased levels may be noted.

Urine Sulkowitch test: Shows heavy precipitate.

Urine calcium: Increased.

Urine osmolality: Decreased.

Urine specific gravity: Decreased.

X-ray: May reveal evidence of bone cavitation, pathologic fracture, osteoporosis, urinary calculi.

ECG changes: Shortened Q-T interval, inverted T waves. In severe deficit, QRS may widen, P-R interval lengthen, and ventricular prematurities develop.

1075

ACTIONS/INTERVENTIONS	RATIONALE
Independent	
Monitor cardiac rate/rhythm. Be aware that cardiac arrest can occur in hypercalcemic crisis.	Overstimulation of cardiac muscle occurs with resultant dysrhythmias and ineffective cardiac contraction. Sinus bradycardia, sinus dysrhythmias, wandering pacemaker, and AV block may be noted. Hypercalcemia creates a predisposition to cardiac arrest.
Assess level of consciousness and neuromuscular status, e.g., muscle movement, strength, tone.	Nerve and muscle activity is depressed. Lethargy and fatigue can progress to convulsion/coma.
Monitor I&O; calculate fluid balance.	Efforts to correct original condition may result in secondary imbalances/complications.
Encourage fluid intake of 3–4 L/d, including sodium-containing fluids, (within cardiac tolerance) and use of acid–ash juices, e.g., cranberry and prune if kidney stones present or suspected.	Reduces dehydration, encourages urinary flow and clearance of calcium, reduces risk of stone formation. *Note:* Sodium favors calcium excretion and can be used if not contraindicated by other conditions.
Strain urine if flank pain occurs.	Large amount of calcium present in kidney parenchyma may lead to stone formation.
Auscultate bowel sounds.	Hypotonicity leads to constipation when the smooth muscle tone is inadequate to produce peristalsis.
Maintain bulk in diet.	Constipation may be a problem because of decreased GI tone.
Turn frequently and do ROM and/or muscle-setting exercises with caution. Encourage ambulation if able.	Muscle activity may reduce calcium shifting from the bones that occurs during immobilization. *Note:* Increased risk for pathologic fractures exists due to calcium shifts out of the bones.
Provide safety measures, e.g., gentle handling when moving/transferring patient.	Reduces risk of injury/pathologic fractures.
Review drug regimen, noting use of calcium elevating drugs, e.g., heparin, tetracyclines, methicillin, phenytoin.	May affect drug choice or require reduction in oral sources of calcium.
Identify/restrict sources of calcium intake, e.g., dairy products, eggs, and spinach; calcium-containing antacids (Titralac, Dicarbosil, Tums).	Foods or drugs containing calcium may need to be limited in chronic conditions causing hypercalcemia.
Collaborative	
Assist with identification/treatment of underlying cause.	Refer to listing of predisposing/contributing factors.
Monitor laboratory studies, e.g., calcium, magnesium, phosphate.	Monitors therapy needs/effectiveness. *Note:* Phosphate levels may be low when parathyroid hormone inversely promotes calcium uptake and calcium competes with phosphate for absorption/transport with vitamin D.
Administer isotonic saline and sodium sulfate IV/orally.	Emergency measures in severe hypercalcemia used to dilute extracellular calcium concentration and inhibit tubular reabsorption of calcium, thereby increasing urinary excretion.

ACTIONS/INTERVENTIONS	RATIONALE
Collaborative	
Administer medications as indicated:	
Diuretics, e.g., furosemide (Lasix);	Diuresis promotes renal excretion of calcium and reduces risks of fluid excess from isotonic saline infusion.
Sodium bicarbonate;	Induces alkalosis, thereby reducing the ionized calcium fraction.
Phosphate;	Rapid-acting agent that induces calcium excretion and inhibits resorption of bone.
Glucocorticoid therapy;	Inhibits intestinal absorption of calcium and reduces inflammation and associated stress response that mobilizes calcium from the bone.
Mithramycin (Mithracin);	Antibiotic that lowers serum calcium by inhibiting bone resorption.
Disodium edetate (EDTA);	Chelating action lowers serum calcium level.
Calcitonin;	Promotes movement of serum calcium into bones temporarily reducing serum calcium levels especially in the presence of increased parathyroid hormone.
Neutra-Phos, Fleet Phospho-Soda.	These drugs bind calcium in the GI tract promoting excretion.
Prepare for/assist with hemodialysis.	Rapid reduction of serum calcium may be necessary to correct life-threatening situation.

MAGNESIUM

Magnesium influences carbohydrate metabolism, secretion of parathyroid hormone, sodium/potassium transport across the cell membrane, and synthesis of protein and nucleic acid. Magnesium activates ATP and mediates neural transmission within the CNS. Magnesium deficit is often associated with hypokalemia and promotes intracellular potassium loss and sodium accumulation, altering and exacerbating membrane excitability. Normal serum range is 1.5–2.5 mEq/L or 1.8–3.0 mg/dl.

HYPOMAGNESEMIA (MAGNESIUM DEFICIT)

PREDISPOSING/CONTRIBUTING FACTORS

GI losses: Biliary/intestinal fistula; surgery (bowel resection, small-bowel bypass), severe, protracted diarrhea, laxative abuse, impaired GI absorption/malabsorption syndrome, gastric/colon cancer, prolonged gastric suction.
Protein/calorie malnutrition. Feeding (enteral or parenteral) without adequate magnesium replacement.
Prolonged IV infusion of magnesium-free solutions.
Chronic alcoholism, alcohol withdrawal.
Toxemia of pregnancy.
Renal losses: Severe renal disease/diuretic phase of ARF; vigorous and/or prolonged diuresis with mercurial thiazides or loop diuretics; SIADH.
Drugs that affect magnesium balance: Aminoglycosides (gentamicin, tobramycin), antifungals (amphotericin B); chemotherapy agents (cisplatin); antirejection agents (cyclosporine), and excessive doses of calcium or vitamin D.

1077

Diabetic ketoacidosis, malignancies causing hypercalcemic states, severe burns, sepsis, hypothermia.
Acute pancreatitis, hypoparathyroidism, multiple transfusions of citrated blood.
Primary hyperaldosteronism, hypercalcemia, hyperthyroidism.

PATIENT ASSESSMENT DATA BASE

ACTIVITY/REST

May report:	Generalized weakness, insomnia.
	Ataxia, vertigo.

CIRCULATION

May exhibit:	Tachycardia, dysrhythmias.
	Hypotension (vasodilation); occasional hypertension.

FOOD/FLUID

May report:	Anorexia, nausea/vomiting, diarrhea.

NEUROSENSORY

May report:	Paresthesia (legs, feet).
	Vertigo.
May exhibit:	Nystagmus.
	Musculoskeletal fasciculations/tremors, neuromuscular irritability/spasticity, spontaneous carpopedal spasms, hyperactive deep-tendon reflexes, clonus.
	Tetany, convulsions; positive Babinski's, Chvostek's, and Trousseau's signs.
	Disorientation, apathy, depression, irritability, agitation, hallucinations/pschoses, coma.

TEACHING/LEARNING

	Refer to predisposing/contributing factors.
Discharge Plan Considerations:	**DRG projected mean length of stay: 4.1 days.**
	May require assistance with changes in therapeutic regimen, dietary management.

DIAGNOSTIC STUDIES

Serum magnesium: Decreased, less than 1.5 mEq/L or 1.8 mg/dl. *Note:* Usually symptoms do not appear until level is less than 1 mEq/L.

Calcium: May be decreased, unless there is a hypercalcemic condition causing the magnesium deficit.

ECG: Prolonged P-R and Q-T intervals, T-wave inversion, ST-segment depression.

ACTIONS/INTERVENTIONS	RATIONALE
Independent	
Monitor cardiac rate/rhythm, noting tachydysrhythmias and characteristic ECG changes.	Magnesium influences sodium/potassium transport across the cell membrane and affects excitability of cardiac tissue.

ACTIONS/INTERVENTIONS	RATIONALE

Independent

Monitor for signs of digitalis intoxication when used (e.g., reports of nausea/vomiting, blurred vision; increasing atrial dysrhythmias and heart block).

Magnesium deficit may precipitate digitalis toxicity.

Assess level of consciousness and neuromuscular status, e. g., movement, strength, reflexes/tone; note presence of Chvostek's/Trousseau's signs.

Confusion, irritability, and psychosis may occur. However, more common manifestations are muscular, e.g., hyperactive deep-tendon reflexes, muscle tremors, spasticity, generalized tetany.

Take seizure/safety precautions, e.g., side rails, bed in low position, frequent observation.

Changes in mentation or the development of seizures increases the risk of patient injury.

Provide quiet environment and subdued lighting.

Reduces extraneous stimuli; promotes rest.

Provide ROM exercises as tolerated.

Reduces deleterious effects of muscle weakness/spasticity.

Place footboard/cradle on bed.

Elevation of linens may reduce spasms.

Auscultate bowel sounds.

Muscle weakness/spasticity may reduce peristalsis and bowel function.

Encourage intake of dairy products, whole grains, green leafy vegetables, meat, and fish.

Provides oral replacement of mild magnesium deficits; may prevent recurrence.

Observe for signs of magnesium toxicity during replacement therapy, e.g., thirst, feeling hot and flushed, diaphoresis, anxiety, drowsiness, hypotension, increased muscular and nervous system irritability, loss of patellar reflex.

Rapid, excessive IV replacement may lead to toxicity and life-threatening complications.

Collaborative

Assist with identification/treatment of underlying cause.

Refer to listing of predisposing/contributing factors.

Monitor laboratory studies, e.g., serum magnesium, calcium, and potassium levels.

Evaluates therapy needs/effectiveness. *Note:* These electrolytes are interrelated, symptoms may be similar, and deficits of more than one may be present.

Administer medications as indicated:

Magnesium sulfate or magnesium chloride IV:

IV replacement is preferred in severe deficit because absorption of magnesium from intestinal tract varies inversely with calcium absorption. *Note:* Calcium gluconate is the antidote should hypermagnesemia occur as evidenced by depressed deep-tendon reflexes or respiratory depression and hypotension (late sign).

Magnesium sulfate IM, or magnesium hydroxide PO.

May be given for mild deficit or in nonemergent situations. Injections should be deep IM because they may be painful.

Magnesium-based antacids, e.g., Mylanta, Maalox, Gelusil, Riopan.

Can supplement dietary replacement. *Note:* Use of these products may cause diarrhea, which can be alleviated by concurrent use of aluminum-containing products, e.g., Amphojel, Basaljel.

1079

HYPERMAGNESEMIA (MAGNESIUM EXCESS)

PREDISPOSING/CONTRIBUTING FACTORS

Reduced renal function (e.g., acute processes or age), chronic renal disease/failure; or dialysis with hard water.

Excessive intake/absorption: e.g., too rapid replacement of magnesium; excessive use of magnesium-containing drugs/products, e.g., Maalox, Milk of Magnesia, Epsom salts.

Untreated diabetic ketoacidosis.

Hyperparathyroidism, aldosterone deficiency, adrenal insufficiency.

Extracellular fluid volume depletion (e.g., after diuretic abuse).

Salt-H_2O near-drowning, hypothermia, shock.

Chronic diarrhea; diseases that interfere with gastric absorption.

PATIENT ASSESSMENT DATA BASE

ACTIVITY/REST

May report:	Generalized weakness, lethargy.
May exhibit:	Drowsiness, lethargy, stupor.

CIRCULATION

May exhibit:	Hypotension (mild to severe).
	Pulses weak/irregular, bradycardia, cardiac arrest.

FOOD/FLUID

May report:	Nausea/vomiting.

NEUROSENSORY

May exhibit:	Skin flushing, sweating.
	Depressed deep tendon reflexes progressing to flaccid paralysis.
	Decreased level of consciousness, lethargy progressing to coma.
	Slurred speech.

RESPIRATION

May exhibit:	Hypoventilation progressing to apnea.

TEACHING/LEARNING

	Refer to predisposing/contributing factors.
Discharge Plan Considerations:	**DRG projected mean length of stay: 4.1 days.**
	May require assistance with changes in therapeutic regimen, dietary management.

DIAGNOSTIC STUDIES

Serum magnesium: Symptomatic levels greater than 3 mEq/L (increase to 10–20 mEq/L results in respiratory depression, coma, and cardiac arrest).

ECG: Prolonged P-R and Q-T intervals, wide QRS, elevated T waves, development of heart block, cardiac arrest.

ACTIONS/INTERVENTIONS	RATIONALE
Independent	
Monitor cardiac rate/rhythm.	Bradycardia and heart block may develop progressing to cardiac arrest as a direct result of hypermagnesemia on cardiac muscle.
Monitor BP.	Hypotension unexplained by other causes is an early sign of toxicity.
Assess level of consciousness and neuromuscular status, e.g., reflexes/tone, movement, strength.	CNS and neuromuscular depression can cause decreasing level of alertness, progressing to coma, and depressed muscular responses, progressing to flaccid paralysis.
Monitor respiratory rate/depth/rhythm. Encourage cough/deep-breathing exercises. Elevate head of bed as indicated.	Neuromuscular transmissions are blocked by magnesium excess, resulting in respiratory muscular weakness and hypoventilation, which may progress to apnea.
Encourage increased fluid intake if appropriate.	Increased hydration enhances magnesium excretion, but fluid intake must be cautious in event of renal/cardiac failure.
Monitor urinary output and 24-hour fluid balance.	Renal failure is the primary contributing factor in hypermagnesemia; and if present, fluid excess can easily occur.
Promote bedrest, assist with personal care activities as needed.	Flaccid paralysis, lethargy, and decreased mentation reduce activity tolerance/ability.
Recommend avoidance of magnesium-containing antacids e.g., Maalox, Mylanta, Gelusil, Riopan, in patient with renal disease.	Limits oral intake to help prevent hypermagnesemia.
Collaborative	
Assist with identification/treatment of underlying cause.	Refer to lising of predisposing/contributing factors.
Monitor laboratory studies as indicated: serum magnesium and calcium levels.	Evaluates therapy needs/effectiveness.
Administer IV fluids and thiazide diuretics as indicated.	Promotes renal clearance of magnesium (if renal function is normal).
Administer 10% calcium chloride or gluconate IV.	Antagonizes action/reverses symptoms of magnesium toxicity to improve neuromuscular transmission.
Assist with dialysis as needed.	In the presence of renal disease/failure, dialysis may be needed to lower serum levels.

Acid/Base Imbalances

The body has the remarkable ability to maintain plasma pH within the narrow range of 7.35–7.45. It does so by means of chemical buffering mechanisms by the kidneys and the lungs. Although single acid/base (e.g., respiratory acidosis) imbalances do occur, mixed acid/base imbalances are more common (e.g., metabolic acidosis/respiratory acidosis as occurs with cardiac arrest).

RELATED CONCERNS

Plans of care specific to predisposing factors.
Fluid and Electrolyte Imbalances, p 1054
Renal Dialysis, p 646

NURSING PRIORITIES

1. Achieve homeostasis.
2. Prevent/minimize complications.
3. Provide information about condition/prognosis and treatment needs as appropriate.

DISCHARGE GOALS

1. Physiologic balance restored.
2. Free of complications.
3. Condition, prognosis, and treatment needs understood.

METABOLIC ACIDOSIS (PRIMARY BASE BICARBONATE DEFICIT)

Reflects an excess of acid (hydrogen) and a deficit of base (bicarbonate) resulting from acid overproduction, loss of intestinal bicarbonate, inadequate conservation of bicarbonate, and excretion of acid, or anaerobic metabolism. Metabolic acidosis is characterized by normal or high anion gap situations. If the primary problem is direct loss of bicarbonate, gain of chloride or decreased ammonia production, the anion gap will be within normal limits. If the primary problem is the accumulation of organic anions (such as ketones or lactic acid), the condition is known as high anion gap acidosis. Compensatory mechanisms to correct this imbalance include an increase in respirations to blow off excess CO_2, an increase in ammonia formation, and acid excretion (H+) by the kidneys, with retention of bicarbonate and sodium.

High anion gap acidosis: Diabetic ketoacidosis, starvational or alcoholic lactic acidosis, renal failure, high-fat diets/lipid administration. Poisoning, e.g., salicylate intoxication (after initial stage), paraldehyde intoxication, and drug therapy, e.g., Diamox, NH_4Cl.

Normal anion gap acidosis: Loss of bicarbonate from the body as may occur in renal tubular acidosis, hyperalimentation, vomiting/diarrhea, small-bowel/pancreatic fistulas, and ileostomy. Use of IV sodium chloride in presence of preexisting kidney dysfunction.

Systemic infections/sepsis, liver failure.

Use of carbonic anhydrase inhibitors or anion-exchange resins, e.g., cholestyramine (Questran).

PATIENT ASSESSMENT DATA BASE (Dependent on underlying cause)

ACTIVITY/REST

May report: Lethargy, fatigue; muscle weakness.

CIRCULATION

May exhibit: Hypotension, wide pulse pressure.

Pulse may be weak, irregular (dysrhythmias).

1082

ELIMINATION

May report: Diarrhea.

May exhibit: Dark/concentrated urine.

FOOD/FLUID

May report: Anorexia, nausea/vomiting.

May exhibit: Poor skin turgor, dry mucous membranes.

NEUROSENSORY

May report: Headache, drowsiness, decreased mental function.

May exhibit: Changes in sensorium, e.g., stupor, confusion, lethargy, depression, delirium, coma.

RESPIRATION

May report: Dyspnea on exertion.

May exhibit: Hyperventilation, Kussmaul's respirations (deep, rapid breathing).

TEACHING/LEARNING

Refer to predisposing/contributing factors.

Discharge Plan Considerations: **DRG projected mean length of stay: 4.1 days.**

May require change in therapies for underlying disease process/condition.

DIAGNOSTIC STUDIES

Arterial pH: Decreased, less than 7.35.

Bicarbonate: Decreased, less than 22 mEq/L.

$PaCO_2$: Less than 35–40 mm Hg.

Base excess: Decreased or absent.

Anion gap: Greater than 14 mEq/L (high anion gap) or no greater than 10 to 14 mEq/L (normal anion gap).

Serum potassium: Increased.

Serum chloride: Increased.

Serum glucose: May be decreased or increased dependent on etiology.

Serum ketones: Increased in DM, starvation, alcohol intoxication.

Plasma lactic acid: Elevated in lactic acidosis.

Urine pH: Decreased, less than 4.5 (in absence of renal disease).

ECG: Cardiac dysrhythmias (bradycardia) and pattern changes associated with hyperkalemia, e.g., tall T

ACTIONS/INTERVENTIONS	RATIONALE
Independent	
Monitor BP.	Arteriolar dilation/decreased cardiac contractility, (e.g., sepsis) and hypovolemia (e.g., ketoacidosis) occurs resulting in systemic shock, e.g., hypotension and tissue hypoxia.

1083

ACTIONS/INTERVENTIONS	RATIONALE
Independent	
Assess level of consciousness and note progressive changes in neuromuscular status, e.g., strength, tone, movement.	Decreased mental function, confusion, seizures, weakness, flaccid paralysis can occur due to hypoxia, hyperkalemia, and decreased pH of CNS fluid.
Provide seizure/coma precautions, e.g., bed in low position, use of side rails, frequent observation.	Protects patient from injury resulting from decreased mentation/convulsions.
Monitor heart rate/rhythm.	Acidemia may be manifested by changes in ECG configuration and presence of tachydysrhythmias or bradydysrhythmias as well as increased ventricular irritability (signs of hyperkalemia). Life-threatening cardiovascular collapse may also occur due to vasodilation and decreased cardiac contractility.
Observe for altered respiratory excursion, rate, and depth.	Deep, rapid respirations (Kussmaul's) may be noted as a compensatory mechanism to eliminate excess acid. However, as potassium shifts out of cell in an attempt to correct acidosis, respirations may become depressed. Transient respiratory depression may be the result of overcorrection of metabolic acidosis with sodium bicarbonate.
Assess skin temperature, color, capillary refill.	Evaluates circulatory status, tissue perfusion, effects of hypotension.
Auscultate bowel sounds; measure abdominal girth as indicated.	In the presence of coexisting hyperkalemia, GI distress (e.g., distention, diarrhea, and colic) may occur.
Monitor I&O closely and weigh daily.	Marked dehydration may be present due to vomiting, diarrhea. Therapy needs are based on underlying cause and fluid balance.
Test/monitor urine pH.	Kidneys attempt to compensate for acidosis by excreting excess hydrogen in the form of weak acids and ammonia. Maximum urine acidity is pH of 4.0.
Provide oral hygiene with sodium bicarbonate washes, lemon/glycerine swabs.	Neutralizes mouth acids and provides protective lubrication.
Collaborative	
Assist with identification/treatment of underlying cause.	Refer to listing of predisposing/contributing factors.
Monitor/graph serial ABGs.	Evaluates therapy needs/effectiveness. Blood bicarbonate and pH should slowly increase toward normal levels.
Monitor serum electrolytes, e.g., potassium.	As acidosis is corrected, serum potassium deficit may occur as potassium shifts back into the cells.
Replace fluids, as indicated depending on underlying etiology, e.g., D5W/saline solutions.	Choice of solution varies with cause of acidosis, e.g., DKA. *Note:* Lactate-containing solutions may be contraindicated in the presence of lactic acidosis.

ACTIONS/INTERVENTIONS	RATIONALE
Collaborative	
Administer medications as indicated, e.g.:	
Sodium bicarbonate/lactate or saline IV;	Corrects bicarbonate deficit, but is used cautiously to correct severe acidosis (pH less than 7.2) because sodium bicarbonate can cause rebound metabolic alkalosis.
Potassium chloride;	May be required as potassium reenters the cell, causing a serum deficit.
Phosphate;	May be administered to enhance acid excretion in presence of chronic acidosis with hypophosphatemia.
Calcium.	May be given to improve neuromuscular conduction/function.
Modify diet as indicated, e.g., low-protein, high-carbohydrate diet in presence of renal failure or ADA diet for diabetic.	Restriction of protein may be necessary to decrease production of acid waste products, whereas addition of complex carbohydrates will correct acid production from the metabolism of fats in the diabetic.
Administer exchange resins and/or assist with dialysis as indicated.	May be desired to reduce acidosis by decreasing excess potassium and acid waste products if pH less than 7.1 and other therapies are ineffective, or CHF develops.

METABOLIC ALKALOSIS (PRIMARY BASE BICARBONATE EXCESS)

Metabolic alkalosis is characterized by a high pH (loss of hydrogen ions) and high plasma bicarbonate caused by excessive intake of sodium bicarbonate, gastric/intestinal loss of acid, renal excretion of hydrogen and chloride, prolonged hypercalcemia, hypokalemia, and hyperaldosteronism. Compensatory mechanisms include slow, shallow respirations to increase CO_2 level and an increase of bicarbonate excretion and hydrogen reabsorption by the kidneys.

PREDISPOSING/CONTRIBUTING FACTORS

Prolonged vomiting, gastric lavage; diarrhea (if it has a high chloride content).
Use of potent diuretics (e.g., thiazides, Lasix, ethacrynic acid) with acid loss (hydrogen and potassium).
Excessive use of salt, laxatives, antacids/baking soda, licorice.
Excessive/overzealous correction of metabolic acidosis with sodium bicarbonate.
Administration of potassium-free IV solutions, citrated blood.
Primary and secondary hyperaldosteronism.
Adrenocortical hormone disease, e.g., Cushing's syndrome or corticosteroid therapy.
Prolonged hypercalcemia (nonparathyroid), hypokalemia.

PATIENT ASSESSMENT DATA BASE (Dependent on underlying cause)

CIRCULATION

May exhibit:　　Tachycardia, irregularities/dysrhythmias.
　　　　　　　　　Cyanosis.

1085

ELIMINATION

May report: Diarrhea.

FOOD/FLUID

May report: Nausea/vomiting, diarrhea.
High salt intake.

NEUROSENSORY

May report: Tingling of fingers and toes; circumoral paresthesia.
Dizziness.

May exhibit: Hypertonicity of muscles, tetany, tremors, convulsions.
Confusion, irritability, restlessness, belligerence, apathy, coma.
Picking at bedclothes.

RESPIRATION

May exhibit: Hypoventilation (increases PCO_2 and conserves carbonic acid), periods of apnea.

TEACHING/LEARNING

Refer to predisposing/contributing factors.

Discharge Plan   **DRG projected mean length of stay: 4.1 days.**
Considerations: May require change in therapy for underlying disease process/condition.

DIAGNOSTIC STUDIES

Arterial pH: Increased, greater than 7.45.

Bicarbonate: Increased, greater than 26 mEq/L (primary).

$PaCO_2$: Slightly increased, greater than 45 mm Hg (compensatory).

Base excess: Increased.

Serum chloride: Decreased, less than 98 mEq/L (if alkalosis is hypochloremia) disproportionately to serum sodium decreases.

Serum potassium: Decreased.

Serum calcium: Usually decreased.

Urine pH: Increased, greater than 7.0.

Urine chloride: Less than 10 mEq/L suggests chloride responsive alkalosis, whereas levels greater than 20 mEq/L suggest chloride resistance.

ECG: May show hypokalemic changes including peaked P waves, flat T waves, depressed ST segment, low T wave merging to P wave, and elevated U waves.

ACTIONS/INTERVENTIONS	RATIONALE
Independent	
Monitor respiratory rate, rhythm, and depth.	Hypoventilation is a compensatory mechanism to conserve carbonic acid and represents definite risks to the individual, e.g., hypoxemia and respiratory failure.

ACTIONS/INTERVENTIONS	RATIONALE
Independent	
Assess level of consciousness and neuromuscular status, e.g., strength, tone, movement; note presence of Chvostek's/Trousseau's signs.	The CNS may be hyperirritable (increased pH of CNS fluid), resulting in tingling, numbness, dizziness, restlessness, or apathy and confusion. Hypocalcemia may contribute to tetany (although occurrence is rare).
Monitor heart rate/rhythm.	Atrial/ventricular ectopics and tachydysrhythmias may develop.
Record amount and source of output. Monitor intake and daily weight.	Helpful in identifying source of ion loss; e.g., potassium and HCl are lost in vomiting and GI suctioning.
Restrict oral intake and reduce noxious environmental stimuli; use intermittent/low suction during NG suctioning; irrigate gastric tube with isotonic solutions, rather than water.	Limits gastric losses of hydrochloric acid, potassium, and calcium.
Provide seizure/safety precautions as indicated, e.g., padded side rails, airway protection, bed in low position, frequent observation.	Changes in mentation and CNS/neuromuscular hyperirritability may result in patient harm, especially if tetany/convulsions occur.
Encourage intake of foods and fluids high in potassium and possibly calcium (dependent on blood level), e.g., canned grapefruit and apple juices, bananas, cauliflower, dried peaches, figs, and wheat germ.	Useful in replacing potassium losses when oral intake permitted.
Review medication regimen for use of diuretics (thiazides, Lasix, ethacrynic acid); and cathartics.	Discontinuation of these potassium-losing drugs may prevent recurrence of imbalance.
Instruct patient to avoid use of excessive amounts of sodium bicarbonate.	Ulcer patients can cause alkalosis by taking baking soda and Milk of Magnesia in addition to prescribed alkaline antacids.
Collaborative	
Assist with identification/treatment of underlying disorder.	Refer to listing of predisposing/contributing factors.
Monitor laboratory studies as indicated, e.g., ABGs/pH, serum electrolytes (especially potassium), and BUN.	Evaluates therapy needs/effectiveness and monitors renal function.
Administer medications as indicated, e.g.;	
Sodium chloride PO/Ringer's solution IV unless contraindicated;	Correcting sodium, water, and chloride defects may be all that is needed to permit kidneys to excrete bicarbonate and correct alkalosis but must be used with caution in patients with CHF or renal insufficiency.
Potassium chloride;	Hypokalemia is frequently present. Chloride is needed so kidney can absorb Na with chloride, enhancing excretion of bicarbonate.
Ammonium chloride or arginine hydrochloride;	Increases amount of circulating hydrogen ions. Monitor administration closely to prevent too rapid a decrease in pH, hemolysis of RBCs. *Note:* May cause rebound metabolic acidosis and is usually contraindicated in patients with renal/hepatic failure.

1087

ACTIONS/INTERVENTIONS	RATIONALE
Collaborative	
Acetazolamide (Diamox);	A carbonic anhydrase inhibitor that increases renal excretion of bicarbonate.
Spironolactone (Aldactone).	Effective in treating chloride-resistant alkalosis, e.g., Cushing's syndrome.
Avoid/limit use of sedatives or hypnotics.	If respirations are depressed, may cause hypoxia/ respiratory failure.
Encourage fluids IV/PO.	Replaces extracellular fluid losses, and adequate hydration facilitates removal of pulmonary secretions to improve ventilation.
Administer supplemental O_2 as indicated and respiratory treatments to improve ventilation.	Respiratory compensation for metabolic alkalosis is hypoventilation, which may cause decreased PaO_2 levels/hypoxia.
Assist with dialysis as needed.	Useful when renal dysfunction prevents clearance of bicarbonate.

RESPIRATORY ACIDOSIS (PRIMARY CARBONIC ACID EXCESS)

Represents an elevation of $PaCO_2$ with resultant excess of carbonic acid (H_2CO_3) due to primary defects in lung function or changes in normal respiratory pattern. The condition may be acute or chronic. Compensaory mechanisms include an increased respiratory rate; Hb buffering carbonic acid, forming bicarbonate ions and deoxygenated Hb; and an increased renal formation of ammonia acid excretions, with reabsorption of bicarbonate.

PREDISPOSING/CONTRIBUTING FACTORS

Acute respiratory acidosis: Associated with acute pulmonary edema, aspiration of foreign body, overdose of sedatives, anesthesia, barbiturate poisoning, smoke inhalation, acute laryngospasm, hemothorax/ pneumothorax, atelectasis, ARDS, mechanical ventilators, or Pickwickian syndrome; excessive CO_2 intake, e.g., use of rebreathing mask, CVA therapy.
Chronic respiratory acidosis is associated with emphysema, asthma, bronchiectasis, neuromuscular disorders, such as Guillain-Barré syndrome and myasthenia gravis, botulism, spinal cord injuries.
Hypoventilation associated with decreased function of respiratory center, such as with head trauma, oversedation, general anesthesia, metabolic alkalosis.

PATIENT ASSESSMENT DATA BASE (Dependent on underlying cause)

ACTIVITY/REST

May report:	Fatigue.
May exhibit:	Generalized weakness, ataxia, loss of coordination (chronic).

CIRCULATORY

May exhibit:	Hypertension.
	Bounding pulses, pinkish color, warm skin associated with hypotension reflects vasodilation (severe acidosis).

Tachycardia, dysrhythmias.
Diaphoresis, pallor, and cyanosis (late stage of hypoxia).

FOOD/FLUID

May report: Nausea/vomiting.

NEUROSENSORY

May report: Feeling of fullness in head (acute; associated with vasodilation).
                    Dull headache, dizziness, visual disturbances.

May exhibit: Confusion, apprehension, agitation, restlessness, somnolence, coma (acute).
                    Tremors, decreased reflexes.

RESPIRATORY

May report: Dyspnea with exertion.

May exhibit: Increased respiratory effort with nasal flaring/yawning.
                    Decreased respiratory rate.
                    Crackles, wheezes, stridor.

TEACHING/LEARNING

Refer to predisposing/contributing factors.

Discharge Plan Considerations: **DRG projected mean length of stay: 4.1 days.**
May require assistance with changes in therapies for underlying disease process/condition.

DIAGNOSTIC STUDIES

Arterial pH: Decreased, less than 7.35.

Bicarbonate: Normal or increased, greater than 26 mEq/L (in chronic stage).

PaCO$_2$: Increased, greater than 45 mm Hg (primary).

PO$_2$: Normal or decreased.

O$_2$ saturation: Decreased.

Urine pH: Decreased, 6.0.

Serum potassium: Normal or increased.

Serum calcium: Increased.

Serum chloride: Decreased.

Lactic acid: Elevated.

ACTIONS/INTERVENTIONS	RATIONALE
Independent	
Monitor respiratory rate, depth, and effort. Note pulse oximetry readings.	Hypoventilation and associated hypoxemia leads to respiratory distress/failure. Use of pulse oximetry can identify progression of hypoxia/response to therapy before other signs or symptoms are observed.
Auscultate breath sounds.	Identifies area(s) of decreased ventilation/airway obstruction and therapy needs/effectiveness.

ACTIONS/INTERVENTIONS	RATIONALE
Independent	
Assess for decreased level of consciousness.	Signals severe acidotic state, which requires immediate attention. Sensorium clears slowly because it takes longer for hydrogen ions to clear from CSF.
Monitor heart rate/rhythm.	Tachycardia develops in an attempt to increase O_2 delivery to the tissues. Dysrhythmias may occur due to hypoxia (myocardial ischemia) and electrolyte imbalances.
Note skin color, temperature, moisture.	Diaphoresis, pallor, cool/clammy skin are associated with hypoxemia.
Encourage/assist with turning, coughing and deep breathing. Place in semi-Fowler's position. Suction as necessary. Provide airway adjunct as indicated.	These measures improve ventilation and prevent airway obstruction or decreased alveolar diffusion/perfusion.
Collaborative	
Assist with identification/treatment of underlying cause.	Refer to listing of predisposing/contributing factors.
Monitor/graph serial ABGs; serum electrolyte levels.	Evaluates therapy needs/effectiveness.
Administer O_2 as indicated by mask, cannula, or mechanical ventilation. Increase respiratory rate or tidal volume of ventilator.	Prevents/corrects hypoxemia and respiratory failure. *Note:* Must be used with caution in presence of emphysema/COPD because respiratory depression/failure may result.
Administer medications as indicated, e.g.:	
Naloxone hydrochloride (Narcan);	May be useful in arousing patient and stimulating respiratory function in presence of drug sedation.
Sodium bicarbonate;	Given in emergent situations to correct acidosis if pH is less than 7.25 and hyperkalemia coexists. *Note:* Rebound alkalosis or tetany may occur.
IV solutions of Ringer's lactate or 0.6 M solution of Na lactate.	May be useful in nonemergent situations to help control acidosis, until underlying respiratory problem can be corrected.
Potassium chloride;	Acidosis shifts potassium out of cells and hydrogen into cells. Correction of acidosis may then cause serum hypokalemia as potassium reenters the cell. Either imbalance can impair neuromuscular/respiratory function.
Limit use of hypnotic sedatives or tranquilizers.	In the presence of hypoventilation, respiratory depression can occur with the use of sedatives, and CO_2 narcosis may develop.
Maintain hydration (IV/PO)/provide humidification.	Assists in thinning/mobilization of secretions.
Provide aggressive chest physiotherapy, including postural drainage.	Aids in clearing secretions which may improve ventilation, allowing excess CO_2 to be eliminated.
Assist with ventilatory aids, e.g., IPPB in conjunction with bronchodilators.	Increases lung expansion and opens airways to improve ventilation preventing respiratory failure.

RESPIRATORY ALKALOSIS (PRIMARY CARBONIC ACID DEFICIT)

There is a decrease in PCO_2 with a deficit of carbonic acid (H_2CO_3) due to a marked increase in the rate of respirations. Compensatory mechanisms include decreased respiratory rate (if the body is able to respond to the drop in PCO_2) to retain CO_2, increased renal excretion of bicarbonate, and retention of hydrogen.

PREDISPOSING/CONTRIBUTING FACTORS

Hyperventilation caused by nervousness, anxiety, intentional overbreathing, hysteria/extreme emotions; fever; sepsis (usually gram-negative organism), meningitis; severe pain; brain trauma/lesions; multiple pulmonary emboli; or mechanical ventilators.

Restrictive problems, such as asthma, pulmonary fibrosis, pregnancy (abdominal distention with elevation of diaphragm).

O_2 lack, such as high-altitude sickness, severe anemia, hypoxemia.

CHF, alcoholic intoxication, cirrhosis/hepatic failure, thyrotoxicosis.

Paraldehyde, epinephrine, or early salicylate intoxication.

Rapid correction of metabolic acidosis, e.g., peritoneal dialysis.

PATIENT ASSESSMENT DATA BASE (Dependent on underlying cause)

CIRCULATION

May exhibit: Hypotension.

Tachycardia.

Pulse irregular if dysrhythmias present.

FOOD/FLUID

May report: Dry mouth.

Nausea/vomiting.

NEUROSENSORY

May report: Headache, tinnitus.

Numbness/tingling of face, hands, and toes; circumoral paresthesia.

Syncope, blurred vision, vertigo, palpitations.

May exhibit: Confusion, restlessness, anxiety, obtundation, coma.

Muscle weakness, hyperreflexia, positive Chvostek's sign, tetany, seizures.

PAIN/COMFORT

May report: Muscle cramps, epigastric pain.

RESPIRATION

May exhibit: Tachypnea, rapid shallow breathing, dyspnea. Intermittent periods of apnea.

TEACHING/LEARNING

Refer to predisposing/contributing factors.

Discharge Plan Considerations: **DRG projected mean length of stay: 4.1 days.**

May require change in treatment/therapy of underlying disease process/condition.

1091

DIAGNOSTIC STUDIES

Arterial pH: Greater than 7.45 (may be near normal in chronic stage).

Bicarbonate: Normal or decreased, less than 22 mEq/L (compensatory).

PaCO$_2$: Decreased, less than 35 mm Hg (primary).

Serum potassium: Decreased.

Serum chloride: Increased.

Serum calcium: Decreased.

Urine pH: Increased, greater than 7.0.

ACTIONS/INTERVENTIONS	RATIONALE
Independent	
Monitor respiratory rate, depth, and effort; ascertain cause for hyperventilation if possible, e.g., anxiety, pain, improper ventilator settings.	Identifies alterations from usual breathing pattern and influences choice of intervention.
Assess level of consciousness and note neuromuscular status, e.g., strength, tone, reflexes, and sensation.	Decreased mentation, and tetany or convulsions may occur.
Demonstrate appropriate breathing patterns and review/assist with ordered treatments, e.g., rebreathing mask/bag.	Decreasing the rate of respirations will elevate PCO$_2$ level.
Provide support by a calm manner and voice.	May help reassure and calm the agitated patient, thereby aiding in reduction of respiratory rate.
Provide safety/seizure precautions, e.g., bed in low position, padded side rails, frequent observation.	Changes in mentation or CNS and neuromuscular hyperirritability may result in patient harm, especially if tetany/convulsions occur.
Collaborative	
Assist with identification/treatment of underlying cause.	Refer to listing of predisposing/contributing factors.
Monitor/graph serial ABGs.	Identifies therapy needs/effectiveness.
Monitor serum potassium. Replace as indicated.	Hypokalemia may occur as potassium is lost (urine) or shifted into the cell in exchange for hydrogen in an attempt to correct alkalosis.
Provide sedation, as indicated.	May be required to reduce psychogenic cause.
Administer CO$_2$, or use rebreathing mask as indicated. Reduce respiratory rate/tidal volume, or add additional dead space (tubing) to mechanical ventilator.	Increasing CO$_2$ retention may correct carbonic acid deficit.

Bibliography

General References

Bellak, JP and Bamford, PA: Nursing Assessment: A Multidimensional Approach. Jones & Bartlett, Boston, 1987.
Berkow, R (ed): The Merck Manual, ed 15. Merck Sharp & Dohme Research Laboratories, Rahway, NJ, 1987.
Cella, JH and Watson, J: Nurse's Manual of Laboratory Tests. FA Davis, Philadelphia, 1989.
Condon, RE and Nyhus, LM (eds): Manual of Surgical Therapeutics, ed 7. Little, Brown & Co, Boston, 1988.
Deglin, JH and Vallerand, AH: Davis's Drug Guide for Nurses, ed 3. FA Davis, Philadelphia, 1992.

Diseases and Disorders Handbook, ed 3. Springhouse Corp, Springhouse, PA, 1989.
Doenges, ME and Moorhouse, MF: Nurse's Pocket Guide: Nursing Diagnoses with Interventions, ed 3. FA Davis, Philadelphia, 1991.
Dunagan, WC and Ridner, ML (eds): Manual of Medical Therapeutics, ed 26. Little, Brown & Co, Boston, 1989.
Fischbach, F: A Manual of Laboratory and Diagnostic Tests, ed 4. JB Lippincott, Philadelphia, 1992.
Guyton, AC: Textbook of Medical Physiology, ed 8. WB Saunders, Philadelphia, 1991.
Kuhn, MM: Pharmacotherapeutics: A Nursing Process Approach, ed 2. FA Davis, Philadelphia, 1991.
Professional Guide to Diseases, ed 3. Springhouse Corp, Springhouse, PA, 1989.
Suddarth, DS (ed): The Lippincott Manual of Nursing Practice, ed 5. JB Lippincott, Philadelphia, 1991.
Thomas, CL (ed): Taber's Cyclopedic Medical Dictionary, ed 17. FA Davis, Philadelphia, 1993.
Thompson, JM, et al: Mosby's Manual of Clinical Nursing, ed 2. CV Mosby, St Louis, 1989.

Books

Acute Pain Management: Operative or Medical Procedures and Trauma. Clinical Practice Guidelines. US Dept of Health and Human Services. US Government Printing Office, Washington, D.C., Feb 1992.
Christensen, AB and Harrity, AS: Parenting Guidelines for Substance Abuse Prevention. Overland Community Task Force For Alcohol/Drug Youth. 1985.
Depressants. Channing L. Bete Co, South Deerfield, MA, 1988.
Metheny, NM: Fluid and Electrolyte Balance: Nursing Considerations, ed 2. JB Lippincott, Philadelphia, 1992.
Townsend, M: Psychiatric/Mental Health Nursing, FA Davis, Philadelphia, 1993.

Articles

Anderson, AR: Are your IV chemo skills up-to-date? RN 52(1): 40, 1989.
Anderson, S: ABGs—six easy steps to interpreting blood gases. AJN 90(8):42, 1990.
Andresen, GP: A fresh look at assessing the elderly. RN 52(6): 28, 1989.
Andresen, GP: How to assess the older mind. RN 52(7): 34, 1992.
Behner, N and Hageratt, J: A proposal for change to achieve competence in long-term psychosocial nursing care. J Psychosoc Nurs 29(8):30, 1991.
Bolgiano, CS et al: Administering oxygen therapy: What you need to know. Nursing90 20(6):47, 1990.
Cahill-Wright, C: Managing postoperative pain. Nursing91 21(12):42, 1991.
Camp-Sorrell, D: Controlling adverse effects of chemotherapy. Nursing91 21(4):34, 1991.
Campbell, A and Johnston, CA: OR-PACU reports: What they should tell you about your postoperative patient. Nursing91 21(10):49, 1991.
Cuzzell, JZ and Stotts, NA: Wound care: Trial and error yields to knowledge. AJN 20(10):53, 1990.
Dang, S: When the patient is out of control. RN 53(10): 57, 1990.
Dellasaga, C: Coping with caregiving-stress management for caregivers of the elderly. J Psychosoc Nurs 28(1):15, 1990.
Dudjak, LA and Fleck, AE: BRMs: New drug therapy comes of age. RN 54(10):42, 1991.
Durhan, E and Frost-Hartzer, P: Relaxation therapy works. RN 54(8):40, 1991.
Ferrell, BR: Managing pain with long-acting morphine. Nursing91 21(10):34, 1991.
Greifzu, S, Radjeski, D, and Winnick, B: Oral care is part of cancer care. RN 53(6):43, 1990.
Gallagher, M and Kahn, C: Lasers: Scalpels of Light, RN 53(5):46, 1990.
Gribbin, ME: Could you detect these oncological crises? RN 53(6):36, 1990.
Handerhan, B: Computing the ion gap. RN 54(7):30, 1991.
Heath, I: Pain hugs, PRN. AJN 92(4):120, 1992.
Heater, BS, Olson, RK, and Becker, AM: Helping patients recover faster. AJN 90(10):19, 1990.
House, MA: Cocaine. AJN 90(4):40, 1990.
Hutchison, CP and Bahr, RT: Types and meanings of caring behaviors among elderly nursing home residents. J Nurs Scholarship 23(2):85, 1991.
Hussar, DA: Drug update92. Nursing92 92(5):55, 1992.
Janusek, LW: Metabolic acidosis. Nursing90 20(7):52, 1990.
Joel, LP and Patterson, JE: Nursing homes can't afford cheap nursing care. RN 53(4):57, 1990.
Katzin, L: Chronic illness and sexuality. AJN January: 56, 1992.
McCaffery, M: Pain management: Nurses lead the way to new priorities. AJN 20(10):45, 1990.
McCaffery, M and Ferrell, BR: Pain-control vignettes: How vital are vital signs. Nursing92 22(1):43, 1992.
McGowan, KL: Radiation therapy: Saving your patient's skin. RN 52(6):24, 1989.
Meddaugh, DI: Reactance—understanding aggressive behavior in long-term care. J Psychosoc Nurs 1990 28(4):28, 1990.
Meyer, C: Nurses vote for the most valuable new drugs. AJN 91(9):33, 1991.
Mims, BS: Interpreting ABGs. RN 54(3): 42, 1991.
Oleander, L: Why tube feeding may be the wrong answer. RN 52(6):43, 1989.

Pavia, Z: Sundown syndrome. RN 53(7):46, 1990.

Povenmire, KI and House, MA: Acute crack cocaine intoxication: A case study. Focus on Crit Care 16(2):112, 1989.

Povenmire, KI and House, MA: Recognizing the cocaine addict. Nursing90 20(5):46, 1990.

Powell, AE: Alcohol withdrawal syndrome. AJN 88(3):312, 1988.

Rowland, MA: Myths and facts about postop discomfort. AJN 90(5):60, 1990.

Sonnesso, G: Are you ready to use pulse oximetry? Nursing92 21(8):60, 1991.

Stotts, NA: Seeing red and yellow and black: The three-color concept of wound care. Nursing90 20(2):59, 1990.

Strong, B: The view from the mattress. Nursing92 92(5):47, 1992.

Taylor, DL: Respiratory alkalosis. Nursing90 20(8):60, 1990.

Taylor, DL: Respiratory acidosis. Nursing90 20(9):52, 1990.

Uretsky, ST: New drugs: The class of 1991. AJN 92(12):40, 1991.

Vanete, SM and Saunders, JM: Dealing with serious depression in cancer patients. Nursing89 19(2):44, 1989.

Walters, P: Chemo: A nurse's guide to action administration and side effects. RN 53(2):52, 1990.

Waltman, RE: Dealing with older patients and their families. Nursing91 21(10):66, 1991.

Weber, BA: Timely tips on adhesive tape. Nursing91 21(10):52, 1991.

Wickland, S and Devroye, M: Nurses' drug alert. AJN 12(3):329, 1988.

Wickland, S and Green, D: TPN in patients receiving chemotherapy. Nurses' drug alert. AJN 13(7):957, 1989.

Wild, L and Coyne, C: The basics and beyond: Epidural analgesia. AJN 92(4):26, 1992.

Wroblewski, B and Young, LS: Topics in parenteral nutrition for the 1990s. Focus on Crit Care 18(4):276, 1991.

Yarnell, RP and Craig, MP: Detecting hypomagnesemia: The most overlooked electrolyte imbalance. Nursing91 21(7):55, 1991.

Young, CK and White, S: Preparing patients for tube feeding at home. AJN 92(4):46, 1992.

APPENDIX

Key to Abbreviations _____

A-a DO$_2$ ratio: Alveolar to arterial oxygen gradient
ABG: arterial blood gas
a.c.: before meals
ACE: angiotension converting enzyme
ACh RAb: acetylcholine receptor antibody
ACT: activated clotting time
ACTH: adrenocorticotropic hormone
AD: autonomic dysreflexia
ADA: American Diabetes Association
ADH: antidiuretic hormone
ADLs: activities of daily living
ADRDA: Alzheimer's Disease and Related Disorders Association
AED: antiepileptic drug
AF: atrial fibrillation
AI: aortic valve insufficiency
AICD: Automatic implantable cardioverter defibrillator
AIDS: acquired immunodeficiency syndrome
ALS: amyotrophic lateral sclerosis
ALT: alanine aminotransferase (equivalent SGPT)
ANA: nuclear antibody
AntiDNA: deoxyribonuclease
AP: anterior-posterior
APTT: activated partial thromboplastic time
AR: aortic valve regurgitation
ARDS: adult respiratory distress syndrome
ARF: acute renal failure
AS: aortic valve stenosis
ASA: acetylsalicylic acid
ASI: addiction severity index
ASHD: arteriosclerotic heart disease
ASL: antistreptolysin
ASO: antistreptolysin-O titer
AST: aspartate aminotransferase (equivalent SGOT)
ATN: acute tubular necrosis
AV: aortic valve: atrioventricular; arteriovenous

AVF: augmented unipolar foot lead of electrocardiogram
BAERs: brainstem auditory evoked responses
BBB: bundle branch block
BEAM: brain electrical activity map
BEE: basal energy expenditure
BFP: biologically false positive
b.i.d.: twice a day
BKA: below-knee amputation
BM: bowel movement
BMR: basal metabolic rate
B&O: belladonna and opium
BP: blood pressure
BPM: beats per minute
BSP: bromsulphalein
BUN: blood urea nitrogen

C: centigrade
Ca^{++}: calcium
CABG: coronary artery bypass graft
CAD: coronary artery disease
CAPD: continuous ambulatory peritoneal dialysis
CAVH: continuous arteriovenous hemofiltration
CBC: complete blood count
cc: cubic centimeters
CCPD: continuous cycling peritoneal dialysis
CEA: carcinogenic embryonic antigen
CHF: congestive heart failure
CHI: creatinine height index
CI: cardiac index
Cl$^-$: chloride
cm: centimeter
CMV: cytomegalovirus
CNS: central nervous system
CO: cardiac output; carbon monoxide
CO$_2$: carbon dioxide
COHbg: carboxyhemoglobin

1095

COPD: chronic obstructive pulmonary disease
CPB: cardiopulmonary bypass (machine)
CPK: creatinine phosphokinase
CPK-MB: creatinine phosphokinase isoenzyme
CPP: cerebral perfusion pressure
CPR: cardiopulmonary resuscitation
CPT: chest physiotherapy
Cr: creatinine
CRF: chronic renal failure
CRP: c-reactive protein
C&S: culture and sensitivities
CSF: cerebrospinal fluid
CT: computerized axial tomography
CTZ: chemoreceptor trigger zone
cu: cubic
CVA: cerebrovascular accident; costovertebral angle
CVP: central venous pressure

DAT: dementia of the Alzheimer's type
DI: diabetes insipidus
DIC: disseminated intravascular coagulation
DIPs: distal interphalangeal joints
DKA: diabetic ketoacidosis
dl: decaliter
DM: diabetes mellitus
D&C: dilation and curettage
DOB: date of birth
DOM: dimethoxymethylamphetamine, STP (used as street drug)
DRG: diagnosis-related group
DSA: digital subtraction antiography
DST: dexamethasone suppression test
DT: delirium tremens
DTIC: dicarbazine (synthetic chemotherapeutic agent)
DTRS: deep-tendon reflexes
DUI: driving under the influence
D5W: dextrose 5% water
DVT: deep vein thrombosis

EACA: epsilon aminocaproic acid
ECF: extracellular fluid
ECG: electrocardiogram
ECT: electroconvulsive therapy
EEG: electroencephalogram
ENG: electromyogram
ELISA: enzyme-linked immunosorbent assay
ESR: erythrocyte sedimentation rate
ESWL: extracorporeal shock-wave lithrotripsy
ET: endotracheal tube

F: Fahrenheit
FAS: fetal alcohol syndrome
FBS: fasting blood sugar
FEV_1: forced expiratory volume in 1 second
FFP: fresh frozen plasma

FIO_2: fraction of inspired oxygen
FRC: functional reserve capacity
FVC: forced vital capacity

GF: glomerular filtration
GFR: glomerular filtration rate
GH: growth hormone
GI: gastrointestinal
Gly-Hb: glycosylated hemoglobin
g: gram
GU: genitourinary

H: hydrogen
HAA: hepatitis associated antigen
HAV: hepatitis A virus
Hb: hemoglobin
Hb/Hct: hemoglobin and hematocrit
HBIg: hepatitis B immunoglobulin
HBsAg: hepatitis B surface antigen
HCG: human chorionic gonadotropin
HCl: hydrochloric acid
HCO_2: carbonate
HCO_3: bicarbonate
Hct: hematocrit
Hg: mercury
HHNC: hyperglycemic, hyperosmotic nonketotic coma
HIV: human immunodeficiency virus
HOB: head of bed
HNP: herniated nucleus pulposus
H_2O: water
HR: heart rate
HS: hour of sleep
HSV: herpes simplex virus

IABP: intraaortic balloon pump
ICF: intracellular fluid
ICP: intracranial pressure
ICU: intensive care unit
ID: iron deficiency (anemia)
I&D: incision and drainage
IDDM: insulin-dependent diabetes mellitus
I:E: inspiratory/expiratory ratio
Ig: immune globulin
IHSS: idiopathic hypertrophic subaortic stenosis
IICP: increased intracranial pressure
IM: intramuscular
IMV: intermittent mandatory ventilation
I&O: intake and output
IOL: intraocular lens
IOP: intraocular pressure
IP: identified patient
IPPB: intermittent positive pressure breathing
IV: intravenous
IVP: intravenous pyelogram

JVD: jugular vein distention

K+: potassium
kg: kilogram
KS: Kaposi's sarcoma
KUB: kidneys, ureters, bladder

l/L: liter
LAP: leucine aminopeptidase
LDH: lactate dehydrogenase
LE cell: neutrophil
LOC: level of consciousness
LP: lumbar puncture
LR: lactated Ringer's
LSD: D-lysergic acid (used as street drug)
LTC: long-term care
LUQ: left upper quadrant
LV: left ventricle
LVEDP: left ventricular end-diastolic pressure
LVF: left ventricular failure

MAO: monoamine oxidase inhibitors
MAP: mean arterial pressure
MAT: multiple atrial tachycardia
MCL$_1$: Modified chest lead (V$_1$)
MCL$_6$: Modified chest lead (V$_6$)
MCT: medium chain triglycerides
MCV: mean corpuscular volume
MDA: methylenedioxymethamphetamine
MDF: myocardial depressant factor
mEq: milliequivalent
Mg++: magnesium
mg: milligram
MG: myasthenia gravis
MI: myocardial infarction, mitral valve insufficiency
min: minute
ml: milliliter
mm: millimeter
mOsm: milliosmol
MR: mitral regurgitation
MRI: magnetic resonance imaging
MS: mitral valve stenosis; multiple sclerosis
MSG: monosodium glutamate
MSH: melanocyte-stimulating hormone
MTM: Modified-Thayer-Martin (culture media for gonococcus)
MUGA: multigated acquisition (radioactive heart scan)
MV: mitral valve
MVP: mitral valve prolapse

Na+: sodium
NaHCO$_3$: sodium bicarbonate
NG: nasogastric
NIDDM: non-insulin-dependent diabetes mellitus
NMR: nuclear magnetic resonance
NPO: nothing by mouth
NS: normal saline

NSAID: nonsteroid anti-inflammatory drugs
NSR: normal sinus rhythm
NSU: nonspecific urethritis
NTG: nitroglycerin
n/v: nausea/vomiting

O$_2$: oxygen
OR: operating room
Osm: osmolality
OTC: over-the-counter (drugs)
OT: occupational therapy

PA: posterior-anterior
PAC: premature atrial contraction
PaCO$_2$: arterial carbon dioxide pressure
PAO$_2$: alveolar oxygen pressure
PaO$_2$: arterial oxygen pressure
PAP: pulmonary artery pressure
PAT: paroxysmal atrial tachycardia
PAWP: pulmonary artery wedge pressure
pc/hs: after meals and at bedtime
PCA: patient-controlled analgesia
PCO$_2$: partial pressure of carbon dioxide
PCP: *Pneumocystis carinii* pneumonia; phencyclidine (used as street drug)
PCWP: pulmonary capillary wedge pressure
PE: pulmonary embolus; physical examination
PEEP: positive end-expiratory pressure
PET: positron emission tomography
PG: phostidylglycerol
pH: acid base
PI: phosphotidylinositol, pulmonary insufficiency
PIPs: proximal interphalangeal joints
PJC: premature junctional contraction
PMI: point of maximal impulse
PNO: paroxysmal nocturnal dyspnea
PO: per os (by mouth)
PO$_2$: partial pressure of oxygen
PO$_4$: phosphate
PPD: purified protein derivative
p.r.n.: as necessary
PS: pulmonary valve stenosis
PT: prothrombin time; physical therapy
PTCA: percutaneous transluminal coronary angioplasty
PTH: parathyroid hormone
PTT: partial thromboplastin time
PTU: propylthiouracil
PUL: percutaneous ultrasonic lithotripsy
PVC: premature ventricular contractions
PWP: pulmonary wedge pressure

q.i.d.: four times a day
QP/QS: shunt measurement pulmonary vs systemic flow
QS/QT: shunt measure-quality shunted/quantity total (respiratory)

1097

QRS: electrocardiogram measure of electrical activity of ventricle

R: electrocardiogram wave representing ventricular innervation
RA: rheumatoid arthritis
Rad: right axis deviation; radiation dosage
RAI: radioactive iodine
RAP: right atrial pressure
RBC: red blood cell
RCVA: right cerebral vascular accident
REM: rapid eye movement
RIA: radioimmunoassay
RL: renal electrolytes
ROM: range of motion
RPR: rapid plasma reagin (serologic test)
RUQ: right upper quadrant
RV: right ventricle
RVF: right ventricular failure

S_1, S_2, S_3, S_4: heart sounds
SA: sinoatrial
SB: sinus bradycardia
SC: subcutaneous
SCI: spinal cord injury
sec: second
SGOT: serum glutamic-oxaloacetic transaminase
SGPT: serum glutamic pyruvic transaminase
SIADH: syndrome of inappropriate antidiuretic hormone
SIMV: synchronized intermittent mandatory ventilation
SLE: systemic lupus erythematosus
SMA: serum chemistry profile
SO: significant other(s)
SPF: sun protective factor
SR: sinus rhythm
ST: sinus tachycardia, electrocardiographic wave representing ventricular repolarization
STD: sexually transmitted disease
STP: (serendipity, tranquility, peace) dimethoxy-methylamphetamine (used as a street drug)
ST/T: segment/interval measure on ECG
SVO_2: systemic venous oxygen
SVR: systemic vascular resistance

T_3: triiodothyronine
T_4: thyroxine
TB: tuberculosis
TBSA: total body surface area
TCDB: turn, cough, deep breath
TENS: transcutaneous electrical nerve stimulator
THC: tetrahydrocannabinol (used as a street drug)
TI: tricuspid valve insufficiency
TIA: transient ischemic attacks
TIBC: total iron binding capacity
t.i.d.: three times a day
TKO: to keep open
TLC: total lung capacity
TMJ: temporomandibular joint
TPN: total parenteral nutrition
TRF: thyrotropin-releasing factor
TRH: thyrotropin-releasing hormone
TS: tricuspid stenosis
TSH: thyroid-stimulating hormone
TUR: transurethral resection
TVC: true vomiting center
T-tube: T-shaped drainage tube generally for the common bile duct

UA: urinalysis
UC: ulcerative colitis
UO: urinary output
URI: upper respiratory infection
UTI: urinary tract infection

V, V_1, V_5, V_6: electrocardiogram chest leads
$\dot{V}_E$: minute ventilation
VC: vital capacity
VCU: voiding cystourethrogram
V_D/V_T: dead space/tidal volume
VF: ventricular fibrillation
VMA: vanillylmandelic acid
VNA: visiting nurse association
VPD: ventricular premature depolarization
V/Q: ventilation/perfusion
VS: vital signs
V_T: tidal volume
VT: ventricular tachycardia

WBC: white blood cell
WNL: within normal limits

Taxonomy 1R

Conceptual base for identifying and classifying nursing diagnoses.

1. **EXCHANGING;** A human response pattern involving mutual giving and receiving.
   1.1. Alterations in Nutrition
   1.1.1. (Cellular)*
   1.1.2. (Systemic)*
   1.1.2.1. More than body requirements
   1.1.2.2. Less than body requirements
   1.1.2.3. Potential for more than body requirements
   1.2. (Alterations in Physical Regulation)*
   1.2.1. (Immune)*
   1.2.1.1. Potential for Infection
   1.2.2. Alteration in Body Temperature
   1.2.2.1. Potential
   1.2.2.2. Hypothermia
   1.2.2.3. Hyperthermia
   1.2.2.4. Ineffective Thermoregulation
   1.2.3. (——)*
   1.2.3.1. Dysreflexia
   1.3. Alterations in Elimination
   1.3.1. Bowel
   1.3.1.1. Constipation
   1.3.1.1.1. Perceived Constipation
   1.3.1.1.2. Colonic Constipation
   1.3.1.2. Diarrhea
   1.3.1.3. Bowel Incontinence
   1.3.2. Altered Patterns of Urinary Elimination
   1.3.2.1. Incontinence
   1.3.2.1.1. Stress
   1.3.2.1.2. Reflex
   1.3.2.1.3. Urge
   1.3.2.1.4. Functional
   1.3.2.1.5. Total
   1.3.2.2. Retention [Acute/Chronic]
   1.3.3. (Skin)*
   1.4. (Alterations in Circulation)*
   1.4.1. (Vascular)*
   1.4.1.1. Tissue Perfusion
   1.4.1.1.1. Renal
   1.4.1.1.2. Cerebral
   1.4.1.1.3. Cardiopulmonary
   1.4.1.1.4. Gastrointestinal
   1.4.1.1.5. Peripheral
   1.4.1.2. Fluid Volume
   1.4.1.2.1. Excess
   1.4.1.2.2.1. Deficit (1) and (2)
   1.4.1.2.2.2. Potential
   1.4.2. (Cardiac)*
   1.4.2.1. Decreased Cardiac Output
   1.5. (Alterations in Oxygenation)*
   1.5.1. (Respiration)*
   1.5.1.1. Impaired Gas Exchange
   1.5.1.2. Ineffective Airway Clearance
   1.5.1.3. Ineffective Breathing Pattern
   1.5.1.3.1. Inability–Spontaneous Ventilation
   1.5.1.3.2. Dysfunctional Ventilation Weaning
   1.6. (Alterations in Physical Integrity)*
   1.6.1. Potential for Injury
   1.6.1.1. Potential for Suffocating
   1.6.1.2. Potential for Poisoning
   1.6.1.3. Potential for Trauma
   1.6.1.4. Potential for Aspiration
   1.6.1.5. Potential for Disuse Syndrome
   1.6.2. Impairment
   1.6.2.1. Tissue Integrity
   1.6.2.1.1. Oral Mucous Membrane
   1.6.2.1.2.1. Skin Integrity
   1.6.2.1.2.2. Potential
2. **COMMUNICATING:** A human response pattern involving sending messages.
   2.1 Alterations in Communication
   2.1.1. Verbal
   2.1.2.1. Impaired
   2.1.2. (Nonverbal)*
3. **RELATING:** A human response pattern involving establishing bonds.
   3.1. (Alterations in Socialization)*
   3.1.1. Impaired Social Interaction
   3.1.2. Social Isolation
   3.2. (Alterations in Role)*
   3.2.1. Altered Role Performance
   3.2.1.1.1. Altered Parenting
   3.2.1.1.2. Potential
   3.2.1.2. Sexual
   3.2.1.2.1. Dysfunction
   3.2.1.3. (Work)*
   3.2.2. Family Processes
   3.2.2.1. Caregiver Role Strain
   3.2.2.2. High Risk Caregiver Role
   3.2.3. Parental Role Conflict
   3.3. Altered Sexuality Patterns
4. **VALUING:** A human response pattern involving the assigning of relative worth.
   4.1. Alterations in Spiritual State
   4.1.1. Distress
5. **CHOOSING:** A human response pattern involving the selection of alternatives.
   5.1. Alterations in Coping
   5.1.1. Individual
   5.1.1.1. Ineffective
   5.1.1.1.1. Impaired Adjustment
   5.1.1.1.2. Defensive Coping
   5.1.1.1.3. Ineffective Denial

5.1.2. Family
  5.1.2.1. Ineffective
    5.1.2.1.1. Disabled
    5.1.2.1.2. Compromised
  5.1.2.2. Potential for Growth
5.1.3. (Community)*
5.2. (Alterations in Participation)*
  5.2.1. Therapeutic Regimen
    5.2.1.1. Noncompliance
  5.2.2. (Family)*
  5.2.3. (Community)*
    5.3.1.1. Decisional Conflict (specify)
5.4. Health Seeking Behaviors (specify)

6. **MOVING:** A human response pattern involving activity
6.1. (Alterations in Activity)*
  6.1.1. Physical Mobility
    6.1.1.1. Impaired
      6.1.1.1.1. HR Peripheral Neurovascular
    6.1.1.2. Activity Intolerance
      6.1.1.2.1. Fatigue
    6.1.1.3. Potential Activity Intolerance
  6.1.2. (Social Mobility)*
6.2. (Alterations in Rest)*
  6.2.1. Sleep Pattern Disturbance
6.3. (Alterations in Recreation)*
  6.3.1. Diversional Activity
    6.3.1.1. Deficit
6.4. (Alterations in Activities of Daily Living)*
  6.4.1. Home Maintenance Management
    6.4.1.1. Impaired
  6.4.2. Health Maintenance
6.5. Alterations in Self-Care
  6.5.1. Feeding
    6.5.1.1. Impaired Swallowing
    6.5.1.2. Ineffective Breast Feeding
      6.5.1.2.1. Interrupted Breast Feeding
    6.5.1.3. Ineffective Infant Feeding
  6.5.2. Bathing/Hygiene
  6.5.3. Dressing/Grooming
  6.5.4. Toileting
6.6. Altered Growth and Development
6.7. Relocation Stress

7. **PERCEIVING:** A human response pattern involving the reception of information.

7.1. Alterations in Self-Concept
  7.1.1. Disturbance in Body Image
  7.1.2. Disturbance in Self-Esteem
    7.1.2.1. Chronic Low Self-Esteem
    7.1.2.2. Situational Low Self-Esteem
  7.1.3. Disturbance in Personal Identity
7.2. Sensory/Perceptual Alteration
  7.2.1. Visual
    7.2.1.1. Unilateral Neglect
  7.2.2. Auditory
  7.2.3. Kinesthetic
  7.2.4. Gustatory
  7.2.5. Tactile
  7.2.6. Olfactory
7.3. (Alterations in Meaningfulness)*
  7.3.1. Hopelessness
  7.3.2. Powerlessness

8. **KNOWING:** A human response pattern involving the meaning associated with information.
8.1. Alterations in Knowledge
  8.1.1. Deficit
8.2. (Alterations in Learning)*
8.3. Alterations in Thought Processes
  8.3.1. (Confusion)*

9. **FEELING:** A human response pattern involving the subjective awareness of information.
9.1. Alterations in Comfort
  9.1.1. Pain
    9.1.1.1. Chronic
    9.1.1.2. Acute
  9.1.2. (Discomfort)*
9.2. (Alterations in Emotional Integrity)*
  9.2.1. Grieving
    9.2.1.1. Dysfunctional
    9.2.1.2. Anticipatory
  9.2.2. Potential for Violence: self-directed or directed at others
    9.2.2.1. HR Self-Mutilation
  9.2.3. Post-Trauma Response
    9.2.3.1. Rape Trauma Syndrome
      9.2.3.1.1. Compound Reaction
      9.2.3.1.2. Silent Reaction
  9.3.1. Anxiety
  9.3.2. Fear

---

* Recommended by The Taxonomy Committee but not yet approved by NANDA.

Diagnosis Qualifiers

ACTUAL

(Label): This part provides a name for the diagnosis, a concise phrase or term which represents a pattern of related cues.

HIGH RISK NURSING DIAGNOSIS (FORMERLY POTENTIAL)

(Label): This part provides a name for the diagnosis, a concise phrase or term which represents a pattern of related cues.

Diagnostic labels may include but are not limited to the following qualifiers:

Impaired: Made worse, weakened; damaged, reduced; deteriorated.

Depleted: Emptied wholly or partially; exhausted of.

Deficient: Inadequate in amount, quality, or degree; defective; not suffficient; incomplete.

Excessive: Characterized by an amount or quantity that is greater than is necessary, desirable or useable.

Dysfunctional: Abnormal; impaired or incompletely functioning.

Disturbed: Agitated; interrupted, interfered with.

Acute: Severe but of short duration.

Chronic: Lasting a long time; recurring; habitual; constant.

Intermittent: Stopping and starting again at intervals; periodic; cyclic.

INDEX OF NURSING DIAGNOSES

Cardiac output, decreased: Addison's disease (adrenal insufficiency/crisis) and, 713; alcoholism [acute]: intoxication/overdose and, 964; angina pectoris and, 74; cardiac surgery; coronary artery bypass graft; valve replacement (postoperative care) and, 116; congestive heart failure: chronic and, 51; digitalis toxicity and, 64; dysrhythmias and, 96; hypertension and, 37; hyperthyroidism (thyrotoxicosis, Graves' disease) and, 721; inflammatory cardiac conditions; pericarditis, myocarditis, endocarditis and, 130; myocardial infarction and, 88; renal failure: acute and, 624; renal failure: chronic and, 635; stimulants (amphetamines, cocaine, caffeine, tobacco): intoxication/overdose and, 985; valvular heart disease and, 105

Caregiver role strain: psychosocial aspects of acute care and, 909; substance dependence/abuse rehabilitation and, 1007; substance dependence/abuse rehabilitation and, 1007

Communication, impaired verbal: cerebrovascular accident/stroke and, 297; long-term care and, 945; radical neck surgery: laryngectomy (postoperative care) and, 206; reconstructive facial surgery (intermaxillary fixation, facial fractures) and, 794; thyroidectomy and, 732; ventilatory assistance (mechanical) and, 231

Constipation: Alzheimer's disease (non-substance-induced organic mental disorders) and, 385; anemias (iron deficiency, pernicious, aplastic, hemolytic) and, 582; cancer and, 1033; disk surgery and, 332; fecal diversions: postoperative care of ileostomy and colostomy and, 494; Guillain-Barré syndrome (acute polyneuritis) and, 366; hysterectomy and, 756; intestinal surgery without diversion and, 506; long-term care and, 954; renal dialysis and, 650; spinal cord injury (acute rehabilitative phase) and, 350

Coping, ineffective, individual: headache and, 258; Coping, individual, ineffective: herniated nucleus pulposus (ruptured intervertebal disk) and, 323; hypertension and, 42; inflammatory bowel disease: ulcerative colitis, regional enteritis, (Crohn's disease, ileocolitis) and, 483; multiple sclerosis and, 400; psychosocial aspects of acute care and, 907; substance dependence/abuse rehabilitation and, 1001

Decisional conflict (specify): psychosocial aspects of acute care and, 907

Denial, ineffective: substance dependence/abuse rehabilitation and, 1001

Diarrhea: anemias (iron deficiency, pernicious, aplastic, hemolytic) and, 582; cancer and, 1033; fecal diversions: postoperative care of ileostomy and colostomy and, 494; hysterectomy and, 756; inflammatory bowel disease: ulcerative colitis, regional enteritis, (Crohn's disease, ileocolitis) and, 475; intestinal surgery without diversion and, 506; long-term care and, 954; obesity: surgical interventions (gastric partitioning/gastroplasty, gastric bypass) and, 450

Diversional activity deficit: long-term care and, 956

Dysreflexia: spinal cord injury (acute rehabilitative phase) and, 352

Family coping, compromised: Alzheimer's disease (non-substance-induced organic mental disorders) and, 387; long-term care and, 943; multiple sclerosis and, 402; psychosocial aspects of acute care and, 909; substance dependence/abuse rehabilitation and, 1007

Family coping, disabling: Alzheimer's disease (non-substance-induced organic mental disorders) and, 387; multiple sclerosis and, 402; psychosocial aspects of acute care and, 909; substance dependence/abuse rehabilitation and, 1007

Family coping, potential for growth: psychosocial aspects of acute care and, 911

Family processes, altered: cancer and, 1035; craniocerebral trauma (acute rehabilitative phase) and, 286; eating disorders: anorexia nervosa/bulimia nervosa and, 431

Fatigue: Addison's disease (adrenal insufficiency/crisis) and, 712; AIDS and, 865; cancer and, 1027; diabetes mellitus/diabetic ketoacidosis and, 747; hyperthyroidism (thyrotoxicosis, Graves' disease) and, 724; renal failure: acute and, 627; total nutritional support and, 1050

Fear: adult respiratory distress syndrome (ARDS) (preacute/postacute care) and, 223; AIDS and, 869; alcoholism [acute]: intoxication/overdose and, 970; benign prostatic hyperplasia and, 686; burns: thermal/chemical/electrical (acute and convalescent phase) and, 837; cancer and, 1016; Guillain-Barré syndrome (acute polyneuritis) and, 368; hallucinogens (LSD, PCP, cannabis): intoxication/overdose and, 980; intracranial infections: meningitis, encephalitis, brain abscess and, 316; long-term care and, 939; lung cancer: surgical intervention (postoperative care) and, 191; mastectomy and, 764; myocardial infarction and, 86; peritonitis and, 520; psychosocial aspects of acute care and, 901; pulmonary embolism (PE) and, 180; reconstructive facial surgery (intermaxillary fixation, facial fractures) and, 797; renal dialysis and, 652; stimulants (amphetamines, cocaine, caffeine, tobacco): intoxication/overdose and, 989; surgical intervention and, 921; upper gastrointestinal/esophageal bleeding and, 461; ventilatory assistance (mechanical) and, 232

Fluid volume, altered: fluctuation: total nutritional support: parenteral/enteral feeding and, 1039

Fluid volume deficit [active loss]: peritonitis and, 517; upper gastrointestinal/esophageal bleeding and, 457

Fluid volume deficit, high risk for: acute hemodialysis and, 665 adult respiratory distress syndrome (ARDS) (preacute/postacute care) and, 222; AIDS and, 856; appendectomy and, 511; benign prostatic hyperplasia and, 686; burns: thermal/chemical/electrical (acute and convalescent phase) and, 825; cancer and, 1025; cholecystectomy and, 532; cholecystitis with cholelithiasis and, 527; digitalis toxicity and, 66; eating disorders: anorexia nervosa/bulimia nervosa and, 426; fecal diversions: postoperative care of ileostomy and colostomy and, 491; hepatitis and, 541; inflammatory bowel disease: ulcerative colitis, regional enteritis, (Crohn's disease, ileocolitis) and, 477; intestinal surgery without diversion and, 500; leukemias and, 605; obesity: surgical interventions (gastric partitioning/gastroplasty, gastric bypass) and, 447; pancreatitis and, 565; pneumonia: microbial and, 171; prostatectomy and, 690; renal dialysis: peritoneal and, 658; renal failure: chronic and, 629; sepsis/septicemia and, 894; sickle cell crisis and, 593; surgical intervention and, 930; urolithiasis (renal calculi) and, 702

Fluid volume, excess: acute hemodialysis and, 667; cirrhosis of the liver and, 551; congestive heart failure: chronic and, 55; digitalis toxicity and, 66; myocardial infarction and, 91; renal dialysis: peritoneal and, 657;

renal failure: acute and, 618; valvular heart disease and, 102

Fluid volume excess [regulatory failure]: Addison's disease (adrenal insufficiency/crisis) and, 709; diabetes mellitus/diabetic ketoacidosis and, 740

Gas exchange, impaired: adult respiratory distress syndrome (ARDS) (preacute/postacute) and, 221; AIDS and, 858; chronic obstructive pulmonary disease (COPD) and, 155; congestive heart failure: chronic and, 57; depressants (benzodiazepines, barbiturates, opioids): intoxication/overdose and, 997; fractures and, 779; pneumonia: microbial and, 166; pulmonary embolism (PE) and, 186; pulmonary embolism (PE) and, 177; pulmonary tuberculosis (TB) and, 246; sepsis/septicemia and, 895; sickle cell crisis and, 590

Grieving, anticipatory: Alzheimer's disease (non-substance-induced organic mental disorders) and, 388; cancer and, 1018; long-term care and, 940; spinal cord injury (acute rehabilitative phase) and, 346

Grieving, dysfunctional: psychosocial aspects of acute care and, 903

Health maintenance, altered: Alzheimer's disease (non-substance-induced organic mental disorders) and, 389; long-term care and, 958

Home maintenance management, impaired: Alzheimer's disease (non-substance-induced organic mental disorders) and, 389; rheumatoid arthritis and, 882

Hopelessness: multiple sclerosis and, 399

Hyperthermia: sepsis/septicemia and, 891

Incontinence, functional: Alzheimer's disease (non-substance-induced mental organic disorders) and, 385

Incontinence, reflex: Alzheimer's disease (non-substance-induced organic mental disorders) and, 385

Incontinence, stress: Alzheimer's disease (non-substance-induced organic mental disorders) and, 385

Incontinence, total: Alzheimer's disease (non-substance-induced mental organic disorders) and, 385

Infection, high risk for: AIDS and, 854; amputation and, 805; anemias (iron deficiency, pernicious, aplastic, hemolytic) and, 583; appendectomy and, 510; burns: thermal/chemical/electrical (acute and convalescent phase) and, 827; cancer and, 1028; chronic obstructive pulmonary disease (COPD) and, 158; craniocerebral trauma (acute rehabilitative phase) and, 284; depressants (benzodiazepines, barbiturates, opioids): intoxication/overdose and, 998; diabetes mellitus/diabetic ketoacidosis and, 744; fractures and, 785; hepatitis and, 543; intestinal surgery without diversion and, 503; intracranial infections: meningitis, encephalitis, brain abscess and, 310; leukemias and, 603; obesity: surgical interventions (gastric partitioning/gastroplasty, gastric bypass) and, 450; ocular disorders and, 411; pancreatitis and, 568; peritonitis and, 516; pneumonia: microbial and, 167; prostatectomy and, 692; pulmonary tuberculosis (TB) and, 243; renal dialysis: peritoneal and, 661; renal failure: acute and, 628; sepsis/septicemia and, 889; sickle cell crisis and, 597; stimulants (amphetamines, cocaine, caffeine, tobacco): intoxication/overdose and, 991; surgical intervention and, 925; total joint replacement and, 811; total nutritional support: parenteral/enteral feeding and, 1045; urinary diversions/urostomy (postoperative care) and, 674; ventilatory assistance (mechanical) and, 236

Injury, high risk for: acute hemodialysis and, 664; AIDS and, 859; alcoholism [acute]: intoxication/overdose and, 965; Alzheimer's disease (non-substance-induced organic mental disorders) and, 376; cirrhosis of the liver and, 555; long-term care and, 944; ocular disorders, and, 410; renal failure: chronic and, 636; thyroidectomy and, 733; total nutritional support: parenteral/enteral feeding and, 1047

Knowledge deficit [learning need] specify: Addison's disease (adrenal insufficiency/crisis) and 716; adult respiratory distress syndrome (ARDS) (preacute/postacute care) and, 224; AIDS and, 873; amputation and, 808; anemias (iron deficiency, pernicious, aplastic, hemolytic) and, 584; angina pectoris and, 77; appendectomy and, 513; benign prostatic hyperplasia and, 687; burns: thermal/chemical/electrical (acute and convalescent phase) and, 840; cancer and, 1036; cardiac surgery: coronary artery bypass graft; valve replacement (postoperative care) and, 123; cerebrovascular accident/stroke and, 290; cholecystectomy and, 524; cholecystitis with cholelithiasis and, 529; chronic obstructive pulmonary disease (COPD) and, 159; cirrhosis of the liver and, 559; congestive heart failure: chronic and, 59; craniocerebral trauma (acute rehabilitative phase) and, 288; diabetes mellitus/diabetic ketoacidosis and, 748; digitalis toxicity and, 68; disk surgery and, 334; dysrhythmias and, 100; eating disorders: anorexia nervosa/bulimia nervosa and, 433; eating disorders: obesity and, 442; fecal diversions: postoperative care of ileostomy and colostomy and, 497; fractures and, 787; glaucoma and, 417; Guillain-Barré syndrome and, 370; headache and, 259; hemothorax/pneumothorax and, 201; hepatitis and, 545; herniated nucleus pulposus (ruptured intervertebral disk) and, 325; HIV-positive patient and, 846; hypertension and, 44; hyperthyroidism (thyrotoxicosis, Graves' disease) and, 729; hysterectomy and, 759; inflammatory bowel disease: ulcerative colitis, regional enteritis, (Crohn's disease, ileocolitis) and, 484; inflammatory cardiac conditions: pericarditis, myocarditis, endocarditis and, 133; intestinal surgery without diversion and, 507; intracranial infections: meningitis, encephalitis, brain abscess and, 317; leukemias and, 609; lung cancer: surgical intervention (postoperative care) and, 192; mastectomy and, 770; multiple sclerosis and, 404; myocardial infarction and, 92; obesity: surgical interventions (gastric partitioning/gastroplasty, gastric bypass) and, 451; ocular disorders and, 413; pancreatitis and, 570; peritonitis and, 521; pneumonia: microbial and, 172; prostatectomy and, 695; pulmonary embolism (PE) and, 182; pulmonary tuberculosis (TB) and, 248; radical neck surgery: laryngectomy (postoperative care) and, 215; Raynaud's disease and, 146; reconstructive facial surgery (intermaxillary fixation, facial fractures) and, 798; renal dialysis and, 654; renal failure: acute and, 630; renal failure: chronic and, 641; rheumatoid arthritis and, 883; seizure disorders/epilepsy and, 269; sepsis/septicemia and, 897; sickle cell disease and, 589; spinal cord injury (acute rehabilitative phase) and, 355; substance dependence/abuse rehabilitation and, 1010; subtotal gastrectomy/gastric resection and, 469; surgical intervention and, 920, 936; thrombophlebitis: deep vein thrombosis and, 135; thyroidectomy and, 735; total joint replacement and, 817; total nutritional support: parenteral/enteral feeding, 1039; upper gastrointestinal/esophageal bleeding and, 464; urinary diversions/urostomy (postoperative

1107

CLASSIFICATION OF NANDA NURSING DIAGNOSES BY GORDON'S FUNCTIONAL HEALTH PATTERNS*

HEALTH PERCEPTION—HEALTH MANAGEMENT PATTERN
Altered health maintenance
Ineffective management of therapeutic regimen
Total health management deficit
Health management deficit (specify)
Noncompliance (specify)
High risk for noncompliance (specify)
Health-seeking behaviors (specify)
High risk for infection
High risk for injury (trauma)
High risk for poisoning
High risk for suffocation
Altered protection

NUTRITIONAL-METABOLIC PATTERN
Altered nutrition: potential for more than body requirements or high risk for obesity
Altered nutrition: more than body requirements or exogenous obesity
Altered nutrition: less than body requirements or nutritional deficit (specify)
Ineffective breastfeeding
Effective breastfeeding
Interrupted breastfeeding
Ineffective infant feeding pattern
High risk for aspiration
Impaired swallowing or uncompensated swallowing impairment
Altered oral mucous membrane
High risk for fluid volume deficit
Fluid volume deficit (1)
Fluid volume deficit (2)
Fluid volume excess
High risk for impaired skin integrity or high risk for skin breakdown
Impaired skin integrity
Pressure ulcer (specify stage)
Impaired tissue integrity
High risk for altered body temperature
Ineffective thermoregulation
Hyperthermia
Hypothermia

ELIMINATION PATTERN
Constipation or intermittent constipation pattern
Colonic constipation
Perceived constipation
Diarrhea
Bowel incontinence
Altered urinary elimination pattern
Functional incontinence
Reflex incontinence
Stress incontinence
Urge incontinence
Total incontinence
Urinary retention

ACTIVITY-EXERCISE PATTERN
High risk for activity intolerance
Activity intolerance (specify level)
Fatigue
Impaired physical mobility (specify level)
High risk for disuse syndrome
High risk for joint contractures
Total self-care deficit (specify level)
Self–bathing-hygiene deficit (specify level)
Self–dressing-grooming deficit (specify level)
Self–feeding deficit (specify level)
Selt–toileting deficit (specify level)
Altered growth and development: self-care skills (specify)
Diversional activity deficit
Impaired home maintenance management (mild, moderate, severe, potential, chronic)
Dysfunctional ventilatory weaning response (DVWR)
Inability to sustain spontaneous ventilation
Ineffective airway clearance
Ineffective breathing pattern
Impaired gas exchange
Decreased cardiac output
Altered tissue perfusion (specify)

Dysreflexia
High risk for peripheral neurovascular dysfunction
Altered growth and development

SLEEP-REST PATTERN
Sleep-pattern disturbance

COGNITIVE-PERCEPTUAL PATTERN
Pain
Chronic pain
Pain self-management deficit (acute, chronic)
Uncompensated sensory deficit (specify)
Sensory-perceptual alterations: input deficit or sensory deprivation
Sensory-perceptual alterations: input excess or sensory overload
Unilateral neglect
Knowledge deficit (specify)
Impaired thought processes
Uncompensated short-term memory deficit
High risk for cognitive impairment
Decisional conflict (specify)

SELF-PERCEPTION–SELF-CONCEPT PATTERN
Fear (specify focus)
Anxiety
Mild anxiety
Moderate anxiety
Severe anxiety (panic)
Anticipatory anxiety (mild, moderate, severe)
Reactive depression (situational)
Hopelessness
Powerlessness (severe, low, moderate)
Self-esteem disturbance
Chronic low self-esteem
Situational low self-esteem
Body image disturbance
High risk for self-mutilation
Personal identity confusion

ROLE-RELATIONSHIP PATTERN
Anticipatory grieving
Dysfunctional grieving
Disturbance in role performance
Unresolved independence-dependence conflict
Social isolation or social rejection
Social isolation
Impaired social interaction
Altered growth and development: social skills (specify)
Relocation stress syndrome
Altered family processes
High risk for altered parenting
Altered parenting
Parental role conflict
Parent-infant separation
Weak mother-infant or parent-infant attachment
Caregiver role strain
High risk for caregiver role strain
Impaired verbal communication
Altered growth and development: communication skills (specify)
Potential for violence

SEXUALITY-REPRODUCTIVE PATTERN
Sexual dysfunction (specify type)
Altered sexuality patterns
Rape trauma syndrome
Rape trauma syndrome: compound reaction
Rape trauma syndrome: silent reaction

COPING-STRESS TOLERANCE PATTERN
Coping, ineffective (individual)
Avoidance coping
Defensive coping
Ineffective denial or denial
Impaired adjustment
Post-trauma response
Family coping: potential for growth
Ineffective family coping: compromised
Ineffective family coping: disabling

VALUE-BELIEF PATTERN
Spiritual distress (distress of the human spirit)

---

* Based on Gordon, M: Nursing Diagnosis: Process and Applications. McGraw Hill, New York, 1986, with permission.